Current Clinical Oncology

Maurie Markman, MD, Series Editor

For further volumes:
http://www.springer.com/series/7631

Frank E. Johnson • Yoshihiko Maehara
George P. Browman • Julie A. Margenthaler
Riccardo A. Audisio • John F. Thompson
David Y. Johnson • Craig C. Earle
Katherine S. Virgo
Editors

Patient Surveillance After Cancer Treatment

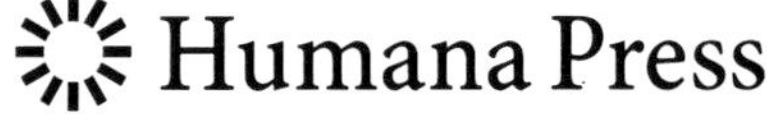

Editors
Frank E. Johnson
Department of Surgery
Saint Louis University
St. Louis, Missouri, USA

George P. Browman
British Columbia Cancer Agency
Vancouver
British Columbia, Canada

Riccardo A. Audisio
Whiston Hospital, Department of Surgery
University of Liverpool
Merseyside, United Kingdom

David Y. Johnson
Department of Internal Medicine
Saint Louis University Medical Center
Saint Louis, Missouri, USA

Katherine S. Virgo
Department of Surgery
St. Louis University
St. Louis, Missouri, USA

Yoshihiko Maehara
Faculty of Medicine, Department of Surgery II
Kyushu University
Fukuoka, Japan

Julie A. Margenthaler
School of Medicine
Washington University
St. Louis, Missouri, USA

John F. Thompson
Sydney Cancer Centre, Sydney Melanoma Unit
Royal Prince Alfred Hospital
Camperdown, New South Wales, Australia

Craig C. Earle
Dana-Farber Cancer Institute
Harvard Medical School
Boston, Massachusetts, USA

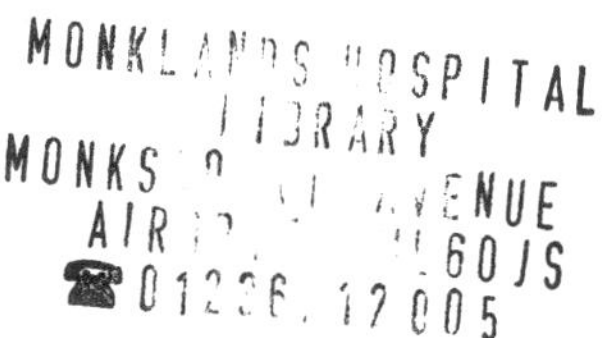

ISBN 978-1-60327-968-0 ISBN 978-1-60327-969-7 (eBook)
DOI 10.1007/978-1-60327-969-7
Springer New York Heidelberg Dordrecht London

Library of Congress Control Number: 2012955411

Printed on acid-free paper

Humana Press is a brand of Springer
Springer is part of Springer Science+Business Media (www.springer.com)

To our families, whose support made the creation of this book feasible.

To our colleagues, whose research findings we incorporated in writing this book.

To our patients, whose care this book is intended to improve.

To Judith Ann Feldworth, the Saint Louis University editor, whose skill, tenacity, and creativity over several years made this book a reality.

Preface

Cancer remains a major cause of death worldwide. With modern therapy, millions of patients can expect (or at least hope) to be cured. With the passage of time, a proportion of these cancer survivors experience recurrence. Some die and some are rescued by further interventions. Some sustain complications of treatment which are merely annoying; others are fatal. These considerations show that cancer patient care is an important topic, but it is presently underresearched and underappreciated. The primary focus of this book is patient surveillance after curative-intent initial treatment. It is my second book devoted to this topic. The format is somewhat different from the first (*Cancer Patient Follow-up*, Mosby, 1997). The secondary focus of the book is to publicize the need for well-designed, adequately powered randomized clinical trials comparing two (or more) surveillance strategies for each type of cancer. Currently the National Institutes of Health and other major sources of funding in America do sponsor research about the clinical course of cancer patients after treatment but do not support such trials. Clinicians, patients, and society as a whole are harmed by this. Clinicians lack high-quality evidence upon which to base surveillance for their patients. Patients are subjected to diagnostic tests that are utilized at remarkably different rates, even by expert physicians. This is prima facie evidence of overuse and/or underuse of resources, with significant risk of misuse as well. In order to rationalize surveillance, we believe that patients, physicians, the public health community, advocacy groups, payers, and others will need to advocate for enabling legislation that requires such trials. The Medical Research Council of the United Kingdom and similar agencies in other European countries have already accepted this premise, and the trial results have changed medical practice. Such trials are expensive. They typically take years to accrue a sufficient number of patients, and several more years to mature and yield results. Successor trials will be required as new salvage therapies enter clinical practice, better methods of prevention and early detection are devised, toxic effects of therapy are avoided or mitigated, and so on.

Saint Louis, MO, USA　　　　Frank E. Johnson, MD

Contents

1 **Overview** 1
David Y. Johnson and Frank E. Johnson

2 **Introduction to Cancer Surveillance Strategies** 9
Brooke Crawford and David D. Greenberg

3 **Using Decision Analysis to Model Cancer Surveillance** 15
Kim E.M. van Kessel, Sandra M.E. Geurts, André L.M. Verbeek, and Ewout W. Steyerberg

4 **Cancer Survivorship: Monitoring the Long-Term and Late Effects of Treatment** 31
Craig C. Earle and Jennifer Deevy

5 **Upper Aerodigestive Tract Carcinoma** 39
David Y. Johnson, Shilpi Wadhwa, and Frank E. Johnson

6 **Upper Aerodigestive Tract Carcinoma Surveillance Counterpoint: Europe** 43
Béatrix Barry and Dominique De Raucourt

7 **Upper Aerodigestive Tract Carcinoma Surveillance Counterpoint: Japan** 47
Torahiko Nakashima, Ryuji Yasumatsu, and Shizuo Komune

8 **Upper Aerodigestive Tract Carcinoma Surveillance Counterpoint: Canada** 51
Richard W. Nason and James B. Butler

9 **Thyroid (Papillary, Follicular, Medullary, Hürthle Cell) Carcinoma** 57
David Y. Johnson, Shilpi Wadhwa, and Frank E. Johnson

10 **Thyroid (Papillary, Follicular, Medullary, Hürthle Cell) Carcinoma Surveillance Counterpoint: Australia** 63
Leigh Delbridge

11 **Thyroid (Papillary, Follicular, Medullary, Hürthle Cell) Carcinoma Surveillance Counterpoint: Japan** 69
Ryuji Yasumatsu, Torahiko Nakashima, and Shizuo Komune

12 **Lung Carcinoma** 71
Shilpi Wadhwa, David Y. Johnson, and Frank E. Johnson

13 **Lung Carcinoma Surveillance Counterpoint: Australia** 75
Michael Boyer and Kate Mahon

14 **Lung Carcinoma Surveillance Counterpoint: Japan** 79
Tokujiro Yano and Yoshihiko Maehara

15 **Lung Carcinoma Surveillance Counterpoint: Canada** 83
Gail Darling, Yee Ung, Peter Ellis, Lorraine Martelli-Reid, and Bill Evans

16 **Esophagus Carcinoma** 93
Shilpi Wadhwa, David Y. Johnson, and Frank E. Johnson

17 **Esophagus Carcinoma Surveillance Counterpoint: Australia** 97
Bernard Mark Smithers, Janine M. Thomas, and Bryan H. Burmeister

18 **Esophagus Carcinoma Surveillance Counterpoint: Japan** 101
Masaru Morita and Yoshihiko Maehara

19 **Stomach** 107
Shilpi Wadhwa, David Y. Johnson, and Frank E. Johnson

20 **Stomach Carcinoma Surveillance Counterpoint: USA** 109
Andrew Coleman and Douglas Tyler

21 **Stomach Carcinoma Surveillance Counterpoint: Japan** 113
Yoshihiro Kakeji, Masaru Morita, and Yoshihiko Maehara

22 **Pancreatic Adenocarcinoma** 121
David Y. Johnson, Shilpi Wadhwa, and Frank E. Johnson

23 **Pancreatic Adenocarcinoma Surveillance Counterpoint: USA** 125
Tanios S. Bekaii-Saab

24 **Pancreatic Adenocarcinoma Surveillance Counterpoint: Europe** 129
Richard A. Smith, Jane V. Butler, and John P. Neoptolemos

25 **Pancreatic Adenocarcinoma Surveillance Counterpoint: Japan** 145
Ken Shirabe and Yoshihiko Maehara

26 **Pancreatic Adenocarcinoma Surveillance Counterpoint: Canada** 149
Malcolm J. Moore and Anastasios Stathis

27 **Liver and Biliary Tract Carcinoma** 153
David Y. Johnson, Shilpi Wadhwa, and Frank E. Johnson

28 **Liver and Biliary Tract Carcinoma Surveillance Counterpoint: Europe** 157
Michele Colledan

29 **Liver and Biliary Tract Carcinoma Surveillance Counterpoint: Australia** 159
Michael D. Crawford

30 **Liver and Biliary Tract Carcinoma Surveillance Counterpoint: Japan** 165
Akinobu Taketomi and Yoshihiko Maehara

31 **Liver and Biliary Tract Carcinoma Surveillance Counterpoint: Canada** 169
Oliver F. Bathe and Kelly Warren Burak

32 **Colon and Rectum Carcinoma** 179
David Y. Johnson, Shilpi Wadhwa, and Frank E. Johnson

33 **Colon and Rectum Carcinoma Surveillance Counterpoint: USA** 185
Mohamedtaki A. Tejani and Steven J. Cohen

34 **Colon and Rectum Carcinoma Surveillance Counterpoint: Australia** 189
Toufic El-Khoury, Michael Solomon, and Jane Young

35 **Colon and Rectum Carcinoma Surveillance Counterpoint: Japan** 195
Yasushi Toh and Yoshihisa Sakaguchi

36 **Colon and Rectum Carcinoma Surveillance Counterpoint: Canada** 199
Marko Simunovic

37 **Anal Carcinoma** 205
David Y. Johnson, Shilpi Wadhwa, and Frank E. Johnson

38 **Anal Carcinoma Surveillance Counterpoint: USA** 207
Jonathan M. Hernandez, Erin M. Siegel, Abby Koch, and David Shibata

39 **Anal Carcinoma Surveillance Counterpoint: Australia** 215
Toufic El-Khoury, Michael Solomon, and Jane Young

40 **Anal Carcinoma Surveillance Counterpoint: Japan** 219
Yoshihisa Sakaguchi and Yasushi Toh

41 **Anal Carcinoma Surveillance Counterpoint: Canada** 223
Natasha Press and John Hay

42 **Soft Tissue Sarcoma** 227
David Y. Johnson, Shilpi Wadhwa, and Frank E. Johnson

43 **Soft Tissue Sarcoma Surveillance Counterpoint: USA** 231
Valeriy Sedov and Janice M. Mehnert

44 **Soft-Tissue Sarcoma Surveillance Counterpoint: Japan** 233
Shuichi Matsuda and Yukihide Iwamoto

45 **Soft Tissue Sarcoma Surveillance Counterpoint: Canada** 235
Lloyd A. Mack and Vivien H.C. Bramwell

46 **Osteogenic Sarcoma and Dedifferentiated Chondrosarcoma** 243
David Y. Johnson, Shilpi Wadhwa, and Frank E. Johnson

47 **Osteogenic Sarcoma and Dedifferentiated Chondrosarcoma Surveillance Counterpoint: Japan** 247
Shuichi Matsuda and Yukihide Iwamoto

48 **Osteogenic Sarcoma and Dedifferentiated Chondrosarcoma Surveillance Counterpoint: Canada** 249
Timothy R. Asmis, Joel Werier, and Shailendra Verma

49 **Cutaneous Melanoma** 251
David Y. Johnson, Shilpi Wadhwa, and Frank E. Johnson

50 **Cutaneous Melanoma Surveillance Counterpoint: USA** 255
Gerald Linette and Lynn A. Cornelius

51 **Cutaneous Melanoma Surveillance Counterpoint: Australia** 265
Michael A. Henderson

52 **Cutaneous Melanoma Surveillance Counterpoint: Japan** 269
Yoichi Moroi

53 **Breast Carcinoma** 273
David Y. Johnson, Shilpi Wadhwa, and Frank E. Johnson

54 **Breast Carcinoma Surveillance Counterpoint: USA** 277
Kelli Pettit and Julie A. Margenthaler

55 **Breast Carcinoma Surveillance Counterpoint: Europe** 281
Stefano Ciatto

56 **Breast Carcinoma Surveillance Counterpoint: Australia** 285
Andrew J. Spillane and Meagan E. Brennan

57 **Breast Carcinoma Surveillance Counterpoint: Japan** 293
Eriko Tokunaga and Yoshihiko Maehara

58 **Endometrial Carcinoma** 297
David Y. Johnson, Shilpi Wadhwa, and Frank E. Johnson

59 **Endometrial Cancer Surveillance Counterpoint: USA** 301
Amit Bhate, Eric Donnelly, John Lurain, Julian Schink, and William Small Jr.

60 **Endometrial Cancer Surveillance Counterpoint: USA** 305
Summer B. Dewdney and Premal H. Thaker

61 **Carcinoma of the Endometrium Surveillance Counterpoint: Japan** 311
Yousuke Ueoka, Hiroaki Kobayashi, and Norio Wake

62 **Endometrial Carcinoma Surveillance Counterpoint: Canada** 317
Michael Fung-Kee-Fung and Thomas K. Oliver

63 **Cervical Carcinoma** 323
David Y. Johnson, Shilpi Wadhwa, and Frank E. Johnson

64 **Cervical Carcinoma Surveillance Counterpoint: USA** 327
Joshua P. Kesterson and Shashikant Lele

65 **Cervical Carcinoma Surveillance Counterpoint: Japan** 335
Kenzo Sonoda, Hiroaki Kobayashi, and Norio Wake

66 **Cervical Carcinoma Surveillance Counterpoint: Canada** 341
Michael Fung-Kee-Fung and Thomas K. Oliver

67 **Vaginal and Vulvar Carcinoma** 349
David Y. Johnson, Shilpi Wadhwa, and Frank E. Johnson

68 **Vaginal and Vulvar Carcinoma Surveillance Counterpoint: Japan** 353
Shinji Ogawa, Hiroaki Kobayashi, and Norio Wake

69 **Ovarian Carcinoma** 357
David Y. Johnson, Shilpi Wadhwa, and Frank E. Johnson

70 **Ovarian Carcinoma Surveillance Counterpoint: USA** 361
Maurie Markman

71 **Ovarian Cancer Surveillance Counterpoint: Europe** 365
Andy Nordin

72 **Ovarian Cancer Surveillance Counterpoint: Japan** 369
Hiroaki Kobayashi and Norio Wake

73 **Renal Carcinoma** 373
Shilpi Wadhwa, David Y. Johnson, and Frank E. Johnson

74 **Renal Carcinoma Surveillance Counterpoint: Europe** 375
Alessandro Antonelli, Claudio Simeone, and Sergio Cosciani Cunico

75 **Renal Carcinoma Surveillance Counterpoint: Japan** ... 381
Masatoshi Eto, Wataru Takahashi, Yoshiaki Kawano, Jiro Honda, Juro Nakanishi, and Yoshihiro Wada

76 **Renal Carcinoma Surveillance Counterpoint: Canada** ... 383
Michael Leveridge, Robert Abouassaly, and Michael A.S. Jewett

77 **Urinary Bladder Carcinoma** ... 387
David Y. Johnson, Shilpi Wadhwa, and Frank E. Johnson

78 **Urinary Bladder Carcinoma Surveillance Counterpoint: Japan** ... 393
Kentaro Kuroiwa

79 **Urinary Bladder Carcinoma Surveillance Counterpoint: Canada** ... 395
Faysal A. Yafi and Wassim Kassouf

80 **Prostate Carcinoma** ... 399
David Y. Johnson, Shilpi Wadhwa, and Frank E. Johnson

81 **Prostate Carcinoma Surveillance Counterpoint: USA** ... 403
Angela Smith and Raj Pruthi

82 **Prostate Cancer Surveillance Counterpoint: USA** ... 411
Erik T. Goluboff and Matthew Wosnitzer

83 **Prostate Carcinoma Surveillance Counterpoint: Europe** ... 421
Stefano Ciatto

84 **Prostate Carcinoma Surveillance Counterpoint: Japan** ... 423
Akira Yokomizo

85 **Prostate Carcinoma Surveillance Counterpoint: Canada** ... 427
Andrew Loblaw and Colin Tang

86 **Testicle Carcinoma** ... 437
David Y. Johnson, Shilpi Wadhwa, and Frank E. Johnson

87 **Testicle Carcinoma Surveillance Counterpoint: USA** ... 443
Ian M. Thompson III and Sam S. Chang

88 **Testicle Carcinoma Surveillance Counterpoint: Australia** ... 449
Michael Boyer and Kate Mahon

89 **Testicle Carcinoma Surveillance Counterpoint: Japan** ... 453
Narihito Seki

90 **Lymphoma** ... 457
David Y. Johnson, Shilpi Wadhwa, and Frank E. Johnson

91 **Lymphoma Surveillance Counterpoint: USA** ... 461
Kenneth R. Carson and Nancy L. Bartlett

92 **Lymphoma Surveillance Counterpoint: Japan** ... 467
Kenjiro Kamezaki

93 **Lymphoma (Following Autologous Stem Cell Transplant)** ... 469
Shilpi Wadhwa, David Y. Johnson, and Frank E. Johnson

94 **Lymphoma (Following Autologous Stem Cell Transplant) Surveillance Counterpoint: Japan** ... 471
Toshihiro Miyamoto

95 Leukemia 475
David Y. Johnson, Shilpi Wadhwa, and Frank E. Johnson

96 Leukemia Surveillance Counterpoint: USA 479
Olalekan Oluwole, Susan Greenhut, Bipin N. Savani, and Nishitha Reddy

97 Leukemia Surveillance Counterpoint: Japan 485
Koji Nagafuji

98 Multiple Myeloma 487
Shilpi Wadhwa, David Y. Johnson, and Frank E. Johnson

99 Multiple Myeloma Surveillance Counterpoint: USA 489
Niyati Modi, G. David Roodman, and Suzanne Lentzsch

100 Multiple Myeloma Surveillance Counterpoint: Australia 493
Liane Khoo and Douglas Joshua

101 Multiple Myeloma Surveillance Counterpoint: Japan 501
Katsuto Takenaka

102 Multiple Myeloma Surveillance Counterpoint: Canada 503
Matthew C. Cheung and Kevin R. Imrie

103 Glioma of the Central Nervous System 511
David Y. Johnson, Shilpi Wadhwa, and Frank E. Johnson

104 Glioma of the Central Nervous System Surveillance Counterpoint: Europe 515
Wolfgang Grisold, Stefan Oberndorfer, and Eefje Sizoo

105 Glioma of the Central Nervous System Surveillance Counterpoint: Australia 517
Margot Lehman and Michael Barton

106 Glioma of the Central Nervous System Surveillance Counterpoint: Japan 521
Masahiro Mizoguchi, Koji Yoshimoto, and Tomio Sasaki

Index 525

Contributors

Robert Abouassaly University of Toronto, Toronto, ON, Canada

Division of Urology, Department of Surgical Oncology, Princess Margaret Hospital and the University Health Network, University of Toronto, Toronto, ON, Canada

Alessandro Antonelli Department of Urology, University of Brescia, Brescia, Italy

Timothy R. Asmis The Ottawa Hospital Regional Cancer Centre, Ottawa, ON, Canada

Béatrix Barry Service Otorhinolaryngologie et Chirurgie Cervico-faciale, Hôpital Bichat-Claude Bernard, Paris, France

Nancy L. Bartlett Siteman Cancer Center, Washington University, Washington, MO, USA

Michael Barton Liverpool Cancer Therapy Centre, Liverpool, BC, Australia

Oliver F. Bathe Division of Surgical Oncology, Tom Baker Cancer Centre, Calgary, AB, Canada

Tanios S. Bekaii-Saab James Cancer Hospital, The Ohio State University, Columbus, OH, USA

Amit Bhate Department of Radiation Oncology, The Robert H. Lurie Comprehensive Cancer Center of Northwestern University, DeKalb, IL, USA

Michael Boyer Department of Medical Oncology, Sydney Cancer Centre, Royal Prince Albert Hospital, Camperdown, Australia

Vivien H.C. Bramwell Department of Medicine, Alberta Health Services—Cancer Care, Tom Baker Cancer Centre, University of Calgary, Calgary, AB, Canada

Division of Medical and Radiation Oncology, Alberta Health Services, Calgary Zone, 1, Calgary, AB, Canada

Meagan E. Brennan The University of Sydney, Northern Clinical School, Sydney, Australia

Mater Hospital, The Poche Centre, North Sydney, NSW, Australia

Kelly Warren Burak Southern Alberta Liver Transplant Clinic, University of Calgary Liver Unit, Calgary, AB, Canada

Bryan H. Burmeister Department of Radiation Oncology, Princess Alexandra Hospital, University of Queensland, Woolloongabba, QLD, Australia

James B. Butler Department of Radiation Oncology, CancerCare Manitoba, MB, Canada

Jane V. Butler Division of Surgery and Oncology, The Owen and Ellen Evans Chair of Cancer Studies, School of Cancer Studies, Royal Liverpool University Hospital, University of Liverpool, Liverpool, UK

Kenneth R. Carson Section of Medical Oncology, Washington University School of Medicine, St. Louis, MO, USA

Sam S. Chang Department of Urologic Surgery, Vanderbilt University Medical Center, Nashville, TN, USA

Matthew C. Cheung Odette Cancer Centre, Sunnybrook Health Sciences, Toronto, ON, Canada

Department of Medicine, Division of Hematology/Medical Oncology, University of Toronto, Toronto, ON, Canada

Stefano Ciatto ISPO—Istituto per lo Studio e la Prevenzione Oncologica, Florence, Italy

Steven J. Cohen Fox Chase Cancer Center, Philadelphia, PA, USA

Andrew Coleman Duke University School of Medicine, Durham, NC, USA

Michele Colledan Ospedali Riuniti di Bergamo, Bergamo, Italy

Lynn A. Cornelius Department of Dermatology, Washington University School of Medicine, St. Louis, MO, USA

Brooke Crawford Department of Orthopaedic Surgery, Saint Louis University School of Medicine, St. Louis, MO, USA

Michael D. Crawford Royal Prince Alfred Medical Centre, Newtown, Australia

Sergio Cosciani Cunico Department of Urology, University of Brescia, Brescia, Italy

Gail Darling University Health Network and University of Toronto, Toronto, ON, Canada

Jennifer Deevy Institute for Clinical Evaluative Sciences, Sunnybrook Health Sciences Centre, Toronto, ON, Canada

Leigh Delbridge University of Sydney Endocrine Surgical Unit, Sydney, Australia

Department of Endocrine and Oncology Surgery, Royal North Shore Hospital, Sydney, Australia

Summer B. Dewdney Department of Obstetrics and Gynecology, Rush University Medical Center, Chicago, IL, USA

Eric Donnelly Department of Radiation Oncology, The Robert H. Lurie Comprehensive Cancer Center of Northwestern University, DeKalb, IL, USA

Craig C. Earle Dana-Farber Cancer Institute Harvard Medical School, Boston, Massachusetts, USA

Toufic El-Khoury Surgical Outcome Research Centre (SOuRCe), Royal Prince Alfred Hospital Sydney, University of Sydney, Sydney, Australia

Peter Ellis Juravinski Cancer Centre and McMaster University, Hamilton, ON, Canada

Masatoshi Eto Department of Urology, Kumamoto University, Kumamoto, Japan

Bill Evans Juravinski Cancer Centre and McMaster University, Hamilton, ON, Canada

Michael Fung-Kee-Fung Division of Gynecologic Oncology Surgical Oncology Program, Department of Obstetrics and Gynecology, Ottawa Hospital/University of Ottawa, Ottawa, ON, Canada

Sandra M.E. Geurts Department of Epidemiology, Biostatistics and HTA, Radboud University Nijmegen Medical Centre, Nijmegen, The Netherlands

Erik T. Goluboff Beth Israel Medical Center, New York, NY, USA

David D. Greenberg Department of Orthopaedic Surgery, Saint Louis University School of Medicine, St. Louis, MO, USA

Susan Greenhut Department of Medicine, Division of Hematology/Oncology, Hematology and Stem Cell Transplantation Section, Vanderbilt University Medical Center, Nashville, TN, USA

Wolfgang Grisold Department of Neurology, Kaiser-Franz-Josef-Spital Hospital, Ludwig Boltzmann Institute for Neuro-Oncology, Vienna, Austria

John Hay Radiation Oncologist, British Columbia Cancer Agency, Vancouver Cancer Centre, University of British Columbia, Vancouver, BC, Canada

Michael A. Henderson Division of Cancer Surgery, Peter MacCallum Cancer Center, East Melbourne, Australia

Jonathan M. Hernandez Department of Surgery, University of South Florida, Tampa, FL, USA

Department of Gastrointestinal Oncology, H. Lee Moffitt Cancer Center and Research Institute, Tampa, FL, USA

Jiro Honda Department of Urology, Kumamoto University, Kumamoto, Japan

Kevin R. Imrie Department of Medicine, Sunnybrook Health Sciences Center, University of Toronto, Toronto, ON, Canada

Department of Medicine, Division of Hematology/Medical Oncology, University of Toronto, Toronto, ON, Canada

Yukihide Iwamoto Department of Orthopaedic Surgery, Kyushu University, Fukuoka, Japan

Michael A.S. Jewett Division of Urology, University of Toronto, Toronto, ON, Canada

David Y. Johnson Department of Internal Medicine, Saint Louis University Medical Center, Saint Louis, MO, USA

Frank E. Johnson Saint Louis University Medical Center and Saint Louis Veterans Affairs Medical Center, Saint Louis, MO, USA

Douglas Joshua Institute of Haematology, Royal Prince Alfred Hospital, Camperdown Sydney, Australia

Kenjiro Kamezaki Medicine and Biosystemic Science, Graduate School of Medical Sciences, Kyushu University, Fukuoka, Japan

Yoshihiro Kakeji Department of Surgery and Science, Graduate School of Medical Sciences, Kyushu University, Fukuoka, Japan

Wassim Kassouf Division of Urology, McGill University Health Center, Montreal, QC, Canada

Yoshiaki Kawano Department of Urology, Kumamoto University, Kumamoto, Japan

Kim E.M. van Kessel Department of Public Health, Erasmus University, Rotterdam, The Netherlands

Joshua P. Kesterson Division of Gynecologic Oncology, Roswell Park Cancer Institute, Buffalo, NY, USA

Liane Khoo Institute of Haematology, Royal Prince Alfred Hospital, Camperdown, Sydney, NSW, Australia

Hiroaki Kobayashi Department of Obstetrics and Gynecology, Graduate School of Medical Sciences, Kyushu University, Fukuoka, Japan

Abby Koch Department of Cancer Epidemiology and Genetics, Risk Assessment, Detection & Intervention Program, H. Lee Moffitt Cancer Center and Research Institute, Tampa, FL, USA

Shizuo Komune Department of Otorhinolaryngology, Graduate School of Medical Sciences, Kyushu University, Fukuoka, Japan

Kentaro Kuroiwa Department of Urology, Graduate School of Medical Sciences, Kyushu University, Fukuoka, Japan

Shashikant Lele Division of Gynecologic Oncology, Roswell Park Cancer Institute, Buffalo, NY, USA

Margot Lehman Princess Alexandra Hospital, Woolloongabbo, Australia

Suzanne Lentzsch Multiple Myeloma Program, Division of Hematology/Oncology, University of Pittsburgh, Pittsburgh, PA, USA

Michael Leveridge University of Toronto, Toronto, ON, Canada

Department of Urology, Queen's University, Kingston, ON, Canada

Gerald Linette Department of Medical Oncology, Washington University School of Medicine, St. Louis, MO, USA

Andrew Loblaw Department of Radiation Oncology, Odette Cancer Centre, Sunnybrook Health Sciences Centre, Toronto, ON, Canada

John Lurain Department of Obstetrics and Gynecology, Division of Gynecologic Oncology, The Robert H. Lurie Comprehensive Cancer Center, Northwestern University Feinberg School of Medicine, Chicago, IL, USA

Lloyd A. Mack Department of Surgical Oncology, Alberta Health Services—Cancer Care, Tom Baker Cancer Centre, University of Calgary, Surgical, Oncologist, Calgary, AB, Canada

Yoshihiko Maehara Department of Surgery and Science, Graduate School of Medical Sciences, Kyushu University, Fukuoka, Japan

Kate Mahon Garvan Institute, Sydney, NSW, Australia

Julie A. Margenthaler Department of Surgery, Washington University School of Medicine, Siteman Cancer Center, St. Louis, MO, USA

Maurie Markman Department of Gynecologic Medical Oncology, The University of Texas, M.D. Anderson Cancer Center, Houston, TX, USA

Lorraine Martelli-Reid Juravinski Cancer Centre and McMaster University, Hamilton, ON, Canada

Shuichi Matsuda Department of Orthopaedic Surgery, Kyushu University, Fukuoka, Japan

Janice M. Mehnert Melanoma and Soft Tissue Oncology, The Cancer Institute of New Jersey, New Brunswick, NJ, USA

Toshihiro Miyamoto Department of Medicine and Biosystemic Science, Graduate School of Medical Sciences, Kyushu University, Fukuoka, Japan

Masahiro Mizoguchi Department of Neurosurgery, Graduate School of Medical Sciences, Kyushu University, Fukuoka, Japan

Niyati Modi Department of Medicine, West Penn Allegheny Health System, Pittsburgh, PA, USA

Malcolm J. Moore Division of Medical Oncology and Hematology, Princess Margaret Hospital, Toronto, ON, Canada

Masaru Morita Department of Surgery and Science, Graduate School of Medical Sciences, Kyushu University, Fukuoka, Japan

Yoichi Moroi Department of Dermatology, Graduate School of Medical Science, Kyushu University, Fukuoka, Japan

Koji Nagafuji Department of Medicine, Division of Hematology, Kurume University School of Medicine, Kurume, Japan

Juro Nakanishi Department of Urology, Kumamoto University, Kumamoto, Japan

Torahiko Nakashima Department of Otorhinolaryngology, Graduate School of Medical Sciences, Kyushu University, Fukuoka, Japan

Richard W. Nason Department of Surgical Oncology, CancerCare Manitoba, MB, Canada

Andy Nordin Cancer Services Collaborative, National Clinical Lead For Gynaecology, East Kent Gynaecological Oncology Centre, Queen Elizabeth The Queen Mother Hospital, University College London, Kent, UK

John P. Neoptolemos Division of Surgery and Oncology, The Owen and Ellen Evans Chair of Cancer Studies, School of Cancer Studies, Royal Liverpool University Hospital, University of Liverpool, Liverpool, UK

Stefan Oberndorfer Department of Neurology, Kaiser-Franz-Josef-Spital Hospital, Ludwig Boltzmann Institute for Neuro-Oncology, Vienna, Austria

Shinji Ogawa Department of Obstetrics and Gynecology, Graduate School of Medical Sciences, Kyushu University, Fukuoka, Japan

Thomas K. Oliver Department of Oncology, McMaster University, Hamilton, ON, Canada

Kelli Pettit Department of Surgery, Washington University School of Medicine, Siteman Cancer Center, St. Louis, MO, USA

Natasha Press Division of Infectious Diseases, University of British Columbia, Vancouver, BC, Canada

Raj Pruthi Division of Urologic Surgery, University of North Carolina, Chapel Hill, NC, USA

Dominique De Raucourt Service Chirurgie Tête et Cou, Centre François Baclesse, Caen, France

Nishitha Reddy Department of Medicine, Division of Hematology/Oncology, Hematology and Stem Cell Transplantation Section, Vanderbilt University Medical Center, Nashville, TN, USA

G. David Roodman University of Pittsburgh School of Medicine, Pittsburgh, PA, USA

UPMC Health System, VA Pittsburgh Healthcare System, Research and Development, Pittsburgh, PA, USA

Yoshihisa Sakaguchi Department of Gastroenterological Surgery, National Kyushu Cancer Center, Fukuoka, Japan

Tomio Sasaki Department of Neurosurgery, Graduate School of Medical Sciences, Kyushu University, Fukuoka, Japan

Bipin N. Savani Department of Medicine, Division of Hematology/Oncology, Hematology and Stem Cell Transplantation Section, Vanderbilt University Medical Center, Nashville, TN, USA

Valeriy Sedov Melanoma and Soft Tissue Oncology, The Cancer Institute of New Jersey, New Brunswick, NJ, USA

Julian Schink Department of Obstetrics and Gynecology, Division of Gynecologic Oncology, The Robert H. Lurie Comprehensive Cancer Center, Northwestern University Feinberg School of Medicine, Chicago, IL, USA

Narihito Seki Department of Urology, Graduate School of Medical Sciences, Kyushu University, Fukuoka, Japan

David Shibata Department of Gastrointestinal Oncology, H. Lee Moffitt Cancer Center and Research Institute, Tampa, FL, USA

Ken Shirabe Department of Surgery and Science, Graduate School of Medical Sciences, Kyushu University, Fukuoka, Japan

Erin M. Siegel Department of Cancer Epidemiology and Genetics,33Risk Assessment, Detection & Intervention Program, H. Lee Moffitt Cancer Center and Research Institute, Tampa, FL, USA

Claudio Simeone Department of Urology, University of Brescia, Brescia, Italy

Marko Simunovic Department of Surgery, McMaster University, Hamilton, ON, Canada

Surgical Oncologist, Juravinski Cancer Centre, Hamilton Health Sciences, Hamilton, ON, Canada

Eefje Sizoo Department of Neurology, Vrije Universiteit Medical Center, Amsterdam, The Netherlands

William Small Jr. Department of Radiation Oncology, The Robert H. Lurie Comprehensive Cancer Center of Northwestern University, Chicago, IL, USA

Angela Smith Division of Urologic Surgery, University of North Carolina, Chapel Hill, NC, USA

Richard A. Smith Division of Surgery and Oncology, The Owen and Ellen Evans Chair of Cancer Studies, School of Cancer Studies, Royal Liverpool University Hospital, University of Liverpool, Liverpoo1, UK

Bernard Mark Smithers Upper Gastrointestinal and Soft Tissue Unit, Princess Alexandra Hospital, University of Queensland, Woolloongabba, QLD, Australia

Michael Solomon Surgical Outcome Research Centre (SOuRCe), Royal Prince Alfred Hospital Sydney, University of Sydney, Sydney, Australia

Kenzo Sonoda Department of Obstetrics and Gynecology, Graduate School of Medical Sciences, Kyushu University, Fukuoka, Japan

Andrew J. Spillane The University of Sydney, Northern Clinical School, Sydney, Australia

Mater Hospital, The Poche Centre, North Sydney, NSW, Australia

Royal North Shore Hospital, St. Leonards, Sydney, Australia

Sydney Cancer Centre, Royal Prince Alfred Hospital, Camperdown, NSW, Australia

Anastasios Stathis Drug Development Program, Princess Margaret Hospital, Toronto, ON, Canada

Ewout W. Steyerberg Department of Public Health, Erasmus University, Rotterdam, The Netherlands

Wataru Takahashi Department of Urology, Kumamoto University, Kumamoto, Japan

Akinobu Taketomi Department of Surgery and Science, Graduate School of Medicine, Kyushu University, Fukuoka, Japan

Katsuto Takenaka Medicine and Biosystemic Science, Kyushu University Graduate School of Medical Sciences, Maidashi, Fukuoka, Japan

Colin Tang Department of Radiation Oncology, Calvary Mater Newcastle Hospital, Waratah, NSW, Australia

Mohamedtaki A. Tejani Fox Chase Cancer Center, Philadelphia, PA, USA

Premal H. Thaker Division of Gynecologic Oncology, Department of Obstetrics and Gynecology, Washington University School of Medicine, Campus, St. Louis, MO, USA

Janine M. Thomas Upper Gastrointestinal and Soft Tissue Unit, Princess Alexandra Hospital, Woolloongabba, QLD, Australia

Ian M. Thompson III Department of Urologic Surgery, Vanderbilt University Medical Center, Nashville, TN, USA

Yasushi Toh Department of Gastroenterological Surgery, National Kyushu Cancer Center, Fukuoka, Japan

Eriko Tokunaga Department of Surgery and Science, Graduate School of Medical Sciences, Kyushu University, Fukuoka, Japan

Douglas Tyler Department of Surgery, Duke University Medical Center, Durham, NC, USA

Yousuke Ueoka Hamanomachi Hospital, Fukuoka, Japan

Yee Ung Odette Cancer Centre and University of Toronto Sunnybrook Health Sciences Centre, Toronto, ON, Canada

André L.M. Verbeek Department of Epidemiology, Biostatistics and HTA, Radboud University, Nijmegen Medical Centre, Nijmegen, The Netherlands

Shailendra Verma The Ottawa Hospital Regional Cancer Centre, Ottawa, ON, Canada

Yoshihiro Wada Department of Urology, Kumamoto University, Kumamoto, Japan

Shilpi Wadhwa Department of Internal Medicine, Saint Louis University Medical Center, Saint Louis, MO, USA

Norio Wake Department of Obstetrics and Gynecology, Graduate School of Medical Sciences, Kyushu University, Fukuoka, Japan

Joel Werier The Ottawa Hospital Regional Cancer Centre, Ottawa, ON, Canada

Matthew Wosnitzer Beth Israel Medical Center, New York, NY, USA

Faysal A. Yafi Division of Urology, McGill University Health Center, Montreal, QC, Canada

Tokujiro Yano Department of Surgery, Beppu Medical Center, Uchikamado, Beppu, Japan

Ryuji Yasumatsu Department of Otorhinolaryngology, Graduate School of Medical Sciences, Kyushu University, Fukuoka, Japan

Akira Yokomizo Department of Urology, Graduate School of Medical Sciences, Kyushu University, Fukuoka, Japan

Koji Yoshimoto Department of Neurosurgery, Graduate School of Medical Sciences, Kyushu University, Fukuoka, Japan

Jane Young Surgical Outcome Research Centre (SOuRCe), Royal Prince Alfred Hospital Sydney, University of Sydney, Sydney, Australia

Overview

1

David Y. Johnson and Frank E. Johnson

Keywords
AHCPR • Cancer • Guidelines • Postoperative surveillance • Protocol

Self-awareness is a particularly human trait. When it evolved, proto-humans became aware that they were destined to die. When language evolved, they were able to share this understanding with others. When written languages were developed, their thoughts about mortality were recorded in permanent form. The documents that have survived to the present convincingly demonstrate that humans have sought to understand why they become ill and die for a very long time. Cancer, in its many forms, is featured in the earliest of these documents [1]. It is feared and many forms of treatment have been employed throughout the ages, almost all of which were unsuccessful. By the nineteenth century, with the introduction of effective anesthesia, relatively safe major surgery became feasible. As a result, for the first time in history some patients with cancer were cured [2]. This created a cohort of cancer survivors. Shortly thereafter, it became clear that this population is prone to recurrence of the index cancer and/or new primary cancers and/or adverse effects of therapy. Treatments often failed, however, and major medical texts in the early-twentieth century made no mention of second primary cancers [3,4] but adverse effects of therapy were well known. This soon led to the concept of postoperative surveillance. This was facilitated in the late nineteenth century by the development of diagnostic x-rays [5]. Cancer patients also benefited by the introduction of radiation as a powerful treatment. Its hazards soon were recognized and those who had received radiation therapy as the initial treatment were soon candidates for surveillance. Relapse often occurred, as for those treated with surgery. Effective systemic therapy (oophorectomy for metastatic breast cancer) had its start in the late nineteenth century also [6]. The complications of this operation were presumably infrequent and manageable, but surveillance was probably carried out to determine how useful this novel form of therapy would be—since the concept of "chemical messengers" (hormones) was unknown until secretin was discovered in 1906 [7,8]. By the time effective systemic cytotoxic therapy was introduced into practice in the mid-twentieth century, the idea that it might eventually be curative was imagined by the few medical oncologists of that time and became a reality shortly thereafter, providing another cohort of survivors. The use of cytotoxic chemotherapy was regulated by regimen-specific drug administration protocols and institutional review boards (both novel concepts at that time). The post-treatment course was carefully documented. Documentation of initial disease status and estimation of prognosis were improved by the introduction of systematic staging methods such as the Federation Internationale de Gynecologie et d'Obstetrique and American Joint Committee on Cancer-Union for International Cancer Control systems. These common descriptors improved data collection and analysis. Introduction of new diagnostic testing modalities (serologic tumor marker measurement, computer-assisted tomography, magnetic resonance imaging, monoclonal antibody-based cellular stains, and the like) found immediate application in surveillance.

Medical practice, including cancer screening, diagnosis, staging, treatment, and posttreatment management, became rather complex in the twentieth century. The complexity led to

D.Y. Johnson
Department of Internal Medicine, Saint Louis University Medical Center, Saint Louis, MO, USA
e-mail: djohns69@slu.edu

F.E. Johnson, M.D., FACS (✉)
Saint Louis University Medical Center and Saint Louis Veterans Affairs Medical Center, Saint Louis, MO, USA
e-mail: frank.johnson1@va.gov

F.E. Johnson et al. (eds.), *Patient Surveillance After Cancer Treatment*, Current Clinical Oncology,
DOI 10.1007/978-1-60327-969-7_1, © Springer Science+Business Media New York 2013

increasing reliance on guidelines. From the time of the Edwin Smith Papyrus [1], informal health-related guidelines, often generated by untrained citizens and promoted by churches, schools, government agencies, and the like, have been used. These included advice about diet, behavior, hazardous materials, and so on. In recent times, guideline development has become much more rigorous and evidence-based. The U.S. Institute of Medicine published a book about this topic in 1990 [9]. It provided advice to the U.S. Agency for Health Care Policy and Research (AHCPR), particularly its Forum for Quality and Effectiveness in Health Care. The AHCPR and many other interested parties helped another Institute of Medicine committee formulate ways to develop guidelines [10]. This included methods to precisely define relevant terms, estimation of strengths and weaknesses of guideline development efforts, and so on. The books were produced by outstanding groups of experts who recognized that clinical practice guidelines had been used in various ways by some organizations to consider "costs, quality, access, patient empowerment, professional autonomy, medical liability, rationing, competition, benefit design, utilization variation, bureaucratic micromanagement of health care, and more" [11]. The authors intended to utilize a systematic approach, consider the evidence base, and evaluate the processes, structures, and incentives that contribute to the effectiveness and periodic evaluation of such guidelines. The 1992 book detailed desirable attributes of clinical practice guidelines: validity, reliability, reproducibility, clinical applicability, clinical flexibility, clarity, a multidisciplinary development process, scheduled review, documentation of the process of guideline development, sensitivity, specificity, patient responsiveness, readability, minimum obtrusiveness, feasibility, computer compatibility, and appeals criteria [12]. All medical guidelines available today fail to possess some of these attributes; many fail to possess most of them. The Institute of Medicine experts exerted much effort to evaluate the state of the evidence supporting medical care. David Eddy, a very influential thought leader and a member of the Institute of Medicine, recognized three levels of appropriate medical care, related directly to the importance of the outcomes to patients and the persuasiveness and clarity of the evidence. In his analysis, when the evidence in favor of a particular course of care is very strong, the course can be termed a "standard" and recommended to all patients with only a few exceptions. When the evidence is not very strong, the course can be termed a "guideline." A guideline applies in most situations but with more exceptions than are warranted for standards. The term "option" refers to a course of management in which the evidence does not warrant specific recommendations [13]. The Institute of Medicine committee also explained the meaning of terms such as "strong evidence," "strong consensus," and the like. They recognized that consensus statements generated by experts have some value.

Table 1.1 Hypothetical distribution of evidence and consensus for all health services and patient management strategies

Strength of evidence	Strength of consensus	Percentage of all services
++	++	2
++	+	2
++	0	0
+	++	20
+	+	25
+	0	0
0	++	20
0	+	25
0	0	6

++ = strong evidence or consensus
+ = modest evidence or consensus
0 = very weak or no evidence or consensus
From Ref. [15]

The reliability of consensus-based guidelines has increasingly been questioned, however. A major reason is the near-inevitability of conflict of interest among those who create guidelines of most sorts. Those who create guidelines are always well-informed about the topic at hand. They usually have carried out research about that particular topic. They have often served as paid consultants to for-profit companies. Some have participated in industry-sponsored research. Even if these individuals agree to abstain from voting on guidelines during the process of creating them, their comments during the development process are often quite persuasive [14]. The committee also recognized that many courses of care in medical practice are not supported by good evidence. The committee estimated how evidence of variable quality and consensus of variable strength are distributed among all courses of care in healthcare systems [15] (Table 1.1).

Since publication of these two very influential books, interest in guidelines has increased. There has also been an explosion in the number of guidelines. Floyd Bloom, in his presidential address at the 2003 meeting of the American Association for the Advancement of Science, noted that there were at that time 10,000 medicines, >100,000 described diseases and conditions, thousands of guidelines, and millions of rules covering various aspects of medical care delivery [16]. Since then, the number of guidelines has increased. They guide medical practice in virtually all countries and some have quasi-legal status. In response to these daunting statistics (among other things), the Institute of Medicine sought to help society know what works in medical care. One early step was to decide whether to consider costs. This is a central component of healthcare economics among most governments in the world but, in the U.S., the consideration of cost in government health policy about insurance coverage decisions is often absent, sporadic, or irrational. Because of this, the committee chose not to make recommendations about the role of cost in evaluating the value of clinical services, focusing instead on effectiveness [17]. This Institute of Medicine report noted that guideline development in the U.S. is somewhat disorganized, resulting in gross duplication of efforts in some areas and minimal efforts in others. At the time when the committee was deliberating (2006–2008), the National Guideline Clearinghouse of AHCPR received guidelines from >350 organizations. This clearinghouse contained >450 guidelines related to high blood pressure and >250 related to stroke—but few related to patient surveillance after curative-intent therapy for cancer patients, for example [18]. In contrast, in the United Kingdom (where considerations of cost are explicit), a single entity, the National Institute for Health and Clinical Excellence (NICE), is charged with generating clinical guidelines and providing guidance about public health issues, including health technologies for the National Health Service in England, Northern Ireland, and Wales. A similar entity creates separate guidelines for Scotland [19]. In the opinions of the authors of this chapter, these systems are the best of their kind in the world. However, they have produced few guidelines about surveillance for patients after initial therapy for most types of cancer.

The process of guideline development was reassessed by the Institute of Medicine in 2011 [20]. The committee concluded that trustworthy guidelines should be based on a systematic review of existing evidence; be developed by a knowledgeable, multidisciplinary group of experts and representatives from key affected groups; consider important patient subgroups and patient preferences, as appropriate; be based on an explicit and transparent process that minimizes distortions, biases, and conflicts of interest; provide a clear explanation of the logical relationships between alternative care options and health outcomes, and provide ratings of both the quality of evidence and the strength of the recommendations; and be reconsidered and revised as appropriate when important new evidence warrants modification of recommendations.

The concept of patient surveillance after cancer treatment is clearly here to stay. There are many types of cancer, many forms of treatment, and many surveillance tools. Curative-intent primary therapy can be delivered to many patients with most types of cancer. Surveillance is felt to be warranted for virtually all such patients, even those in whom cure is not possible, but this book is primarily concerned with those treated with curative intent. In such patients, surveillance is felt by most patients and most caregivers to be valuable. It is regularly carried out, at least in wealthy countries. There have been few large, well-controlled trials of posttreatment surveillance strategies published in the relevant literature for most types of cancer at present. There are many reasons for this evidence deficit and the consequences are important for payers, physicians and other caregivers, patients, and their friends and families.

As an alternative approach, the authors of this book have attempted to collect and summarize succinctly the guidelines that have been generated by reputable professional societies, nonprofit groups, and relevant government agencies for many common cancers. To this end, we searched for guidelines generated by nine relevant professional groups, nonprofit organizations, and government agencies and also available on the internet: the National Comprehensive Cancer Network (NCCN, www.nccn.org), the American Society of Clinical Oncology (ASCO, www.asco.org), the European Society for Medical Oncology (ESMO, www.esmo.org), the European Society of Surgical Oncology (ESSO, www.essoweb.org), the National Institute for Health and Clinical Excellence (NICE, www.nice.org.uk) of the United Kingdom, the National Guideline Clearinghouse (NGC, www.guideline.gov), the Cochrane Collaboration (TCC, www.cochrane.org), the Society of Surgical Oncology (SSO, www.surgonc.org), and Cancer Care Ontario (CCO, www.cancercare.on.ca) in 2007–2008 and 2011–2012. Evaluation of the two searches revealed that there are few guidelines from these sources that even make specific recommendations about how frequently the available surveillance modalities (office visit, blood tests, imaging studies, etc.) should be recommended. In addition, there have been few changes between the two sets of guidelines, indicating that little new evidence has been introduced concerning patient surveillance over this period. Many clinicians refer to the NCCN guidelines when inquiring about posttreatment follow-up recommendations for their patients, in large part, apparently, because they make fairly specific recommendations.

We recognized the lack of high-quality data on this topic about 20 years ago, the subsequent vagueness of most guidelines and the weakness of the evidence base underpinning NCCN and ESMO guidelines. We set out to determine how experts around the world conduct such surveillance. The experts were all from wealthy industrial democracies and leaders in their fields. The results were published in 1995 [21]. The practices these experts recommended were often quite complex, related largely to estimated risk of recurrence. However, they were not congruent, which was not surprising in retrospect, given the minimal available evidence about the utility of any surveillance strategy and the variability among institutions, payers, treatment philosophies of the various experts, and the populations served.

We next attempted to quantify the actual practices of clinicians who treated patients with a particular form of cancer, provided posttreatment surveillance, and were members of their main professional organization. To accomplish this, we relied on custom-made survey instruments that were sent by conventional mail or email. An example is surveillance after treatment for soft-tissue sarcoma. The survey featured four brief vignettes, succinctly describing generally healthy sarcoma patients with different prognoses. It revealed dramatic variation in the self-reported actual practice of these experts [22]. Realizing that variation is a measure of quality [23] and that unwarranted variation is prima facie evidence of overuse and/or underuse and/or misuse of scarce medical resources, we next sought to determine the source of this variation [24]. We analyzed the role of physician age in the observed variation and found that, although significant variation attributable to surgeon age was present, it was much too small to account for the overall variation previously documented [25]. We estimated the effect of the size and grade of the sarcoma on the overall surveillance variability; again significant variation was documented but it was too small to be considered a major source of the previously observed variation [26]. We evaluated the effect of the geographic location of the surgeon, which would incorporate factors such as the presence of a nearby academic center and managed care organization penetration rate. This complex analysis showed again that, though significant variability was attributable to these factors, they could not explain the overall variation we had earlier noted [27]. In an attempt to understand the motivation of the clinicians, we inquired about this directly [28]. We estimated the costs of posttreatment surveillance strategies recommended for soft-tissue sarcoma patients in an earlier textbook devoted to this topic and found 25-fold variation among the five institutions represented, based on Medicare-allowed charges [29,30]. One might presume that even greater differences among clinicians might have been detected if we had asked more experts about their strategies. Many other factors play major roles in determining surveillance intensity utilized by experts, even though we have only indirect evidence for this. Such factors include patient income, patient insurance status, patient expectations, and societal expectations. All of these differ according to the patient population served. For example, a physician caring for a cancer patient in a public safety-net hospital typically has stringent limits placed on patient-care resources. Patients who live in middle- and low-income countries, even those with national health care systems, can also be assumed to have limited resources. Even in low-income countries, of course, some citizens are wealthy and can afford excellent medical attention, often delivered in a wealthy, technologically advanced country. Failed states such as present-day Somalia are typically chaotic and basic medical care, even for simple illnesses, is often unavailable or inaccessible because of armed conflict.

Because the goals of surveillance are not well circumscribed, explicit, and generally accepted, uniformity of surveillance practice will presumably be difficult to attain. Detection of recurrence of the index cancer is a major goal in the opinions of most clinicians, followed by detection of second cancers and detection of adverse effects of treatment. Other goals are discussed in more detail elsewhere [31] but one (detection of other medically significant conditions) deserves attention here. This invites screening for hypertension and dyslipidemia, lung cancer in tobacco abusers, and the like—all of which are usually the responsibility of the patient's primary-care provider [13]. We presume that this accounts for the inclusion of tests such as liver function tests, complete blood count, urinalysis, and the like in surveillance test strategies, although they are rather unlikely to diagnose recurrent cancer, a new primary cancer, or adverse effects of initial therapy [19]. The goal of detecting other medically important conditions opens a very wide door and invites marked variability among surveillance strategies. Other likely causes of variation in surveillance strategies will be apparent to most readers of this textbook.

At present, we consider that the variation in surveillance practice for most patients after primary curative-intent therapy largely results from the belief that surveillance is worthwhile, based primarily on intuition and anecdotal evidence, the current willingness of payers in wealthy countries to pay for surveillance testing, and the lack of rigorous clinical evidence to support any particular strategy for most types of cancer.

There is some evidence derived from registry data that posttreatment surveillance can be limited in some instances. Siva et al. showed that cervix cancer patients treated with radiation and chemotherapy with a complete metabolic tumor response on posttreatment 18F-fluorodeoxyglucose positron emission tomography (FDG-PET) were quite likely to be cured and advocated low-intensity surveillance based largely on FDG-PET scans for such patients [32]. Buchler et al. also using registry data, documented low utility of a common surveillance strategy for certain patients treated for testicular cancer and recommended that surveillance intensity should be minimal [33]. In general, patients estimated to have a very low risk of recurrence are good candidates for low-intensity surveillance. Those designing surveillance strategies should limit or abandon use of modalities with low utility.

Considering costs is rational in designing surveillance protocols. Effectiveness of testing modalities using epidemiological principles is also rational [34]. Each modality that deserves a place in a strategy in which a main goal is detection of recurrence while the recurrence is still asymptomatic can be considered a screening test. Pertinent criteria for an acceptable screening test include validity, reliability, yield, and likelihood ratios. The proposed frequency of screening using any modality that meets such criteria should probably incorporate human factors such as the preference of the doctor and the preference of the patient, although increased testing frequency could reasonably impose direct patient costs. To establish a rational screening program, consideration of the receiver operating characteristic curve, thresholds for instituting treatment, and the thresholds for testing are required (but infrequently done).

Clinicians, administrators, and other contributors in any rigorous analysis of the costs of surveillance testing must contend with limited resources and increasing demand. This reflects, to some extent, the excellence of modern diagnostic testing techniques and the excellence of modern treatment which renders so many patients free of evident cancer at the termination of initial therapy. Rigorous analysis of costs, benefits, quality, available resources, and the like is beyond the scope of this chapter but can be found in modern books about epidemiology, business, and medical care [35–47].

It should now be quite clear that devising a cost-effective strategy means one thing to the average clinician caring for a cancer patient and quite another to a health economist, insurance analyst, or technical advisor to a politician deciding whether to vote for or against a proposal to alter a national health care system. Data permitting rigorous creation of a cost-effective strategy for surveillance of cancer patients after curative-intent treatment simply do not exist in the U.S. The National Clinical Guideline Centre of the United Kingdom has created a rigorous process on behalf of NICE to develop evidence-based guidelines in which cost-effectiveness is also weighed [48]. As mentioned before, the authors of this chapter consider this process to be the best of its kind in the world at present.

The conduct of posttreatment surveillance has changed over time. A recent innovation is the patient treatment plan [49]. This is designed to enable the battery of doctors, physical therapists, and others who have been caring for a cancer patient to transfer responsibility for care to others. The plan is a written document explaining pertinent details about the patient's cancer, the initial management plan devised by the team involved in the initial work-up, diagnosis, and treatment, and elements of the treatment course that are noteworthy. The patient treatment plan informs the intended primary-care physician (and others, as appropriate) of the recommendations of the team involved in the initial care for the remainder of the patient's life. This includes such items as the schedules of diagnostic testing for recurrence of the index neoplasm and second primary neoplasms, genetic testing of relatives, as indicated, advice about appropriate management of treatment-related disabilities, and the like. The formal written treatment plan may contain a wealth of other useful information such as the contact information of those involved in primary treatment of the cancer, relevant support groups, and so on. Expected ill effects or toxicities of the treatments are often enumerated. Recommended behavioral changes (smoking cessation, avoidance of excessive sun exposure, etc.) are often included. The treatment plan has not been widely adopted, however, for practical reasons. It takes considerable effort to compile the elements and organize them in an understandable format. The physician often simply does not have enough time to create this document, so a nurse or secretary often assembles the main elements and gives the physician that draft to work with. However, lack of reimbursement is currently a major impediment. Health care systems are likely to value these plans but will presumably have to provide payment to those who create them. Computerized medical records will certainly aid in this process. The available evidence indicates that survivorship care plans are highly valued by primary-care providers [50]. They help educate these providers and influence their management of the cancer patient. However, the limited evidence to date does not suggest that such documents markedly improve patient outcomes [51].

Medical care is famously complex. It has been compared in difficulty to being a parent. The authors of this chapter feel that nihilism about the apparently illogical features of current posttreatment surveillance is unacceptable. This is why the status quo has been maintained even for medical practice guidelines that are merely based on expert consensus. The relevance of such guidelines erodes with time as new diagnostic criteria are introduced, new risk-estimation tools are devised and validated, new salvage therapies for local and distant relapse replace old therapies, and new treatments for incurable disease enter the clinical armamentarium. These considerations apply to all varieties of cancer.

The importance of posttreatment surveillance for all types of life-threatening chronic disorders (such as cancer) is under-appreciated and under-researched. For example, the two large, very influential randomized trials of breast cancer surveillance [52,53] are nearly two decades old and no longer fully relevant to the practice of breast cancer management. New diagnostic modalities, new treatments for relapse, and new methods of primary breast cancer therapy are available. New trials are needed, although they are difficult and expensive to carry out. Surely patient surveillance for all forms of cancer after initial therapy deserves to be established by such trials, if feasible. Phelps and Parente have estimated that the economic returns on high-quality clinical trials exceed expenditures by one to two orders of magnitude [54]. Such trials should determine whether current guideline-compliant patient surveillance represents best medical practice.

At present, although the National Institutes of Health and other relevant funding entities consider posttreatment patient surveillance as falling within their realm [55], they do not support comparative trials of a particular surveillance strategy with an alternative strategy. The public health community has long recognized that "if we want more evidence-based practice, we need more practice-based evidence" [56]. Presumably, the community of patients, insurers, advocacy groups, health care professionals, and others will also have to advocate for adoption of enabling language in legislation to change the status quo. This is likely to be difficult. However, unless we can improve the evidence based upon which medical practice is founded, the current marked variation in practice is not likely to improve. Constraints on physician practices, based largely on cost, by medical management systems is another potential approach to decrease such variation but one that has proven to be unpopular with physicians and patients. Such constraints, if they are not based mainly on clinical data, are likely to be sources of overuse, underuse, or misuse of resources.

References

1. Breasted JH. The Edwin Smith surgical papyrus. Vol. 1. Hieroglyphic transliteration, translation, and commentary. Chicago, IL: University of Chicago Press; 1930. p. 324–7.
2. Wangensteen OH, Wangensteen SD. The rise of surgery: from empiric craft to scientific discipline. Minneapolis, MN: University of Minnesota Press; 1978. p. 567–72.
3. Cecil RL, Loeb RF, Gutman AB, McDermott W, Wolf HG, editors. Textbook of medicine. 10th ed. Philadelphia, PA: WB Saunders Company; 1959.
4. Bell ET. Tumors. In: Bell ET, editor. Textbook of pathology. 3rd ed. Philadelphia, PA: Lea & Fabiger; 1938. p. 232–371.
5. Roentgen WC. On a new kind of rays (translation). Br J Radiol. 1931;4:32.
6. Beatson GT. On the treatment of inoperable cases of carcinoma of the mamma: suggestions for a new method of treatment. Lancet. 1896;2:104–7.
7. Bayliss WM, Starling EH. On the causation of the so-called 'peripheral reflex secretion' of the pancreas. Proc R Soc Lond [Biol]. 1902;69:352.
8. Yamada T, Alpers DH, Kaplowitz N, Laine L, Owyang C, Powell DW. Textbook of gastroenterology. 4th ed. Philadelphia, PA: Lippincott, Williams and Wilkins; 2003. p. 67.
9. Field MJ, Lohr KN, editors. Clinical practice guidelines: directions for a new program. Washington, DC: The National Academies Press; 1990.
10. Field MJ, Lohr KN, editors. Guidelines for clinical practice: from development to use. Washington, DC: The National Academies Press; 1992.
11. Field MJ, Lohr KN, editors. Guidelines for clinical practice: from development to use. Washington, DC: The National Academies Press; 1992. p. 23.
12. Field MJ, Lohr KN, editors. Guidelines for clinical practice: from development to use. Washington, DC: The National Academies Press; 1992. p. 8–9.
13. Eddy D. Designing a practice policy—standards, guidelines, and options. JAMA. 1990;263:3077–84.
14. Wilson D. Conflicts on health guideline panels. The New York Times: B1, B6. 3 Nov 2011.
15. Field MJ, Lohr KN, editors. Guidelines for clinical practice: from development to use. Washington, DC: The National Academies Press; 1992. p. 32–5.
16. Bloom F. Science as a way of life: perplexities of a physician–scientist. Science. 2003;300:1680–5.
17. Eden J, Wheatley B, McNeil B, Sox H, editors. Knowing what works in health care. Washington, DC: The National Academies Press; 2008. p. 19.
18. Eden J, Wheatley B, McNeil B, Sox H, editors. Knowing what works in health care. Washington, DC: The National Academies Press; 2008. p. 8.
19. Hill J, Bullock I, Alderson P. A summary of the methods that the National Clinical Guideline Centre uses to produce clinical guidelines for The National Institute for Health and Clinical Excellence. Ann Intern Med. 2011;154:752–7.
20. Committee on standards for developing trustworthy clinical practice guidelines. Clinical practice guidelines we can trust. Washington, DC: The National Academies Press; 2011 (available in electronic form at www.iom.edu).
21. O'Donnell RJ, Bruckner JD, Conrad EU. Soft tissue sarcoma. In: Johnson FE, Virgo KS, Edge SB, Pellegrini CA, Poston GJ, Schantz SP, Tsukamoto N, editors. Cancer patient follow-up. St. Louis: Mosby; 1995. p. 238–67.
22. Beitler AL, Virgo KS, Johnson FE, Gibbs J, Kraybill WG. Current follow-up strategies after potentially curative resection of extremity sarcomas: results of a survey of the members of the Society of Surgical Oncology. Cancer. 2000;88:777–85.
23. Wennberg J, Gittelson A. Small area variations in health care delivery. Science. 1973;182:1102–8.
24. Chassin MR, Galvin RW, The National Roundtable on Health Care Quality. The urgent need to improve health care quality: Institute of Medicine National Roundtable on Health Care Quality. JAMA. 1998;280:1000–5.
25. Sakata K, Beitler AL, Gibbs JF, Kraybill WG, Virgo KS, Johnson FE. How surgeon age affects surveillance strategies for extremity soft tissue sarcoma patients after potentially curative treatment. J Surg Res. 2002;108:227–34.
26. Sakata K, Johnson FE, Kraybill WG, Virgo KS. Extremity soft tissue sarcoma patient follow-up: tumor grade and size affect surveillance strategies after potentially curative surgery. Int J Oncol. 2003;22:1335–43.
27. Johnson FE, Sakata K, Sarkar S, Audisio RA, Kraybill WG, Gibbs JF, et al. Patient surveillance after treatment for soft-tissue sarcoma. Int J Oncol. 2011;38:233–9.
28. Johnson FE, Sakata K, Kraybill WG, Gibbs JF, Beitler AL, Sarkar S, et al. Long-term management of patients after potentially curative treatment of extremity soft tissue sarcoma: practice patterns of members of the Society of Surgical Oncology. Surg Oncol. 2005;14:33–40.
29. Virgo KS, Johnson FE. Costs of surveillance after potentially curative treatment for cancer. In: Cancer patient follow-up. St. Louis, MO: Mosby; 1995. chapter 3.
30. Goel A, Christy MEL, Virgo KS, Kraybill WG, Johnson FE. Costs of follow-up after potentially curative treatment for extremity soft-tissue sarcoma. Int J Oncol. 2004;25:429–35.
31. Johnson FE. Overview. In: Johnson FE, Virgo KS, Edge SB, Pellegrini CA, Poston GJ, Schantz SP, Tsukomoto N, editors. Cancer patient follow-up. St. Louis, MO: Mosby; 1995. chapter 1.
32. Siva S, Herschtal A, Thomas JM, Bernshaw DM, Gill S, Hicks R, et al. Impact of post-therapy positron emission tomography on prognostic stratification and surveillance after chemoradiotherapy for cervical cancer. Cancer. 2011;117:3981–8.
33. Buchler T, Kubankova P, Boublikova L, Donatova Z, Foldyna M, Kanakova J, et al. Detection of second malignancies during long-term follow-up of testicular cancer survivors. Cancer. 2011;117:4212–8.
34. Virgo KS, Johnson FE. Costs of surveillance after potentially curative treatment for cancer. In: Johnson FE et al., editors. Cancer patient follow-up. St. Louis, MO: Mosby; 1995. chapter 3.
35. Mausner JS, Kramer S. Epidemiology—an introductory text. 2nd ed. Philadelphia, PA: WB Saunders Company; 1985.
36. Feinstein AR. Clinical epidemiology: the architecture of clinical research. Philadelphia, PA: WB Saunders Company; 1985.
37. Sox HC, Blatt MA, Higgins MC, Marton KI. Medical decision making. Boston, MA: Butterworths; 1988.
38. Warner KE, Luce BR. Cost–benefit and cost-effectiveness analysis in health care. Ann Arbor, MI: Health Administration Press; 1982.
39. Drummond MF, Stoddart GL, Torrance GW. Methods for the economic evaluation of health care programmes. Oxford, UK: Oxford Medical Publications; 1987.
40. Weinstein MC. Foundations of cost-effectiveness analysis for health and medical practices. N Engl J Med. 1977;296:716–21.
41. Dasgupta AK, Pearce DW. Cost–benefit analysis: theory and practice. London, UK: Macmillan; 1972.

42. Mishan EJ. Cost–benefit analysis. London, UK: George Allen and Unwin; 1975.
43. Sugden R, Williams AH. The principles of practical cost–benefit analysis. Oxford, UK: Oxford University Press; 1979.
44. Eastaugh SR. Medical economics and health finance. Dover, MA: Auburn House Publishing Company; 1981.
45. Jacobs P. The economics of health and medical care. Rockville, MD: Aspen Publishers, Inc.; 1987.
46. Weinstein MC. Principles of cost-effective resource allocation in health care organizations. Int J Technol Assess Health Care. 1990; 6:93–103.
47. Wonderling D, Sawyer L, Fenu E, Lovibond K, Laramée P. National Clinical Guideline Centre cost-effectiveness assessment for the National Institute for Health and Clinical Excellence. Ann Intern Med. 2011;154:758–65.
48. Robinson R. Cost-effectiveness analysis. Br Med J. 1993;307(c): 793–5.
49. Hewitt M, Greenfield S, Stovall E, editors. From cancer patient to cancer survivor—lost in transition. Washington, DC: The National Academies Press; 2006. p. 151–63.
50. Shalom MM, et al. Do survivorship care plans make a difference? A primary care provider perspective. J Oncol Pract. 2011;7:314–8.
51. Grunfeld E, Julian JA, Pond G, et al. Evaluating survivorship care plans: results of a randomized clinical trial of patients with breast cancer. J Clin Oncol. 2011;36:4755–62.
52. The GIVIO Investigators. Impact of follow-up testing on survival and health-related quality of life in breast cancer patients: a multicenter randomized controlled trial. JAMA. 1994;271:1587–92.
53. Rosselli Del Turco M, Palli D, Cariddi A, et al. Intensive diagnostic follow-up after treatment of primary breast cancer: a randomized trial. JAMA. 1994;271:1593–7.
54. Phelps CE, Parente ST. Priority setting in medical technology and medical practice assessment. Medical Care. 1990;28:703–23.
55. NCI Expands Office of Cancer Survivorship Website. http://www.cancer.gov/newscenter/pressreleases/1999/survivorship [Accessed Jun 2012]
56. Green LW, Glasgow RE. Evaluating the relevance, generalization, and applicability of research: issues in external validation and translation methodology. Eval Health Prof. 2006;29:126–53.

Introduction to Cancer Surveillance Strategies

2

Brooke Crawford and David D. Greenberg

Keywords
Survivorship • Surveillance • Treatment • Medicolegal • Costs

Introduction

In recent decades, detection and treatment of cancer has become increasingly successful. Cure is possible and, even if it is not, therapies can lead to remission of and survival with the disease for years. In the United States alone, there are greater than 12 million cancer survivors [1]. With this number of patients experiencing what has come to be known as cancer survivorship, a need has arisen for the process of surveillance—monitoring cancer survivors for recurrence of disease. Beyond recurrence, surveillance also encompasses posttreatment complications as well as the diagnosis and treatment of secondary malignancies that can arise from initial treatment.

A patient's cancer and his or her response to treatment are unique, which leads to the question of how surveillance should be implemented. Ideally, medical practice is based on clinical and/or scientific evidence. However, this is not always feasible and, in terms of cancer survivorship, there is often insufficient evidence to generate complete surveillance strategies. Cancer societies and committees attempt to fill the void by recommending surveillance protocols based on multiple factors.

In the following chapters, guidelines for specific surveillance strategies will be outlined. Here, we attempt to explain what considerations go into choosing surveillance strategies.

First, the options for strategies have to be considered, and these vary based on the disease process. Certain cancers have specific serum markers which can be useful after treatment to detect recurrence. Imaging studies such as PET, CT, and MRI scans are available to detect metastases or local recurrence. These modalities have different sensitivities based on the cancer and organ system. Although these technologies continue to advance, the dilemma of unnecessary tissue biopsies is based on them. The primary malignancy often dictates the timing and location of recurrence and these factors should direct surveillance. If lung metastases are common, chest imaging will clearly be part of the surveillance protocol. If local recurrence is the most likely complication of the malignancy, perhaps clinical examination or local imaging is all that is needed. Delayed treatment effects and complications are a separate, but equally important, concern to the treating oncologist and patient. Lymphedema after mastectomy and axillary dissection, osteonecrosis from corticosteroids, and secondary malignancies from radiation therapy are just a few examples.

Although the prevalence of cancer survivors continues to increase, two key factors have led to a substantial lack of evidence on which to base a surveillance strategy. First of all, while standard treatment protocols are certainly in place for a majority of malignancies, individual patients continue to experience unique clinical courses based on their response. These treatment variations (i.e., whether or not a patient receives radiation, organ systems affected, chemotherapy regimens selected, and treatment complications) impact surveillance. Secondly, survivorship is still a relatively young concept and long-term data are limited. Even when evidence does exist for certain strategies, such as using prostate-specific antigen (PSA) for monitoring prostate cancer recurrence, the evidence, and therefore the recommendations, evolve as long-term follow-up becomes available. Yes, an elevated serum PSA level in a previously "cured" prostate

B. Crawford, M.D. • D.D. Greenberg, M.D. (✉)
Department of Orthopaedic Surgery, Saint Louis University School of Medicine, 3635 Vista Ave, 7th Floor Desloge Towers, St. Louis, MO 63110, USA
e-mail: bcrawfo5@slu.edu; dgreenb5@slu.edu

F.E. Johnson et al. (eds.), *Patient Surveillance After Cancer Treatment*, Current Clinical Oncology,
DOI 10.1007/978-1-60327-969-7_2,

cancer patient is concerning for a recurrence. But does everyone get surveillance PSA tests? If they are normal, how long does the patient need to be monitored? What will the treatment be if a recurrence is diagnosed?

After treatment of any type of malignancy, the goals that should direct surveillance include the following:

1. The interval between examinations and duration of testing should be consistent with time of maximal risk of recurrence and the natural course of the tumor.
2. Tests should focus on the most likely recurrence locations and have high positive and negative predictive values.
3. There should be a possibility of cure, prolongation of life, or palliation of symptoms. Earlier treatment should improve outcome compared to treatment started based on symptoms.
4. Risk of secondary malignancy should guide the ordering of tests. Treatment should be performed with frequency and duration consistent with nature of the malignant and nonmalignant complications of said treatment [2,3].

An Example

Prostate cancer is the most common non-skin cancer in men in the United States [4]. In 1986, the FDA approved screening—in healthy, asymptomatic patients—for the disease by using the PSA test, on the premise that prostate cancer causes elevations in the serum PSA level [4]. Unfortunately, cancer is not the only condition that leads to elevations in PSA: prostatitis, urinary tract infection, and benign prostatic hypertrophy can all cause abnormally high PSA levels. Also, up to 90% of the time, prostate cancer is a low-grade process and, in the majority of older men, does not progress fast enough to cause significant effects on their health [5]. In 2002, the US Preventive Task Force (USPSTF) found that, although PSA screening can detect early stage prostate cancer, health outcomes remained unchanged [4]. This called into question the utility of the PSA test as a screening tool [6,7]. In 2011, the USPSTF issued an update on their 2008 PSA recommendation, stating that healthy men of any age, race, or family history need not undergo routine PSA screening. In 2012, the American Academy of Family Physicians made the same recommendation, based on the extensive body of literature regarding PSA screening that shows 90% of men with PSA-detected prostate cancer undergo treatment. For surgical patients, 5 out of 1,000 will die within 1 month of the operation due to complications, and 200–300 out of 1,000 will suffer urinary incontinence or impotence [8,9]. These numbers indicated to the Task Force that the risk of screening outweighs the benefit. Other evidence contradicts the endpoints the USPSTF used for its recommendation. Schroder recently published his 11-year follow-up of the European Randomized Study of Screening for Prostate Cancer, and showed that, although PSA screening does not decrease overall mortality, there is a significant 21% risk reduction in mortality from prostate cancer specifically, likely due to early detection and a less severe disease state at the time of diagnosis [10].

Despite the heated debate about prostate cancer screening, PSA testing has found great utility as a surveillance tool. If an otherwise healthy man in his 70s has a known prostate cancer diagnosis, there are many options for treatment. First, if the cancer is considered low-grade, the condition can simply be monitored, as low-grade disease does not progress rapidly [11]. If there is concern that the disease is more advanced, options range from chemotherapy and brachytherapy to radical prostatectomy and radiation. In all instances, the serum PSA level provides a tool to follow the disease. Levels that are consistent imply no progression or regression, falling levels suggest successful treatment, and rising levels are interpreted as progression or possibly recurrence. For most patients, serial PSA levels are necessary to follow the course of the prostate cancer.

Patient Concerns

Let us assume that the patient has made one of the following decisions on how to handle his diagnosis. In scenario 1, it is found to be low-grade, and he chooses to simply have it followed with serial PSA tests. In scenario 2, he decides to have surgery. There are other therapeutic options to consider, but none eliminate the possibility that his cancer may progress or recur. Combine the potential for recurrence with the morbidity intervention, and the emotional toll becomes quite high. These scenarios demonstrate some of the patient concerns that must be considered when considering surveillance strategies, specifically: anxiety, morbidity, cost, and convenience.

Anxiety is present in at least 20% of patients just related to keeping their clinic appointments [12]. Some fear venipuncture or claustrophobia during a CT scan or an MRI [12]. Invasive tests can be perceived as painful—another strong deterrent. This physical pain is in addition to a patient's fear of discovering cancer relapse with each office visit or test. The emotional stress and anxiety the surveillance generates for the patient can lead to noncompliance, and has to be considered in surveillance strategies.

Whether or not procedures are considered successful in treating cancer, none are entirely benign. Going back to our example of prostate cancer, prostatectomies are major abdominal operations, which have risks such as bowel perforation, urinary tract injuries, impotence, infection, etc. Radiation, an increasingly utilized tool in the cancer treatment armamentarium, is associated with significant potential morbidity. Decreased healing potential in the irradiated field, scarring, neuropathy, and edema are just some of the adverse effects. Radiation also can lead to secondary malignancies [13]. Chemotherapy has its own associated morbidities. Androgen deprivation, frequently used in the treatment of prostate cancer, can lead to osteoporosis, gynecomastia, and muscle mass loss.

Chemotherapy-related malignancies are potentially lethal and must be considered during follow-up [2,14]. These treatment-associated morbidities occur within the surveillance time frame, and the surveillance strategy chosen must incorporate these potential issues. Late-effects clinics and evaluations are becoming part of the routine global care of cancer patients.

Cost is another consideration and one that cannot be ignored given today's economic climate. Patients with healthcare coverage are keenly aware of the required co-pays for office visits, diagnostic imaging, and laboratory tests. A false sense of security can develop for the patient after successful treatment of his or her cancer. The potential to save money by foregoing the anxiety-provoking surveillance testing weighs heavily in a patient's decision-making. Returning to our patient with prostate cancer, if he loses his job (or his health insurance), it is possible that he will forego further PSA testing, unknowingly allowing a potential recurrence to progress. Alternatively, he can demand unnecessary testing, regardless of cost, requiring the physician to allow defensive medicine to dictate his or her decision-making.

Along with cost comes convenience. Although traditional cancer centers exist within academic centers in urban settings, many cancer patients are from rural areas. Patients often lament having to travel far from home for treatment, let alone surveillance. Depending on the patient's state of health, transportation may not be possible without assistance. Ideally, surveillance should be simple, inexpensive, and available to all patients locally, but for multiple reasons this is often not the case. Nevertheless, these criteria should be considered when devising a successful surveillance strategy.

Physician Concerns

Physicians have a slightly different perspective, but within it the patient concerns must be considered and weighed against compliance issues, quality of life, and whether effective treatment can be had should surveillance detect a recurrence.

An accurate form of surveillance is the most important concern. Medical and surgical oncologists recommend treatment plans based on medical information, and they want that information to be reliable. Optimal lung surveillance for metastatic disease is an applicable example. The decision whether to undergo the more expensive PET scan or the lower-cost but higher radiation standard chest CT is challenging. Pros and cons exist for both, but knowing the more accurate test facilitates the decision, as accuracy remains the most important consideration [15]. A valid test must be accurate, but a physician should also be familiar with a test's sensitivity, specificity, and other performance parameters. The PSA test, as mentioned above, is not specific for prostate cancer. If a patient's PSA starts rising, even with his known prostate cancer, he likely will need to be evaluated for other potential causes of the elevation.

An accurate surveillance test that detects local or systemic recurrence when the patient cannot receive curative-intent or palliative treatment is of little clinical benefit. The strategy selected must detect local or systemic recurrence early enough to allow the physician to offer treatment. Furthermore, the goal should be for the patient to survive the treatment without devastating morbidity and to recover from it enough to maintain some quality of life.

Cost is not only a concern for the patient, but for the physician and society as a whole. Some patients are adamant about wanting a treatment that does not apply to their situation—a radical prostatectomy in a patient with low-grade prostate cancer—and spending healthcare dollars because of sympathy, patient demand, or fear of medicolegal issues, places an enormous strain on healthcare costs. Doctors must also be aware that what is best for an individual patient may not fit the cost–benefit analysis applied to the entire population. A fine balance between the individual patient and society as a whole—both in terms of cost and success—must be reached for a successful surveillance strategy when considering a disease as broad-reaching as cancer.

The Disease

A number of factors are used to determine the appropriate treatment for a patient with cancer. Standard treatment alternatives, in addition to investigational trials, exist. Along with the patient's overall health, treatment is dependent on factors such as location, stage, size, and type of cancer. The TNM staging system is the one most commonly used [16]. The reason to stage cancer is twofold. First, the stage helps to determine appropriate treatment; and second, the stage provides a statistical prognosis.

How does this relate to surveillance? Generally, with a more aggressive tumor (higher stage), the likelihood for recurrence is higher and the prognosis is poorer. Surveillance may need to be more frequent for a higher stage tumor. In addition, the stage may dictate the extent of surveillance. While most malignant tumors can spread systemically, higher grade cancers have greater metastatic potential. For example, grade I chondrosarcomas have low (<10%) metastatic potential and long-term survival in as much as 90% of patients. This is in contrast to a 40–60% survival rate with intermediate- and high-grade tumors. Local recurrence is the primary concern in a patient with a grade I chondrosarcoma whereas pulmonary surveillance is essential with higher grade tumors

[17–19]. In this example, a surveillance strategy cannot ignore the metastatic potential in low-grade chondrosarcomas, but certainly the emphasis is altered. For a number of other tumors, the TNM stage-specific variation in surveillance strategy has been documented [20].

A similar rationale applies when considering the tumor location and method selected for local control. The surgeon's ability to obtain adequate resection margins is affected by tumor location and invasiveness into vital structures such as vessels and nerves. Surgical margins are classified as clear R0 (microscopically uninvolved), RI (microscopically involved), or R2 (macroscopically involved) [21]. This classification scheme and the margin achieved not only help determine the need for adjuvant treatment (for, example, radiation therapy) but also the risk of recurrence and therefore surveillance intensity. Once again returning to our patient with prostate cancer, if he elects to be treated with radiotherapy, such knowledge is instrumental for surveillance. PSA levels are expected to fall to very low levels after surgery, but not after radiotherapy due to residual prostate tissue [11]. A normalization of PSA after radiotherapy is expected; elevations of his PSA after normalization are indicative of relapse.

Duration of Surveillance

How often should a prostate cancer patient have his PSA checked? When would he be considered "cured"? If the PSA levels start rising again, what would be the next step? In the field of oncology, many solid tumors do not recur after 5 years, and patients who are disease free after 5 years are often considered cured [12]. However, a number of cancers recur frequently after 5 years [2]. Patients with localized prostate cancer are at risk of relapse for more than 10 years despite treatment [13,22]. A surveillance strategy should be most intensive during the time when risk of recurrence is greatest and then taper off. In order to develop such a strategy, the individual patient's risk of recurrence must be known, as outlined above. For PSA surveillance after primary treatment of prostate malignancy, every 6 months for 5 years with a yearly digital rectal exam is recommended, followed by yearly PSA checks after 5 years [23–25]. These recommendations have the advantage of providing general guidelines for physicians to follow. Such recommendations are often formulated by expert opinion or committee consensus as opposed to level-one evidence. Unfortunately, until additional evidence is obtained, these guidelines provided by societies such as the American Society of Clinical Oncology and the Children's Oncology Group are often the best available. Certain types of cancer, sarcomas for example, unfortunately lack even these organizational guidelines, leaving individual physicians to devise surveillance strategies based on their training, communication with colleagues, or local standards. Even worse, without standardization, the individual's protocol may be dictated by his or her insurance company and what it will approve. A transition from cost-based surveillance strategies determined by insurance organizations to evidence-based strategies will only occur with clinical trials and scientific data.

The word "cure" is not often used in the field of oncology. "In remission" or "latent" are more commonly used as "cure" suggests that there is no chance of recurrence. There is an ongoing debate as to whether, since the term cure cannot accurately be applied to cancer, surveillance should ever cease. Lifelong follow-up is probably appropriate for certain cancers. For others, a strong argument can be made that patients do not need continued surveillance after a set amount of time has passed. Returning to the previous example of chondrosarcoma, these malignancies, due to their relatively slow growth, require ongoing surveillance for decades. On the other hand, conventional osteosarcoma rarely recurs beyond 5 years. Counter to such reasoning are the numerous case reports and anecdotal evidence of recurrence after decades of remission.

Summary

Cancer surveillance is an evolving area in the medical field as cancer treatments continue to become more effective and patients are surviving longer. Ideally, surveillance should be developed like any other medical protocol: based on evidence. As tumor registries and databases continue to become standard, the challenges of acquiring enough data on individual malignancies and long enough follow-up on individual patients will ease. This will pave the way for the evidence required to develop standard surveillance strategies. The most persuasive evidence comes from randomized control trials, however, and these are very costly to carry out and take many years to complete.

Some tumors produce serological markers such as PSA for prostate cancer and carcinoembryonic antigen for colorectal cancer; serum levels vary with disease burden. Other cancers do not and clinicians must rely on symptoms, nonspecific laboratory abnormalities, and/or imaging studies for detection and monitoring.

The concerns outlined above will continue to exist despite the best evidence. Patients who have a cancer diagnosis and undergo surveillance will have to deal with the possibility of recurrence and the anxiety of follow-up. Cost is an issue that will remain on the forefront of healthcare reform for the foreseeable future. Cancer treatments are often very extensive, both in complexity and duration. The cost of surveillance, while formidable, must be viewed relative to the costs, financial and emotional, of recurrence. Tumor staging, disease burden, and treatment are other factors that must be taken into consideration when deciding on a strategy for surveillance. When treatment is successful, duration of surveillance comes into question.

Currently, possible approaches that a clinician could utilize to determine how to choose a surveillance strategy for a particular patient with a particular type of cancer after completing a particular type of therapy include:

1. Examining journal articles describing how clinical experts (such as members of relevant professional organizations such as the Society of Gynecologic Oncologists, American Society of Clinical Oncology [ASCO], Society of Surgical Oncology, etc.) follow their own patients with particular cancers after primary curative-intent therapy.
2. Find online resources or society websites for suggested guidelines related to posttreatment surveillance. For example, ASCO, the American Head and Neck Society, the European Society for Medical Oncology, the National Comprehensive Cancer Network, and the National Institute for Health and Clinical Excellence of the UK have developed such guidelines.
3. Devise a strategy based on fellowship training and/or local standards.
4. Devise a strategy based on what the patient or his/her insurance organization can afford or approve, compliance issues, overall health status, and likelihood of quality of life improvement if an issue is discovered in the surveillance period.

Specific tumors and their surveillance strategies will be discussed in detail in the following chapters. These strategies were devised by considering the patient, the physician, and the disease and interfacing these complex components with somewhat limited evidence as guidance. The authors believe that, despite the continued complexity, clinical research will provide clarity on the optimal choice.

References

1. Cancer Survivors-United States. 2007. http://wwwcdc.gov/cancer/dcpc/research/articles/survivors.htm. Accessed Jun 2012
2. Edelman MJ, Meyers FJ, Siegel D. The utility of follow-up testing after curative cancer therapy. J Gen Intern Med. 1997;12:318–31.
3. Early Breast Cancer Trialists' Collaborative Group. Systemic treatment of early breast cancer by hormonal, cytotoxic, or immune therapy. Lancet. 1992;339:1–15. 71–85.
4. Lin K, Lipsitz R, Miller T, Janakiraman S. Benefits and harms of prostate-specific antigen screening for prostate cancer: an evidence update for the U.S. Preventive Services Task Force. Ann Intern Med. 2008;149:192–9.
5. Simon H, MD. Prostate cancer. http://www.lifespan.org/adam/indepthreports/10/000033.html. Accessed Jun 2012
6. Brown, Matt. AAF, USPSTF issue final recommendation against routine PSA-based screening for prostate cancer. http://www.aafp.org/online/en/home/publications/news/news-now/health-of-the-public/20120522psascreenrec.html. Accessed Jun 2012
7. Moyer VA, on behalf of USPSTF. Screening for prostate cancer: US preventive services task force recommendation statement. Ann Intern Med. 2012;157(2):120–34.
8. Stenger M. Study shows continued benefit of PSA screening in reducing prostate cancer mortality. The ASCO Post. 15 May 2012. p. 20–21.
9. Hayes JH, Ollendorf DA, Pearson SD, et al. Active surveillance compared with initial treatment for men with low-risk prostate cancer: a decision analysis. JAMA. 2010;304:2373–80.
10. Sandblom G, Varenhorst E, Rosell J, Lofman O, Carlsson P. Randomised prostate cancer screening trial: 20 year follow-up. BMJ. 2011;342:d1539.
11. Klotz L. Active surveillance for prostate cancer: patient selection and management. Curr Oncol. 2010;17 Suppl 2:S11–7.
12. Johnson FE. How are surveillance strategies chosen? In: Johnson FE, Virgo KS, Audisio RA, et al., editors. Patient surveillance after cancer treatment. Berlin: Springer; 2012. p. 48–54. Chapter 4. ISBN 978-1-60327-968-0.
13. Hanks GE, Hanlon A, Schultheiss T, Corn B, Shipley WU, Lee R. Early prostate cancer: the national results of radiation treatment from the patterns of care and radiation therapy oncology group studies with prospects for improvement with conformal radiation and adjuvant androgen deprivation. J Urol. 1994;152:1775–80.
14. Sill H, Olipitz W, Zebisch A, Schulz E, Wolfler A. Therapy-related myeloid neoplasms: pathobiology and clinical characteristics. Br J Pharmacol. 2011;162:792–805.
15. Lin P, Koh ES, Lin M, Vinod SK, Ho-Shon I, Yap J, et al. Diagnostic and staging impact of radiotherapy planning FDG-PET-CT in non-small-cell lung cancer. Radiother Oncol. 2011;101:284–90.
16. Cancer staging. http://www.cancer.gov/cancertopics/factsheet/detection/staging. Accessed Jun 2012
17. Aaron C, Potter BK, Adams SC, Pitcher JD, Temple HT. Extended intralesional treatment versus resection of low-grade chondrosarcomas. Clin Orthop Relat Res. 2009;467:2105–11.
18. Donati D, Colangeli S, Colangeli M, Di Bella C, Bertoni F. Surgical treatment of grade I central chondrosarcoma. Clin Orthop Related Res. 2009;468:581–9.
19. Mohler DG, Chiu R, McCall DA, Avedian RS. Curettage and cryosurgery for low-grade cartilage tumors is associated with low recurrence and high function. Clin Orthop Relat Res. 2010;468:2765–73.
20. Naunheim KS, Virgo KS, Coplin MA, Johnson FE. Clinical surveillance testing after lung cancer operations. Ann Thorac Surg. 1995;60:1612–6.
21. Goda JS, Ferguson PC, O'Sullivan B, Catton CN, Griffin AM, Wunder JS, et al. High-risk extracranial chondrosarcoma. Cancer. 2011;117:2513–9.
22. Zincke H, Oesterling JE, Blute ML, Bergstralh EJ, Myers RP, Barrett DM. Long-term (15 years) results after radical prostatectomy for clinically localized (stage T2c or lower) prostate cancer. J Urol. 1994;152:1850–7.
23. Freedland SJ, Humphreys EB, Mangold LA, et al. Risk of prostate cancer-specific mortality following biochemical recurrence after radical prostatectomy. JAMA. 2005;294:433–9.
24. McIntosh HM, Neal RD, Rose P, et al. Follow-up care for men with prostate cancer and the role of primary care: a systematic review of international guidelines. Br J Cancer. 2009;100:1852–60.
25. Pound CR, Partin AW, Eisenberger MA, Chan DW, Pearson JD, Walsh PC. Natural history of progression after PSA elevation following radical prostatectomy. JAMA. 1999;281(17):1591–7.

Using Decision Analysis to Model Cancer Surveillance

3

Kim E.M. van Kessel, Sandra M.E. Geurts, André L.M. Verbeek, and Ewout W. Steyerberg

Keywords
Models • Analysis • Surveillance strategies • CEA • Decision node

Cancer management includes surveillance of patients after treatment. Such programs become increasingly important since chances of survival after cancer treatment and, thus, disease-free survival rates are continuing to increase. Surveillance programs are also time-consuming and, in addition, a very expensive component of clinical activity since frequent testing is often involved. The choice of a surveillance program is complex and should ideally consider aspects of survival, quality of life, the burden of surveillance tests, and financial costs. As for all clinical decisions, the choice involves a condition of uncertainty. This uncertainty originates from relationships between diagnostic information and the presence of disease, uncertainty about the effects of early treatment, and ambiguity in clinical information [1].

Decision analysis is a systematic approach to decision making under conditions of uncertainty. It enables a systematic and explicit comparison of clinical strategies with respect to their benefits for the patient. Decision analysis is, therefore, potentially an important method in the development of surveillance programs for cancer. In this chapter we first provide a brief review of decision analytic patient models in the recent medical literature. We then go through some of the characteristics of the main types of decision analytic models that have been used to evaluate cancer surveillance. Finally, a framework to model cancer surveillance is discussed using ovarian cancer as an example.

Surveillance

Surveillance after treatment of cancer can be seen as a form of screening in which the aim of surveillance is early detection and treatment of recurrent disease to improve survival [2]. It may also be beneficial for a variety of other reasons, including assessment of the morbidity of treatment, rehabilitation and psychological support of patients (e.g., reassurance) and, especially for less common cancer types, gaining an understanding of the clinical course of the disease [3]. In addition, a surveillance strategy may be favored for quality control.

The main issues regarding surveillance programs are:

1. What type(s) of test(s) to include?
2. At what interval (frequency) should follow-up visits take place?

Recurrences should be detected in an early asymptomatic phase, enabling better treatment than waiting for symptoms to occur (clinical suspicion). On the other hand, surveillance should not be too burdensome for patients and the health care system. One should hence try to balance burden and benefit. When analyzing different strategies, a number of alternative surveillance programs should be considered. We may include a "no surveillance" strategy as a reference, reflecting the natural course of disease.

To answer above-mentioned questions, or to model these issues, empirical data is needed. It can be obtained by means of randomized controlled trials, observational studies, or

K.E.M. van Kessel • E.W. Steyerberg (✉)
Department of Public Health, Erasmus University,
P.O. Box 2040, 3000 CA, Rotterdam, The Netherlands
e-mail: kimvkessel@gmail.com; e.steyerberg@erasmusmc.nl

S.M.E. Geurts • A.L.M. Verbeek
Department of Epidemiology, Biostatistics and HTA,
Radboud University Nijmegen Medical Centre,
P.O. Box 9101, 6500 HB Nijmegen, The Netherlands
e-mail: S.Geurts@ebh.umcn.nl; A.Verbeek@ebh.umcn.nl

F.E. Johnson et al. (eds.), *Patient Surveillance After Cancer Treatment*, Current Clinical Oncology,
DOI 10.1007/978-1-60327-969-7_3,

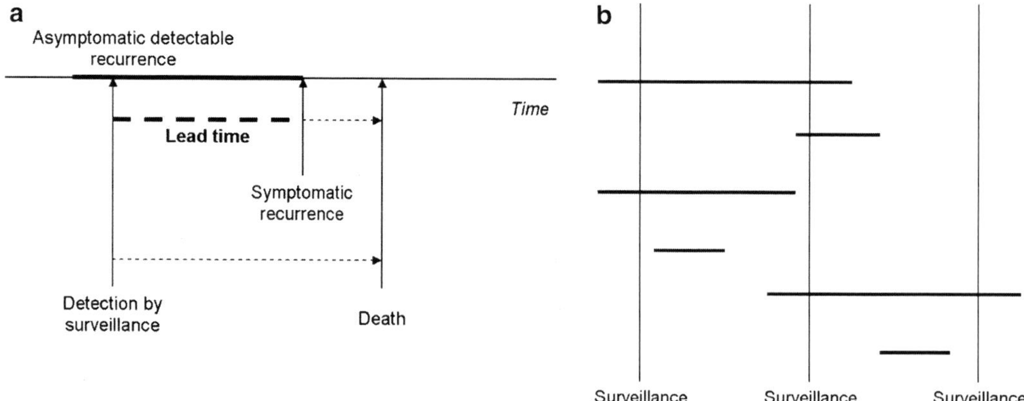

Fig. 3.1 (**a**) Illustration of lead time bias. The increased duration of survival time reflects the longer time that a recurrent cancer was known. (**b**) Illustration of length time bias. The duration of the asymptomatic phase for six patients with recurrent cancer is shown. Recurrences with a longer detectable asymptomatic phase, thus slow-growing recurrent tumors, are more likely to be detected asymptomatically than fast-growing recurrent tumors which have a short asymptomatic phase

clinical experience. To determine whether early treatment leads to improved survival, a randomized controlled trial is ideal. Such a trial might include one group strictly followed according to the surveillance guideline and a control group receiving no surveillance. However, this is generally not considered ethical since surveillance is generally assumed to be beneficial. Therefore, randomized controlled trials evaluating the effect of routine surveillance on survival often include randomization of routinely used diagnostic tests and alternative surveillance schemes [4, 5].

Example: In oncology, specific tumor markers are measured routinely to diagnose recurrence in an early phase. An example in ovarian cancer is tumor marker CA125. To measure the effect of CA125 monitoring on survival, one could think of randomization of treatment initiated at the time CA125 is elevated versus blinding for CA125, but with the other surveillance examinations remaining [5]. These trials are useful to obtain insight into the impact of certain diagnostic tests on survival, but are unsuitable to study a wide range of alternative surveillance scenarios.

Observational follow-up studies may also be useful to evaluate post-cancer surveillance [6, 7]. We may compare patients with their recurrences detected early, without symptoms, to patients with their recurrent cancer detected in presence of symptoms. The rationale is that routine surveillance failed with respect to early recurrence detection in the latter case. In these studies recurrence patterns are determined as well as hard endpoints, such as progression and survival. The cohorts in these studies are often evaluated using Kaplan–Meier curves and Cox proportional hazard regression models. The probability of survival or recurrence rate can then be calculated. Extrapolation to estimate long-term outcome is, however, problematic because only small numbers of patients remain at risk at the long term [8]. Another problem is that the effect of a different surveillance strategy than what was followed in the study can only be speculated about.

Biases

Important biases may be present in observational studies on surveillance, which need to be considered in the analyses. Biases include lead time, length time, and self-selection bias.

- *Lead time bias* is confounding of the results due to the time it takes for an asymptomatic recurrence to become symptomatic, i.e., the increased duration of survival only reflects a longer time that recurrent cancer was known (Fig. 3.1a). This bias is present if date of recurrence detection is defined as the start of survival analysis. Adjustment for lead time bias can be done in the data analysis by defining the start of follow-up as start for survival analysis.
- To perform a valid survival comparison between patients with asymptomatic and symptomatic detected recurrences, prognosis at start of follow-up should be equal. Slow-growing tumor recurrences have a better prognosis compared to fast-growing recurrences. In addition, slow-growing tumors are more likely to be detected in the asymptomatic phase, which leads to *length time bias* (Fig. 3.1b). Length time bias may partly be corrected for by adjustment for known prognostic factors like age or tumor stage, histology, or grade.
- The third surveillance specific bias is caused by *self-selection*. Patients with their recurrence detected at interval visits (between scheduled visits) may bias the effect of

Table 3.1 Decision analytic models for surveillance of cancer published between 1990 and 2010

Type of cancer		First author, year	Research question	Model
1	Colorectal cancer	Hassan 2009 [14]	Standard vs. early surveillance	Decision tree
2		Park 2009 [13]	Eight different surveillance protocols	Markov model
3		Borie 2004 [9]	Standard vs. simplified surveillance	Markov model
4		Park 2001 [12]	Standard vs. modified surveillance: addition of a test	Decision tree
5		Michel 1999 [11]	Surveillance in different patient age categories vs. no surveillance	Decision tree
6		Kievit 1990 [10]	Standard vs. modified surveillance: addition of a test	Markov model
7	Bladder cancer	de Bekker-Grob 2009 [15]	Standard vs. modified surveillance: addition of a test	Markov model
8		Lotan 2002 [17]	Standard vs. modified surveillance: addition of a test	Decision tree
9		Nam 2000 [18]	Standard costs vs. modified surveillance costs: replacement of the standard test	Decision tree
10		Lachaine 2000 [16]	Standard vs. modified surveillance: addition of a test	Decision tree
11	Breast cancer	Lee 2002 [24]	Surveillance vs. adjuvant therapy and surveillance	Markov model
12		Jacobs 2001 [23]	Standard surveillance vs. no surveillance vs. perfect surveillance	Markov model
13		Hayman 1998 [22]	Surveillance vs. adjuvant therapy and surveillance	Markov model
14	Testicular cancer	Spermon 2005 [20]	Surveillance protocol 1 vs. surveillance protocol 2 vs. shorter duration of surveillance	Markov model
15		Stiggelbout 1996 [21]	Surveillance vs. adjuvant therapy and surveillance	Decision tree
16		Munro 1991 [19]	Seven different surveillance protocols vs. no surveillance	Markov model
17	Hodgkin lymphoma	Das 2006 [25]	Surveillance vs. no surveillance	Markov model
18		Guadagnolo 2006 [26]	Different tests: CT vs. non-CT modalities Different duration of CT surveillance: 5 years vs. 10 years	Markov model
19	Lung cancer	Van Loon 2010 [30]	Different tests: PET-CT vs. CT vs. X-ray	Markov model
20		Kent 2005 [29]	Surveillance vs. no surveillance	Markov model
21	Melanoma	Krug 2010 [28]	Different tests: PET-CT vs. whole-body CT	Markov model
22		Hengge 2007 [27]	Standard surveillance vs. reduced surveillance	Markov model
23	Laryngeal cancer	Ritoe 2007 [31]	Standard surveillance vs. no surveillance vs. perfect surveillance	Markov model
24	Ovarian cancer	Hopkins 2007 [32]	Standard vs. modified surveillance: addition of a test	Markov model

routine surveillance on survival. The degree of confounding can be studied by sensitivity analysis: in- and excluding interval recurrences.

Decision analytic models go a step further than empirical studies. Long-term outcome after the end of follow-up in a study (e.g., life expectancy) may be estimated using the empirical data as input data for the decision model. More importantly, different surveillance strategies can systematically be compared.

Literature Review

We searched the Medline database with the terms "cost-benefit analysis [MesH]," "decision support techniques [MesH]," "decision trees [MesH]," "Markov," "surveillance," "cancer," and "follow-up." We extended the search using cross-references. The search was limited to the English language and studies concerning humans. A total of 24 studies were identified that used decision analysis to model cancer surveillance (Table 3.1). Of these, six studies modeled surveillance of colorectal cancer [9–14], four modeled surveillance of bladder cancer [15–18], three testicular cancer [19–21], three modeled breast cancer [22–24], two modeled Hodgkin's lymphoma [25, 26], two melanoma [27, 28], two lung cancer [29, 30], and other studies modeled laryngeal cancer [31] and ovarian cancer [32].

Different research questions were answered: which test to use during surveillance, which patients to include, at what duration, and if the current surveillance strategy is beneficial over no surveillance. To answer these questions, some researchers used a decision tree as a model, while others used a Markov model. These modeling techniques will be discussed next.

The fundamental analytic tool for decision analysis is the decision tree. A decision tree represents, in a logical sequence, the series of chance events and decisions over time. Its construction commonly entails a number of steps, as listed below [33]. Subsequently, a more detailed description of the steps is given.

1. *Definition of the clinical problem.* This should include the characteristics of the type of patient for whom the decision is analyzed, possible diagnostic and therapeutic

actions (decision alternatives), and possible short- and long-term outcomes.

The clinical problem should then be structured as a decision tree that typically includes decision nodes and chance nodes. The decision node (□) reflects a point in time at which several options (e.g., surveillance alternatives) are possible; the decision maker is in control of the decision. A chance node (○) reflects a point in time at which the outcome occurs

Example: In Fig. 3.2a, an example of a decision tree is given similar to a tree seen in the literature [18]. Two surveillance regimens of bladder cancer were compared: a standard care regimen (cystoscopy) and a modified care regimen (urinary markers). The outcome of the decision tree was detection of disease recurrence. Input data used in this example are fictional.

2. *Quantification of the decision tree.* Two aspects towards quantification are important: probabilities (at chance nodes) and utilities or relative value judgments of the outcomes of interest (at terminal nodes).

After defining a structure for the tree, we need to fill in the relevant probabilities. Probabilities are a quantitative manner to express the relative frequency of occurrence (chances) for possible outcome categories, ranging from 0 to 1, from impossible to certain [34].

Probabilities in the decision tree may relate to tests (e.g., a positive test result when the disease is present, or sensitivity), therapies (e.g., the risk of short-term complications, the probability of long-term success), and prognosis (e.g., expected outcome without treatment). Therapeutic effects are ideally determined from randomized clinical trials, which enable unbiased comparisons between alternative treatments. Prognostic estimates might be obtained from a follow-up study in a well-defined cohort. In the absence of empirical data, assumptions based on, for instance, personal or expert experience have to be made. The probability estimates may thus come from (a combination of) personal or expert experience, empirical data, and understanding of the different disease processes.

Outcome can be measured in absolute quantities, for example, life expectancy (years), survival (0–1), or financial costs. But decision analyses often use utility values to indicate the relative desirability of an outcome (e.g., disability or malfunctioning on a scale that ranges from dead (valued as 0) to well (valued as 1)). Utilities can be obtained in a variety of ways. Common techniques for eliciting utilities are specialized assessments such as "standard gamble," "time trade-off," or the "visual analogue scale" [35, 36]. Utility estimates are also frequently based on quality-of-life questionnaires (e.g., SF-36 [37] or EuroQol [38]) and instruments like the "Health Utility Index" [39]. If all utilities are measured in consistent units, the values of the outcome can be compared and ordered.

Effectiveness (or health benefit) can be summarized in quality-adjusted life years (QALYs). QALYs hence incorporate both survival and morbidity aspects (malfunctioning) in a single measure [40].

Example: In Fig. 3.2b, the decision tree is quantified. The probabilities are filled in at the chance nodes, the costs, and QALYs (as value judgment of the outcome of interest) at the terminal nodes. The result is shown as total cost/total QALY.

3. *Calculation of the preferred clinical strategy.* The contribution of each of the terminal branches to the value of a particular course of action (decision) is equal to the product of the utility of that branch and the probability of its occurrence [41]. Based on the decision tree, the average outcome value that can be expected (the expected value) for each choice hence can be calculated.

For all possible options at the decision node, the best option is determined. If a positive outcome value has been used (e.g., survival, life expectancy, or utility), the expected value must be maximized. If a negative outcome value has been used (e.g., mortality or costs), the expected value must be minimized. This process of removing less optimal alternatives from further consideration is called "folding back." Finally, a decision will be made to which surveillance method would, on average, be favorable. Averaging out and folding back are together referred to as "rolling back" [34]. Rolling back can readily be done by modern computer software. However, to gain confidence about this final decision, we need to explore how assumptions affect the decision.

Example: In Fig. 3.2c, the decision tree is rolled back. The standard regimen (cystoscopy) is pointed out as the most cost-effective option (the preferred strategy).

4. *Evaluation of uncertainty with sensitivity analyses.* The term "sensitivity analysis" refers to a technique that tests the stability and robustness of the conclusions of an analysis. This is relevant for decision analysis, as the results of the analysis are only as robust as the quality of the data on which the analysis is based [35]. Considerable uncertainty may be present in the preferred clinical strategy because of limited available data or poor quality data on which the probabilities and/or utilities are based.

In a sensitivity analysis, the value of one or more parameters in a model is varied to study the effect on the preferred decision. These parameter variations are based on a range of likely probabilities and utilities, e.g., a 95 % confidence interval, a 20 % difference range, or a halving and doubling of parameter values. If the variation has small effects, the

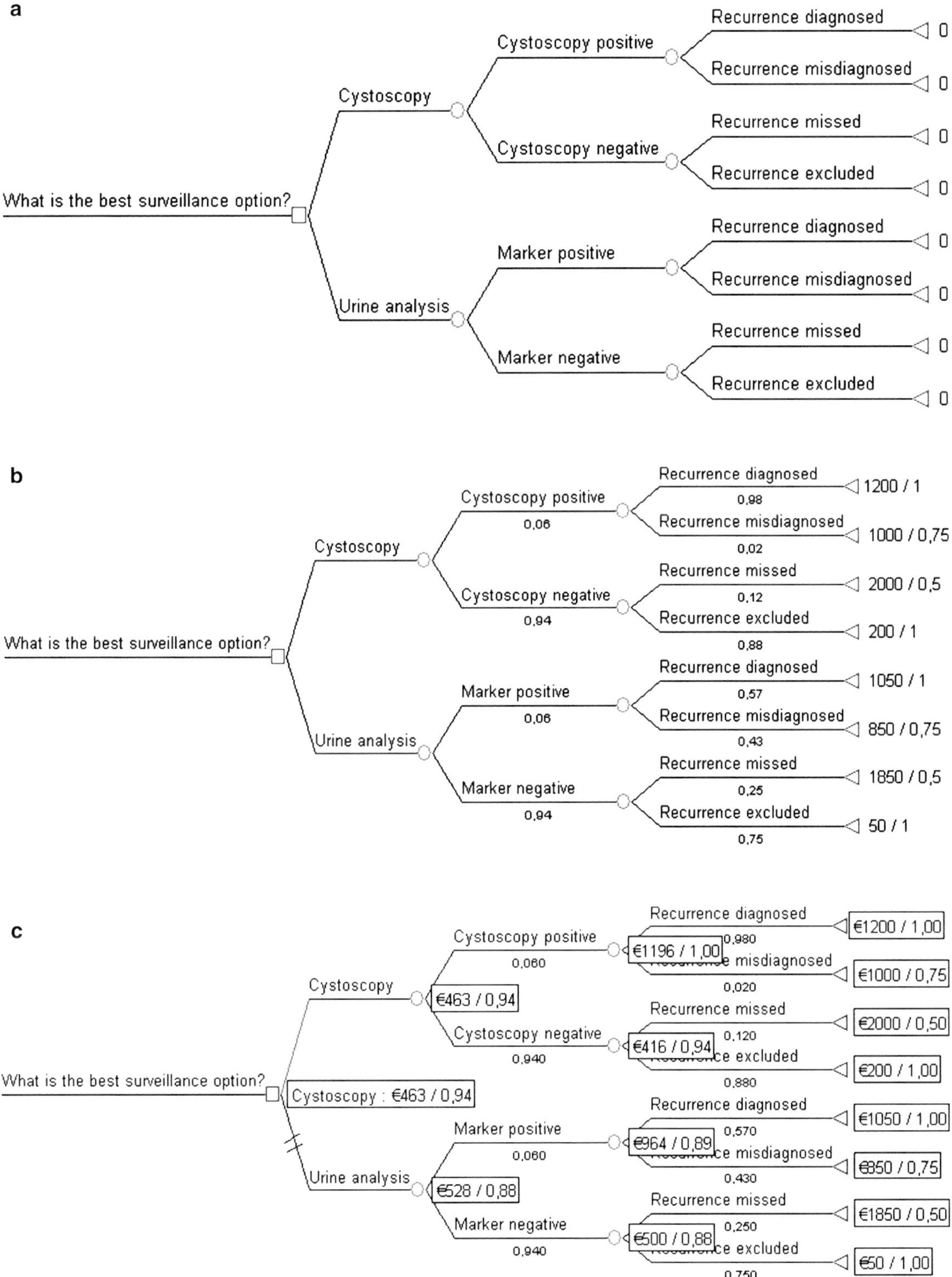

Fig. 3.2 (**a**) Basic diagnostic decision tree comparing cystoscopy with urine analysis in surveillance of bladder cancer patients. (**b**) Quantification of the basic decision tree for bladder cancer. Six percent of all patients are expected to have a positive test result with each test. The result is shown as total cost/total QALY. (**c**) Rolling back the basic decision tree for bladder cancer. Cystoscopy is both less costly and more effective (higher number of QALYs gained)

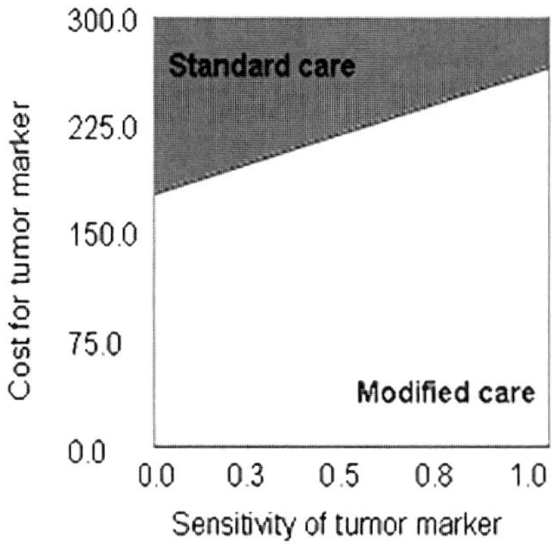

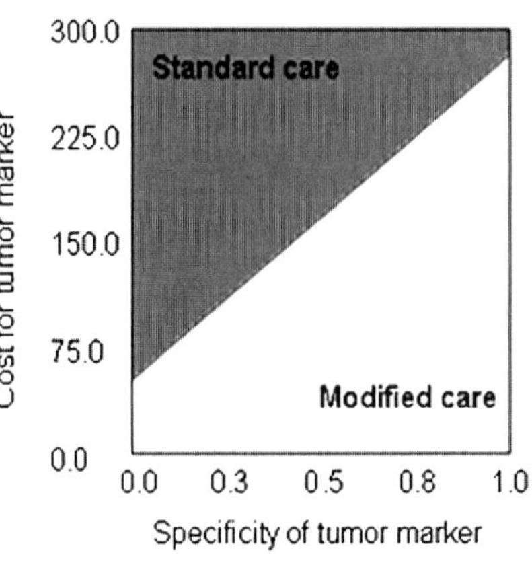

Fig. 3.3 Two-way sensitivity analysis to study the influence of tumor marker costs, sensitivity, and specificity variation on the decision to use either standardized (cystoscopy + cytology every 3 months) or modified (tumor marker test every 3 months) care in the surveillance of bladder cancer patients

uncertainty in the value of the parameter is said to be relatively unimportant (the decision is not sensitive to that factor). If such variations cause large changes in the results from the analysis, the parameter is important and needs to be considered carefully in the interpretation of the results.

When the value of one parameter is varied, while the others are kept constant, the sensitivity analysis is called one-way. To evaluate the effect of simultaneous changes in two or more variables, a two-way or *n*-way sensitivity analysis can be performed [34].

Example: In the study of Lotan and Roehrborn, the standard care surveillance protocol of bladder cancer was compared to a modified care protocol [17]. The modified care protocol consisted of alternating a tumor marker test with cystoscopy at months intervals and the standard care protocol consisted of cystoscopy and cytology every 3 months. To compare the costs of the modified and standard care protocols, a two-way sensitivity analysis was performed using varying sensitivities and specificities of the tumor marker test.

Figure 3.3 shows a plot of the threshold variables. The modified care protocol was less costly than the standard care protocol unless the tumor marker was more expensive than $168, regardless of the sensitivity of the test. Further, the tumor marker test should have a specificity greater than 50 % at $168 to remain less costly than the standard care protocol.

5. *Presentation in a clinically useful way*. The decision tree may need simplification for presentation, and qualitative and quantitative results should be presented such that they are easily understandable.

Steps 1–5 do not need to be followed in a strict order. For example, quantification of a highly realistic, detailed tree may be problematic (step 2), leading to a revision with simplifying assumptions (step 1). Internal and external validation may suggest some alterations. Also, sensitivity analysis may reveal a large influence of variation in some parameters (step 4) which hence need further study to obtain a more reliable estimate of probabilities and utilities (step 2) [33].

In a cost-effectiveness analysis (CEA), costs of different surveillance strategies are related to their medical effects. A strategy can sometimes be eliminated based on its relative cost and effectiveness compared to another strategy. An option is said to be "dominated" (never the best option) if it both costs more and is less effective than a comparator.

An incremental cost-effectiveness ratio (ICER) can be calculated when comparing two non-dominated options. The ICER is the ratio of additional costs to additional benefits and is often expressed as the cost per additional year of life saved or the cost per QALY saved [34]. This ICER can, for instance, be used to determine if the next more effective option exceeds a threshold ICER. This threshold is sometimes referred to as the willingness to pay or ceiling ratio [40]. As for all decision analyses, CEA should also contain sensitivity analysis that tests the robustness of the results given plausible ranges for important parameter values.

Next we describe the Markov models. Events and decisions are chronologically ordered from left to right in a conventional decision tree (e.g., events on the right side of the tree happen after events on the left side of the tree). A Markov model can, however, account for events that involve risk over time and events that happen more than once. Instead of modeling uncertain events at chance nodes, the uncertain events are modeled as transitions between defined health states. These are called

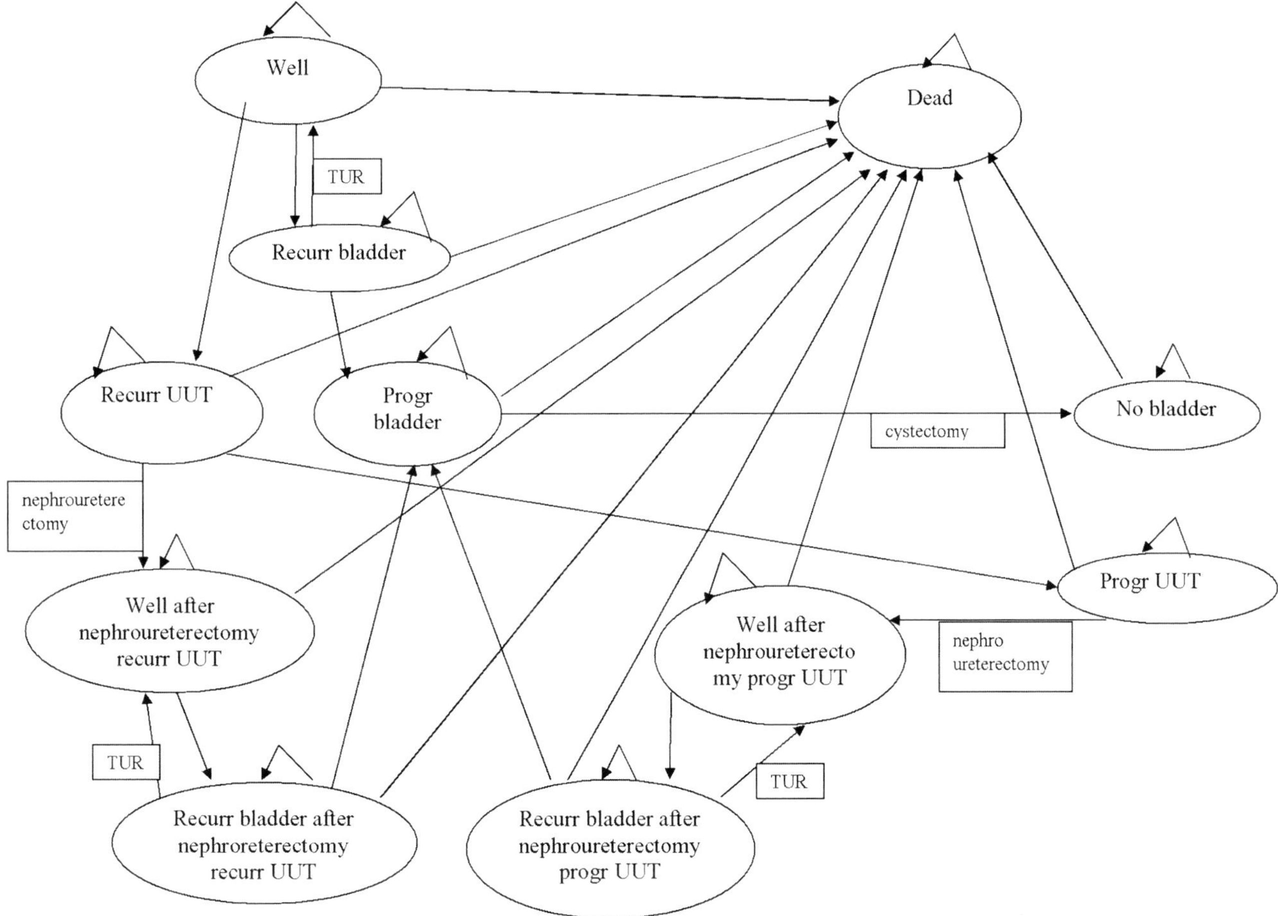

Fig. 3.4 Influence diagram representing a Markov model for surveillance of bladder cancer patients [15]. The influence diagram can readily portray the relationships between factors included in the decision model

Markov states. The model assumes that a patient is always in one of these finite number of Markov states.

A time horizon is chosen (depending on the available data) and is divided into discrete increments of time. These increments of time are referred to as Markov cycles. During each cycle, the patient may make a transition from one state to another. Events can, however, occur only once during a cycle (one transition per cycle). A matrix of one-cycle transition probabilities, applied in each successive cycle, defines the possible changes in state. One-cycle transition probabilities may be constant throughout many cycles (stationary Markov model, Markov chain) or may depend on time and thus change from cycle to cycle (a semi-Markov model) [34, 42]. An important feature of the Markov model is that it has "no memory." This absence of memory in the Markov process is known in mathematics as the Markov assumption: the transition risk only depends on the current health state and not on previous states or transitions.

The Markov states and possible transitions can be represented by an influence diagram.

Example: In Fig. 3.4, a rather complex example of such an influence diagram is shown that represents a Markov model for bladder cancer [15]. Using this model, two surveillance strategies were compared. Recurrences in the bladder, as well as progression and recurrences in the upper urinary tract, were taken into account. All patients start in the Well state and, as time progresses, the patients move to different health states. In such complex decision problems, the Markov decision tree is far too large to fit on a single-printed page. The influence diagram can portray more clearly the factors to consider and how those factors are related.

Constant transition probabilities are used in a Markov chain. Constant transition probabilities are, however, only realistic for a short-time horizon. In calculations using a longer time horizon (such as cancer surveillance), or more chronic conditions, time-dependent probabilities are usually necessary [43].

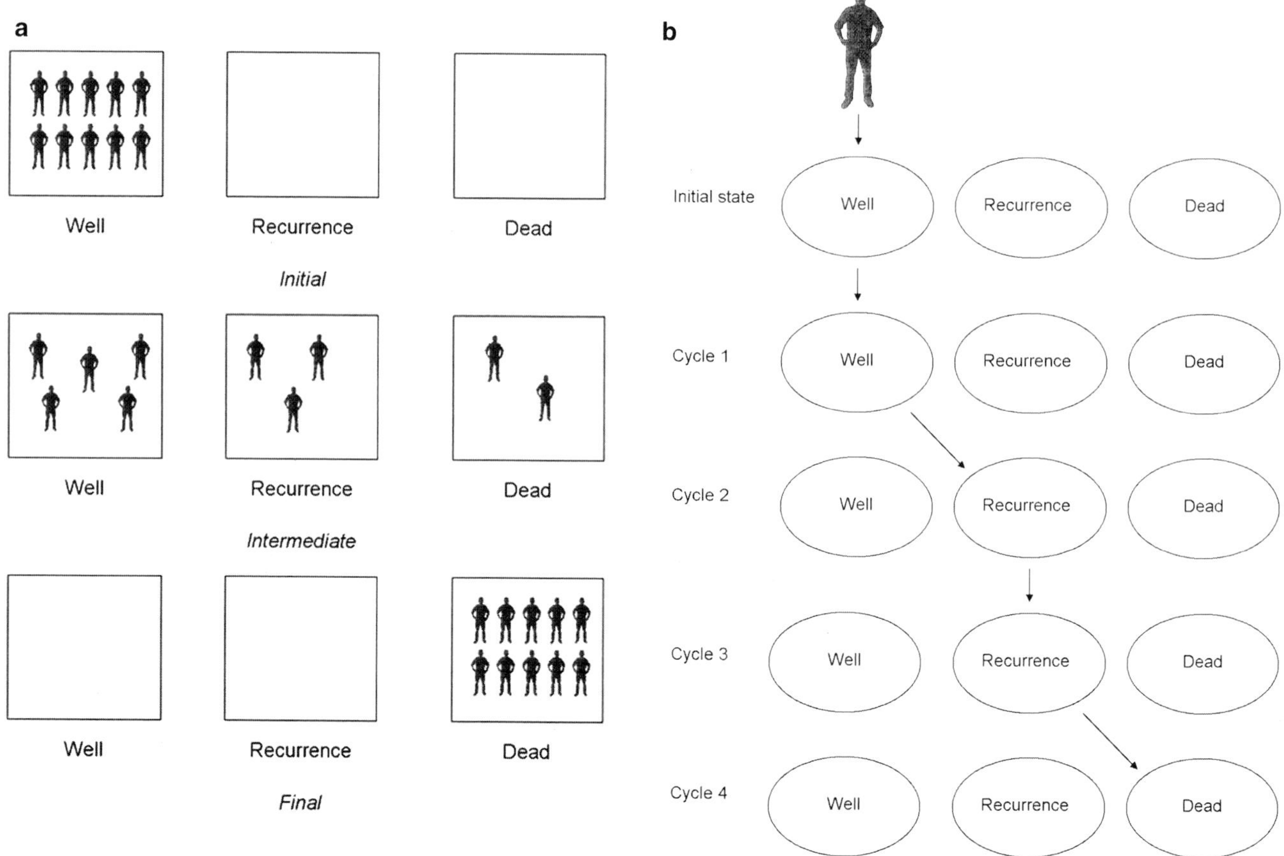

Fig. 3.5 (**a**) Schematic representation of a Markov cohort analysis. (**b**) Schematic representation of a Monte Carlo simulation

The probability of recurrence of cancer, for example, will generally decrease with surveillance time. The risk of death from other causes increases as patients grow older. So, if the time horizon for the analysis is long, the mortality rate will increase during later Markov cycles. There are two ways of handling such changing probabilities. One is with a continuous function. For each cycle, the appropriate mortality rate is calculated from a formula and converted to a transition probability. Some rates are, however, not easily described as a simple function. One example is the recurrence rate of tumors, which may initially be higher than later during follow-up. In such cases, the necessary rates (or corresponding probabilities) may be stored in a table, indexed by cycle number, and retrieved as the Markov model is evaluated. Current computer software provides facilities for constructing and using such tables [42].

Moreover, to retain and recall detailed memory of patient history (e.g., an event), special variables, called tracker variables, can be used. With tracker variables, model transition probabilities are allowed to depend on the states experienced in previous cycles [34]. The use of tracker variables is beyond the scope of this chapter but, fortunately, modern decision-making computer software can be used in the evaluation of such more complex Markov models.

Utilities can be assigned to each Markov state. The contribution of this utility to the total sum (e.g., QALY) depends on the length of time, number of cycles, spent in each specific state. When performing cost-effectiveness analysis, costs may be specified separately for each state to represent the cost of being in that state for one cycle. The model is then evaluated separately for costs and survival [42].

There are three general methods for evaluating a Markov model; Fundamental matrix solution, Markov cohort analysis, and Monte Carlo simulation. We will further discuss the latter two, since they were used in the recent literature considering surveillance of cancer.

For an analysis of expected outcomes, the percentage of a hypothetical cohort (group of patients) in a state during a cycle is multiplied by the cost and/or utility associated with that state. These products are summed over all states and all cycles.

The cohort begins in an initial distribution of states, and at each cycle the entire cohort is reallocated to states according to the transition probabilities (Fig. 3.5a). In the cohort analysis two values are kept for each state at each cycle: the number of patients currently in the state and the total number of patient-cycles in the state. When a Markov cohort analysis is terminated, the total number of patient-cycles for each state is divided by the size of the original cohort, yielding the expected time that each individual member will spend in each state. For example; life expectancy is the sum of these expected values. The Markov cohort analysis is a simulation, although it does not follow patients as individuals [43].

For greater flexibility, analyses can be performed via Monte Carlo microsimulation. The Monte Carlo simulation determines the prognoses of a large number of individual patients. Each patient begins in the starting state (e.g., the well state), and at the end of each cycle, a random number generator is used together with the transition probabilities to determine in which state the patient will begin the next cycle (Fig. 3.5b) [42]. Just as for the cohort simulation, the patient is given credit for each cycle spent in a specific state and for each state expected utility, and expected costs can be calculated. When the patient enters the ("absorbing") dead-state, the simulation for that individual is stopped. The process is repeated many times. The appropriate number of simulated patients depends on the magnitudes of the transition probabilities in the model (smaller probabilities of rare events necessitate more simulations) and on the size of the difference between intervention strategies that is expected to be found. It is not uncommon for Monte Carlo simulation models to require 50,000–1,000,000 fictive patients [34].

Each series of cycles (trial) generates a quality-adjusted survival time. After a large number of trials, these constitute a distribution of survival values. The mean value of this Monte Carlo-derived distribution will be similar to the expected value (e.g., utility) obtained by a cohort simulation. However, in addition to the mean survival, statistical measures such as variance and standard deviation of the expected utility may be determined from the Monte Carlo-derived distribution [42].

A Framework to Model Cancer Surveillance: Ovarian Cancer

In this section, we will describe a step by step approach to model surveillance after treatment for ovarian cancer, which can also be used for other malignancies. Outcomes of interest can be overall survival, disease-specific survival, quality of life, and cost-effectiveness. In this example, we will focus on the effect of surveillance on overall survival. There is no single best way to model surveillance, but the main steps taken in this example are important for all modeling approaches. The results are for illustrative purpose only.

The important first step in studying the effect of surveillance on survival is to obtain an impression of the possible benefit of early treatment. For ovarian cancer, overall survival of patients with an early detected, asymptomatic recurrence is significantly better than in patients with a symptomatic recurrence (Fig. 3.6). However, as stated earlier in this chapter, this difference may be explained in part or fully by lead time bias, length time bias, and self-selection bias. Survival analysis alone cannot give the effect estimate for "current surveillance" vs. "no surveillance."

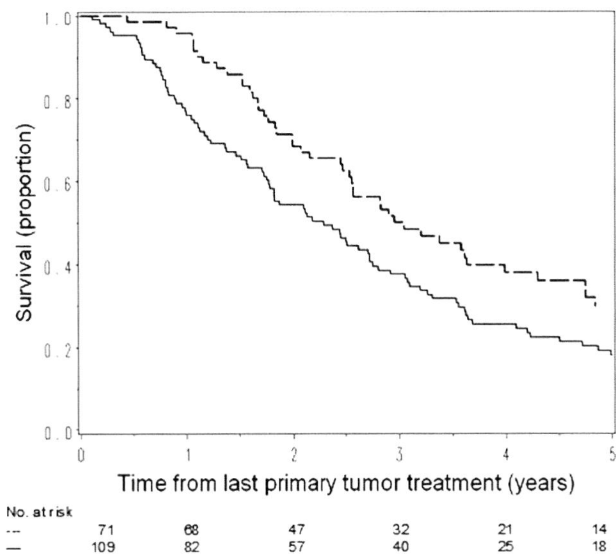

Fig. 3.6 Survival in 180 patients with recurrent ovarian cancer detected asymptomatically (*dashed line*) and symptomatically (*straight line*)

The question "what is the effect of surveillance on life-expectancy?" can be rephrased into a decision-analytical problem: "With respect to survival, should we continue the current routine surveillance protocol trying to detect a recurrence as early as possible, should we abolish early recurrence detection, or should we implement a more stringent surveillance protocol in patients treated for ovarian cancer with curative intent?" Ovarian cancer may reoccur over time; therefore, Markov-modeling is a suitable method to model the natural history and clinical progress of ovarian cancer. A Markov-model can simulate the effect of different surveillance programs to detect cancer recurrence early on life expectancy.

Next, we will propose a framework to model the effectiveness of cancer surveillance. The successive steps are: (1) model the natural history of disease, (2) assess model parameters (transition probabilities) for the natural history model, (3) validate the results of the model with information from the literature, (4) sensitivity analysis of the key parameters used in the model, and (5) simulate the effect of alternative surveillance scenarios on survival.

Step 1 Model Current Cancer Surveillance

According to the European guideline for medical oncologists, the recommended frequency of surveillance after treatment for ovarian cancer is every 3 months the first 2 years, every 4 months the third year, and every 6 months during year 4 and 5. These follow-up visits consist of medical history taking, physical examination, and tumor marker measurement. If a recurrent ovarian cancer is suspected, additional diagnostic tests may be performed like a CT-scan or ultrasound [44].

In routine surveillance, patients can be diagnosed with recurrent disease based on clinical symptoms or based on diagnostic tests alone. The effect of surveillance is hidden in the observed difference in survival between patients with asymptomatic and symptomatic recurrences. Therefore, the Markov model basically consists of three health states—curatively treated, asymptomatic recurrence, and symptomatic recurrence—and one absorbing state-death from all causes. This Markov model is illustrated in Fig. 3.7. The entire simulation cohort will start in the "curatively treated" state. The start of the simulation (t_0) is defined as the last date of primary tumor treatment which is equal to the start of surveillance.

Note: A different approach is to design a more biologically based surveillance model. In theory, all patients with recurrent disease enter the preclinical asymptomatic phase and will become symptomatic as the recurrence progresses (Fig. 3.8) [23]. The problem with this approach is that the transition from asymptomatic recurrence to symptomatic recurrence is unknown and the effect of early recurrence treatment is hidden in this parameter. Due to the difficulty to assess this parameter, it will yield a large uncertainty.

In addition, recurrences can be distinguished into locoregional recurrence, distant metastasis, and second primary tumors (Fig. 3.8).

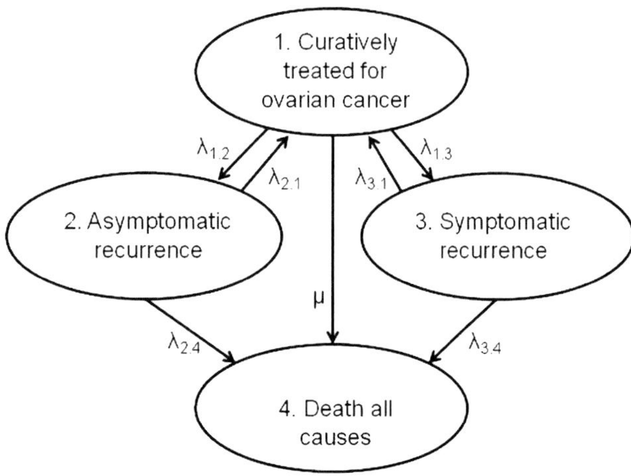

Fig. 3.7 Basic Markov model representing the course of curatively treated ovarian cancer patients across four disease states, λ indicates a transition rate between two health states

Step 2 Model Parameters for Current Cancer Surveillance

The transition probabilities can be estimated based on empirical data or expert experience. We analyzed data from a cohort of 594 ovarian cancer patients diagnosed between 1996 and 2006 in four hospitals in the Netherlands (Fig. 3.6).

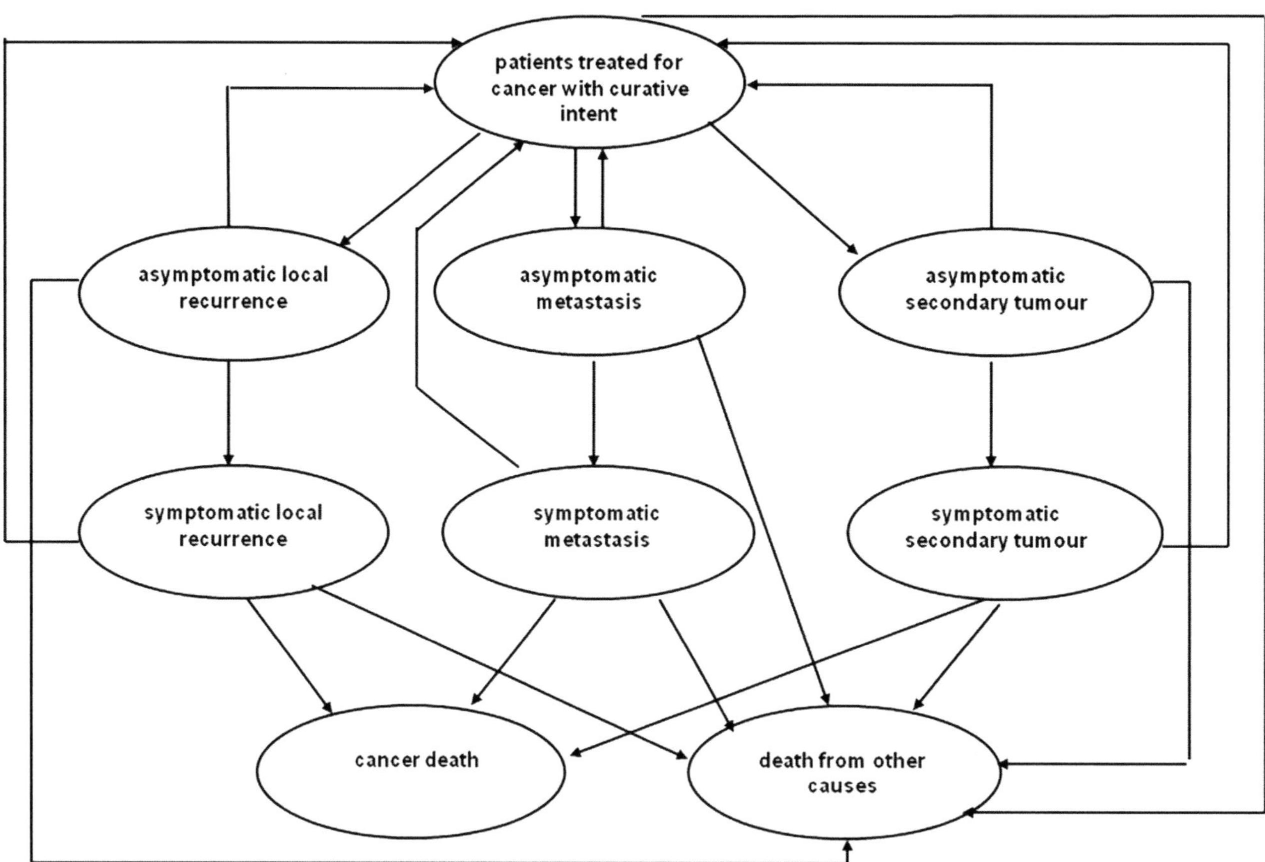

Fig. 3.8 Extended Markov model for surveillance of patients curatively treated for cancer

Table 3.2 Three-monthly transition probabilities for current routine follow-up and one-way sensitivity analyses

Transition	Best estimate	Sensitivity analysis—based on limits of the 95 % confidence interval			
		Lower limit	Life expectancy (change),[a] years	Upper limit	Life expectancy (change),[a] years
Curatively treated to asymptomatic state ($\lambda_{1,2}$)	0.03	0.02	6.0 (+0.2)	0.05	5.4 (−0.4)
Curatively treated to symptomatic state ($\lambda_{1,3}$)	0.07	0.05	6.7 (+1.2)	0.09	4.9 (−0.9)
Asymptomatic state to curatively treated ($\lambda_{2,1}$)	0.13	0.09	5.8 (+0.0)	0.18	5.7 (−0.1)
Symptomatic state to curatively treated ($\lambda_{3,1}$)	0.15	0.10	5.3 (−0.5)	0.20	6.2 (+0.4)
Asymptomatic state to death ($\lambda_{2,4}$)	0.08	0.04	6.0 (+0.2)	0.12	5.5 (−0.3)
Symptomatic state to death ($\lambda_{3,4}$)	0.20	0.14	6.9 (+1.1)	0.25	5.1 (−0.7)

[a]Compared to best estimate resulting in a life expectancy of 5.8 years

Table 3.3 Internal and external validation of the model to simulate ovarian cancer surveillance

	Markov model	Cohort data	CCCS, 2006 (%)	Heintz [47] (%)
Life expectancy (months)	69	80		
Median survival (months)	54	31		
Five-year survival	44 %	22.4 %	23–27	49.7

CCCS Comprehensive Cancer Centre South, the Netherlands (source: http:\\www.ikcnet.nl, accessed June 20, 2011)

The transition probabilities (λ_{ij}) are defined as the transition from health state *i* to state *j* (Fig. 3.7). Transition probabilities are defined as the proportion of patients who transfer from one to the other state during a three-month interval (cycle length), corresponding to the routine surveillance interval in practice. We assume constant transition probabilities for first, second, etc., ovarian cancer recurrences.

The transition probabilities for the current surveillance protocol are presented in Table 3.2. A detailed description on how these transition probabilities are calculated can be found in the Appendix.

Step 3 Validate Current Cancer Surveillance Model

Internal validation means that the life expectancy derived from the model should be similar to the overall survival retrieved from the primary data [45]. We externally validated the model based on national and international registry data [45–47]. The model overestimates the median and 5-year survival and slightly underestimates life expectancy (Table 3.3).

If the model estimates do not resemble the estimates from the primary data source and literature, it is necessary to rethink steps 1 and 2. Possible actions may be to adjust the model and/or reconsider the assumptions made to a more realistic situation, for example by including time-dependent probabilities for recurrence risks.

Step 4 Sensitivity Analysis for Current Cancer Surveillance Model

The next step is to assess the stability and robustness of the model. As an illustration, we will evaluate the impact of varying the transition probabilities using the 95 % confidence intervals on life expectancy. Uncertainties in the transition probabilities for symptomatic recurrence have a larger impact on life expectancy than the transition probabilities for asymptomatic recurrence (Table 3.2). The transition probabilities for symptomatic recurrence are thus less stable than the transition probabilities for asymptomatic recurrence.

Step 5 Simulate Alternative Scenarios

The final step is to compare different surveillance strategies with respect to life expectancy. Absence of surveillance is equal to monitoring the natural history, which means that all recurrences are diagnosed based on clinical symptoms. In ovarian cancer, the tumor marker CA125 is able to detect recurrences before symptoms arise in approximately 80 % of the cases, so in perfect surveillance 80 % of the patients with recurrent disease will be treated in the asymptomatic phase [48] (Fig. 3.9). We also simulated the situation in which all recurrences are detected in the asymptomatic phase (Table 3.4). According to the current model, current surveillance increases life expectancy with 0.5 year. In the most ideal situation, all recurrences are detected in the asymptomatic phase, which would increase life expectancy with 3.3 years. This difference remains when performing one-way sensitivity analysis on the transition probabilities, with the exception of the asymptomatic and symptomatic mortality rate (Fig. 3.10).

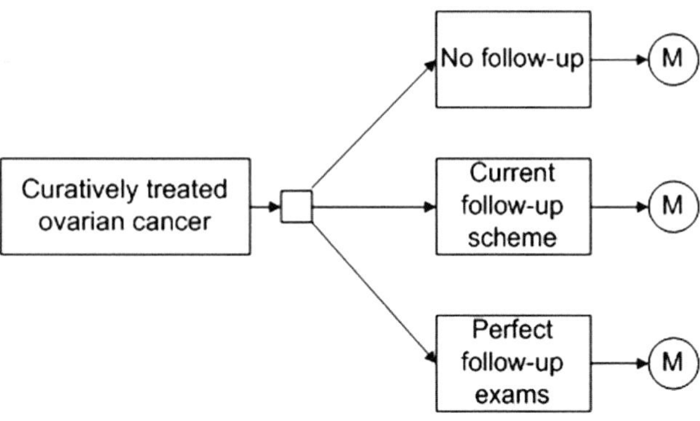

Fig. 3.9 Schematic decision tree for ovarian cancer surveillance, with *M* indicating the Markov model

Table 3.4 Life expectancy (LE) after current routine follow-up compared with alternative scenarios

Alternatives	Assumptions	LE (change) (years)
No follow-up	All recurrences symptomatic ($\lambda_{1,2}=0$, $\lambda_{1,3}=0.10$)	5.3 (–0.5)
Current follow-up	According to the data ($\lambda_{1,2}=0.03$, $\lambda_{1,3}=0.07$)	5.8
Perfect CA125 testing	80% asymptomatic ($\lambda_{1,2}=0.08$ $\lambda_{1,3}=0.02$)	8.1 (+2.3)
Perfect follow-up	All recurrences asymptomatic ($\lambda_{1,2}=0.10$, $\lambda_{1,3}=0$)	9.1 (+3.3)

Discussion

In this chapter we discussed various issues regarding decision modeling, with a focus on surveillance strategies in patients treated for cancer. Next we will reflect on some issues in such decision modeling.

The principal reason for surveillance is detection of recurrent disease in an early phase. Yet the value of surveillance programs after potentially curative treatment of cancer remains controversial. Is it truly beneficial to detect asymptomatic recurrences? Why not wait till clinical suspicion?

Clearly, as explained in this chapter, observed gain in survival time through early recurrence detection may be biased. Furthermore, research has shown that, for a number of cancer types, early detection was not associated with a gain in survival duration. It has, therefore, been suggested that perhaps for some cancers with limited evidence on the effectiveness of early recurrence detection, surveillance should be abolished entirely or could be replaced by psychosocial care alone [2].

To evaluate the cancer-specific effectiveness of routine surveillance, an essential first question is: what is the benefit for patients in whom recurrences are detected in an early asymptomatic phase compared to treatment initiated when patients present with symptoms? Empirical evidence for this benefit is hard to obtain. Ideally, evidence would come from a randomized controlled trial. Such randomized controlled trials would, for instance, compare consequences (e.g., survival or progression of disease) of different surveillance strategies, (e.g., no surveillance, current surveillance, or a more intensive surveillance).The contrast between such surveillance strategies may be rather small, requiring excessive patient numbers for a reliable evaluation. In addition, conducting a no surveillance regime would be often considered unethical.

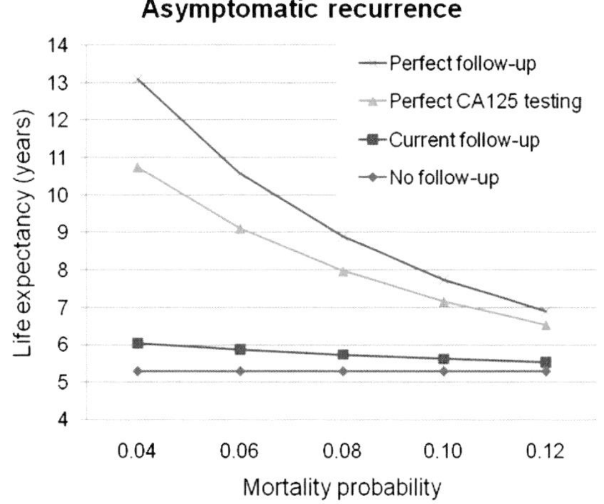

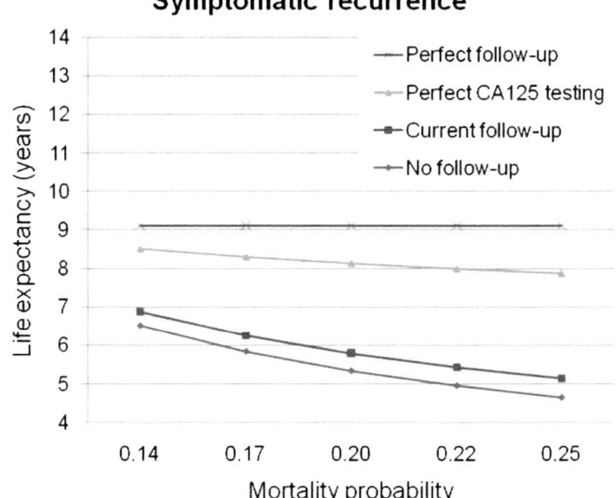

Fig. 3.10 One-way sensitivity analyses for the mortality probability in ovarian cancer patients with asymptomatic recurrence (point estimate = 0.08) and symptomatic recurrence (point estimate = 0.20) and the effect on life expectancy for the range of follow-up alternatives

A second question is: If there is a benefit, at what interval should surveillance take place and which diagnostic tests should be included in this surveillance protocol? To answer this question, empirical evidence on test characteristics is required, which can become available from diagnostic evaluations.

The Health Council of the Netherlands concluded in 2007 that there is a need for more research to unravel the effectiveness of routine surveillance to support evidence-based surveillance programs [49]. As these research data become more available, decision analysis will increasingly be a valid method to develop evidence-based surveillance programs and play a central role in this process.

Decision analysis enables a systematic and clear comparison of surveillance strategies. Surprisingly, decision modeling is as yet only a small part of the literature on surveillance programs. Reasons include the limited acquaintance of decision analyses methods in clinical practice and the lack of empirical data to define key probabilities related to the benefit of early treatment and test characteristics. However, if we make certain assumptions, for example, that survival depends only on the stage of disease (which is generally more favorable with surveillance), surveillance strategies can be evaluated. By use of sensitivity analyses, we can analyze the impact of these assumptions on model outcomes.

Decision analysis of surveillance strategies is especially relevant in patients treated for cancers which are mostly curable, where patients attend surveillance programs during a long time and as cancer incidence increases (given the costs of these surveillance programs). This may explain the fact that most decision analyses of surveillance programs were for colon cancer (very frequent), bladder cancer (mostly not lethal, costly because of long surveillance), testicular cancer (mostly not lethal, costly because of long surveillance, but less frequent than bladder cancer), and breast cancer (very frequent).

Recommendations on Modeling Cancer Surveillance

Regarding the type of model, the decision model should arguably only be as complex as is necessary to adequately answer the research question. Another consideration is the quality and extent of available input data. It makes no sense to develop a detailed decision model if the required detailed knowledge is not available.

In the literature, for example, we identified a number of studies including different bladder cancer models, all addressing the same decision problem, i.e., the role of a new urinary marker test in surveillance [15–18]. One of these studies used the simplest model, a conventional decision tree which represented a single follow-up visit at 3-month intervals [18]. This simple model was sufficient to answer the research question, i.e., which strategy was most cost-effective.

In another bladder cancer study, a more detailed way of representing the surveillance schedule was chosen. It modeled a one- and two-year surveillance schedule per three months, with a chance node every 3 months to account for a possibly detected recurrence [17]. Therefore, a more detailed decision tree model was needed to be able to answer the question of which strategy was best. Yet, a different bladder cancer study applied a Markov model for each trimester separately [15]. Many possible diagnostic test outcomes and consequences were taken into account, requiring a more advanced modeling technique.

In summary, conventional decision trees are most appropriate when clinically important events happen within a relatively short, fixed period of time following the decision, when each event can occur only once, and when the probability of experiencing each event is constant over time. In situations where events can reoccur over time and where timing of events is important, a Markov model is more appropriate. In cancer, surveillance risk of recurrence is likely to vary over time and can occur more than once. A Markov model is, therefore, often the natural choice to model cancer surveillance programs.

Future research should focus on better estimating underlying transition probabilities to improve the quality of the decision analytic models. Decision analysis can then better be used to explore the potential impact of new developments, e.g., in treatment and diagnostic testing. Moreover, patient heterogeneity needs to be taken into account, e.g., in the difference in risk for recurrence or other outcomes.

Implementation

A practical challenge is how to implement decision analysis in real-world decision making. A complex decision model may not convince physicians to let go of a standard surveillance regimen. The decision model must, therefore, often be simplified to make it more understandable. When the decision model results in different sufficient surveillance programs, a possible next step is to conduct randomized controlled trials to compare these programs. The contrast may, however, be small, leading to large sample size requirements. Applications of decision analyses to support an individual patient's decision making are currently less prominent. Several practical barriers (e.g., how well do patients anticipate the impact of disease symptoms and adverse effects on their quality of life) must be addressed to bring decision analysis into the clinic to facilitate shared decision making by patients and physicians [35].

Appendix for the Ovarian Cancer Case Study

The transition rate is equal to the hazard rate underlying the survival curve: transition rate = $-(1/t) \times \ln(t - \text{survival})$, where t is defined as a period of 3 months. The Markov model requires probabilities, which can be converted from rates by the formula: probability = 1 − exp(−rate).

- From curatively treated condition to asymptomatic recurrence ($\lambda_{1.2}$)
  This transition represents the risk for asymptomatic recurrence. The state curatively treated includes both time from last primary tumor treatment as well as time from curatively treated recurrences, since recurrences may reoccur. Patients may, therefore, be included more than once under the assumption that the recurrence rate is constant over time. The transition rate can be determined using Kaplan-Meier survival analysis, with asymptomatic recurrence as event, and death, symptomatic recurrence, or lost to follow-up considered as censored. Risk for asymptomatic recurrence follows an exponential declining function, so $\lambda_{1.2} = -(1/t) \times \ln(R(t_1)/R(t_0))$, where R = 1–risk for asymptomatic recurrence and $t = t_1 - t_0$, time per 3 months.
  $\lambda_{1.2} = -(1/t) \times \ln(\mathrm{R}(t1)/\mathrm{R}(t0)) = -(1/12) \times \ln(0.6788) = 0.03$ → probability = 0.03
- From curatively treated to symptomatic recurrence (l1.3).
- This transition represents the risk for symptomatic recurrence. This is calculated similar to $\lambda_{1.2}$, with symptomatic recurrence as event, and death, asymptomatic recurrence, or lost to follow-up considered as censored.
  $\lambda_{1.3} = -(1/t) \times \ln(\mathrm{R}(t_1)/\mathrm{R}(t_0)) = -(1/12) \times \ln(0.4291) = 0.07$ → probability = 0.07
- From asymptomatic recurrence to death from ovarian cancer ($\lambda_{2.4}$)
- The mortality rate for patients with asymptomatic recurrent disease includes both ovarian cancer-specific and overall mortality. The date of asymptomatic recurrence detection is defined as the start of surveillance. Mortality rate is calculated using Kaplan-Meier survival analysis with mortality as event, and response to recurrence treatment and lost to follow-up considered as censored. Survival rate follows an exponential declining function, so $\lambda_{2.4} = -(1/t) \times \ln(\mathrm{S}(t_1)/\mathrm{S}(t_0))$, where S = 1 − mortality rate, $t = t_1 - t_0$, time per three months.
  $\lambda_{2.4} = -(1/t) \times \ln(\mathrm{S}(t_1)/\mathrm{S}(t_0) = -(1/4) \times \ln(0.7187) = 0.08$ → probability = 0.08
- From symptomatic recurrence to death from ovarian cancer ($\lambda_{3.4}$)
  This calculation is similar as for $\lambda_{2.1}$. Including all symptomatic recurrences.
  $\lambda_{3.4} = -(1/t) \times \ln(\mathrm{S}(t_1)/\mathrm{S}(t_0) = -(1/4) \times \ln(0.4185) = 0.22$ → probability = 0.20
- From asymptomatic recurrence to curatively treated ($\lambda_{2.1}$)
  If asymptomatic recurrent disease responds to treatment, treatment duration is defined as the time between asymptomatic recurrence diagnosis and the first surveillance visit following asymptomatic recurrence diagnosis. If consecutive surveillance visits are missing, transition to curatively treat is defined as date of asymptomatic recurrence detection plus six months of treatment (two Markov cycles). Using Kaplan-Meier survival analysis, the transition rate to curatively treat is calculated. If patients with asymptomatic recurrence progress during recurrence treatment, death or last surveillance date is considered as censored. Response rate is derived from an exponentially declining function, so $\lambda_{2.1} = -(1/t) \times \ln(\mathrm{RR}(t_1)/\mathrm{RR}(t_0))$, where RR = 1 − response rate, $t = t_1 - t_0$, time per three months.
  $\lambda_{2.1} = -(1/t) \times \ln(\mathrm{S}(t_1)/\mathrm{S}(t_0) = -(1/2) \times \ln(0.7500) = 0.14$ → probability = 0.13
- *From symptomatic recurrence to curatively treated* ($\lambda_{3.1}$)
  This transition is calculated similar to $\lambda_{2.1}$, including all symptomatic recurrences. Response rate follows an exponential declining function, so $\lambda_{3.1} = -(1/t) \times \ln(\mathrm{RR}(t_1)/\mathrm{RR}(t_0))$, where RR = 1 − response rate, $t = t_1 - t_0$, time per three months.
  $\lambda_{3.1} = -(1/t) \times \ln(\mathrm{S}(t_1)/\mathrm{S}(t_0) = -(1/2) \times \ln(0.7229) = 0.16$ → probability = 0.15
- Age-specific mortality (μ)
  Age-specific survival rates for women can, in this case, be acquired from Statistics Netherlands. The cohort of ovarian cancer patients will be used to determine the age distribution. This age distribution is used for the age of the Markov simulation cohort, and m is based on this aging population.

References

1. Weinstein M, Fineberg H. Clinical decision analysis. Philadelphia: Saunders; 1980.
2. Brada M. Is there a need to follow-up cancer patients? Eur J Cancer. 1995;31A:655–7.
3. Dewar JA, Kerr GR. Value of routine follow up of women treated for early carcinoma of the breast. Br Med J (Clin Res Ed). 1985;291:1464–7.
4. Roselli Del Turco M, Palli D, Cariddi A, Ciatto S, Pacini P, Distante V. The efficacy of intensive follow-up testing in breast cancer cases. Ann Oncol. 1995;6 Suppl 2:37–9.
5. Rustin GJS, van der Burg MEL, Griffin CL, et al. Early versus delayed treatment of relapsed ovarian cancer (MRC OV05/EORTC 55955): a randomised trial. Lancet. 2010;376:1155–63.
6. Joseph E, Hyacinthe M, Lyman GH, et al. Evaluation of an intensive strategy for follow-up and surveillance of primary breast cancer. Ann Surg Oncol. 1998;5:522–8.
7. Warde P, Specht L, Horwich A, et al. Prognostic factors for relapse in stage I seminoma managed by surveillance: a pooled analysis. J Clin Oncol. 2002;20:4448–52.
8. Steyerberg EW. Clinical prediction models, a practical approach to development, validation, and updating. New York, NY: Springer; 2009.
9. Borie F, Combescure C, Daures JP, Tretarre B, Millat B. Cost-effectiveness of two follow-up strategies for curative resection of colorectal cancer: comparative study using a Markov model. World J Surg. 2004;28:563–9.

10. Kievit J, van de Velde CJ. Utility and cost of carcinoembryonic antigen monitoring in colon cancer follow-up evaluation. A Markov analysis. Cancer. 1990;65:2580–2.
11. Michel P, Merle V, Chiron A, et al. Postoperative management of stage II/III colon cancer: a decision analysis. Gastroenterology. 1999;117:784–93.
12. Park KC, Schwimmer J, Shepherd JE, et al. Decision analysis for the cost-effective management of recurrent colorectal cancer. Ann Surg. 2001;233:310–9.
13. Park SM, Kim SY, Earle CC, Jeong SY, Yun YH. What is the most cost-effective strategy to screen for second primary colorectal cancers in male cancer survivors in Korea? World J Gastroenterol. 2009;15:3153–60.
14. Hassan C, Pickhardt PJ, Zullo A, et al. Cost-effectiveness of early colonoscopy surveillance after cancer resection. Dig Liver Dis. 2009;41:881–5.
15. de Bekker-Grob EW, van der Aa MNM, Zwarthoff EC, et al. Non-muscle invasive bladder cancer surveillance in which cystoscopy is partly replaced by microsatellite analysis on urine: a cost-effective alternative? (CEFUB-trial). BJU Int. 2009;104:41–7.
16. Lachaine J, Valiquette L, Crott R. Economic evaluation of NMP22 in the management of bladder cancer. Can J Urol. 2000;7:974–80.
17. Lotan Y, Roehrborn CG. Cost-effectiveness of a modified care protocol substituting bladder tumor markers for cystoscopy for the followup of patients with transitional cell carcinoma of the bladder: a decision analytical approach. J Urol. 2002;167:75–9.
18. Nam RK, Redelmeier DA, Spiess PE, Sampson HA, Fradet Y, Jewett MA. Comparison of molecular and conventional strategies for followup of superficial bladder cancer using decision analysis. J Urol. 2000;163:752–7.
19. Munro AJ, Warde PR. The use of a Markov process to simulate and assess follow-up policies for patients with malignant disease: surveillance for stage I nonseminomatous tumors of the testis. Med Decis Making. 1991;11:131–9.
20. Spermon JR, Hoffmann AL, Horenblas S, Verbeek AL, Witjes JA, Kiemeney LA. The efficacy of different follow-up strategies in clinical stage I non-seminomatous germ cell cancer: a Markov simulation study. Eur Urol. 2005;48:258–67; discussion 67–8.
21. Stiggelbout AM, Kiebert GM, de Haes JC, et al. Surveillance versus adjuvant chemotherapy in stage I non-seminomatous testicular cancer: a decision analysis. Eur J Cancer. 1996;32A:2267–74.
22. Hayman JA, Hillner BE, Harris JR, Weeks JC. Cost-effectiveness of routine radiation therapy following conservative surgery for early-stage breast cancer. J Clin Oncol. 1998;16:1022–9.
23. Jacobs HJ, van Dijck JA, de Kleijn EM, Kiemeney LA, Verbeek AL. Routine follow-up examinations in breast cancer patients have minimal impact on life expectancy: a simulation study. Ann Oncol. 2001;12:1107–13.
24. Lee JH, Glick HA, Hayman JA, Solin LJ. Decision-analytic model and cost-effectiveness evaluation of postmastectomy radiation therapy in high-risk premenopausal breast cancer patients. J Clin Oncol. 2002;20:2713–25.
25. Das P, Ng AK, Earle CC, Mauch PM, Kuntz KM. Computed tomography screening for lung cancer in Hodgkin's lymphoma survivors: decision analysis and cost-effectiveness analysis. Ann Oncol. 2006;17:785–93.
26. Guadagnolo BA, Punglia RS, Kuntz KM, Mauch PM, Ng AK. Cost-effectiveness analysis of computerized tomography in the routine follow-up of patients after primary treatment for Hodgkin's disease. J Clin Oncol. 2006;24:4116–22.
27. Hengge UR, Wallerand A, Stutzki A, Kockel N. Cost-effectiveness of reduced follow-up in malignant melanoma. J Dtsch Dermatol Ges. 2007;5:898–907.
28. Krug B, Crott R, Roch I, et al. Cost-effectiveness analysis of FDG PET-CT in the management of pulmonary metastases from malignant melanoma. Acta Oncol. 2010;49:192–200.
29. Kent MS, Korn P, Port JL, Lee PC, Altorki NK, Korst RJ. Cost effectiveness of chest computed tomography after lung cancer resection: a decision analysis model. Ann Thorac Surg. 2005;80:1215–22; discussion 1222–3.
30. van Loon J, Grutters JP, Wanders R, et al. 18FDG-PET-CT in the follow-up of non-small cell lung cancer patients after radical radiotherapy with or without chemotherapy: an economic evaluation. Eur J Cancer. 2010;46:110–9.
31. Ritoe SC, de Vegt F, Scheike IM, et al. Effect of routine follow-up after treatment for laryngeal cancer on life expectancy and mortality: results of a Markov model analysis. Cancer. 2007;109:239–47.
32. Hopkins ML, Coyle D, Le T, Fung MF, Wells G. Cancer antigen 125 in ovarian cancer surveillance: a decision analysis model. Curr Oncol. 2007;14:167–72.
33. Habbema JD, Bossuyt PM, Dippel DW, Marshall S, Hilden J. Analysing clinical decision analyses. Stat Med. 1990;9:1229–42.
34. Hunink M, Glasziou P. Decision making in health and medicine: integrating evidence and values. Cambridge, UK: Cambridge University Press; 2001.
35. Elkin EB, Vickers AJ, Kattan MW. Primer: using decision analysis to improve clinical decision making in urology. Nat Clin Pract Urol. 2006;3:439–48.
36. Torrance GW. Utility approach to measuring health-related quality of life. J Chronic Dis. 1987;40:593–603.
37. Ware Jr JE, Sherbourne CD. The MOS 36-item short-form health survey (SF-36). I. Conceptual framework and item selection. Med Care. 1992;30:473–83.
38. EuroQol-a new facility for the measurement of health-related quality of life. The EuroQol Group. Health Policy. 1990;16:199–208.
39. Feeny D, Furlong W, Boyle M, Torrance GW. Multi-attribute health status classification systems. Health utilities index. Pharmacoeconomics. 1995;7:490–502.
40. Gold M, Siegel J, Russell L, Weinstein M. Cost-effectiveness in health and medicine. New York, NY: Oxford University Press; 1996.
41. Pauker SG, Kassirer JP. Therapeutic decision making: a cost-benefit analysis. N Engl J Med. 1975;293:229–34.
42. Sonnenberg FA, Beck JR. Markov models in medical decision making: a practical guide. Med Decis Making. 1993;13:322–38.
43. Beck JR, Pauker SG. The Markov process in medical prognosis. Med Decis Making. 1983;3:419–58.
44. Aebi S, Castiglione M, Group EGW. Newly and relapsed epithelial ovarian carcinoma: ESMO clinical recommendations for diagnosis, treatment and follow-up. Ann Oncol. 2009;20 Suppl 4:21–3.
45. Iagaru AH, Mittra ES, McDougall IR, Quon A, Gambhir SS. 18F-FDG PET/CT evaluation of patients with ovarian carcinoma. Nucl Med Commun. 2008;29:1046–51.
46. Greuter MJ, Jansen-van der Weide MC, Jacobi CE, et al. The validation of a simulation model incorporating radiation risk for mammography breast cancer screening in women with a hereditary-increased breast cancer risk. Eur J Cancer. 2010;46:495–504.
47. Heintz AP, Odicino F, Maisonneuve P, et al. Carcinoma of the ovary. FIGO 6th annual report on the results of treatment in gynecological cancer. Int J Gynaecol Obstet. 2006;95 Suppl 1:S161–92.
48. Rustin GJ, Nelstrop AE, Tuxen MK, Lambert HE. Defining progression of ovarian carcinoma during follow-up according to CA 125: a North Thames ovary group study. Ann Oncol. 1996;7:361–4.
49. Health Council of the Netherlands. Follow-up in oncology. Identify objectives, substantiate actions. The Hague: Health Council of the Netherlands; 2007.

4 Cancer Survivorship: Monitoring the Long-Term and Late Effects of Treatment

Craig C. Earle and Jennifer Deevy

Keywords
Surveillance protocols • Therapies • Late-term effects • Survivorship • Care plan

The majority of this text is focused on protocols for surveillance of cancer recurrence and new primary cancers. Optimal care of the cancer survivor involves dealing with many other issues, however. In its 2005 report *From cancer patient to cancer survivor: Lost in transition* [1], the Institute of Medicine (IOM) noted in its first recommendation that survivorship should be considered a distinct entity with cross-cutting issues. Indeed, while the details of surveillance might be specific to the site and stage of cancer a patient had, all survivors are concerned about the possibility of recurrence. Moreover, the effects of a history of cancer on insurance, employment, and relationships are remarkably similar almost regardless of the specific cancer diagnosis. This chapter outlines the general approach we took to survivorship care at the Lance Armstrong Foundation Adult Survivorship Clinic at Dana-Farber Cancer Institute in Boston, MA.

The IOM's second recommendation was that, at the conclusion of any primary, potentially curative treatment for cancer patients should be provided with a summary of the care they received and a plan for how their care should be managed going forward. Table 4.1 summarizes the recommended content of the treatment summary and care plan. Table 4.6 is an example of a generic template for such a plan, created by the American Society of Clinical Oncology (ASCO). In particular, a comprehensive care plan prompts recognition of elements of care that go beyond the medical monitoring of cancer. Examples include routine age-related screening for cancers other than the index cancer (e.g., cervical, breast, and colorectal cancer screening), screening for diabetes, hypertension, and dyslipidemia, and attention to routine health maintenance such as smoking cessation, weight management, exercise, and immunizations. It also prompts consideration of referral for genetic testing in patients who are unusually young or have a strong family history of cancer. Moreover, there may be issues surrounding changes in body image, roles, relationships, lifestyle, occupation, stigma, and discrimination, as well as the common fears around recurrence and death for which counseling may help.

Long-Term and Late Effects

The focus of this chapter is recommendations for surveillance for long-term and late effects of cancer treatment. Treatment of these effects is usually the same as when they are due to noncancer-related causes. Detailed discussion of management of these effects is beyond the chapter's scope. Long-term effects are those that first occur during cancer treatment and persist after completion of primary therapy, like functional disability from surgery. Late effects, on the other hand, are those that were not apparent during primary treatment but become apparent at some later time, such as sacral fracture following pelvic radiation [2]. Unfortunately, evidence on which to base firm surveillance guidelines is generally lacking beyond a few notable exceptions, and there are not even comprehensive consensus guidelines for monitoring or managing long-term and late effects of cancer therapy for survivors of adult cancer. The Children's Oncology Group has developed consensus guidelines for the surveillance and management of survivors of childhood cancer, however, which can be found at www.survivorshipguidelines.org and

C.C. Earle, M.D., M.Sc., FRCP(C) (✉) • J. Deevy
Institute for Clinical Evaluative Sciences, Sunnybrook Health Sciences Centre, 2075 Bayview Avenue, G Wing 106, Toronto, ON M4N 3M5, Canada
e-mail: craig.earle@ices.on.ca

F.E. Johnson et al. (eds.), *Patient Surveillance After Cancer Treatment*, Current Clinical Oncology,
DOI 10.1007/978-1-60327-969-7_4,

Table 4.1 The Institute of Medicine Treatment Summary and Survivorship Care Plan

Upon discharge from cancer treatment, including treatment of recurrences, every patient should be given a record of all care received and important disease characteristics. This should include, at a minimum
Diagnostic tests performed and results Tumor characteristics (e.g., site(s), stage and grade, hormone receptor status, marker information) Dates of treatment initiation and completion Surgery, chemotherapy, radiotherapy, transplant, hormonal therapy, or gene or other therapies provided, including agents used, treatment regimen, total dosage, identifying number and title of clinical trials (if any), indicators of treatment response, and toxicities experienced during treatment Psychosocial, nutritional, and other supportive services provided Full contact information on treating institutions and key individual providers Identification of a key point of contact and coordinator of continuing care
Upon discharge from cancer treatment, every patient and his/her primary health care provider should receive a written follow-up care plan incorporating available evidence-based standards of care. This should include, at a minimum
The likely course of recovery from acute treatment toxicities, as well as the need for ongoing health maintenance or adjuvant therapy A description of recommended cancer screening and other periodic testing and examinations, and the schedule on which they should be performed (and who should provide them) Information on possible late and long-term effects of treatment and symptoms of such effects Information on possible signs of recurrence and second tumors Information on the possible effects of cancer on marital/partner relationship, sexual functioning, work, and parenting, and the potential future need for psychosocial support Information on the potential insurance, employment, and financial consequences of cancer and, as necessary, referral to counseling, legal aid, and financial assistance Specific recommendations for healthy behaviors (e.g., diet, exercise, healthy weight, sunscreen use, immunizations, smoking cessation, osteoporosis prevention). When appropriate, recommendations that first-degree relatives be informed about their increased risk and the need for cancer screening (e.g., breast cancer, colorectal cancer, prostate cancer) As appropriate, information on genetic counseling and testing to identify high-risk individuals who could benefit from more comprehensive cancer surveillance, chemoprevention, or risk-reducing surgery As appropriate, information on known effective chemoprevention and behavioral strategies for secondary prevention (e.g., tamoxifen in women at high risk for breast cancer; smoking cessation after lung cancer) and monitoring of adherence to these recommendations Referrals to specific follow-up care providers (e.g., rehabilitation, fertility, psychology), support groups, and/or the patient's primary care provider A listing of cancer-related resources and information (e.g., Internet-based sources and telephone listings for major cancer support organizations)

Source: Adapted from the IOM Report: From Cancer patient to Cancer Survivor: Lost in Transition, Box 3-16, pp. 152-3, which was adapted from the President's Cancer Panel (2004)

from which an approach to the major issues can be extrapolated. In most cases, at this point in time, surveillance for long-term and late effects consists only of awareness on the part of cancer survivors and physicians of potential risks based on exposure and the elicitation of targeted symptoms and signs during the clinical encounter to guide further investigation. For example, while it would be nice to have a cardiac screening protocol to apply to patients 20 years out from mantle radiation for Hodgkin's disease, there is not an evidence based on which to make such a recommendation [3]. Instead, awareness of the risk leads to recommendations for an otherwise heart-healthy lifestyle (diet, exercise, control of comorbid conditions like hypertension and diabetes) and an appropriately high index of suspicion to investigate chest pain in such a patient who might otherwise not appear to be at high risk.

Surgical long-term effects (Table 4.2) generally stem from direct damage to local tissues sustained in the course of surgery.

Table 4.2 Common long-term and late effects of cancer surgery

Surgery
• Cosmetic effects
• Functional disability from removal of a limb or organ
• Damage to an organ (bowel, bladder, sexual organs)
• Pain
• Scarring/adhesions
• Incisional hernia
• Lymphedema
Systemic effects (e.g., removal of endocrine organs, infection risk postsplenectomy)

Systemic effects are also possible, however, through mechanisms like the removal of endocrine glands or the spleen. Similarly, radiation late effects (Table 4.3) are usually local and due to fibrosis, lymphedema, and ongoing radiation-induced inflammation. The risk of these effects depends on a

Table 4.3 Common long-term and late effects of radiation

General (any site)
• Second malignancies
Bone radiation
• Marrow insufficiency
• Bone fractures
Skin radiation
• Hair loss (which may be permanent), pigmentation, thickening, or scarring in the radiation field
Delayed wound healing
• Skin cancer
• Lymphedema
Cranial radiation
• Neurocognitive deficits
• Cataracts
• Xerophalmia, rarely painful
• Rare gradual visual loss
• Rare pituitary abnormalities
Head and neck radiation
Xerostomia, dental caries, periodontal disease
• Hypothyroidism
• Inflammation and swelling of neck muscles
• Voice alterations
• Changes in taste, smell, or hearing
• Increased stroke risk (carotid stenosis)
Chest radiation
• Pneumonitis, pulmonary fibrosis
• Accelerated coronary artery disease, valvular damage, conduction abnormalities, cardiomyopathy, and pericardial inflammation and scarring.
• Esophageal stricture
• L'Hermitte's syndrome, rare damage to spinal cord and nerves
• Breast cancer
• Lung cancer
Abdominal radiation
• Bowel stricture, fistula
• Gastric ulceration
• Hyposplenism
• Renal insufficiency
• Radiation hepatitis
• Biliary stricture
Pelvic radiation
• Infertility, premature menopause
• Radiation proctitis
• Bladder inflammation or scarring
• Erectile dysfunction
• Decreased vaginal secretions and vaginal scarring
• Gonadal failure/osteopenia, osteoporosis
• Hip or sacral fractures in radiation field
Limb radiation
• Scarring of muscle limiting function

host of factors such as the radiation dose and the presence of any preexisting organ or tissue damage. Radiation-induced cancer can occur in any radiated tissue, especially at the edge of a radiation field, and typically around 7 years post-exposure. Lymphedema most commonly follows limb, head and neck, or pelvic radiation. There are also less well-understood systemic complaints, however, such as persistent fatigue and depression, which may be due to circulating chronic inflammatory mediators.

Systemic therapy can have an array of long-term and late effects, some localized to particular organs, and some more constitutional. Table 4.4 lists some of the common toxicities associated with certain drug exposures. Several long-term and late effects are cross-cutting. For example, almost any chemotherapy drug can be associated with gonadal failure, although the alkylating agents are most strongly associated. Fatigue is another common but generally nonspecific complaint. Anemia, hypothyroidism, and depression must be ruled out as causes. "Chemobrain" is a term that has come to mean a variety of neurocognitive symptoms that can occur following chemotherapy, such as impaired concentration, word-finding problems, and forgetfulness. While any chemotherapy exposure can be associated with this, it is most commonly associated with breast cancer and intrathecal chemotherapies.

Graft versus host disease following allogeneic bone marrow transplant for hematological malignancies bears special mention as it comes about as a result of treatment other than chemotherapy or radiation but rather is an immune reaction related to the graft. It can affect many parts of the body, including the skin, mucosa, lungs, liver, connective tissues, and exocrine glands. Importantly, immune function may be compromised, making immunization and prompt treatment of infections crucial.

Lastly, Table 4.5 gives some examples of surveillance interventions beyond targeted history and physical examination that may be required for certain long-term and late effects, regardless of which treatment modality is responsible. From this rather short list it is clear that a research priority in the field of survivorship is to identify and test surveillance strategies that have the potential to decrease the burden of late toxicity through early detection and intervention. Until then the state of the science dictates a parsimonious approach grounded in awareness of these effects and routine but targeted clinical evaluation.

Other Survivorship Resources

Books

- Cured II—LENT cancer survivorship research and education: late effects on normal tissues. Editors P. Rubin, L.S. Constine, L.B. Marks, and P. Okunieff, Springer 2008.
- Cancer survivors: today and tomorrow. Editor P. Ganz, Springer 2007.

Table 4.4 Common long-term or late effects of systemic therapy

Drug	Cardiac muscle damage	Pulmonary fibrosis	Peripheral neuropathy	Hearing loss	Renal damage	Hepatic toxicity	Ocular toxicity	MDS/ Leukemia	Infertility	Other
Adriamycin	X									
Bleomycin		X								Raynaud's syndrome
Bortezomib			X							
Busulfan		X	X				Cataracts	X	X	
Carboplatin			X	X						
Carmustine (BCNU)		X			X	X	Retinal damage	X	X	
Chlorambucil								X	X	
Cisplatin			X	X	X				X	Dyslipidemia
Cyclophosphamide	X								X	
Daunorubicin	X									
Denileukin							X			
Docetaxel			X							
Doxorubicin	X									
Epirubicin	X							X		
Etoposide								X		
Ifosfamide					X				X	Bladder toxicity
Lapatinib	X	X								
Lomustine (CCNU)		X			X		Optic atrophy	X	X	
Mechlorethamine (Nitrogen Mustard)					X			X	X	
Melphalan								X	X	
Methotrexate		X			X	X				
Mitomycin		X			X		X			
Mitoxantrone	X									
Oxaliplatin			X							
Paclitaxel			X							
Procarbazine			X					X	X	
Rituxumab							X			
Sorafenib	X									
Steroids							X			Osteopenia
Tamoxifen										Osteopenia, Uterine cancer
Thalidomide			X							
Toremifine							X			
Traztuzumab	X									
Vincristine			X							Constipation
Vinblastine			X						X	
Vinorelbine			X							

MDS Myelodysplastic syndrome

Table 4.5 Surveillance for late effects, beyond targeted history and physical examination

Risk	Surveillance
Skin cancer	Periodic skin examination in radiation field
	Screening for sun exposure practices
Neurocognitive deficits	Consider neuropsychiatric testing and depression screening if symptomatic
Xerostomia, dental disease	Regular dental evaluation, cleaning, fluoride
	Screen for oral hygiene practices, tobacco use
Hypothyroidism	Annual TSH monitoring
Increased cardiovascular risk	Screen for other modifiable risk factors: tobacco use, obesity, inactivity, poor diet
	Annual blood pressure, serum glucose, and lipid monitoring
	Annual influenza vaccination status
	If the heart was directly radiated, for example, in mantle radiation, consider baseline stress test and echocardiogram 10 years post-radiotherapy, then as indicated[a]
Breast cancer	Annual mammography or breast MRI in women who had chest irradiation between ages 10 and 30 starting 8–10 years post-RT or at age 40, whichever comes first[a]
Lung cancer	Controversial: Annual chest imaging[a]
Pulmonary toxicity	Annual influenza vaccination
Renal insufficiency	Monitor blood pressure
Hyposplenism	Screen for pneumococcal vaccination and re-vaccination every 5–7 years, as well as meningococcal and *H. influenzae* vaccinations
Uterine cancer	Annual gynecologic exam
Osteopenia/osteoporosis	Screen for other modifiable risk factors: tobacco use, inactivity, poor calcium intake
	Periodic bone densitometry (e.g., every 1–2 years while on hormone therapy)

[a]Based on consensus guidelines from the National Comprehensive Cancer Network, available at www.nccn.org

- Handbook of cancer survivorship. Editor M. Feuerstein, Springer 2007.
- From cancer patient to cancer survivor: Lost in transition. Editors M. Hewitt, S. Greenfield, and E. Stovall, National Academies Press 2005.

Journals

- Journal of Cancer Survivorship www.springer.com/public+health/journal/11764

Websites

- National Coalition for Cancer Survivorship www.canceradvocacy.org.
- Lance Armstrong Foundation www.laf.org.
- American Cancer Society Cancer Survivors' Network www.csn.cancer.org.
- Children's Oncology Group www.survivorshipguidelines.org.

Table 4.6 The American Society of Clinical Oncology template for a treatment summary and survivorship care plan

[Insert Practice Name/Info Here]

The Treatment Plan and Summary is a brief record of major aspects of cancer treatment. This is not a complete patient history or comprehensive record of intended therapies.

Patient name:	**Patient ID:**
Medical oncology provider name:	**PCP:**
Patient DOB: (__/__/__) **Age:**	**Patient phone**:
Support contact name:	
Support contact relationship:	**Support contact phone**:

BACKGROUND INFORMATION

Symptoms/signs:

Family history/predisposing conditions:

Major co-morbid conditions:

Tobacco use: □ No □ Yes, past □ Yes, current **(If current, cessation counseling provided?**: □ Yes □ No**)**

Cancer type/location: **Diagnosis date:** (__/__/____)

Is this a new cancer diagnosis or recurrence?: □ New □ Recurrence (date: __/__/____)

Surgery: □ None □ Diagnosis only □ Palliative resection □ Curative resection

Surgical procedure/location/findings:

Tumor type/histology/grade:

STAGING

Study	Date	Findings

T stage : □ T1 □ T2 □ T3 □ T4 □ Not applicable	**N stage:** □ N0 □ N1 □ N2 □N3 □ Not applicable
M stage: □ M0 □ M1 □ Not applicable	**Tumor markers:**
Stage: □ I__ □ II__ □ III__ □ IV__ □ Recurrence	Alternative staging system: ________________

Location(s) of metastasis or recurrence (if applicable):

TREATMENT PLAN	**TREATMENT SUMMARY**
White sections to be completed prior to chemotherapy administration, shaded sections following chemotherapy	
Height: in/cm **Pre-treatment weight:** lb/kg	**Post-treatment weight:** lb/kg
Pre-treatment BSA: **Treatment on clinical trial:** □ Yes □ No	
Name of chemotherapy regimen:	
Chemotherapy start date: (__/__/____)	**Chemotherapy end date:** (__/__/____)
Chemotherapy intent: □ Curative, adjuvant or neoadjuvant □ Disease or symptom control	
ECOG performance status at start of treatment: □ 0 □ 1 □ 2 □ 3 □ 4	**ECOG performance status at end of treatment:** □ 0 □ 1 □ 2 □ 3 □ 4

Chemotherapy Drug Name	Route	Dose mg/m^2	Schedule	Dose reduction	# cycles administered
				□ Yes _____% □ No	
				□ Yes _____% □ No	
				□ Yes _____% □ No	
				□ Yes _____% □ No	
				□ Yes _____% □ No	
				□ Yes _____% □ No	

Major side effects of this regimen: □ Hair loss □ Nausea/Vomiting □ Neuropathy □ Low blood count □ Fatigue □ Menopause symptoms □ Cardiac □ Other ____________________

Available at www.ASCO.org

Important caution: this is a *summary* document whose purpose is to review the *highlights* of the cancer treatment for this patient. This does not replace information available in the medical record, a complete medical history provided by the patient, examination and diagnostic information, or educational materials that describe strategies for coping with cancer and cancer therapies in detail. Both medical science and an individual's health care needs change, and therefore this document is current only as of the date of preparation. This summary document does not prescribe or recommend any particular medical treatment or care for cancer or any other disease and does not substitute for the independent medical judgment of the treating professional

References

1. Institute of Medicine. From cancer patient to cancer survivor: lost in transition. Washington: National Academies Press; 2005.
2. Baxter NN, Habermann EB, Tepper JE, Durham SB, Virnig BA. Risk of pelvic fractures in older women following pelvic irradiation. JAMA. 2005;294:2587–93.
3. Carver JR, Shapiro CL, Ng A, Jacobs L, Schwartz C, Virgo KS, et al. American Society of Clinical Oncology clinical evidence review on the ongoing care of adult cancer survivors: cardiac and pulmonary late effects. J Clin Oncol. 2007;25:3991–4008.

Upper Aerodigestive Tract Carcinoma

5

David Y. Johnson, Shilpi Wadhwa, and Frank E. Johnson

Keywords
Aerodigestive tract • Guidelines • Surveillance • Cancer • Cancer incidence

The International Agency for Research on Cancer (IARC), a component of the World Health Organization (WHO), estimated that there were 484,628 new cases of upper aerodigestive tract carcinoma worldwide in 2002 [1]. The IARC also estimated that there were 261,784 deaths due to this cause in 2002 [1].

The American Cancer Society estimated that there were 36,700 new cases and 7,700 deaths due to this cause in the USA in 2007 [2]. The estimated five-year survival rate (all races) in the USA in 2007 was 65 % for larynx cancer and 60 % for oral cavity cancer [2]. Survival rates were adjusted for normal life expectancies and were based on cases diagnosed from 1996 to 2002 and followed through 2003.

The dominant known etiologic factors for carcinoma of most upper aerodigestive tract sites are tobacco use and alcohol use [3]. Viral infections are important causative agents, particularly for carcinoma of the nasopharynx. Certain occupations are hazardous and genetic predisposition factors, such as Li-Fraumeni syndrome, are known [4].

Geographic Variation Worldwide

There is considerable geographic variation in the incidence of head and neck cancer. In western countries such as the USA and the United Kingdom, oral cancer accounts for 2–5 % of all cancers. The incidence is much higher in Sri Lanka and India [5]. The Indian subcontinent accounts for one-third of the world burden. The incidence and mortality from oral cancer is rising in several regions of Europe, Japan, and Australia [6]. Nasopharyngeal cancer is very common in Southeast Asia, with incidence rates many times higher than in other areas. Geographic variation in the USA is also pronounced [7].

Surveillance Strategies Proposed by Professional Organizations or National Government Agencies and Available on the Internet

National Comprehensive Cancer Network (NCCN, http://www.nccn.org)

NCCN guidelines were accessed on 1/28/12 (Table 5.1). There were minor qualitative changes compared to the guidelines accessed on 4/10/07.

American Society of Clinical Oncology (ASCO, http://www.asco.org)

ASCO guidelines were accessed on 1/28/12. No quantitative guidelines exist for upper aerodigestive tract cancer surveillance, including when first accessed on 10/31/07.

The Society of Surgical Oncology (SSO, http://www.surgonc.org)

SSO guidelines were accessed on 1/28/12. No quantitative guidelines exist for upper aerodigestive tract cancer surveillance, including when first accessed on 10/31/07.

European Society for Medical Oncology (ESMO, http://www.esmo.org)

ESMO guidelines were accessed on 1/28/12 (Table 5.2 and 5.3). There are new quantitative guidelines compared to the qualitative guidelines accessed on 10/31/07.

D.Y. Johnson • S. Wadhwa
Department of Internal Medicine, Saint Louis University Medical Center, Saint Louis, MO, USA

F.E. Johnson, M.D., FACS (✉)
Saint Louis University Medical Center and Saint Louis Veterans Affairs Medical Center, Saint Louis, MO, USA
e-mail: frank.johnson1@va.gov

F.E. Johnson et al. (eds.), *Patient Surveillance After Cancer Treatment*, Current Clinical Oncology,
DOI 10.1007/978-1-60327-969-7_5, © Springer Science+Business Media New York 2013

Table 5.1 Obtained from NCCN (http://www.nccn.org) on 1-28-12 Head and Neck Cancers

	Years posttreatment[a]					
	1	2	3	4	5	>5
Office visit[b]	4–12	3–6	2–3	2–3	2–3	1–2
Serum TSH level[c]	1–2	1–2	1–2	1–2	1–2	1–2

- Posttreatment baseline imaging of primary (and neck if treated) recommended within 6 months of treatment.[d, e]
- Chest imaging as clinically indicated.
- Speech/hearing and swallowing evaluation and rehabilitation as clinically indicated.
- Smoking cessation and alcohol counseling as clinically indicated.
- Dental evaluation.[f]
- Consider Epstein-Barr virus (EBV) monitoring for nasopharynx.

[a]The numbers in the table indicate the number of times the modality is recommended during the indicated year posttreatment.
[b]For mucosal melanoma, physical examination should include endoscopic inspection for paranasal sinus disease.
[c]If neck has been irradiated.
[d]For cancer of the oropharynx, hypopharynx, glottic larynx, supraglottic larynx, and nasopharynx: imaging recommended for T3-4 or N2-3 disease only.
[e]Further reimaging as indicated based on signs/symptoms; not routinely recommended for asymptomatic patients.
[f]Recommended for oral cavity cancer. As indicated for oropharynx, hypopharynx, and nasopharynx cancer. As indicated for other sites, if significant intraoral radiation.
NCCN guidelines were accessed on 1/28/12. There were minor qualitative changes compared to the guidelines accessed on 4/10/07.

Table 5.2 Obtained from ESMO (http://www.esmo.org) on 1-28-12 Squamous Cell Carcinoma of the Head and Neck

	Years posttreatment[a]					
	1	2	3	4	5	>5
Office visit[b]	1	1	1	1	1	1
Chest X-ray	1	1	1	1	1	1
Serum TSH level	1	1	0	0	1	0

- CT scan or MRI of head and neck may be indicated depending on initial procedure.
- FDG-PET (or PET-CT) may be used to evaluate the response to radiotherapy or concomitant chemoradiotherapy at the neck level to decide usefulness of neck node dissection.

[a]The numbers in the table indicate the number of times the modality is recommended during the indicated year posttreatment.
[b]Chest X-ray and TSH level were the only quantitative recommendations given. We inferred that office visit would be recommended as frequently as these.
ESMO guidelines were accessed on 1/28/12. These are new quantitative guidelines compared to the qualitative guidelines accessed on 10/31/07.

European Society of Surgical Oncology (ESSO, http://www.esso-surgeonline.org)

ESSO guidelines were accessed on 1/28/12. No quantitative guidelines exist for upper aerodigestive tract cancer surveillance, including when first accessed on 10/31/07.

Cancer Care Ontario (CCO, http://www.cancercare.on.ca)

CCO guidelines were accessed on 1/28/12 (Table 5.4). There are new quantitative guidelines compared to no guidelines found on 10/31/07.

National Institute for Health and Clinical Excellence (NICE, http://www.nice.org.uk)

NICE guidelines were accessed on 1/28/12. No quantitative guidelines exist for upper aerodigestive tract cancer surveillance, including when first accessed on 10/31/07.

The Cochrane Collaboration (CC, http://www.cochrane.org)

CC guidelines were accessed on 1/28/12. No quantitative guidelines exist for upper aerodigestive tract cancer surveillance, including when first accessed on 10/31/07.

American Head and Neck Society (AHNS, http://www.headandneckcancer.org)

AHNS guidelines were accessed on 1/28/12. No quantitative guidelines exist for upper aerodigestive tract cancer surveillance, including when first accessed on 10/31/07.

The M.D. Anderson Surgical Oncology Handbook also has surveillance guidelines, proposed by authors from a single National Cancer Institute-designated Comprehensive Cancer Center, for many types of cancer [8]. Some are detailed and quantitative, others qualitative.

Table 5.3 Obtained from ESMO (http://www.esmo.org) on 1-28-12Nasopharyngeal Cancer

	Years posttreatment[a]					
	1	2	3	4	5	>5
Office visit[b]	1–2	1–2	1–2	0	1	0
MRI[c]	1–2	1–2	1–2	0	0	0
Serum TSH level	1	1	0	0	1	0

- Surveillance includes periodic examination of nasopharynx and neck, cranial nerve function, and evaluation of systemic complaints to identify distant metastasis.
- MRI to evaluate response to radiotherapy or chemoradiotherapy.

[a]The numbers in the table indicate the number of times the modality is recommended during the indicated year posttreatment.
[b]MRI and TSH level were the only quantitative recommendations given. We inferred that office visit would be recommended as frequently as these.
[c]ESMO recommends that, for T3 and T4 tumors, MRI might be used on a 6- to 12-month basis to evaluate the nasopharynx and base of the skull at least for the first few years after treatment. We inferred that this would apply to the first 3 years.
ESMO guidelines were accessed on 1/28/12. These are new quantitative guidelines compared to the qualitative guidelines accessed on 10/31/07.

Table 5.4 Obtained from CCO (http://www.cancercare.on.ca) on 1-28-12. Head and Neck Cancer

	Years posttreatment[a]					
	1	2	3	4	5	>5
Office visit	4	3	2	0	0	0

- Assessment of the late complications of treatment is an important component of the surveillance of patients treated for head and neck cancer.
- Surveillance imaging should be symptom directed and not part of routine screening.
- Psychosocial support.[b]
- Patients receiving oral surgery or radiotherapy to the mouth (with or without adjuvant chemotherapy) should have posttreatment dental rehabilitation.
- Lifelong dental follow-up and dental rehabilitation.
- Dental extractions in irradiated jaws should be carried out in hospital by a dental oncologist or oral surgeon.
- Hyperbaric oxygen facilities should be available for selected patients.

[a]The numbers in the table indicate the number of times the modality is recommended during the indicated year posttreatment.
[b]Assessment of distress, anxiety, and coping should be included in routine assessments.
CCO guidelines were accessed on 1/28/12. These are new quantitative guidelines compared to no guidelines found on 10/31/07.

Summary

This is a common cancer with significant variability in incidence worldwide. We found consensus-based guidelines but none based on high-quality evidence.

References

1. Parkin DM, Whelan SL, Ferlay J, Teppo L, Thomas DB. Cancer incidence in five continents. Vol. VIII. International Agency for Research on Cancer, 2002. (IARC Scientific Publication 155). Lyon, France: IARC Press
2. Jemal A, Seigel R, Ward E, Murray T, Xu J, Thun MJ. Cancer Statistics, 2007. CA Cancer J Clin. 2007;57:43–66.
3. Schottenfeld D, Fraumeni JG. Cancer epidemiology and prevention. 3rd ed. New York, NY: Oxford University Press; 2006.
4. DeVita VT, Hellman S, Rosenberg SA. Cancer. 7th ed. Philadelphia, PA: Lippincott Williams & Wilkins; 2005.
5. CDC: National Center for Chronic Disease Prevention and Health Promotion Oral Health Resources. Resource library fact sheet. Oral cancer: deadly to ignore. February 2002. Available at http://www.cdc.gov/OralHealth/factsheets/oc-facts.htm. Accessed May 2012
6. International Agency for Research on Cancer IARC Screening Group. Lancet 2005: 365:1927–33. Available online at http://www.screening.iarc.fr/oralindex.php Accessed May 2012
7. Devesa SS, Grauman DJ, Blot WJ, Pennello GA, Hoover RN, Fraumeni JF Jr. Atlas of cancer mortality in the United States. National institutes of health, national cancer institute. NIH Publication No. 99–4564; September 1999.
8. Feig BW, Berger DH, Fuhrman GM. The M.D. Anderson Surgical Oncology Handbook. 4th ed. Philadelphia, PA: Lippincott Williams & Wilkins; 2006 (paperback).

6 Upper Aerodigestive Tract Carcinoma Surveillance Counterpoint: Europe

Béatrix Barry and Dominique De Raucourt

Keywords
Laryngeal cancer • Surveillance strategies • Survival • Head and neck carcinoma • Spread

Head and neck cancer is frequent in Europe, especially in Southern and Western Europe. Squamous cell carcinoma is the most frequent histological type. It is mainly a disease of men and is associated with alcohol and tobacco abuse. The estimated incidence of oral cavity and pharyngeal cancer in Europe in 2008 was 92,000 [1]. Western and Southern Europe are areas with a high incidence of oral cavity cancers (10 per 100,000) [2]. Laryngeal cancer is common also, particularly in Southern Europe (France, Spain, and Italy) and Eastern Europe (Russia, Ukraine).

Recently human papilloma virus (HPV) has been shown to be a cause of upper aerodigestive tract cancer. This could explain the increasing incidence of carcinoma of the tonsil and base of tongue in nontobacco and nonalcohol exposed populations [3]. The prevalence of HPV infection is very high in Western Europe (over 50 %).

The major sites of head and neck cancer are larynx, oral cavity, hypopharynx, and oropharynx. The presence of lymph nodes metastases (especially with extranodal spread) is an important poor prognostic factor [4].

Treatment is based on surgery, irradiation, or both. Exclusive single-modality therapy can be used in small cancers, but both modalities are used in T3 or T4 lesions. Recently the notion of laryngeal preservation has been introduced and induction chemotherapy is often used to avoid total laryngectomy. In the last 10 years the use of adjuvant chemotherapy has proven to significantly improve local control and survival. It is now used as single-modality primary therapy or as postoperative adjuvant therapy. Of particular interest in squamous cell carcinoma of the head and neck is the frequency of second primary tumors in the head and neck, esophagus, and lung with an annual frequency of 3–7 % [5]. The follow-up of patients with head and neck carcinomas is highly variable and depends on the doctor's habits. It has many goals and detection of local relapse is only one of them. Another main goal is rehabilitation, which is usually necessary for patients who have undergone extensive surgery and/or chemoradiation. The detection of new tumors has unfortunately had limited success as further curative local therapy is restricted.

The "Société Française d'oto-rhino-laryngologie" proposed clinical recommendations for surveillance based on relevant literature [6]. However, most recommendations were based on professional consensus because of the lack of evidence derived from controlled clinical trials of alternative surveillance strategies. Most recurrences occur in the 3 years after the initial treatment. This justifies regular clinical examinations. Patients who might benefit from curative treatment of recurrence should have extensive surveillance. This should be done by an ENT specialist. Office visit should consist of a weight check and questioning the patient about recent changes in swallowing, voice or pain. It should also include a clinical examination of the mucosa using a flexible nasopharyngoscope and neck palpation. The use of panendoscopy and radiologic procedures such as tomodensitometry or MRI is not indicated unless the patient examination is very difficult or if there is a clinical suspicion of recurrence. A baseline radiological exam (CT or MRI) is useful, especially in case of nonsurgical initial treatment. The optimal

B. Barry (✉)
Chef de Service Otorhinolaryngologie et Chirurgie Cervico-faciale, Hôpital Bichat-Claude Bernard, 46 rue Henri Huchard, 75877 Cedex 18 Paris, France
e-mail: beatrix.barrry@bch.aphp.fr

D. De Raucourt
Chef de Département, Service Chirurgie Tête et Cou, Centre François Baclesse, 3 avenue Général Harris, BP 5026 14076 cedex 05 Caen, France
e-mail: d.de.raucourt@baclesse.fr

F.E. Johnson et al. (eds.), *Patient Surveillance After Cancer Treatment*, Current Clinical Oncology,
DOI 10.1007/978-1-60327-969-7_6, © Springer Science+Business Media New York 2013

Table 6.1 Surveillance after curative-intent initial therapy for patients with upper aerodigestive tract squamous cell carcinoma by otolaryngologists at Hôpital Bichat-Claude Bernard and Centre François Baclesse

	Posttreatment year					
Modality	1	2	3	4	5	>5
Office visit[a]	6	4	3	2	2	2
Chest X-ray	1	1	1	1	1	1
Serum thyroid stimulating hormone level	2	2	1	1	1	1

Smoking-cessation and alcohol-cessation programs are offered at each office visit
Treatment-related effects are evaluated at each office visit and managed as clinically indicated
[a]Endoscopy, if indicated clinically
Dental care is recommended two times each year in patients who received radiation therapy
The numbers in each cell indicate the number of times a particular modality is recommended in a particular posttreatment year

time for this is around the fourth month after the end of the treatment. Blood tests are not necessary in the absence of validated serological markers for recurrence.

The office visits should be done every 2 months in the first year, every 3 months in the second year and every 4 months in the third year. After the third year, a visit every sixth month is useful for patients whose index cancer is related to tobacco and alcohol consumption. For those patients the risk of a second cancer remains high for the remainder of life (Table 6.1). It is important to inform the patients of symptoms and signs that could indicate tumor recurrence or new primary cancer so that an early medical examination can be done. The patient's general practitioner must be clearly informed about those suspected symptoms and signs.

Distant metastases occur in about 20 % of patients after curative-intent primary treatment. This risk is particularly high in the first 2 years following the treatment. The risk of second primary upper aerodigestive tract cancers remains rather high for patients with tobacco or alcohol consumption. Patients should be informed and educated about lung and esophageal cancer symptoms also.

Blood tests are not necessary. An X-ray of the chest is recommended every year and a tomodensitometry is indicated when there is an abnormality. Bone and liver metastases usually present with clinical symptoms or signs. The detection of esophageal and pulmonary tumors is of little benefit with only 2–3 % survival [7, 8]. Surveillance tomodensitometry has not been shown to increase survival rate [9–11].

Head and neck cancer patients who later develop esophageal cancer have a poor survival rate. Esophageal cancer can be detected at an early stage by endoscopy with color enhancement, but a significant survival benefit has not been proven. It should therefore not be a standard procedure but can be proposed every 2 years, especially in patients with hypopharyngeal cancer who are at high risk of developing a second primary cancer of the eosophagus.

An important goal of surveillance is to detect functional disabilities due to the primary treatment. This includes problems with pain, shoulder function, speech, and swallowing. Collaboration with dieticians, speech therapists, and physiotherapists is usually required. A weight check at each office visit is standard.

The patient should be offered help with smoking and alcohol cessation. The psychological consequences of treatment must be taken into account and counseling may be useful. Hypothyroidism is a frequent complication after neck radiotherapy (15–20 % with radiotherapy alone and 40–60 % after combined surgery and radiotherapy). It can appear many years after treatment. It is best detected by a yearly serum thyroid stimulating hormone level. Dental problems occur often after radiotherapy. Dental examinations are recommended every 6 months for the duration of life. Fluoride should be offered at each consultation.

Patients with head and neck cancer, especially those who have a tobacco and alcohol abuse history, often have other related illnesses that should be managed by their primary care practitioner or specialist(s).

Few professional organizations and government agencies have been able to propose surveillance strategies for head and neck cancer. Practice care guidelines of the British Association of Head and Neck Oncologists [12] advise a 4–6-week follow-up schedule in the first 2 years, 3-monthly follow-up in year 3, and 6-monthly for years 4 and 5. These and our recommendations are similar to the National Comprehensive Cancer Network (NCCN) guidelines [13, 14]. There are no randomized clinical trials comparing a high-intensity strategy with a low-intensity strategy.

Many factors influence surveillance, which explains why guidelines vary. In France, and probably in most other countries, most radiation oncologists follow their patients only once a year and most of the burden of surveillance is assumed by the head and neck specialists. The ENT specialist is usually the doctor who detected the tumor and announced the disease. Most patients consider the ENT surgeon as their doctor and return to him or her after their treatment for care.

Most guidelines propose a simple clinical examination and regular endoscopic and regular endoscopic and radiological investigations. The results of studies about the results are contradictory. DeVisscher et al. (1994) [15] in a prospective survey of 428 patients showed that routine follow up provides significantly better survival than self-referral. This result was not observed in a similar prospective study conducted with more than 600 patients by Boysen et al. [16]. The importance of surveillance is certainly greater for patients for whom a salvage treatment option exists. The stage of the tumor and the modality of treatment modify clinical strategy. For example, when the primary tumor was small, without involved lymph nodes, and when a single treatment modality was used, the doctor is often tempted to propose a close follow-up regimen. Conversely, patients who presented with very advanced disease and were treated with combined surgery and radiotherapy usually have a lot of treatment aftereffects and these require frequent recurrent office visits. Their symptoms tend to be frequent and, as the examination is often difficult, the temptation to use radiological investigations is high. These considerations are supported by studies with patients who received combined modality treatment for advanced upper aerodigestive tract carcinoma. Most conclude that surveillance is important for emotional support and evaluation of treatment results as well as improving survival duration [13].

Residual and recurrent head and neck cancer is difficult to detect in a postirradiation neck. Mucosal examination is often difficult in an irradiated larynx or hypopharynx. On CT scan a tumor is often difficult to differentiate from edema. PET/CT is associated with good specificity (85 %) and a 100 % negative predictive value but it is very expensive [17]. Screening for lung cancer is not currently recommended because it has not been shown to increase survival rate. A recent trial NLST (National Lung Screening Trial) showed a 20 % decrease in deaths from lung cancer in a high-risk group of patients undergoing screening with low-dose computed tomography of the chest compared with chest radiography. The high-risk group comprised more than 53,000 asymptomatic patients aged 55–74 years, with smoking history of at least 30 pack-years. Participants received baseline and annual screening for 2 additional years and were followed for a median of 6.5 years [18]. This 20 % decrease is the most dramatic decrease ever reported for deaths from lung cancer and strongly advocates discussing screening in our ENT patients who fit the risk profile.

The authors believe a large well-controlled study of alternative surveillance strategies is clearly indicated in order to rationalize clinical care. Such trials are difficult to carry out and are very expensive but usually result in changes in practice.

References

1. Ferlay J, Parkin DM, Bray F, Steliarova-Foucher E. Estimates of cancer incidence and mortality in 2008. Eur J Cancer. 2010;46:765–81.
2. Parkin DM, Bray F, Ferlay J, Pisani P. Global cancer statistics 2002. CA Cancer J Clin. 2005;55:74–108.
3. D'Souza G, Kreimer AR, Viscidi R, et al. Case-control study of human papillomavirus and oropharyngeal cancer. N Engl J Med. 2007;356:1944–56.
4. Layland MK, Sessions DG, Lenox J. The influence of lymph node metastasis in the treatment of squamous cell carcinoma of the oral cavity, oropharynx, larynx, and hypopharyn: N0 versus N+. Laryngoscope. 2005;115:6329–39.
5. Wynder EL, Munshinski MH, Spivak JC. Tobacco and alcohol consumption in relation to the development of multiple primary cancers. Cancer. 1977;40:1872–8.
6. Barry B, De Raucourt D, Société française d'ORL. Suivi post-thérapeutique des carcinomes épidermoïdes des voies aéro-digestives supérieures de l'adulte. Ann Otolaryngol Chir Cervicofac. 2006;123:240–79.
7. Schwartz LH, Ozsahin M, Zhang GN, et al. Synchronous and metachronous head and neck carcinomas. Cancer. 1994;74: 1933–8.
8. Rennemo E, Zätterström U, Boysen M. Impact of second primary tumors on survival in head and neck cancer: an analysis of 2,063 cases. Laryngoscope. 2008;118:1350–6.
9. Henschke CI, McCauley DI, Yankelevitz DF, et al. Early lung cancer action project: overall design and findings from baseline screening. Lancet. 1999;354:99–105.
10. Henschke CI, Naidich DP, Yankelevitz DF, et al. Early lung cancer action project initial findings on repeat screening. Cancer. 2001;92:153–9.
11. Strauss GM. Measuring effectiveness of lung cancer screening: from consensus to controversy and back. Chest. 1997;112: 216S–28.
12. British Association of Head and Neck Oncologists. Practice care guidance for clinicians participating in the management of head and neck cancer patients in the UK. Drawn up by a consensus group of practicing clinicians. Eur J Surg Oncol. 2001;27(Suppl A):S1–17.
13. Cooney TR, Poulsen MG. Is routine follow-up useful after combined modality therapy for advanced head and neck cancer? Arch Otolaryngol Head Neck Surg. 1999;125:379–82.
14. Manikantan K, Khode S, Dwivedi C, et al. Making sense of post-treatment surveillance in head and neck cancer: when and what of follow up. Cancer Treat Rev. 2009;35:744–53.
15. DeVisscher AV, Manni JJ. Routine long-term follow-up in patients treated with curative intend for squamous cell carcinoma of the larynx pharynx and oral cavity. Arch Otolaryngol Head Neck Surg. 1994;120:934–9.
16. Boysen M, Lovdal O, Tausjo j, Winther F. The value of follow up in patients treated for squamous cell carcinomas of the head and neck. Eur J Cancer. 1992;28:426–30.
17. Abgral R, Querellou S, Potard G, et al. Does 18FDG PET/CT improve the detection of posttreatment recurrence of head and neck squamous cell carcinoma in patients negative for disease on clinical follow-up? J Nucl Med. 2009;50:24–9.
18. Aberle DR, Adams AM, Berg CD, et al. Reduced lung-cancer mortality with low-dose computed tomographic screening. N Engl J Med. 2011;365:395–409.

7 Upper Aerodigestive Tract Carcinoma Surveillance Counterpoint: Japan

Torahiko Nakashima, Ryuji Yasumatsu, and Shizuo Komune

Keywords
Modalities • Cancer • Japan • Cancer rates • Treatment

In Japan, head and neck cancer comprises 5–6 % of all cancer patients. The major sites of head and neck cancer are oral cavity, oropharynx, hypopharynx, and larynx. Squamous cell carcinoma is the most common histological type and the age-standardized incidence rates for tongue, oropharyngeal, hypopharyngeal cancer are now steadily increasing [1]. Age-standardized mortality rates for oral and pharyngeal cancer had been low compared to the US, UK, France, and Italy, but are now both increasing [2]. The age-standardized mortality rate for laryngeal cancer in Japan is also lower than in other countries; it is decreasing, especially in females [3]. The incidence of maxillary sinus cancer had been high compared to the western countries (comprising approximately 7 % of head and neck cancers in Japan). This is related to the high incidence of chronic maxillary sinusitis. However, due to improved nutrition and the decreasing incidence of maxillary sinusitis, the incidence of maxillary sinus cancer is decreasing.

Until recently, surgery and radiotherapy had been the standard treatment modalities. Partial glossectomy or brachytherapy is still often chosen for early tongue cancer. Intraoral laser resection, partial laryngectomy, or radiation therapy is often chosen for early glottic laryngeal cancer. However, since the combination of chemotherapy and radiation (chemoradiation) has been shown in multiple meta-analyses to improve both locoregional control and prognosis of head and neck cancer patients, many hospitals are utilizing chemoradiation as the standard treatment method for both early-stage and advanced-stage head and neck cancer.

New modalities, such as intra-arterial high-dose chemotherapy and stereotactic radiotherapy (e.g., Cyberknife radiotherapy), are also used in many Japanese institutions and proton or carbon-beam radiotherapy is available in selected hospitals.

As recognized worldwide, second primary cancers are also frequently observed in Japanese head and neck cancer patients (Table 7.1). This has slowed the improvement in prognosis. The remaining high frequency of smoking (male: 39.9 %, female: 10 %) is a cause of field cancerization and the increasing rate of second primary cancers.

Surveillance includes not only the early detection of the recurrence of the primary cancer but also the early detection of second primary cancer. For this reason, endoscopic surveillance is routine. Lugol dye staining and narrow band imaging endoscopy is widely applied during esophagoscopy. Positron emission tomography (PET) is also useful for detecting second primary cancers [4]. Patients who continue to smoke and drink make the assessment of recurrence more difficult due to continuous laryngeal/pharyngeal edema. Guiding the patient to moderate alcohol intake and to quit smoking is an important goal of the surveillance program.

The pattern of recurrence of head and neck cancer can be local, within regional neck nodes, or in distant metastatic sites. The risk for locoregional recurrence following definitive treatment of head and neck cancer is high within the first 2 years after the initial therapy so we intensively follow patients within this period. Surveillance should continue for at least 5 years. Routine physical examination by inspection and palpation form the basis of surveillance. Multiple imaging methods [ultrasonography (US), computed tomography (CT), magnetic resonance imaging (MRI)] are also used. F18-fluorodeoxyglucose

T. Nakashima, M.D., Ph.D (✉) • R. Yasumatsu, M.D., Ph.D
• S. Komune, M.D., P.D
Department of Otorhinolaryngology, Graduate School of Medical Sciences, Kyushu University, 3-1-1 Maidashi, Higashi-ku, Fukuoka 812-8582, Japan
e-mail: nakatora@qent.med.kyushu-u.ac.jp; yasuryuj@qent.med.kyushu-u.ac.jp; komu@qent.med.kyushu-u.ac.jp

F.E. Johnson et al. (eds.), *Patient Surveillance After Cancer Treatment*, Current Clinical Oncology,
DOI 10.1007/978-1-60327-969-7_7,

Table 7.1 Surveillance after curative-intent treatment for Upper Aerodigestive Tract at Kyushu University Hospital

	Posttreatment year				
Follow-up modality	1	2	3	4	5
Office visit	12	6	4	3	2
CBC+LFTs+RFTs	12	6	4	3	2
Ultrasonography (neck)	6	6	4	3	2
CT (neck+chest)	2	2	2	1	1
Positron emission tomography	1	1	1	1	1
Thyroid function tests[a]	1	1	1	1	1
Tumor markers[b]	3	3	1	0	0

[a]for patients who have received therapeutic neck irradiation
[b]Serum SCC Antigen and Cyfra 2 levels
CBC=complete blood count, LFTs=liver function tests, RFTs=renal function tests
The number in each cell indicates the number of times a particular modality is recommended in a particular posttreatment year

positron emission tomography (FDG-PET) is widely used and provides early information about recurrent cancer and second primary cancer. In addition, some serological biomarkers, such as the SCC Antigen and Cyfra 21 are reported to be useful for detecting recurrent disease [5, 6] and used during surveillance in many Japanese institutions. In our institution, the patients visit the clinic at least once a month for the first year and at least once every 2 months through the second year. Patients with low risk of recurrence (early-stage glottic laryngeal cancer treated by surgery or radiation) may be followed more infrequently but most patients with advanced disease are followed intensively. A baseline CT scan and FDG-PET scan is performed 4–6 weeks after definitive initial treatment. Local inspection and palpation of the neck is routinely performed in the clinic at every visit and US examination of the neck is performed at least every 2 months during the first 2 years. Thyroid function tests including TSH should be performed every year for all patients who received radiation to the neck. For laryngeal or hypopharyngeal cancer patients, examination using a laryngeal mirror or a flexible laryngeal endoscope is also performed. Stroboscopic assessment is also useful for the early detection of recurrent glottic cancer in patients treated with radiation [7].

Patients who were treated by chemoradiation for cure must be carefully evaluated to be certain that they have achieved a complete response. The methodology for evaluating neck nodes following definitive chemoradiotherapy is being intensively discussed and the necessity of a planned neck dissection is still controversial [8, 9]. We are determining the effect of chemoradiation with the combination of US, CT, MRI, and FDG-PET (usually PET-CT). Laryngeal/pharyngeal and cervical edema following definitive chemoradiotherapy makes it difficult to detect persistent disease. We allow at least 4–6 weeks after definitive chemoradiotherapy before performing CT or PET scan as a follow-up examination. CT scans from above the primary region through the neck to the chest is performed every 6 months for the first 2 years and a PET or PET-CT scan is performed at least once a year for 5 years.

Some patients who receive intensive chemoradiotherapy to the pharynx or esophagus develop chronic swallowing disturbance due to secondary fibrosis. We evaluate for recurrence by esophagoscopy and, if a benign stricture is noted, dilatation procedures may be necessary. Oral and dental care for patients who received oral or oropharyngeal radiation is also mandatory to evaluate and cope with side effects such as dry mouth, stomatitis, and the development of osteoradionecrosis. The goals of our surveillance program include not only detection of recurrence of the primary tumor, detection of new primary lesions but also a detection of treatment-related problems. This helps us maintain the quality of life of our patients.

References

1. Ioka A, Tsukuma H, Ajiki W, Oshima A. Trends in head and neck cancer incidence in Japan during 1965-1999. Jpn J Clin Oncol. 2005;35:45–7.
2. Tanaka S, Sobue T. Comparison of oral and pharyngeal cancer mortality in five countries: France, Italy, Japan, UK and USA from the WHO Mortality Database (1960-2000). Jpn J Clin Oncol. 2005;35:488–91.
3. Sano H, Hamashima C. Comparison of laryngeal cancer mortality in five countries: France, Italy, Japan, UK and USA from the WHO mortality database (1960-2000). Jpn J Clin Oncol. 2005;35:626–9.
4. Bold B, Piao Y, Murata Y, Kishino M, Shibuya H. Usefulness of PET/CT for detecting a second primary cancer after treatment for squamous cell carcinoma of the head and neck. Clin Nucl Med. 2008;33:831–3.
5. Wollenberg B, Jan V, Schmit UM, Hofmann K, Stieber P, Fateh-Moghadam A. CYFRA 21-1 is not superior to SCC antigen and CEA in head and neck squamous cell cancer. Anticancer Res. 1996;16:3117–24.
6. Kandiloros D, Eleftheriadou A, Chalastras T, Kyriou L, Yiotakis I, Ferekidis E. Prospective study of a panel of tumor markers as

prognostic factors in patients with squamous cell carcinoma of head and neck. Med Oncol. 2006;23:463–70.
7. Matsubara N, Umezaki T, Adachi K, Tomita E, Matsuyama K, Nakagawa T, et al. Multidimensional voice evaluation in pretreatment glottic carcinoma. Folia Phoniatr Logop. 2005;57:173–80.
8. Rogers JW, Greven KM, McGuirt WF, Keyes Jr JW, Williams 3rd DW, Watson NE, et al. Can post-RT neck dissection be omitted for patients with head-and-neck cancer who have a negative PET scan after definitive radiation therapy? Int J Radiat Oncol Biol Phys. 2004;58:694–7.
9. Pellitteri PK, Ferlito A, Rinaldo A, Shah JP, Weber RS, Lowry J, et al. Planned neck dissection following chemoradiotherapy for advanced head and neck cancer: is it necessary for all? Head Neck. 2006;28:166–75.

Upper Aerodigestive Tract Carcinoma Surveillance Counterpoint: Canada

8

Richard W. Nason and James B. Butler

Keywords
Head and neck • Modality • PET • Surveillance • Treatment outcome

The number of new mucosal cancers of the upper aerodigestive tract in Canada each year exceeds 4,500 cases, with about 700 deaths [1] (2.8 % of new cancer cases and 2.3 % of cancer-related deaths). The estimated age standardized incidence for oral cancer by Province ranges from 9 to 14 per 100,000 population for males and 4 to 6 per 100,000 for females. Larynx is the single most common site. The incidence across provinces varies from 3 to 8 per 100,000. There appears to be a relatively higher incidence of these cancers in the Atlantic Provinces, Quebec, and Manitoba. Higher historical smoking rates have been documented for Quebec and the Atlantic Provinces. The annual incidence of laryngeal cancer is declining for both males and females by 3.6–3.4 % annually, and the mortality rate among males is decreasing [1].

In Canada the majority of these patients are managed through provincially based cancer treatment facilities. In Manitoba, 95 % of all registered head and neck cancer patients are managed through a Multidisciplinary Head and Neck Clinic at CancerCare Manitoba, Winnipeg. The Head and Neck Team manages approximately 150–200 new cases annually. The heterogeneous nature of these tumors needs to be emphasized. There are five different regions based on anatomic and clinical-pathologic behavior of the tumors: oral cavity, pharynx, larynx, nasal cavity, and paranasal sinuses. The oral cavity alone has six subsites [2]. Each region has its own set of rules for staging. Moving only several centimeters along the upper aerodigestive tract can influence disease presentation, staging system, treatment approach, and outcome.

Despite the heterogeneity of this anatomic region there are general patterns to the treatment plans. Early stage disease (I and II) is treated by a single modality (surgery or radiotherapy). Advanced-stage disease (stages III and IV) is approached with multimodality treatment plans that can incorporate surgery and/or radiotherapy and chemotherapy. Selection of modalities is negotiated with the patient and is based on predicted treatment response and functional outcome. The treatment plans in Manitoba conform to the treatment guidelines developed and supported by the American Head and Neck Society (AHNS) [3].

Overall survival for patients with squamous cell cancer of the upper aerodigestive tract is determined by events such as recurrent disease, second primary tumors, and intercurrent medical comorbid conditions.

The incidence of recurrence following treatment with curative intent ranges from 19 to 50 %, depending on disease stage, primary site, and other factors such as the initial treatment modality [4–8]. The predominant sites of recurrence are the primary site and neck (regional lymph nodes). Distant metastases at diagnosis are reported in 6–8 % of this population [4–6, 9]. In a series of 2,600 patients, those with early stage oral and oropharyngeal cancer treated surgically [5] experienced a recurrence rate of 29 %; while for those with advanced stages of oropharyngeal cancer treated primarily with radiotherapy, the recurrence rate was 80 %. Histopathologic features of the primary tumor such as the nature of the tumor–host interface [10–12], tumor thickness [13, 14], and the status of the surgical margin on permanent

R.W. Nason, M.D. (✉)
Department of Surgical Oncology, CancerCare Manitoba,
ON 3274-675 McDermot Ave, Winnipeg, MB, Canada R3E 0V9
e-mail: nasonrw@cc.umanitoba.ca

J.B. Butler
Department of Radiation Oncology, CancerCare Manitoba,
ON 3274-675 McDermot Ave, Winnipeg, MB, Canada R3E 0V9
e-mail: Jim.Butler@cancercare.mb.ca

F.E. Johnson et al. (eds.), *Patient Surveillance After Cancer Treatment*, Current Clinical Oncology,
DOI 10.1007/978-1-60327-969-7_8, © Springer Science+Business Media New York 2013

section [15, 16] also have an important impact on recurrence. The incidence of distant metastases as an initial site of treatment failure has been increasing as local–regional control improves [4]. Distant metastases are related to advanced stages of disease at presentation [5, 8, 9] and are most frequently observed with hypopharyngeal tumors [8]. The majority of all treatment failures are identified within 24–36 months of treatment [8, 17–21].

Second primary tumors are defined as those arising at a different site in the aerodigestive tract within 5 years of treatment of the index tumor, or at the same location as the index tumor after 5 years. In contrast to recurrences, second primary cancers tend to occur at a rate of 2.7–6 % per year for the life of the patient [22, 24]. Second primary tumors are most significant in patients with early stage disease [25, 26]. Patients with carcinoma of the larynx have a higher incidence of second primaries in the lung [22]. After 36 months the appearance of a second primary tumor is the most common cause of treatment failure [8, 22, 24].

The ability to cure patients with new tumor events (i.e., recurrence or second primary) is generally poor. For patients with recurrence, only 14–26 % experience a disease-free period of 2 years or more following treatment [8, 18, 27, 28]. In a pooled analysis of 488 patients treated for recurrence from 28 institutions, the weighted average percent survival at 5 years was 39 % [29]. In another review of 377 patients with recurrent squamous cell carcinoma [28], all patients that were successfully salvaged following recurrence were amenable to a complete surgical resection, but the mean survival duration for patients treated with nonsurgical methods was 6 months, with no survivors at 5 years. The majority had advanced disease and were not amenable to further treatment. Ritoe [21] reported that only 27.5 % of patients with recurrent disease after total laryngectomy were candidates for salvage treatment. Surgical salvage has a higher chance of success in patients with early stage index tumors [8, 29] and is most effective for recurrent early stage laryngeal cancer, with survival rates consistently greater than 50 % at 5 years [8, 19, 30–32]. Salvage treatment is least effective for recurrent cancer of the hypopharynx [30, 32]. Patients with isolated neck recurrences have a poor prognosis despite salvage treatment. Patients with recurrence who have had a previous neck dissection are generally not candidates for salvage treatment. Distant metastases from squamous cell carcinoma of the head and neck can rarely be cured [21, 28, 33].

For second primaries, the success of treatment is similar to that described for recurrence [22, 34]. Survival tends to be better for a second primary in the head and neck region with successful treatment reported in 20 % [23]. The prognosis for a second primary in the lung is poor [23, 35]. In one series [8], the occurrence of distant metastases or second primary tumors outside the head and neck region was associated with mean survival duration of less than 2 years after detection. Continued use of tobacco and alcohol has an adverse impact on the outcome and treatment of second primary cancers [23].

Survival for squamous cell head and neck cancer is generally reported in relation to site and stage of disease. Reported percent survival for early stage oral cancer is in the range of 66–78 % at 5 years [36–39]. Percent survival for early stage laryngeal cancer is consistently higher, between 88 and 97 % [40, 41]. Percent survival for advanced-stage disease at all sites is poor, ranging from 33 to 47 % at 5 years [42–44].

In Manitoba, our cancer care system allows us to report on survival data from a provincial population perspective as opposed to a narrower institutional perspective. The data relating to squamous cell carcinoma of the upper aerodigestive tract in Manitoba are consistent with data reported above. In an historical cohort of 700 patients with oral cancer at all stages, 625 were treated with curative intent. Persistent disease was observed in 50 patients; the majority of these treated with radiotherapy as a single treatment modality. Of the 575 patients who were rendered disease-free, 190 (30 %) experienced recurrence. The documented site of initial treatment failure was the primary site and neck in 117 and 82 patients, respectively. Distant metastases were observed at the time of initial treatment failure in 24 patients (3.8 %). Fifty-four patients (28 %) were rendered disease-free with further treatment. One hundred fifty-seven second primary tumors were identified in 146 patients. The most frequent site was the head and neck ($n = 100$), followed by lung ($n = 50$) and esophagus ($n = 7$). Overall and cause-specific mortality rates due to cancer at 5 years were 49 % and 37 %. Overall percent survival by stage of disease was 74 %, 59 %, 52 %, and 29 % at 5 years, for stages I–IV. Among 379 deaths observed in this cohort the cause was documented in 336. Death was attributed to the initial disease in 186, new primary tumors in 70, and other causes in 80 patients.

The relatively high incidence of new tumors in patients with squamous cell carcinoma of the upper digestive tract seems to justify aggressive surveillance [20, 45] based on the assumption that identifying and treating a new tumor event at an early and asymptomatic stage may allow for appropriate therapeutic options, improve survival, and reduce cancer-specific morbidity [7, 20], although data from well-controlled studies are not avaialble to support this.

The frequency and duration of surveillance testing has been a matter of preference and common acceptance. In 1993, Marchant and coworkers [45] reported the results of a survey of 290 members of the American Society for Head and Neck Surgery. Patients were followed monthly for the first year by 73 % of respondents and then every 2–3 months in the second postoperative year by 90 % of respondents. Patients were seen every 4–6 months in postoperative years 3–5 by 97 % of respondents. All respondents reported seeing the patients either annually or semiannually for the remainder of their lives. Eighty percent advocated use of screening chest radiographs.

Table 8.1 Surveillance after curative-intent treatment for upper aerodigestive tract carcinoma at CancerCare Manitoba

	Year					
Modality	1	2	3	4	5	>5
Office visit[a]	6–8	4–6	3–4	3–4	3–4	1–2
Serum TSH level[b]	1–2	1–2	1–2	1–2	1–2	1–2
CT/MRI[c]	1–2	[d]	[d]	[d]	[d]	[d]

[a]Visit includes needs assessment performed by nursing staff; completion of quality of life survey; evaluation of upper aerodigestive tract by physician with fiberoptic endoscopy as indicated; evaluation and intervention of speech language pathology, nutrition, physiotherapy, psychosocial oncology per needs assessment
[b]Patients with neck irradiation or thyroidectomy
[c]Initial imaging study 6 weeks posttreatment. Second study performed 6–12 weeks later to establish stability of post treatment changes
[d]As clinically indicated
The number in each cell is the number of times a particular modality is recommended in a particular posttreatment year

The majority reserved head and neck imaging studies such as CT scans and endoscopic examination under anesthetic for symptomatic patients. In 1996 the American Society of Head and Neck Surgery and the Society of Head and Neck Surgery collaborated to form a clinical guidelines task force resulting in a booklet of consensus guidelines [46]. Surveillance guidelines are provided for the major tumor sites in the head and neck. These guidelines are now published as part of the NCCN Clinical Practice Guidelines in Oncology [3] and are endorsed by the AHNS. These guidelines form the basis of surveillance for the Head and Neck Team at CancerCare Manitoba (Table 8.1). The pattern of surveillance is similar for all sites and initial stages. Patients with advanced stages of disease have a higher frequency of visits driven by the symptomatic consequences of treatment.

Evaluation of the efficacy of surveillance is limited to several general [6–8, 19, 47] and site-specific [20, 21, 48, 49] descriptive studies. The assumption challenged in these studies is that rigid scheduled surveillance can reduce cancer-related mortality from new tumors by identifying patients at an early and asymptomatic stage. The balance of opinion suggests that the use of routine and rigid schedules is of limited benefit [7, 8, 20, 21]. In these studies, 40–60 % of the recurrences were symptomatic [8, 19, 49] and patients with symptomatic recurrences tended to present on a self-referred basis outside of scheduled visits. Two studies [20, 49] showed no difference in survival duration between patients presenting with symptoms and asymptomatic patients identified at the time of routine visit. In contrast, de Visscher and Manni [47] reported improved survival duration in patients with asymptomatic recurrences identified at the time of a scheduled visit. It is noted, however, that these authors measured survival time from the time of treatment of the recurrence and not the time of treatment of the index tumor. This therefore confounded the results with lead-time bias [49]. It is estimated that only 2–3 % of patients with asymptomatic recurrences benefit from the exercise of routine office visits [7, 49]. These studies again emphasized that the limited treatment success observed was restricted to patients with early stage disease treated with a single modality. This subset of patients tended to be amenable to further treatment options. In patients with advanced disease, the probability of survival following a recurrence is negligible as a consequence of no available effective treatment options [7, 19–21, 49]. The majority of the investigators questioned the necessity of surveillance after 3 years and particularly beyond 5 years.

The use of chest x-rays on a routine basis during surveillance has recently been questioned. Ritoe et al. [50] performed 2008 routine chest radiographs in high-risk laryngeal cancer patients, which yielded 11 patients in whom a curative-intent resection could be offered, with three experiencing long term survival. Additional studies have shown no benefit from routine chest radiographs [51, 52].

The role of routine surveillance in patients with squamous cell carcinoma of the upper aerodigestive tract at CancerCare Manitoba has not been systematically evaluated. It is our clinical impression that the majority of patients with recurrence are symptomatic. The poor outcomes of patients with recurrent disease has been demonstrated in our historical cohort of oral cancer patients.

Conclusion and Future Directions

The objectives of surveillance after treatment of squamous cell carcinoma of the upper aerodigestive tract extend beyond simply decreasing morbidity and mortality rates. Requirements for rehabilitation are a major component of follow-up visits. Surveillance is also important to document outcomes, which should be the evidence base for our therapeutic decisions.

Surveillance of head and neck cancers posttreatment should continue using the guidelines that have been presented. We do, however, feel that there is a need to clearly identify the goals and possibly shift the emphasis of certain tasks away from physicians. In the majority of patients the intent of follow-up should be care and not cure [7, 49]. All patients require monitoring for complications of treatment such as hypothyroidism in patients in whom the neck is irradiated. Most patients require involvement with speech and language therapists, nutritionists, physiotherapists, and dental specialists [53]. The psychosocial consequences of treatment of head and neck cancer are recognized [54]. In patients with early stage disease who are treated with a single modality, surveillance is appropriate to identify recurrences that are potentially treatable. In patients with advanced-stage disease, the emphasis needs to be on managing and minimizing the consequences of recurrent disease. Surveillance of patients beyond 2–3 years has the advantage of documenting treatment outcomes.

The emphasis of follow-up should shift from a physician-centric event to a multidisciplinary exercise that addresses the needs and expectations of the patient. The multidisciplinary team should educate patients about the signs and symptoms of recurrent disease and align the expectations of the patients appropriately in the event of a new tumor event.

It is the authors' opinion that recurrent disease very often indicates aggressive disease. There is a reasonable chance that even with earlier diagnosis the ultimate outcome will not change. It needs to be emphasized that the studies presented are based on identification of recurrence of physical findings and there is evidence that physical examination is inferior to imaging in certain aspects. The sensitivity of physical examination in identifying cervical lymph nodes is about 50–60 %. Imaging studies, including MR, CT, and ultrasound, are all superior to physical examination, identifying 75–80 % of patients with metastatic disease in the neck [55]. Nieuwenhuis and coworkers [56] evaluated the use of ultrasound-guided cytological assessment of sentinel nodes in the management of the N0 neck. Ultrasound was used as part of the follow-up process. During the follow-up period 34 of 161 (21 %) patients developed lymph node metastases. These authors reported a salvage rate of 79 %, which is two to three times higher than that observed in our own series. This suggests that these investigators were able to identify cervical node metastases when they were more amenable to salvage treatment. There have been qualitative assessments of the use of positron emission tomography (PET) in the follow-up of patients with advanced head and neck cancer [57, 58]. Current evidence suggests that PET is useful in identifying residual or recurrent head and neck cancer. In our opinion, imaging needs to be introduced in a formal fashion into our follow-up protocols. This aspect of surveillance would be amenable to a systematic assessment.

The outcome of patients with squamous cell carcinoma of the upper aerodigestive tract is predominantly determined by the biology of the tumor. Treatment can modify the course of the illness. The ability to predict treatment outcome based on the biology of the tumor would facilitate planning for surveillance. At the present time the ability to stratify the patients into high and low risk groups based on clinical and histopathologic parameters does not permit refinements of surveillance schedules [48]. Cancer is a consequence of genetic and epigenetic alterations at the cellular level. The use of molecular techniques to describe tumor specific characteristics to predict the tumor phenotype would be of obvious benefit. This science is in its infancy. The study of DNA microarrays and genomic hybridization shows promise. At the present time, however, there is no single marker, technique, or group of parameters that are sufficiently reproducible and sensitive for clinical use [59]. The use of structured surveillance programs will, however, be necessary to evaluate the benefit of new prognostic indices.

In summary, structured surveillance visits following treatment of carcinoma of the upper aerodigestive tract are justified. The emphasis for most patients needs to shift from cure to care. Surveillance, as currently performed, does not appear to have a significant impact on improving survival. Rehabilitation, identification and management of symptoms, and documentation of treatment outcomes are the major reasons for structured programs. The modulation of intensity of follow-up relative to site and stage of disease, the role of the physician versus team-based evaluation, and the integration of modern imaging techniques into surveillance plans need to be formally evaluated within the context of clinical trials.

References

1. Canadian Cancer Statistics. 2008. http://www.cancer.ca. Accessed 18 Nov 2008.
2. Edge SB, Byrd DR, Compton CC, Fritz AG, Greene FL, Trotti A (Eds). AJCC Cancer Staging Handbook 7th ed. USA: Springer 2010
3. NCCN clinical practice guidelines in oncology. 2008. http://www.nccn.org. Accessed 18 Nov 2008
4. Taneja C, Allen H, Koness RJ, Radie-Keane K, Wanebo HJ. Changing patterns in failure of head and neck cancer. Arch Otolaryngol Head Neck Surg. 2002;128:324–7.
5. Carvalho AL, Magrin J, Kowalski LP. Sites of recurrence in oral and oropharyngeal cancers according to the treatment approach. Oral Dis. 2003;9:112–8.
6. Grau JJ, Cuchi A, Traserra J, Fírvida JL, Arias C, Blanch JL, et al. Follow-up study in head and neck cancer: cure rate according to tumor location and stage. Oncology. 1997;54(1):38–42.
7. Cooney TR, Poulsen MG. Is routine follow-up useful after combined-modality therapy for advanced head and neck cancer? Arch Otolaryngol Head Neck Surg. 1999;125:379–82.
8. Haas I, Hauser U, Ganzer U. The dilemma of follow-up in head and neck cancer patients. Eur Arch Otorhinolaryngol. 2001;258:177–83.
9. Spector JG, Sessions DG, Haughey BH, Chao KS, Simpson J, El Mofty S, et al. Delayed regional metastases, distant metastases, and second primary malignancies in squamous cell carcinomas of the larynx and hypopharynx. The Laryngoscope 2001;111(6):1079–87.
10. Anneroth G, Hansen LS, Silverman Jr S. Malignancy grading in oral squamous cell carcinoma. I. Squamous cell carcinoma of the tongue and floor of mouth: histologic grading in the clinical evaluation. J Oral Pathol. 1986;15(3):162–8.
11. Bryne M, Koppang HS, Lilleng R, Stene T, Bang G, Dabelsteen E. New malignancy grading is a better prognostic indicator than Broders' grading in oral squamous cell carcinomas. J Oral Pathol Med. 1989;18(8):432–7.
12. Brandwein-Gensler M, Teixeira MS, Lewis CM, Lee B, Rolnitzky L, Hille JJ, et al. Oral squamous cell carcinoma: histologic risk assessment, but not margin status, is strongly predictive of local disease-free and overall survival. Am J Surg Pathol. 2005;29(2):167–78.
13. Spiro RH, Huvos AG, Wong GY, Spiro JD, Gnecco CA, Strong EW. Predictive value of tumor thickness in squamous carcinoma confined to the tongue and floor of the mouth. Am J Surg. 1986;152(4):345–50.
14. Po WY, Lam KY, Lam LK, Ho CM, Wong A, Chow TL, et al. Prognostic factors of clinically stage I and II oral tongue carcinoma-A comparative study of stage, thickness, shape, growth pattern,

invasive front malignancy grading, Martinez-Gimeno score, and pathologic features. Head and Neck. 2002;24(6):513–20.

15. Sutton DN, Brown JS, Rogers SN, Vaughan ED, Woolgar JA. The prognostic implications of the surgical margin in oral squamous cell carcinoma. Int J Oral Maxillofac Surg. 2003;32(1): 30–4.
16. Binahmed A, Nason RW, Abdoh AA. The clinical significance of the positive surgical margin in oral cancer. Oral Oncol. 2007;43(8): 780–4.
17. Kowalski LP. Results of salvage treatment of the neck in patients with oral cancer. Arch Otolaryngol Head Neck Surg. 2002;128:58–62.
18. Schwartz GJ, Mehta RH, Wenig BL, Shaligram C, Portugal LG. Salvage treatment for recurrent squamous cell carcinoma of the oral cavity. Head and Neck. 2000;22(1):34–41.
19. Boysen M, Lovdal O, Tausjo J, Winther F. The value of follow-up in patients treated for squamous cell carcinoma of the head and neck. Eur J Cancer. 1992;28(2–3):426–30.
20. Merkx MA, van Gulick JJ, Marres HA, Kaanders JH, Bruaset I, Verbeek A, et al. Effectiveness of routine follow-up of patients treated for T1-2N0 oral squamous cell carcinomas of the floor of mouth and tongue. Head and Neck. 2006;28(1):1–7.
21. Ritoe SC, Bergman H, Krabbe PFM, Kaanders JH, van den Hoogen FJ, Verbeek AL, et al. Cancer recurrence after total laryngectomy: treatment options, survival, and complications. Head and Neck. 2006;28(5):383–388.
22. Dhooge IJ, De Vos M, Van Cauwenberge PB. Multiple primary malignant tumors in patients with head and neck cancer: results of a prospective study and future perspectives. Laryngoscope. 1998;108(2):250–6.
23. Schwartz LH, Ozsahin M, Zhang GN, Touboul E, De Vataire F, Andolenko P, et al. Synchronous and metachronous head and neck carcinomas. Cancer. 1994;74(7):1933–8.
24. Vikram B. Changing patterns of failure in advanced head and neck cancer. Arch Otolaryngol Head Neck Surg. 1984;110(9):564–5.
25. Lippman SM, Hong WK. Second malignant tumors in head and neck squamous cell carcinoma: the overshadowing threat for patients with early-stage disease. Int J Radiat Oncol Biol Phys. 1989;17(3):691–4.
26. Licciardello JT, Spitz MR, Hong WK. Multiple primary cancer in patients with cancer of the head and neck: second cancer of the head and neck, esophagus, and lung. Int J Radiat Oncol Biol Phys. 1989;17(3):467–76.
27. Gleich LL, Ryzenman J, Gluckman JL, et al. Recurrent advanced (T3 or T4) head and neck squamous cell carcinoma. Arch Otolaryngol Head Neck Surg. 2004;130:35–8.
28. Wong LY, Wei WI, Lam LK, Yuen APW. Salvage of recurrent head and neck squamous cell carcinoma after primary curative surgery. Head Neck. 2003;25(11):953–9.
29. Goodwin Jr WJ. Salvage surgery for patients with recurrent squamous cell carcinoma of the upper aerodigestive tract: when do the ends justify the means? Laryngoscope. 2000;110 Suppl 93:1–18.
30. Stoeckli SJ, Pawlik AB, Lipp M, Huber A, Schmid S. Salvage surgery after failure of nonsurgical therapy for carcinoma of the larynx and hypopharynx. Arch Otolaryngol Head Neck Surg. 2000;126: 1473–1477.
31. Ganly I, Patel SG, Matsuo J, Singh B, Kraus DH, Boyle JO, et al. Results of surgical salvage after failure of definitive radiation therapy for early-stage squamous cell carcinoma of the glottic larynx. Arch Otolaryngol Head Neck Surg. 2006;132:59–66.
32. Arnold DJ, Goodwin WJ, Weed DT, Civantos FJ. Treatment of recurrent and advanced stage squamous cell carcinoma of the head and neck. Semin Radiat Oncol. 2004;14(2):190–5.
33. Calhoun KH, Fulmer P, Weiss R, Hokanson JA. Distant metastases from head and neck squamous cell carcinomas. Laryngoscope. 1994;104(10):1199–205.
34. Geurts TW, Balm AJM, van Velthuysen MLF, van Tinteren H, Burgers JA, van Zandwijk N, et al. Survival after surgical resection of pulmonary metastases and second primary squamous cell lung carcinomas in head and neck cancer. Head Neck. 2009;31(2): 220–6.
35. Douglas WG, Rigual NR, Loree TR, Wiseman SM, Al-Rawi S, Hicks WL Jr. Current concepts in the management of a second malignancy of the lung in patients with head and neck cancer. Curr Opin Otolaryngol Head Neck Surg. 2003 Apr;11(2):85–8. Review.
36. Nason RW, Sako K, Beecroft WA, Razack MS, Bakamjian VY, Shedd DP. Surgical management of squamous cell carcinoma of the floor of the mouth. Am J Surg. 1989;158:292–6.
37. Lee WR, Mendenhall WM, Parsons JT, Million RR, Cassisi NJ, Stringer SPl. Carcinoma of the tonsillar region: a multivariate analysis of 243 patients treated with radical radiotherapy. Head and Neck. 1993;15:283–8.
38. Rodgers LW, Stringer SP, Mendenhall WM, Parsons JT, Cassisi NJ, Million RR. Management of squamous cell carcinoma of the floor of mouth. Head and Neck. 1993;15:16–9.
39. Sessions DG, Spector GJ, Lenox J, Haughey B, Chao C, Marks Jl. Analysis of treatment results for oral tongue cancer. Laryngoscope. 2002;112(4):616–25.
40. Mendenhall WM, Parsons JT, Stringer SP, Cassisi NJ. Management of Tis, T1, and T2 squamous cell carcinoma of the glottic larynx. Am J Otolaryngol. 1994;15(4):250–7.
41. Spector GJ, Sessions DG, Chao KSC, Haughey BH, Hanson JM, Simpson JR, et al. Stage I (T1 N0 M0) squamous cell carcinoma of the laryngeal glottis: therapeutic results and voice preservation. Head and Neck. 1999;21(8):707–17.
42. Gleich LL, Collins CM, Gartside PS, Gluckman JL, Barrett WL, Wilson KM, et al. Therapeutic decision making in stage III and IV head and neck squamous cell carcinoma. Arch Otolaryngol Head Neck Surg. 2003;129(1):26–35.
43. Spector GJ, Sessions DG, Lenox J, Newland D, Simpson J, Haughey BH. Management of stage IV glottic carcinoma: therapeutic outcomes. Laryngoscope. 2004;114(8):1438–46.
44. Sessions DG, Lenox J, Spector GJ, Chao C, Chaudry OA. Analysis of treatment results for base of tongue cancer. Laryngoscope. 2003;113(7):1252–61.
45. Marchant FE, Lowry LD, Moffitt JJ, Sabbagh R. Current national trends in the posttreatment follow-up of patients with squamous cell carcinoma of the head and neck. Am J Otolaryngol. 1993;14(2):88–93.
46. Clinical practice guidelines for the diagnosis and management of cancer of the head and neck. The American Society for Head and Neck Surgery and American Head and Neck Society 1995, http://www.ahns.info/clinicalresources/.
47. De Visscher AV, Manni JJ. Routine long-term follow-up in patients treated with curative intent for squamous cell carcinoma of the larynx, pharynx, and oral cavity. Does it make sense? Arch Otolaryngol Head Neck Surg. 1994;120(9):934–9.
48. Ritoe SC, Verbeek ALM, Krabbe PFM, Kaanders JH, van den Hoogen FJ, Marres HA. Screening for local and regional cancer recurrence in patients curatively treated for laryngeal cancer: definition of a high-risk group and estimation of the lead time. Head and Neck. 2007;29(5):431–8.
49. Ritoe SC, Krabbe PF, Kaanders JH, van den Hoogen FJ, Verbeek AL, Marres HA. Value of routine follow-up for patients cured of laryngeal carcinoma. Cancer. 2004;101(6):1382–9.
50. Ritoe SC, Krabbe PF, Jansen MM, Festen J, Joosten FB, Kaanders JH, et al. Screening for second primary lung cancer after treatment of laryngeal cancer. Laryngoscope. 2002;112(11):2002–8.
51. Merkx MA, Boustahji AH, Kaanders JH, Joosten F, Marres HA, Bruaset I, et al. A half-yearly chest radiograph for early detection of lung cancer following oral cancer. Int J Oral Maxillofac Surg. 2002;31(4):378–82.

52. Shah SI, Applebaum EL. Lung cancer after head and neck cancer: role of chest radiography. Laryngoscope. 2000;110(12):2033–6.
53. Van der Molen L, van Rossum M, Burkhead L, Smeele LE, Hilgers FJ. Functional outcomes and rehabilitation strategies in patients treated with chemoradiotherapy for advanced head and neck cancer: a systematic review. Eur Arch Otorhinolaryngol. 2009;266(6): 889–900. Epub 2008 Sep 30.
54. Geurts TW, Ackerstaff AH, Van Zandwijk, Hart AA, Hilgers FJ, Balm AJ. The psychological impact of annual chest X-Ray follow-up in head and neck cancer. Acta Otolaryngol. 2006;126(12):1315–20.
55. Van den Brekel MW, Castelijns JA, Snow GB. Diagnostic evaluation of the neck. Otolaryngol Clin North Am. 1998;31(4):601–20.
56. Nieuwenhuis EJ, Castelijns JA, Pijpers R, van den Brekel MW, Brakenhoff RH, van der Waal I, et al. Wait-and-see policy for the N0 neck in early-stage oral and oropharyngeal squamous cell carcinoma using ultrasonography-guided cytology: is there a role for identification of the sentinel node? Head and Neck. 2002:24(3): 282–9.
57. Goerres GW, Schmid DT, Bandhauer F, Huguenin PU, von Schulthess GK, Schmid S, et al. Positron emission tomography in the early follow-up of advanced head and neck cancer. Arch Otolaryngol Head Neck Surg. 2004;130:105–9.
58. Isles MG, McConkey C, Mehanna HM. A systematic review and meta-analysis of the role of positron emission tomography in the follow up of head and neck squamous cell carcinoma following radiotherapy or chemotherapy. Clin Otolaryngol. 2008;33:210–22.
59. Cheng AC, Schmidt BL. Management of the N0 neck in oral squamous cell carcinoma. Oral Maxillofac Surg Clin N Am. 2008;40(3):477–97.

9 Thyroid (Papillary, Follicular, Medullary, Hürthle Cell) Carcinoma

David Y. Johnson, Shilpi Wadhwa, and Frank E. Johnson

Keywords
Follicular carcinoma • Thyroid • Hürthle cell • Variability • Survival rate

The International Agency for Research on Cancer (IARC), a component of the World Health Organization (WHO), estimated that there were 141,013 new cases of thyroid (papillary, follicular, Hürthle cell) carcinoma worldwide in 2002 [1]. The IARC estimated that there were 35,375 deaths due to this cause in 2002 [1].

The American Cancer Society estimated that there were 33,550 new cases and 1,530 deaths due to this cause in the USA in 2007[2]. The estimated 5-year survival rate (all races) in the USA in 2007 was 97 % for thyroid cancer [2]. Survival rates were adjusted for normal life expectancies and were based on cases diagnosed from 1996 to 2002 and followed through 2003.

The best-documented risk factor is exposure to ionizing radiation. The incidence in females is approximately three times that in males [3]. A family history or papillary of follicular carcinoma is a major risk factor; specific syndromes and specific chromosomal and gene linkages have been described [4]. For medullary carcinoma, radiation does not seem to be an important risk factor [4]. Mutations in the RET gene are a dominant cause of medullary carcinoma although sporadic cases still account for 60–70 % of the total [4].

D.Y. Johnson • S. Wadhwa
Department of Internal Medicine, Saint Louis University Medical Center, Saint Louis, MO, USA
e-mail: dyjohnson@gmail.com; shilpi_wadhwa@unc.edu; swadhwa@gmail.com; mini.mermaid@gmail.com

F.E. Johnson, M.D., FACS (✉)
Saint Louis University Medical Center and Saint Louis Veterans Affairs Medical Center, Saint Louis, MO, USA
e-mail: frank.johnson1@va.gov

Geographic Variation Worldwide

The incidence of thyroid cancer varies among different ethnic groups, suggesting a role for environmental factors. A higher incidence of papillary cancer is found in regions with high dietary iodine intake such as the Pacific rim and Iceland. In contrast, follicular cancer is more prevalent in iodine-deficient countries [5]. Adequate data is not available to document geographic variation of thyroid cancer incidence in the USA [6].

Surveillance Strategies Proposed by Professional Organizations or National Government Agencies and Available on the Internet

National Comprehensive Cancer Network (www.nccn.org)

National Comprehensive Cancer Network (NCCN) guidelines were accessed on 1/28/12 (Tables 9.1 and 9.2). There were major quantitative and qualitative changes compared to the guidelines accessed on 4/10/07.

F.E. Johnson et al. (eds.), *Patient Surveillance After Cancer Treatment*, Current Clinical Oncology, DOI 10.1007/978-1-60327-969-7_9, © Springer Science+Business Media New York 2013

Table 9.1 Thyroid carcinoma: papillary, follicular, Hürthle cell carcinoma

	Years posttreatment[a]					
	1	2	3	4	5	>5
Office visit	1–2	1	1	1	1	1
Serum thyroid-stimulating hormone, thyroglobulin, and antithyroglobulin antibody levels	1–2	1	1	1	1	1
Radioactive iodine imaging[b]	0.5–1	0.5–1	0.5–1	0.5–1	0.5–1	0.5–1
• Periodic neck ultrasound[c]						
• Consider thyroid-stimulating hormone (TSH) stimulated thyroglobulin (Tg) measurement in patients previously treated with radioactive iodine (RAI) and with negative TSH-suppressed Tg and anti-Tg antibodies[d]						
• Consider TSH-stimulated RAI imaging in high-risk patients, patients with previous RAI avid metastases, or patients with abnormal Tg levels (either TSH-suppressed or TSH-stimulated), abnormal anti-Tg antibodies, or abnormal ultrasound during surveillance						
• If ^{131}I scans negative and stimulated serum Tg level >2–5 ng/mL, consider additional non-RAI imaging (e.g., neck ultrasound, neck CT, FDG-PET ± CT if serum Tg level ≥10 ng/mL)						

Obtained from NCCN (www.nccn.org) on 1/28/12

NCCN guidelines were accessed on 1/28/12. There were major quantitative and qualitative changes compared to the guidelines accessed on 4/10/07

[a]The numbers in the table indicate the number of times the modality is recommended during the indicated year posttreatment

[b]If detectable thyroglobulin or distant metastases or soft tissue invasion on initial staging, radioiodine imaging every 12–24 months until no clinically significant response is seen to RAI treatment in iodine responsive tumors (following either withdrawal of thyroid hormone or recombinant human TSH (rhTSH)). If there is a high likelihood of RAI therapy, thyroid hormone withdrawal suggested; if not, suggest using rhTSH

[c]A subgroup of low-risk patients may only require an ultrasound if there is a reasonable suspicion for recurrence

[d]In selected patients who may be at level risk for residual/recurrent disease (e.g., N1 patients), obtain a stimulated Tg and consider concomitant diagnostic RAI imaging. With a positive stimulated Tg, concomitant RAI imaging may help determine whether treatment with RAI is indicated (i.e., RAI is often beneficial in iodine-avid disease but not in non-iodine avid disease)

Table 9.2 Thyroid carcinoma: medullary carcinoma

	Years posttreatmenta					
	1	2	3	4	5	>5
Office visit[b]	1	1	1	1	1	1
Serum calcitonin, carcinoembryonic antigen levels	1	1	1	1	1	1
• Consider neck ultrasound						
• Additional studies or more frequent testing if significantly rising serum calcitonin or carcinoembryonic antigen (CEA) levels						
• No additional imaging required if calcitonin and CEA levels stable						
• For MEN 2A or 2B, annual screening for pheochromocytoma and hyperparathyroidism (MEN 2A)						

Obtained from NCCN (www.nccn.org) on 1/28/12

NCCN guidelines were accessed on 1/28/12. There were minor qualitative changes compared to the guidelines accessed on 4/10/07

[a]The numbers in the table indicate the number of times the modality is recommended during the indicated year posttreatment

[b]Serum calcitonin and CEA levels were the only quantitative recommendations given. We inferred that office visit would be recommended as frequently as these

American Society of Clinical Oncology (www.asco.org)

American Society of Clinical Oncology (ASCO) guidelines were accessed on 1/28/12. No quantitative guidelines exist for thyroid cancer surveillance including when first accessed on 10/31/07.

The Society of Surgical Oncology (www.surgonc.org)

The Society of Surgical Oncology (SSO) guidelines were accessed on 1/28/12. No quantitative guidelines exist for thyroid cancer surveillance including when first accessed on 10/31/07.

Table 9.3 Thyroid cancer: differentiated thyroid cancer

	Years posttreatment[a]					
	1	2	3	4	5	>5
Office visit[b]	1–2	1–2	1–2	1–2	1–2	1–2
Neck ultrasound	1–2	1–2	1–2	1–2	1–2	1–2
Thyroglobulin on levothyroxine	1–2	1–2	1–2	1–2	1–2	1–2

- Two to three months after initial treatment, thyroid function tests (free T3, free T4, thyroid-stimulating hormone) should be obtained to check the adequacy of levothyroxine (LT4) suppressive therapy
- For very low-risk patients, stimulated thyroglobulin (Tg) is not useful. For low- and high-risk patients, stimulated Tg at 12 months if Tg on LT4 is undetectable
- For very low-risk patients, diagnostic whole-body scan (WBS) is not useful. For low-risk patients, diagnostic WBS is not required if stimulated Tg is undetectable. For high-risk patients, diagnostic WBS may be helpful
- Patients with evidence of persistent disease, or with detectable levels of serum Tg increasing with time, require imaging techniques for localization of disease and appropriate treatment; consider FDG-PET

Obtained from ESMO (www.esmo.org) on 1/28/12

ESMO guidelines were accessed on 1/28/12. These are new quantitative guidelines compared to no guidelines found on 10/31/07

[a]The numbers in the table indicate the number of times the modality is recommended during the indicated year posttreatment

[b]Tg on LT4 and neck ultrasound were the only quantitative recommendations given. We inferred that office visit would be recommended as frequently as these

Table 9.4 Head and neck cancers: thyroid cancer

	Years posttreatment[a]					
	1	2	3	4	5	>5
Office visit	≥1	≥1	≥1	≥1	≥1	≥1

- Serum thyroid hormone and calcium levels should be monitored regularly
- Serum thyroglobulin level should be monitored in patients with differentiated thyroid cancer, and serum calcitonin level should be monitored in those with medullary cancer

Obtained from NICE (www.nice.org.uk) on 1/28/12

NICE guidelines were accessed on 1/28/12. There were no significant changes compared to the guidelines accessed on 10/31/07

[a]The numbers in the table indicate the number of times the modality is recommended during the indicated year posttreatment

European Society for Medical Oncology (www.esmo.org)

European Society for Medical Oncology (ESMO) guidelines were accessed on 1/28/12 (Table 9.3). There are new quantitative guidelines compared to no guidelines found on 10/31/07.

European Society of Surgical Oncology (www.esso-surgeonline.org)

European Society of Surgical Oncology (ESSO) guidelines were accessed on 1/28/12. No quantitative guidelines exist for thyroid cancer surveillance including when first accessed on 10/31/07.

Cancer Care Ontario (www.cancercare.on.ca)

Cancer Care Ontario (CCO) guidelines were accessed on 1/28/12. No quantitative guidelines exist for thyroid cancer surveillance including when first accessed on 10/31/07.

National Institute for Health and Clinical Excellence (www.nice.org.uk)

National Institute for Health and Clinical Excellence (NICE) guidelines were accessed on 1/28/12 (Table 9.4). There were no significant changes compared to the guidelines accessed on 10/31/07.

The Cochrane Collaboration (CC, www.cochrane.org)

CC guidelines were accessed on 1/28/12. No quantitative guidelines exist for thyroid cancer surveillance including when first accessed on 11/24/07.

American Head and Neck Society (www.headandneckcancer.org)

American Head and Neck Society (AHNS) guidelines were accessed on 1/28/12. No quantitative guidelines exist for thyroid cancer surveillance including when first accessed on 12/13/07.

Table 9.5 Papillary thyroid microcarcinoma

	Years posttreatment[a]					
	1	2	3	4	5	>5
Office visit	1	1	1	1	1	0
Cervical ultrasound[b]	1	1	1	1	1	0

- More extensive surveillance is necessary for patients with findings indicative of more aggressive disease

Obtained from ATA (www.thyroid.org) on 1/28/12
ATA guidelines were accessed on 1/28/12. These are new quantitative guidelines compared to the qualitative guidelines accessed on 10/31/07
[a]The numbers in the table indicate the number of times the modality is recommended during the indicated year posttreatment
[b]Special attention to lymph nodes

Table 9.6 Medullary thyroid cancer

	Years posttreatment[a]					
	1	2	3	4	5	>5
Office visit	1–2	1–2	1–2	1–2	1–2	1–2
Serum carcinoembryonic antigen and calcitonin levels[b]	1–2	1–2	1–2	1–2	1–2	1–2

- If calcitonin or carcinoembryonic antigen (CEA) rises substantially since the previous anatomic imaging evaluation, a neck ultrasound should be performed

Obtained from ATA (www.thyroid.org) on 1/28/12
ATA guidelines were accessed on 1/28/12. These are new quantitative guidelines compared to the qualitative guidelines accessed on 10/31/07
[a]The numbers in the table indicate the number of times the modality is recommended during the indicated year posttreatment
[b]After thyroidectomy and no evidence of persistent or recurrent medullary thyroid carcinoma, annual measurement of basal serum calcitonin level without measurement of serum CEA level should be considered. Less frequent testing may be considered if there is no evidence of disease after prolonged follow-up

Table 9.7 Differentiated thyroid cancer

	Years posttreatment[a]					
	1	2	3	4	5	>5
Office visit	1–2	1–2	1–2	1–2	1–2	1–2
Serum thyroglobulin level	1–2	1–2	1–2	1–2	1–2	1–2

- Periodic serum thyroglobulin (Tg) level measurements and neck ultrasonography should be considered during surveillance of patients with differentiated thyroid cancer who have undergone less than total thyroidectomy, and in patients who have had a total thyroidectomy but not radioactive iodine ablation
- In low-risk patients who have had remnant ablation and negative cervical ultrasound and undetectable thyroid-stimulating hormone (TSH) suppressed Tg within the first year after treatment, serum Tg should be measured after thyroxine withdrawal or recombinant human TSH stimulation approximately 12 months after the ablation to verify the absence of disease

Obtained from ATA (www.thyroid.org) on 1/28/12
ATA guidelines were accessed on 1/28/12. These are new quantitative guidelines compared to the qualitative guidelines accessed on 10/31/07
[a]The numbers in the table indicate the number of times the modality is recommended during the indicated year posttreatment

American Thyroid Association (www.thyroid.org)

American Thyroid Association (ATA) guidelines were accessed on 1/28/12 (Tables 9.5, 9.6, and 9.7). There are new quantitative guidelines compared to the qualitative guidelines accessed on 10/31/07.

The M.D. Anderson Surgical Oncology Handbook also has surveillance guidelines, proposed by authors from a single National Cancer Institute-designated Comprehensive Cancer Center, for many types of cancer [7]. Some are detailed and quantitative, others are qualitative.

Summary

This is a relatively uncommon cancer with significant variability in incidence worldwide based on dietary iodine intake. We found consensus-based guidelines but none based on high-quality evidence.

References

1. Parkin DM, Whelan SL, Ferlay J, Teppo L, Thomas DB. Cancer incidence in five continents, Vol. VIII, International Agency for Research on Cancer. (IARC Scientific Publication 155). Lyon, France: IARC Press; 2002. ISBN 92-832-2155-9.
2. Jemal A, Seigel R, Ward E, Murray T, Xu J, Thun MJ. Cancer statistics, 2007. CA Cancer J Clin. 2007;57:43–66.
3. Schottenfeld D, Fraumeni JG. Cancer epidemiology and prevention. 3rd ed. New York, NY: Oxford University Press; 2006. ISBN 13:978-0-19-514961-6.
4. DeVita VT, Hellman S, Rosenberg SA. Cancer. 7th ed. Philadelphia, PA: Lippincott Williams & Wilkins; 2005. 0-781-74450-4.
5. Abeloff MD, Armitage JO, Niederhuber JE, Kastan MB, McKenna WG. Clinical oncology. 3rd ed. Philadelphia, PA: Elsevier Churchill Livingstone; 2004. ISBN 0-443-06629-9.
6. Devesa SS, Grauman DJ, Blot WJ, Pennello GA, Hoover RN, Fraumeni JF Jr. Atlas of Cancer Mortality in the United States. National Institutes of Health, National Cancer Institute. NIH Publication No. 99-4564; Sep 1999.
7. Feig BW, Berger DH, Fuhrman GM. The M.D. Anderson Surgical Oncology Handbook. 4th ed. Philadelphia, PA: Lippincott Williams & Wilkins; 2006. ISBN 0-7817-5643-X (paperback).

10 Thyroid (Papillary, Follicular, Medullary, Hürthle Cell) Carcinoma Surveillance Counterpoint: Australia

Leigh Delbridge

Keywords

Papillary thyroid cancer • Follicular thyroid cancer • Hurthle-cell thyroid cancer • Medullary thyroid cancer • Thyroidectomy • Cervical lymph node dissection • Serum thyroglobulin • Thyroid autoantibodies • Serum calcitonin • Radioiodine ablative therapy

Thyroid cancer arises from follicular cells, giving rise to several types of cancer (papillary, follicular, Hurthle cell, and anaplastic thyroid cancer), C-cells, giving rise to medullary cancer, or lymphocytes and stromal cells, giving rise to thyroid lymphoma or sarcoma. This counterpoint will summarize the Australian practice of surveillance for patients with well-differentiated thyroid cancer of follicular cell origin and medullary thyroid cancer treated surgically with curative intent.

There are three significant features which differentiate surveillance for well-differentiated thyroid cancer of follicular cell origin from that of most other malignancies. First, it has an excellent overall prognosis for most patients. Over 85% of patients have Stage 1 papillary carcinoma, which has an overall 5-year survival rate of 97.2% (95% CI: 96.7 –97.7) [1]. Thus, the vast majority of patients with thyroid cancer receive treatment with curative intent and remain well. Second, tumor recurrence, particularly local recurrence, may occur decades after initial therapy. Third, there are highly sensitive and highly specific tests for tumor recurrence in the form of radioactive iodine scintigraphy and serum thyroglobulin measurement, both of which can detect subclinical disease very early. As such, a major goal of follow-up for patients with well-differentiated thyroid cancer is prompt attention to local recurrence in patients thought to be free of disease, rather than the detection of distant metastases [2].

Recently there have been major changes in the techniques used for surveillance. Previously, the mainstay of long-term follow-up was radioiodine scintigraphy following thyroxine withdrawal, together with measurement of serum thyroglobulin level on and off thyroxine therapy. The increasing accuracy of cervical ultrasound examination has led to a greater appreciation of importance of local recurrence in central cervical lymph node compartments. Most patients with low-risk differentiated thyroid cancer that does recur have detectable disease in the central lymph node compartment [3]. Radioactive iodine scans are particularly unreliable in detecting recurrent disease in this area. Associated with that change has been a paradigm shift in the surgical management of lymph nodes in differentiated thyroid cancer, with a current recommendation for routine prophylactic central lymph node clearance in patients without preoperative evidence of nodal involvement [4].

A further change has been made possible by the ready availability of recombinant thyroid-stimulating hormone. Now a period of thyroxine withdrawal, with its attendant symptoms of hypothyroidism, is no longer required for diagnostic tests. Regular measurement of recombinant thyroid-stimulating hormone-stimulated serum thyroglobulin level for long-term follow-up is now standard practice [5].

Surveillance of medullary thyroid cancer differs markedly from that of differentiated thyroid cancer. First, it has a worse outlook in terms of both survival duration and recurrence rate, and the majority of patients are not rendered disease-free by initial surgery. Second, it does not respond to radioiodine ablation, so surgery alone is the mainstay of

L. Delbridge, M.D., F.R.A.C.S. (✉)
University of Sydney Endocrine Surgical Unit, Sydney, Australia

Department of Endocrine and Oncology Surgery, Royal North Shore Hospital, St Leonards, NSW 2065, Sydney, Australia
e-mail: leigh.delbridge@sydney.edu.au

F.E. Johnson et al. (eds.), *Patient Surveillance After Cancer Treatment*, Current Clinical Oncology,
DOI 10.1007/978-1-60327-969-7_10,

treatment. The one similarity is that there is also a highly sensitive and highly specific marker of tumor recurrence in the form serum calcitonin measurement [6].

It is estimated that, in Australia, 1 in 92 women and 1 in 280 males will develop thyroid cancer by age 75 [7]. Furthermore, the incidence of thyroid cancer in Western societies appears to have risen faster than almost any other cancer over the last decade. For example, in Australia, the incidence of thyroid cancer is rising more rapidly than any other cancer in females. The incidence of thyroid cancer in the state of New South Wales has increased by 40% in males and 84% in females in the last 10 years [7]. On the other hand, there has not been any increase in thyroid cancer-related deaths in any study, raising the possibility that the current "epidemic" of thyroid cancer may well be due to increased detection [8]. Whatever the cause, the major economic implications for the management of thyroid cancer relate not to hospital treatment or palliation of patients with metastatic disease, but to the long-term follow-up of increasing numbers of patients who are most likely disease-free.

Long-term surveillance of both differentiated thyroid cancer and medullary thyroid cancer requires a multidisciplinary approach [9]. Ideally, this involves having experienced thyroid specialists in surgery, pathology, endocrinology, nuclear medicine, and radiation oncology all within the same center. In our unit, the initial point of contact for long-term surveillance is the endocrinologist on the team. He or she sees the patient for all scheduled follow-up visits. However, close liaison with all team members is maintained with appropriate cross-referral, whenever indicated. Such a system works very well as it minimizes the number of patient visits as well as costs. We find it a very satisfactory system from both the patient and physician perspectives.

Within our unit an important aspect of the management of thyroid cancer is that long-term surveillance commences with the initial management plan agreed to by the multidisciplinary team. The operative approach is planned largely with a view to facilitation of long-term surveillance, based on the philosophy that effective follow-up is critically dependent upon appropriate initial surgical management.

For decades, surgeons and endocrinologists have argued the relative merits of the differing initial surgical approaches to differentiated thyroid cancer, namely thyroid lobectomy alone, total thyroidectomy with or without radioiodine remnant ablation, or total thyroidectomy with prophylactic central lymph node dissection, also with or without radioiodine remnant ablation. This issue is particularly pertinent to patients at low risk, particularly those with papillary carcinoma, which constitutes the majority of patients with differentiated thyroid cancer overall. For these patients, proponents of thyroid lobectomy alone point out that no significant long-term survival advantage to total thyroidectomy when compared to unilateral surgery has ever been demonstrated. The problem with thyroid lobectomy, however, is that there has been demonstrated a significant increase in local recurrence in the central lymph node compartment (19% vs. 8%) [10]. More importantly, in patients who have had a thyroid lobectomy alone, measurement of the serum thyroglobulin level cannot be used as a marker of recurrence since thyroglobulin is secreted by both the remaining thyroid and thyroid cancer. Such patients can never be assured of disease-free status and can only be provided with the statistical reassurance that their chances of long-term survival are very good indeed. Total thyroidectomy significantly reduces the risk of local recurrence. However, the same argument as above applies if total thyroidectomy is utilized without routine radioiodine remnant ablation. Even in the most capable hands, total thyroidectomy often leaves behind residual normal thyroid tissue which continues to secrete thyroglobulin. Remnant ablation with radioiodine is effective in achieving undetectable thyroglobulin levels in patients who have had total thyroidectomy and are clinically disease-free. This provides an effective baseline for long-term surveillance, as patients who remain thyroglobulin-negative in the absence of antithyroglobulin antibodies have a high assurance of disease free-status [11]. More recently, attention has focused on routine prophylactic central node dissection. Although there are no data to demonstrate any benefits in terms of long-term survival and local recurrence, there are data to demonstrate that prophylactic unilateral node dissection reduces postoperative thyroglobulin levels and the number of radioiodine ablative doses required [4].

In our unit, therefore, the initial approach to a patient with a preoperative diagnosis of differentiated thyroid cancer is to assess tumor extent and lymph node status. The critical imaging study is an ultrasound examination of the thyroid gland and cervical lymph nodes. This not only guides the anatomical extent of surgical dissection [12] but, equally important, also provides a baseline study to facilitate long-term surveillance ultrasound scans. We perform this study as clinical surgeons, as we believe that clinician-performed ultrasound examinations provide more relevant anatomical information than third-party ultrasound examinations, both preoperatively and during follow-up surveillance. For differentiated thyroid cancer which has been diagnosed preoperatively on fine-needle cytological examination, if the tumor appears confined to the thyroid gland and there is no clinical or radiological evidence of lymph node involvement, our initial approach is total thyroidectomy, prophylactic unilateral central lymph node dissection, and routine recombinant thyroid-stimulating hormone-stimulated radioiodine remnant ablation. Patients with locally advanced disease, e.g., those with tracheal or oesophageal involvement, require more extensive local surgery. Patients with lymph node involvement require a selective node dissection tailored to the particular lymph node level involved, most commonly levels

IIB, III, and IV, less commonly level V or level VII. Patients diagnosed following a diagnostic lobectomy should be managed based on exactly the same principles at completion thyroidectomy. The above approach is supported in all the various published guidelines, including the American Thyroid Association [2], the British Thyroid Association [9], and the European Consensus guidelines [13].

There is a greater degree of consensus in the initial management of medullary thyroid cancer. For patients to be managed with an expectation of being rendered disease-free, the tumor needs to be confined to the central neck compartment. Initial surgery comprises total thyroidectomy and central node dissection. Indications for including an ipsilateral lateral node dissection include extracapsular extension of the tumor, large tumor size (>4 cm), or clinical involvement of the cervical lymph nodes. Although more extensive resections, such as contralateral node dissection or mediastinal node dissection, may be undertaken to reduce the burden of tumor, there is no expectation of achieving disease-free status once the cancer is beyond the central nodal compartment.

Planning for follow-up surveillance is then dependent upon whether or not patients are classified as being at low, intermediate, or high risk of having persistent or recurrent disease [2]. While staging based on the American Joint Committee on Cancer stage is valuable in estimating prognosis, it is important to realize that this system was developed principally to predict death from metastatic disease, not risk of local recurrence. However, as noted earlier, the main goal of long-term surveillance for the majority of patients with well-differentiated thyroid cancer is the detection of local recurrence in those thought to be free of disease; hence, a classification system to estimate risk of local recurrence is also relevant. There are numerous systems proposed for this. We employ a system based on the American Thyroid Association guidelines [2] that propose a three-level stratification determined after initial surgery and remnant ablation.

Low-risk patients have complete tumor resection at surgery with no locoregional invasion, absence of aggressive histology (e.g., tall cell, insular or columnar cell carcinoma), absence of vascular invasion, and absence of uptake outside the thyroid bed on remnant ablation. Intermediate-risk patients have either microscopic invasion of tumor into perithyroidal tissues, aggressive histology, or vascular invasion. High-risk patients have macroscopic tumor invasion, incomplete tumor resection, uptake outside the thyroid bed on remnant ablation, or distant metastases.

We prefer this system to others as it simplifies management. The European guidelines [13] also have a three-tier system. However, these are based on the American Joint Committee on Cancer system, with very low risk being unifocal T1N0M0 and no extension beyond the thyroid capsule, low risk being T1N0M0 or T2N0M0 or multifocal T1N0M0, and high risk being any T3, any T4, or any T, N1, or any M1. We find this system limited for the reasons noted above. However, in patients with medullary thyroid cancer, the American Joint Committee on Cancer TNM system does more accurately reflect long-term risk of recurrence.

Over 85% of patients with well-differentiated thyroid cancer have papillary thyroid carcinoma and are classified as low risk [14]. The majority are likely to be disease-free following initial therapy. Criteria for the absence of disease are based upon three criteria: no clinical evidence of tumor; no imaging evidence of tumor; and undetectable serum thyroglobulin levels (since we routinely carry out total thyroidectomy and radioactive iodine ablation). Clinical evidence of tumor recurrence is based upon a careful history and clinical examination, including an assessment of all the cervical node groups.

Imaging for locally recurrent disease is now best undertaken with cervical ultrasound scans. Previously, long-term surveillance was based upon repeated thyroid-stimulating hormone-stimulated diagnostic whole-body radioiodine scans but there is now extensive data to demonstrate that, after effective remnant ablation, diagnostic whole-body radioiodine scans have a low sensitivity, especially in thyroglobulin-negative patients. The requirement for periods of hypothyroidism and repeated radiation exposure poses an added risk. Radionuclide scans are now considered unnecessary for surveillance in low-risk patients with undetectable thyroglobulin and a negative cervical ultrasound examination [15]. The ultrasound scan, on the other hand, is highly sensitive in the detection of local recurrence and cervical node metastases [16]. Cervical nodal metastases may even be detected with ultrasound in the presence of an undetectable serum thyroglobulin level [17]. We prefer to have the sonogram performed by the surgeon. If a third-party ultrasound is undertaken, it is important that this be done by an experienced radiologist with knowledge of the clinical findings at surgery and previous imaging studies.

Thyroglobulin is secreted by both normal and malignant thyroid cells. The measurement of serum levels of thyroglobulin is central to long-term follow-up surveillance of patients with well-differentiated thyroid cancer. Following total thyroidectomy and radioiodine remnant ablation, the serum thyroglobulin level has a very high sensitivity and specificity for detection of tumor recurrence. This can be done while patients remain on thyroxine although, with a suppressed thyroid stimulating hormone, small remnants of tumor may not be detected. Sensitivity is significantly increased with an elevated thyroid-stimulating hormone level, achieved either by thyroxine withdrawal or recombinant thyroid-stimulating hormone-stimulation, although recombinant thyroid-stimulating hormone is not funded in Australia for this purpose. One significant additional factor which needs to be taken into account when assessing serum thyroglobulin levels is

Table 10.1 Surveillance after curative-intent treatment for well-differentiated thyroid carcinoma at Royal North Shore Hospital

	Years posttreatment					
	1	2	3	4	5	≥5
Office visit	2	1	1	1	1	1
Serum thyroglobulin and antithyroglobulin antibody levels	2[a]	1	1	1	1	1
Thyroid function tests	1	1	1	1	1	1
Cervical ultrasound scan	1	1	1	1	1	1
Radioiodine diagnostic whole body scan	1[b]	0	0	0	0	0

The number in each cell indicates the number of times a particular modality is recommended in a particular posttreatment year

[a]Unstimulated serum thyroglobulin level is measured at 6 months. Both stimulated and serum thyroglobulin levels are measured at 12 months

[b]If the radioactive iodine scan at 12 months is negative and the stimulated serum thyroglobulin level is <1 ng/mL, then long-term follow-up can consist of annual cervical ultrasound scan and unstimulated serum thyroglobulin level measurement

the presence of antithyroglobulin antibodies, which have been reported to occur in up to 25% of thyroid cancer patients [18]. In the presence of such antibodies, serum thyroglobulin measurement may fail to detect clinically significant tumor recurrence, even in patients with an elevated thyroid-stimulating hormone level. For this reason, antithyroglobulin antibodies should always be measured at the same time as measurement of serum thyroglobulin. Given the biological variation in these measurements, it is also preferable to measure both serum thyroglobulin and antithyroglobulin antibodies in the same laboratory using the same assay at each office visit. A progressively rising serum thyroglobulin level indicates subclinical disease [19]. The other reason that an elevated serum thyroglobulin level may not be detected in patients with clinically significant recurrent disease is that the tumor may have dedifferentiated and may no longer be producing thyroglobulin.

The timing of routine follow-up for well-differentiated thyroid cancer varies among published guidelines. Our own unit's practice for low-risk patients is summarized in Table 10.1. Low-risk patients are those who have had a total thyroidectomy and recombinant thyroid-stimulating hormone-stimulated radioiodine remnant ablation. The initial post-ablation diagnostic scan is likely to show uptake in the thyroid bed. At 6 months following initial treatment, the patient then has a clinical examination and an unstimulated thyroglobulin level is measured. If that is negative, then at 12 months a more intensive assessment is undertaken, including clinical examination, cervical ultrasound scan, whole body diagnostic radioiodine scan with thyroxine withdrawal, and measurement of the serum thyroglobulin level both on and off thyroxine. If these studies verify the absence of disease, then a program of long-term follow-up surveillance is instituted. This consists solely of yearly clinical examination, cervical ultrasound examination, and measurement of the unstimulated serum thyroglobulin level.

Long-term follow-up surveillance for patients with well-differentiated thyroid cancer who are at intermediate or high risk, or who were at low risk but who have subsequently demonstrated recurrent disease, follow the same overall principles but with varying recommendations, depending on the results of extent-of-disease investigations. Patients with a positive cervical ultrasound scan, or with clinical evidence of local disease recurrence, require assessment to determine resectability. If so, then surgery is the appropriate first-line therapy with consideration of subsequent radioiodine administration. If the cervical ultrasound scan is negative but the serum thyroglobulin level is >1 ng/mL, then a whole body diagnostic radioiodine scan is indicated, with subsequent ablation of any detectable disease. In a patient with a negative whole body scan but a rising thyroglobulin level, a chest CT (without contrast agent) may provide evidence of metastatic disease. Empirical radioiodine ablation could also be considered.

In addition to the foregoing investigations, the other important aspect of long-term follow-up surveillance of patients with well-differentiated thyroid cancer is to ensure appropriate levels of thyroxine suppression. This requires regular thyroid function tests, including serum thyroid-stimulating hormone and free serum T4 levels. There is good data that long-term thyroid-stimulating hormone suppression by thyroxine therapy is associated with a significant reduction in tumor recurrence risk [20]. There is, however, some controversy as to the degree of suppression needed. The American Thyroid Association guidelines [2] recommend that low-risk patients who are felt to be free of disease should have their thyroid-stimulating hormone kept within the low normal range (0.3–2 mU/L). High-risk patients who are clinically free of disease should have sufficient suppressive therapy to maintain levels in the range of 0.1–0.5 mU/L. Patients with persistent or recurrent disease should have a level >0.1 mU/L.

Table 10.2 Surveillance after curative-intent treatment for medullary thyroid carcinoma at Royal North Shore Hospital

	Years posttreatment				
	1	2	3	4	≥5
Office visit	2	1	1	1	1
Serum calcitonin level	2	1	1	1	1
[a]Cervical ultrasound scan	1	0	0	0	0

Additional imaging modalities such as CT, MRI, or PET scan are only indicated if the serum calcitonin level becomes detectable and rises in a patient with a negative cervical ultrasound examination

The number in each cell indicates the number of times a particular modality is recommended in a particular posttreatment year

[a]Baseline postoperative cervical ultrasound scan should be performed at 6 months. If clear, then long-term follow-up can consist of lifelong annual serum calcitonin measurement

There is no role for nonspecific tests such as blood counts, liver function tests, etc., in a patient without evidence of clinical disease. Imaging studies such as CT or MRI are limited to the delineation of suspected or known metastatic disease in the bone, lungs, or brain, as noted above.

The sole modalities for long-term follow-up of patients with medullary thyroid carcinoma are the office visit and measurement of the serum calcitonin level (Table 10.2). Serum carcinoembryonic antigen level is also raised in patients with medullary thyroid cancer but it is not as reliable a marker for surveillance. A patient who is disease-free following surgery has an undetectable calcitonin level. The presence of a detectable level following initial curative-intent surgery always indicates recurrent or persistent disease. The serum calcitonin level, as well as its rate of rise, correlates with tumor bulk [21]. A postoperative cervical ultrasound scan at 6 months provides useful baseline information. If the serum calcitonin level is undetectable, with no abnormality noted on the cervical sonogram, then long-term surveillance can consist solely of annual serum calcitonin measurement. There is no role for other imaging studies (CT, MRI, PET) as a screening tool. If the serum calcitonin level becomes detectable and continues to rise, targeted imaging should be undertaken. The cervical ultrasound examination detects recurrence in cervical lymph nodes. This is the most common site of recurrence. CT scans and MRI are useful for evaluating other sites. Positron emission tomography is also a sensitive imaging modality.

Given the already excellent prognosis of well-differentiated thyroid cancer, and the long-time frame for detection of recurrence over decades, it is unlikely that any multi-institutional prospective trials will ever be sufficiently powered to demonstrate significant improvements to current follow-up and treatment programs. There are no particular avenues for molecular biology approaches in long-term surveillance of patients thought to be disease-free, but targeted therapies for patients with otherwise untreatable metastatic follicular or medullary thyroid cancer appear to be feasible.

References

1. Greene F, Page D, Fleming I, et al. Thyroid tumors. In: Greene F, Page D, Fleming I, et al., editors. AJCC cancer staging manual. New York: Springer; 2002. p. 77–87.
2. Cooper DS, Doherty GM, Haugen BR, et al. Management guidelines for patients with thyroid nodules and differentiated thyroid cancer (American Thyroid Association). Thyroid. 2006;16:109–42.
3. Shah MD, Hall FT, Eski SJ, Witterick IJ, Walfish PG, Freeman JL. Clinical course of thyroid carcinoma after neck dissection. Laryngoscope. 2003;113:2102–7.
4. Sywak M, Cornford L, Roach P, Stalberg P, Sidhu S, Delbridge L. Routine ipsilateral level VI lymphadenectomy reduces postoperative thyroglobulin levels in papillary thyroid cancer. Surgery. 2006;140:1000–5.
5. Schlumberger M, Ricard M, De Pouvourville G, Pacini F. How the availability of recombinant human TSH has changed the management of patients who have thyroid cancer. Nat Clin Pract Endocrinol Metab. 2007;3:641–50.
6. Roman S, Mehta P, Sosa JA. Medullary thyroid cancer: early detection and novel treatments. Curr Opin Oncol. 2009;21:5–10.
7. Stavrou E, Baker D, McElroy H, Bishop J. Thyroid cancer in NSW. NSW Cancer Institute. Sydney, Australia: NSW Cancer Institute; 2008. p. 9–10.
8. Grodski S, Brown T, Sidhu S, Gill A, Robinson B, Learoyd D, Sywak M, Reeve T, Delbridge L. Increasing incidence of thyroid cancer is due to increased pathologic detection. Surgery. 2008;144:1038–43.
9. Perros P, Clarke SE, Franklyn J, et al. Guidelines for the management of thyroid cancer (British Thyroid Association). 2nd ed. Suffolk: Lavenham Press, Royal College of Physicians of London; 2007.
10. Hay ID, Grant CS, Bergstralh EJ, Thompson GB, van Heerden JA, Goellner JR. Unilateral total lobectomy: is it sufficient surgical treatment for patients with AMES low-risk papillary thyroid carcinoma? Surgery. 1998;124:958–64.
11. Mazzaferri EL, Robbins RJ, Spencer CA, et al. A consensus report on the role of serum thyroglobulin as a monitoring method for low-risk patients with papillary thyroid cancer. J Clin Endocrinol Metab. 2003;88:1433–41.
12. Lee L, Steward DL. Sonographically-directed neck dissection for recurrent thyroid carcinoma. Laryngoscope. 2008;118:991–4.
13. Pacini F, Schlumberger M, Dralle H, et al. European consensus for the management of patents with differentiated thyroid carcinoma of the follicular epithelium. Eur J Endocrinol. 2006;154:787–803.
14. Schlumberger M, Berg G, Cohen O, et al. Follow-up of low-risk patients with differentiated thyroid carcinoma: a European perspective. Eur J Endocrinol. 2004;150:105–12.

15. Pacini F, Capezzone M, Elisei R, et al. Diagnostic 131-iodine whole body scan may be avoided in thyroid cancer patients who have undetectable stimulated serum thyroglobulin after initial treatment. J Clin Endocrinol Metab. 2002;87:1499–501.
16. Pacini F, Molinaro E, Castagna MG. Recombinant human thyrotropin-stimulated serum thyroglobulin combined with neck ultrasonography has highest sensitivity in monitoring differentiated thyroid carcinoma. J Clin Endocrinol Metab. 2003;88:3668–73.
17. David A, Blotta A, Rossi R, et al. Clinical value of different responses of serum thyroglobulin in the follow-up of patients with differentiated thyroid carcinoma. Thyroid. 2005;15:267–73.
18. Spencer CA. Challenges of serum thyroglobulin (thyroglobulin) measurement in the presence of thyroglobulin autoantibodies. J Clin Endocrinol Metab. 2004;89:3702–4.
19. Baudin E, Do Czao C, Cailleux AF, et al. Positive predictive value of different responses of serum thyroglobulin to recombinant human thyrotropin in the follow-up of patients with differentiated thyroid carcinoma. J Clin Endocrinol Metab. 2003;88: 1107–11.
20. McGriff NJ, Csako G, Gourgiotos L, Lori CG, Pucino F, Sarlis NJ. Effects of thyroid hormone suppression therapy on adverse clinical outcomes in thyroid cancer. Ann Med. 2002;34:554–64.
21. Machens A, Schneyer U, Holzhausen H, Dralle H. Prospects of remission in medullary thyroid carcinoma according to basal calcitonin level. J Clin Endocrinol Metab. 2005;90:2029–34.

11 Thyroid (Papillary, Follicular, Medullary, Hürthle Cell) Carcinoma Surveillance Counterpoint: Japan

Ryuji Yasumatsu, Torahiko Nakashima, and Shizuo Komune

Keywords
Thyroid • Thyroidectomy • TG • Recurrence • Resection

Thyroid nodules are common but the rate of malignancy is only 4–5% [1, 2]. From 1975 to 2001, the incidence of thyroid cancer in Japan slightly and consistently increased, from 0.5 per 100,000 to 1.7 in men and from 2.1 per 100,000 to 5.9 in women [3]. A careful history is important because it can reveal information that immediately stratifies a patient into a high-risk category. High-risk factors include ionizing radiation to the neck during childhood [4], a history of benign goiter and thyroid nodules [5], and a family history of thyroid cancer. The risk of thyroid cancer in first-degree relatives of patients with differentiated thyroid cancer has been shown to be six times that of the general population [6].

Surgery is the primary treatment for differentiated papillary or follicular carcinoma and medullary carcinoma, and complete resection offers the best chance of cure. Surgical options have included nodulectomy, hemithyroidectomy, subtotal thyroidectomy, and total thyroidectomy. The high rate of recurrence associated with nodulectomy has confirmed that this approach is inadequate. Although there has been a trend toward more aggressive surgical resection, based on the well-documented multicentric nature of the disease, there are still some surgeons who insist that a partial thyroidectomy is sufficient for some patients. The AGES and the AMES classification systems are commonly used to classify patients into high-risk or low-risk groups. It has been suggested that low-risk patients can be managed with a thyroid lobectomy whereas high-risk patients are better managed with a total thyroidectomy. Most surgeons in Japan perform total thyroidectomy for high-risk patients. Controversy still exists for the low-risk patient group.

Suppression of thyrotropin (TSH) by administration of exogenous thyroid hormone has been reported to prevent recurrences after surgery and to result in temporary and occasionally permanent regression of metastatic well-differentiated papillary and follicular thyroid carcinoma [7]. In patients who have remaining functional thyroid tissue, thyroid hormone is administered for its TSH-suppressive effect.

The definitive diagnosis of follicular thyroid carcinoma can be made only by pathological examination of permanent sections. Once the diagnosis of follicular carcinoma has been confirmed, the decision to proceed with thyroidectomy, or to follow the patient, is based on a variety of factors, including risk-group analysis. Most Japanese surgeons agree that high-risk patients require a total thyroidectomy. Not only does a total thyroidectomy improve prognosis but it is also very helpful in surveillance by facilitating radioactive iodine-^{131}I administration and permitting thyroglobulin (TG) monitoring.

After total thyroidectomy, remnant ablation with ^{131}I is performed in patients <70 years of age to decrease the risk of recurrence in Kyushu University Hospital. The rate of a response of pulmonary metastasis to ^{131}I is related to the size of the lesion, the age of the patient, and the avidity of the lesion for ^{131}I. Bone metastases tend to be less responsive to ^{131}I.

Patients with thyroid cancer require long-term monitoring as thyroid cancer can recur many years after the initial treatment. For at least two decades after presentation, patients with thyroid cancer should undergo routine

R. Yasumatsu, M.D. (✉) • T. Nakashima, M.D. (✉) • S. Komune, M.D.
Department of Otorhinolaryngology, Graduate School of Medical Sciences, Kyushu University, 3-1-1 Maidashi, Higashi-ku, Fukuoka 812- 8582, Japan
e-mail: yasuryuj@qent.med.kyushu-u.ac.jp; nakatora@qent.med.kyushu-u.ac.jp; komu@qent.med.kyushu-u.ac.jp

F.E. Johnson et al. (eds.), *Patient Surveillance After Cancer Treatment*, Current Clinical Oncology,
DOI 10.1007/978-1-60327-969-7_11,

Table 11.1 Follow-up of patients with well-differentiated thyroid cancer: Department of Otorhinolaryngology, Head and Neck Surgery, Kyushu University Hospital

	Years posttreatment					
	1	2	3	4	5	>5
Office visit	4	4	2	1	1	1
Serum TSH level and antithyroglobulin antibody level	2	2	1	1	1	1
RAI scan or FDG-PET CT scan[a]	1	1	1	1	1	1
Periodic neck ultrasound sonography	2	2	1	1	1	1

The numbers in each cell indicate the number of times a particular modality is recommended during a particular posttreatment year

[a] *RAI* radioactive iodine

physical examination, thyroid function tests, and serum tumor marker level determinations (thyroglobulin for patients with well-differentiated papillary or follicular carcinoma and calcitonin for patients with medullary carcinoma). The schedule of follow-up is shown in Table 11.1. Occasionally, patients with diffuse pulmonary metastases or with early locoregional recurrence have tumors too small or too inaccessible to be detected on routine chest X-ray or by clinical examination. ^{131}I scan and FDG-PET CT scan are useful in monitoring patients at high risk of developing recurrence. FDG-PET CT is used primarily in the setting of non-iodine-avid tumors. The role of FDG-PET CT in the postoperative surveillance of differentiated thyroid carcinoma is in large part related to the inverse relationship between 18F fluorodeoxyglucose avidity of the tumor and its ability to concentrate iodine [8]. These scans are done annually until the tenth year. At each follow-up visit, examination of the neck is performed. Thyroid hormone and TSH levels are monitored to ensure that the proper dose of thyroid hormone is being prescribed and that adequate suppression has been achieved. After total thyroidectomy has been performed for differentiated cancer, the thyroglobulin (TG) level is the most predictive marker for tumor presence. A rising serum TG level suggests recurrent cancer in patients who received ablative or therapeutic doses of ^{131}I or in those who are fully suppressed on thyroid hormone therapy [9]. It has been reported that the elevation of serum TG is highly sensitive (97%) and specific (100%) for thyroid cancer recurrence [10]. When there is evidence of recurrence, examination of neck using ultrasonography, contrast-enhanced CT, and FDG-PET CT scan are performed. An undetectable TG level in a patient with papillary carcinoma who is on thyroid hormone therapy may be falsely negative but it has been shown to have a very low false-negative rate in patients with follicular carcinoma. TG is being used in some studies to identify proper suppressive doses of thyroid hormone in patients with thyroid cancer.

References

1. Lin JD, Chao TC, Huang BY, Chen ST, Chang HY, Hsueh C. Thyroid cancer in the thyroid nodules evaluated by ultrasonography and fine-needle aspiration cytology. Thyroid. 2005;15(7):708–17.
2. Rojeski MT, Gharib H. Nodular thyroid disease. Evaluation and management. N Engl J Med. 1985;313(7):428–36.
3. Center for Cancer Control and Information Services, National Cancer Center. Cancer incidence (1975–2001). Center for Cancer Control and Information Services, National Cancer Center, Japan; 2006.
4. Cardis E, Kesminiene A, Ivanov V, et al. Risk of thyroid cancer after exposure to 131I in childhood. J Natl Cancer Inst. 2005;97(10): 724–32.
5. Franceschi S, Preston-Martin S, Dal Maso L, et al. A pooled analysis of case-control studies of thyroid cancer. IV. Benign thyroid diseases. Cancer Causes Control. 1999;10(6):583–95.
6. Handkiewcz-Junak D, Banasik T, Kolosza Z, et al. Risk of malignant tumors in first-degree relatives of patients with differentiated thyroid cancer—a hospital based study. Neoplasma. 2006;53(1):67–72.
7. Crile Jr G. Treatment of carcinomas of the thyroid. In: Young S, Inman DR, editors. Thyroid neoplasia. London, UK: Academic; 1968. p. 39–50.
8. Lazar V, Bidart JM, Caillou B, et al. Expression of the Na+/I- symporter gene in human thyroid tumors: a comparison study with other thyroid-specific genes. J Clin Endocrinol Metab. 1999;84(9): 3228–34.
9. Ozata M, Suzuki S, Miyamoto T, Liu RT, Fierro-Renoy F, DeGroot LJ. Serum thyroglobulin in the follow-up of patients with treated differentiated thyroid cancer. J Clin Endocrinol Metab. 1994;79(1): 98–105.
10. van Sorge-van Boxtel RA, van Eck-Smit BL, Goslings BM. Comparison of serum thyroglobulin, 131I and 201Tl scintigraphy in the postoperative follow-up of differentiated thyroid cancer. Nucl Med Commun. 1993;14(5):365–72.

Lung Carcinoma

12

Shilpi Wadhwa, David Y. Johnson, and Frank E. Johnson

Keywords
Lung cancer • Guidelines • Smoking • Death rates • Pollution

The International Agency for Research on Cancer (IARC), a component of the World Health Organization (WHO), estimated that there were 1,352,132 new cases of lung carcinoma worldwide in 2002 [1]. The IARC also estimated that there were 1,178,918 deaths due to this cause in 2002 [1].

The American Cancer Society estimated that there were 213,380 new cases and 160,390 deaths due to this cause in the USA in 2007 [2]. The estimated 5-year survival rates (all races) in the USA in 2007 was 16 % for lung and bronchial carcinoma [2]. Survival rates were adjusted for normal life expectancies and were based on cases diagnosed from 1996 to 2002 and followed through 2003.

The dominant cause of lung carcinoma is tobacco smoking, including passive or second-hand smoking. The incidence in males is higher than in females, generally by at least twofold, but this is largely due to the higher prevalence of smoking in men. Occupational exposure to arsenic, asbestos, silica, chromium, and several organic chemicals is an important cause [3]. Ionizing radiation, arising from products of atomic bomb blasts, diagnostic and therapeutic medical radiation, radon gas and its daughter products, and other sources, is an important cause [3]. Chemicals in air pollution, particularly polycyclic aromatic hydrocarbons, are well-documented causative agents [3]. Various chronic benign lung disorders, such as tuberculosis, increase the risk as well. The genetic causes of lung cancer are undoubtedly multiple [4] and many more will presumably be detected in the near future.

S. Wadhwa • D.Y. Johnson
Department of Internal Medicine, Saint Louis University Medical Center, Saint Louis, MO, USA
e-mail: shilpi_wadhwa@unc.edu; swadhwa@gmail.com; mini.mermaid@gmail.com; dyjohnson@gmail.com

F.E. Johnson, M.D., FACS (✉)
Saint Louis University Medical Center and Saint Louis Veterans Affairs Medical Center, Saint Louis, MO, USA
e-mail: frank.johnson1@va.gov

Geographic Variation Worldwide

Lung cancer is the only major cancer with equal incidence in both developed and developing countries [5]. However, trends in lung cancer death rates vary widely among countries, according to the stage of the tobacco epidemic. In Eastern and Southern Europe, where tobacco use is still increasing, death rates have climbed in men, and are now rising in women [5]. In men, lung cancer remains the dominant cancer in large parts of Europe, Cuba, Asian countries, such as Pakistan, China, Russia, North Korea, and Mongolia, parts of the African subcontinent such as Morocco, Algeria, and Tunisia, and South American countries, particularly Argentina and Uruguay [5]. Geographic variation in the USA is also pronounced [6].

Surveillance Strategies Proposed by Professional Organizations or National Government Agencies and Available on the Internet

National Comprehensive Cancer Network (www.nccn.org)

National Comprehensive Cancer Network (NCCN) guidelines were accessed on 1/28/12 (Tables 12.1 and 12.2). There were minor quantitative and qualitative changes compared to the guidelines accessed on 4/10/07.

F.E. Johnson et al. (eds.), *Patient Surveillance After Cancer Treatment*, Current Clinical Oncology,
DOI 10.1007/978-1-60327-969-7_12, © Springer Science+Business Media New York 2013

Table 12.1 Non-small cell lung cancer

	Years posttreatment[a]					
	1	2	3	4	5	>5
Office visit	1–2	1–2	1	1	1	1
Chest CT[b]	1–2	1–2	1	1	1	1
• Smoking cessation advice, counseling, and pharmacotherapy						
• PET or brain MRI is not indicated for routine follow-up						

Obtained from NCCN (www.nccn.org) on 1/28/12

NCCN guidelines were accessed on 1/28/12. There were minor quantitative and qualitative changes compared to the guidelines accessed on 4/10/07

[a]The numbers in the table indicate the number of times the modality is recommended during the indicated year posttreatment

[b]Chest CT ± contrast for 2 years, non-contrast-enhanced chest CT thereafter

Table 12.2 Small cell lung cancer

	Years posttreatment[a]					
	1	2	3	4	5	>5
Office visit	3–4	3–4	2	2	2	1
• At every office visit: H&P, chest imaging, bloodwork as clinically indicated						
• New pulmonary nodule should initiate workup for potential new primary						
• Smoking cessation intervention						
• PET/CT is not recommended for routine follow-up						

Obtained from NCCN (www.nccn.org) on 1/28/12

NCCN guidelines were accessed on 1/28/12. There were minor quantitative and qualitative changes compared to the guidelines accessed on 4/10/07

[a]The numbers in the table indicate the number of times the modality is recommended during the indicated year posttreatment

American Society of Clinical Oncology (www.asco.org)

American Society of Clinical Oncology (ASCO) guidelines were accessed on 1/28/12. No quantitative guidelines exist for lung cancer surveillance, although they did exist when first accessed on 10/31/07.

The Society of Surgical Oncology (www.surgonc.org)

The Society of Surgical Oncology (SSO) guidelines were accessed on 1/28/12. No quantitative guidelines exist for lung cancer surveillance, including when first accessed on 10/31/07.

European Society for Medical Oncology (www.esmo.org)

European Society for Medical Oncology (ESMO) guidelines were accessed on 1/28/12 (Table 12.3). There were major quantitative and qualitative changes compared to the guidelines accessed on 10/31/07.

European Society of Surgical Oncology (www.esso-surgeonline.org)

European Society of Surgical Oncology (ESSO) guidelines were accessed on 1/28/12. No quantitative guidelines exist for lung cancer surveillance, including when first accessed on 10/31/07.

Cancer Care Ontario (CCO, www.cancercare.on.ca)

SSO guidelines were accessed on 1/28/12. No quantitative guidelines exist for lung cancer surveillance, including when first accessed on 10/31/07.

National Institute for Clinical Excellence (www.nice.org.uk)

National Institute for Clinical Excellence (NICE) guidelines were accessed on 1/28/12. No quantitative guidelines exist for lung cancer surveillance, although they did exist when first accessed on 10/31/07.

Table 12.3 Early stage and locally advanced (non-metastatic) non-small-cell lung cancer

	Years posttreatment[a]					
	1	2	3	4	5	>5
Office visit	2	2	1	1	1	1
CT scan	2	2	1	1	1	1

- Treatment complications related to surgery, adjuvant chemotherapy, or radiotherapy should be carefully evaluated for a frame time of 3–6 months
- PET/CT is not recommended
- Patients treated with curative intent should be encouraged and sustained in programs to quit smoking

Obtained from ESMO (www.esmo.org) on 1/28/12

ESMO guidelines were accessed on 1/28/12. There were major quantitative and qualitative changes compared to the guidelines accessed on 10/31/07

[a]The numbers in the table indicate the number of times the modality is recommended during the indicated year posttreatment

Table 12.4 Lung cancer

	Years posttreatment[a]					
	1	2	3	4	5	>5
Office visit	2	2	1	1	1	1
Chest X-ray or CT Scan	2	2	1	1	1	1

- Surveillance for complications related to the curative-intent therapy should be managed by the appropriate specialist and should probably last at least 3–6 months
- All patients should be counseled on symptom recognition and be advised to contact their physician if worrisome symptoms are recognized
- Use of blood tests, PET scanning, sputum cytology, tumor markers, and fluorescence bronchoscopy is not currently recommended for surveillance
- Patients who smoke should be strongly encouraged to stop smoking, and offered pharmacotherapeutic and behavioral therapy, including follow-up

Obtained from ACCP (www.chestjournal.org) on 1/28/12

ACCP guidelines were accessed on 1/28/12. There were no significant changes compared to the guidelines accessed on 10/31/07

[a]The numbers in the table indicate the number of times the modality is recommended during the indicated year posttreatment

The Cochrane Collaboration (CC, www.cochrane.org)

CC guidelines were accessed on 1/28/12. No quantitative guidelines exist for lung cancer surveillance, including when first accessed on 11/24/07.

The American College of Chest Physicians (www.chestjournal.org)

The American College of Chest Physicians (ACCP) guidelines were accessed on 1/28/12 (Table 12.4). There were no significant changes compared to the guidelines accessed on 10/31/07.

The M.D. Anderson Surgical Oncology Handbook also has follow-up guidelines, proposed by authors from a single National Cancer Institute-designated Comprehensive Cancer Center, for many types of cancer [7]. Some are detailed and quantitative, others are qualitative.

Summary

This is a common cancer with significant variability in incidence worldwide. We found consensus-based guidelines but none based on high-quality evidence.

References

1. Parkin DM, Whelan SL, Ferlay J, Teppo L, Thomas DB. Cancer incidence in five continents, Vol. VIII, International Agency for Research on Cancer. (IARC Scientific Publication 155). Lyon, France: IARC Press; 2002. ISBN 92-832-2155-9.
2. Jemal A, Seigel R, Ward E, Murray T, Xu J, Thun MJ. Cancer statistics, 2007. CA Cancer J Clin. 2007;57:43–66.
3. Schottenfeld D, Fraumeni JG. Cancer epidemiology and prevention. 3rd ed. New York, NY: Oxford University Press; 2006. ISBN 13:978-0-19-514961-6.
4. DeVita VT, Hellman S, Rosenberg SA. Cancer. 7th ed. Philadelphia, PA: Lippincott Williams & Wilkins; 2005. ISBN 0-781-74450-4.
5. Mackay J, Jemal A, Lee NC, Parkin M. The Cancer Atlas. 2006 American Cancer Society 1599 Clifton Road NE, Atlanta, Georgia 30329, USA. Can also be accessed at www.cancer.org. ISBN 0-944235-62-X.

6. Devesa SS, Grauman DJ, Blot WJ, Pennello GA, Hoover RN, Fraumeni JF Jr. Atlas of Cancer Mortality in the United States. National Institutes of Health, National Cancer Institute. NIH Publication No. 99-4564; Sep 1999.
7. Feig BW, Berger DH, Fuhrman GM. The M.D. Anderson Surgical Oncology Handbook. 4th ed. Philadelphia, PA: Lippincott Williams & Wilkins; 2006. ISBN 0-7817-5643-X (paperback).

Lung Carcinoma Surveillance Counterpoint: Australia

13

Michael Boyer and Kate Mahon

Keywords
Lung carcinoma • NSCLC • SCLC • Tumors • Therapy

Lung carcinoma is the most common cancer worldwide, accounting for 12% of all new cancer diagnoses [1]. It remains the leading cause of cancer-specific mortality, responsible for 18% of cancer deaths internationally [1] and 19% in Australia [2]. Following potentially curative therapy for lung cancer, patients remain at high risk of recurrence and second malignancy. Despite this, posttreatment surveillance remains poorly defined and controversial.

Non-small cell lung cancer (NSCLC) comprises around 85% of lung cancer diagnoses. The most common pathological variants included in this group are adenocarcinoma, squamous cell carcinoma, and large cell carcinoma, though rare forms, such as adenosquamous carcinoma and those with sarcomatoid differentiation, are also seen.

Treatment options and prognosis are dependent on the stage of disease at diagnosis as well as pulmonary function and comorbid conditions. Following intended curative resection of stage I disease, reported 5-year survival rates are around 60% with a 10% risk of local recurrence. Even for early stage disease, distant recurrence rates are relatively high at 15% (stage IA, T1N0M0) and 30% (stage IB T2N0M0). Stage IIIA disease, following surgery alone, has a 5-year survival rate of 25%, local recurrence rate of 15%, and a high likelihood of distant metastatic relapse (60%) [3]. The recent addition of adjuvant chemotherapy in patients with stages II and III disease has improved long-term survival by 4–15%, predominantly by reducing the risk of distant relapse [3]. In inoperable stage III disease following definitive concurrent chemoradiotherapy, 3-year survival rates are around 15–30% [4, 5].

Surveillance after potentially curative therapy for NSCLC is aimed at detecting posttreatment complications, recurrence of disease and new primary malignancies. Postthoracotomy complications include hospital readmission, loss of lung function, and pain. Up to 20% of patients require readmission to hospital within 3 months of surgery, predominantly for respiratory and infectious complications [6]. Loss of lung function may also be clinically significant with an average reduction in FEV1 of 10–15% following lobectomy and 25–35% following pneumonectomy. In up to 60% of postpneumonectomy patients, exercise is limited by dyspnea [7]. Postthoracotomy pain is common, occurring in 55% of patients over a year following surgery. Pain may be disabling, with 10% of patients requiring significant intervention, including narcotic analgesia or nerve blocks [8]. Following thoracic radiotherapy, complications include pulmonary toxicity and injury to surrounding structures such as esophagus, heart, spinal cord, and skin. Acute radiation pneumonitis may occur in up to 50% of patients, but severe pneumonitis is less common (13%) [9]. Pneumonitis usually occurs within 3 months of treatment and often presents with cough and dyspnea. It may be steroid responsive. Irreversible pulmonary fibrosis complicates curative-intent radiotherapy in approximately 8% of patients, presenting up to 2 years after treatment [10]. Chemotherapy-related complications tend to occur during treatment. Peripheral neuropathy is the predominant long-term complication seen in this population due to the use of platinum-containing vinca alkaloid and taxane compounds. Consensus recommendations advise surveillance for posttreatment complications for at least 3–6 months following completion of therapy [11].

M. Boyer, MBBS, PhD, FRACP(✉) • K. Mahon, BSc, MBBS, FRACP
Department of Medical Oncology, Sydney Cancer Centre,
Royal Prince Alfred Hospital, Missenden Road, Camperdown,
NSW 2050, Australia
e-mail: michael.boyer@lifehouserpa.org.au; drkatemahon@gmail.com; k.mahon@garvan.org.au

F.E. Johnson et al. (eds.), *Patient Surveillance After Cancer Treatment*, Current Clinical Oncology,
DOI 10.1007/978-1-60327-969-7_13,

Table 13.1 Surveillance after curative-intent primary therapy for TNM stage I, II, and IIIA non-small cell lung carcinoma at the Sydney Cancer Centre

	Year posttreatment					
Modality	1	2	3	4	5	>5
Office visit	4	2	2	1	1	1
CXR	2	2	1	1	1	1
CT chest and upper abdomen	1	0	0	0	0	0

The number in each cell is the number of times a particular modality is recommended in a particular posttreatment year

Table 13.2 Surveillance after curative-intent primary therapy for TNM stage IIIB non-small cell lung carcinoma at the Sydney Cancer Centre

	Years posttreatment					
Modality	1	2	3	4	5	>5
Office visit	4	2	2	1	1	1
CXR	2	1	1	1	1	1
CT chest and upper abdomen	1	0	0	0	0	0

The number in each cell is the number of times a particular modality is recommended in a particular posttreatment year

Table 13.3 Surveillance after curative-intent primary therapy for small-cell lung carcinoma (limited stage) at the Sydney Cancer Centre

	Years posttreatment					
Modality	1	2	3	4	5	>5
Office visit	4	3	2	1	1	1
CXR	2	1	1	1	1	1
CT chest and upper abdomen	1	0	0	0	0	0

The number in each cell is the number of times a particular modality is recommended in a particular posttreatment year

Most recurrences of NSCLC are extrathoracic [3]. Treatment of distant metastases remains palliative in intent. Early detection while the patient remains asymptomatic does not alter outcome. Therefore, strategies to search for systemic recurrence are not recommended. The risk of locoregional recurrence is highest up to 2 years following initial treatment and our surveillance strategy reflects this. However, local recurrence is infrequently amenable to curative surgery [12, 13]. Treatment most commonly involves radiotherapy and/or chemotherapy. Survival rates are poor. Following treatment for locoregional recurrence, 1 year disease-free survival probability approaches 20% [13]. Surveillance for recurrence using positron emission tomography (PET) scans has been investigated. While the sensitivity is high (96%), false positives are often seen. Interpretation of posttreatment PET scans is often difficult, particularly in the first 6 months, due to inflammation at the surgical site, radiation pneumonitis, and uptake in the non-irradiated pleura [14]. As it is unlikely to change outcomes for recurrent disease, routine PET scanning for surveillance is not recommended [11].

The risk of developing a new primary malignancy, particularly of the aerodigestive tract, is high following curative-intent treatment for NSCLC. The risk of a new primary lung cancer is estimated at 1–2% per patient per year. There is a suggestion that this risk increases with time and imparts a cumulative risk of 13–20% at 8 years following treatment [15]. The median survival duration of patients diagnosed with a second primary lung cancer is only 1–2 years with a 5-year survival probability on the order of 20%. This reflects the fact that half of all second primary lung malignancies are deemed unresectable, in most cases due to poor pulmonary reserve or extent of disease [15]. For those with resectable disease, surgery is less successful than with the initial lung cancer with 5-year survival probability in several series ranging from 25 to 53% [11]. As curative resection may be an option for new primary lung cancers diagnosed at an early stage, surveillance strategies have been primarily aimed at detecting these.

While many studies investigating surveillance schedules have been published, there is no evidence based on randomized trials to guide management. A retrospective study of

358 patients who underwent complete resection of NSCLC examined the difference in outcomes according to symptom status at diagnosis of a recurrence or new primary malignancy [16]. These patients had follow-up on various undefined schedules. While a quarter of patients were diagnosed with asymptomatic disease, only one-third of these were later treated with curative intent. Asymptomatic patients were diagnosed earlier, with a 9-month lead time bias. However, on multivariate analysis there was no difference in overall survival duration or mode of treatment, with 70% of patients in both groups being treated with palliative intent. Another retrospective study of 130 patients compared a strict surveillance schedule (clinic visits and CXR every 2–3 months, thoracic and upper abdominal CT scans every 6 months, liver function tests yearly) vs. a symptom-led regimen (maximum of three clinic visits per year with investigations for symptoms only) [17]. There was no difference in survival duration from diagnosis of recurrence (median survival 7 months). However, more patients on the symptom led regimen were diagnosed in the emergency department and required inpatient treatment. Even allowing for this, the cost analysis revealed that the strict regimen was twice as expensive as the symptom-led regimen. This study also highlighted the poor outcome after recurrence of lung cancer, with a 2-year overall survival probability of 9%. The authors concluded that regular clinic visits and CXRs are an appropriate compromise.

In a prospective study, 563 completely resected lung cancer patients on a specific surveillance schedule were followed for 10 years [18]. The surveillance involved four clinic visits and chest X-rays over the first 2 years. This decreased to twice a year for the following 3 years and then annually until year 10. Recurrence or new primary malignancy was diagnosed in 239 patients, but only 23 of these went on to have a further curative-intent resection. Twenty-one of the resected group had metachronous tumors and two had recurrent local disease. Most patients (over 70%) with recurrent or new primary disease were diagnosed in the first 2 years; 93% were diagnosed within 5 years. The authors suggested that outcomes would not be significantly different if surveillance was reduced to clinic visits and CXR every 6 months for the first 5 years. In another prospective trial, 192 patients had an intensive surveillance schedule of clinic visits and CXR every 3 months in conjunction with chest CT scans and bronchoscopies every 6 months for 3 years [19]. The frequency of these investigations was then halved until year 7. There were 136 recurrences, 35 of which were asymptomatic and detected by a scheduled investigation. Around one-third were identified by each investigation modality (physical examination+CXR, CT, or bronchoscopy). Eighty percent of the asymptomatic recurrences were intrathoracic and almost half underwent curative-intent treatment (compared with only 21% of the whole recurrent group). In the asymptomatic group, 3-year survival probability (from detection of recurrence) was impressive at 31%. However, this study has been criticized because of lead time bias [11]. A randomized trial is now underway to compare this surveillance strategy with a less intense schedule. Until there is evidence from a well-controlled trial to suggest that an intensive surveillance program improves survival or quality of life it should not be considered standard practice.

Recent evidence from population-based screening studies of people at increased risk of lung cancer suggests that low-dose helical CT scanning detects lung malignancy at earlier stages than CXR. The Early Lung Cancer Action Project compared CXR and helical CT surveillance. Of 1,000 people, CT detected malignancy in 27 while CXR identified only 7 of these [20]. It has been suggested that helical CT scans may detect up to 85% of stage I lung malignancies. While the cost of this improved sensitivity is higher radiation exposure, low-dose spiral CT scans provide 1/16th of the radiation dose of a conventional CT scan or tenfold of that of a CXR [21]. While helical CT scanning may be useful in surveillance of patients following curative treatment for lung cancer in the future, its use for this purpose remains investigational at present.

Small-cell lung carcinoma (SCLC) comprises about 15% of lung cancer diagnoses. It has a dismal prognosis with a 7% 2-year overall survival probability [15]. Around 40% of patients present with limited disease, making concurrent chemoradiotherapy a treatment option [22]. The disease initially responds well to chemotherapy and radiotherapy (with response rates over 80%) but it recurs very frequently. The median survival duration with limited stage SCLC following concurrent chemoradiotherapy is up to 20 months with 5-year survival probability around 15% [23]. Recurrent SCLC has limited treatment options and a very poor prognosis.

For patients who survive over 2 years from the diagnosis of lung cancer, the risk of a new primary lung cancer is significant. The average risk of a new cancer is 6% per patient per year (pt/yr). This risk increases from 2% pt/yr initially to 10% pt/yr at 10 years. This represents a cumulative second malignancy risk of 30% at 12 years after treatment. This risk is significantly reduced by smoking cessation with a fourfold reduction in relative risk in those who quit smoking at initial diagnosis. Seventy percent of metachronous lung cancers following SCLC are squamous cell carcinomas and less than 20% are deemed resectable [15]. Due to small numbers of such patients, there is minimal data on survival following resection of second primary tumors after small cell lung cancer.

There are no comparative studies of surveillance strategies following SCLC and current practice is not well documented. In view of the high risk of second malignancies, a surveillance strategy to detect new primary lung cancers in patients who have survived SCLC is reasonable.

References

1. Ferlay JBF, Pisani P, Parkin DM. GLOBOCAN 2002. Cancer incidence, mortality and prevalence worldwide. IARC CancerBase No.5, Version 2.0. Lyon: IARC Press; 2004.
2. Tracey E, Baker D, Bishop J, et al. Cancer in New South Wales: incidence, mortality and prevalence report 2005. Sydney: Cancer Institute NSW; 2007.
3. Pisters KMW, Le Chevalier T. Adjuvant chemotherapy in completely resected non-small-cell lung cancer. J Clin Oncol. 2005;23:3270–8.
4. Gandara DR, Chansky K, Albain KS, et al. Consolidation docetaxel after concurrent chemoradiotherapy in stage IIIB non-small-cell lung cancer. Phase II Southwest Oncology Group Study S9504. J Clin Oncol. 2003;21:2004–10.
5. Bedano PM, Neubauer M, Ansari R, et al. Phase III study of cisplatin plus etoposide with concurrent chest radiation followed by docetaxel vs. observation in patients with stage III non-small cell lung cancer: an interim toxicity analysis of consolidation therapy. J Clin Oncol. 2006;24:374s (suppl; abstr 7043).
6. Handy JR, Child AI, Grunkemeier GL, et al. Hospital readmission after pulmonary resection: prevalence, patterns, and predisposing characteristics. Ann Thorac Surg. 2001;72:1855–9.
7. Nezu K, Kushibe K, Tojo T, et al. Recovery and limitation of exercise capacity after lung resection for lung cancer. Chest. 1998; 113:1511–6.
8. Dajczman E, Gordon A, Kreisman H, et al. Long term post-thoracotomy pain. Chest. 1991;99:270–4.
9. Inoue A, Kunitoh H, Sekine I. Radiation pneumonitis in lung cancer patients. Int J Radiat Oncol Biol Phys. 2001;49:649–55.
10. Cox JD, Azarnia N, Byhardt RW. A randomized phase I/II trial of hyperfractionated radiation therapy with total doses of 60.0 Gy to 79.2 Gy. J Clin Oncol. 1990;8:1543–55.
11. Rubins J, Unger M, Colice G. Follow-up and surveillance of the lung cancer patient following curative intent therapy. Chest. 2007;132:355S–67.
12. Martini N, Bains MS, Burt ME, et al. Incidence of local recurrence and second primary tumours in resected stage I lung cancer. J Thorac Cardiovasc Surg. 1995;109:120–9.
13. Lamont JP, Kakuda JT, Smith D, et al. Systematic postoperative radiologic follow-up in patients with non-small cell lung cancer for detecting second primary lung cancer in stage IA. Arch Surg. 2002;137:935–8.
14. Inoue T, Kim EE, Komaki R, et al. Detecting recurrent or residual lung cancer with FDG-PET. J Nucl Med. 1995;36:788–93.
15. Johnson BE. Second lung cancers in patients after treatment for an initial lung cancer. J Nat Cancer Inst. 1998;90:1335–45.
16. Walsh GL, O'Connor M, Willis KM, et al. Is follow-up of lung cancer patients after resection medically indicated and cost-effective? Ann Thorac Surg. 1995;60:1563–70.
17. Younes RN, Gross JL, Deheinzelin D. Follow-up in lung cancer. How often and for what purpose? Chest. 1999;115:1494–9.
18. Egermann U, Jaeggi K, Habicht JM, et al. Regular follow-up after curative resection of non-small cell lung cancer: a real benefit for patients? Eur Respir J. 2002;19:464–8.
19. Westeel V, Choma D, Clement F, et al. Relevance of an intensive postoperative follow-up after surgery for non-small cell lung cancer. Ann Thorac Surg. 2000;70:1185–90.
20. Porter JC, Spiro SG. Detection of early lung cancer. Thorax. 2000;55:S56–62.
21. Kaneko M, Eguchi K, Ohmatsu H, et al. Peripheral lung cancer: screening and detection with low-dose spiral CT versus radiography. Radiology. 1996;201:798–802.
22. Govindan R, Page N, Morgensztern D, et al. Changing epidemiology of small-cell lung cancer in the United States over the last 30 years: analysis of the surveillance, epidemiologic, and end results database. J Clin Oncol. 2006;24:4539–44.
23. Socinski MA, Bogart JA. Limited-stage small-cell lung cancer: the current status of combined-modality therapy. J Clin Oncol. 2007;25:4137–45.

Lung Carcinoma Surveillance Counterpoint: Japan

14

Tokujiro Yano and Yoshihiko Maehara

Keywords

Non-small cell lung cancer • Japan • Local recurrence • Postoperative adjuvant chemotherapy • Never smokers

Introduction

In Japan, primary lung cancer has been the leading cause of cancer death since 1998, and is still increasing both in prevalence and mortality. In 2006, the number of deaths due to primary lung cancer was approximately 63,000, including 46,000 males and 17,000 females in Japan. Despite the progress of both radiotherapy and chemotherapy, surgical resection remains the first choice of treatment for locally limited (stage I to IIIA) non-small cell lung cancer (NSCLC). Although the surgical results for NSCLC have improved, it is mostly attributed to improvements in diagnostic techniques and early detection of the disease. In fact, the prognosis of patients with locally advanced stages (II or IIIA) is still not satisfactory, even if a complete resection can be performed. According to the current Japanese registry database, the 5-year-survival rate after complete resection is 83.3% for IA disease, 66.4% for IB, 60.1% for IIA, 47.2% for IIB, and 32.8% for IIIA [1]. In order to improve the surgical results, both efficient postoperative surveillance and adjuvant chemotherapy are necessary.

The clinical guidelines for primary lung cancer from the Japan Lung Cancer Society do not recommend postoperative surveillance after a complete resection of NSCLC, based on the lack of worldwide evidence for its survival benefit. However, in Japan, periodical surveillance is conducted with various imaging modalities for several reasons. First, regardless of whether postoperative surveillance yields a survival benefit, the cost of periodical surveillance including both hematological and imaging examinations is mostly covered by the public insurance in Japan. Second, the earlier detection of recurrence is believed to result in better prognosis by both most patients and some thoracic surgeons. Third, most importantly, there is no active evidence to break off the practice of periodical surveillance after a complete resection of NSCLC. Therefore, periodical postoperative follow-up, including tumor marker tests (CEA, CYFRA) and imaging examinations, as shown in Table 14.1 is routinely conducted following resection of NSCLC.

Even after a complete resection of NSCLC, postoperative recurrence occurs in about 45% of the patients [2]. Information on the first recurrent site is useful for an efficient postoperative follow-up. The mode of recurrence dose not differ among pathologic stages of the disease at surgery. The recurrent site is distant organs in 73.4%, locoregional sites in 19.0%, and combined sites in 7.6% [3]. The common sites of distant metastasis are the brain, bone, and lung. Recently, both brain magnetic resonance imaging (MRI) and whole body positron emission tomography (PET) are used for meticulous preoperative screening. Consequently, the incidence of distant metastasis after surgery has decreased due to the accurate preoperative staging and proper selection of surgical patients, and thus the incidence of distant metastasis seems to be similar to that of local recurrence.

Postoperative pulmonary metastasis is more prevalent in patients with pN2 disease than in those with pN0 disease,

T. Yano, MD (✉)
Department of Surgery, Beppu Medical Center, Uchikamado 1473, Beppu Japan
e-mail: tokujiro@beppu.hosp.go.jp

Y. Maehara, MD
Department of Surgery and Science, Graduate School of Medical Sciences, Kyushu University, Maidashi 3-1-1, Higashi-ku, Fukuoka, Japan

F.E. Johnson et al. (eds.), *Patient Surveillance After Cancer Treatment*, Current Clinical Oncology, DOI 10.1007/978-1-60327-969-7_14,

Table 14.1 Surveillance of patients with completely resected non-small cell lung cancer

	Years after operation				
	1	2	3	4	5
Office visit	4	4	2–3	2–3	2–3
Complete blood count	4	4	2–3	2–3	2–3
Blood chemistry[a]	4	4	2–3	2–3	2–3
Serum tumor marker levels[b]	4	4	2–3	2–3	2–3
Chest X-ray	3	3	2–3	2–3	1–2
Chest and upper abdominal CT[c]	1	1	0	0	1
Bone scintigraphy	1	1	0	0	1

The number in each cell indicates the number of times a particular modality is recommended in a particular post-treatment year

[a] Blood chemistry includes serum levels of total protein, albumin, total bilirubin, asparatate aminotransferase, alanine, lactate dehydrogenase, alkaline phosphatase, creatinine, plus blood urea nitrogen.

[b] *CEA* (carcinoembryonic antigen); *CYFRA* (cytokeratin fragments)

[c] *CT* computed tomography

because of the presence of drainage routes from the N2 nodes (superior mediastinal lymph nodes) into the superior vena cava [3]. It is important to differentiate pulmonary lesions appearing after surgery into hematogenous distant metastasis, locoregional recurrence at the surgical margin, or second primary carcinoma. Recurrence at the surgical margin is more frequent in a limited operation such as a wedge resection or segmentectomy than a standard lobectomy [4]. From an anatomic aspect, the lungs would not likely be the first site of hematogenous metastasis in patients with pN0 disease. On the other hand, pulmonary metastasis is prevalent in patients with pN2 disease. Accordingly, when a new solitary lesion develops in the residual lung after a standard operation, then pulmonary metastasis is suspected in patients with pN2 disease and a second primary cancer is suspected in patients with pN0 disease [3]. Serial imaging examinations, including plain chest X-ray and computed tomography are helpful to determine the strategy for treatment of newly appearing pulmonary lesions.

Detecting locoregional spread is critical and local control is important even if it is temporary. In terms of survival, local treatment with radiation is also beneficial for local recurrence after a complete resection. In one study [2], half of the patients who received radiation treatment achieved a good local response which resulted in prolonged survival with a median survival time of 27 months. The median survival time of patients with uncontrolled disease was only 6 months. The potential of radiotherapy to control a localized lesion is naturally best against less extensive disease. However, early locoregional recurrence, especially hilar and mediastinal lymph node recurrence is rarely detected by an incidental plain chest X-ray. Therefore, in addition to chest X-rays, chest CT should be performed annually for the first 2 years of postoperative surveillance.

Postoperative adjuvant chemotherapy has been recommended in the clinical guideline edited by the Japan Lung Cancer Society since 2005, in order to improve results for patients with resected stage IB, II and IIIA lesions. Therefore, except for stage IA patients, most patients with good performance status receive adjuvant chemotherapy after surgery in Japan. For those patients, periodical systemic screening for the disease recurrence is needed using both chest CT and bone scintigraphy annually for the first 2 years. Adjuvant chemotherapy must be discontinued as soon as possible in the event that it fails.

The Japanese postoperative adjuvant chemotherapy guideline is based on recent well-designed phase III trials which demonstrate positive results with platinum-based doublet regimens [5–7]. The survival benefits are small, while grades 3 or 4 toxic adverse events occurred in a considerable number of patients (about 80%) with a treatment-related mortality of 0.8–2.0%.

In Japan, UFT, an oral DPD-inhibitory 5-fluorouracil compound of uracil and tegafur, has been demonstrated to be effective in the postoperative adjuvant setting for NSCLC, especially for stage IB disease [8]. S-1, another oral DPD-inhibitory 5-fluorouracil compound of tegaful, gimeracil, and oteracil potassium, yields a higher response rate against metastatic NSCLC than UFT [9]. The long-term (for 1 or 2 years) administration of oral DPD-inhibitory 5-fluorouracil drugs such as UFT and S-1 in the outpatient setting is now common in Japan. These regimens require office visits every 3 months for the first 2 years after surgery to monitor compliance and adverse events.

A recent increase of primary lung cancer in never-smokers has been observed despite the increase in smoking in wealthy countries. The proportion of never-smoking patients with surgical NSCLC has been steadily increasing over time

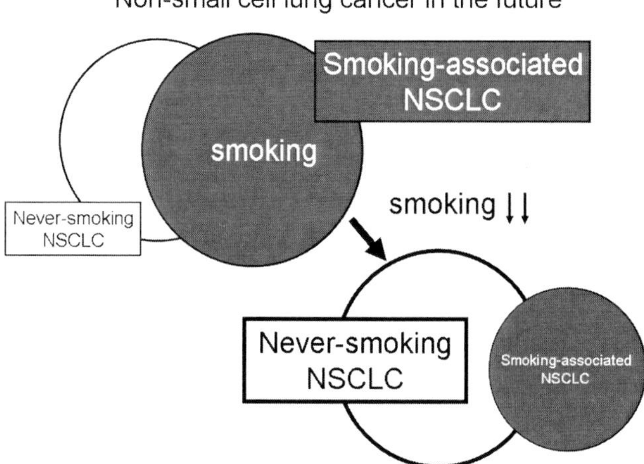

Fig. 14.1 Non-small lung cell cancer in the future

at the Kyushu University Hospital, from 15.9% in the 1970s, 25.8% in the 1980s, 30.4% in the 1990s, and 32.8% in the 2000s. The never-smoking NSCLC cohort is characterized by an increased incidence in females, a higher occurrence of adenocarcinoma, and a better postoperative prognosis in comparison to the smoking NSCLC group [10]. NSCLC in never-smokers is thus considered an etiologically separate entity from smoking-associated lung cancer (Fig. 14.1).

Multiple small-sized lesions (less than 1 cm in diameter) often coexist in never-smoking NSCLC patients. Most are pathologically atypical adenomatous hyperplasia (AAH) or early bronchioloalveolar cell carcinoma (BAC). Therefore, when either AAH or early BAC is suspected, periodical CT follow-up is needed after resection of the NSCLC. Cases without AAH or BAC may require less postoperative follow-up because the postoperative prognosis of never-smoking NSCLC is likely better than that of smoking-related NSCLC [10]. Further investigation concerning the nature of never-smoking NSCLC should therefore help determine the best surveillance strategy for postoperative patients in the near future.

References

1. Goya T, Asamura H, Yoshimura H, et al. Prognosis of 6644 resected non-small cell lung cancers in Japan: a Japanese lung cancer registry study. Lung Cancer. 2005;50:227–34.
2. Yano T, Hara N, Ichinose Y, et al. Local recurrence after complete resection for non-small-cell carcinoma of the lung: significance of local control by radiation treatment. J Thorac Cardiovasc Surg. 1994;107:8–12.
3. Yano T, Yokoyama H, Inoue T, et al. The first site of recurrence after complete resection in non-small-cell carcinoma of the lung. J Thorac Cardiovasc Surg. 1994;108:680–3.
4. Lung Cancer Study Group. Randomized trial of lobectomy versus limited resection for T1N0 non-small cell lung cancer. Ann Thorac Surg. 1995;60:615–23.
5. The International Adjuvant Lung Cancer Trial Collaborative Group. Cisplatin-based adjuvant chemotherapy in patients with completely resected non-small-cell lung cancer. N Engl J Med. 2004;350:351–60.
6. Winton T, Livingston R, Johnson D, et al. Vinorelbine plus Cisplatin vs. observation in resected non-small-cell-lung cancer. N Engl J Med. 2005;352(25):2589–97.
7. Douillard JY, Rosell R, De Lena M, et al. Adjuvant vinorelbine plus cisplatin versus observation in patients with completely resected stage IB-IIIA non-small cell lung cancer (Adjuvant Navelbine International Trialist Association. [ANITA]): A randomized controlled trial. Lancet Oncol. 2006;7:719–27.
8. Kato H, Ichinose Y, Ohta M, et al. A randomized trial of adjuvant chemotherapy with uracil-tegafur for adenocarcinoma of the lung. N Engl J Med. 2004;350:1713–21.
9. Kawahara M, Furuse K, Segawa Y, et al. Phase II study of S-1, a novel oral fluorouracil, in advanced non-small-cell lung cancer. Br J Cancer. 2001;85:939–43.
10. Yano T, Miura N, Takenaka T, et al. Never-smoking non-small cell lung cancer as a separate entity—the clinico-pathologic features and survival. Cancer. 2008;113:1012–8.

15 Lung Carcinoma Surveillance Counterpoint: Canada

Gail Darling, Yee Ung, Peter Ellis, Lorraine Martelli-Reid, and Bill Evans

Keywords
5A model • Canada • Radical radiotherapy • Recurrence • Treatment modality

There were approximately 23,900 new cases of lung cancer in Canada in 2008 and 20,200 deaths [1]. Between 1995 and 2004, age-standardized incidence and mortality rates decreased for men but have increased for women (Table 15.1) [2]. Non-small cell histology makes up over 80% of lung cancer and the remainder is largely small cell lung cancer (SCLC), a disease which typically spreads early and is treated using nonsurgical approaches [3]. Patients with stage I or II and highly selected patients with stage IIIA non-small cell lung cancer (NSCLC) are potential candidates for resection [3]. Only about 12% of patients have stage I disease and 6% have stage II. Approximately 30% of patients present with locally advanced disease and are not candidates for curative resection. However, a subset of these patients with good performance status, minimal or no weight loss, and nonbulky disease are candidates for combined modality therapy consisting of chemotherapy and radical radiation administered with curative intent.

Edelman et al. have set out principles for the use of diagnostic tests in the evaluation of patients after delivery of any potentially curative therapy [4]. These are: (a) the interval between examinations and the duration of testing should be consistent with an understanding of the natural history of the tumor, including its growth rate and the time frame in which the risk for disease recurrence is most likely; (b) tests should be directed at the most likely sites of recurrence and should have high enough positive and negative predictive values to be clinically useful; (c) therapy should be available that will result in cure, significant prolongation of life or symptom control; (d) initiation of earlier therapy should improve outcome; (e) increased risk of second malignancies should guide tests. These guiding principles are useful to consider in the context of recommendations for the follow-up of lung cancer patients treated with curative intent.

In this chapter on posttreatment surveillance for lung cancer patients, Canadian authors describe the rationale and frequency of surveillance following the surgical management of early-stage NSCLC, as well as following combined modality therapy for locally advanced NSCLC and limited stage (LS) SCLC, where the goal of treatment also is cure. As smoking is responsible for most cases of lung cancer, it is extremely important that surveillance be used as an opportunity to ensure that the lung cancer survivor does not resume smoking and that members of the patient's family are counseled not to smoke. Guidance is provided on the most appropriate strategies for health care providers to use during surveillance to assist patients and family members to abstain from smoking.

Surveillance Following Surgical Resection for Cure

Surgery is the modality of treatment most commonly used for the treatment of early-stage NSCLC. Depending on stage and histology, the 5-year survival rate can be as high as 70%.

G. Darling, M.D., F.R.C.S.C.
University Health Network and University of Toronto,
200 Elizabeth Street, 9N-955, Toronto, ON, Canada M5G 2C4
e-mail: gail.darling@uhn.on.ca

Y. Ung, M.D., F.R.C.P.C.
Odette Cancer Centre and University of Toronto Sunnybrook Health Sciences Centre, 2075 Bayview Avenue, Toronto, ON, Canada M4N 3M5
e-mail: yee.ung@sunnybrook.ca

P. Ellis, M.B.B.S., M.Med. (Clin Epi) Ph.D., F.R.A.C.P., F.R.C.P.C.
• L. Martelli-Reid, R.N.(EC), M.N. • B. Evans, M.D., F.R.C.P.C(✉)
Juravinski Cancer Centre and McMaster University,
699 Concession Street, Hamilton, ON, Canada, L8V 5C2
e-mail: peter.ellis@jcc.hhsc.ca; lorraine.martelli-reid@jcc.hhsc.ca; bill.evans@jcc.hhsc.ca

F.E. Johnson et al. (eds.), *Patient Surveillance After Cancer Treatment*, Current Clinical Oncology,
DOI 10.1007/978-1-60327-969-7_15,

Table 15.1 Average annual percent change in age-standardized incidence and mortality rates for lung cancer in Canada 1995–2004 [2]

	Incidence	Mortality
Males	−2.5	−2.1
Females	1.2	1.2

However, despite surgical resection, many patients develop recurrent disease. More than 70% of recurrences occur in the first 2 years after resection and 93% occur within the first 5 years [5]. The overall 5-year survival rates for resected patients with stages I and II NSCLC are 45% and 40%, respectively [3]. If recurrence develops, it may be limited to the chest, but more commonly occurs in distant sites such as the brain, bone, adrenals, and liver.

Smoking is the single most important risk factor for the development of lung cancer and continued smoking also increases the risk of cancer recurrence. Furthermore, patients who have had a lung cancer resection are at increased risk for developing a second lung primary, as well as other primary cancers of the aerodigestive tract. Smoking cessation reduces the relative risk of a second primary lung cancer [6].

Recurrent lung cancer may be local, regional, distant, or any combination thereof. Local recurrence refers to recurrence in the operative field such as in the bronchial stump, pulmonary parenchymal staple line, or within the same hemithorax. This distinction is important as such recurrences may be amenable to potentially curative therapy either with further surgery or radical radiation. Following complete resection, the rate of local recurrence varies depending on the stage of disease and also the extent of resection. For stage I NSCLC, the rate of isolated local recurrence is 10–30% over 5 years [7–9] but is doubled for sublobar resection (either wedge excision or segmentectomy) as compared to lobectomy [10].

Regional recurrence generally refers to recurrence in the lymphatic drainage basins either within the chest or neck. Such disease may be amenable to radical radiotherapy and is potentially curable but this presentation is more often the harbinger of more widespread disease.

Distant recurrence develops in two-thirds of patients after lung cancer resection. In most patients, these metastases present in multiple sites but in 7% of cases, isolated metastases occur. Rarely such isolated metastases may be amenable to surgical resection or radical radiotherapy. For example, resected isolated brain metastases may be associated with a 15–20% 5-year survival [11]. Although distant recurrence is generally not curable, prompt treatment is important for the palliation of symptoms and for improved health-related quality of life [12].

In contrast to the high recurrence rate after surgery, which declines over time, the rate of development of second primary lung cancer is constant at 1–2% per year [7]. When a new lesion develops in the lung following a previous lung cancer resection, it is important to determine if it is a recurrence or a new primary. If the two lesions have different histologies, they are separate primaries. If the histology is the same, other factors have to be considered, such as whether the second tumor is in the contralateral lung, or there is a long time interval between the two tumors. Both of these situations favor a metachronous tumor. Many times, however, it is impossible to be certain, although modern molecular genomic analytical techniques hold promise in this area. In such cases, the patient should be given the benefit of the doubt and the second tumor treated with curative intent assuming that there is no evidence of regional or distant disease and the patient is fit for the proposed treatment. Similarly, if other primary tumors of the aerodigestive tract develop, they should be treated with curative intent if there is no evidence of metastatic disease either related to the original lung cancer or the new second cancer.

There is general agreement among Canadian thoracic surgeons regarding the interval between surveillance visits, although local practice may vary. Following lung cancer surgery, patients are generally assessed by their surgeon 3–4 weeks postoperatively to ensure satisfactory recovery from their surgical procedure. Subsequently, they are seen every 3 months for the first 2 years, then every 4 months for the following year and then every 6 months until 5 years postresection. They are assessed annually thereafter. The interval between visits is shorter in the first 2–3 years as recurrences are most common in the first 2 years [13]. Five years following lung cancer surgery, the patient is considered cured of his/her primary lung cancer and the main purpose of subsequent visits is to assess for the development of second cancers.

As there is no high-quality evidence to support one surveillance schedule over any other, there is some variability in the guideline recommendations from different organizations (Table 15.2). Most recommend more frequent surveillance visits in the first 2 years following surgery in order to detect recurrences. Our Canadian recommendations most closely parallel those of the Association of Community Cancer Centres (ACCC) [14], American Society of Clinical Oncology (ASCO) [15], and the European Society of Medical Oncology (ESMO) [16] which all recommend follow-up every 3 months in the first 2 years. The low frequency of follow-up in the 5 years following curative intent therapy recommended by the American College of Chest Physicians (ACCP) [17] would be less likely to detect either an early recurrence or new primary.

Canadian surgeons tend toward a focused history and physical examination at each visit as well as a plain chest radiograph (Table 15.2). To date, no serum markers or routine blood tests have been shown to be useful for the purpose of screening for recurrence. Chest CT is not routine in Canadian practice and generally only performed if clinically

Table 15.2 Recommendations for surveillance in patients with NSCLC following curative intent therapy

Guideline/source	Test	Year 1	Year 2	Year 3	Year 4	Year 5	>5 years
ACCC [14]	Visits (H&P)	4	4	2	2	2	1
	Chest CT						
ACCP [17]	Visits (H&P)	2	2	1	1	1	1
	CXR or chest CT						
ACR [18]	Visits (H&P)	3–6	3–6	2	2	2	1
	CXR						
	Chest CT	1	1	1	1	1	1
ASCO [15]	Visits (H&P)	4	4	2	2	2	1
ESMO [16]	Visits (H&P)	4	4	2	2	2	2
NCCN [19]	Visits (H&P)	2	2	1	1	1	1
	Chest CT						
Canadian	Visits (H&P)	4	4	3	2	2	1
	CXR						

H&P = history and physical examination
CXR = chest x-ray
ACCC = Association of Community Cancer Centres; ACCP = American College of Chest Physicians; ACR = American College of Radiology; ASCO = American Society of Clinical Oncology; ESMO = European Society of Medical Oncology; NCCN = National Community Cancer Network
The number in each cell indicates the number of times a particular modality is recommended in a particular posttreatment year

indicated. On the other hand ACCC, the American College of Radiology [18], and National Comprehensive Cancer Network (NCCN) [19] all recommend a chest CT at each visit. It is clear that CT is more sensitive than plain chest x-ray in detecting "abnormalities" [20]. However, most abnormalities are not cancer. Korst and colleagues demonstrated the importance of involving the treating surgeon in the review of follow-up CT scans. Among 140 patients, 105 of 168 CT scans were reported as abnormal by the radiologist, of which only 32 were considered suspicious by the surgeon. Further evaluation diagnosed new or recurrent lung cancer in 16 of these cases [21]. Bronchoscopy is not routinely performed but is used in specific situations where the surgeon is concerned about the possibility of recurrence in the bronchus, dysplasia at the bronchial resection margin or multifocal squamous cancers. Similarly, routine sputum cytology is not performed as there is no evidence that the routine use of cytology confers a survival benefit and many patients are unable to produce an adequate sample. There is some evidence that autofluorescence bronchoscopy may detect endobronchial disease at an earlier stage, but there is no evidence at this time of a survival benefit from routine surveillance using this technology [22]. In addition, more intensive investigations are also more costly [23, 24]. In summary, intensive surveillance is not supported by the available evidence; therefore, the current practice in Canada has followed the schedule and level of testing described above.

This approach may need to be reconsidered in light of a recent study utilizing routine CT scans for surveillance, in which 78% of first recurrences were intrathoracic [25]. Of the intrathoracic recurrences detected by surveillance, 32% (16 patients) were amenable to potentially curative resection, which is higher than previously reported. Another study utilizing bronchoscopy and CT scans every 6 months in 192 patients with predominantly squamous cell cancer (76%), detected 85 recurrences, of which 36 were asymptomatic at the time of scheduled follow-up [26]. Of the asymptomatic recurrences, approximately one-third were detected by one of either physical examination or chest x-ray, CT scan, and bronchoscopy. Curative intent surgery was performed in 15 (43%) of the asymptomatic patients and 7 (14%) of the symptomatic patients. Survival at 3 years was 31% among asymptomatic patients, 10% among the symptomatic patients detected at routine follow-up, and 4% among symptomatic patients detected by an unscheduled procedure. There was no difference in disease-free interval between asymptomatic and symptomatic patients, suggesting that lead time bias did not account for improved survival. Also, 22 new second cancers were found, 17 in the aerodigestive tract. Previous studies have not reported a survival advantage with more intensive surveillance procedures and have suggested that it only increased costs [27–30].

Lung cancer patients are generally followed by their treating surgeon, although some patients may be followed by their primary care physician. This latter approach may be desirable if the patient has to travel long distances to see the surgical specialist. Patient preference and low risk of recurrence (disease-free postresection for 5 or more years) are other reasons for primary care physician follow-up. There is no evidence that follow-up with a surgeon impacts on survival whereas follow-up by a family physician may reduce costs [27].

In summary, routine surveillance of postresection NSCLC patients is reasonable in the frequency shown in Table 15.2 in order to detect recurrent disease or new primaries, particularly as most recurrences develop within 2 years of lung cancer surgery. Although most recurrences are symptomatic and are detected by history alone, a significant number are asymptomatic and will be detected by physical examination and/or plain chest x-ray. Routine CT scanning may detect more abnormalities but it has yet to be determined whether this will improve survival. There is no evidence that other tests (blood work, other imaging tests, bronchoscopy) improve survival and, therefore, these investigations are not performed routinely in Canada.

Surveillance Following Radical Radiation Therapy for Lung Cancer

Radiation therapy is a highly specialized treatment modality which has an important role in the management of lung cancer. In Canada, radiation therapy services are publically financed, government regulated, and delivered through regional cancer centers that provide expertise in consultation, treatment planning, and the delivery of radiation therapy to patients in geographically defined areas. Larger centers generally organize their services around disease site teams (i.e., tumor groups). For lung cancer, the team consists of thoracic surgeons, medical and radiation oncologists, nurses and supportive care workers who interact through tumor boards and multidisciplinary clinics to make treatment recommendations and to promote research. Radiation oncologists are particularly interested in implementing and evaluating technical innovations for the delivery of radiation. Because of the specialized nature of radiotherapy and the medical community's general lack of familiarity with its early and late side-effects, follow-up care is often conducted at the regional cancer center.

Consensus guidelines have been developed by a variety of professional organizations for surveillance following curative intent therapy, including radical radiotherapy. These guidelines include those of the NCCN [19], ASCO [15], ESMO [16], National Institute of Health and Clinical Excellence [31], and the ACCP [17]. In examining the evidence base for these guideline recommendations, it is clear that there is not yet convincing evidence that frequent follow-up with intensive imaging alters survival in patients with recurrent NSCLC, but there may be some benefit from the earlier detection of second primaries that are amenable to curative treatment. The majority of published studies have focused on resected early-stage NSCLC [7, 17, 19, 30] but a recent study has evaluated follow-up in advanced lung cancer [31]. There is no data on the role of surveillance for patients with medically inoperable early-stage lung cancer treated with radical radiation therapy or stereotactic radiation.

While there is a lack of high-quality evidence to show that intensive follow-up alters the outcome of lung cancer patients treated with radical radiation therapy and curative intent, clinical experience allows two general recommendations to be made. First, adequate follow-up is required to manage potential complications of aggressive therapy and this is the responsibility of the radiation oncologist. The growing use of image-guided radiation therapy utilizing intensity-modulated radiation therapy and stereotactic body radiation has made it possible to deliver focused higher dose intense treatment to the primary tumor site. However, these techniques result in more low-dose scatter radiation to surrounding normal tissues and the implications for late effects are as yet unknown. Ongoing follow-up and monitoring for delayed toxicity and second malignancies is, therefore, important.

Secondly, surveillance can detect local recurrences or a second primary tumor which may still be amenable to effective treatment. With the availability of high-precision radiation therapy, it is now technically possible to retreat the primary tumor site and to deliver very intense focused doses of potentially curative radiation (stereotactic radiotherapy or intensity-modulated radiotherapy, IMRT). The availability of these radiotherapy approaches provides a rationale for more frequent follow-up in the first 2 years of follow-up when both local recurrence and distant metastases are most likely to appear. Long-term data on the outcomes from the treatment of oligometastases are still too preliminary but hold promise [32, 33].

A systematic review of the literature undertaken by the ACCPs on the role of follow-up and surveillance of lung cancer patients following curative intent therapy makes particular reference to surveillance for the toxicities of therapy [17]. Complications related to the delivery of radiation therapy can be divided into acute and late side-effects. The acute side-effects of radical radiation therapy include fatigue, esophagitis, acute radiation pneumonitis, as well as some minor effects on the skin and surrounding critical structures (e.g., heart, spinal cord) that usually do not have any acute clinical manifestations. Acute radiation pneumonitis can occur up to 3 months after treatment and generally only requires intervention with steroids if the patient becomes symptomatic with low-grade fever, cough, and dyspnea. Rarely, patients may require oxygen. However, the incidence of acute radiation pneumonitis may increase as combined modality therapy with concurrent chemotherapy and radical radiation are increasingly used for locally advanced disease. The reported incidence of grade 3 or higher acute radiation pneumonitis varies from 11 to 13% in recent clinical trials [34–36]. Radiation induced pulmonary fibrosis is a late effect that can occur from 3 to 24 months after treatment. There is no effective treatment for radiation fibrosis. Consequently, some deterioration of the patient's pulmonary function can be expected with some degree of late recovery [37–40].

An important consideration in the follow-up of radically treated lung cancer patients is the need to evaluate local control and patterns of relapse. Currently with high-precision radiation dose escalation, it is critical that the target volume be carefully defined and that geographic misses be avoided. Image-guided radiation therapy now routinely uses

Table 15.3 Recommended frequency of visits and tests during follow-up for non-small cell lung carcinoma after radical radiation

Guideline source	Test	Year 1	Year 2	Year 3	Year 4	Year 5	>5 years
ACCC [14]	Visits (H&P)	4	4	2	2	2	1
	CXR	4	4	2	2	2	1
	CBC and chemistry	4	4	2	2	2	1
ACCP [17]	Visits (H&P)	2	2	1	1	1	1
	CXR or chest CT	2	2	1	1	1	1
ACR [18]	Visits (H&P)	3–6	3–6	2	2	2	1
	CXR	2	2	2	2	2	1
	Chest CT	2	2	2	2	2	1
ASCO [15]	Visits (H&P)	4	4	2	2	2	1
ESMO [16]	Visits (H&P)	2–4	2–4	2	2	2	2
NICE [30]	Visits (H&P)	2	2	2	2	2	0
	CXR	2	2	2	2	2	0
	Smoking cessation counseling	2	2	2	2	2	0
NCCN [19]	Visits (H&P)	2–3	2–3	1	1	1	1
	Chest CT	2–3	2–3	1	1	1	1
	Smoking cessation counseling	2–3	2–3	1	1	1	1
Odette Cancer Centre (Academic Centre)	Visits (H&P)	4	3	2	2	2	1
	CXR	4	3	2	2	2	1
	Chest CT	2	2	2	2	2	1
	CBC and chemistry	4	3	2	2	2	1

ACCC = Association of Community Cancer Centres; ACCP = American College of Chest Physicians; ACR = American College of Radiology Committee on Appropriateness Criteria; ASCO = American Society of Clinical Oncology; ESMO = European Society of Medical Oncology; NICE = National Institute for Clinical Excellence; NCCN = National Community Cancer Network; H&P = history and physical exam; CXR = chest radiograph; CBC = complete blood count; Chemistry = liver and renal profile

The number in each cell indicates the number of times a particular modality is recommended in a particular posttreatment year

multimodality imaging with CT often supplemented with positron emission tomography. However, there continues to be a great deal of variation in the definition of the target volume and very little pathological validation of the accuracy of these newer treatment targeting methods [41–46]. Rigorous follow-up with evaluation of the site(s) of local recurrence will, over time, improve the radiation oncologist's ability to precisely define the tumor volume and accurately plan the radiation fields.

Unfortunately, most recurrences following combined modality therapy occur outside the thorax and, at present, therapy is very rarely curative once metastatic disease occurs. Metachronous cancers either of the lung or aerodigestive tract can occur after curative intent treatment and some metachronous cancers are still amenable to curative treatment [47]. Therefore, surveillance for the early detection of potentially curable metachronous cancers is an important reason for follow-up of these patients.

In an academic setting, such as the Odette Cancer Centre in Toronto, Ontario, where patterns of recurrence are being evaluated after intensity-modulated radiation therapy as part of a research protocol, the frequency of surveillance may need to be greater in order to document the initial site(s) of recurrence (Table 15.3). However, for routine follow-up, the frequency of visits and test procedures shown in Table 15.4 would be considered reasonable in Canada as there is no evidence that intensive follow-up alters survival. It is recommended that patients be seen at 3-month intervals for the first 2 years after treatment as that is the time frame during which they are at highest risk for recurrence. Subsequent follow-up up to 5 years is generally at the same frequency as for surgical follow-up for the assessment of local or distant recurrence, late toxicities, and second malignancies (Table 15.2). These recommendations are consistent with the guideline recommendations from various guideline developers, as summarized in Table 15.3.

Table 15.4 Usual surveillance protocol in Canada for non-small cell lung carcinoma and small cell lung carcinoma after radical radiation

	Years posttreatment					
	1	2	3	4	5	>5
Number of office visits	4	3	2	2	2	1
CXRs	4	3	2	2	2	1
CT chest and upper abdomen	4	3	2	2	2	0
Blood work[a]	4	3	2	2	2	1

[a]Complete blood counts, liver, and renal function profile
The number in each cell indicates the number of times a particular modality is recommended in a particular posttreatment year

Surveillance Following Combined Modality Therapy for SCLC

SCLC represents approximately 15% of incident cases of lung cancer [48]. At the time of diagnosis, two-thirds of cases are extensive stage (disease outside of one hemithorax) where the goals of care are not curative. The remaining cases are classified as LS disease [49]. Patients with LS SCLC are generally treated with curative intent. Treatment, including platinum-based chemotherapy, thoracic radiation, and prophylactic cranial radiation, results in 5-year survival rates approaching 25% [50, 51]. The schedule of follow-up for this group of patients is influenced both by the risk and timing of recurrent disease as well as the risk of developing second primary lung cancers.

Recurrent Disease

The majority of patients undergoing curative treatment for LS SCLC will ultimately suffer a recurrence of their disease and most of the recurrences occur early. Only about 25% of patients remain recurrence free at 2 years [51]. However, early detection of recurrent disease may be beneficial given that second-line treatment for recurrent disease has been shown to improve survival [52, 53].

Second Primary Cancers

Patients with LS SCLC also have a significant risk of second primary malignancies [54–56]. Tucker et al. reviewed the records of 611 patients with SCLC surviving more than 2 years [56]. They observed a 3.5-fold increase in the risk of all second cancers relative to the general population. These were primarily NSCLCs. The observed risk was higher among smokers and patients who had received thoracic radiation. Similar findings have been observed among Japanese patients with SCLC [55].

In a review reported by Johnson, the average risk of second primary lung cancers among survivors of SCLC was noted to be approximately 6% per year [54]. The risk increases from approximately 2% per patient-year at 2 years to as high as 10% per patient-year by 10 years of follow-up.

Recommendations for Follow-up of LS SCLC

Consensus recommendations from Cancer Care Ontario [57], the NCCN [58], ESMO [59], and ACCPs [17] are summarized in Table 15.4. These recommendations are based on very limited evidence.

The only study identified in the literature on the follow-up of SCLC has significant methodological limitations. Sugiyama et al. [60] evaluated an intensive schedule of follow-up in patients achieving a partial or complete response to initial chemotherapy. The intensive follow-up consisted of bimonthly chest x-ray, CT chest/abdomen, MRI brain and bone scan for 6 months, then quarterly for 1.5 years. History and physical examination were performed monthly for 2 years, then bimonthly for another 3 years in both groups. Sixty-two patients were followed intensively and 32 received less intensive follow-up. It is unclear how patients were allocated to intensive or non-intensive follow-up as there is no mention of randomization. There are significant baseline imbalances between the two groups, with a greater proportion of patients with LS SCLC in the intensive follow-up group. The median time to recurrence was similar (intensive 5 months vs. non-intensive 7 months, $p=0.25$). Median overall survival was longer in the intensive follow-up group (20 months vs. 13 months, $p=0.04$). More patients in the intensive follow-up group were well enough for salvage therapy (91% vs. 72%, $p=0.03$).

Our recommendations (Juravinski Cancer Centre, Hamilton, Ontario) for follow-up of LS SCLC are summarized in Table 15.5. Current data support regular follow-up of patients with LS SCLC for the early detection of second primary cancers. In addition, lower level evidence suggests that early detection of recurrent disease may increase the proportion of SCLC patients eligible for second-line therapy. We recommend follow-up visits every 3 months in the first 2 years, every 6 months in year 3, and then yearly thereafter. History and physical examination (including smoking cessation counseling) are done at every visit. CT chest ± abdomen are recommended every 6 months in the first 2 years, with CXR on alternating visits. Annual CXR is recommended from year 4 onward.

Smoking Cessation and Surveillance

Tobacco use is the main cause of lung cancer [61]. Although smoking rates in Canada have dropped significantly since 1985 (35.1%), and especially after 1991, it is estimated in 2001 that approximately 20% of males and 17% of females were current smokers, and 31% and 23% respectively were

Table 15.5 Recommendations for surveillance following treatment of limited SCLC

Organization	Test	Year 1	Year 2	Year 3	Year 4	Year 5	>5 years
NCCN [58]	Visit (H&P)[a]	4–5	3–4	3–4	2–3	2–3	1
	Chest imaging[b]	4–5	3–4	3–4	2–3	2–3	1
Cancer Care Ontario [57]	Visit (H&P)	2	2	1	1	1	1
	Chest imaging[b]	2	2	1	1	1	1
ACCP [17]	Visit (H&P)	4	4	2	2	2	1
	CXR	4	4	2	2	2	1
ESMO [59]	Follow-up for second primary	NS[c]					
Juravinski Cancer Centre	Visit (H&P)[a]	4	4	2	1	1	1
	CXR	2	2	2	1	1	1
	Alternating with CT	2	2				

Superscript indicates the number of times per year:
[a]Smoking cessation at every visit
[b]Chest x-ray or chest CT
[c]Follow-up recommended because of risk of second primary, but frequency of visits and tests not specified
The number in each cell indicates the number of times a particular modality is recommended in a particular posttreatment year

former smokers [62]. Despite a diagnosis of lung cancer, many people continue to smoke or take up smoking again after a period of stoppage during treatment [63]. As well, many family members and friends of lung cancer patients are also smokers or former smokers. Therefore, during surveillance it is important that care providers be aware of the information that links continued smoking to worse treatment outcomes and the increased risk of second primaries, as well as the strategies that can lead smokers to smoking cessation, whether they have a diagnosis of cancer or are close friends and family of the lung cancer patient.

The link between smoking as a cause for all histological subtypes of lung cancer has been well established. Smoking reduction, however, can reduce the risk of lung cancer. A decrease of approximately 60% in the amount smoked can result in close to a 30% reduction in the risk of lung cancer [64]. Additionally, smoking cessation after the completion of treatment for LS SCLC results in fewer smoking-related second primary cancers [64]. So smoking cessation can reduce the risk of developing lung cancer and for those who have been treated for lung cancer, smoking cessation reduces the risk of a second primary.

Many studies have shown that continued smoking after a diagnosis of lung cancer can further worsen one's health and interfere with the response to cancer treatment. For lung cancer patients who have undergone surgical resection but continue to smoke, their relapse rates are higher than for nonsmokers in the first year following resection [63, 65–67]. Continued smoking after surgery is also associated with significantly lower 5- and 10-year survival rates (34% and 23.7%) compared with nonsmokers (56.2% and 44.1%) [68]. In a multivariate analysis in surgically resected patients, smoking was a significant independent prognostic factor. Compared with nonsmokers, the relative risk of mortality was 1.70 for former smokers and 1.99 for current smokers [68]. Current smokers also have a higher incidence of death related to pulmonary disease, heart disease, and surgery-related events [68].

Numerous studies assessing patients with a variety of different cancers have shown that continued smoking during treatment can impair the response to cancer treatment [69–71]. In lung cancer patients undergoing radiation treatment, continued smoking increases the probability of developing radiation pneumonitis by 20% [72]. In patients with LS SCLC, smoking during radiation has been shown to decrease median survival and overall survival rates at 5 and 10 years [73]. Smoking during radiation treatment for NSCLC has been shown to be associated with higher rates of locoregional recurrence [74].

Smoking can also interfere with the effectiveness of chemotherapy. In patients with stage III/IV NSCLC, treated with chemotherapy, the 1-year overall survival rate was significantly greater for never-smokers and former smokers compared with current smokers [74]. Never-smokers also had higher response rates (19%) to chemotherapy than former (8%) and current (12%) smokers as well as lower disease progression rates (49% vs. 65% and 66%, respectively) [74].

Because tobacco dependence is a chronic disease, which typically persists for many years with multiple periods of remission and relapse, clinicians must recognize the need for continued education, counseling, and advice over time. Brief advice from a variety of health care professionals and an appropriate approach to smoking cessation can be successful in increasing long-term quit rates [75].

At the Juravinski Cancer Centre in Hamilton Ontario, we have implemented the 5A model of Minimal Contact Intervention which is recognized internationally as an evidence-based approach to smoking cessation [76]. All health care providers have received education on how to provide the brief interventions that are part of the Minimal Contact Intervention and carry a pocket card/ring with the 5A prompts (Asking, Advising, Assessing, Assisting, and Arranging) (Fig. 15.1). A sign in every patient waiting room highlights the commitment of the organization to smoking prevention

5A Tobacco Use Intervention

ASK About Tobacco Use at Every Visit

- Implement an office system that ensures that, for every patient at every visit, tobacco use status is queried and documented.

ADVISE All Tobacco Users to Quit

- Urge every tobacco user to quit in a way that is personally relevant.

ASSESS Tobacco User's Readiness to Quit

- Ask every tobacco user if they are ready to make a quit attempt at this time.
- Assess how important it is for them, and how confident and ready they are to make a change (see reverse for *Readiness Ruler*).

ASSIST Tobacco Users in Quitting

- Build motivation to change (see reverse for *Decisional Balance*).
- Help the patient make a quit plan.
  - ✓ Set a quit date within two weeks.
  - ✓ Discuss stop smoking medications.
  - ✓ Review past quit experiences.
  - ✓ Identify triggers and brainstorm strategies.
  - ✓ Discuss alcohol and other drug use.
  - ✓ Assist patient to identify social support.

ARRANGE Follow-Up or Referral

For cessation services and other tobacco-related information:
- Public Health Tobacco Hotline 905-540-5566

For telephone counselling/online support:
- Smokers' Helpline 1-877-513-5333/www.smokershelpline.ca

Helpful Counselling Tools

Readiness Ruler

How ***important*** is it for you to quit/cut down?
0 1 2 3 4 5 6 7 8 9 10

How ***confident*** are you about making this change?
0 1 2 3 4 5 6 7 8 9 10

How ***ready*** are you to make this change?
0 1 2 3 4 5 6 7 8 9 10

Follow-Up Questions:
- Why are you at (current score) and not zero?
- What would it take for you to get to a higher score?

Decisional Balance

	If you continue to smoke	If you quit/ cut back
Positives		
Negatives		

Points to cover:
- Encourage the patient to state why quitting is personally relevant.
- Ask the patient to identify potential negative consequences of use.
- Ask the patient to identify potential benefits of quitting.
- Ask the patient to identify barriers to quitting, and discuss options to address those barriers.

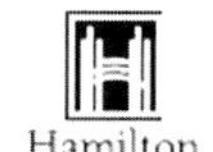

City of Hamilton
Public Health Services
Tobacco Control Program
Tobacco Hotline (905) 540-5566
www.hamilton.ca/tobacco

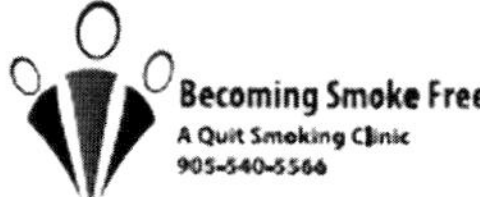

Adapted from: University of Massachusetts Medical School and Centre for Addiction and Mental Health

Fig. 15.1 5A model of minimal contact intervention adopted at the Juravinski Cancer Centre, Hamilton, ON

and cessation and informs the patient that they will be asked at every visit about their smoking status. At each follow-up visit, every patient is asked whether they are a current smoker, ex-smoker, or never smoker. Referral to a smoking cessation clinic is offered to current smokers who live locally. Out-of-town patients and family members are offered the Fax Referral program with Smokers Helpline who will contact them directly to work on a quit attempt or help them find resources that are available in their local community. Self-help books and materials are given to the patients and families and are also available in all waiting rooms. The smoking status of the patient, the healthcare provider who uses the 5A intervention and the steps implemented are all documented in the patient's chart. This intervention is delivered in less than 3 min and has been easily incorporated into each patient follow-up visit.

Although the number of Canadians who continue to smoke has sharply decreased in the last 20 years, many continue to smoke and more than half will be diagnosed with a smoking-related cancer. Smoking continues to be a critical public health issue and primary prevention must remain a priority. As part of surveillance following a diagnosis of lung cancer, smoking cessation must be encouraged.

References

1. Canadian Cancer Society. Canadian cancer statistics. 2008. http:\\www.cancer.ca. Accessed 8 Feb 2009.
2. Marrett LD, De P, Airia P. Dryer D for the steering committee of Canadian Cancer Statistics 2008. CMAJ. 2008;179:1163–70.
3. Xie L, Ugnat A-M, Moriss J, Semenciw R, Mao Y. Histology related variation in the treatment and survival of patients with lung carcinoma in Canada. Lung Cancer. 2003;42:127–39.
4. Edelman MJ, Meyer FJH, Siegel D. The utility of follow-up testing after curative cancer therapy. A critical review and economic analysis. J Gen Intern Med. 1997;12:318–37.
5. Egermann U, Jaeggi K, Habicht JM, Perruchoud AP, Dalquen P, Soler M. Regular follow-up after curative resection of non small cell lung cancer: a real benefit for patients? Eur Respir J. 2002;19:464–8.
6. Richardson GE, Tucker MA, Venzon DJ, Linnoila RI, Phelps R, Phares JC, et al. Smoking cessation after successful treatment of

small cell lung cancer is associated with fewer smoking related second primary cancers. Ann Intern Med. 1993;119:383–90.
7. Martini N, Bains MS, Burt ME, et al. Incidence of local recurrence and second primary tumors in resected stage I lung cancer. J Thorac Cardiovasc Surg. 1995;109:120–9.
8. Ludwig Lung Cancer Study Group. Patterns of failure in patients with resected stage I and II non small carcinoma of the lung. Ann Surg. 1987;205:67–71.
9. Feld R, Rubinsein LV, Weisenberger TH, The Lung Cancer Study Group. Sites of recurrence in resected stage I nonsmall cell lung cancer; a guide for future studies. J Clin Oncol. 1984;2:1352–8.
10. Ginsberg RJ, Rubinstein L. Randomized trial of lobectomy versus limited resection for T1N0 nonsmall cell lung cancer. Ann Thorac Surg. 1995;60:615–23.
11. Burt M, Wronski M, Arbit E, Balicich JH, The Memorial Sloan Kettering Cancer Center thoracic surgical staff. Resection of brain metastases for non small cell lung carcinoma: results of therapy. J Thorac Cardiovasc Surg. 1992;103:399–410.
12. Fairchild A, Harris K, Barnes E, Wong R, Lutz S, Bezjak A, et al. Palliative thoracic radiotherapy for lung cancer: a systematic review. J Clin Oncol. 2008;26:4001–11.
13. Downey RJ, Martini N, Ginsberg RJ. Bronchogenic carcinoma. In: Johnson FE, Virgo KS, editors. Cancer patient follow-up. St Louis: Mosby; 1997. p. 226–30.
14. Association of Community Cancer Network. Oncology patient management guidelines version 3.0. Rockville, MD: Association of Community Oncology Centres; 2000.
15. Pfister DG, Johnson DH, Azzoli CG, Sause W, Smith TJ, Baker S Jr, et al. American Society of Clinical Oncology treatment of unresectable non-small cell lung cancer guideline: update 2003. J Clin Oncol. 2004;22:330–53.
16. D'Addario G, Felip E, ESMO Guidelines Working Group. Non-small-cell lung cancer: ESMO clinical recommendations for diagnosis, treatment and follow-up. Ann Oncol. 2008;19 Suppl 2:ii39–40.
17. Rubins J, Unger M, Colice GL, American College of Chest Physicians. Follow-up and surveillance of the lung cancer patient following curative intent therapy. ACCP evidence-based clinical practice guidelines (2nd ed.). Chest. 2007;132 Suppl 3:355s–67s.
18. Follow-up of non-small cell lung cancer: American College of Radiology appropriateness criteria. 2005. http:\\www.acr.org. Accessed 8 Feb 2009.
19. National Comprehensive Cancer Network. Practice guidelines for non-small cell lung cancer. Rockledge, PA: National Comprehensive Network; 2000.
20. Henschke CI, McCauley DI, Yankelevitz DF, Naidich DP, McGuinness G, Mitettinen OS, et al. Early Lung Cancer Action Project: overall design and findings from baseline screening. Lancet. 1999;354:99–105.
21. Korst RJ, Gold HT, Kent MS, Port JL, Lee PC, Altorki NK. Surveillance computed tomography after complete resection for non small cell lung cancer: results and costs. J Thorac Cardiovasc Sur. 2005;129:652–60.
22. Weigel TL, Yousem S, Dacic S, Kosco PJ, Siegfried J, Luketich JD. Fluorescence bronchoscopic surveillance after curative surgical resection for nonsmall cell lung cancer. Ann Surg Oncol. 2000;7:176–80.
23. Smith TJ. Evidence based follow-up of lung cancer patients. Sem Oncol. 2003;30:361–8.
24. Korst RJ, Kansler AL, Port JL, Lee PC, Altorki NK. Accuracy of Surveillance Computed tomography in detecting recurrence of new primary lung cancer in patients with completely resected lung cancer. Ann Thorac Surg. 2006;82:1009–15.
25. Westeel V, Choma D, Clement F, Woronoff-Lemsi M-C, Pujol J-F, Dubiez A, et al. Relevance of an intensive postoperative follow-up after surgery for nonsmall cell lung cancer. Ann Thorac Surg. 2000;70:1185–90.
26. Gilbert S, Reid KR, Lam MY, Petsikas D. Who should follow-up lung cancer patients after operation? Ann Thorac Surg. 2000;69: 1696–700.
27. Virgo KS, Naunheim KS, McKirgan LW, Kissling ME, Lin JC, Johnson FE. Cost of patient follow-up after potentially curative lung cancer treatment. J Thorac Cardiovasc Surg. 1996;112: 356–63.
28. Walsh GL, O'Connor M, Willis KM, Milas M, Wong RS, Nesbitt JC, et al. Is follow-up of lung cancer patients after resection medically indicated and cost effective? Ann Thorac Surg. 1995;60:1563–72.
29. Younes RN, Gross JL, Deheinzelin D. Follow-up of lung cancer: How often and for what purpose? Chest. 1999;115:1494–9.
30. National Institute for Clinical Excellence: the diagnosis and treatment of lung cancer: methods, evidence and guidance. 2005. http://www.nice.org.uk/nicemedia/pdf/CG024niceguideline.pdf. Accessed 8 Feb 2009.
31. Benamore R, Shepherd FA, Leighl N, Pintikie M, Patel M, Feld R, et al. Does intensive follow-up alter outcome in patients with advanced lung cancer? J Thorac Oncol. 2007;2:273–81.
32. Kavanagh BD, McGarry RD, Timmerman RD. Extracranial radiosurgery (stereotactic body radiation) for oligometastases. Semin Radiat Oncol. 2006;16:77–84.
33. Pastorini U, Buyse M, Griedel G, Ginsberg RJ, Girard P, Goldstraw P, et al. Long-term results of lung metastatectomy: prognostic analysis based on 5206 cases. J Thorac Cardiovasc Surg. 1997;113:37–49.
34. Curran WJ, Scott CB, Langer CJ, Komaki R, Lee J, Hauser S, et al. Long-term benefit is observed in a phase III comparison of sequential versus concurrent chemoradiation for patients with unresectable stage III non-small cell lung cancer: RTOG 9410. Proc Am Soc Clin Oncol. 2003;22:621. Abst. #2499.
35. Gandara DR, Chansky K, Albain KS, Leigh BR, Gaspar LE, Lara PN, et al. Consolidation docetaxel after concurrent chemoradiotherapy in stage IIIB non-small cell lung cancer: Phase II SWOG S9504. J Clin Oncol. 2003;21:2004–10.
36. Kelly K, Chanksy K, Gaspar LE, Albain KS, Jett J, Ung YC, et al. Phase III trial of maintenance gefitnib or placebo after concurrent chemoradiotherapy and docetaxel consolidation in inoperable stage III non-small cell lung cancer: SWOG S0023. J Clin Oncol. 2008;26:2450–6.
37. Choi NC, Kanarek DJ. Toxicity of thoracic radiotherapy on pulmonary function in lung cancer. Lung Cancer. 1994;10 Suppl 1:S219–30.
38. Rodrigues G, Lock M, D'Souza D, Yu E, Van Dyk J. Prediction of radiation pneumonitis by dose-volume histogram parameters in lung cancer: a systematic review. Radiother Oncol. 2004;71:127–38.
39. Miller KL, Shafman TD, Marks LB. A practical approach to pulmonary risk assessment in the radiotherapy of lung cancer. Semin Radiat Oncol. 2004;14:298–307.
40. Miller KL, Zhour SM, Barrier RC, Shafman T, Golz RJ, Clough RW, et al. Long-term changes in pulmonary function tests after definitive radiotherapy for lung cancer. Int J Radiat Oncol Biol Phys. 2003;56:611–5.
41. Mah K, Caldwell CB, Ung YC, Danjoux CE, Balogh JM, Ganguli SN, et al. The impact of 18FDG PET on target and critical organs in CT-based treatment planning of patients with poorly defined non-small cell lung carcinoma: a prospective study. Int J Radiat Oncol Biol Phys. 2002;52:339–50.
42. Caldwell CB, Mah K, Ung YC, Danjoux CE, Balogh JM, Ganguli SN, et al. Observer variation in contouring gross tumor volume in patients with poorly defined non-small cell lung tumors on CT: the impact of 18FDG-Hybrid PET fusion. Int J Radiat Oncol Biol Phys. 2001;51:923–31.

43. Ashmalla H, Rafla S, Parikh K, Mokhtar B, Goswami G, Kambam S, et al. The contribution of integrated PET/CT to the evolving definition of treatment volumes in radiation treatment planning in lung cancer. Int J Radiat Oncol Biol Phys. 2005;63:1016–23.
44. Dahele MR, Ung YC. 18FDG PET in planning radiation treatment of non-small cell lung cancer: Where exactly is the tumor? J Nucl Med. 2007;48:1402.
45. Stroom J, Blaauvgeers H, van Baardwuk A, Boersma L, Lebesque J, Theuws J, et al. Feasibility of pathology correlated lung imaging for accurate target definition of lung tumors. Int J Radiat Oncol Biol Phys. 2007;69:267–75.
46. Dahele M, Hwang D, Peressotti C, Sun L, Kusano M, Okhai S, et al. Developing a methodology for 3-D correlation of PET-CT images and whole mount histopathology in non-small cell lung cancer. Curr Oncol. 2008;15:62–9.
47. Ponn RB. Lightning can strike twice: second primary lung cancers. Chest. 2000;118:1526–9.
48. Greenlee RT, Murray T, Bolden S, Wingo PA. Cancer statistics, 2000. CA Cancer J Clin. 2000;50:7–33.
49. Ellis PM, Delaney G, Della-Fiorentina S, Moylan E. Assessing outcomes of cancer care: lessons to be learned from a retrospective review of the management of small cell lung cancer at the Cancer Therapy Centre, Liverpool Hospital, January 1996–July 2000. Australas Radiol. 2004;48(3):364–70.
50. Murray N, Coy P, Pater JL, Hodson I, Arnold A, Zee BC, et al. Importance of timing for thoracic irradiation in the combined modality treatment of limited-stage small-cell lung cancer. The National Cancer Institute of Canada Clinical Trials Group. J Clin Oncol. 1993;11:336–44.
51. Turrisi 3rd AT, Kim K, Blum R, Sause WT, Livingston RB, Komaki R, et al. Twice-daily compared with once-daily thoracic radiotherapy in limited small-cell lung cancer treated concurrently with cisplatin and etoposide. N Eng J Med. 1999;340:265–71.
52. O'Brien ME, Ciuleanu TE, Tsekov H, Shparyk Y, Cuceviá B, Juhasz G, et al. Phase III trial comparing supportive care alone with supportive care with oral topotecan in patients with relapsed small-cell lung cancer. J Clin Oncol. 2006;24:5441–7.
53. von Pawel J, Schiller JH, Shepherd FA, Fields SZ, Kleisbauer JP, Chrysson NG, et al. Topotecan versus cyclophosphamide, doxorubicin, and vincristine for the treatment of recurrent small-cell lung cancer. J Clin Oncol. 1999;17:658–67.
54. Johnson BE. Second lung cancers in patients after treatment for an initial lung cancer. J Natl Cancer Inst. 1998;90:1335–45.
55. Kawahara M, Ushijima S, Kamimori T, Kodam N, Ogawara M, Matsui K, et al. Second primary tumours in more than 2-year disease-free survivors of small-cell lung cancer in Japan: the role of smoking cessation. Br J Cancer. 1998;78:409–12.
56. Tucker MA, Murray N, Shaw EG, Ettinger DS, Mabry M, Huber MH, et al. Second primary cancers related to smoking and treatment of small-cell lung cancer. Lung Cancer Working Cadre. J Natl Cancer Inst. 1997;89:1782–8.
57. Cancer Care Ontario. Cross-sectional diagnostic imaging in lung cancer: a Cancer Care Ontario recommendations report. 2006. http://www.cancercare.on.ca/pdf/pebcdilungf.pdf. Accessed 8 Feb 2009.
58. National Comprehensive Cancer Network (NCCN). Clinical practice guidelines in oncology: small cell lung cancer. V.2. 2009. http://www,nccn.org/professionals/physician_gls/PDF/sclc.pdf. Accessed 8 Feb 2009.
59. Sorensen M, Felip E, ESMO Guidelines Working Group. Small-cell lung cancer: ESMO clinical recommendations for diagnosis, treatment and follow-up. Ann Oncol. 2008;19 Suppl 2:ii41–2.
60. Sugiyama T, Hirose T, Hosaka T, Kusumoto S, Nakashima M, Yamaoka T, et al. Effectiveness of intensive follow-up after response in patients with small cell lung cancer. Lung Cancer. 2008;59: 255–61.
61. Stewart BW, Kleihues P, editors. World cancer report. Lyon: IARC Press; 2003.
62. Gilmore J. Report on smoking in Canada, 1985 to 2001 (Statistics Canada, Catalogue 82F0077XIE). 2002.
63. Walker MS, Larsen RJ, Zona DM, Govindan R, Fisher EB. Smoking urges and relapse among lung cancer patients: findings from a preliminary retrospective study. Prev Med. 2004;39:449–57.
64. Godtfredsen NS, Prescott E, Osler M. Effect of smoking reduction on lung cancer risk. JAMA. 2005;294:1505–10.
65. Richardson GE, Tucker MA, Venzon DJ, Linnoila RI, Phelps R, Phares JC, et al. Smoking cessation after successful treatment of small-cell lung cancer is associated with fewer smoking-related second primary cancers. Ann Intern Med. 2005;119:383–90.
66. Gritz ER, Nisenbaum R, Elashoff RE, Holmes EC. Smoking behavior following diagnosis in patients with stage I non-small cell lung cancer. Cancer Causes Control. 1991;2:105–12.
67. Davison AG, Duffy M. Smoking habits of long-term survivors of surgery for lung cancer. Thorax. 1982;37:331–3.
68. Nakamura H, Haruki T, Adachi Y, Fujioka S, Miwa K, Taniguchi Y. Smoking affects prognosis after lung cancer surgery. Surg Today. 2008;38:227–31.
69. Browman GP, Wong G, Hodson I, Sathya J, Russell R, McAlpine L, et al. Influence of cigarette smoking on the efficacy of radiation therapy in head and neck cancer. N Engl J Med. 1993;328:159–63.
70. Yu GP, Ostroff JS, Zhang ZF, Tang J, Schantz SP. Smoking history and cancer patient survival: a hospital cancer registry study. Cancer Detect Prev. 1997;21:497–509.
71. Fleshner N, Garland J, Moadel A, Herr H, Ostroff J, Trambert R, et al. Influence of smoking status on the disease-related outcomes of patients with tobacco-associated superficial transitional cell carcinoma of the bladder. Cancer. 1999;86:2337–45.
72. Monson JM, Stark P, Reilly JJ, Sugarbaker DJ, Strauss GM, Swanson SJ, et al. Clinical radiation pneumonitis and radiographic changes after thoracic radiation therapy for lung carcinoma. Cancer. 1998;82:842–50.
73. Videtic GMM, Stitt LW, Dar AR, Kocha WI, Tomiak AT, Truong PT, et al. Continued cigarette smoking by patients receiving concurrent chemoradiotherapy for limited-stage small-cell lung cancer is associated with decreased survival. J Clin Oncol. 2003;21:1544–9.
74. Tsao AS, Liu D, Lee JJ, Spitz M, Hong WK. Smoking affects treatment outcome in patients with advanced non small cell lung cancer. Cancer. 2006;106:2428–36.
75. Fiore MC, Jaen CR, Baker TB, Bailey WC, Benowitz NL, Curry SJ, et al. Treating tobacco use and dependence: 2008 update. Rockville, MD: Public Health Service, US Department of Health and Human Services; 2008. http://www.surgeongeneral.gov/tobacco/treating_tobacco_use08.pdf. Accessed 8 Feb 2009.
76. U.S. Department of Health and Human Services. Clinical practice guideline: treating tobacco use and dependence. 2000. http://www.surgeongeneral.gov/tobacco/treating_tobacco_use.pdf. Accessed 8 Feb 2009.

16 Esophagus Carcinoma

Shilpi Wadhwa, David Y. Johnson, and Frank E. Johnson

Keywords
Esophagus • Surveillance • Esophageal cancer • Squamous cell carcinoma • Risk factors

The International Agency for Research on Cancer (IARC), a component of the World Health Organization (WHO), estimated that there were 462,117 new cases of esophageal cancer worldwide in 2002 [1]. The IARC also estimated that there were 385,892 deaths due to this cause in 2002 [1].

The American Cancer Society estimated that there were 15,560 new cases and 13,940 deaths due to this cause in the USA in 2007 [2]. The estimated 5-year survival rate (all races) in the USA in 2007 was 16% for esophageal cancer [2]. Survival rates were adjusted for normal life expectancies and are based on cases diagnosed from 1996 to 2002 and followed through 2003.

Many studies of esophageal carcinoma do not distinguish among the several subtypes. Since the most common (>90%) histological variety is squamous cell carcinoma in most populations around the world, the epidemiology of esophageal cancer is heavily influenced by this subset. Geographic factors are well established [3]. Consumption of tobacco products (smoked or chewed), alcohol, opium, and betel products increases risk markedly. Certain pickled vegetables [3], bracken fern ingestion, ionizing radiation, asbestos, various mycotoxins, and other less well-documented agents are probably causative agents. Low socioeconomic status is associated with increased risk of both squamous cell carcinoma and adenocarcinoma [4].

S. Wadhwa • D.Y. Johnson
Department of Internal Medicine, Saint Louis University Medical Center, Saint Louis, MO, USA

F.E. Johnson (✉)
Saint Louis University Medical Center and Saint Louis Veterans Affairs Medical Center, Saint Louis, MO, USA
e-mail: frank.johnson1@va.gov

Gastroesophageal reflux disease is a major risk factor for adenocarcinoma. Prior upper aerodigestive tract cancer is a very powerful risk factor [4]. As with most types of cancers, some genetic risk factors have been described and many more seem likely to be discovered in the near future.

Geographic Variation Worldwide

Esophageal cancer is a common cancer in the developing countries and the incidence varies considerably according to the geographic location. The incidence is highest in East Africa and Asia, including China and Central Asia [5]. In the USA the geographic variation for esophageal cancer is more pronounced among males than females and among whites than among blacks. In Washington, DC, and coastal areas of South Carolina, the rates are especially high in blacks. The incidence among white males is highest in Connecticut and Seattle [6].

Surveillance Strategies Proposed by Professional Organizations or National Government Agencies and Available on the Internet

National Comprehensive Cancer Network (www.nccn.org)

National Comprehensive Cancer Network (NCCN) guidelines were accessed on 1/28/12 (Table 16.1). There were minor quantitative and qualitative changes compared to the guidelines accessed on 4/10/07.

F.E. Johnson et al. (eds.), *Patient Surveillance After Cancer Treatment*, Current Clinical Oncology,
DOI 10.1007/978-1-60327-969-7_16, © Springer Science+Business Media New York 2013

Table 16.1 Esophageal and esophagogastric junction cancer

	Years posttreatment[a]					
	1	2	3	4	5	>5
Office visit	2–4	2–4	1–2	1–2	1–2	1
• Chemistry profile and CBC, as clinically indicated						
• Imaging as clinically indicated						
• Upper GI endoscopy and biopsy as clinically indicated						
• Dilatation for anastomotic stenosis						
• Nutritional counseling						
• Confirm HER2-neu testing has been done if metastatic disease was present at diagnosis						

Obtained from NCCN (www.nccn.org) on 1/28/12
NCCN guidelines were accessed on 1/28/12. There were minor quantitative and qualitative changes compared to the guidelines accessed on 4/10/07
[a]The numbers in the table indicate the number of times the modality is recommended during the indicated year posttreatment

American Society of Clinical Oncology (www.asco.org)

American Society of Clinical Oncology (ASCO) guidelines were accessed on 1/28/12. No quantitative guidelines exist for esophagus cancer surveillance, including when first accessed on 10/31/07.

The Society of Surgical Oncology (www.surgonc.org)

The Society of Surgical Oncology (SSO) guidelines were accessed on 1/28/12. No quantitative guidelines exist for esophagus cancer surveillance, including when first accessed on 10/31/07.

European Society for Medical Oncology (www.esmo.org)

European Society for Medical Oncology (ESMO) guidelines were accessed on 1/28/12. No quantitative guidelines exist for esophagus cancer surveillance, including when first accessed on 10/31/07.

European Society of Surgical Oncology (www.esso-surgeonline.org)

European Society of Surgical Oncology (ESSO) guidelines were accessed on 1/28/12. No quantitative guidelines exist for esophagus cancer surveillance, including when first accessed on 10/31/07.

Cancer Care Ontario (www.cancercare.on.ca)

Cancer Care Ontario (CCO) guidelines were accessed on 1/28/12. No quantitative guidelines exist for esophagus cancer surveillance, including when first accessed on 10/31/07.

National Institute for Clinical Excellence (www.nice.org.uk)

National Institute for Clinical Excellence (NICE) guidelines were accessed on 1/28/12. No quantitative guidelines exist for esophagus cancer surveillance, including when first accessed on 10/31/07.

The Cochrane Collaboration (CC, www.cochrane.org)

CC guidelines were accessed on 1/28/12. No quantitative guidelines exist for esophagus cancer surveillance, including when first accessed on 11/24/07.

Society for the Surgery of the Alimentary Tract (www.ssat.com)

Society for the Surgery of the Alimentary Tract (SSAT) guidelines were accessed on 1/28/12. No quantitative guidelines exist for esophagus cancer surveillance, including when first accessed on 12/18/07

The M.D. Anderson Surgical Oncology Handbook also has follow-up guidelines, proposed by authors from a single National Cancer Institute-designated Comprehensive Cancer Center, for many types of cancer [7]. Some are detailed and quantitative, others are qualitative.

Summary

This is a common cancer with significant variability in incidence worldwide. We found consensus-based guidelines but none based on high-quality evidence.

References

1. Parkin DM, Whelan SL, Ferlay J, Teppo L, Thomas DB. Cancer incidence in five continents, Vol. VIII, International Agency for Research on Cancer. (IARC Scientific Publication 155). Lyon, France: IARC Press; 2002. ISBN 92-832-2155-9.

2. Jemal A, Seigel R, Ward E, Murray T, Xu J, Thun MJ. Cancer statistics, 2007. CA Cancer J Clin. 2007;57:43–66.
3. Schottenfeld D, Fraumeni JG. Cancer epidemiology and prevention. 3rd ed. New York, NY: Oxford University Press; 2006. ISBN 13:978-0-19-514961-6.
4. DeVita VT, Hellman S, Rosenberg SA. Cancer. 7th ed. Philadelphia, PA: Lippincott Williams & Wilkins; 2005. ISBN 0-781-74450-4.
5. Mackay J, Jemal A, Lee NC, Parkin M. The Cancer Atlas. 2006 American Cancer Society 1599 Clifton Road NE, Atlanta, Georgia 30329, USA. Can also be accessed at www.cancer.org. ISBN 0-944235-62-X.
6. Devesa SS, Grauman DJ, Blot WJ, Pennello GA, Hoover RN, Fraumeni JF Jr. Atlas of Cancer Mortality in the United States. National Institutes of Health, National Cancer Institute. NIH Publication No. 99-4564; Sep 1999.
7. Feig BW, Berger DH, Fuhrman GM. The M.D. Anderson Surgical Oncology Handbook. 4th ed. Philadelphia, PA: Lippincott Williams & Wilkins; 2006. ISBN 0-7817-5643-X (paperback).

Esophagus Carcinoma Surveillance Counterpoint: Australia

17

Bernard Mark Smithers, Janine M. Thomas, and Bryan H. Burmeister

Keywords
Esophageal cancer • Esophagectomy • Definitive chemoradiation therapy • Dysphagia • Australia

The demographics of esophageal cancer in Australia reflect those of other Western countries [1] with a rising incidence in adenocarcinoma of the lower esophagus and esophagogastric junction. However, in Western countries we still see patients with squamous cell carcinoma of the thoracic and cervical esophagus. The other change over the last 20 years has been an evolution of the use of the combination of chemotherapy with radiation therapy in the management of patients with esophageal cancer. Traditionally, resection was the definitive curative therapy, with radiation therapy used for patients who were not medically fit or who refused resection. However, the combination of chemoradiation therapy without resection was shown to offer a greater potential for cure for patients with squamous cell carcinoma, when compared with radiation therapy alone [2]. Thus, the recent trend has been to use concurrent chemoradiation therapy as definitive treatment or as neoadjuvant therapy for those patients having a resection [3, 4]. Recently, two randomized studies have supported the use of definitive chemoradiation therapy instead of esophageal resection in medically fit patients with squamous cell carcinoma [5, 6]. The role for definitive chemoradiation therapy in patients with adenocarcinoma of the esophagus is not clear, as most trials have had a predominance of squamous cell carcinoma. At this time the gold standard is still resection for locally advanced disease with the use of preoperative chemotherapy or chemoradiation therapy, given the survival benefits shown in meta-analyses [7]. There are some data to suggest that neoadjuvant chemoradiation therapy results in downstaging and improves resectability [8, 9].

The outcomes from the management of patients with esophageal cancer are typically poor. There are no directed systemic therapies for metastatic disease such that the value of regular surveillance in patients treated with curative intent may be questioned. The early detection of metastatic disease offers little benefit to the patient. As with other cancers with a similar outcome profile, regular surveillance throughout offers the patient psychosocial support and recognition of the very small cohort for whom treatment offers improved quality of life or even prolongs survival. However, in the early posttreatment period, there are benefits from follow-up to the patient relating to the assessment and management of the functional problems that may occur after an esophageal resection or definitive chemoradiation therapy.

Following an esophagectomy, there is little to no potential for resection of recurrent disease. There are a few patients who may develop isolated locoregional recurrence who may be amenable to definitive radiation therapy with or without concurrent chemotherapy. We reported 14 patients from 525 resections that were able to undergo salvage definitive

B.M. Smithers (✉)
Upper Gastrointestinal and Soft Tissue Unit, Princess Alexandra Hospital, University of Queensland, Ipswich Road, Woolloongabba, Brisbane, QLD 4102, Australia
e-mail: m.smithers@uq.edu.au

J.M. Thomas
Upper Gastrointestinal and Soft Tissue Unit, Princess Alexandra Hospital, Ipswich Road, Woolloongabba, Brisbane, QLD 4102, Australia
e-mail: janine1972@hotmail.com

B.H. Burmeister
Department of Radiation Oncology, Princess Alexandra Hospital, University of Queensland, Ipswich Road, Woolloongabba, Brisbane, QLD 4102, Australia
e-mail: Bryan_Burmeister@health.qld.gov.au

F.E. Johnson et al. (eds.), *Patient Surveillance After Cancer Treatment*, Current Clinical Oncology, DOI 10.1007/978-1-60327-969-7_17,

chemoradiation therapy with a 2-year survival rate of 21% [10]. These patients present with symptoms that direct the investigations. A few patients who have undergone definitive chemoradiation therapy have persistent or recurrent disease localized to the primary site. Salvage esophagectomy offers a potential for cure [11]. However, the number suitable for this therapy is likely to be small because, generally, the patients are offered chemoradiation therapy as they are not medically fit or are not suitable for resection for other reasons. In a randomized trial of definitive chemoradiation therapy compared with resection alone for squamous cell carcinoma of the esophagus, Chui et al. reported that, when patients medically fit for resection were randomized to resection or definitive chemoradiation therapy, 5 of 36 (14%) required a salvage esophagectomy in the median follow-up period of 2 years [6]. That figure is likely to increase with longer follow-up. Thus, in deciding upon a suitable follow-up regimen for our patients, we used our own experience as a guide. With knowledge of the rate at which recurrence occurs, our regimen allows us to deal with the functional problems that exist after an esophageal resection or treatment with definitive chemoradiation therapy.

Between January 1994 and December 2008 our unit assessed 1,534 patients with carcinoma of the esophagus or esophagogastric junction. There were 984 (62%) who were offered curative treatment. Treatment consisted of surgery alone in 385 (39%), neoadjuvant therapy followed by resection in 297 (30%), definitive chemoradiation therapy in 277 (28%), and radiation therapy alone in 5 (1%). Definitive chemoradiation therapy was followed by salvage resection in 20 (2%). There were 553 (56%) patients who developed recurrence after a median follow-up period of 13 months (range 3–167). The number of patients who have been able to be treated with curative intent following recurrent disease is 35 (6%); 22 patients had salvage definitive chemoradiation therapy after resection and 13 patients had salvage esophagectomy after definitive chemoradiation therapy.

The patients who had preoperative therapy had typically been enrolled in trials using a combination of a single cycle of cisplatin and 5-fluorouracil with radiation therapy to 35 Gy [12] and more recently a local phase II randomized trial of two cycles of cisplatin and 5-fluorouracil with and without the same dose of radiation therapy.

One would expect that the pattern of recurrence would be different, depending upon the modality of curative therapy. Patients having resection may recur in the locoregional area but more commonly present with distant recurrences. Those patients having definitive chemoradiation therapy are more likely to have persistent or recurrent disease at the primary site. We systematically record the first site of recurrence of disease. This is typically discovered from directed imaging studies performed due to the patient's symptoms.

In our series, the majority of systemic and locoregional recurrences occurred in the first 2 years for patients in both the resection (79%) and definitive chemoradiation therapy (83%) groups. The large majority of the recurrences that ever develop will occur by 5 years (Tables 17.1 and 17.2). For those patients surviving beyond 5 years, recurrent disease may still occur. In our group of patients treated with curative intent, there were 135 patients (surgery 114, chemoradiation therapy 21) alive after 5 years; 21 (15%) developed clinical evidence of recurrence later—16 (14%) in the surgery group; and 5 (24%) in the chemoradiation therapy group. We have seen recurrence beyond 10 years in 3 of the 18 (16%) patients who survived beyond that time.

When we examine the timing and the pattern of recurrence in relation to the role of neoadjuvant chemoradiotherapy, or chemotherapy alone, and surgery alone, the time to first symptomatic recurrence was similar among the groups (Table 17.1). Table 17.1 also shows that the majority of locoregional recurrences became evident in the first 3 years after treatment no matter what preoperative therapy was used.

If definitive chemoradiation therapy was performed on a patient who would otherwise have been fit for resection, there is the potential to consider an operation if this patient suffers a recurrence or persisting disease at the primary site. Thus, in this subgroup of patients, the assessment of the primary site using endoscopy is appropriate. When specifically assessed for this site of recurrence after definitive chemoradiation therapy, 73% of the patients had a recurrence at the primary site within 2 years and 98% by 5 years (Table 17.2). However, in our dataset, the majority of these patients were subsequently proven to have other locoregional and/or systemic disease with further imaging. Other patients presented with recurrent dysphagia but, because of their poor medical status, no investigations were performed to define the site of other disease unless clinically indicated.

Following an esophagectomy, functional problems may be short or long term. The most common short-term problem is an anastomotic stricture. This is more common in patients with an anastomosis in the neck than those with an intrathoracic anastomosis. Thus, early clinical assessment the patient's ability to swallow is important. Significant dysphagia is assessed by endoscopy with dilation of the stricture, if confirmed. Patients may require a series of dilations at regular short intervals until the scarring at the anastomosis has matured.

The long-term functional problems that may occur relate to the disturbance of the normal anatomy and physiology of the upper gastrointestinal tract. Typically, a gastric tube is used as a replacement for the resected esophageal segment. The problems that may require attention include gastroparesis and poor emptying (postvagotomy effect), dumping syndrome, symptoms of abdominal colic, lightheadedness and epigastric discomfort, as well as diarrhea, requiring regular medications. The majority of the functional symptoms improve over the first 9 months [13], but it is our experience that a small number of patients continue to complain of prob-

Table 17.1 Percentage annual esophageal cancer recurrence post-curative surgery

	Year				
	1	2	3	4	5
Surgery alone (*n* = 183)					
Percentage of recurrence	48%(88)	79%(145)	92%(168)	96%(175)	96%(176)
Local/regional	9%(16)	14%(26)	16%(29)	17%(31)	17%(31)
Distant	36%(67)	61%(112)	71%(130)	74%(135)	74%(136)
Combination	3%(5)	4%(7)	5%(9)	5%(9)	5%(9)
Chemotherapy and surgery (*n* = 40)	43%(17)	85%(34)	93%(37)	98%(39)	98%(39)
Percentage of recurrence	3%(1)	5%(2)	8%(3)	8%(3)	8%(3)
Local/regional	25%(10)	55%(22)	60%(24)	65%(26)	65%(26)
Distant	15%(6)	25%(10)	25%(10)	25%(10)	25%(10)
Combination	–	–	–	–	–
CXRT and surgery (*n* = 92)					
Percentage of recurrence	51%(47)	76%(70)	85%(78)	91%(84)	92%(85)
Local/regional	4%(4)	8%(7)	9%(8)	12%(11)	12%(11)
Distant	41%(38)	58%(53)	64%(59)	67%(62)	67%(62)
Combination	6%(5)	10%(9)	12%(11)	12%(11)	13%(12)

The annual cumulative recurrence rate for the 315 recurrences among 682 patients who had an esophageal resection. The median follow-up time was 16 months for the surgery-alone group and 13 months for the group who had neoadjuvant therapy
CXRT chemotherapy in combination with radiation therapy

Table 17.2 Percentage annual esophageal cancer recurrence post-curative-intent chemoradiation therapy

	Year				
n = 181	1	2	3	4	5
Overall recurrence	51% (92)	83% (150)	93% (168)	96% (174)	97% (175)
Recurrence at primary site	39% (71)	73% (157)	87% (157)	92% (167)	98% (177)

The annual cumulative recurrence rate for the 181 recurrences that occurred in 277 patients treated with definitive chemoradiation. Median follow-up time was 11 months

lems with eating, reflux, and loose bowel motions long term. Assessing the functional outcomes and quality of life in a group of 5-year survivors following resection for esophageal cancer, one group reported that the most common symptoms in these patients were reflux, shortness of breath, pain, and appetite loss [14].

The most common early problem following definitive chemoradiation therapy is a stricture at the primary cancer site. As well, there is the potential for persistence of the disease at this site. Our experience has been that 72 patients (24%) have required endoscopic dilatation of a stricture after definitive chemoradiation therapy. This may require a series of endoscopies until the stricture has stabilized. We usually perform the first endoscopy 4–6 weeks posttherapy, allowing the inflammation to settle. We do not perform a dilatation inside of that time period, although there is no evidence to suggest that this might lead to major problems. In the long term, patients may have mild stable dysphagia related to a disturbance in esophageal motility. However, if significant dysphagia develops after a period of normal swallowing, the most likely diagnosis is a recurrence of the malignancy. Thus, endoscopy is the first choice investigation.

Some patients develop radiation pneumonitis after definitive chemoradiation. This may be nondetectable on CT imaging but is detectable on respiratory function tests following the onset of dyspnea. This is frequently related to poor pretreatment lung function. This late effect is manageable with the use of intermittent steroids in most cases. Less commonly, patients with preexisting osteoporosis develop compression fractures of the spinal vertebrae within the radiation field. This is manageable with the use of bisphosphates and support garments. Significant damage to other organs, such as the heart, spinal cord, or bone marrow from radiation therapy is exceptionally rare. We do not schedule any specific tests to detect complications of chemotherapy or radiation therapy but rely on clinical symptoms and signs to trigger investigations.

In summary, following an esophageal resection the majority of the major functional problems occur in the first year and cancer recurrence in the first 2 years. Thus, we perform clinical assessment with symptom-directed investigations every 3 months for the first year, every 4 months in the second year, every 6 months in postsurgery years 3 and 4, moving to annual assessment from that time onwards (Table 17.3). The assessment encompasses the functional status. Our examination

Table 17.3 Surveillance after curative-intent surgery

	Year					
Modality	1	2	3	4	5	>5
Office visit	4	3–4	2	2	1	1

Other modalities as clinically indicated only
The number in each cell is the number of times an office visit is recommended in a particular posttreatment year

Table 17.4 Surveillance after curative-intent chemotherapy and radiation therapy

	Year					
Modality	1	2	3	4	5	>5
Office visit	4	3	2	2	1	1
Endoscopy	4	3	2	2	1	1

Blood tests/X-rays/other investigations are ordered as clinically indicated only
Office visit includes assessment of the ability to swallow
The number in each cell is the number of times a particular modality is recommended in a particular posttreatment year

includes the patient's weight and a general examination of the neck, chest, and abdomen. Because a number of our patients live a significant distance from our center, the assessment is often done on the telephone with the patient seeing his or her local doctor for the physical examination.

Patients who have had definitive chemoradiation therapy have an endoscopy 4–6 weeks posttherapy. Biopsies are directed to proliferative areas. Typically, in the first 3–4 months, there is some persistent ulceration that shows changes consistent with radiation effect if biopsied. If the patient is considered a surgical candidate, clinical review and endoscopic surveillance continues every 3–4 months in the first 2 years, every 6 months in years 3 and 4, and annually after that time (Table 17.4). If the patient is not fit for resection, endoscopy is not routine (although a number of patients will request the study) but is the investigation of choice if dysphagia develops. Clinical review is performed without any specific protocol at the discretion of the treating doctor following discussion with the patient. Many patients with esophageal cancer have unrelated medical problems. Additional office visits and various tests may be required to manage these problems.

The treating surgeon follows the patients who have had a resection. When recurrence occurs, referral to an appropriate oncologist is arranged and the management is taken over by this group. Patients who have had definitive chemoradiation therapy are followed by the treating radiation oncologist in liaison with the surgeons in the unit who perform endoscopy when required or indicated.

When our protocol is compared with the recommended follow-up published by the National Comprehensive Cancer Network [15], we are in concordance with the timing of patient review and the need for clinically directed investigations rather than routine tests or images. The protocol we use has been well accepted by the members of our unit and the members of the multidisciplinary clinic in which our patients are routinely discussed.

References

1. Pohl H, Welch G. The role of over-diagnosis and reclassification in the marked increase of esophageal adenocarcinoma incidence. J Natl Cancer Inst. 2005;97:142–6.
2. Herskovic A, Martz K, Al-Sarraf MV, et al. Combined chemotherapy and radiotherapy compared with radiotherapy alone in patients with cancer of the oesophagus. N Engl J Med. 1992;326:1593–8.
3. Geh JI. The use of chemoradiotherapy in oesophageal cancer. Eur J Cancer. 2002;38:300–13.
4. Geh JI, Crellen AM, Glynne-Jones R. Preoperative (neoadjuvant) chemoradiotherapy in oesophageal cancer. Br J Surg. 2001;88: 338–56.
5. Stahl M, Stuschke M, Lehmann N, et al. Chemoradiation with and without surgery in patients with locally advanced squamous cell carcinoma of the esophagus. J Clin Oncol. 2005;23:2310–7.
6. Chui P, Chan A, Leung S, et al. Multicenter prospective randomized trial comparing standard esophagectomy with chemoradiotherapy for treatment of squamous oesophageal cancer: early results from the Chinese University Research Group for Esophageal Cancer (CURE). J Gastrointest Surg. 2005;9:794–802.
7. Gebski V, Burmeister B, Smithers BM, et al. Survival benefits from neoadjuvant chemoradiotherapy or chemotherapy in oesophageal cancer: a meta-analysis. Lancet Oncol. 2007;8:226–34.
8. Burmeister B, Smithers BM, Thomas J, et al. A randomized phase II trial comparing pre-operative chemotherapy with pre-operative chemoradiation therapy for localised carcinoma of the oesophagus. Eur J Cancer 2011;47:354–60.
9. Stahl M, Walz MK, Stuschke M, et al. Phase II comparison of pre-operative chemotherapy compared with chemoradiotherapy in patients with locally advanced adenocarcinoma of the esophago-gastric junction. J Clin Oncol. 2009;27:851–6.
10. Baxi SN, Burmeister B, Harvey JA, et al. Salvage definitive chemoradiotherapy for locally recurrent oesophageal carcinoma after primary surgery; retrospective review. J Med Imaging Radiat Oncol. 2008;52:1–5.
11. Smithers BM, Cullinan M, Thomas JM, et al. Outcomes from salvage esophagectomy post definitive chemoradiotherapy compared with resection following preoperative neoadjuvant chemoradiotherapy. Dis Esophagus. 2007;20:471–7.
12. Burmeister BH, Smithers BM, Gebski V, et al. A randomised phase III study comparing surgery alone with chemoradiation therapy followed by surgery for resectable carcinoma of the oesophagus: an intergroup study of the Trans-Tasman Radiation Oncology Group (TROG) and the Australasian Gastro-Intestinal Trials Group (AGITG). Lancet Oncol. 2005;6:659–68.
13. Conroy T, Marchal F, Blazeby JM. Quality of life in patients with oesophageal and gastric cancer: an overview. Oncology. 2006;70:391–402.
14. Hallas CN, Patel N, Oo A, et al. Five-year survival following oesophageal cancer resection: psychological functioning and quality of life. Psychol Health Med. 2001;6:684–94.
15. National Comprehensive Cancer Network. Practice Guidelines in Oncology: Esophageal Cancer: Version 1. Available: http://www.nccn.org (2009).

Esophagus Carcinoma Surveillance Counterpoint: Japan

18

Masaru Morita and Yoshihiko Maehara

Keywords
Japan • Esophagus • Recurrence • Radiation • Curative operation

Cancer has been the leading cause of death in Japan since 1981. The number of cancer deaths in Japan in 2010 was approximately 353,500, and about 11,900 patients were due to esophageal cancer, thus making it the sixth most common cause of cancer death [1]. In Western countries the incidence of adenocarcinoma of the esophagus is increasing and the site is typically the lower esophagus or the esophagogastric junction [2]. In Japan, 89% of esophageal carcinomas are of the squamous cell variety and 47% of all esophageal carcinomas are located in the midthoracic esophagus [3].

The Annual Review of 2010 performed by the Japanese Association for Thoracic Surgery revealed that 59% of patients had conventional surgical resections, and 18% of patients had endoscopic resections. Resection was not performed in the remaining 29% [4]. Control of lymph node metastases has been emphasized in Japan. Radical lymphadenectomy, especially of the upper mediastinal lymph nodes around the recurrent laryngeal nerves, is considered very important. Resection of the cervical lymph nodes, including paraesophageal and supraclavicular nodes, is frequently added. Lymphadenectomy of cervical, mediastinal, and abdominal nodes is known as a "three-field" dissection [5]. Esophagectomy via cervical, right thoracic, and abdominal approaches with a radical lymphadenectomy is currently the standard operation for thoracic esophageal cancer in Japan. As a result, 5-year survival rates of more than 40% have been reported [5, 6]. A recent review of 1,000 consecutive patients with esophageal cancer who underwent esophagectomy in our institution over two decades showed remarkable improvement in patient prognosis as well as decreased operative mortality and morbidity [7].

Although the prognosis of patients with esophageal cancer has markedly improved, especially in high-volume centers in Japan, a recent nationwide review revealed that the 5-year relative survival is only 33.2% [1]. Even when curative resections are performed, recurrence is frequently experienced fairly soon after surgery.

From 1998 to 2006, 255 patients with esophageal cancer underwent a surgical resection at Kyushu University. Among these patients, curative resections (R0) were achieved in 219 (86%). After excluding 11 patients who could not be followed up, the clinical course of the remaining 208 patients was analyzed. Among these patients, recurrence was recognized in 61 patients (29%) and recurrence patterns were evident in 56 patients. Recurrence was diagnosed within 1 year after surgery in 40 patients (71%) and within 2 years in 47 patients (84%). Locoregional recurrence was observed in 30 patients (54%), including lymphatic recurrence (27 patients) and local recurrence (3 patients). The upper mediastinal nodal area was the most frequent recurrence site. Abdominal recurrence was mainly in the celiac and para-aortic lymph nodes. Hematogenous recurrence was recognized in 20 patients (36%), while mixed-type recurrence (locoregional recurrence plus hematogenous recurrence) was recognized in 6 patients (8%). The most frequent site of initial hematogenous recurrence was the lungs, followed by liver, bone, and skin [8].

Table 18.1 indicates the characteristics of recurrence after a curative operation reported in Japan [9–18]. The distribution of locoregional recurrence and distant recurrence varies among institutions. The incidence of locoregional recurrence ranged from 22 to 56%. The upper mediastinum is the most

M. Morita, M.D., Ph.D., F.A.C.S. (✉) • Y. Maehara, M.D., Ph.D., F.A.C.S.
Department of Surgery and Science, Graduate School of Medical Sciences, Kyushu University, 3-1-1 Maidashi, Higashi-ku, Fukuoka 812-8582, Japan
e-mail: masarum@surg2.med.kyushu-u.ac.jp

F.E. Johnson et al. (eds.), *Patient Surveillance After Cancer Treatment*, Current Clinical Oncology,
DOI 10.1007/978-1-60327-969-7_18, © Springer Science+Business Media New York 2013

Table 18.1 Characteristics of recurrence after a curative resection for esophageal cancer in Japan [8–17]

Year reported	Lymph node dissection	Recurrence/Total	Incidence of each recurrence pattern: Locoregional Lymphatic	Locoregional Local	Distant Hematogenous	Mixed	Recurrence time after surgery
1994	Two-field	95/187 (51%)	48%	4%	24%	23%	56% within 1 year 84% within 2 year
1996	Three-field	83/230 (36%)	42%		46%	12%	
1996	Three-field	33/115 (29%)	27%	21%	33%	4%	11.1 months (mean) for pT3 tumor
1997	Three-field	39/90 (43%)	49%	51%			10.5 months (mean) for locoregional rec 11.4 months (mean)for distant recurrence
2003	Three-field	41/151 (27%)	42%	22%	37%		19 months (median) for locoregional rec 8.4 months (median) for distant recurrence
2003	Three-field	98/246 (40%)	21%	11%	68%		83% within 2 years
2004	Three-field	74/171 (43%)	48%	6%	38%	8%	17.5 months (median) for locoregional recurrence 8.0 months (median) for distant recurrence
2005	Two-field or Three-field	59/160 (37%)	22%		51%	27%	18.8 months (mean) for locoregional recurrence 13.9 months (mean)for hematogenous recurrence 8.4 months (mean) for mixed recurrence
2006	Two-field or three-field	131/367 (36%)	33%	3%	34%	31%	
2006	Two-field or three-field	90/270 (33%)	48%	8%	31%	13%	
2008 Current review	Two-field or three-field	61/208 (29%)	48%	5%	36%	11%	71% within 1 year 84% within 2 years

common site and abdominal lymph node recurrences are also common. The incidence of recurrence in the cervical lymph node seems to depend on the extent of lymph node dissection. Lung and liver are the most frequent sites of distant recurrence. Even after a curative esophagectomy associated with radical lymph node dissection, recurrence is recognized within 2 years in more than 80% of the patients who ever experience recurrence. This suggests the importance of strict follow-up during this period. Some authors report that distant metastasis, especially mixed-type recurrence, occurs earlier than locoregional recurrence [2, 15, 16]. Others report little difference in the disease-free interval between patients with distant metastasis as the first evidence of recurrence and those with locoregional metastasis as the first evidence of recurrence [12].

It is important to identify the patients at high risk of recurrence when a follow-up schedule is chosen in order to control costs as well as to detect recurrence promptly. Both the depth of invasion at the primary site and lymph node metastasis are predictors of poor prognosis. The number of histologically positive lymph nodes is considered to be the most powerful prognostic factor according to studies of patients receiving three-field dissection. Shimada, et al. [19], reported that the number of positive nodes was associated with the 5-year survival rate as follows: node negative 60%; single node involved 65%; two nodes involved 51%; ≥three nodes 20%. Igaki et al. [20], examined the results of a three-field lymphadenectomy for pT1/T2 esophageal cancer. The 5-year survival rates of patients with 0–4 positive nodes were 74% in pT1 and 55% in pT2. All patients with five or more positive nodes died of cancer within 5 years, even those with pT1 or 2 tumors.

Intramural spread is considered to be another important prognostic factor. One study reported that 14.4% of patients with esophageal cancer have intramural metastasis [21]. The prognosis of these patients is significantly worse than the prognosis of those without intramural metastasis. Multivariate analysis revealed that depth of invasion, tumor length, and intramural metastasis are all independent prognostic factors [21]. Another study revealed that intramural metastasis was found in 5% of patients with submucosal cancer, while a multivariate analysis revealed the independent prognostic factors of patents with submucosal esophageal cancer to be intramural metastasis, vessel invasion, and lymph node metastasis [22].

Osugi et al. emphasized the prognostic significance of vessel invasion after an extended lymphadenectomy and concluded that lymphatic vessel invasion is the only independent prognostic factor in patients with no evidence of node metastasis [23]. The type of vessel invasion is closely related to the recurrence pattern. Lymphatic vessel invasion predicts lymphatic recurrence, while blood vessel invasion predicts hematogenous recurrence [9]. Consequently, patients at high risk for recurrence are those with pStage III/IV cancer, those with ≥four nodex with metastases, intramural metastasis, or marked vessel invasion [24].

Table 18.2 Follow-up after curative-intent esophagectomy in patients at low or medium risk for recurrence (pStage 0–II esophageal cancer histologically associated with neither marked vessel penetration, four or more lymph node metastases, nor intramural metastasis) Kyushu University, Japan

	Year after surgery				
Modality	1	2	3	4	5
Office visit	12	12	4	2	2
Complete blood count and liver/renal function	12	12	4	2	2
Tumor markers (CEA, SCC)	12	12	4	2	2
Computed tomography (Cervical + chest + abdominal)	2	2	2	1	1
Chest X-ray	1	1	1	1	1
Esophagoscopy	1	1	1	1	1

The number in each cell indicates the number of times a particular modality is recommended in a particular year

Positron emission tomography and laryngoscopy (by otolaryngologists) are performed as clinically indicated

What liver function tests?

What renal function tests?

CEA serum carcinoembryonic antigen level

SCC serum squamous cell carcinoma antigen level

Patients with esophageal cancer frequently have second extraesophageal malignancies. Sato et al. [25] examined the cause of death among thoracic esophageal cancer patients without nodal metastasis and concluded that a second malignancy is a major cause of death. Gastric cancer and head and neck cancer are the most frequent sites. The early diagnosis of carcinoma that develops in the gastric tube after an esophagectomy permits less invasive endoscopic treatment. Curative treatment is more difficult when gastric cancer in the gastric tube is advanced. Therefore, a strict follow-up using endoscopy is recommended.

Squamous cell carcinoma frequently develops multicentrically in the upper aerodigestive tract including esophageal and head and neck cancer. Patients with multifocal esophageal carcinoma often develop head and neck cancer as well [26]. Both cigarette smoking and alcohol consumption are closely associated with the development of multiple cancers in the upper aerodigestive tract [27, 28]. Therefore, in patients with concomitant with esophageal and head and neck cancers, as well as those with multifocal esophageal cancer, strict follow-up is essential for the detection of second cancers. Both laryngoscopy performed by otolaryngologists and esophagoscopy using Lugol staining [29] are recommended for the early detection of these cancers.

Tables 18.2 and 18.3 indicate our principal follow-up schedules after curative esophagectomy. Since recurrence frequently develops within 2 years after an operation, both office visits and measurement of tumor markers are performed every month during this period. Lymph node recurrence frequently

Table 18.3 Follow-up after curative-intent esophagectomy in patients at high risk for recurrence (either pStage III esophageal cancer or tumor histologically associated with marked vessel penetration, four or more lymph node metastases, or intramural metastasis) at Kyushu University, Japan

	Year after surgery				
Modality	1	2	3	4	5
Office visit	12	12	6	2	2
Complete blood count and liver/ renal function	12	12	6	2	2
Tumor markers (CEA, SCC)	12	12	6	2	2
Computed tomography (Cervical + chest + abdominal)	3	2	2	1	1
Chest X-ray	1	1	1	1	1
Esophagoscopy	1	1	1	1	1

The number in each cell indicates the number of times a particular modality is recommended in a particular year
Positron emission tomography and laryngoscopy (by otolaryngologists) are performed as clinically indicated
What liver function tests?
What renal function tests?
CEA serum carcinoembryonic antigen level
SCC serum squamous cell carcinoma antigen level

Table 18.4 Follow-up after curative-intent endoscopic mucosal resection for superficial esophageal cancer

	Year after endoscopic mucosal resection				
Modality	1	2	3	4	5
Office visit	3	2	2	2	2
Tumor markers (CEA, SCC)	3	2	2	2	
Computed tomography (Cervical + chest + abdominal)	1	1	1	#	#
Esophagoscopy	3	2	2	2	2
Laryngoscopy (by otolaryngologists)	#	#	#	#	#

The number in each cell indicates the number of times a particular modality is recommended in a particular year.
Positron emission tomography and laryngoscopy (by otolaryngologists) are performed as clinically indicated.
CEA serum carcinoembryonic antigen level
SCC serum squamous cell carcinoma antigen level
As clinically indicated only

develops in the neck and abdomen as well as the upper mediastinum, while hematogenous recurrence frequently develops in the lungs or liver. Since computed tomography (CT) is a reliable tool to detect these metastases, scanning from the neck to the upper-abdomen are performed at least two times per year within this period. Positron emission tomography is also useful for detecting recurrence [30]. Combined PET–CT is performed 1 year after an operation for high-risk patients. Once recurrence is suspected by some other examination, PET–CT is aggressively performed. Endoscopy is performed annually to detect anastomotic recurrence as well as second primary cancers, particularly head and neck cancer. Laryngoscopy by an otolaryngologist is employed in cases with multiple cancers in the upper aerodigestive tract. Lugol staining is routinely applied for detection of the minute lesions in the remnant esophagus [29] and gastric tube.

Endoscopic mucosal resection is effective treatment for superficial esophageal cancer without lymph node metastasis. After this treatment, detection of local recurrence is extremely important. Local recurrence is seen within 1 year after initial treatment, but may occur many years later [31]. Esaki et al. [32] reported that local recurrence was detected in 14 of 64 patients with superficial esophageal cancer between 3 and 36 months resection. Lymph node recurrence and distant organ recurrence are often >3 years after primary therapy. Detecting second cancers is just as important in patients receiving endoscopic mucosal resection as in those receiving radical surgery. Endoscopy with Lugol staining is performed 3, 6, and 12 months after an endoscopic mucosal resection. Subsequently, patients are followed twice a year. Computed tomography is also conducted annually for 3 years after endoscopic surgery distant recurrence (Table 18.4).

A review of the clinical course of 56 patients with recurrence after a curative operation showed that most (26) patients with distant recurrence died within 1 year after the detection of the recurrence. One patient with a chest wall recurrence treated by a surgical resection was still alive after more than 3 years. In the 30 patients with locoregional recurrence, the median survival time was 16.1 months after detection. This is consistent with other reports [14, 16].

Patients with recurrence treated by multimodal therapy, including radiation or surgery combined with systemic chemotherapy, survive longer than patients who receive systemic chemotherapy alone for recurrent disease (median survival times: 16.1 months and 8.4 months, respectively). Nine patients with recurrence who were not treated died within 10 months after the recurrence. These results are also quite similar to other reports [16, 17]. Multimodal treatment including surgical resection and chemotherapy for solitary cervical lymph node recurrence is reported to improve survival [18, 33]. Few patients with recurrence are candidates for a surgical resection. These findings suggest that multimodal treatment including chemoradiotherapy and, if possible, a surgical resection should be undertaken for localized recurrence after a curative-intent esophagectomy.

In this counterpoint, the recurrence patterns after curative operation in our institute were summarized and reports from other Japanese institutions were reviewed. Even when curative resections with radical lymphadenectomies are performed, recurrences are found to develop in approximately one-third to one-half of the patients. The prognosis of patients with recurrent esophageal cancer is generally poor. Surveillance after curative-intent resection is therefore essential for the early detection of recurrence as well as second primary carcinoma.

References

1. National Cancer Center. Cancer Statistics in Japan-2011. http://ganjoho.ncc.go.jp/public/statistics/backnumber/2011_en.html
2. Stein HJ, Siewert JR. Improved prognosis of resected esophageal cancer. World J Surg. 2004;28:520–5.
3. Ozawa S, Tachimori Y, Baba H, Fujishiro M, Matsubara H, Numasak H, Oyama T, Shinoda M, Takeushi H, Teshima T, Udagawa H, Uno T, Barron P. Comprehensive registry of esophageal cancer in Japan. Esophagus. 2012;9:75–78.
4. Ueda Y, Fujii Y, Udagawa H. Thoracic and cardiovascular surgery in Japan during 2006. Annual report by the Japanese Association for Thoracic Surgery. Gen Thorac Cardiovasc Surg. 2008;56:365–88.
5. Akiyama H, Tsufumaru M, Udagawa H, Kajiyama Y. Radical lymph node dissection for thoracic esophagus. Ann Surg. 1994;220:364–73.
6. Ando N, Ozawa S, Kitagawa Y, Shinozawa Y, Kitajima M. Improvement in the results of surgical treatment of advanced squamous esophageal carcinoma during 15 consecutive years. Ann Surg. 2000;232:225–32.
7. Morita M, Yoshida R, Ikeda K, Egashira A, Oki E, Sadanaga N, Kakeji Y, Yamanaka T, Maehara Y. Advance in esophageal cancer surgery in Japan: an analysis of 1000 consecutive patients treated at a single institute. Surgery. 2008;143:499–508.
8. Sugiyama M, Morita M, Yoshida R, Ando K, Egashira A, Takefumi O, Saeki H, Oki E, Kakeji Y, Sakaguchi Y, Maehara Y. Patterns and time of recurrence after complete resection of esophageal cancer. Surg Today. 2012;42 (8):752–758.
9. Morita M, Kuwano H, Ohno S, Furusawa M, Sugimachi K. Characteristics and sequence of the recurrent patterns after curative esophagectomy for squamous cell carcinoma. Surgery. 1994;116:1–7.
10. Matsubara Matsubara T, Ueda M, Takahashi T, Nakajima T, Nishi M. Matsubara T, Ueda M, Takahashi T, Nakajima T, Nishi M. J Am Coll Surg. 1996;182:340–6.
11. Kato H, Tachimori Y, Watanabe H, Igaki H, Nakanishi Y, Ochiai A. Recurrent esophageal carcinoma after esophagectomy with three-field lymph node dissection. J Surg Oncol. 1996;61(4):267–72.
12. Bhansali MS, Fujita H, Kakegawa T, Yamana H, Ono T, Hikita S, Toh Y, Fujii T, Tou U, Shirouzu K. Pattern of recurrence after extended radical esophagectomy with three-field lymph node dissection for squamous cell carcinoma in the thoracic esophagus. World J Surg. 1997;21:275–81.
13. Kiazanos Kyriazanos ID, Tachibana M, Shibakita M, Yoshimura H, Kinugasa S, Dhar DK, Nakamoto T, Fujii T, Nagasue N. Pattern of recurrence after extended esophagectomy for squamous cell carcinoma of the esophagus. Hepatogastroenterology. 2003;50:115–20.
14. Osugi H, Takemura M, Higashino M, Takada N, Lee S, Ueno M, Tanaka Y, Fukuhara K, Hashimoto Y, Fujiwara Y, Kinoshita H. Causes of death and pattern of recurrence after esophagectomy and extended lymphadenectomy for squamous cell carcinoma of the thoracic esophagus. Oncol Rep. 2003;10(1):81–7.
15. Nakagawa S, Kanda T, Kosugi S, Ohashi M, Suzuki T, Hatakeyama K. Recurrence pattern of squamous cell carcinoma of the thoracic esophagus after extended radical esophagectomy with three-field lymphadenectomy. J Am Coll Surg. 2004;198(2):205–11.
16. Kato H, Fukuchi M, Miyazaki T, Nakajima M, Kimura H, Faried A, Sohda M, Fukai Y, Masuda N, Manda R, Ojima H, Tsukada K, Kuwano H. Classification of recurrent esophageal cancer after radical esophagectomy with two- or three-field lymphadenectomy. Anticancer Res. 2005;25(5):3461–7.
17. Natsugoe S, Okumura H, Matsumoto M, Uchikado Y, Setoyama T, Uenosono Y, Ishigami S, Owaki T, Aikou T. The role of salvage surgery for recurrence of esophageal squamous cell cancer. Eur J Surg Oncol. 2006;32(5):544–7.
18. Motoyama S, Kitamura M, Saito R, Maruyama K, Okuyama M, Ogawa J. Outcome and treatment strategy for mid- and lower-thoracic esophageal cancer recurring locally in the lymph nodes of the neck. World J Surg. 2006;30(2):191–8.
19. Shimada H, Okazumi S, Matsubara H, Nabeya Y, Shiratori T, Shimizu T, Shuto K, Hayashi H, Ochiai T. Impact of the number and extent of positive lymph nodes in 200 patients with thoracic esophageal squamous cell carcinoma after three-field lymph node dissection. World J Surg. 2006;30(8):1441–9.
20. Igaki H, Kato H, Tachimori Y, Nakanishi Y. Prognostic evaluation of patients with clinical T1 and T2 squamous cell carcinomas of the thoracic esophagus after 3-field lymph node dissection. Surgery. 2003;133(4):368–74.
21. Kuwano H, Watanabe M, Sadanaga N, Kamakura T, Nozoe T, Yasuda M, Mimori K, Mori M, Sugimachi K. Univariate and multivariate analyses of the prognostic significance of discontinuous intramural metastasis in patients with esophageal cancer. J Surg Oncol. 1994;57:17–21.
22. Watanabe M, Kuwano H, Araki K, Kawaguchi H, Saeki H, Kitamura K, Ohno S, Sugimachi K. Prognostic factors in patients with submucosal carcinoma of the oesophagus. Br J Cancer. 2000;83:609–13.
23. Osugi H, Takemura M, Takada N, Hirohashi K, Kinoshita H, Higashino M. Prognostic factors after oesophagectomy and extended lymphadenectomy for squamous oesophageal cancer. Br J Surg. 2002;89:9009–13.
24. Japan Esophageal Society. Japanese classification of esophageal cancer. 10th ed. Tokyo, Japan: Kanehara & Co. Ltd.; 2008.
25. Sato Y, Motoyama S, Maruyama K, Okuyama M, Ogawa J. A second malignancy is the major cause of death among thoracic squamous cell esophageal cancer patients negative for lymph node involvement. J Am Coll Surg. 2005;201(2):188–93.
26. Kuwano H, Morita M, Tsutsui S, Kido Y, Mori M, Sugimachi K. Comparison of characteristics of esophageal squamous cell carcinoma associated with head and neck cancer and those with gastric cancer. J Surg Oncol. 1991;46:107–9.
27. Morita M, Kuwano H, Ohno S, Sugimachi K, Seo Y, Tomoda H, Furusawa M, Nakashima K. Multiple occurrence of carcinoma in the upper aerodigestive tract associated with esophageal cancer: reference to smoking, drinking and family history. Int J Cancer. 1994;58:207–10.
28. Morita M, Araki K, Saeki H, Sakaguchi Y, Baba H, Suginmachi K, Yano K, Sugio K, Yasumoto K. Risk factors for multicentric occurrence of carcinoma in the upper aerodigestive tract—analysis with a serial histologic evaluation of the whole resected-esophagus including carcinoma. J Surg Oncol. 2003;3:216–21.
29. Sugimachi K, Ohno S, Matsuda H, Mori M, Kuwano H. Lugol-combined endoscopic detection of minute malignant lesions of the thoracic esophagus. Ann Surg. 1988;208:179–83.
30. Kato H, Miyazaki T, Nakajim M, Fukuchi M, Manda R, Kuwano H. Value of positron emission tomography in the diagnosis of recurrent oesophage4al carcinoma. Br J Surg. 2004;91:1004–9.
31. Kuwano H, Nishimura Y, Ohtsu A, Kato H, Tamai S, Toh Y, Matsubata H. Guidelines for diagnosis and treatment of carcinoma of the esophagus. April 2007 edition: part II edited by the Japan Esophageal Society. Esophagus. 2008;117–32.
32. Esaki M, Matsumoto T, Hirakawa K, Nakamura S, Umeno J, Koga H, Yao T, Iida M. Risk factors for local recurrence of superficial esophageal cancer treatment by endoscopic mucosal resection. Endoscopy. 2007;39:41–5.
33. Nakamura T, Ota M, Narumiya K, Sato T, Ohki T, Yamamoto M, Mitsuhashi N. Multimodal treatment for lymph node recurrence of esophageal carcinoma after curative resection. Ann Surg Oncol. 2008;15:2451–7.

19 Stomach

Shilpi Wadhwa, David Y. Johnson, and Frank E. Johnson

Keywords
Gastric cancer • Environment • Surveillance • ACS • Variability

The International Agency for Research on Cancer (IARC), a component of the World Health Organization (WHO), estimated that there were 938,937 new cases of gastric cancer worldwide in 2002 [1]. The IARC also estimated that there were 700,349 deaths due to this cause in 2002 [1].

The American Cancer Society estimated that there were 21,600 new cases and 4,600 deaths due to this cause in the USA in 2007 [2]. The estimated 5-year survival rate (all races) in the USA in 2007 was 24 % for gastric cancer [2]. Survival rates were adjusted for normal life expectancies and were based on cases diagnosed from 1996 to 2002 and followed through 2003.

Migration studies have suggested that environmental factors play an important role in causation of gastric cancer, particularly carcinoma. The male sex and advancing age are well-documented risk factors. Certain occupations confer increased risks, as do race and ethnic factors [3]. Gastric polyps, particularly adenomatous polyps, are premalignant lesions. Prior to radiation, chronic gastritis (particularly atrophic gastritis), intestinal metaplasia, cigarette smoking, and consumption of certain salty foods or foods containing nitrates, nitrites and *N*-nitroso compounds, are all strongly associated with gastric carcinoma. *H. pylori* infection is strongly carcinogenic. Familial clustering of gastric carcinoma is observed in 12–25 % of cases and genetic factors have been described [4].

Geographic Variation Worldwide

In men, gastric cancer remains the dominant cancer in Cuba, South American countries such as Ecuador and Chile, and Asian countries such as South Korea, Japan, Oman, Afghanistan, Iran, and Tajikistan. In women, the incidence of gastric cancer is highest in Ecuador and Peru among South American nations, and in Asian countries, mainly Japan and South Korea [5]. In the USA, the highest incidence of gastric cancer is found among northeastern and north central states, especially in urban areas. Rates are also elevated in some southwestern states but are generally low in the southeast [6].

Surveillance Strategies Proposed by Professional Organizations or National Government Agencies and Available on the Internet

National Comprehensive Cancer Network (NCCN, www.nccn.org)

NCCN guidelines were accessed on 1/28/12 (Table 19.1). There were minor quantitative and qualitative changes compared to the guidelines accessed on 4/10/07.

American Society of Clinical Oncology (ASCO, www.asco.org)

ASCO guidelines were accessed on 1/28/12. No quantitative guidelines exist for stomach cancer surveillance, including when first accessed on 10/31/07.

S. Wadhwa • D.Y. Johnson
Department of Internal Medicine, Saint Louis University Medical Center, Saint Louis, MO, USA

F.E. Johnson (✉)
Saint Louis University Medical Center and Saint Louis Veterans Affairs Medical Center, Saint Louis, MO, USA
e-mail: frank.johnson1@va.gov

F.E. Johnson et al. (eds.), *Patient Surveillance After Cancer Treatment*, Current Clinical Oncology,
DOI 10.1007/978-1-60327-969-7_19, © Springer Science+Business Media New York 2013

Table 19.1 Gastric cancer

	Years posttreatment[a]					
	1	2	3	4	5	>5
Office visit	2–4	2–4	1–2	1–2	1–2	1
CBC and chemistry profile as indicated						
Radiologic imaging or endoscopy, as clinically indicated						
Monitor for nutritional deficiency in surgically resected patients and treat as indicated						
Confirm that HER2-neu testing has been done if metastatic disease was present at diagnosis						

[a]The numbers in the table indicate the number of times the modality is recommended during the indicated year posttreatment

Obtained from NCCN (www.nccn.org) on 1-28-12

NCCN guidelines were accessed on 1/28/12. There were minor quantitative and qualitative changes compared to the guidelines accessed on 4/10/07

The Society of Surgical Oncology (SSO, www.surgonc.org)

SSO guidelines were accessed on 1/28/12. No quantitative guidelines exist for stomach cancer surveillance, including when first accessed on 10/31/07.

European Society for Medical Oncology (ESMO, www.esmo.org)

ESMO guidelines were accessed on 1/28/12. No quantitative guidelines exist for stomach cancer surveillance, including when first accessed on 10/31/07.

European Society of Surgical Oncology (ESSO, www.esso-surgeonline.org)

ESSO guidelines were accessed on 1/28/12. No quantitative guidelines exist for stomach cancer surveillance, including when first accessed on 10/31/07.

Cancer Care Ontario (CCO, www.cancercare.on.ca)

CCO guidelines were accessed on 1/28/12. No quantitative guidelines exist for stomach cancer surveillance, including when first accessed on 10/31/07.

National Institute for Clinical Excellence (NICE, www.nice.org.uk)

NICE guidelines were accessed on 1/28/12. No quantitative guidelines exist for stomach cancer surveillance, including when first accessed on 10/31/07.

The Cochrane Collaboration (CC, www.cochrane.org)

CC guidelines were accessed on 1/28/12. No quantitative guidelines exist for stomach cancer surveillance, including when first accessed on 10/31/07.

Society for the Surgery of the Alimentary Tract (SSAT, www.ssat.com)

SSAT guidelines were accessed on 1/28/12. No quantitative guidelines exist for stomach cancer surveillance, including when first accessed on 10/31/07.

The M.D. Anderson Surgical Oncology Handbook also has follow-up guidelines, proposed by authors from a single National Cancer Institute-designated Comprehensive Cancer Center, for many types of cancer [7]. Some are detailed and quantitative, others are qualitative.

Summary

This is a common cancer with significant variability in incidence worldwide. We found consensus-based guidelines but none based on high-quality evidence.

References

1. Parkin DM, Whelan SL, Ferlay J, Teppo L, Thomas DB. Cancer incidence in five continents, Vol. VIII. Lyon, France: International Agency for Research on Cancer; 2002 (IARC Scientific Publication 155). ISBN 92-832-2155-9.
2. Jemal A, Seigel R, Ward E, Murray T, Xu J, Thun MJ. Cancer Statistics, 2007. CA Cancer J Clin. 2007;57:43–66.
3. Schottenfeld D, Fraumeni JG. Cancer epidemiology and prevention. 3rd ed. New York, NY: Oxford University Press; 2006. ISBN 13:978-0-19-514961-6.
4. DeVita VT, Hellman S, Rosenberg SA. Cancer. 7th ed. Philadelphia, PA: Lippincott Williams & Wilkins; 2005. ISBN 0-781-74450-4.
5. Mackay J, Jemal A, Lee NC, Parkin M. The Cancer Atlas; 2006. American Cancer Society 1599 Clifton Road NE, Atlanta, Georgia 30329, USA. Can also be accessed at www.cancer.org. ISBN 0-944235-62-X.
6. Devesa SS, Grauman DJ, Blot WJ, Pennello GA, Hoover RN, Fraumeni JF Jr. Atlas of Cancer Mortality in the United States. National Institutes of Health, National Cancer Institute; September 1999 (NIH Publication No. 99-4564).
7. Feig BW, Berger DH, Fuhrman GM. The M.D. Anderson surgical oncology handbook. 4th ed. Philadelphia, PA: Lippincott Williams & Wilkins; 2006 (paperback). ISBN 0-7817-5643-X.

Stomach Carcinoma Surveillance Counterpoint: USA

20

Andrew Coleman and Douglas Tyler

Keywords
Survival rate • Gastric cancer • Gastrectomy • Lymphatic • Peritoneal • Hematogenous • Spread

The combined 5-year survival rate for all newly diagnosed gastric cancer patients in the United States is about 24 % [1]. The mortality rate is high because two-thirds of Americans initially present with TNM stage III–IV disease, not only making it more difficult to achieve resection with uninvolved margins, but also increasing the probability of systemic spread. Cure is only achieved through a combination of gastrectomy and lymphadenectomy with or without neo-adjuvant and/or perioperative chemotherapy. In the USA, only about one-quarter of newly diagnosed patients undergo curative-intent resection [2]. Though this intervention undoubtedly improves the prognosis, it is by no means a panacea, as the 5-year survival rate of patients treated with curative intent is 47–60 % and recurrence occurs in 15–37 % [3] (Table 20.1).

Resection of gastric adenocarcinoma, as demonstrated by these statistics, is often incomplete. We have few tools with which to combat recurrence. Surveillance after initial treatment is controversial, largely driven by individual opinion and anecdotal experience. In the following pages, we review the patterns of recurrence, the prognostic factors for recurrence, and evidence supporting the use of various tests and procedures in the process of monitoring for recurrence. Finally, we conclude with our own recommendations as to how to follow patients after gastrectomy depending on their likelihood of recurrence (Table 20.2).

Of the three patterns of spread—lymphatic, peritoneal, and hematogenous—there is significant variation in the literature as to which recurrence route is most common. Japanese studies demonstrate a predilection toward peritoneal and hematogenous spread [4–6], while the American experience suggests that lymphatic spread is more frequent [6]. There is some evidence that this difference is due to the common practice in Japan of performing a D2 lymphadenectomy, thus lessening the chances of local recurrence [7]. The recurrence pattern also seems to depend on its timing: early recurrence (<2 years from surgery) is usually due to lymphatic metastasis. Late recurrence is usually due to peritoneal implants or distant disease [8].

In a retrospective observational study of 308 Chinese patients with early gastric cancer, Wu et al. found an average time to recurrence of 4 years following margin-negative (R0) resection [5]. In contrast, a Memorial Sloan-Kettering group followed 1,172 patients prospectively and found a median time to recurrence of 10.8 and 12.4 months for symptomatic and asymptomatic patients, respectively. According to this same study, of the patients who recurred, 79 % did so within 2 years and 95 % did so within 4 years [9]. In a review of the literature, Whiting et al. found that two-thirds of patients with early gastric cancer who developed recurrence did so within 3 years and that fewer than 10 % had relapse beyond 5 years [7]. Although this data is not perfectly consistent, especially with respect to the approximate time to recurrence, it is informative in its provision of a time line of the natural history of recurrence. Such data help clinicians devise surveillance strategies.

Numerous studies have dealt with prognostic factors for gastric cancer recurrence following gastrectomy. There is a

A. Coleman (✉)
Duke University School of Medicine,
100 Remington Cir, Durham, NC 27705, USA
e-mail: andrew.coleman@duke.edu

D. Tyler, M.D. (✉)
Department of Surgery, Duke University Medical Center,
Box 3118, Durham, NC 27710, USA
e-mail: doug.tyler@duke.edu

F.E. Johnson et al. (eds.), *Patient Surveillance After Cancer Treatment*, Current Clinical Oncology,
DOI 10.1007/978-1-60327-969-7_20, © Springer Science+Business Media New York 2013

Table 20.1 Surveillance after curative-intent treatment for patients with gastric carcinoma (preoperative TNM stages I–II) at Duke University Medical Center

	Years posttreatment					
Modality	1	2	3	4	5	>5
Office visit and blood tests[a]	3	3	3	2	2	1

[a]CBC, metabolic panel (electrolytes, liver function tests, renal function tests) Serum CEA level, serum CA 19-9 level, chest X-ray, esophagogastroduodenoscopy, CT scan as clinically indicated
The number in each cell is the number of times a particular modality is recommended in a particular posttreatment year

Table 20.2 Surveillance after curative-intent treatment for patients with gastric carcinoma (preoperative TNM stage III) at Duke University Medical Center

	Years posttreatment					
Modality	1	2	3	4	5	>5
Office visit and blood tests[a]	4	4	4	3	3	1

[a]CBC, metabolic panel (electrolytes, liver function tests, renal function tests)
Serum CEA level, serum CA 19-9 level, chest X-ray, esophagogastroduodenoscopy, CT scan as clinically indicated
The number in each cell is the number of times a particular modality is recommended in a particular posttreatment year

consensus within the literature that the extent of lymphatic spread is the most important prognostic factor for recurrence and survival [2, 8, 10, 11]. A study by Sakar et al. further elucidated the temporal characteristics of lymph node metastasis. He divided 142 patients who developed recurrence following R0 resection into an early recurrence group (less than 2 years out from surgery) and a late group (2 years and beyond). Early recurrence was associated with TNM stage [8]. Deng et al. reviewed 6,309 lymph nodes harvested from 308 patients undergoing R0 resection and found a threshold of nine positive lymph nodes to be a significant prognostic factor for recurrence. No patients in the study with nine or more positive lymph nodes survived more than 5 years. Patients with four or fewer, however, had a 62 % 5-year survival rate [10]. Marchet et al. studied the ratio of metastatic to total lymph nodes harvested during R0 resection—a parameter termed N-ratio. They found the N-ratio, but not the TNM N-category, to be an independent prognostic factor for survival [11]. Serosal invasion and liver metastasis are important prognostic factors [12]. Finally, Marrelli et al. used multivariate linear regression analysis to develop a model to predict recurrence. Using a number of parameters including gender, age, tumor size, depth of invasion and location, Lauren histotype, nodal status, and type of gastrectomy and lymphadenectomy, they were able to correctly predict 227 of 272 recurrences (sensitivity, 83.5 %) and 214 of 264 non-recurrences (specificity, 81.1 %) [13].

There are several useful serological tests, each with a unique sensitivity and specificity profile. The most studied of the tumor markers in the setting of gastric cancer recurrence is the serum carcinoembryonic antigen (CEA) level. It has a relatively good specificity profile (79–100 %), depending on the patient population, but a poor sensitivity profile (16–65.8 %). [14–16]. Shimizu et al. studied the accuracy of the CEA level when combined with the immunosuppressive antigen marker, and found an increased (but still suboptimal) sensitivity of 69.2 % and a specificity of 96.7 %. Interestingly, the combination assay had a sensitivity and specificity of 100 % in cases of hepatic metastasis. The combined assay performed poorly in cases of peritoneal dissemination, as is the case with all other tumor markers or combinations thereof [17].

A well-known tumor marker for pancreatic cancer, CA19-9, can also be elevated in the setting of gastric cancer. Like CEA, the sensitivity of the serum CA 19-9 level is mediocre (33.3–56 %). The specificity is 74–93.3 % [14, 15]. In a recent prospective study from Japan, sensitivity was improved by combining the CA 19-9 assay with the CEA assay. A sensitivity of 85 % was attained when serum levels of CEA, CA 19-9, or both were interpreted as positive [16]. The serum level of CA 72-4, a more recently studied tumor marker, is one of the best for detecting gastric cancer. Its sensitivity is on par with CEA and CA 19-9, but its specificity has been shown to be 97 % in one study and 100 % in another [14, 15]. In a small study by Joypaul et al., the CA 72-4 levels rose to diagnostic levels six months prior to clinical diagnosis [18].

Recent research has implicated E-cadherin as an important contributor to gastric carcinogenesis and metastasis. The cadherin proteins play a major role in cell adhesion and, consequently, metastasis and invasion. Notably, the majority of gastric carcinomas contain methylated E-cadherin proteins and many contain mutated forms of the protein. Chan et al. recently assayed soluble E-cadherin and CEA levels in 69 patients undergoing gastrectomy for gastric cancer during the preoperative and postoperative periods. In patients who did not experience recurrence, E-cadherin levels did not become elevated at any time following gastrectomy relative to their preoperative baselines. An elevated E-cadherin level preceded the diagnosis of recurrence in all patients who experienced recurrence by a median time of 13 months (range, 3–20 months). In comparison, CEA elevation preceded the diagnosis of recurrence by a median of only 4 months (range, 1–20 months). Overall, the optimal sensitivity and specificity (59 % and 75 %, respectively) was determined to occur at an E-cadherin level of 10,000 ng/mL [19].

It is generally accepted in the wealthy Western democracies that patients in whom a new diagnosis of gastric cancer is suspected should be worked up with computed tomography, chest X-ray, esophagogastroduodenoscopy (EGD) and often positron emission tomography (PET) scan if metastatic involvement is suspected [20]. What is controversial, however, is how these imaging modalities should be used after surgery. There are few data pertaining to the use of these imaging modalities in surveillance. The exception is FDG-PET (or PET-CT) imaging. In a recent report, PET had a specificity of 70 % (14/20 patients) and sensitivity of 69 % (9/13 patients) in detecting recurrent gastric carcinoma. Though the authors did not suggest PET as a screening tool, they did conclude that the technology was helpful in determining a prognosis, as patients with PET-negative recurrences lived longer than patients with PET-positive recurrences (mean ± SD, 21.9 ± 19.0 months and 9.2 ± 8.2 months, respectively; $P=0.01$) [21]. A study by Yoshioka and colleagues confirmed these sensitivity and specificity results. In addition, the authors analyzed PET accuracy in relation to recurrence site. They concluded that FDG-PET performed best in detecting recurrence in the liver, lymph nodes, and lungs, with a minimum lesion size resolution of 0.5 cm. In cases of ascites, peritonitis, pleuritis, carcinomatosis, locoregional lymph node, or bone metastases, however, the accuracy was poor [22]. To our knowledge, there are no good studies on the role of EGD in the post-gastrectomy setting. However, a number of groups have adopted the use of endoscopy in their surveillance strategies for asymptomatic patients [5].

A number of randomized controlled trials and meta-analyses have demonstrated a survival benefit associated with intensive surveillance in patients with colon cancer [23]. Surveillance for gastric cancer, on the other hand, has been studied only in small, non-blinded, nonrandomized trials. Tan et al. separated 102 patients into two groups: a regular follow-up group in which 53 patients were studied with yearly physical examinations, serum tumor marker tests, and CT scans and an intensive group, in which multiple CT scans were performed each year in addition to the physical examination and serum marker tests. The authors found that recurrence was detected earlier in the intensive surveillance group (11.5 months vs. 19.2 months), but there was no difference in overall survival duration between the groups [6]. Bohner et al. found that the survival rate of patients whose recurrence was detected by follow-up studies did not differ from the survival rate of patients whose recurrence was discovered after development of clinical symptoms [24]. A study by Kodera et al. reported a similar result. Early detection increased the post-detection survival interval, but the overall survival duration was the same [25].

Should we use expensive medical resources to monitor for gastric cancer recurrence if we are unable to demonstrate survival benefit? The authors of this counterpoint feel that surveillance for gastric cancer recurrence is useful not only for patients who wish to know their present prognosis, but also because we can potentially offer novel treatments through phase I/II trials to patients in whom recurrence is identified. To these ends, we believe it is reasonable to adopt a surveillance strategy consisting of frequent physician contact during the first year after surgery. In the subsequent years, as recurrence becomes less likely, the frequency of physician visits can be reduced in the absence of symptoms suggestive of recurrence. Based on evidence suggesting that the odds of recurrence increase with increasing TNM stage, we also suggest stratifying patients based on their preoperative TNM stage into two different intensities of surveillance: a less-intensive version for TNM stage I and II patients and a more intensive version for TNM stage III patients.

We agree with the recommendations of the National Comprehensive Cancer Network (NCCN): a history and physical and complete blood count with complete metabolic panel should be performed during each physician visit. We agree that tumor assays, radiologic imaging, and EGD should be reserved for cases in which recurrence is suspected (the patient describes changes in bowl habits, melena, hematemesis, weight loss, or anorexia; physical examination reveals the presence of ascites, abdominal mass, hepatomegaly, lymphadenopathy, or other signs of metastasis; or the lab values demonstrate anemia or serum transaminase elevation). Using this strategy, we feel that patient surveillance is not compromised and that limited medical resources are utilized as effectively as possible.

Well-designed clinical trials of low-intensity vs. high-intensity surveillance strategies are clearly needed. Such trials are certain to be expensive. They will require many years to accrue patients and permit long-term results to be determined. Such trials have currently been designed, funded, and reported from European countries through their national medical systems.

Currently the US National Institutes of Health carries out studies concerning patients with cancer after treatment but does not fund clinical trials of surveillance. In order to fund such trials, enabling legislation is likely to be required. Professional medical organizations, patient support groups, the public health community, and payers should advocate for funding and performance of such clinical trials. Without them, continued marked variation in surveillance intensity among clinicians is inevitable.

References

1. Jemal A, Siegel R, Ward E, Hao Y, Xu J, Murray T, et al. Cancer statistics 2008. CA Cancer J Clin. 2008;2:71–96.
2. Wanebo HJ, Kennedy BJ, Chmiel J, Steele Jr G, Winchester D, Osteen R. Cancer of the stomach. A patient care study by the American College of Surgeons. Ann Surg. 1993;5:583–92.
3. Samson PS, Escovidal LA, Yrastorza SG, Veneracion RG, Nerves MY. Re-study of gastric cancer: analysis of outcome. World J Surg. 2002;26:428–33.
4. Nashimoto A, Yabusaki H, Nakagawa S. Evaluation and problems of follow-up surveillance after curative gastric cancer surgery. Nippon Geka Gakkai Zasshi. 2007;108:120–4.

5. Wu B, Wu D, Wang M, Wang G. Recurrence in patients following curative resection of early gastric carcinoma. J Surg Oncol. 2008;98:411–4.
6. Tan IT, So BYJ. Value of intensive follow-up of patients after curative surgery for gastric carcinoma. J Surg Oncol. 2007;96:503–6.
7. Whiting J, Sano T, Saka M, Fukagawa T, Katai H, Sasako M. Follow-up of gastric cancer: a review. Gastric Cancer. 2006;9:74–81.
8. Sakar B, Karagol H, Gumus M, Basaran M, Kaytan E, Argon A, et al. Timing of death from tumor recurrence after curative gastrectomy for gastric cancer. Am J Clin Oncol. 2004;27:205–9.
9. Bennett JJ, Gonen M, D'Angelica M, Jaques DP, Brennan MF, Coit DG. Is detection of asymptomatic recurrence after curative resection associated with improved survival in patients with gastric cancer? J Am Coll Surg. 2005;201:503–10.
10. Deng JY, Liang H, Sun D, Zhan H, Wang X. The most appropriate category of metastatic lymph nodes to evaluate overall survival of gastric cancer following curative resection. J Surg Oncol. 2008;98:343–8.
11. Marchet A, Mocellin S, Ambrosi A, De Manzoni G, Di Leo A, Marrelli D, et al. The prognostic value of N-ratio in patients with gastric cancer: validation in a large, multicenter series. Eur J Surg Oncol. 2008;34:159–65.
12. Shiraishi N, Sato K, Yasuda K, Inomata M, Kitano S. Multivariate prognostic study on large gastric cancer. J Surg Oncol. 2007;96:14–8.
13. Marrelli D, De Stefano A, De Manzoni G, Morgagni P, Di Leo A, Roviello F. A scoring system obtained from a prospective multicenter study. Ann Surg. 2005;241:247–55.
14. Marrelli D, Pinto E, De Stafano A, Farnetani M, Garosi L, Roviello F. Clinical utility of CEA, CA 19-9, and CA 72-4 in the follow-up of patients with resectable gastric cancer. Am J Surg. 2001;181:16–9.
15. Patriti A, Graziosi L, Baffa N, Pacifico E, Lamprini P, Valiani S, et al. Postoperative follow-up of gastric adenocarcinoma with neoplastic markers and 18-FDG-PET/CT. Ann Ital Chir. 2007;78:481–5.
16. Takahashi Y, Takeuchi T, Sakamoto J, Touge T, Mai M, Ohkura H, et al. The usefulness of CEA and/or CA 19-9 in monitoring for recurrence in gastric cancer patients: a prospective clinical study. Gastric Cancer. 2003;6:142–5.
17. Shimizu N, Yamashiro H, Murakami A, Hamazoe R, Maeta M. Diagnostic accuracy of a combination of assays for immunosuppressive acidic protein and carcinoembryonic antigen in detection of recurrence of gastric cancer. Eur J Cancer. 1991;27:190–3.
18. Joypaul B, Browning M, Newman E, Byrne D, Cuschieri A. Comparison of serum CA 72-4 and CA 19-9 levels in gastric cancer patients and correlation with recurrence. Am J Surg. 1995;169:595–9.
19. Chan AOO, Chu K, Lam SK, Cheung KL, Law S, Kwok K, et al. Early prediction of tumor recurrence after curative resection of gastric carcinoma by measuring soluble E-cadherin. Cancer. 2005;104:740–6.
20. National Comprehensive Cancer (#6) AND (specificity[Title/Abstract]) AND (gastric[title]) Network (2009) Gastric Cancer *NCCN Clinical Practice Guidelines in Oncology* v.2.2009.
21. De Potter T, Flamen P, Van Cutsem E, Penninckx F, Filez L, Bormans G, et al. Whole-body PET with FDG for the diagnosis of recurrent gastric cancer. Eur J Nucl Med. 2002;29:525–9.
22. Yoshioka T, Yamaguchi K, Kubota K, Saginoya T, Yamazaki T, Ido T, et al. Evaluation of ^{18}F-FDG PET in patients with advanced, metastatic, or recurrent gastric cancer. J Nucl Med. 2003;44:690–9.
23. Renehan AG, Egger M, Saunders MP, O'Dwyer ST. Impact on survival of intensive follow up after curative resection for colorectal cancer: a systematic review and meta-analysis of randomized trials. Br Med J. 2002;324:813–6.
24. Bohner H, Zimmer T, Hopfenmuller W, Berger G, Buhr HJ. Detection and prognosis of recurrent gastric cancer—is routine follow-up after gastrectomy worthwhile? Hepatogastroenterology. 2000;47:1489–94.
25. Kodera Y, Ito S, Yamamura Y, Mochizuki Y, Fujiwara M, Hibi K, et al. Follow-up surveillance for recurrence after curative gastric cancer surgery lacks survival benefit. Ann Surg Oncol. 2003;10:898–902.

21 Stomach Carcinoma Surveillance Counterpoint: Japan

Yoshihiro Kakeji, Masaru Morita, and Yoshihiko Maehara

Keywords
Nonresectable tumor • Japan • Surveillance • Endoscopy • RecurrenceIntroduction

Gastric cancer was overtaken by lung cancer as the leading cause of cancer-related death in Japan in 1999. In 2007, it still accounted for 50,597 deaths (15 % of all deaths from cancer) [1]. The proportion of gastric cancers that are detected early through screening measures is now around 60 % in Japan. These patients require limited surveillance after primary treatment. A large proportion of patients still present with nonresectable tumors at the time of surgery. Those with advanced tumors resected with curative intent are the target of close follow-up.

Helicobacter pylori (*H. pylori*) is a major cause of type B chronic atrophic gastritis and intestinal metaplasia [2], a precursor of gastric carcinoma. Nobuta et al. [3] evaluated *H. pylori* infection in two areas in Japan with different incidences of gastric carcinoma. The standardized mortality rate in males in Niigata in 1995 (in northeastern Honshu Island) was 52.3/100,000 and that in Okinawa (the southernmost island of Japan) was 24.9/100,000. Although there was no significant difference in *H. pylori* prevalence among the persons in Niigata (50 %) and Okinawa (42 %), the prevalence of *H. pylori* strains with the cytotoxin-associated gene A (CagA) in these populations was significantly different, at 41 % and 26 %, respectively (odds ratio 1.98, 95 % confidence interval 1.33–2.95, $P<0.01$). Thus, the difference in gastric carcinoma mortality rates is strongly associated with the prevalence of CagA-positive strains but not to the overall prevalence of *H. pylori* infection between the two areas. *H. pylori* is now well known as an important pathogen related to the development of gastric cancer [4]. A previous nonrandomized study [5] and recent open-label randomized controlled trial [6] showed that *H. pylori* eradication after endoscopic resection for early gastric cancer could prevent the development of metachronous gastric cancer. The guideline by the Japanese Society for Helicobacter Research has been updated, and *H. pylori* eradication is recommended at the highest level (i.e., based on strong scientific evidence) for all patients with *H. pylori* infection [4]. Other factors, such as diet, host factors (including genetic makeup), and acid secretion status, also affect the development of both atrophic gastritis and gastric cancer.

The Japanese Gastric Cancer Association first issued its gastric cancer treatment guidelines in March 2001 [7]. The second version was published in 2004 [8]. These guidelines provide standard indications for available treatments according to the initial clinical stage. They are expected to reduce variability in treatment, improve treatment results by eliminating improper treatments, and improve understanding of the disease and its treatment. Unlike the situation in Western countries, these guidelines do not primarily aim to reduce costs in the national health care system, but expect financial improvement as the result of proper acceptance of guidelines as they lead to better health for patients. Table 21.1 shows treatment indications according to the initial clinical stage [7]. The guidelines represent a consensus among gastroenterologists, surgeons, radiation oncologists, and medical oncologists. As for postoperative follow-up, the guidelines state that patients undergoing gastrectomy should be followed systematically for treatment of postoperative symptoms, lifestyle guidance, and early detection of recurrence or second cancer, depending on risk of recurrence with endoscopy, US, and CT scan [7].

Y. Kakeji, MD, PhD, FACS (✉) • M. Morita • Y. Maehara
Department of Surgery and Science, Graduate School of Medical Sciences, Kyushu University, Fukuoka, Japan
e-mail: kakeji@surg2.med.kyushu-u.ac.jp

F.E. Johnson et al. (eds.), *Patient Surveillance After Cancer Treatment*, Current Clinical Oncology,
DOI 10.1007/978-1-60327-969-7_21, © Springer Science+Business Media New York 2013

Table 21.1 Clinical treatment options by stage [8]

Stage	T and N Factor	Treatment
Early gastric cancer		
IA	T1(m)N0	EMR, Modified surgery
	T1(sm)N0	Modified surgery
IB	T1(m,sm)N1	Modified surgery, standard surgery
	T2N0	Standard surgery
II	T1(m,sm)N2	Standard surgery
IV	T1(m,sm)N3	Extended surgery, palliative surgery, chemotherapy, radiation therapy, palliative care
Advanced gastric cancer		
IB	T2N0	Standard surgery
II	T2N1	Standard surgery
	T3N0	Standard surgery
IIIA	T2N2	Standard surgery
	T3N1	Standard surgery
	T4N0	Extended surgery
IIIB	T3N2	Standard surgery
	T4N1	Extended Surgery
IV	anyT N3	Extended surgery, palliative surgery, chemotherapy, radiation therapy, palliative care
	H1,P1,CY1,M1	Extended surgery, palliative surgery, chemotherapy, radiation therapy, palliative care

EMR: endoscopic mucosal resection
EMR is recommended for differentiated type, ≤2 cm in diameter, no ulceration in cases of depressed type.
Depth of tumor invasion (t)
T1: Tumor invasion of mucosa and/or muscularis mucosa (m) or submucosa (sm)
T2: Tumor invasion of muscularis propria (mp) or subserosa (ss)
T3: Tumor penetration of serosa (se)
T4: Tumor invasion of adjacent structures (si)
Extent of lymph node metastasis (N)
N0: No evidence of lymph node metastasis
N1: Metastasis to Group 1 lymph nodes, but no metastasis to Groups 2 or 3 lymph nodes
N2: Metastasis to Group 2 lymph nodes, but no metastasis to Group 3 lymph nodes
N3: Metastasis to Group 3 lymph nodes
Liver metastasis (H)
H0: No liver metastasis
H1: Liver metastasis
Peritoneal Metastasis (P)
P0: No peritoneal metastasis
P1: Peritoneal metastasis
Peritoneal cytology (cy)
CY0: Benign/indeterminate cells on peritoneal cytology
CY1: Cancer cells on peritoneal cytology
Lymph node dissection (D)
D0: No dissection or incomplete dissection of the Group 1 nodes
D1: Dissection of all the Group 1 nodes
D2: Dissection of all the Group 1 and Group 2 nodes
D3: Dissection of all the Group 1, Group 2, and Group 3 nodes
1. Modified Surgery-A and -B: resection less than standard surgery (see 2 below). This includes an omentum-preserving procedure, omission of omento-bursectomy, pylorus-preserving gastrectomy, and a vagus-preserving procedure. According to the extent of lymph node dissection, modified surgery is classified into surgery-A ($D1+\alpha$ dissection) and surgery-B ($D1+\beta$ dissection).
Dissected lymph nodes for α: site 7 (LN along the left gastric artery) [35] irrespective of the location of the gastric carcinoma lesion, and additionally No.8a (LN along the common hepatic artery) in cases with lesions located in the lower third of the stomach.
Dissected lymph nodes for β: No.7, 8a, 9 (LN around the celiac artery)
2. Standard surgery: resection of two thirds of the stomach with D2 dissection
3. Extended surgery (combined resection): standard surgery with combined resection of involved organs
4. Treatment options by stage are based on macroscopic staging during surgery. If there is any doubt about an indication for modified surgery, standard surgery is recommended.

At 5 years or later after surgery, basic checkups are recommended every year. The guidelines also require treatment or prevention of postoperative disorders such as macrocytic and megaloblastic anemia following total gastrectomy.

The guidelines [8] of the Japanese Gastric Cancer Association do not specify treatment for individual patients. They do not discuss the technical aspects of each treatment option. To show the rationale of the various treatments, the role of each treatment is discussed in relation to the biology of gastric cancer. To the extent possible, evaluation of treatment efficacy is evidence-based. Treatment results are evaluated primarily by overall survival duration, though symptom relief, tumor shrinkage, and improvement in quality of life are also evaluated. Currently available treatments are emphasized, but promising experimental treatments are also included (Table 21.1).

Early Gastric Cancer

The comparatively good overall results of treatment in Japan are considered to be attributable to the large proportion diagnosed at an early stage. Endoscopic mucosal resection (EMR) is an established method for treating small mucosal cancers with a low risk of lymph node metastasis. Endoscopic mucosal resection is adequate treatment for intestinal-type mucosal cancer less than 2 cm in diameter [7]. Conventional endoscopic mucosal resection is performed using strip biopsy, but local recurrence sometimes occurs, as this is a type of piecemeal resection. Endoscopic submucosal dissection is now performed in Japan using new devices such as an insulation-tip diathermic knife [9]. A recent study of a large cohort of patients with early gastric carcinoma treated with conventional radical surgery has shown that intramucosal differentiated adenocarcinoma of any size without ulceration or lymphatic/venous invasion, and intramucosal well-differentiated adenocarcinomas ≤30 mm in diameter with ulceration but without lymphatic/venous invasion are not associated with nodal metastases [10]. Such patients are good candidates for endoscopic treatment. In evaluating patients who have been treated with endoscopic mucosal resection or endoscopic submucosal dissection, an accurate histological evaluation of resected specimens is useful to prevent recurrence in tumors that should be curable. Patients who have had endoscopic treatment but have unfavorable pathology reports are often cured by subsequent conventional radical surgery. Patients who benefit from endoscopic mucosal resection or endoscopic submucosal dissection account for 15 % of all patients with early gastric cancer, and this percentage is increasing.

The indications for laparoscopic surgery for gastric cancer differ in each hospital depending on their experience with laparoscopic surgery [11]. In most hospitals, it is mainly applied only for early distal gastric cancer, in which a distal gastrectomy with limited lymph node dissection is the standard. In some hospitals, the indications are extended to a small subgroup of advanced gastric cancers, in which D2 (extensive) lymph node dissection is the standard. The indications for laparoscopic surgery are generally considered in accordance with The Gastric Cancer Treatment Guidelines [7, 8]. A recent report [12] showed that a total of 21,048 laparoscopic gastrectomies were performed between 1991 and 2007. The number of laparoscopic gastrectomies has increased gradually, and 24.5 % of gastric cancer resections in 2007 in Japan were done laparoscopically.

The Japanese Gastric Cancer Association Registration Committee reported the treatment results and causes of death of patients with primary gastric cancer treated in 1991 at leading hospitals in Japan [13]. Data on 8,851 patients with primary gastric cancer were collected from 113 hospitals, and data on 7,935 patients with gastric resection were analyzed. Of 3,871 patients with early gastric cancer, 84 (2.2 %) died from cancer recurrence, and 161 (4.2 %) died from other diseases. Lymph node metastasis is the strongest prognostic factor for patients with early gastric cancer [14]. The incidence of recurrence was 20 % in patients with lymph node metastasis and 1.2 % in those without nodal metastases. The outcome for patients with early gastric cancer who developed recurrence was as poor as that for patients with advanced gastric cancer [15], highlighting the importance of lymph node metastasis. The predominant mode of recurrence was hematogenous metastasis, most frequently to the liver [14]. Recurrent tumors developed within 5 years in 77 % of the recurrent cases and after more than 5 years in 23 %.

After an endoscopic mucosal resection or endoscopic submucosal dissection, follow-up endoscopic examinations are performed to check for recurrence every 3 months during the first year, and annually thereafter [9]. Biopsies of the postresection scar are necessary for detection of possible residual malignant cells. A gastrectomy is recommended for patients with local recurrence at the primary site. Another endoscopic mucosal resection or endoscopic submucosal dissection is one of the treatment options for a second lesion distant from the original primary site.

The possibility of recurrence is small after a gastrectomy with no histological evidence of node involvement. Follow-up examinations are performed annually for this patient subset with a favorable natural history (Table 21.2). The current surveillance strategy has evolved by consensus among surgeons, gastroenterologists, and medical oncologists. The main purpose of annual surveillance in these patients is to screen for other malignancies. Chest radiography, esophagogastroscopy, abdominal ultrasound, abdominal computed tomography, and blood tests, including serum tumor markers, carcinoembryonic antigen (CEA) and CA 19-9, are performed. A barium enema study or colonoscopy is also recommended to look for

Table 21.2 Surveillance after curative-intent treatment for early gastric cancer without nodal metastasis at Kyushu University Hospital, Japan

	Year					
Modality	1	2	3	4	5	>5
Office visit	1	1	1	1	1	1
Blood tests[a]	1	1	1	1	1	1
Chest x-ray	1	1	1	1	1	1
Abdominal ultrasound examination	1	1	1	1	1	1
Abdominal computered tomography	1	1	1	1	1	1
Esophagogastroscopy	1	1	1	1	1	1
Barium enema/colonoscopy	0	1	0	1	0	0

The number in each cell indicates the number of times a particular modality is recommended in a particular posttreatment year.
[a](complete blood count, serum chemistry (includes total protein, albumin, creatinine, blood urea nitrogen, uric acid, sodium, potassium, chloride, alkaline phosphatase, bilirubin, glucose, lactic dehydrogenase, phosphorus), serum CEA level, serum CA 19-9 level)

colorectal cancer every other year. Yamamoto et al. [16] investigated 671 patients with early gastric cancer and reported that the lifetime rate of recurrence in patients treated for early gastric cancer was 2.1 %, and the lifetime incidence of second primary cancers of any sort was 4.8 %, with an associated cancer-specific death rate of 3.3 %. Most multiple primary cancer cases involved the colorectum and lung. The mean interval (± standard deviation) from surgery to diagnosis of recurrence was 3.4±2.1 years. The mean interval from resection to detection of peritoneal recurrence was shorter than the mean interval to detection of hematogenous recurrence ($P<0.05$). The mean interval (± standard deviation) from the diagnosis of early gastric cancer to the diagnosis of a second primary cancer was 7.1±4.6 years.

A closer follow-up is necessary for patients with nodal metastases (about 10 % of all early gastric cancer). Abdominal and thoracic imaging studies are recommended every 3–6 months for the first 3 years, and every 6 months for years 4 and 5. Follow-up of early gastric cancer should be continued for more than 5 years, since one fourth of patients with recurrence die more than 5 years after initial surgery.

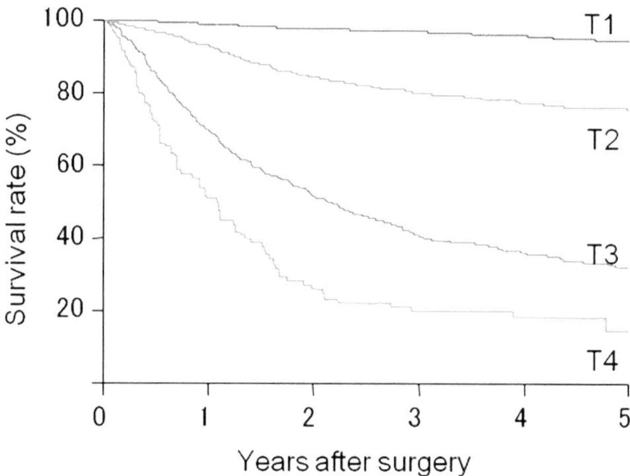

Fig. 21.1 Survival curves after resection of gastric cancer. According to the depth of invasion. The 5-year survival rates of T1 (n=2027), T2 (n=764), T3 (n=699), T4 (n=120) are 94.3 %, 75.8 %, 32.1 %, 14.5 %, respectively. (Data from the cancer registry database of the Cancer Institute Hospital, Tokyo, Japan, 1990–2004) [21]

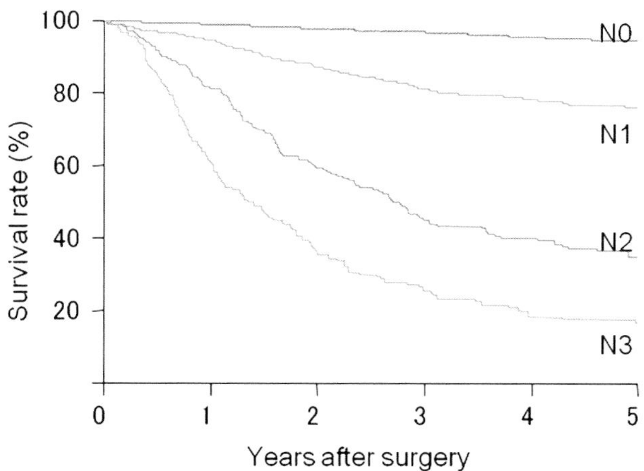

Fig. 21.2 Survival curves after resection of gastric cancer. According to nodal status (by Japanese classification). The 5-year survival rates of N0 (n=1988), N1 (n=671), N2 (n=239), N3 (n=189) are 94.2 %, 75.9 %, 35.1 %, 16.8 %, respectively. (Data from the cancer registry database of the Cancer Institute Hospital, Tokyo, Japan, 1990–2004) [21]

Advanced Gastric Cancer

A radical gastrectomy with an extended (D2) removal of the regional lymph nodes has long been the standard for treatment of curable gastric cancer in Japan [17]. The final results of a multi-institutional, randomized, controlled trial by the Japan Clinical Oncology Group (JCOG 9501) concluded that treatment with a D2 lymphadenectomy plus para-aortic nodal dissection does not improve the survival rate in curable gastric cancer, in comparison to a D2 lymphadenectomy alone [17]. Thus, for all patients with potentially curable lesions, D2 gastrectomy remains standard, except for those who are candidates for minimally invasive surgery.

S-1 is a novel oral anticancer drug, which was developed based on the biochemical modulation of Tegafur by 5-chloro-2, 4-dihydroxypyridine and potassium oxonate in a molar ratio of 1:0.4:1 [18]. In Japan, S-1 has been in common use in clinical practice since 1999 and now is the key drug for the treatment of advanced or recurrent gastric cancer. S-1 is an effective adjuvant treatment for East Asian patients who have undergone a D2 dissection for locally advanced (stage II and III) gastric cancer [19].

The number of metastatic lymph nodes (N stage) and the depth of the primary tumor (T stage) are currently considered the most reliable prognostic indicators for patients with radically

Table 21.3 Surveillance after curative-intent treatment for patients with nodal metastases at Kyushu University Hospital, Japan

	Year					
Modality	1	2	3	4	5	>5
Office visit	4	4	4	2	2	2
Blood tests[a]	4	4	4	2	2	2
Chest x-ray	2	2	2	1	1	1
Abdominal ultrasound examination	2–4	2–4	2–4	2	2	2
Abdominal computered tomography	2–4	2–4	2–4	2	2	2
Esophagogastroscopy	1	1	1	1	1	1
Barium enema/colonoscopy	0	1	0	1	0	0

The number in each cell indicates the number of times a particular modality is recommended in a particular posttreatment year.
[a](complete blood count, serum chemistry (includes total protein, albumin, creatinine, blood urea nitrogen, uric acid, sodium, potassium, chloride, alkaline phosphatase, bilirubin, glucose, lactic dehydrogenase, phosphorus), serum CEA level, serum CA 19-9 level)

Table 21.4 Surveillance after curative-intent treatment for patients with advanced gastric cancer at Kyushu University Hospital, Japan

	Year					
Modality	1	2	3	4	5	>5
Office visit	4	4	4	2	2	2
Blood tests[a]	4	4	4	2	2	2
Chest x-ray	2	2	2	1	1	1
Abdominal ultrasound examination	2–4	2–4	2–4	2	2	2
Abdominal computered tomography	2–4	2–4	2–4	2	2	2
Esophagogastroscopy	1	1	1	1	1	1
Barium enema/colonoscopy	0	1	0	1	0	0

The number in each cell indicates the number of times a particular modality is recommended in a particular posttreatment year.
[a](complete blood count, serum chemistry (includes total protein, albumin, creatinine, blood urea nitrogen, uric acid, sodium, potassium, chloride, alkaline phosphatase, bilirubin, glucose, lactic dehydrogenase, phosphorus), serum CEA level, serum CA 19-9 level)

resected gastric cancer [20]. Figs. 21.1 and 21.2 show survival curves after resection of gastric cancer in the Cancer Institute Hospital, Tokyo, Japan [21], from 1990 to 2004. The histological type of tumor was significantly related to the mode of recurrence. Hematogenous metastases predominated in differentiated-type tumors, while peritoneal dissemination was frequently seen in undifferentiated-type tumors (poorly differentiated, signet-ring cell, and mucinous carcinomas). Undifferentiated-type gastric cancer characterized by diffuse infiltration often obstructs the urinary tracts or the rectosigmoid colon and sometimes involves the ovaries in females. Bone metastasis is uncommon in patients with poorly differentiated carcinoma.

Anastomotic or stump recurrence is rather uncommon among Japanese patients because the resection margin is generally sufficiently distant from the macroscopic edge of the tumor [22]. Sometimes, in cases with an infiltrative growth pattern, intraoperative pathological confirmation of the surgical margins helps determine the resection line. Local recurrence is also uncommon after thorough clearance of the regional lymph nodes and peritoneal disease.

Death from recurrent gastric carcinoma mainly occurs within 2 years after gastrectomy (75 %) [23]. Death from recurrence occurring >5 years after gastrectomy is rare (6 %).

The basic surveillance schedule for patients with advanced gastric cancer at Kyushu University Hospital is shown in Tables 21.3 and 21.4. This represents a consensus among clinicians commonly treating these patients and is based on the analysis of tumor biology and treatment results. Postoperative follow-up is usually carried out by the surgeon in charge of the patient and in the hospital where surgeons, medical oncologists, and radiation oncologists are all present. All examinations are covered by insurance in Japan. Follow-up methods and intervals are individualized according to the pathological factors in each patient. The depth of invasion, nodal status, and histological type are important in determining the strategy. For example, in T2 differentiated-type tumors, surveillance is focused on liver metastasis; in T3 undifferentiated-type tumors, peritoneal dissemination is the most probable pattern of failure. Lymphatic or vascular invasion are also useful in the evaluation for nodal metastasis and hematogenous metastasis, respectively. After 5 years, annual checkups are recommended.

Monitoring of carcinoembryonic antigen (CEA) and carbohydrate antigens of the sialyl-Lewis A group (CA19-9) after operation is useful to predict recurrence of gastric cancer, especially in patients with high preoperative levels of these markers. A prospective study [24] of 321 Japanese patients with advanced gastric carcinoma showed that the serum CEA level was elevated preoperatively in 28 % of cases and the serum CA19-9 level was elevated preoperatively in 29 %. One or both were elevated in 45 %. The sensitivities of CEA and CA19-9, and combinations of the two markers, for indicating recurrence after curative-intent treatment were 66 %, 55 %, and 85 %, respectively. The levels of these markers were usually elevated before the detection of recurrence by an imaging modality.

Knowledge of the recurrence pattern (local, regional distant) by computed tomography can help in determining the proper patient management [25]. Though the whole-body 18-fluorodeoxyglucose positron emission tomography (FDG-PET) for gastric cancer is not currently covered by Japanese insurance, it is useful and can provide information on recurrence site when computed tomography is non-diagnostic [26]. Barium enema is useful in detecting peritoneal involvement. Esophagogastroscopy is performed only every other year because recurrence of the original cancer and development of a second primary cancer are both rare. When available, abdominal ultrasonography facilitates the detection of liver metastasis, minimal ascites, and mild hydronephrosis.

Although salvage therapy is usually not possible, early detection of recurrence may be beneficial under limited conditions. In some patients with recurrence, surgical treatment may enhance the quality of life, but does not increase survival duration. However, a hepatic resection for liver metastases is reasonable if a complete resection seems feasible after careful preoperative staging, and sometimes results in long-term survival [27]. Liver metastases from gastric cancer are frequently multiple and associated with concurrent peritoneal disease. A hepatic resection should therefore be considered as an option when the primary gastric tumor does not penetrate the gastric serosa with no lymphatic or venous capillary invasion. A surgical resection for liver metastasis may be indicated in patients with unilobar metastasis and/or tumors less than 4 cm in diameter [28]. Synchronous metastasis is not a contraindication for a hepatectomy.

Systemic chemotherapy is usually indicated for recurrent tumors. S-1 is significantly better than 5-FU, as measured by survival duration [29]. In addition, a randomized phase III study suggested that S-1 plus cisplatin confers longer median overall survival duration than S-1 alone [30]. Theoretically, early detection of recurrence would allow systemic therapy to begin when the tumor volume is minimal, thereby producing maximal therapeutic effects.

When patients are fully informed of the risk of recurrence, particularly the decreasing risk over time, negative results during periodic checkups are reassuring. When asymptomatic recurrence is detected by surveillance examination, this early diagnosis allows the patient time to make important decisions and preparations for further treatment.

Presently, no evidence-based guidelines for the follow-up of patients after surgery for gastrointestinal cancer are available in Japan. Follow-up after gastric cancer surgery focuses on finding recurrent disease and metachronous lesions in the remnant stomach or other organs. Follow-up strategies differ among hospitals, depending on the preferences of physicians or surgeons. Multi-institution prospective trials of follow-up strategies have not been done in Japan.

Molecular biology approaches in the follow-up of gastric cancer are not sufficiently developed to predict its role in the future. Vascular endothelial growth factor (VEGF) is an angiogenic factor in human tissues including cancer. Patients with VEGF-positive gastric cancers have more hematogenous metastases than patients with VEGF-negative cancers [31]. Cancer cells producing VEGF-C induce proliferation and dilation of lymphatic vessels, resulting in entry of cancer cells into lymphatic vessels and lymph nodes metastasis [32]. Transforming growth factor beta (TGF-beta) may contribute, in part, to the variations in histogenesis and to the prevalence of peritoneal dissemination in gastric carcinoma [33]. Protein expression profiling using the tissue array method provides a limited means for the molecular classification of gastric cancer into survival-predictive subgroups [34]. This molecular classification can predict lymph node metastasis and prognosis in patients with early stage gastric cancer. Molecular biology approaches in follow-up for gastric cancer are certain to be more sophisticated in the future.

References

1. Ministry of Health, Labor and Welfare, Japan. Figure for vital statistics in 2007. Available at: (http://www.mhlw.go.jp/toukei/saikin/hw/jinkou/kakutei07/hyo7.html) Accessed Jun 2011
2. Craanen ME, Dekker W, Blok P, Ferwerda J, Tytgat GN. Intestinal metaplasia and Helicobacter pylori: an endoscopic bioptic study of the gastric antrum. Gut. 1992;33:16–20.
3. Nobuta A, Asaka M, Sugiyama T, et al. Helicobacter pylori infection in two areas in Japan with different risks for gastric cancer. Aliment Pharmacol Ther. 2004;20 Suppl 1:1–6.
4. Suzuki H, Iwasaki E, Hibi T. Helicobacter pylori and gastric cancer. Gastric Cancer. 2009;12:79–87.
5. Uemura N, Mukai T, Okamoto S, et al. Effect of Helicobacter pylori eradication on subsequent development of cancer after endoscopic resection of early gastric cancer. Cancer Epidemiol Biomarkers Prev. 1997;6:639–42.
6. Fukase K, Kato M, Kikuchi S, et al. Effect of eradication of Helicobacter pylori on incidence of metachronous gastric carcinoma after endoscopic resection of early gastric cancer: an open-label, randomised controlled trial. Lancet. 2008;372:392–7.
7. The Japanese Gastric Cancer Association (JGCA). The first version of gastric cancer treatment guidelines. Available at: (http://www.jgca.jp/PDFfiles/E-guideline.PDF)
8. The Japanese Gastric Cancer Association. Guidelines for diagnosis and treatment of carcinoma of the stomach. April 2004 ed. Available at: (http://www.jgca.jp/PDFfiles/Guidelines2004_eng.pdf)
9. Shimura T, Sasaki M, Kataoka H, et al. Advantages of endoscopic submucosal dissection over conventional endoscopic mucosal resection. J Gastroenterol Hepatol. 2007;22:821–6.
10. Gotoda T, Yanagisawa A, Sasako M, et al. Incidence of lymph node metastasis from early gastric cancer: estimation with a large number of cases at two large centers. Gastric Cancer. 2000;3:219–25.
11. Kojima K, Yamada H, Inokuchi M, Hayashi M, Kawano T, Sugihara K. Current status and evaluation of laparoscopic surgery for gastric cancer. Dig Endosc. 2008;20:1–5.
12. Japan Society for Endoscopic Surgery. A questionnaire survey for endoscopic surgery. The report of the 9th meeting. J Jpn Soc Endosc Surg. 2008;13:525–529.
13. The Japanese Gastric Cancer Association Registration Committee. Gastric cancer treated in 1991 in Japan: data analysis of nationwide registry. Gastric Cancer. 2006;9:51–66.
14. Ikeda Y, Saku M, Kishihara F, Maehara Y. Effective follow-up for recurrence or a second primary cancer in patients with early gastric cancer. Br J Surg. 2005;92:235–9.
15. Maehara Y, Tomisaki S, Emi Y, et al. Clinicopathological features of patients who died with second primary cancer after curative resection for gastric cancer. Anticancer Res. 1995;15:1049–54.
16. Yamamoto M, Yamanaka T, Baba H, et al. Postoperative recurrence and the occurrence of second primary carcinomas in patients with early gastric carcinoma. J Surg Oncol. 2008;97:231–5.
17. Sano T, Yamamoto S, Kurokawa Y, et al. D2 lymphadenectomy alone or with para-aortic nodal dissection for gastric cancer new eng. J Med. 2008;359:453.
18. Shirasaka T, Nakano K, Takechi T, et al. Antitumor activity of 1 M tegafur- 0.4 M 5-chloro-2,4-dihydroxy-pyridine- 1 M potassium oxonate (S-1) against human colon carcinoma orthotopically implanted into nude rats. Cancer Res. 1996;56:2602–6.

19. Sakuramoto S, Sasako M, Yamaguchi T, et al. Adjuvant chemotherapy for gastric cancer with S-1, an oral fluoropyrimidine. N Engl J Med. 2007;357:1810.
20. Dicken BJ, Bigam DL, Cass C, Mackey JR, Joy AA, Hamilton SM. Gastric adenocarcinoma: review and considerations for future directions. Ann Surg. 2005;241:27–39.
21. Nakajima T, Yamaguchi T (eds). The gastric cancer registry database 1946-2004 (Cancer Institute Hospital gastric cancer database 1946–2004), Tokyo: Kanehara & Co., Ltd; 2006
22. Maehara Y, Hasuda S, Koga T, Tokunaga E, Kakeji Y, Sugimachi K. Postoperative outcome and sites of recurrence in patients following curative resection of gastric cancer. Br J Surg. 2000;80:353–7.
23. Shiraishi N, Inomata M, Osawa N, Yasuda K, Adachi Y, Kitano S. Early and late recurrence after gastrectomy for gastric carcinoma. Univariate and multivariate analyses. Cancer. 2000;89:255–61.
24. Takahashi Y, Takeuchi T, Sakamoto J, et al. The usefulness of CEA and/or CA19-9 in monitoring for recurrence in gastric cancer patients: a prospective clinical study. Gastric Cancer. 2003;6:142–5.
25. Kim BS, Namkung S, Kim HC, Hwang IK, Hwang WC, Bae SH. CT findings of recurrent gastric carcinoma. Radiol. 2004;11:55–61.
26. Chen J, Cheong JH, Yun MJ, et al. The role of whole-body positron emission tomography with 18-fluorodeoxyglucose in recurrent gastric cancer. J Clin Oncol. 2004;22(14S):4065.
27. Cheon SH, Rha SY, Jeung HC, et al. Survival benefit of combined curative resection of the stomach (D2 resection) and liver in gastric cancer patients with liver metastases. Ann Oncol. 2008;19:1146–53.
28. Sakamoto Y, Sano T, Shimada K, et al. Favorable indications for hepatectomy in patients with liver Metastasis from gastric cancer. J Surg Oncol. 2007;95:534–9.
29. Boku N, Yamamoto S, Shirao K, et al. Randomized phase III study of 5-fluorouracil (5-FU) alone versus combination of irinotecan and cisplatin (CP) versus S-1 alone in advanced gastric cancer (JCOG9912). Japan clinical oncology group trial. Proc Am Soc Clin Oncol. 2007;25:LBA4513 (abst)
30. Koizumi W, Narahara H, Hara T, et al. S-1plus cisplatin versus S-1 alone for first-line treatment of advanced gastric cancer (SPIRITS trial): a phase III trial. Lancet Oncol. 2008;9(3):215–21.
31. Kakeji Y, Maehara Y, Sumiyoshi Y, et al. Angiogenesis as a target for gastric cancer. Surgery. 2002;131:S48–54.
32. Yonemura Y, Fushida S, Bando E, et al. Lymphangiogenesis and the vascular endothelial growth factor receptor (VEGFR)-3 in gastric cancer. Eur J Cancer. 2001;37:918–23.
33. Niki M, Toyoda M, Nomura E, et al. Expression of transforming growth factor beta (TGF-beta) may contribute, in part, to the variations in histogenesis and the prevalence of peritoneal dissemination in human gastric carcinoma. Gastric Cancer. 2000;3:187–92.
34. Lee HS, Cho SB, Lee HE, et al. Protein expression profiling and molecular classification of gastric cancer by the tissue array method. Clin Cancer Res. 2007;13:4154–63.
35. The Japanese Gastric Cancer Association. Japanese classification of gastric carcinoma-2nd english edition-gastric cancer. 1998;1:10–24

22 Pancreatic Adenocarcinoma

David Y. Johnson, Shilpi Wadhwa, and Frank E. Johnson

Keywords
Prior cholecystectomy • Diabetes mellitus • Cirrhosis • Pancreatic cancer • Variation

The International Agency for Research on Cancer (IARC), a component of the World Health Organization (WHO), estimated that there were 232,306 new cases of pancreatic cancer worldwide in 2002 [1]. The IARC also estimated that there were 227,023 deaths due to this cause in 2002 [1].

The American Cancer Society has estimated that there were 37,170 new cases and 33,370 deaths due to this cause in the USA in 2007 [2]. The estimated 5-year survival rate (all races) in the USA in 2007 was 5 % for pancreatic cancer [2]. Survival rates were adjusted for normal life expectancies and were based on cases diagnosed from 1996 to 2002 and followed through 2003.

Tobacco smoking, prior cholecystectomy, diabetes mellitus, cirrhosis, high fat diet, obesity, and advanced age are risk factors for development of pancreatic cancer. Various ethnic and racial groups are at increased risk, including African-American men and Ashkenazi Jews. Exposure to several organic compounds, nickel and chromium compounds, and silica has been identified as risk factor. It is currently believed that genetic factors are responsible for 10–20 % of instances; this is an active area of research and additional genetic factors are likely to be described in the future [3]. Males are more frequently affected than females [4].

Geographic Variation Worldwide

There is a marked (30-fold) variation in the incidence of pancreatic cancer around the world [4]. The incidence is highest in industrialized countries and lowest in African and Asian countries, suggesting that Western lifestyle substantially increases the risk of pancreatic cancer [5, 6]. High incidence rates observed in African Americans as opposed to low rates observed in African countries strongly suggest a role of environmental factors in the causation of this cancer. In the USA, pancreatic cancer occurs more frequently in blacks than in the whites (relative risk, 2:1) and may be somewhat less common in Asians than in whites (relative risk, 0.7:1) [7]. Geographic variation for this cancer in the USA is less pronounced than for most other cancers [8].

Surveillance Strategies Proposed by Professional Organizations or National Government Agencies and Available on the Internet

National Comprehensive Cancer Network (NCCN, www.nccn.org)

NCCN guidelines were accessed on 1/28/12 (Table 22.1). There were minor quantitative and qualitative changes compared to the guidelines accessed on 4/10/07.

D.Y. Johnson, M.D. • S. Wadhwa
Department of Internal Medicine, Saint Louis University Medical Center, Saint Louis, MO, USA

F.E. Johnson, M.D., F.A.C.S. (✉)
Saint Louis University Medical Center and Saint Louis Veterans Affairs Medical Center, Saint Louis, MO, USA
e-mail: frank.johnson1@va.gov

F.E. Johnson et al. (eds.), *Patient Surveillance After Cancer Treatment*, Current Clinical Oncology,
DOI 10.1007/978-1-60327-969-7_22, © Springer Science+Business Media New York 2013

Table 22.1 Pancreatic adenocarcinoma. Obtained from NCCN (www.nccn.org) on 1/28/12

	Years posttreatment[a]					
	1	2	3	4	5	>5
Office visit	2–4	2–4	1	1	1	1
Serum CA 19-9 level	2–4	2–4	1	1	1	1
CT scan	2–4	2–4	1	1	1	1

NCCN guidelines were accessed on 1/28/12. There were minor quantitative and qualitative changes compared to the guidelines accessed on 4/10/07

[a]The numbers in the table indicate the number of times the modality is recommended during the indicated year posttreatment

Table 22.2 Pancreatic cancer. Obtained from ESMO (www.esmo.org) on 1/28/12

	Years posttreatment[a]					
	1	2	3	4	5	>5
Office visit[b]	6	6	6	6	6	6
Serum CA 19-9 level[c]	4	4	0	0	0	0
Abdominal CT scan[c]	2	2	2	2	2	2

- Clinical benefit and CA 19-9 may be useful tools to assess the course of disease in the metastatic setting
- Imaging procedures such as CT scan may be indicated mainly in locally advanced disease in order to rule out the presence of metastases and to add radiotherapy to the treatment plan
- There is no possibility of cure, even for recurrences diagnosed early, so a follow-up schedule should be discussed with the patient and designed to avoid emotional stress and economic burden for the patient

ESMO guidelines were accessed on 1/28/12. These are new quantitative guidelines compared to the qualitative guidelines accessed on 10/31/07

[a]The numbers in the table indicate the number of times the modality is recommended during the indicated year posttreatment

[b]Patients should be followed at each cycle of chemotherapy for toxicity and evaluated for response to chemotherapy every 2 months

[c]In the case of elevated preoperative CA 19-9 levels

American Society of Clinical Oncology (ASCO, www.asco.org)

ASCO guidelines were accessed on 1/28/12. No quantitative guidelines exist for pancreatic cancer surveillance, including when first accessed on 10/31/07.

The Society of Surgical Oncology (SSO, www.surgonc.org)

SSO guidelines were accessed on 1/28/12. No quantitative guidelines exist for pancreatic cancer surveillance, including when first accessed on 10/31/07.

European Society for Medical Oncology (ESMO, www.esmo.org)

ESMO guidelines were accessed on 1/28/12 (Table 22.2). There are new quantitative guidelines compared to the qualitative guidelines accessed on 10/31/07.

European Society of Surgical Oncology (ESSO, www.esso-surgeonline.org)

ESSO guidelines were accessed on 1/28/12. No quantitative guidelines exist for pancreatic cancer surveillance, including when first accessed on 10/31/07.

Cancer Care Ontario (CCO, www.cancercare.on.ca)

CCO guidelines were accessed on 1/28/12. No quantitative guidelines exist for pancreatic cancer surveillance, including when first accessed on 10/31/07.

National Institute for Clinical Excellence (NICE, www.nice.org.uk)

NICE guidelines were accessed on 1/28/12. No quantitative guidelines exist for pancreatic cancer surveillance, including when first accessed on 10/31/07.

The Cochrane Collaboration (CC, www.cochrane.org)

CC guidelines were accessed on 1/28/12. No quantitative guidelines exist for pancreatic cancer surveillance, including when first accessed on 10/31/07.

Society for the Surgery of the Alimentary Tract (SSAT, www.ssat.com)

SSAT guidelines were accessed on 1/28/12. No quantitative guidelines exist for pancreatic cancer surveillance, including when first accessed on 12/18/07.

The M.D. Anderson Surgical Oncology Handbook also has follow-up guidelines, proposed by authors from a single National Cancer Institute-designated Comprehensive Cancer Center, for many types of cancer [9]. Some are detailed and quantitative, others are qualitative.

Summary

This is a moderately common cancer with low variability in incidence worldwide. We found consensus-based guidelines but none based on high-quality evidence.

References

1. Parkin DM, Whelan SL, Ferlay J, Teppo L, Thomas DB. Cancer incidence in five continents, vol. VIII. Lyon: IARC Press; 2002. International Agency for Research on Cancer (IARC Scientific Publication 155). ISBN 92-832-2155-9.
2. Jemal A, Seigel R, Ward E, Murray T, Xu J, Thun MJ. Cancer statistics, 2007. CA Cancer J Clin. 2007;57:43–66.
3. Schottenfeld D, Fraumeni JG. Cancer epidemiology and prevention. 3rd ed. New York, NY: Oxford University Press; 2006. ISBN 13:978-0-19-514961-6.
4. DeVita VT, Hellman S, Rosenberg SA. Cancer. 7th ed. Philadelphia, PA: Lippincott Williams & Wilkins; 2005. ISBN 0-781-74450-4.
5. Howe GR. Epidemiology of cancer of the pancreas. In: Cameron JL, editor. Pancreatic cancer. London: BC Decker; 2001. p. 1–2.
6. Akoi K, Ogawa H. Cancer of the pancreas: international mortality trends. World Health Stat Q. 1978;31(1):2–27.
7. Abeloff MD, Armitage JO, Niederhuber JE, Kastan MB, McKenna WG. Clinical oncology. 3rd ed. Philadelphia, PA: Elsevier Churchill Livingstone; 2004. ISBN 0-443-06629-9.
8. Devesa SS, Grauman DJ, Blot WJ, Pennello GA, Hoover RN, Fraumeni JF Jr. Atlas of cancer mortality in the United States. National Institutes of Health, National Cancer Institute. NIH Publication No. 99-4564; 1999.
9. Feig BW, Berger DH, Fuhrman GM. The M.D. Anderson surgical oncology handbook (paperback). 4th ed. Philadelphia, PA: Lippincott Williams & Wilkins; 2006. ISBN 0-7817-5643-X.

Pancreatic Adenocarcinoma Surveillance Counterpoint: USA

23

Tanios S. Bekaii-Saab

Keywords
Adjuvant • 5-Fluorouracil • Gemcitabine • Resection • Radiation • Chemotherapy • Surveillance • CA19-9

Pancreas cancer remains a formidable challenge with an overall 5-year survival rate of <5 % [1]. Patients typically present with advanced disease at diagnosis which precludes potentially curative therapy. Only 10–12 % of patients present with localized disease and eventually undergo surgery with curative intent [2]. Although the primary aim of surgical resection is cure, only 9.8 % of patients who undergo curative-intent surgery survive >5 years; by 10 years, >3 % are survivors [3]. By observing continued patient attrition with longer follow-up, Trede et al. state that ductal adenocarcinoma of the pancreas is an incurable disease [4]. As such, pancreaticoduodenectomy for adenocarcinoma of the pancreas appears to be a palliative procedure which confers survival advantage in comparison to other available options. This is my opinion, as well, since we rarely see long-term survivors. Survival is dependent on multiple factors, including the biology of the disease, the success of the surgical intervention, and the choice of appropriate adjuvant therapy. Surgical intervention is likely to be more successful in prolonging life if an R0 resection (complete resection with no microscopic residual tumor) is achieved with minimal morbidity [5]. The more experienced the center where the surgery is performed, the higher the likelihood of minimal morbidity and maximal survival benefit [6]. Regionalization of care (referring patients to high-volume centers) represents a strategy that could improve outcome for patients with localized pancreas cancer.

T.S. Bekaii-Saab, M.D. (✉)
James Cancer Hospital, The Ohio State University,
B407 Starling Loving Hall, 320 West 10th Avenue, Columbus,
OH 43210, USA
e-mail: Tanios.Bekaii-Saab@osumc.edu

The role of adjuvant therapy is continuously being redefined. An initial analysis of 100,313 US patients with pancreas cancer in the National Cancer Database revealed that 9,044 patients (9 %) had a pancreatectomy, but only about 40 % received adjuvant therapy (6.5 % radiation alone, 5.1 % chemotherapy alone, and 28.3 % chemotherapy plus radiation) [7]. The 5-year survival rate was 23.3 % for the observation-only group and 13–17 % for the other three groups. However, numerous randomized studies for the last three decades have established the role of adjuvant therapy by consistently showing an advantage for therapy versus observation alone [8].

Pancreas cancer is likely a systemic disease from diagnosis with locoregional and systemic patterns of recurrence occurring at equal rates [9, 10]. There is no universally accepted standard approach to date. Current options include chemotherapy plus radiation or chemotherapy alone, which is now favored. Most studies available until recently were small, underpowered, and inconclusive. One large well-designed Phase 3 study suggests a benefit from adjuvant gemcitabine (Charité Onkologie-001 or CONKO-001) [11]. There are also data supporting the use of 5-fluorouracil (European Study Group for Pancreatic Cancer-1 or ESPAC-1) [12]. The results of the ESPAC-3 trial were presented at the American Society of Clinical Oncology meeting in 2009. This showed that both bolus 5-fluorouracil and gemcitabine have similar benefits, as measured by survival duration and disease-free survival duration in patients with resected pancreas cancer, although the toxicity profile favored gemcitabine [13]. The role of chemoradiation in the adjuvant setting in pancreas cancer remains very controversial. Both the ESPAC-1 study and a recent meta-analysis indicated a detrimental effect for radiation therapy when compared to

F.E. Johnson et al. (eds.), *Patient Surveillance After Cancer Treatment*, Current Clinical Oncology,
DOI 10.1007/978-1-60327-969-7_23, © Springer Science+Business Media New York 2013

Table 23.1 Historical comparison of the gemcitabine containing arms of the CONKO-01 [11] and the Radiation Therapy Oncology Group 9704 [14] studies

Parameter	CONKO-01 Gemcitabine[a]	Radiation Therapy Oncology Group 9704 Gemcitabine→5FU+Radiation→Gemcitabine[b]
Median overall survival duration	22.1 months	20.6 months
Median progression-free survival duration	13.4 months	11.2 months
3-year overall survival duration	36 %	32 %
Grades 3/4 toxicities	4 %	80 %

[a]Represents all patients. 81 % had R0 resection (19 % had R1). Gemcitabine was given at 1,000 mg/m^2 once weekly for 3 weeks, then every 4 weeks for a total of six cycles
[b]Represents pancreatic head cancer patients only. 66 % had R0 resection (34 % had R1). Gemcitabine was given at 1,000 mg/m^2 once weekly for 3 weeks, followed by a continuous infusion of 250 mg/m^2 of fluorouracil daily throughout radiation therapy (50.4 Gy), then gemcitabine at 1,000 mg/m^2 once weekly for 3 weeks, then every 4 weeks for three more cycles

observation alone [12–14]. The Radiation Therapy Oncology Group 9704 study suggested a clinical benefit from one adjuvant chemotherapy and radiation regimen, as compared to another, in patients with pancreatic head carcinoma [15]. The median disease-free survival duration for pancreatic head tumors (a group with typically a more favorable outcome than body and tail tumors) in both arms on this study was less than 12 months which is comparable to results obtained using gemcitabine alone (13.4 months) [15]. The rest of the efficacy parameters were very similar as well (see Table 23.1). However, there was a large difference between the rate of grades 3 and 4 toxicities favoring chemotherapy alone. Therefore, taking all this together and based on historical comparisons (with all its limitations) between the Radiation Therapy Oncology Group and CONKO studies, radiation does not seem to add to the efficacy of chemotherapy but seems to worsen toxicity in patients with resected pancreas cancer. The ESPAC-1 trial confirmed this [12]. At The Ohio State University, all patients with an R0-resected pancreas cancer are considered for adjuvant therapy with chemotherapy alone (gemcitabine, preferably, although 5-fluorouracil is an acceptable alternative). Patients with an R1 (microscopic residual disease) or R2 (macroscopic residual disease) resection are considered for either gemcitabine alone (preferably) or gemcitabine for three to four months followed by 5-fluorouracil-based chemoradiation if there is no further clinical or radiographic evidence of systemic disease.

Since this disease is so lethal, postoperative surveillance should be cost-effective relative to the potential benefit. Early detection is unlikely to change the outcome or improve the chances of palliation. Therefore, intensive amplified surveillance regimens will not offer the patients any short- or long-term benefit and thus should be avoided.

There is very little evidence that history and physical examination is sensitive enough to detect early recurrence. Typical symptoms include unexplained weight and appetite loss, abdominal pain, and fatigue. The occurrence of new symptoms should prompt the initiation of further diagnostic workup and, if needed, closer follow-up.

Routine laboratory testing should be done at every visit including complete blood count and liver function tests. More importantly, the serum CA 19-9 level, which is highly sensitive and specific [16], should be tested at every visit. In addition to being a marker for early recurrence, it is also a prognostic marker. The post-resection serum CA 19-9 level is a predictor of overall survival in patients with pancreas cancer treated with adjuvant therapy; postoperative levels ≥180 U/mL are associated with worse survival outcome compared to levels <180 U/mL [16, 17].

Since early detection, especially in the absence of symptoms, is unlikely to change the outcome, or improve the chances of palliation, routine radiographic imaging plays no role in the follow-up of these asymptomatic patients. Computed tomograms (CTs) of the chest and abdomen are only recommended in a few situations: prior to initiating adjuvant therapy to help restage patients following surgery and ensure the adequacy of the treatment offered; before any planned radiation (if indicated in R1 or R2 patients); and when clinical suspicion of recurrence is raised during routine clinical evaluation.

Because of potential early perioperative complications, patients with resected pancreas cancer should be followed up very closely in the immediate postoperative period by a multidisciplinary team including a medical oncologist, a surgeon, a nutritionist, and others, as deemed necessary. During receipt of adjuvant therapy, patients are followed up as per routine institutional protocols for patients receiving chemotherapy (and/or radiation if indicated). Following that period, patients are followed by the primary oncologist for life. Survivors should also see their primary care physician as needed and for nononcologic medical issues. The European Society for Medical Oncology clinical guidelines suggest limiting follow-up to health and physical examination at intervals of three to six months depending on the presence or absence of symptoms [18]. As mentioned in the primary chapter, the National Comprehensive Cancer Network recommends surveillance (health and physical examination) every three to six months for two years, then annually [19]. CT scans and CA19-9 levels are considered low yield by the National Comprehensive Cancer Network panel and therefore have a category 2B designation. (The recommendation is based on lower level evidence and there is nonuniform National Comprehensive Cancer Network consensus but no major

Table 23.2 Follow-up of patients with resected pancreas cancer following completion of adjuvant therapy at The Ohio State University

	Years					
Modality	1	2	3	4	5	>5
History and physical examination	4	4	3	2	2	2
Complete blood count	4	4	3	2	2	2
Liver function tests[a]	4	4	3	2	2	2
Serum CA19-9 level	4	4	3	2	2	2

Imaging studies are obtained as clinically indicated only
The number in each cell indicates the number of times a particular modality is recommended in a particular posttreatment year
[a]Serum SGOT, SGPT, alkaline phosphatase, and bilirubin levels

disagreement.) Our current guidelines for the surveillance of patients with resected pancreatic cancer following completion of adjuvant therapy at the Ohio State University are summarized in Table 23.2. It follows the spirit of the National Comprehensive Cancer Network guidelines, although we chose a slightly more intense surveillance schema to allow early identification of recurrence, given the breadth of our pancreas cancer research program. Since this is an incurable disease for most patients, they should be followed for the rest of their lives. It is difficult to assess the cost-effectiveness of our surveillance strategy; however, patients with pancreas cancer seem to prefer close follow-up.

Given that the number of patients who undergo a curative-intent resection is small, trials to assess the costs and benefits of surveillance programs are not feasible. As suggested above, there is no recognized optimal strategy. Molecular and genetic approaches to diagnosis and treatment are likely to create improved surveillance strategies in the future.

References

1. Jemal A, Siegel R, Ward E, et al. CA Cancer J Clin. 2008;58:71–96.
2. Ries LAG, Eisner MP, Kosary CL, et al., editors. SEER cancer statistics review, 1975–2002. National Cancer Institute. Bethesda, MD, 2004. http://seer.cancer.gov/csr/1975_2002/
3. Bradley 3rd EL. Long-term survival after pancreatoduodenectomy for ductal adenocarcinoma: the emperor has no clothes? Pancreas. 2008;37:349–51.
4. Trede M, Richter A, Wendl K. Personal observations, opinions, and approaches to cancer of the pancreas and the periampullary area. Surg Clin North Am. 2001;81:595–610.
5. Howard TJ, Krug JE, Yu J, et al. A margin-negative R0 resection accomplished with minimal postoperative complications is the surgeon's contribution to long-term survival in pancreatic cancer. J Gastrointest Surg. 2006;10:1338–45.
6. Birkmeyer JD, Sun Y, Wong SL, Stukel TA. Hospital volume and late survival after cancer surgery. Ann Surg. 2007;245:777–83.
7. Sener SF, Fremgen A, Menck HR, Winchester DP. Pancreatic cancer: a report of treatment and survival trends for 100,313 patients diagnosed from 1985–1995, using the National Cancer Database. J Am Coll Surg. 1999;189:1–7.
8. Kosuri K, Muscarella P, Bekaii-Saab TS. Updates and controversies in the treatment of pancreatic cancer. Clin Adv Hematol Oncol. 2006;4:47–54.
9. Johnstone PA, Sindelar WF. Patterns of disease recurrence following definitive therapy of adenocarcinoma of the pancreas using surgery and adjuvant radiotherapy: correlations of a clinical trial. Int J Radiat Oncol Biol Phys. 1993;27:831–4.
10. Sperti C, Pasquali C, Piccoli A, Pedrazzoli S. Recurrence after resection for ductal adenocarcinoma of the pancreas. World J Surg. 1997;21:195–200.
11. Oettle H, Post S, Neuhaus P, et al. Adjuvant chemotherapy with gemcitabine vs. observation in patients undergoing curative-intent resection of pancreatic cancer: a randomized controlled trial. JAMA. 2007;297:267–77.
12. Neoptolemos JP, Stocken DD, Friess H, et al. European Study Group for Pancreatic Cancer. A randomized trial of chemoradiotherapy and chemotherapy after resection of pancreatic cancer. N Engl J Med. 2004;350:1200–10.
13. Neoptolemos J, Büchler M, Stocken DD, et al. ESPAC-3(v2): a multicenter, international, open-label, randomized, controlled phase III trial of adjuvant 5-fluorouracil/folinic acid (5-FU/FA) versus gemcitabine (GEM) in patients with resected pancreatic ductal adenocarcinoma. J Clin Oncol. 2009;27:18s(suppl; abstr LBA4505).
14. Stocken DD, Buchler MW, Dervenis C, et al. Pancreatic Cancer Meta-analysis Group. Meta-analysis of randomised adjuvant therapy trials for pancreatic cancer. Br J Cancer. 2005;92:1372–81.
15. Regine WF, Winter KA, Abrams RA, et al. Fluorouracil vs. gemcitabine chemotherapy before and after fluorouracil-based chemoradiation following resection of pancreatic adenocarcinoma: a randomized controlled trial. JAMA. 2008;299:1019–26.
16. Boeck S, Stieber P, Holdenrieder S, Wilkowski R, Heinemann V. Prognostic and therapeutic significance of carbohydrate antigen 19-9 as tumor marker in patients with pancreatic cancer. Oncology. 2006;70:255–64.
17. Berger AC, Garcia Jr M, Hoffman JP, et al. Postresection CA 19-9 predicts overall survival in patients with pancreatic cancer treated with adjuvant chemoradiation: a prospective validation by Radiation Therapy Oncology Group 9704. J Clin Oncol. 2008;26:5918–22.
18. Herrmann R, Jelic S, ESMO Guidelines Working Group. Pancreatic cancer: ESMO clinical recommendations for diagnosis, treatment and follow-up. Ann Oncol. 2008;19 Suppl 2:ii25–6.
19. Tempero M, Arnoletti JP, Ben-Josef E, et al. Pancreatic adenocarcinoma. Clinical Practice Guidelines in Oncology. J Natl Compr Canc Netw. 2007;5:998–1033.

Pancreatic Adenocarcinoma Surveillance Counterpoint: Europe

24

Richard A. Smith, Jane V. Butler, and John P. Neoptolemos

Keywords
United Kingdom • Exocrine • Signet ring cell carcinoma • Penetrance • Pancreatoduodenectomy

Introduction

Exocrine pancreatic cancer accounts for almost a quarter of a million deaths worldwide each year with approximately one third arising in Europe [1, 2]. Despite being only the thirteenth most common malignancy worldwide, it is the eighth most frequent cause of cancer mortality [2]. The singularly aggressive nature of this disease is further underlined by the fact that mortality rates continue to approximate the incidence [3]. There has been a marginal decline in both age-standardised incidence and mortality rates over the past 20 years [3, 4].

Pancreatic ductal adenocarcinoma accounts for almost 90 % of all malignant neoplasms of the exocrine pancreas. Variants of this tumour type exist, including mucinous non-cystic adenocarcinoma, signet-ring cell carcinoma and mixed-ductal endocrine carcinoma. They exhibit similar histological characteristics and clinical outcomes. This group of exocrine tumours is commonly collectively referred to as "pancreatic cancer".

Understanding the aetiology of this group of cancers continues to improve, aided by numerous studies which have been undertaken to examine the significance of various environmental and disease-derived risk factors. One risk factor is advancing age; this is reflected in epidemiological data [5–7]. The US National Cancer Institute Surveillance Epidemiology and End Results (SEER) data from the period 2002–2006 identified that only 0.4 % of exocrine cancers of the pancreas occur within the 20–34-year age group. In contrast, 26.1 % of diagnoses occurred within the 65–74-year age group and 29.4 % were in the 75–84-year age group. The median age of onset of exocrine cancer of the pancreas was 72 years during this time period [5]. The increasing incidence of pancreatic adenocarcinoma seen with advancing age in the United States is reflected in worldwide data factors [6, 7]. In addition to the trend of increasing incidence seen in the older population, there is evidence of a male preponderance. The SEER data recorded an incidence of 13.1 per 100,000 in US males compared to 10.1 per 100,000 in females for the period 2002–2006 [5]. Variation in risk has also been observed between those of different racial and ethnic origins. Data from the SEER analysis relating to pancreatic adenocarcinoma diagnoses according to race identified an increased incidence in the black population within the United States. The incidence within the black male population was the highest observed among any group at 16.6 per 100,000 [5]. An elevated rate of pancreatic cancer is also seen within the Ashkenazi Jewish population. This inherited predisposition to pancreatic carcinoma is usually associated with an inherited genetic alteration, for example, a BRCA2 mutation.

In addition to the presence of certain patient-derived risk factors, there are a number of environmental exposures which also have a recognised role in the aetiology of this cancer. There is a clear association between tobacco smoking and pancreatic cancer. Numerous studies have examined this relationship and have reported a 2 to 5-fold dose-dependent increased risk associated with tobacco smoking [6–11]. The evidence for an aetiological role of high body mass index, lack of physical activity and dietary factors such as alcohol, coffee, tea and red meat intake has been proposed, but these data are

R.A. Smith • J.V. Butler • J.P. Neoptolemos, FMedSci (✉)
Division of Surgery and Oncology, The Owen and Ellen Evans Chair of Cancer Studies, School of Cancer Studies, Royal Liverpool University Hospital, University of Liverpool, 5th Floor UCD Building, Daulby Street, Liverpool, L69 3GA, UK
e-mail: j.p.neoptolemos@liverpool.ac.uk

F.E. Johnson et al. (eds.), *Patient Surveillance After Cancer Treatment*, Current Clinical Oncology,
DOI 10.1007/978-1-60327-969-7_24,

less conclusive [6–10, 12, 13]. Certain medical conditions have been reported as conferring an increased risk for the development of pancreatic cancer. For example, a diagnosis of diabetes mellitus has been identified as a risk factor for pancreatic adenocarcinoma by several authors, although controversy remains as to whether this phenomenon is due to cause or effect [6, 7, 14, 15]. Other medical conditions implicated as risk factors include chronic pancreatitis which has been reported to confer an increased lifetime risk of 15 % [16]. Previous cholecystectomy [7, 14] has also been mentioned as a risk factor, although this association has not been consistently demonstrated.

Although the vast majority of pancreatic cancers arise sporadically, it is estimated that approximately 10 % of cases have an underlying genetic cause. Hereditary pancreatitis is an autosomal dominant condition with incomplete penetrance which confers an estimated cumulative lifetime risk for the development of pancreatic adenocarcinoma in the region of 35–40 % [17, 18]. Certain other cancer syndromes are associated with an elevated risk of pancreatic cancer, such as mutations of the BRCA2 gene and of the p53 tumour suppressor gene (Li-Fraumeni syndrome). Peutz-Jeghers, hereditary non-polyposis colorectal cancer syndrome (HNPCC) and familial multiple mole melanoma syndrome (FAMMM) all confer an increased lifetime risk for the development of a number of malignancies, including pancreatic adenocarcinoma. Even in the absence of a confirmed cancer syndrome, a family history of pancreatic cancer is also a significant risk factor. The US National Familial Pancreas Tumor Registry reported a 6.4-fold increased risk of development of pancreatic cancer in a cohort of individuals with two affected first-degree relatives. The risk increased to 32-fold in the event of there being three or more affected first-degree relatives within a family [19]. In view of the evidence highlighting the increased risk in the presence of a family history of the condition, a number of registries across the United States and Europe offer surveillance to individuals whose families demonstrate an autosomal dominant pattern of inheritance for pancreatic cancer.

The recognition and assessment of lifestyle and disease-derived risk factors offers an important opportunity for health education and risk modification in addition to assessing the indication for surveillance in those deemed to be at particularly high risk. Only through screening in such high-risk populations, with the resulting early identification of cancers at an asymptomatic stage, can hope be offered of improved survival outcomes from this lethal malignancy.

Radical surgery for pancreatic cancer is only possible for around 20 % of patients due to the frequency of vascular involvement and distant metastases at presentation [20]. Significant perioperative mortality rates coupled with overall five-year survival rates of less than 1 % have historically resulted in an outlook of therapeutic nihilism amongst many clinicians with a consequent belief that radical intervention for pancreatic cancer could not be justified [21, 22]. This view, however, has been largely abandoned over the past 20 years as centralisation of pancreatic surgery has resulted in dramatic improvements in perioperative management with operative mortality rates of between 1 and 4 % now typical of most high-volume specialist centres [23–26]. Significant improvements in resectability rates, morbidity and late postoperative survival are also associated with greater caseloads [27]. A definitive role for adjuvant chemotherapy has been firmly established in randomised trials with reported five-year survival rates of 20–30 % [28, 29]. Coupled with a rapidly expanding range of potential therapeutic adjuncts to chemotherapy and an increasing understanding of the molecular basis of pancreatic carcinogenesis, there is every reason for optimism that patient outcomes can continue to improve in the near future.

Improvements in postoperative outcomes place an increasing importance on adopting a rational and evidence-based approach to the follow-up of patients undergoing resection for pancreatic adenocarcinoma. In this chapter, we will discuss the relevant issues and challenges associated with the follow-up of this patient group.

There are a number of key considerations in the follow-up of patients undergoing resection for pancreatic cancer: diagnosis and management of potential intermediate and late complications associated with pancreatic resection, administration of adjuvant chemotherapy, identification of tumour recurrence and provision of second-line chemotherapy and providing appropriate psychological support to patients and their families.

Due to the preponderance of adenocarcinomas which arise in the head of the pancreas, partial pancreatoduodenectomy accounts for between 80 and 90 % of all radical operations performed for this patient group [23] (Fig 24.1). Pylorus-preserving procedures have been widely adopted due to the associated preservation of gastrointestinal function and comparable oncological radicality when compared with a classical approach in previous randomised trials [30, 31], providing the remaining duodenal margin is viable and tumour-free. Despite early reports suggesting that extended lymphadenectomy may improve survival outcomes [32], subsequent randomised controlled trials have failed to demonstrate any survival advantage associated with extended lymphadenectomy and have indicated the potential for additional morbidity when compared with standard surgery [33, 34]. Venous resection may be appropriate for a sub-group of tumours exhibiting involvement of the hepatic, portal or superior mesenteric vein, providing adequate macroscopic tumour clearance can be achieved [35, 37].

The most clinically important early surgical complications associated with partial pancreatoduodenectomy include anastomotic leak with intra-abdominal collections, pancreatic fistula, primary and secondary haemorrhage, delayed gastric emptying and wound infection [38]. Most operative mortali-

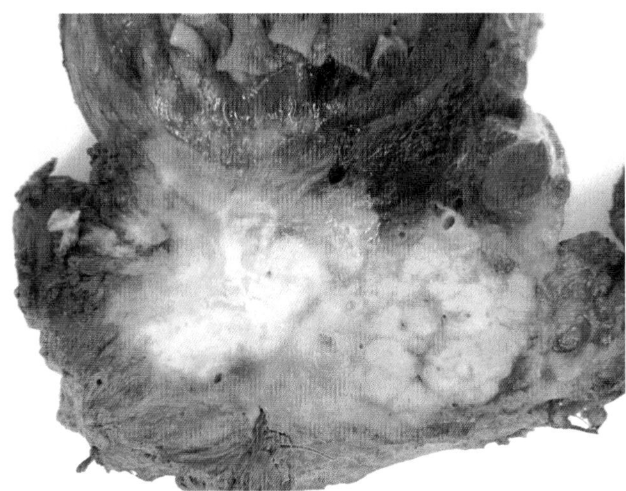

Fig. 24.1 Macroscopic appearance of pancreatoduodenectomy specimen following axial slicing demonstrating pancreatic ductal adenocarcinoma

ties, however, are generally the result of systemic rather than surgical complications [39], and this spectrum of potential morbidity is invariably apparent prior to discharge from hospital. Potential intermediate and late complications of partial pancreatoduodenectomy include nutritional impairment, exocrine and endocrine insufficiency, anastomotic stricture, gastritis and ulceration. In the 10–20 % of patients who require a total or distal pancreatectomy for pancreatic adenocarcinoma, post-splenectomy complications represent an additional consideration during the follow-up if splenectomy is undertaken alongside the pancreatic resection.

Patients undergoing total pancreatectomy inevitably develop exocrine insufficiency and require oral pancreatic enzyme supplementation [40]. Around 50 % of patients undergoing partial pancreatoduodenectomy for cancer also experience significant symptoms due to lipid malabsorption following surgery [41, 42]. Malabsorption of fats and fat-soluble vitamins commonly results in steatorrhoea and abdominal pain; this may significantly contribute to nutritional impairment. Significant pancreatic exocrine insufficiency according to the coefficient of fat absorption or faecal elastase is typically reported in 80–90 % of patients following partial pancreatoduodenectomy for malignancy. This is believed to be related to the degree of co-existing chronic pancreatitis which develops secondary to malignant obstruction of the proximal pancreatic duct [43, 44]. Given the high incidence of exocrine insufficiency in pancreatic cancer patients following resection, clinicians should have a low threshold for commencing early pancreatic enzyme supplementation to facilitate restoration of the patient's postoperative nutritional status and to ameliorate the unpleasant symptoms associated with malabsorption.

The association between diabetes and pancreatic cancer may reflect a causal or consequential one. Previous meta-analyses have suggested that both type I and type II diabetes are associated with an approximately twofold increased risk of developing pancreatic cancer [45–47]. Recently diagnosed diabetics exhibit the greatest risk [46, 48]. These observations may mean that diabetes is an aetiological factor or that it simply represents an early symptom of pancreatic cancer. Although relatively few patients undergoing resection for pancreatic and periampullary malignancy have a formal diagnosis of diabetes prior to surgery, abnormal glucose metabolism is identified in up to 80 % of patients prior to resection [49]. The early postoperative period is often characterised by an improvement in endocrine function [50, 51] (especially in patients with recent-onset diabetes [51]) and this may reflect an underlying role for tumour-derived diabetogenic peptides, resulting in systemic insulin resistance [52]. Despite this phenomenon of early improvement in endocrine function following resection for pancreatic cancer, around 40 % of patients will either develop diabetes or remain diabetic postoperatively [41, 51]. These observations underline the importance of appropriate diabetic monitoring and endocrinology input, where required, for resected pancreatic cancer patients during the follow-up period.

The incidence of anastomotic ulceration following partial pancreatoduodenectomy has previously been reported in up to 10 % of cases [53–55]. Increasing use of proton-pump inhibitors in the postoperative setting, however, is likely to have reduced the incidence of ulceration and related complications over recent years. Pylorus-preserving pancreatoduodenectomy may be associated with a marginally increased risk of anastomotic ulceration when compared with classical Kausch-Whipple procedures, depending on the method of reconstruction [56]. Gastrojejunostomy commonly results in some degree of gastritis and jejunitis following pancreatoduodenectomy due to the nonanatomical arrangement of the pancreatic remnant in relation to the gastric outlet, the reduction in bicarbonate secretion and lower levels of inhibitory gastrointestinal hormones. Patients often benefit symptomatically from administration of a proton-pump inhibitor during the postoperative period. There is no definitive evidence, however, to support the prophylactic use of any anti-ulcer therapy in this setting. Increased acidity in the proximal intestinal lumen also predisposes to early degradation of pancreatic enzymes (especially lipases) [57]. Therefore, use of proton-pump inhibitors may also contribute to improving symptoms associated with exocrine insufficiency [58]. Alkaline gastritis associated with biliary reflux may be more difficult to manage medically and occasionally necessitates reoperation for revision of the jejunal loop.

The hepatojejunostomy represents the most common site for postoperative benign anastomotic stricture following partial pancreatoduodenectomy. Between 5–10 % of patients undergoing pancreatoduodenectomy for benign disease develop a stricture of the hepatojejunostomy within 5 years of surgery, requiring endoscopic, percutaneous or surgical reintervention [59]. Due to the unfavourable long-term survival associated with resected pancreatic cancer, benign anastomotic strictures arising during the follow-up period are relatively uncommon in this patient group. Gallstone formation in the bile duct remnant, intrapancreatic ductal stones and progressive chronic pancreatitis in the pancreatic remnant represent other unusual causes for late reintervention during the follow-up period [60]. Hepatojejunostomy may also be associated with either recurrent acute or chronic cholangitis due to reflux of intraluminal small bowel fluid into the distal bile duct remnant. This may necessitate extended courses of antibiotics and prokinetic therapy in a sub-group of patients.

The majority of patients who present with pancreatic cancer exhibit some degree of nutritional compromise in the preoperative setting even in the absence of locally advanced or disseminated disease. This may be attributable to the association between systemic inflammation and cancer-related anorexia [61] along with the fact that the majority of patients present with obstructive jaundice resulting in hepatic impairment. Over a third of pancreatic cancer patients exhibit hypoalbuminaemia prior to surgery which may represent a marker of unfavourable early survival [62]. A recent study has indicated that the addition of certain nutritional supplements during the preoperative period may yield significant improvements in early postoperative outcomes for patients undergoing major pancreatic resections [63]. Occult exocrine insufficiency and insulin resistance represent additional contributory factors to weight loss during both the pre- and postoperative periods while the spectrum of potential abdominal symptoms associated with a diagnosis of pancreatic cancer may also contribute to a reduced dietary intake and consequent weight loss prior to surgery.

Significant micronutrient deficiencies in iron, selenium, vitamin A, vitamin D and vitamin E may arise during the postoperative period in patients undergoing partial pancreatoduodenectomy [64, 65] and body weight typically takes 4–6 months to return to preoperative levels following surgery [66]. Pancreatic resection can be associated with a spectrum of persistent abdominal symptoms including pain, bloating, early satiety, nausea and reduced appetite. All may have a significant impact on quality of life [41]. This underlines the importance of symptom control and dietary advice during the early postoperative period which may require use of appropriate analgesia, prokinetics, antiemetics and dietary supplements. Patients may also benefit from specialist dietetic input during the initial follow-up period.

The first study to suggest that external-beam radiation therapy might have a beneficial effect on survival when used alongside concomitant cytotoxic therapy in pancreatic cancer was published by Moertel et al. in 1969 [67]. A regimen of external-beam radiotherapy and 5-fluorouracil (5-FU) was shown to be associated with a superior median survival over external-beam radiotherapy alone (10.4 months vs. 6.3 months respectively) in 64 patients with advanced pancreatic adenocarcinoma. This study provided the first clinical evidence to demonstrate a radiosensitising effect of 5-FU and established the basis for chemoradiotherapy as a treatment modality for pancreatic cancer.

The findings of the Gastrointestinal Tumour Study Group #9173 trial [68], published in 1985, formed the basis on which adjuvant chemoradiotherapy came into widespread use for resected pancreatic cancer, particularly in the USA. This randomised controlled trial was conducted between 1974 and 1982 and recruited 43 patients undergoing radical resection for pancreatic adenocarcinoma with subsequent histological evidence of clear resection margins. Participants were randomised to either a treatment arm of split course external-beam radiotherapy (40 Gy) with 5-FU radiosensitisation and subsequent weekly systemic 5-FU administration for 2 years (or until relapse) or an observation arm. Median survival was demonstrated to be significantly improved in the treatment arm when compared with observation (21 months vs. 10.9 months respectively—$p = 0.03$).

The Gastrointestinal Tumour Study Group trial was widely criticised following its publication due to the poor patient accrual rate with less than half of the originally planned 100 patients recruited to the trial in total. The outcomes of a further 30 cases undergoing adjuvant therapy according to the same treatment regimen were subsequently published in an attempt to expand on the results from the original cohort [69]. The outcomes from this additional group of nonrandomised cases largely mirrored those of the original trial. However, the results clearly remained underpowered and no conclusions could be drawn from the Gastrointestinal Tumour Study Group findings as to whether the observed clinical benefit associated with chemoradiotherapy was entirely attributable to combination therapy or whether the chemotherapy or radiotherapy in isolation was actually responsible for the more favourable survival outcome. The UK Pancreatic Cancer Group Study (UKPACA-1) [70] was conducted in an attempt to reproduce the Gastrointestinal Tumour Study Group trial findings by utilising the same adjuvant chemoradiotherapy and follow-on chemotherapy regimen as the original Gastrointestinal Tumour Study Group protocol in 34 patients with pancreatic cancer and six patients with ampullary cancer. Broadly comparable two- and five-year survival rates were obtained by the UKPACA-1 study when compared with the Gastrointestinal Tumour Study Group results. However, the overall median survival of 13.2 months for the 34 pancreatic cancer patients was notably less than the 21 month median survival quoted for the Gastrointestinal Tumour Study Group treatment cohort. This study underlined the requirement for a large randomised controlled trial to clearly establish the roles of adjuvant chemotherapy and chemoradiotherapy in the management of pancreatic cancer. It paved the way for the European Study Group for Pancreatic Cancer (ESPAC-1) trial.

The European Organisation for Research and Treatment of Cancer (EORTC) Cooperative Group conducted a multicentre phase III trial [71] comparing adjuvant chemoradiotherapy and observation in 114 patients undergoing resection for ductal adenocarcinoma of the pancreatic head and 93 cases of periampullary malignancy (i.e. ampullary, duodenal and distal common bile duct adenocarcinoma). Patients with second order nodal involvement were excluded from participation. However, negative resection margins were not a prerequisite for inclusion. Patients were recruited from 29 centres across Europe between 1987 and 1995. The treatment regimen differed from that used in the Gastrointestinal Tumour Study Group trial in that no maintenance chemotherapy was given and 5-FU was delivered as a continuous rather than bolus infusion. When analysing only those patients with adenocarcinoma of the pancreatic head, a trend towards more favourable survival in the treatment group was observed (17.1 months vs. 12.6 months); however, the result was not significant ($p=0.099$). No survival advantage was demonstrated for chemoradiotherapy in the periampullary tumour group. These findings cast doubt on the effectiveness of adjuvant chemoradiotherapy and the EORTC authors concluded that the combination of adjuvant 5-FU and radiotherapy could not be considered as standard treatment following resection for pancreatic cancer. Despite the clearly superior sample sizes compared with the Gastrointestinal Tumour Study Group study, it was generally concluded that the EORTC trial was still underpowered and the question of whether adjuvant chemotherapy in isolation might prove a more beneficial treatment modality remained unanswered. Analysis of the long-term survival data from this trial returned the same conclusions as the original study, indicating no significant survival advantage of chemoradiotherapy over observation [72].

ESPAC-1 was a randomised controlled trial conducted between 1994 and 2000, recruiting 541 patients with resected pancreatic ductal adenocarcinoma from 61 centres in 11 European countries. Two hundred and eighty-five patients were formally randomised into a two-by-two factorial study design whereby participants received chemoradiotherapy, chemotherapy, chemoradiotherapy with follow-up chemotherapy or observation. Chemotherapy consisted of bolus 5-FU and folinic acid given over five consecutive days every 28 days for six cycles. The chemoradiotherapy regimen consisted of a 20 Gy dose given in 10 daily fractions over a two-week period along with a bolus of 5-FU. Analysis was conducted on an intention-to-treat basis and the preliminary results were published in 2001 [73]. The mature trial results were published in 2004 [28]. A total of 147 patients randomised to receive chemotherapy had a median survival of 20.1 months compared with 15.5 months in 142 patients who did not receive chemotherapy ($p=0.009$). Chemotherapy was associated with a five-year survival rate of 21 % compared with 8 % for patients not receiving chemotherapy.

Chemoradiotherapy was shown to be associated with a deleterious survival outcome with 145 patients assigned to receive chemoradiotherapy exhibiting a median survival of 15.9 months compared with 17.9 months in 144 patients not receiving chemoradiotherapy ($p=0.05$). In order to evaluate the findings of ESPAC-1 alongside the existing evidence base for use of adjuvant therapy in pancreatic cancer, a meta-analysis of all randomised adjuvant therapy trials was undertaken and published in 2005 [74]. This analysis included the survival data from Gastrointestinal Tumour Study Group [68, 69], EORTC [71], ESPAC-174 and two studies evaluating adjuvant chemotherapy regimens vs. observation (Bakkevold et al. [75] and Takada et al. [76]). There were 875 patients included in the overall analysis. The findings largely mirrored those of ESPAC-1 with chemoradiotherapy being shown to be associated with no survival advantage while patients receiving chemotherapy continued to exhibit a significantly improved survival.

This current dichotomy in adjuvant therapy practice for pancreatic cancer between Europe and the United States is reflected in the design of the two most recently conducted multicenter randomised trials in each continent. ESPAC-3 was opened in 2000 and aims to assess whether gemcitabine is superior to 5-FU/folinic acid in the adjuvant management of pancreatic cancer, originally comparing both groups against a control group undergoing surgery alone [77]. The study design was amended in 2003 to remove the observation arm following the availability of the mature ESPAC-1 follow-up results. The trial was closed in 2007 having recruited over 1000 participants and the results are due to be published in 2009. In contrast, the most recently conducted US phase III randomised controlled trial (RTOG 97-04) aimed to identify whether the addition of gemcitabine to 5-FU-based chemoradiotherapy is superior to 5-FU when given pre- and postchemoradiotherapy in 538 patients with resected pancreatic cancer. The results of this trial suggested a trend towards more favourable median survival associated with the use of gemcitabine (20.5 months) when compared with 5-FU (16.9 months) in the sub-group of patients with adenocarcinoma arising in the pancreatic head [78]. However, this observation failed to reach significance on either univariate or multivariate analysis.

Other than ESPAC-1, relatively few studies [75, 76, 79–81] have been conducted which have investigated the role of systemic adjuvant chemotherapy in isolation. Splinter et al. [79] conducted a study comparing three-year survival rates of 16 patients (seven with periampullary cancers) undergoing postoperative chemotherapy with 5-FU, doxorubicin and mitomycin C against a group of 36 historical controls. No significant difference in three-year survival was observed between the two groups. Bakkevold et al. [75] reported the results of the first multicentre randomised controlled trial in this setting which recruited 61 patients undergoing radical resection to an adjuvant treatment arm with 5-FU, doxorubicin and mitomycin C or a control arm with no additional postoperative therapy. Both groups included patients with both pancreatic ductal adenocarcinoma and ampullary tumours. Median survival duration in the treatment group (23 months) was significantly greater compared with the control group (11 months). However, no significant improvement in long-term survival was observed. The inclusion of ampullary cancers in the analyses of both of the above studies inevitably impairs the validity of the results. Significant toxicities were also reported in both series. This was largely attributed to doxorubicin.

Takada et al. [76] conducted a multicentre randomised controlled trial recruiting 508 patients following resections for pancreatic, ampullary, biliary and gallbladder carcinomas. Patients were randomised to an adjuvant treatment arm with 5-FU and mitomycin C or a control arm with no additional postoperative treatment. Results for those patients undergoing resections for pancreatic ductal adenocarcinomas ($n=158$) demonstrated a shorter five-year survival in the treatment group (11.5 %) compared with the control group (18 %), but the difference was not significant. The chemotherapy regimen was generally well tolerated with no serious adverse drug reactions reported. The initial 5-FU was administered as a slow intravenous infusion over two courses during weeks 1 and 3 postoperatively. The maintenance 5-FU was administered orally from the fifth postoperative week onwards and the resultant unpredictable absorption and poor efficacy of oral 5-FU may account for the disappointing results in the treatment arm of this study.

More recently Oettle et al. [29] published the results of the CONKO-01 study, a multicentre randomised controlled trial evaluating adjuvant gemcitabine versus no adjuvant therapy in 368 patients undergoing radical resection for pancreatic ductal adenocarcinoma. A significantly improved disease-free interval in the adjuvant treatment arm (13.4 months) over the observation arm (6.9 months) was demonstrated. However, the difference in median overall survival rates between the two groups did not reach significance (22.1 vs. 20.2 months respectively: $p=0.06$). Despite this finding, the five-year survival rates associated with the treatment and control groups in this study (22.5 % and 11.5 % respectively) are consistent with those reported in ESPAC-1 (21 % and 8 % respectively). The gemcitabine regimen used in the CONKO-01 study was associated with a favourable toxicity profile.

The current evidence indicates that adjuvant chemotherapy represents the gold standard of management for patients undergoing resection for pancreatic cancer. The pending results of ESPAC-3 will clarify whether use of gemcitabine should replace 5-FU as the chemotherapeutic agent of choice in this setting. There remains no definitive evidence to support the routine use of adjuvant chemoradiotherapy for pancreatic cancer patients.

The identification of factors which predict survival in pancreatic cancer is important for a number of reasons. Factors which are demonstrated to directly influence disease progression (e.g. molecular markers expressed in tumour material) may provide insight into tumour biology and reveal potential therapeutic targets. The identification of standardised prognostic factors allows meaningful comparisons of outcome between different studies which may exhibit significant differences in case mix. Furthermore, risk stratification as part of clinical trials is important in identifying whether certain sub-groups of patients are more or less likely to benefit from specific treatment modalities. The ability to provide an accurate and honest appraisal of prognosis is also important in patient counselling whether in a pre- or postoperative setting.

Although numerous single-centre studies have reported the prognostic impact of histological tumour characteristics in the setting of resected pancreatic cancer, relatively few published studies incorporate sizeable patient numbers to generate suitably powered analyses. Two such studies, using data from the Johns Hopkins School of Medicine [82] and the ESPAC-1 trial [83] have analysed the prognostic value of tumour histology in large cohorts of resected pancreatic cancer patients ($n=905$ and $n=418$, respectively). Both have demonstrated that tumour size, differentiation and nodal involvement represent independent prognostic factors for overall survival following surgery. Both studies failed to demonstrate a significant independent association between resection margin status and survival on multivariate analysis. This finding has also been mirrored in a recent meta-analysis using data from four randomised trials [84]. Although other tumour characteristics, such as perineural invasion, vascular invasion and tumour size, are often also reported as potential prognostic factors, these usually fail to exhibit any significant prognostic value in larger patient cohorts [82]. The ratio of involved lymph nodes to sampled lymph nodes in resected pancreatic cancer specimens provides superior prognostic information to overall nodal status [82, 85], as in other gastrointestinal malignancies [86, 87]. Thus, tumour size, differentiation and lymph node ratio represent the most informative histopathological prognostic factors in resected pancreatic cancer.

Two recent studies have suggested that margin involvement of the resected pancreatic cancer specimen on microscopic histopathological examination (R1) is commonly under-reported [88, 89]. These demonstrated R1 rates of 85 % [88] and 76 % [89] respectively when using the Royal College of Pathologists guidelines [90], which stipulate that tumour involvement within 1 mm of a resection margin on microscopic assessment should be considered as incompletely excised (R1). This criterion for microscopic R1 classification has been demonstrated to have a significant impact on the proportion of cases classified as R1 [91]. These studies provide increasing evidence to suggest that R1 resection rates for pancreatoduodenectomy may be more indicative of histopathological practice than operative expertise.

p53 is a tumour suppressor gene located on chromosome 17 which codes for a protein with a central role in inducing growth arrest and apoptosis in cells which sustain DNA damage. In normal cells, p53 is bound to MDM2 which maintains p53 in its inactive form. DNA damage initiates cell cycle checkpoint proteins to phosphorylate p53 into its active form which also results in a significant increase in its half-life. The active form of p53 binds to DNA which in turn activates expression of p21 with consequent inhibition of cyclin-dependent kinases, resulting in cell cycle arrest leading to subsequent DNA repair or apoptosis. Point mutations of p53 result in a more stable form of the protein which is unable to bind to DNA and activate p21, allowing the cell to escape growth arrest. Around 50 to 75 % of pancreatic cancers exhibit p53 mutations, most commonly in exons 5 to 8 [92]. Nuclear accumulation of p53 detected by immunohistochemistry has been widely investigated as a potential prognostic factor in resected pancreatic cancer. However, only a relatively small number of studies report a significant relationship between overexpression of p53 and less favourable survival [93, 94]. p21 expression has not been demonstrated to have any significant prognostic value in pancreatic cancer [95, 96].

The smad4 (or DPC4) gene codes for a protein which is involved in the intracellular signalling pathway of transforming growth factor β (TGF-β). The smad4 protein forms heterodimers in the cytoplasm with smad proteins 1, 2 and 3. These translocate to the nucleus, activating gene transcription. Loss of smad4 expression, therefore, inhibits TGF-β signalling with consequent loss of its inhibitory effect on cell proliferation. Loss of smad4 expression is observed in approximately 50 % of resected pancreatic cancers [97]. Contradictory evidence exists with regard to whether loss of smad4 expression in resected pancreatic cancer has an adverse [97] or beneficial effect [98] on patient survival. However, the majority of published studies indicate that loss of smad4 expression results in unfavourable survival post-resection [99–101].

The ability of cancer cells to evade apoptotic pathways is believed to be an important mechanism in the pathogenesis of pancreatic cancer [102]. The bcl-2 family of apoptotic genes codes for a number of proteins (including bcl-2, bcl-x, bax and bak) which exert either a pro-apoptotic or anti-apoptotic effect. These proteins mediate release of mitochondrial cytochrome C into the cytoplasm. This binds to APAF-1 and activates the effector caspases 3 and 9. These trigger breakdown of the intracellular cytoskeleton and the subsequent sequence of events resulting in apoptotic cell death. In pancreatic cancer, bcl-2 expression is variably reported to be a predictor of more favourable survival following resection [103, 104] and this survival pattern is similarly reported for bax immunoreactivity [105]. In contrast, bcl-x expression has been demonstrated to be a predictor of adverse survival in pancreatic cancer [106].

Epidermal growth factor receptor (EGFR) is the cell surface receptor for a family of extracellular ligands which include EGF and TGF-α and is coded for by the c-erbB1 proto-oncogene. Activation of EGFR stimulates intracellular tyrosine kinase phosphorylation with downstream activation of a number of signalling cascades including the MAPK (mitogen-activated protein kinase) and Akt (protein kinase) pathways which promote cell proliferation [107]. Overexpression of EGFR is reported in between 25 to 70 % of pancreatic cancers and the prognostic value of immunohistochemical EGRF status is also variably reported [108, 109]. Studies investigating the prognostic relevance of EGF ligand expression in resected pancreatic cancer have demonstrated similar results [110, 111].

Vascular endothelial growth factor (VEGF) represents a family of four signalling proteins (VEGF-A, B, C and D) which stimulate angiogenesis, promote chemotaxis of inflammatory cells and increase vascular permeability [112]. These ligands have three transmembrane receptors (VEGF-I, -II and -III) which promote intracellular tyrosine kinase cascades when activated. VEGF is probably the most consistently reproducible immunohistochemical marker of prognostic relevance in resected pancreatic cancer and numerous studies have suggested a significant association between VEGF expression and poorer survival following resection [113–116].

Despite the extensive investigation of various biologically relevant immunohistochemical prognostic markers in resected pancreatic cancer, none of these markers have translated into widespread clinical use. The reasons for this are manifold but include the general prevalence of small retrospective studies in this setting, the often contradictory results among individual reports, the sub-optimal study design and statistical methodology commonly employed and the labour-intensive nature of immunohistochemistry and related scoring. It is likely that focused immunohistochemical analysis of resected tumour material for specific markers predictive of response to individual chemotherapeutic agents will become increasingly important in the future in order to allow tailored selection of adjuvant therapy regimens for individual patients [117].

Carbohydrate antigen 19-9 (CA19-9) is a sialylated Lewis blood group antigen expressed in normal pancreatic ductal cells. It is also secreted in a mucin-bound form by the biliary and gallbladder mucosa and excreted in bile. A serum cut-off level of >37 kU/L is generally used as the optimal point at which pancreato-biliary malignancy can be differentiated from benign disease in symptomatic patients [118]. Normalisation of CA19-9 levels following resection for pancreatic cancer has been shown to be associated with more favourable survival outcomes and serial CA19-9 estimations recorded during the postoperative period exhibit a strong correlation with tumour recurrence [119–121]. Preoperative CA19-9 levels in isolation have also been demonstrated to represent a significant adverse prognostic marker in resected pancreatic cancer patients [122–124] with preoperative levels >150 kU/L being associated with a median survival of 10 months compared with 22 months for patients with preoperative levels ≤150 kU/L [85]. Serum CA19-9 represents the only diagnostic and prognostic biomarker in widespread clinical use in the management of pancreatic cancer but, despite its clinical utility, levels can be spuriously elevated in the presence of obstructive jaundice [125]. Previous studies have suggested that biliary obstruction does not appear to have a significant impact on either the overall diagnostic [126] or prognostic [85] value of preoperative CA19-9 levels in pancreatic cancer. However, caution should be exercised when interpreting levels in the presence of significant obstructive jaundice.

The immune status of patients is increasingly recognised as a key determinant of cancer treatment outcomes. Pancreatic cancer exhibits a number of mechanisms via which the tumour can escape immune surveillance. Inhibition of lymphocyte function secondary to release of the inhibitory cytokines interleukin-10 and TGF-β2 is believed to represent one such mechanism [127]. Pancreatic cancer has been shown to be associated with a more significant lymphocytopaenia when compared with other gastrointestinal malignancies [128] and a low preoperative lymphocyte count has been shown to be an adverse prognostic marker in resected pancreatic cancer [129–131]. Elevated preoperative platelet counts [131–133] and C-reactive protein levels [62, 134] have also been demonstrated to exhibit an adverse association with postoperative survival following resection.

Few patients undergoing resection for pancreatic cancer die from non-cancer-related causes during follow-up. Only 12 of the 237 deaths (5 %) recorded from the ESPAC-1 cohort of patients died from unrelated disease during the follow-up period [28]. Both ESPAC-1 and the CONKO-01 trials reported similar mean disease-free intervals associated with adjuvant chemotherapy (15.3 months and 13.4 months respectively). The overall survival times recorded in each trial were 20.1 months and 24.2 months respectively. The difference in the survival period between onset of recurrence and death reported in each trial may potentially reflect superior efficacy of gemcitabine over 5-FU or differences in the use of salvage chemotherapy.

The overall recurrence rate for resected pancreatic cancer is difficult to reliably determine from published literature as reported rates are influenced by the overall follow-up duration for any one individual patient cohort and the proportion of patients receiving adjuvant therapy. However, data from both multicentre trials [28, 29] and individual specialist units [135, 136] indicate overall recurrence rates between 70 and 90 %. Furthermore, 5-year survival following resection for pancreatic ductal adenocarcinoma cannot be equated to cure. A number of long-term follow-up studies have identified disease recurrence in patients after 5 years of follow-up post-resection [136–139]. The Johns Hopkins group has previously reported that 45 % of resected pancreatic cancer patients surviving beyond 5 years die from recurrent disease during the subsequent 5–10-year follow-up period [137]. Results from the Mayo Clinic have demonstrated similar findings in a recent study of long-term follow-up of pancreatic cancer resections [136]. Of 62 patients surviving beyond 5 years, 16 % died from recurrent disease during the 5–10-year follow-up period. No recurrence-related deaths were recorded after 8 years of follow-up in this patient group.

When considering the patterns of tumour recurrence observed following pancreatic cancer resection, rates of locoregional recurrence are variably reported. Both ESPAC-1 and CONKO-01 reported that locoregional recurrence accounted for 34–41 % of confirmed tumour recurrences during follow-up. However, higher rates of locoregional recurrence are commonly reported in patient cohorts from individual surgical centres [140–142]. Post-mortem studies of resected pancreatic cancer patients indicate that around 75 % of cases exhibit local recurrence at the time of death which is not always evident from computed tomography imaging [143].

The liver and peritoneum represent the most common locations for metastatic disease. Distant metastases accounted for 34 % of all confirmed tumour recurrences in ESPAC-1 with a further 27 % exhibiting concurrent locoregional and distant disease. The CONKO-01 trial reported that metastatic disease accounted for 49–56 % of confirmed tumour recurrences. The RTOG-9704 trial reported that locoregional disease was seen in 30 % of recurrent cases with distant metastases accounting for the remaining 70 %. These data suggest that both adjuvant chemotherapy and chemoradiotherapy are associated with similar patterns of tumour recurrence with no evidence to support the assertion that chemoradiotherapy confers superior local control.

Very limited guidance is currently available to clinicians regarding appropriate surveillance in the postoperative period following resection of pancreatic adenocarcinoma. Recommendations published by the National Comprehensive Cancer Network (NCCN) have proposed a regimen of 3–6 monthly clinical assessments for the immediate 2-year postoperative period. There is no uniform consensus within the NCCN regarding routine CA19-9 levels and CT scans within the postoperative surveillance period. No recommendations have been made by NCCN or any other group regarding post-treatment imaging schedules [144]. The apparent lack of consensus regarding the indication for surveillance imaging following surgery and/or adjuvant therapy for pancreatic cancer results from the current scarcity of evidence to suggest that early identification of recurrent disease confers any patient benefit.

This viewpoint is also reflected in the clinical guidelines published by the European Society for Medical Oncology (ESMO). ESMO suggests that follow-up after radical resection of pancreatic adenocarcinoma should be restricted to history and physical examination in view of the limited effectiveness of treatments available for recurrent disease [145]. Despite the lack of evidence to support the use of any specific surveillance protocol in the postoperative setting for resected pancreatic cancer patients, previous studies have evaluated the effectiveness of helical computed tomography in the identification of recurrent disease with a reported sensitivity of 80–94 % [146–148]. Interpretation of follow-up computed tomography images may be complicated, however, by the presence of postoperative inflammatory changes, reactive regional lymphadenopathy and uncertainty with regard to characterising small hepatic metastases. It has been demonstrated that an elevation of serum CA19-9 levels precedes radiological evidence of tumour recurrence in around 40 % of resected pancreatic cancer patients during the postoperative period [147], indicating that equivocal computed tomography findings are best interpreted alongside a recent CA19-9 result.

Given the limitations of computed tomography in the identification of recurrent disease following pancreatic cancer resection, an increasing number of studies have evaluated the potential of positron emission tomography as an alternative or supplementary imaging modality in this setting [148–150], suggesting an improved sensitivity in the identification of liver metastases for positron emission tomography and positron emission tomography–computed tomography fusion scans when compared with conventional computed tomography in isolation. The effectiveness of positron emission tomography, however, may be significantly compromised by the presence of hyperglycaemia due to competitive inhibition of fluorine-18-fluorodeoxyglucose (FDG) uptake. Furthermore, the ability of positron emission tomography to reliably distinguish neoplastic lesions from inflammatory changes (especially in the presence of chronic pancreatitis in the pancreatic remnant) remains limited [135]. Currently, multidetector-row helical computed tomography remains the most widely utilised modality for the identification of disease recurrence following pancreatic resection.

There is very limited evidence to support a definitive role for surgery as part of the management for recurrent disease following previous resection for pancreatic adenocarcinoma. Initial studies examining the role of hepatectomy for resection of hepatic metastases of pancreatic origin were reported in the early 1980s [152, 153]. In one study of five patients undergoing resection for liver metastases of pancreatic origin, the median survival was only 7 months [154]. More recent reports have suggested that survival times of over 5 years may be achievable following hepatic resection for metastatic pancreatic adenocarcinoma [155]. Survival within this group at 1, 3 and 5 years following hepatectomy were 66.7 %, 33.3 % and 16.7 % respectively. Published series thus far have recorded a variable operative mortality rate associated with hepatectomy of up to 10 % [156, 157]. The procedure of choice is determined by the extent of hepatic involvement with the Couinaud classification defining a major resection as greater than three liver segments [158].

Secondary resection for local recurrence in the remnant pancreas has been reported in isolated cases with variable survival duration of up to 24 months [159–162]. One recent case was reported to have survived 6 years from initial resection and 3 years following a second procedure for local recurrence and excision of a hepatic metastasis [161]. One of the larger series to date analysed outcomes in 30 patients undergoing repeated resection for local recurrence and reported an overall median survival of 29 months [162]. Patients who had survived longer than 9 months from initial resection to recurrence exhibited the greatest survival benefit with median survival duration of 17 months, compared with only 7.4 months in those experiencing disease recurrence within the initial 9-month period following primary resection. Current evidence is limited to individual case reports and small patient series and, at present, secondary resection for local recurrence of pancreatic adenocarcinoma is a potential management option for only a small sub-group of patients.

Systemic gemcitabine is firmly established as the first-line chemotherapeutic agent of choice for locally advanced and metastatic pancreatic cancer, exhibiting a modest but significant improvement in survival over 5-FU [163]. Results from both phase III trials and previous meta-analyses indicate that gemcitabine use alongside capecitabine is superior to gemcitabine in isolation as first-line therapy for advanced disease [164, 165]. There are no current recommendations, however, and a lack of clinical evidence regarding chemotherapy use in the specific setting of recurrent disease following previous radical surgery for pancreatic cancer. In patients who previously received adjuvant chemotherapy, an alternative agent or combination regimen is commonly used in the management of subsequent recurrent disease. Previous studies have investigated the potential utility of various novel agents as second-line drugs for advanced pancreatic cancer refractory to gemcitabine, with mixed results [166–169]. Chemoradiotherapy and follow-on chemotherapy have not been demonstrated to exhibit any significant survival benefit over chemotherapy alone for locally advanced pancreatic cancer [170]. Patient selection for second-line chemotherapy

Table 24.1 Surveillance for patients treated with curative intent for carcinoma of the pancreas at University of Liverpool, UK

Year	1	2	3	4	5	>5
Office visit[a]	5	3	3	3	3	3
CT scan of abdomen and chest	2	1	1	1	1	1

[a]The office visit includes history and physical examination, measurement of serum CA 19-9 level, calcium level, urea level, electrolyte levels, and a random glucose level, as well as liver function tests (serum bilirubin, alkaline phosphatase, alanine aminotransferase, gamma-glutamyl transferase, albumin, total protein levels), and a complete blood count

A fasting serum glucose level should be obtained if there is clinical suspicion of progression to diabetes

CT computed tomography (contrast-enhanced, multidetector row)

The number in each cell indicates the number of times in a particular postoperative year a particular modality is recommended

should be guided by the patient's functional performance status. Various biochemical parameters, including elevated serum CA19-9, hypoalbuminaemia and elevated c-reactive protein levels, remain adverse prognostic factors in the setting of advanced pancreatic cancer [171–173].

Pancreatic adenocarcinoma confers a dismal prognosis and it is, therefore, unsurprising that pancreatic cancer is associated with the highest average scores for depression and anxiety in studies investigating the psychological impact of different malignancies [174]. Other studies recording physical and psychological quality of life scores following pancreatoduodenectomy for benign and malignant disease indicate that pancreatic cancer patients exhibit the lowest postoperative physical and psychological quality of life scores when compared with other periampullary malignancies and patients undergoing similar surgery for benign disease [41].

In view of the complexity of medical and psychological issues often associated with a diagnosis of pancreatic cancer, appropriate patient management demands a multi-disciplinary approach with close liaison across a number of specialties including surgeons, gastroenterologists, oncologists, palliative and primary care physicians, dieticians and specialist nurses. Specialist nurses are commonly the patient's primary point of contact for medical and psychological support in the community, ensuring adequate symptom control and liaising among the various specialists to facilitate provision of a co-ordinated and patient-centred cancer service. Specialist nurses can also provide financial advice and social support by informing patients and their families about relevant statutory benefit entitlements associated with a cancer diagnosis.

Given that the overall median survival duration following resection for pancreatic cancer is typically about 12–18 months, the early follow-up period is clearly of greatest importance in terms of identifying potential morbidity and instituting appropriate management to control symptoms and maximise quality of life for patients. The initial postoperative out-patient visit is usually arranged within the first month following discharge from hospital, depending on individual patient circumstances. The most salient clinical issues addressed during this initial visit include wound assessment, management of any drains remaining in situ following discharge, estimation of baseline postoperative serum CA19-9 levels, the nutritional status of the patient and referral to a medical oncologist for adjuvant therapy. Referral to a medical oncologist is usually arranged between 4 and 6 weeks following surgery, at which point an objective assessment of the patient's functional recovery and suitability for cytotoxic therapy can be made. Our department routinely continues to arrange surgical follow-up for the duration that patients receive adjuvant treatment with close liaison with the medical oncologist in order to avoid duplication of investigations. Specialist nurse input is provided as part of all follow-up visits in order to ensure adequate symptom control, provide additional psychological support and arrange appropriate nursing support in the community when required.

Our unit finds this surveillance regimen acceptable both to members of the multi-disciplinary team involved in delivering care and to our postoperative patients. In our experience, 3–6 monthly follow-up intervals provide continuity of care and an opportunity to discuss any change in clinical condition with the clinician and receive advice and support from members of the multi-disciplinary team.

Table 24.1 outlines the overall follow-up matrix for resected pancreatic cancer patients laid out on a yearly basis. This plan comprises a general 3 monthly follow-up schedule during the first year with 4 monthly visits thereafter. Regular clinical, biochemical and haematological assessment of patients are routinely undertaken as part of each out-patient visit. Computed tomography imaging is routinely performed at 6 and 12 months during the first year and annually thereafter. This schedule is only intended to provide a general guideline and should be modified based on individual patient circumstances and postoperative progress. There is little to no evidence to recommend any one particular follow-up schedule in the setting of resected pancreatic cancer. However, a recent questionnaire-based study from the Netherlands suggested that most pancreatic surgeons review their patients on a 3–4 monthly basis during the first year [175].

Glossary

Ductal adenocarcinoma Carcinoma arising from epithelial cells within the pancreatic duct

Mucinous non-cyctic neoplasm Cysts lined by mucin-producing cells may be unilocular or multilocular

Signet ring cell carcinoma Cancer derived from epithelial cells with a characteristic histological appearance resembling a signet ring

Autosomal dominant Mode of inheritance whereby inheritance of one copy of an abnormal gene from a non-XY chromosome will result in expression of the phenotype

Penetrance (genetics) The proportion of those carrying the gene mutation who express the phenotype, e.g. penetrance is said to be incomplete if a certain proportion of those with the mutation do not exhibit any clinical features of the trait; penetrance is complete of all those individuals carrying the mutation express the trait

Pancreatoduodenectomy Surgical removal of the head of the pancreas and most of the duodenum, usually pylorus preserving

Kausch Whipple Eponymous name associated with pancreatoduodenectomy; Walther Kausch performed the first surgical removal of the duodenum and a portion of the pancreas in a two-stage procedure in 1912: Allen Whipple performed the procedure at a later date before adopting a one-stage technique

Anastomosis A surgical join between two hollow structures; this join may leak (anastomotic leak) and may cause narrowing (anastomotic stricture) in the event of a fibrous scar tissue formation

References

1. http://www-dep.iarc.fr/
2. Parkin DM, Bray F, Ferlay J, Pisani P. Global cancer statistics, 2002. CA Cancer J Clin. 2005;55:74–108.
3. Jemal A, Siegel R, Ward E, et al. Cancer statistics, 2008. CA Cancer J Clin. 2008;58:71–96.
4. Fitzsimmons D, Osmond C, George S, Johnson CD. Trends in stomach and pancreatic cancer incidence and mortality in England and Wales, 1951–2000. Br J Surg. 2007;94:1162–71.
5. Horner MJ, Ries LAG, Krapcho M, et al. (eds). SEER Cancer Statistics Review, 1975-2006, National Cancer Institute. Bethesda MD, http://seer.cancer.gov/csr/1975_2006/, based on November 2008 SEER data submission, posted to the SEER web site, 2009
6. Ansary-Moghaddam A, Huxley R, Barzi F, et al. The effect of modifiable risk factors on pancreatic cancer mortality in populations of the Asia-Pacific region. Cancer Epidemiol Biomarkers Prev. 2006;15:2435–40.
7. Qui D, Kurosawa M, Lin Y, et al. Overview of the epidemiology of pancreatic cancer focusing on the JACC study. J Epidemiology. 2005;15(Suppl II):S157–S167
8. Larsson SC, Permert J, Hakansson N, Näslund I, Bergkvist L, Wolk A. Overall obesity, abdominal adiposity, diabetes and cigarette smoking in relation to the risk of pancreatic cancer in two Swedish population-based cohorts. Br J Cancer. 2005;93:1310–5.
9. Luo J, Iwasaki M, Inuoe M, et al. Body mass index, physical activity and the risk of pancreatic cancer in relation to smoking status and history of diabetes: a large scale population-based cohort study in Japan—the JPHC study. Cancer Causes Control. 2007;18:603–12.
10. Hassan MM, Bondy ML, Wolff R, et al. Risk factors for pancreatic cancer: case-control study. Am J Gastroenterol. 2007;102:2696–707.
11. Iodice S, Gandini S, Maisonneuve P, Lowenfels A. Tobacco and the risk of pancreatic cancer: a review and meta-analysis. Langenbecks Arch Surg. 2008;393:535–45.
12. Michaud DS, Giovannucci E, Willett WC, Colditz GA, Fuchs CS. Dietary meat, dairy products, fat and cholesterol and pancreatic cancer risk in a prospective study. Am J Epidemiol. 2003;157:1115–25.
13. Stolzenberg-Solomon RZ, Cross AJ, Silverman DT, et al. Meat and meat mutagen intake and pancreatic cancer risk in the NIH-AARP cohort. Cancer Epidemiol Biomarkers Prev. 2007;16:2664–75.
14. Silverman DT, Schiffman M, Everhart J, et al. Diabetes mellitus, other medical conditions and family history of cancer as risk factors for pancreatic cancer. Br J Cancer. 1999;80:1830–7.
15. Pannala R, Basu A, Petersen GM, Chari ST. New onset diabetes: a potential clue to then early diagnosis of pancreatic cancer. Lancet Oncol. 2009;10:88–95.
16. Lowenfels AB, Maisonneuve P, Cavallini G, et al. Pancreatitis and the risk of pancreatic cancer. International Pancreatitis Study Group. N Engl J Med. 1993;328:1433–7.
17. Lowenfels AB, Maisonneuve P, DiMagno E, et al. Hereditary Pancreatitis and the risk of pancreatic cancer. J Natl Cancer Inst. 1997;89:442–6.
18. Howes N, Lerch M, Greenhalf W, et al. Clinical and genetic characteristics of hereditary pancreatitis. Clin Gastroenterol Hepatol. 2004;2:252–61.
19. Klein AP, Brune KA, Petersen GM, et al. Prospective risk of pancreatic cancer in familial pancreatic cancer kindreds. Cancer Res. 2004;64:2634–8.
20. Alexakis N, Halloran C, Raraty M, Gbaneh P, Neoptolemos JP. Current standards of surgery for pancreatic cancer. Br J Surg. 2004;91:1410–27.
21. Shapiro TM. Adenocarcinoma of the pancreas: a statistical analysis of biliary bypass vs. Whipple resection in good risk patients. Ann Surg. 1975;182:715–21.
22. Gudjonsson B. Cancer of the pancreas: 50 years of surgery. Cancer. 1987;60:2284–303.
23. Sohn TA, Yeo CJ, Cameron JL, et al. Resected adenocarcinoma of the pancreas - 616 patients: results, outcomes and prognostic indicators. J Gastrointest Surg. 2000;4:567–79.
24. Raut CP, Tseng JF, Sun CC, et al. Impact of resection margin status on pattern of failure after pancreaticoduodenectomy for pancreatic adenocarcinoma. Ann Surg. 2007;246:52–60.
25. van Heek NT, Kuhlmann KF, Schloten RJ, et al. Hospital volume and mortality after pancreatic resection: a systematic review and an evaluation of intervention in the Netherlands. Ann Surg. 2005;242:781–8.
26. Büchler MW, Wagner M, Schmied BM, Uhl W, Friess H, Z'graggen K. Changes in morbidity after pancreatic resection. Arch Surg. 2003;138:1310–4.
27. Birkmeyer JD, Warshaw AL, Finlayson SR, Grove MR, Tosteson AN. Relationship between hospital volume and late survival after pancreaticoduodenectomy. Surgery. 1999;126:178–83.
28. Neoptolemos JP, Stocken DD, Friess H, et al. European Study Group for Pancreatic Cancer. A randomized trial of chemoradiotherapy and chemotherapy after resection of pancreatic cancer. N Engl J Med. 2004;350:1200–10.
29. Oettle H, Post S, Neuhaus P, et al. Adjuvant chemotherapy with gemcitabine vs observation in patients undergoing curative-intent resection of pancreatic cancer: a randomized controlled trial. JAMA. 2007;297:267–77.
30. Seiler CA, Wagner M, Bachmann T, et al. Randomized clinical trial of pylorus-preserving duodenopancreatectomy versus classical Whipple resection-long term results. Br J Surg. 2005;92:547–56.
31. Tran KT, Smeenk HG, van Eijck CH, et al. Pylorus preserving pancreaticoduo-denectomy versus standard Whipple procedure: a prospective, randomized, multicenter analysis of 170 patients with pancreatic and periampullary tumors. Ann Surg. 2004;240:738–45.
32. Pedrazzoli S, DiCarlo V, Dionigi R, et al. Standard versus extended lymphadenectomy associated with pancreatoduodenectomy in the surgical treatment of adenocarcinoma of the head of the pancreas: a

multicenter, prospective, randomized study. Lymphadenectomy Study Group. Ann Surg. 1998;228:508–17.
33. Yeo CJ, Cameron JL, Lillemoe KD, et al. Pancreaticoduodenectomy with or without distal gastrectomy and extended retroperitoneal lymphadenectomy for periampullary adenocarcinoma, part 2: randomized controlled trial evaluating survival, morbidity, and mortality. Ann Surg. 2002;236:355–66.
34. Henne-Bruns D, Vogel I, Luttges J, Klöppel G, Kremer B. Surgery for ductal adenocarcinoma of the pancreatic head: staging, complications and survival after regional versus extended lymphadenectomy. World J Surg. 2000;24:595–601.
35. Bold RJ, Charnsangavej C, Cleary KR, et al. Major vascular resection as part of pancreaticoduodenectomy for cancer: radiologic, intraoperative, and pathologic analysis. J Gastrointest Surg. 1999;3:233–43.
36. van Geenan RC, ten Kate FJ, de Wit LT, van Gulik TM, Obertop H, Douma DJ. Segmental resection and wedge excision of the portal or superior mesenteric vein during pancreatoduodenectomy. Surgery. 2001;129:158–63.
37. Nakagohri T, Kinoshita T, Konishi M, Inoue K, Takahashi S. Survival benefits of portal vein resection for pancreatic cancer. Am J Surg. 2003;186:149–53.
38. Halloran CM, Ghaneh P, Bosonnet L, et al. Complications of pancreatic cancer resection. Dig Surg. 2002;19:138–46.
39. Büchler MW, Wagner M, Schmied BM, et al. Changes in morbidity after pancreatic resection. Arch Surg. 2003;138:1310–4.
40. Müller MW, Friess H, Kleeff J, et al. Is there still a role for total pancreatectomy? Ann Surg. 2007;246:966–74.
41. Huang JJ, Yeo CJ, Sohn TA, et al. Quality of life and outcomes after pancreaticoduodenectomy. Ann Surg. 2000;231:890–8.
42. Rault A, SaCunha A, Klopfenstein D, et al. Pancreaticojejunal anastomosis is preferable to pancreaticogastrostomy after pancreaticoduodenectomy for long-term outcomes of pancreatic exocrine function. J Am Coll Surg. 2005;201:239–44.
43. Tran TCK, van't Hof G, Kazemier G, et al. Pancreatic fibrosis correlates with exocrine insufficiency after pancreatoduodenectomy. Dig Surg. 2008;25:311–8.
44. Halloran CM, Taylor S, Chauhan S, et al. Pancreatic exocrine failure is common following partial pancreatic resection for tumour. (In press)
45. Everhart J, Wright D. Diabetes mellitus as a risk factor for pancreatic cancer. A meta-analysis. JAMA. 1995;273:1605–9.
46. Stevens RJ, Roddam AW, Beral V. Pancreatic cancer in type 1 and young onset diabetes: systematic review and meta-analysis. Br J Cancer. 2007;96:507–9.
47. Huxley R, Ansary-Moghaddam A, de Berrington GA, Barzi F, Woodward M. Type II diabetes and pancreatic cancer: a meta-analysis of 36 studies. Br J Cancer. 2005;92:2076–833.
48. Gullo L, Pezzilli R, Morselli-Labate AM, Italian Pancreatic Cancer Study Group. Diabetes and the risk of pancreatic cancer. N Engl J Med. 1994;331:81–4.
49. Permert J, Ihse I, Jorfeldt L, von Schenk H, Arnqvist HJ, Larsson J. Pancreatic cancer is associated with impaired glucose metabolism. Eur J Surg. 1993;159:101–7.
50. Litwin J, Dobrowolski S, Orłowska-Kunikowska E, Sledziński Z. Changes in glucose metabolism after Kausch-Whipple pancreatectomy in pancreatic cancer and chronic pancreatitis patients. Pancreas. 2008;36:26–30.
51. Pannala R, Leirness JB, Bamlet WR, Ananda B, Peterson GM, Chari ST. Prevalence and clinical profile of pancreatic cancer-associated diabetes mellitus. Gastroenterology. 2008;134:981–7.
52. Basso D, Greco E, Fogar P, et al. Pancreatic cancer-derived S-100A8 N-terminal peptide: a diabetes cause? Clin Chim Acta. 2006;372:120–8.
53. Yeo CJ, Sohn TA, Cameron JL, Hruban RH, Lillemoe KD, Pitt HA. Periampullary adenocarcinoma: analysis of 5-year survivors. Ann Surg. 1998;227:821–31.
54. Braasch JW, Deziel DJ, Rossi RL, Watkins Jr E, Winter PF. Pyloric and gastric preserving pancreatic resection. Experience with 87 patients. Ann Surg. 1986;204:411–8.
55. Grace PA, Pitt HA, Longmire WP. Pylorus preserving pancreatoduodenectomy: an overview. Br J Surg. 1990;77:968–74.
56. Sakaguchi T, Nakamura S, Suzuki S, et al. Marginal ulceration after pylorus-preserving pancreaticoduodenectomy. J Hepatobiliary Pancreat Surg. 2000;7:193–7.
57. Ghaneh P, Neoptolemos JP. Pancreatic exocrine insufficiency following pancreatic resection. Digestion. 1999;60:104–10.
58. Kahl S, Malfertheiner P. Exocrine and endocrine pancreatic insufficiency after pancreatic surgery. Best Pract Res Clin Gastroenterol. 2004;18:947–55.
59. Reid-Lombardo KM, la Ramos-De MA, Thomsen K, Harmsen WS, Farnell MB. Long-term anastomotic complications after pancreaticoduodenectomy for benign diseases. J Gastrointest Surg. 2007;11:1704–11.
60. Fang WL, Su CH, Shyr YM, et al. Functional and morphological changes in pancreatic remnant after pancreaticoduodenectomy. Pancreas. 2007;35:361–5.
61. Laviano A, Meguid MM, Rossi-Fanelli F. Cancer anorexia: clinical implications, pathogenesis, and therapeutic strategies. Lancet Oncol. 2003;4:686–94.
62. Smith RA, Dajani K, Dodd S, et al. Preoperative resolution of jaundice following biliary stenting predicts more favourable early survival in resected pancreatic ductal adenocarcinoma. Ann Surg Oncol. 2008;15:3138–46.
63. Giger U, Büchler M, Farhadi J, et al. Preoperative immunonutrition suppresses perioperative inflammatory response in patients with major abdominal surgery-a randomized controlled pilot study. Ann Surg Oncol. 2007;14:2798–806.
64. Armstrong T, Walters E, Varshney S, Johnson CD. Deficiencies of micronutrients, altered bowel function, and quality of life during late follow-up after pancreaticoduodenectomy for malignancy. Pancreatology. 2002;2:528–34.
65. ArmstrongT,StrommerL,Ruiz-JasbonF,etal.Pancreaticoduodenectomy for peri-ampullary neoplasia leads to specific micronutrient deficiencies. Pancreatology. 2007;7:37–44.
66. Niedergethmann M, Shang E, Farag SM, et al. Early and enduring nutritional and functional results of pylorus preservation vs. classic Whipple procedure for pancreatic cancer. Langenbecks Arch Surg. 2006;391:195–202.
67. Moertel CG, Childs DS, Reitmeier RJ, Colby Jr MY, Holbrook MA. Combined 5-fluorouracil and supervoltage radiation therapy of locally unresectable gastrointestinal cancer. Lancet. 1969;2:865–7.
68. Kalser MH, Ellenberg SS. Pancreatic cancer: adjuvant combined radiation and chemotherapy following curative resection. Arch Surg. 1985;120:899–903.
69. Gastrointestinal Tumour Study Group. Further evidence of effective adjuvant combined radiation and chemotherapy following curative resection of pancreatic cancer. Cancer. 1987;59:2006–10.
70. UK Pancreatic Cancer Group. Adjuvant radiotherapy and follow-on chemotherapy in patients with pancreatic cancer: results of the UK Pancreatic Cancer Group Study (UKPACA-1). GI Cancer. 1998;2:235–45.
71. Klinkenbijl JH, Jeekel J, Sahmoud T, et al. Adjuvant radiotherapy and 5-fluorouracil after curative resection of cancer of the pancreas and periampullary region: Phase III trial of the EORTC Gastrointestinal Tract Cancer Cooperative Group. Ann Surg. 1999;230:776–84.
72. Smeenk HG, van Eijck CH, Hop WC, et al. Long-term survival and metastatic pattern of pancreatic and periampullary cancer after adjuvant chemoradiation or observation: long-term results of EORTC trial 40891. Ann Surg. 2007;246:734–40.

73. Neoptolemos JP, Dunn JA, Stocken DD, et al. Adjuvant chemoradiotherapy and chemotherapy in resectable pancreatic cancer: a randomised controlled trial. Lancet. 2001;358:1576–85.
74. Stocken DD, Büchler MW, Dervenis C, et al. Meta-analysis of randomised adjuvant therapy trials for pancreatic cancer. Br J Cancer. 2005;92:1372–82.
75. Bakkevold KE, Arnesjo B, Dahl O, Kambestad B. Adjuvant combination chemotherapy (AMF) following radical resection of carcinoma of the pancreas and papilla of Vater - results of a controlled, prospective, randomised multicentre study. Eur J Cancer. 1993;29:698–703.
76. Takada A, Amano H, Yasuda H, et al. Is postoperative adjuvant chemotherapy useful for gallbladder carcinoma? A Phase III multicenter prospective randomized controlled trial in patients with resected pancreaticobiliary carcinoma. Cancer. 2002;95:1685–95.
77. ESPAC-3(v2) phase III adjuvant trial in pancreatic cancer comparing 5-FU and D-L-folinic acid vs gemcitabine. National cancer research network trial portfolio (http://www.ncrn.org.uk/)
78. Regine WF, Winter KA, Abrams RA, et al. Flurouracil vs Gemcitabine chemotherapy before and after fluorouracil-based chemoradiation following resection of pancreatic adenocarcinoma: a randomized controlled trial. JAMA. 2008;299:1019–26.
79. Splinter TA, Obertop H, Kok TC, et al. Adjuvant chemotherapy after resection of adenocarcinoma of the periampullary region and the head of the pancreas. A non-randomized pilot study. J Cancer Res Clin Oncol. 1989;115:200–2.
80. Kurosaki I, Hatakeyama K. Adjuvant systemic chemotherapy with gemcitabine for stage IV pancreatic cancer: a preliminary report of initial experience. Chemotherapy. 2005;51:305–10.
81. Kosuge T, Kiuchi T, Mukai K, et al. A multicentre randomized controlled trial to evaluate the effect of adjuvant cisplatin and 5-fluorouracil therapy after curative resection in cases of pancreatic cancer. Jpn J Clin Oncol. 2006;36:159–65.
82. Pawlik TM, Gleisner AL, Cameron JL, et al. Prognostic relevance of lymph node ratio following pancreaticoduodenectomy for pancreatic cancer. Surgery. 2007;141:610–8.
83. Bassi C, Stocken DD, Olah A, et al. European Study Group for Pancreatic Cancer (ESPAC). Influence of surgical resection and post-operative complications on survival following adjuvant treatment for pancreatic cancer in the ESPAC-1 randomized controlled trial. Dig Surg. 2005;22:353–63.
84. Butturini G, Stocken DD, Wente MN, et al. Influence of resection margins and treatment on survival in patients with pancreatic cancer: meta-analysis of randomized controlled trials. Arch Surg. 2008;143:75–83.
85. Smith RA, Bosonnet L, Ghaneh P, et al. Preoperative CA19-9 levels and lymph node ratio are independent predictors of survival in patients with resected pancreatic ductal adenocarcinoma. Dig Surg. 2008;25:226–32.
86. Berger AC, Sigurdson ER, Le Voyer TE, et al. Colon cancer survival is associated with decreasing ratio of metastatic to examined lymph nodes. J Clin Oncol. 2005;23:8706–12.
87. Inoue K, Nakane Y, Iiyama H, et al. The superiority of ratio-based lymph node staging in gastric carcinoma. Ann Surg Oncol. 2002;9:27–34.
88. Verbeke CS, Leitch D, Menon KV, et al. Redefining the R1 resection in pancreatic cancer. Br J Surg. 2006;93:1232–7.
89. Esposito I, Kleeff J, Bergmann F, et al. Most pancreatic cancer resections are R1 resections. Ann Surg Oncol. 2008;15:1651–60.
90. Campbell F, Bennett M, Foulis AJ. Minimum dataset for histopathology reporting of pancreatic, ampulla of Vater and bile duct carcinoma. Royal college of pathologists. 2002; http://www.rcpath.org
91. Campbell F, Smith RA, Whelan P et al. Classification of R1 resections for pancreatic cancer: The prognostic relevance of tumour involvement within 1 mm of a resection margin. (In press)
92. De Braud F, Cascinu S, Gatta G. Cancer of pancreas. Critical Reviews In Oncology/Haematology. 2004;50:147–55.
93. Linder S, Parrado C, Falkmer UG, et al. Prognostic significance of Ki-67 antigen and p53 protein expression in pancreatic duct carcinoma: a study of the monoclonal antibodies MIB-1 and DO-7 in formalin-fixed paraffin-embedded tumour material. Br J Cancer. 1997;76:54–9.
94. DiGiuseppe JA, Hruban RH, Goodman SN, et al. Overexpression of p53 protein in adenocarcinoma of the pancreas. Am J Clin Pathol. 1994;101:684–8.
95. Song MM, Nio Y, Sato Y, et al. Clinicopathological significance of Ki-ras point mutation and p21 expression in beign and malignant tumors of the human pancreas. Int J Pancreatol. 1996;20:85–93.
96. Coppola D, Lu L, Fruehauf JP, et al. Analysis of p53, p21WAF1, and TGF-beta1 in human ductal adenocarcinoma of the pancreas: TGF-beta1 protein expression predicts longer survival. Am J Clin Pathol. 1998;110:16–23.
97. Tascilar M, Skinner HG, Rosty C, et al. The SMAD4 protein and prognosis of pancreatic ductal adenocarcinoma. Clin Cancer Res. 2001;7:4115–21.
98. Biankin AV, Morey AL, Lee CS, et al. DPC4/Smad4 expression and outcome in pancreatic ductal adenocarcinoma. J Clin Oncol. 2002;20:4531–42.
99. Hua Z, Zhang YC, Hu XM, et al. Loss of DPC4 expression and its correlation with clinicopathological parameters in pancreatic carcinoma. World J Gastroenterol. 2003;9:2764–7.
100. Toga T, Nio Y, Hashimoto K, et al. The dissociated expression of protein and messenger RNA of DPC4 in human invasive ductal carcinoma of the pancreas and their implication for patient outcome. Anticancer Res. 2004;24:1173–8.
101. Khorana AA, Hu YC, Ryan CK, et al. Vascular endothelial growth factor and DPC4 predict adjuvant therapy outcomes in resected pancreatic cancer. J Gastrointest Surg. 2005;9:903–11.
102. Hamacher R, Schmid RM, Saur D, et al. Apoptotic pathways in pancreatic ductal adenocarcinoma. Mol Cancer. 2008;7:64.
103. Dong M, Zhou JP, Zhang H, et al. Clinicopathological significance of Bcl-2 and Bax protein expression in human pancreatic cancer. World J Gastroenterol. 2005;11:2744–7.
104. Bold RJ, Hess KR, Pearson AS, et al. Prognostic factors in resectable pancreatic cancer: p53 and bcl-2. J Gastrointest Surg. 1999;3:263–77.
105. Friess H, Lu Z, Graber HU, et al. Bax, but not bcl-2, influences the prognosis of human pancreatic cancer. Gut. 1998;43:414–21.
106. Evans JD, Cornford PA, Dodson A, et al. Detailed tissue expression of bcl-2, bax, bak and bcl-x in the normal human pancreas and in chronic pancreatitis, ampullary and pancreatic ductal adenocarcinomas. Pancreatology. 2001;1:254–62.
107. Ciardello F, Tortora G. EGFR antagonists in cancer treatment. N Engl J Med. 2008;358:1160–74.
108. Bloomston M, Bhardwaj A, Ellison EC, et al. Epidermal growth factor receptor expression in pancreatic carcinoma using tissue microarray technique. Dig Surg. 2006;23:74–9.
109. Smeenk HG, Erdmann J, van Dekken H, et al. Long-term survival after radical resection for pancreatic head and ampullary cancer: a potential role for the EGF-R. Dig Surg. 2007;24:38–45.
110. Gansauge F, Gansauge S, Schmidt E, et al. Prognostic significance of molecular alterations in human pancreatic carcinoma - an immunohistological study. Langenbecks Arch Surg. 1998;383:152–5.
111. Dong M, Nio Y, Guo KJ, et al. Epidermal growth factor and its receptor as prognostic indicators in Chinese patients with pancreatic cancer. Anticancer Res. 1998;18:4613–9.
112. Dallas NA, Fan F, Gray MJ, et al. Functional significance of vascular endothelial growth factor receptors on gastrointestinal cancer cells. Cancer Metastasis Rev. 2007;26:433–41.
113. Seo Y, Baba H, Fukuda T, et al. High expression of vascular endothelial growth factor is associated with liver metastasis and a poor prognosis for patients with ductal pancreatic adenocarcinoma. Cancer. 2000;88:2239–45.

114. Ikeda N, Nakajima Y, Sho M, et al. The association of K-ras gene mutation and vascular endothelial growth factor gene expression in pancreatic carcinoma. Cancer. 2001;92:488–99.
115. Niedergethmann M, Hildenbrand R, Wostbrock B, et al. High expression of vascular endothelial growth factor predicts early recurrence and poor prognosis after curative resection for ductal adenocarcinoma of the pancreas. Pancreas. 2002;25:122–9.
116. Kuwahara K, Sasaki T, Kuwada Y, et al. Expressions of angiogenic factors in pancreatic ductal carcinoma: a correlative study with clinicopathologic parameters and patient survival. Pancreas. 2003;26:344–9.
117. Farrell JJ, Elsaleh H, Garcia M, et al. Human equilibrative nucleoside transporter 1 levels predict response to gemcitabine in patients with pancreatic cancer. Gastroenterology. 2009;136(1):187–95.
118. Goonetilleke KS, Siriwardena AK. Systematic review of carbohydrate antigen (CA 19-9) as a biochemical marker in the diagnosis of pancreatic cancer. Eur J Surg Oncol. 2007;33:266–70.
119. Sperti C, Pasquali C, Catalini S, et al. CA 19-9 as a prognostic index after resection for pancreatic cancer. J Surg Oncol. 1993;52:137–41.
120. Montgomery RC, Hoffman JP, Riley LB, et al. Prediction of recurrence and survival by post-resection CA 19-9 values in patients with adenocarcinoma of the pancreas. Ann Surg Oncol. 1997;4:551–6.
121. Safi F, Schlosser W, Falkenreck S, et al. Prognostic value of CA 19-9 serum course in pancreatic cancer. Hepatogastroenterology. 1998;45:253–9.
122. Lundin J, Roberts PJ, Kuusela P, et al. The prognostic value of preoperative serum levels of CA 19-9 and CEA in patients with pancreatic cancer. Br J Cancer. 1994;69:515–9.
123. Kau SY, Shyr YM, Su CH, et al. Diagnostic and prognostic values of CA 19-9 and CEA in periampullary cancers. J Am Coll Surg. 1999;188:415–20.
124. Ferrone CR, Finkelstein DM, Thayer SP, et al. Perioperative CA19-9 levels can predict stage and survival in patients with resectable pancreatic adenocarcinoma. J Clin Oncol. 2006;24:2897–902.
125. Duraker N, Hot S, Polat Y, et al. CEA, CA19-9 and CA125 in the differential diagnosis of benign and malignant pancreatic disease with or without jaundice. J Surg Oncol. 2007;95:142–7.
126. Kim HJ, Kim MH, Myung SJ, et al. A new strategy for the application of CA19-9 in the differentiation of pancreato-biliary cancer: analysis using a receiver operating characteristic curve. Am J Gastroenterol. 1999;94:1941–6.
127. Bellone G, Turletti A, Artusio E, et al. Tumor-associated transforming growth factor-beta and interleukin-10 contribute to a systemic Th2 immune phenotype in pancreatic carcinoma patients. Am J Pathol. 1999;155:537–47.
128. Romano F, Uggeri F, Crippa S, et al. Immunodeficiency in different histotypes of radically operable gastrointestinal cancers. J Exp Clin Cancer Res. 2004;23:195–200.
129. Yamaguchi K, Noshiro H, Shimizu S, et al. Long-term and short-term survivors after pancreatectomy for pancreatic cancer. Int Surg. 2000;85:71–6.
130. Fogar P, Sperti C, Basso D, et al. Decreased total lymphocyte counts in pancreatic cancer: an index of adverse outcome. Pancreas. 2006;32:22–8.
131. Smith RA, Bosonnet L, Raraty M, et al. Preoperative platelet-lymphocyte ratio is an independent significant prognostic marker in resected pancreatic ductal adenocarcinoma. Am J Surg. 2009;197(4):466–72.
132. Suzuki K, Aiura K, Kitagou M, et al. Platelets counts closely correlate with the disease-free survival interval of pancreatic cancer patients. Hepatogastroenterology. 2004;51:847–53.
133. Brown KM, Domin C, Aranha GV, et al. Increased preoperative platelet count is associated with decreased survival after resection for adenocarcinoma of the pancreas. Am J Surg. 2005;189:278–82.
134. Jamieson NB, Glen P, McMillan DC, et al. Systemic inflammatory response predicts clinical outcome in patients undergoing resection for ductal adenocarcinoma head of pancreas. Br J Cancer. 2005;92:21–3.
135. Nitecki SS, Sarr MG, Colby MG, et al. Long-term survival after resection for ductal adenocarcinoma of the pancreas: is it really improving? Ann Surg. 1995;221:59–66.
136. Schneldorfer T, Ware AL, Sarr MG, et al. Long-term survival after pancreatoduodenectomy for pancreatic adenocarcinoma: is cure possible? Ann Surg. 2008;247:456–62.
137. Riall TS, Cameron JL, Lillemoe KD, et al. Resected periampullary adenocarcinoma: 5-year survivors and their 6- to 10-year follow-up. Surgery. 2006;140:746–72.
138. Richter A, Niedergethmann M, Sturm JW, et al. Long-term results of partial pancreaticoduodenectomy for ductal adenocarcinoma of the pancreatic head: 25 year experience. World J Surg. 2004;27:324–9.
139. Cleary SP, Gryfe R, Guindi M, et al. Prognostic factors in resected pancreatic adenocarcinoma: amalysis of actual 5-year survivors. J Am Coll Surg. 2004;198:722–31.
140. Kayahara M, Nagakawa T, Ueno K, et al. An evaluation of radical resection for pancreatic cancer based on the mode of recurrence as determined by autopsy and diagnostic imaging. Cancer. 1993;72:2118–223.
141. Westerdahl J, Andren-Sandberg A, Ihse I. Recurrence of exocrine pancreatic cancer: local or hepatic? Hepatogastroenterology. 1993;40:384–7.
142. Sperti C, Pasquali C, Piccoli A, et al. Recurrence after resection for ductal adenocarcinoma of the pancreas. World J Surg. 1997;21:195–200.
143. Hishinuma S, Ogata Y, Tomikawa M, et al. Patterns of recurrence after curative resection of pancreatic cancer, based on autopsy findings. J Gastrointest Surg. 2006;10:511–8.
144. National Comprehensive Cancer Network (NCCN) Practice guidelines in oncology: pancreatic adenocarcinoma version 1 2009, 26/03/2009;http://www.nccn.org
145. Hermann R, Jelic S. Pancreatic cancer: ESMO clinical recommendations for diagnosis, treatment and follow-up. Ann Oncol. 2009;20(S4):37–40.
146. Mortele KJ, Lemmerling M, de Hamptinne B, et al. Postoperative findings following the Whipple procedure. Eur Radiol. 2000;10:301–5.
147. Bluemke DA, Abrams RA, Yeo CJ, et al. Reccurrent pancreatic adenocarcinoma: spiral computed tomography evaluation following the Whipple procedure. Radiographics. 1997;17:303–13.
148. Casneuf V, Delrue L, Kelles A, et al. Is combined 18 F-fluorodeoxyglucose-positron emission tomography/computed tomography superior to positron emission tomography or computed tomography alone for diagnosis, staging and restaging of pancreatic lesions? Acta Gastroenterol Belg. 2007;70(4):331–8.
149. Ruff J, Hänninen EL, Oettle H, et al. Detection of recurrent pancreatic cancer: comparison of FDG-PET with CT/MRI. Pancreatology. 2005;5:266–72.
150. Nakamoto Y, Higashi T, Sakahara H, et al. Contribution of positron emission tomography in the detection of liver metastases from pancreatic tumours. Clin Radiol. 1999;54:248–52.
151. Delbeke D, Wright PC. Pancreatic tumors: role of imaging in the diagnosis, staging and treatment. J Hepatobiliary Pancreat Surg. 2004;11:4–10.
152. Morrow CE, Grage TB, Sutherland DE, et al. Hepatic resection for secondary neoplasms. Surgery. 1982;92:610–4.
153. Thompson HH, Tompkins RK, Longmire WP. Major hepatic resection: a 25-year experience. Ann Surg. 1983;197:375–88.
154. Schildberg FW, Meyer G, Piltz S, Koebe HG. Surgical treatment of tumour metastases: general considerations and results. Surg Today. 1995;25:1–10.

155. Yamada H, Hirano S, Tanaka E, et al. Surgical treatment of liver metastases from pancreatic cancer. HPB. 2006;8:85–8.
156. Lindell G, Ohlsson B, Saarela A, et al. Liver resection of noncolorectal secondaries. J Surg Oncol. 1998;69:66–70.
157. Elias D, de Calvacanti AA, Eggenspieler P, et al. Resection of liver metastases from a noncolorectal primary: indications and results based on 147 monocentric patients. J Am Coll Surg. 1998;187:487–93.
158. Hemming AW, Sielaff TD, Gallinger S, et al. Hepatic resection of noncolorectal nonneuroendocrine metastases. Liver Transpl. 2000;6:97–101.
159. Dalla Valle R, Mancini C, Crafa P, et al. Pancreatic carcinoma recurrence in the remnant pancreas after a pancreaticoduodenectomy. JOP. 2006;7(5):473–7.
160. Takamatsu S, Ban D, Irie T, et al. Resection of a cancer developing in the remnant pancreas after a pancreaticoduodenectomy for pancreas head cancer. J Gastrointest Surg. 2005;9:263–9.
161. Tajima Y, Kuroki T, Ohno T, et al. Resectable carcinoma developing in the remnant pancreas 3 years after pylorus-preserving pancreaticoduodenectomy for invasive ductal carcinoma of the pancreas. Pancreas. 2008;36(3):325–6.
162. Kleeff J, Reiser C, Hinz U, et al. Surgery for recurrent pancreatic ductal adenocarcinoma. Ann Surg. 2007;245:566–72.
163. Burris HA, Moore MJ, Andersen J, et al. Improvements in survival and clinical benefit with gemcitabine as first-line therapy for patients with advanced pancreas cancer: a randomised trial. J Clin Oncol. 1997;15:2403–13.
164. Herrmann R, Bodoky D, Ruhstaller T, et al. Gemcitabine plus capecitabine compared with gemcitabine alone in advanced pancreatic cancer: a randomized, multicenter, phase III trial of the Swiss Group for Clinical Cancer Research and the Central European Cooperative Oncology Group. J Clin Oncol. 2007;25:2212–7.
165. Sultana A, Tudur-Smith C, Cunningham D, et al. Meta-analyses of chemotherapy for locally advanced and metastatic pancreatic cancer. J Clin Oncol. 2007;25:2607–15.
166. Kozuch P, Grossbard ML, Barzdins A, et al. Irinotecan combined with gemcitabine, 5-fluorouracil, leucovorin, and cisplatin (G-FLIP) is an effective and non crossresistant treatment for chemotherapy refractory metastatic pancreatic cancer. Oncologist. 2001;6:488–95.
167. Cantore M, Rabbi C, Fiorentini G, et al. Combined irinotecan and oxalipatin in patients with advanced pre-treated pancreatic cancer. Oncology. 2004;67:93–7.
168. Ulrich-Pur H, Raderer M, Kornek GV, et al. Irinotecan plus raltitrexed vs raltitrexed alone in patients with gemcitabine-pretreated advanced adenocarcinoma. Br J Cancer. 2003;88: 1180–4.
169. Reni M, Pasetto L, Aprile G, et al. Raltitrexed-eloxatin salvage chemotherapy in gemcitabine resistant metastatic pancreatic cancer. Br J Cancer. 2006;94:785–91.
170. Sultana A, Tudur-Smith C, Cunningham D, et al. Systematic review, including meta-analyses, on the management of locally advanced pancreatic cancer using radiation/ combined modality therapy. Br J Cancer. 2007;96:1183–90.
171. Stocken DD, Hassan AB, Altman DG, et al. Modelling prognostic factors in advanced pancreatic cancer. Br J Cancer. 2008;99:883–93.
172. Müller MW, Friess H, Könninger J, et al. Factors influencing survival after bypass procedures in patients with advanced pancreatic adenocarcinomas. Am J Surg. 2008;195:221–8.
173. Glen P, Jamieson NB, McMillan DC, et al. Evaluation of an inflammation-based prognostic score in patients with inoperable pancreatic cancer. Pancreatology. 2006;6:450–3.
174. Zabora J, Brintzenhofeszoc K, Curbow B, et al. The prevalence of psychological distress by cancer site. Psychooncology. 2001;10:19–28.
175. Verschuur EM, Steyerberg EW, Kuipers EJ, et al. Follow-up after surgical treatment for cancer of the gastrointestinal tract. Dig Liver Dis. 2006;38:479–84.

25 Pancreatic Adenocarcinoma Surveillance Counterpoint: Japan

Ken Shirabe and Yoshihiko Maehara

Keywords
Pancreatic carcinoma • Japan • Recurrent site • Postoperative adjuvant chemotherapy

The incidence of pancreatic cancer has increased steadily over the last 4 decades. It is now the fifth leading cause of cancer death in Japan. Pancreatic cancer was responsible for the death of more than 22,000 Japanese in 2004 [1]. However, therapeutic modalities for resectable cases vary among institutions throughout the country. More than 90% of the cancers are invasive ductal carcinomas, most of which are advanced. Series published since the year 2000 have exhibited variability in the probability of long-term survival for patients undergoing resection of pancreatic ductal adenocarcinoma. In these series, the probability of 5-year survival ranged from 12 to 32% [2–8].

In several countries, ductal adenocarcinoma of the pancreas is considered a systemic disease at the time of diagnosis. Surgical resection might be beneficial in prolonging survival; in very few patients will the disease be cured radically [9]. A randomized controlled study from our country demonstrated that surgery results in significantly better survival than radiochemotherapy [10]. Therefore, surgery for locally advanced pancreas cancer is the first choice among therapeutic modalities in Japan.

No survival benefit has been shown for extended pancreaticoduodenectomy (PD) as compared to standard PD. A prospective randomized trial [11] and large scale meta-analysis [12] failed to show a survival benefit for extended lymphadenectomy. These results suggest a limitation in radical resection for cure of pancreatic cancer.

K. Shirabe, M.D. (✉) • Y. Maehara, M.D.
Department of Surgery and Science, Graduate School of Medical Sciences, Kyushu University, Maidashi 3-1-1, Higashi-ku, Fukuoka 812-8582, Japan
e-mail: kshirabe@surg2.med.kyushu-u.ac.jp; maehara@surg2.med.kyushu-u.ac.jp

Because standard lymphadenectomy has been established as the preferred option, pylorus-preserving PD (PPPD) has become a standard operation, rather than conventional PD, because of its effect on nutritional status. Niedergethmann et al. [13] showed that there is no significant difference in the disease-free survival of PD and PPPD groups but the preoperative body weight was reached after 4 months in the PPPD group and after 6 months in the PD group. Furthermore, bioelectrical impedance analysis revealed significantly lower total body water and significantly higher total body fat in the PPPD group, compared to the PD group, 24 and 54 months after surgery. These results suggest that pylorus preservation has value in enduring and functional and nutritional status years after surgery for pancreatic cancer.

Postoperative adjuvant chemotherapy, but not radiation therapy, has proven to be effective for improving long-term survival, as Buttrini, et al. [14] demonstrated in a meta-analysis of randomized controlled trials.

The goals of surveillance after treatment are improved quality of life and prolongation of life. Yermilov et al. [15] demonstrated that, of 2,023 patients with pancreas cancer after PD, 1,194 patients (59%) were readmitted to hospital within 1 year. The causes of readmission included progression of the cancer (24%), surgery-related complications (14%), and infection (13%).

The most common reason for readmission within 1 year was recurrent cancer. Therefore, postoperative surveillance should be planned. The most common type of recurrence after radical resection is local recurrence. Other areas of recurrence include the liver, peritoneum, and lymph nodes. Hishimura et al. [16] showed that local recurrence frequently occurs, but is rarely a direct cause of death, and most patients die of metastatic disease. They also concluded that treatment focusing on local recurrence cannot improve the survival of a

F.E. Johnson et al. (eds.), *Patient Surveillance After Cancer Treatment*, Current Clinical Oncology, DOI 10.1007/978-1-60327-969-7_25, © Springer Science+Business Media New York 2013

patient with pancreatic cancer, thus, treatment regimens that are effective against metastasis are needed.

The follow-up of patients with pancreatic ductal adenocarcinoma will be addressed in a review of the Japanese experience. An intensive follow-up strategy is supported by reports of curative surgical treatment of recurrent cases and the potentially beneficial effects of chemotherapy on survival and quality of life.

Adjuvant Therapy

Recently, Oettle et al. [17] showed in a randomized trial that postoperative gemcitabine significantly delays the development of recurrent disease and improves overall survival, compared to observation alone.

Data from the United States often asserts that chemoradiation therapy is an acceptable option for adjuvant therapy [9]. However, a large meta-analysis from Europe failed to prove the beneficial effects of chemoradiation [14].

Intravenous gemcitabine can improve symptoms compared to 5-FU [18]. Now, clinical trials of S-1 for advanced pancreatic cancer have been reported and combination chemotherapy, using gemcitabine and S-1 is employed in Japan. A report about this regimen may be expected [19].

The protocol for adjuvant chemotherapy of patients undergoing curative-intent resection of pancreatic cancer in our institute is based on Oettle et al. [17]. The patients receive adjuvant chemotherapy with six cycles of gemcitabine every 4 weeks. Each chemotherapy cycle consists of three weekly infusions of 1,000 mg/m^2 intravenous gemcitabine infusion during a 30-min period

There are many potential methods of surveillance. History and physical examination are not sensitive for detecting tumor recurrence. Nevertheless, the occurrence of new symptoms can prompt the initiation of further diagnostic steps. Major symptoms and signs of pancreatic cancer recurrence after resection are abdominal pain, weight loss, jaundice, and ascites. Therefore Japanese physicians emphasize careful histories and physical examination.

Radiological examinations are extremely helpful in the surveillance of patients after pancreatic cancer therapy. Among the various diagnostic imaging studies, computed tomography is the most useful. Distant metastasis to the liver or lung is detectable with computed tomography, even if the metastasis is less than 1 cm. Thickening of the intestine, caking of the omentum, and ascites suggests peritoneal recurrence. Ultrasonography of the liver is occasionally helpful in diagnosing metastases, so it is commonly performed alternately with computed tomography. FDG-PET is also useful for detecting the early recurrence of pancreatic cancer [20].

Table 25.1 Surveillance for patients treated with curative intent for pancreatic cancer

	Postoperative year				
Modality	1	2	3	4	5
Office visit	12	6	4	2	2
Complete blood count	12	6	4	2	2
Multichannel blood tests[a]	12	4	4	2	2
Serum CEA level	12	4	2	2	2
Serum CA 19-9 level	12	4	2	2	2
Computed tomography (chest/abdomen/pelvis)	4	2	2	1	1

CEA, Carcinoembryonic antigen. [a]Includes total protein, glutamate-oxaloacetate transaminase, glutamate-pyruvic transaminase, bilirubin, alkaline phosphatase, cholesterol, blood urea nitrogen, and creatinine. The number in each cell indicates the number of times a particular modality is recommended during a particular posttreatment year

In Japan, two commonly used serological tumor markers of pancreatic cancer are CEA and CA 19-9. A combination of CA 19-9, DUPAN-2, and SPAN-1 can be useful for detecting recurrence in more than 80% of patients with pancreatic cancer.

Because it is possible to prolong life and/or improve the quality of life after detecting recurrence, Japanese physicians advocate vigorous surveillance, using the patient's history, physical examination, serum tumor marker levels, and imaging studies such as ultrasound, computed tomography, and magnetic resonance.

We recommend monthly office visits during the first year and every 3 months during the second year. As mentioned previously, readmission within 1 year is quite common. Physicians should continue to follow patients vigorously, aiming for the early detection of recurrence.

The current guidelines for the follow-up of patients with pancreatic cancer at the Department of Surgery and Science, Kyushu University, are presented in Table 25.1.

References

1. Matsuno S, Egawa S, Fukuyama S, et al. Pancreatic cancer registry in Japan. 20 years of experience. Pancreas. 2004;28:219–30.
2. Helm JF, Centeno BA, Coppola D, et al. Outcomes following resection of pancreatic adenocarcinoma: 20-year experience at a single institution. Cancer Control. 2008;15:288–94.
3. Winter JM, Cameron JL, Campbell KA, et al. 1423 pancreaticoduodenectomies for pancreatic cancer: a single-institution experience. J Gastrointest Surg. 2006;10:1199–210.
4. Takai S, Satoi S, Toyokawa H, et al. Clinicopathologic evaluation after resection for ductal adenocarcinoma of the pancreas: a retrospective, single institution experience. Pancreas. 2003;26:243–9.
5. Moon HJ, An JY, Heo JS, et al. Predicting survival after surgical resection for pancreatic ductal carcinoma. Pancreas. 2006;32:37–43.
6. Richter A, Niedergethmann M, Strum JW, et al. Long-term results of partial pancreaticoduodenectomy for ductal adenocarcinoma of the pancreatic head: 25-year experience. World J Surg. 2003;32:271–5.
7. SchmidtCM,PowellES,YiannoutsosCT,etal.Pancreaticoduodenectomy: 20-year experience in 516 patients. Arch Surg. 2004;139:718–25.
8. Han SS, Jang JK, Kim SW, et al. Analysis of long-term survivors after surgical resection for pancreatic cancer. Pancreas. 2006;32:271–5.

9. Iott MJ, Corsini MM, Miller RC. Evidence-based guidelines for adjuvant therapy for resected adenocarcinoma of the pancreas. Clin J Oncol Nurs. 2008;12:599–605.
10. Doi R, Imamura M, Hosotani R, et al. Surgery versus radiochemotherapy for resectable locally invasive pancreatic cancer: final surveillance results of a randomized multi-institutional trial. Surg Today. 2008;38:1021–8.
11. Farnell MB, Pearson RK, Sarr MG, et al. A prospective randomized trial comparing standard pancreatoduodenectomy with pancreatoduodenectomy with extended lymphadenectomy in resectable pancreatic head adenocarcinoma. Surgery. 2005;138:618–28.
12. Iqbal N, Lovegrove RE, Tilney HS, et al. A comparison of pancreaticoduodenectomy with extended pancreaticoduodenectomy: a meta-analysis of 1909 patients. Eur J Surg Oncol. 2009;35: 79–86.
13. Niedergethmann M, Shang E, Farag Soliman M, et al. Early and enduring nutritional and functional results of pylorus preservation vs classic Whipple procedure for pancreatic cancer. Langenbecks Arch Surg. 2006;391(3):195–202.
14. Buttrini G, Stocken DD, Wente MN, et al. Influence of resection margins and treatment on survival in patients with pancreatic cancer: meta-analysis of randomized controlled trials. Arch Surg. 2008;143:75–83.
15. Yermilov I, Bentrem D, Sekeris E, et al. Readmissions following pancreaticoduodenectomy for pancreas cancer: a population-based appraisal. Ann Surg Oncol. 2009;16:554–61.
16. Hishinuma S, Ogata Y, Tomikawa M, et al. Patterns of recurrence after curative resection of pancreatic cancer, based on autopsy findings. J Gastrointest Surg. 2006;10:511–8.
17. Oettle H, Post S, Neuhaus P, et al. Adjuvant chemotherapy with gemcitabine vs observation in patients undergoing curative-intent resection of pancreatic cancer. A randomized controlled trial. JAMA. 2007;297:267–77.
18. Moore MJ. Pancreatic cancer: what the oncologist can offer palliation. Can J Gastroenterol. 2002;16:121–4.
19. Ueno H, Kosuge T. Adjuvant treatments for resectable pancreatic cancer. J Hepatobiliary Pancreat Surg. 2008;15:468–72.
20. Fletcher JW, Djulbegovic B, Soares HP, et al. Recommendations of the use of 18F-FDG PET in oncology. J Nucl Med. 2008;49: 480–509.

Pancreatic Adenocarcinoma Surveillance Counterpoint: Canada

26

Malcolm J. Moore and Anastasios Stathis

Keywords
Ductal adenocarcinoma • Relapse • Pancreatectomy • Chemoradiotherapy • NCCN

Ductal adenocarcinoma accounts for over 90% of pancreatic malignancies. Other less common pancreatic tumors include neuroendocrine cancers, acinar cell carcinoma, pancreatoblastoma, squamous cell carcinoma, and occasional benign conditions. Rarely, the pancreas can be the site of metastases from other solid tumor malignancies (e.g., colon, breast, renal cancer) [1]. Pancreatic adenocarcinoma has a mortality rate virtually identical to that of its incidence with conventional cancer treatments having little impact on long-term survival. In Canada, about 3,800 new cases and about 3,700 deaths from pancreatic cancer occur annually. It is the fourth leading cause of cancer-related death in both males and females (4.6% and 5.6% of cancer-related deaths, respectively) [2].

Advanced disease is incurable with medial survival duration of around 6 months. The 5-year relative survival rate is less than 5% [3, 4]. Only 15–20% of patients present with potentially resectable disease for which surgical resection is the standard of care [5–7]. This was associated with high mortality rates historically; this has now improved and current operative mortality rates are under 5% in high-volume centers [8, 9]. At present there are no guidelines for surveillance after resection and most patients are followed based on individual/center experience and policy.

M.J. Moore, M.D. (✉)
Division of Medical Oncology and Hematology, Princess Margaret Hospital, 610 University Avenue, 5-700, Toronto, ON, Canada M5G 2M9
e-mail: Malcom.moore@uhn.ca

A. Stathis, M.D.
Drug Development Program, Princess Margaret Hospital, 610 University Avenue, 5-700, Toronto, ON, Canada, M5G 2M9

Surgical resection is the only potentially curative therapy. It should be done by an expert team of surgeons in high-volume centers in order to increase resection rates and minimize postoperative morbidity and mortality rates [10]. Almost two-thirds of pancreatic adenocarcinoma arises in the head, neck, or uncinate process of the pancreas. For these tumors a pylorus-preserving pancreaticoduodenectomy is appropriate. In cases of proximal duodenal involvement or location of the tumor close to the pylorus, a classical proximal pancreaticoduodenectomy with antrectomy (Whipple's operation) is indicated. Pancreatic body and tail tumors require a left (distal) pancreatectomy. Involvement of the splenic vessels does not preclude resection. More radical and technically demanding procedures, including portal vein or superior mesenteric vein excision or total pancreatectomy are sometimes necessary in order to obtain resection with microscopically clear margins. Every procedure should include a locoregional lymph node resection, but the benefit of extensive lymphadenectomy has not been demonstrated [11, 12].

There is a high relapse rate after surgery, with a median disease-free interval of 8–13 months, medial survival duration of 11–20 months, and 5-year survival rate of less than 20% [11, 13, 14]. Prognostic factors (stage, nodal, and margin status) have been identified. In view of the high relapse rate, adjuvant therapy has been investigated. In 1985 the Gastrointestinal Tumor Study Group (GITSG) reported that survival of patients after pancreaticoduodenectomy could be prolonged by adjuvant chemotherapy and radiation [15]. However, this was a small study and results were not confirmed in a larger study of similar design conducted by The European Organization for Research and Treatment of Cancer (EORTC) [16]. The European Study Group of Pancreatic Cancer (ESPAC) used a two-by-two factorial design in which patients after surgery were randomized to treatment with chemoradiation

F.E. Johnson et al. (eds.), *Patient Surveillance After Cancer Treatment*, Current Clinical Oncology,
DOI 10.1007/978-1-60327-969-7_26, © Springer Science+Business Media New York 2013

Table 26.1 Patient surveillance after curative-intent treatment for pancreas cancer at Princess Margaret Hospital

	Years Posttreatment					
Modality	1	2	3	4	5	>5
Office visit	2–3	2–3	2–3	1–2	1–2	1–2
Abdominal CT	1	a	a	a	a	a
Routine blood tests[b] plus serum CA 19-9 level	2–3	2–3	2–3	1–2	1–2	1–2

[a]as clinically indicated only. [b]CBC, serum Na, K, Ca, creatinine, total bilirubin, aspartate transaminase, alanine transaminase, alkaline phosphatase, lactic dehydrogenase, glucose levels. The number in each cell indicates the number of times a particular modality is recommended during a particular posttreatment year

alone (20 Gy over a 5-week period plus 5-FU), to chemotherapy alone (5-FU and folinic acid) for 6 months, to both chemoradiotherapy and chemotherapy and to observation alone. The median overall survival rate was 21.1 months for the groups receiving chemotherapy compared with 15.5 months for the groups not receiving chemotherapy, with 5-year survivals of 22% vs. 8%, respectively ($p=-0.009$). Adjuvant chemoradiotherapy actually had a deleterious effect on survival [17]. This trial has been criticized for methodological and statistical flaws and, as such, while it raises questions about current practice, it does not necessarily eliminate 5FU-based chemoradiation as a treatment option [18, 19]. A second trial similarly demonstrated a survival benefit using adjuvant chemotherapy. In the CONKO-001 trial, 368 patients were randomly assigned to adjuvant chemotherapy with gemcitabine for 6 months or observation following resection. Disease-free survival duration (13.4 months vs. 6.9 months, $p<0.001$) and overall survival rate (I<0.005) were significantly increased in the gemcitabine arm with 5-year survival of 21% vs. 9% [20, 21].

For some cancers, surveillance after curative surgical resection may improve survival and quality of life by identifying and managing therapeutic complications, discovery of recurrence at a potentially curable stage or identification of new neoplasms at a preinvasive stage. In pancreatic cancer, recurrence occurs in more than 80% of those resected, most within 2 years following surgery. After recurrence, a second curative-intent procedure is practically never possible. The goal of surveillance after pancreatic surgery is to deal with the sequelae of therapy and to identify problems when treatment can improve symptoms and quality of life. Follow-up studies may include history and physical examination, hematological and biochemical profile, serum CA 19-9 measurements and radiologic evaluations (CT scans or abdominal ultrasound) [22]. There is no evidence that surveillance after surgery can affect survival and guidelines are limited. The frequency and mode of surveillance is based on an individual/center experience and patient requests. The 2008 European Society of Medical Oncology (ESMO) guidelines recommend only history and physical examination but do not specify the frequency [23]. The National Comprehensive Cancer Network (NCCN) recognized that early identification of relapse may facilitate entry into investigational studies and aid in symptom control. NCCN recommends a history and physical examination every 3–6 months for 2 years. The role of CA 19-9 determinations and follow-up CT scans every 3–6 months for 2 years was discussed but, in the absence of data indicating that early treatment of recurrence (using CA 19-9 or CT scans) leads to better patient outcomes, no consensus was reached [24]. No prospective trials of surveillance after surgery have been performed.

Between 1996 and 2006, 1,169 patients with pancreatic adenocarcinoma were seen at Princess Margaret Hospital. Of these, 667 presented at the time of initial diagnosis and 494 (74%) presented with locally advanced or metastatic disease (142 and 352, respectively). There were 174 with resectable disease. During the same period, 402 patients were referred with relapsed or metastatic disease for a second opinion. There has been a steady increase in the number of resectable cases (stages I–II) due to an initiative in Ontario to restrict specialized hepatopancreaticobiliary surgery to high-volume centers. Currently, 80% of surgical resections in Ontario are performed in one of three hospitals. There are 60–70 resections for pancreatic adenocarcinoma every year at the Princess Margaret Hospital in Toronto. Our mortality rate after surgery has been 2% or less on average in the last 10 years. All patients who undergo surgical resection are assessed for suitability for adjuvant therapy and our current standard is gemcitabine for 6 months as was used in the CONKO study. We do not routinely use adjuvant chemoradiation, although patients with a positive margin are considered for radiation at the end of chemotherapy. We monitor CA 19-9 levels monthly during adjuvant chemotherapy and initiate imaging if an elevation is noted. There is no written policy for monitoring after surgery but ongoing surveillance is practiced. Generally, this consists of a clinic assessment every 4–6 months for the first 3 years and every 6–12 months thereafter. We usually obtain routine blood tests and a CA 19-9 level at every visit. Radiologic investigations (CT scans) are performed after recovery from surgery and if symptoms or the CA 19-9 level indicate a need for further assessment (Table 26.1). This surveillance is part of an overall patient care plan to assist patients in dealing with the complications of their treatment and to detect problems at a time when therapy may have a greater chance of success. We feel this is necessary when dealing with a disease which is infrequently managed by family physicians or in smaller volume centers and whose consequences can diminish both the length and quality of life. A high clinical trial activity is present at our institution and many of the patients with relapsed pancreatic adenocarcinoma are treated in the context of one of these trials.

Data on the value of surveillance in patients with resected pancreatic adenocarcinoma is limited and there are no evidence-based guidelines. Given the high rate of relapse after surgery and limited impact of currently available treatments, one would not expect any surveillance policy to impact upon survival. The principal role of surveillance after surgery for pancreatic carcinoma remains patient support and maintenance of quality of life. Surveillance aimed to detect early recurrence after surgery may become important in the future if effective salvage treatments become available.

References

1. De Vita Jr VT, Lawrence T, Rosenberg SA. Cancer. Principles and practice of oncology. 8th ed. Vol. 1. Philadelphia, PA; 2008. p. 1118-1120.
2. Canadian Cancer Society/National Cancer Institute of Canada: Canadian cancer statistics 2007. Toronto, Canada. 2008; ISSN 0835-2976.
3. Kern S, Hruban R, Hollingsworth MA, Brand R, Adrian TE, Jaffae E, et al. A white paper: the product of a pancreas cancer think tank. Cancer Res. 2001;61:4923–32.
4. Jemal A, Siegel R, Ward E, Hao Y, Xu J, Murray T, et al. Cancer statistics 2008. CA Cancer J Clin. 2008;58:71–96.
5. Varadhachary GR, Tamm EP, Abbruzzese JL, et al. Borderline resectable pancreatic cancer: definitions, management and role of preoperative therapy. Ann Surg Oncol. 2006;13:1035–46.
6. Li D, Xie K, Wolff R, Abbruzzese JL. Pancreatic cancer. Lancet. 2004;363:1049–57.
7. Berger HG, Rau B, Gansauge F, et al. Treatment of pancreatic cancer: challenge of the facts. World J Surg. 2003;27:1075–84.
8. Crist DW, Sitzmann JV, Cameron JL. Improved hospital morbidity, mortality and survival after the Whipple procedure. Ann Surg. 1987;206:358–65.
9. Sohn TA, Yeo CJ, Cameron JL, et al. Resected adenocarcinoma of the pancreas-616 patients: results, outcomes, and prognostic indicators. J Gastrointest Surg. 2001;5:681.
10. Birkmeyer JD, Siewers AE, Finlayson EV, et al. Hospital volume and surgical mortality in the United States. N Engl J Med. 2002;346:1128–37.
11. Verslype C, Van Cutsem E, Dicato M, et al. The management of pancreatic cancer. Current expert and recommendations derived from the 8th World Congress on Gastrointestinal Cancer, Barcelona, 2006. Ann Oncol. 2007;18 Suppl 7:vii1–10.
12. Pedrazzoli S, DiCarlo V, Dionigi R, et al. Standard versus extended lymphadenectomy associated with pancreaticoduodenectomy in the surgical treatment of adenocarcinoma of the head of the pancreas: a multicenter, prospective, randomized study. Lymphadenectomy Study Group. Ann Surg. 1998;228:508–17.
13. Alexakis N, Halloran C, Raraty M, Ghaneh P, Sutton R, Neoptolemeos JP. Current standards of surgery for pancreatic cancer. Br J Surg. 2004;91:1410–27.
14. Yeo CJ, Cameron JL, Lillemoe KD, et al. Pancreaticoduodenectomy for cancer of the pancreas. 201 patients. Ann Surg. 1995;22:721–33.
15. Kaiser MH, Ellenberg SS. Pancreatic cancer. Adjuvant combined radiation and chemotherapy following curative resection. Arch Surg. 1985;120:899–903.
16. Klinkerbijl JH, Jeekel J, Sahmoud T, et al. Adjuvant radiotherapy and 5-fluorouracil after resection of cancer of the pancreas and periampullary region: phase III trial of the EORTC gastrointestinal tract cancer group. Ann Surg. 1999;230:776–82. discussion 782–784.
17. Neoptolemos JP, Stocken DD, Friess H, et al. A randomized trial of chemoradiotherapy and chemotherapy after resection of pancreatic cancer. N Engl J Med. 2004;350:1200–10.
18. Heinemann V, Boeck S. Perioperative management of pancreatic cancer. Ann Oncol. 2008;19 Suppl 7:vii273–8.
19. Crane CH, Ben-Losef E, Small Jr W. Chemotherapy for pancreatic cancer. N Engl J Med. 2004;350:2713–5. author reply 2713–1715.
20. Oettle H, Post S, Neuhaus P, et al. Adjuvant chemotherapy with gemcitabine vs. observation in patients undergoing curative-intent resection of pancreatic cancer. JAMA. 2007;297:267–77.
21. Neuhaus P, Riess H, Post S, et al. CONKO-001: final results of the randomized, prospective, multicentre phase III of adjuvant chemotherapy and gemcitabine versus observation in patients with resected pancreatic cancer. ASCO Annual Meeting Proceedings. 2008;26(18S):LBA4504.
22. Rhodes JM. Usefulness of novel tumor markers. Ann Oncol. 1999;10 Suppl 4:S118–21.
23. Hermann R, Jelic S. Pancreatic cancer: ESMO clinical recommendations for diagnosis, treatment and follow-up. Ann Oncol. 2008;19 Suppl 2:ii25–6.
24. NCCN clinical guidelines in oncology. Pancreatic Adenocarcinoma. Version 1.207. www.nccn.org.

27 Liver and Biliary Tract Carcinoma

David Y. Johnson, Shilpi Wadhwa, and Frank E. Johnson

Keywords
Hepatitis B • Infection • Biliary tract cancer • Chemical • Aflatoxins

The International Agency for Research on Cancer (IARC), a component of the World Health Organization (WHO), estimated that there were 626,162 new cases of liver carcinoma worldwide in 2002 [1]. The IARC also estimated that there were 598,321 deaths due to this cause in 2002 [1].

The American Cancer Society estimated that there were 28,410 new cases and 20,030 deaths due to liver, intrahepatic bile duct, gallbladder, and other biliary cancers in the United States in 2007 [2]. The estimated 5-year survival rate (all races) in the United States in 2007 was 10 % for liver and bile duct cancer [2]. Survival rates were adjusted for normal life expectancies and were based on cases diagnosed from 1996 to 2002 and followed through 2003.

About 80 % cases of liver cancer are caused by chronic hepatitis B infection [3]. Advancing age, male sex, chronic hepatitis C infection, cirrhosis, and exposure to aflatoxins (mycotoxins produced by specific fungal species and present on moldy foods) are risk factors. Several chemicals, particularly vinyl chloride, steroid hormones, and iron overload are also implicated [3]. Many genetic disorders cause liver carcinoma [4]. Risk factors for biliary tract cancer include gallstones, liver flukes, ulcerative colitis, prior partial gastrectomy, obesity, certain occupations, number of pregnancies, various congenital anatomic biliary anomalies, and certain occupational exposures. Known genetic risk factors account for a small minority of instances [3].

D.Y. Johnson, M.D. • S. Wadhwa
Department of Internal Medicine, Saint Louis University Medical Center, Saint Louis, MO, USA

F.E. Johnson (✉)
Saint Louis University Medical Center and Saint Louis Veterans Affairs Medical Center, Saint Louis, MO, USA
e-mail: frank.johnson1@va.gov

Geographic Variation Worldwide

The incidence of hepatocellular carcinoma varies greatly around the world. It is uncommon in the western industrial democracies, but very common in east Asia and sub-Saharan Africa. China alone accounts for at least 50 % of liver cancer cases [3]. The geographic variation in biliary tract cancer incidence is also great. Among women, the highest rate in the world for gallbladder cancer is reported in Delhi, India. The highest rates for men are reported from Asia, particularly Korea and Japan, and from Eastern Europe [3]. Geographic variation in the United States is also pronounced [5].

Surveillance Strategies Proposed By Professional Organizations or National Government Agencies and Available on the Internet

National Comprehensive Cancer Network (NCCN, www.nccn.org)

NCCN guidelines were accessed on January 28, 2012 (Tables 27.1 and 27.2). There were minor quantitative and qualitative changes compared to the guidelines accessed on April 10, 2007.

F.E. Johnson et al. (eds.), *Patient Surveillance After Cancer Treatment*, Current Clinical Oncology,
DOI 10.1007/978-1-60327-969-7_27,

Table 27.1 Hepatobiliary cancers: hepatocellular carcinoma. Obtained from NCCN (www.nccn.org) on January 28, 2012

	Years post-treatment[a]					
	1	2	3	4	5	>5
Office visit[b]	2–4	2–4	1–2	1–2	1–2	1–2
Imaging	2–4	2–4	1–2	1–2	1–2	1–2
Serum AFP level[c]	2–4	2–4	1–2	1–2	1–2	1–2

NCCN guidelines were accessed on January 28, 2012. There were minor quantitative and qualitative changes compared to the guidelines accessed on April 10, 2007

[a]The numbers in the table indicate the number of times the modality is recommended during the indicated year post-treatment

[b]Imaging and serum AFP level were the only quantitative recommendations given. We inferred that office visits would be recommended as frequently as these

[c]If initially elevated

Table 27.2 Hepatobiliary cancers: gallbladder cancer, intrahepatic/extrahepatic cholangiocarcinoma. Obtained from NCCN (www.nccn.org) on January 28, 2012

	Years post-treatment[a]					
	1	2	3	4	5	>5
Office visit	2	2	0	0	0	0
Imaging	2	2	0	0	0	0

•There are no data to support aggressive surveillance. There should be a patient/physician discussion regarding appropriate follow-up schedules/imaging.

NCCN guidelines were accessed on January 28, 2012. There were minor quantitative and qualitative changes compared to the guidelines accessed on April 10, 2007

[a]The numbers in the table indicate the number of times the modality is recommended during the indicated year post-treatment

American Society of Clinical Oncology (ASCO, www.asco.org)

ASCO guidelines were accessed on January 28, 2012. No quantitative guidelines exist for liver and biliary cancer surveillance, including when first accessed on October 31, 2007.

The Society of Surgical Oncology (SSO, www.surgonc.org)

ASCO guidelines were accessed on January 28, 2012. No quantitative guidelines exist for liver and biliary cancer surveillance, including when first accessed on October 31, 2007.

European Society for Medical Oncology (ESMO, www.esmo.org)

ESMO guidelines were accessed on January 28, 2012 (Tables 27.3 and 27.4). There are new quantitative guidelines compared to no guidelines found on October 31, 2007.

Table 27.3 Hepatocellular carcinoma with liver resection. Obtained from ESMO (www.esmo.org) on January 28, 2012

	Years post-treatment[a]					
	1	2	3	4	5	>5
Office visit	2–4	2–4	0	0	0	0
Serum AFP level	2–4	2–4	0	0	0	0
Liver imaging	2–4	2–4	0	0	0	0

•The indications for antiviral/interferon therapy for patients positive for HCV and HBV should depend on the degree of hepatitis and/or liver cirrhosis and viral replicative status.

•For other patients, follow-up aims to prevent and/or treat hepatic decompensation.

ESMO guidelines were accessed on January 28, 2012. These are new quantitative guidelines compared to no guidelines found on October 31, 2007

[a]The numbers in the table indicate the number of times the modality is recommended during the indicated year post-treatment

Table 27.4 Hepatocellular carcinoma with liver transplant. Obtained from ESMO (www.esmo.org) on January 28, 2012

	Years post-treatment[a]					
	1	2	3	4	5	>5
Office visit[b]	8	2	2	1	1	1

- Transplanted patients should be followed only in specialized transplant centers.
- Imaging studies should be performed as needed.
- The follow-up is aimed at drug dosage adjustment, early diagnosis of eventual immunosuppression-related infection, early detection of rejection or transplant dysfunction, and later also at detection of immunosuppression-related neoplasia.
- Antiviral therapy should be continued if previously started.

ESMO guidelines were accessed on January 28, 2012. These are new quantitative guidelines compared to no guidelines found on October 31, 2007

[a]The numbers in the table indicate the number of times the modality is recommended during the indicated year post-treatment

[b]Once monthly up to 6 months, then once every 3 months up to 1 year, then twice a year up to 2 years and once a year every year thereafter

European Society of Surgical Oncology (ESSO, www.esso-surgeonline.org)

ESSO guidelines were accessed on January 28, 2012. No quantitative guidelines exist for liver and biliary cancer surveillance, including when first accessed on October 31, 2007.

Cancer Care Ontario (CCO, www.cancercare.on.ca)

CCO guidelines were accessed on January 28, 2012. No quantitative guidelines exist for liver and biliary cancer surveillance, including when first accessed on October 31, 2007.

National Institute for Clinical Excellence (NICE, www.nice.org.uk)

NICE guidelines were accessed on January 28, 2012. No quantitative guidelines exist for liver and biliary cancer surveillance, including when first accessed on October 31, 2007.

The Cochrane Collaboration (CC, www.cochrane.org)

CC guidelines were accessed on January 28, 2012. No quantitative guidelines exist for liver and biliary cancer surveillance, including when first accessed on October 31, 2007.

Society for Surgery of the Alimentary Tract (SSAT, www.ssat.com)

SSAT guidelines were accessed on January 28, 2012. No quantitative guidelines exist for liver and biliary cancer surveillance, including when first accessed on December 18, 2007.

The M.D. Anderson Surgical Oncology Handbook also has follow-up guidelines, proposed by authors from a single National Cancer Institute-designated Comprehensive Cancer Center, for many types of cancer [6]. Some are detailed and quantitative, others are qualitative.

Summary

This is a common cancer with significant variability in incidence worldwide. We found consensus-based guidelines but none based on high-quality evidence.

References

1. Parkin DM, Whelan SL, Ferlay J, Teppo L, Thomas DB. Cancer incidence in five continents, Vol. VIII, International Agency for Research on Cancer (IARC Scientific Publication 155). Lyon, France: IARC Press; 2002. ISBN 92-832-2155-9.
2. Jemal A, Seigel R, Ward E, Murray T, Xu J, Thun MJ. Cancer statistics, 2007. CA Cancer J Clin. 2007;57:43–66.
3. Schottenfeld D, Fraumeni JG. Cancer epidemiology and prevention. 3rd ed. New York, NY: Oxford University Press; 2006. ISBN 13:978-0-19-514961-6.
4. De Vita VT, Hellman S, Rosenberg SA. Cancer. 7th ed. Philadelphia, PA: Lippincott Williams & Wilkins; 2005. ISBN 0-781-74450-4.
5. Devesa SS, Grauman DJ, Blot WJ, Pennello GA, Hoover RN, Fraumeni JF Jr. Atlas of Cancer Mortality in the United States. National Institutes of Health, National Cancer Institute. NIH Publication No. 99-4564; 1999.
6. Feig BW, Berger DH, Fuhrman GM. The M.D. Anderson surgical oncology handbook. 4th ed. Philadelphia, PA: Lippincott Williams & Wilkins; 2006. paperback. ISBN 0-7817-5643-X.

Liver and Biliary Tract Carcinoma Surveillance Counterpoint: Europe

28

Michele Colledan

Keywords
Hepatobiliary cancer • HCC • Italy • OLT • UltrasoundIntroduction

Little or no evidence exists on which criteria for follow-up for postsurgical treatment of hepatobiliary cancer may be based. Therefore, although these cancers are common, current guidelines seldom address this issue and only with generic recommendations. In addition to what was reported in the main chapter, the only guidelines generated in Europe and written in English on the treatment of hepatic and biliary tumors are those published by the British Society of Gastroenterology [1, 2]. However, these report no recommendation about posttreatment surveillance. On the other hand, the Associazione Italiana Studio Fegato (AISF—Italian Association for the Study of the Liver) has published guidelines written in Italian on the management of patients with hepatocellular carcinoma (HCC) which include some recommendations about surveillance [3–5]. These recommendations, currently followed by most Italian institutions, including ours, are summarized here.

Hepatocellular Carcinoma

Epidemiology of HCC in Italy

The great variability in incidence of HCC across continents and even across different areas of large nations is already clearly reported in the main chapter. Europe is no exception to this rule. Among European countries, Italy is one of the most affected countries. This is mainly due to the high prevalence of HBV and HCV hepatitis. In 1999, mortality due to HCC in Italy was reported to be as high as 10.9 per 100,000 people per year.

Less than 5% of HCC develops in a previously healthy liver and little is known about the prognosis of these cases. In all the other cases, the disease develops in the setting of chronic liver disease which, in general terms, is a precancerous lesion [3].

Surveillance After Surgical Resection or Ablation

The incidents of recurrence after surgical resection of HCC in patients with chronic liver disease ranges between 70 and 100% at 5 years. Most recurrences occur in the liver and two different mechanisms are involved: local recurrence of the primary tumor or one of its satellites or a new tumor arising in a different portion of the liver [3]. Recurrence has only a limited tendency to spread to extrahepatic sites. Aggressive treatment, when technically feasible, may therefore be justified. Few investigations are considered useful in surveillance after surgical resection or ablation and are listed here below (Table 28.1):

- Measurement of alpha fetoprotein level in serum may be a useful tool if elevated levels were present before treatment of the primary lesion. It is recommended to repeat the measurement every 3–4 months. However, due to the limited specificity of the test, integration with imaging procedures is necessary.
  Imaging should include:
- Ultrasound examination of the liver every 3–4 months, possibly with color-power Doppler analysis.
- CT with arterial and portal phase acquisitions every 6–8 months. CT may be replaced by dynamic MRI.

M. Colledan (✉)
Ospedali Riuniti di Bergamo, Largo Barozzi 1, 24128 Bergamo, Italy
e-mail: mcolledan@ospedaliriuniti.bergamo.it

F.E. Johnson et al. (eds.), *Patient Surveillance After Cancer Treatment*, Current Clinical Oncology,
DOI 10.1007/978-1-60327-969-7_28, © Springer Science+Business Media New York 2013

Table 28.1 Hepatocellular carcinoma arising in patients with chronic liver disease

	Years posttreatment[a]				
	1	2	3	4	5
Serum AFP level[b]	4	4	4	4	4
Ultrasound (possibly with Power Flow Doppler)	3–4	3–4	3–4	3–4	3–4
Spiral CT with arterial and portal phases (or dynamic MRI)	1–2	1–2	1–2	1–2	1–2

Follow-up after nontransplant surgical resection.
AFP alpha feta protein.
[a]The number in each cell is the number of times in a particular posttreatment year a particular modality is recommended.
[b]If initially elevated.

In case of multifocal lesions, ultrasound may not be adequate. CT or MRI every 3–4 months is preferable.

Surveillance After Orthotopic Liver Transplantation (OLT)

Total hepatectomy with liver transplantation is the most appropriate form of treatment for HCC arising in a setting of chronic liver disease since it treats both the cancer itself and the underlying disease, thus minimizing the risk of new tumors. In most countries, however, organ scarcity imposes a limitation in indications to patients with early stages of the disease. Candidates must satisfy the so-called Milano criteria. They have the lowest risk of recurrence after this treatment [3]. A patient whose explanted native liver has early-stage disease has a probability of recurrence-free survival at 5 years as high as 95%. Sixty to seventy percent of recurrences occur in the first 2 years after transplant. The most common sites of recurrence are the transplanted liver, lung, and bone. Prevention of recurrence may be attempted by selected protocols of immunosuppression. One of the recently introduced immunosuppressive agents (rapamycin) has been reported to reduce the risk of recurrence of HCC after liver transplantation [3] (Table 28.2).

The schedule of follow-up investigations for these patients may vary from center to center. AISF recommendations followed by our group are:

Table 28.2 Hepatocellular carcinoma arising in patients with chronic liver disease

	Years posttreatment[a]				
	1	2	3	4	5
Serum AFP level[b]	4	4	2	2	2
Ultrasound (possibly with Power Flow Doppler)	4	2	2	2	2
Total body CT[c]	1				
Total body bone scintigraphy[c]	1				

Follow-up after liver transplantation.
AFP alpha feta protein.
[a]The number in each cell is the number of times in a particular posttreatment year a particular modality is recommended.
[b]If initially elevated.
[c]In patients with increased risk of recurrence.

- Serum alpha fetoprotein measurement at least every 3 months for the first 2 years and at least every 6 months thereafter.
- Ultrasound of the liver every 3 months in the first year and every 6 months from the second to the fifth year.
- Total body CT and bone scintigraphy in the first year for all the patients with moderate to high risk of recurrence [3].

References

1. Ryder SD. Guidelines for the diagnosis and treatment of hepatocellular carcinoma in adults. Gut. 2003;52(Suppl III):iii1–8.
2. Kahan SA, Davidson BR, Goldin R, et al. Guidelines for the diagnosis and treatment of cholangiocarcinoma: consensus document. Gut. 2002;51(Suppl VI):vi1–9.
3. Ruisultati Commissioni: Epatocarcinoma. http://www.webaisf.org/index.php?option=com_docman&task=doc_view&gid=41&tmpl=component&format=raw&itemid=72&lang=it (2009). Accessed 25 Feb 2009.
4. Risultati Commissioni: Trapianto di fegato non urgente nell'adulto. http://www.webaisf.org/index.php?option=com_docman&task=doc_view&gid=38&tmpl=component&format=raw&itemid=72&lang=it (2009). Accessed 25 Feb 2009.
5. Risultati Commissioni: Trapianto di Fegato. http://www.webaisf.org/index.php?option=com_docman&task=doc_view&gid=52&tmpl=component&format=raw&itemid=72&lang=it (2009). Accessed 25 Feb 2009.

29 Liver and Biliary Tract Carcinoma Surveillance Counterpoint: Australia

Michael D. Crawford

Keywords
Chronic liver injury • Transplantation • Curative surgery • HCC • Cancer death

Carcinoma of the liver and carcinoma of the biliary tract are leading causes of cancer death worldwide. The commoner cancer types include hepatocellular carcinoma (HCC), cholangiocarcinoma and gallbladder carcinoma. The incidence, predisposing factors, treatment and prognosis for these cancers are very different according to tumour type. HCC accounts for the majority worldwide in this group.

As noted elsewhere in this book, screening for recurrent cancer following curative-intent therapy is not supported by high-level evidence. Individual practices vary widely from no surveillance to intensive surveillance. Practices are influenced by available evidence, anecdotes, cost and personal experiences. The aim of this chapter is to describe our standard surveillance strategies for patients with cancer of the liver and biliary tract after curative-intent surgery and to justify the regimens with evidence or empiricism as far as possible.

HCC is a primary cancer of hepatocytes or their stem cells. It generally arises secondary to a chronic liver injury after many years of inflammation when fibrosis or cirrhosis is established. The degree of liver injury and cirrhosis has an impact on both treatment options and survival after the diagnosis. There are large geographical variations in the incidence of HCC worldwide, reflecting differences in the prevalence of viral hepatitis. Pre-disposing factors are hepatitis B, hepatitis C, alcohol abuse, haemochromatosis and other conditions and toxins that cause chronic liver inflammation. Around 10% occur without any apparent chronic inflammatory process or cirrhosis. The progression from adenoma (benign neoplasia of hepatocytes) to carcinoma may account for some of these cases.

The treatment options for a patient with HCC are hierarchical. The hierarchy reflects the evidence for cure and the reported long-term survival probability for each treatment option as well as access to treatment. The evidence-based hierarchy is for surgical removal over ablation (physical destruction without resection), over transhepatic chemoembolization (TACE), over systemic chemotherapy, over other treatments and supportive care. Surgical removal is the only one routinely performed with intent to cure, although occasionally ablation or TACE may in fact be curative. Surgical removal consists of either partial hepatectomy or total hepatectomy with liver transplantation. Most patients presenting with HCC are not suitable for either partial hepatectomy or transplantation, and their management is not with curative intent.

Liver transplantation in a highly selected group of patients offers the best long-term disease-free and disease-specific survival. Partial hepatectomy in similar patients has a 5-year overall survival probability that approaches transplant but poorer disease-free survival probability. Although there are no adequate data available, it is likely that transplantation has a substantial overall survival advantage beyond 5 years. The reason that liver transplant is such a successful strategy is that it removes not only the primary cancer but also the rest of the diseased liver. In doing so, it improves long-term survival probability in three ways over partial hepatectomy. First, it removes not only the primary tumour but also any microscopic intra-hepatic metastases or other primaries. Second, it effectively treats the underlying liver disease and cirrhosis that would otherwise have an impact on survival. Third, it removes the entire inflamed, cirrhotic liver, preventing the development of new primary tumours.

M.D. Crawford, MBBS, FRACS (✉)
Royal Prince Alfred Medical Centre, Suite 314, 100 Carillon Avenue, Newtown, NSW 2042, Australia
e-mail: info@drmichaelcrawford.com.au

F.E. Johnson et al. (eds.), *Patient Surveillance After Cancer Treatment*, Current Clinical Oncology,
DOI 10.1007/978-1-60327-969-7_29, © Springer Science+Business Media New York 2013

There are no randomised studies comparing hepatectomy with liver transplantation for HCC. There are problems comparing transplantation over hepatectomy in non-randomised studies as a result of both selection and lead-time biases. First, the pre-operative work-up for liver transplantation candidates is usually more extensive than for patients scheduled for hepatectomy, ruling out more patients. Second, the time waiting for a liver transplant allows patients with unfavourable tumour biology to declare themselves and not receive a transplant, whereas there is effectively no waiting time for hepatectomy. Third, there is lead-time bias in comparative studies of survival because the time of the actual transplant rather than the time of listing for transplant is used. When intent-to-treat comparison is made between hepatectomy and transplant using assessment as the starting point, the apparent benefits of transplant are less impressive.

Liver transplantation is not available worldwide. In places where it is an option, there are essentially two sources of donors: the deceased donor and the live donor. There is almost always a shortage of deceased donors, and therefore some form of rationing is necessary. This means that, in most parts of the world where transplant is an option, a patient with HCC who is suitable for either deceased donor liver transplantation or partial hepatectomy tends to be offered partial hepatectomy despite a probable long-term survival advantage with transplantation. In places with adult-to-adult live donor liver transplantation, this distinction is less clear, although there are ethical concerns about putting a donor at risk when there is a treatment strategy with similar short- and intermediate-term efficacy available. For patients with advanced cirrhosis, in whom partial hepatectomy would be dangerous, transplantation is the only option available and is recommended when the tumour meets applicable criteria [1, 2] and there is no contra-indication to transplant.

Given that the only treatment options routinely applied with curative intent are partial hepatectomy and transplant, surveillance strategies can be defined for these two groups of patients. The goals should include detection of recurrent or new HCC, complications of treatments, and diseases that are not cancer-related, such as progressive liver disease and non-HCC cancers. For the purposes of this review, only surveillance for the development of recurrent or new HCC is considered.

The purpose of a follow-up programme (outside of clinical trials) to detect recurrent or new HCC should be to identify cancers when they are small enough that early therapies are likely to have an impact on survival and/or quality of life. The schedule and type of follow-up should reflect effectiveness, cost, toxicity and the ability for early intervention to impact outcomes. There are few data to support any particular strategy. The author's follow-up regimens after liver transplant and partial hepatectomy are different and are considered separately. The available surveillance modalities for HCC are clinical examination, serum tumour marker levels and imaging. Clinical examination, with the rare exception of implantation in a wound, biopsy or drain site, only detects recurrence when it is incurable. Clinical examination, however, is cheap and expected by patients and therefore included in any strategy. The tumour markers commonly used are alpha fetoprotein (AFP) and prothrombin induced by vitamin K absence (PIVKA-II) or both. In the western world, AFP is the most accessible and commonly used. The usual imaging modalities are ultrasound (US) and computed tomography (CT).

Surveillance after liver transplantation for HCC is surprisingly simple (Table 29.1). Most patients who receive a liver transplant for HCC within strict criteria [3] are cured of HCC. Most recurrences are not curable; they are metastases and occur in an immunosuppressed patient. The therapeutic strategies available include reduction or change of immunosuppression, systemic chemotherapy, surgical resection, ablation, radiotherapy, supportive and palliative care. The type of therapy that might be implemented in a given patient depends on the timing of recurrence, the site(s) of recurrence, the health of the patient and the presence of symptoms. Given that this book is addressing the surveillance of asymptomatic patients, symptoms should not be relevant here. This contracts the list of options to surgical removal or ablation, systemic chemotherapy, alterations in immunosuppression or a combination of these. While there are anecdotal reports of cures or long-term survival after treatment of recurrent HCC following transplant, they are rare. There are no available data to prove that intervention for recurrence in the asymptomatic patient is better than treating only symptomatic recurrences.

The NCCN guidelines [4] were the only identified guidelines that addressed the issue of follow-up following liver transplant for HCC, and that schedule is described in the first part of this chapter. These are consensus guidelines based on expert opinion. No evidence (randomised or otherwise) was given to support the schedule.

In the author's practise, surveillance (outside of clinical trials) in transplant patients, with evidence of HCC in the native liver, consists of serum AFP levels and clinical examination each time the patient is seen in the office for transplant reasons (Table 29.1). Imaging is ordered on the basis of an abnormal or rising AFP level, abnormality on clinical examination or history or for non-cancer-related reasons. The rationale for this practise is that recurrence after liver transplant is uncommon and usually consists of incurable systemic metastasis. This means that the ability to convert a recurrence, once identified, into a cure is exceptionally unlikely. Isolated resectable metastases may occur, but so infrequently that expensive imaging and therapy are not efficient uses of funds. In fact, more patients may be harmed by a follow-up programme through radiation exposure, investigation and treatment of false positives, surgical or chemotherapy complications, etc. than would benefit.

Table 29.1 Surveillance after curative-intent liver transplantation for hepatocellular carcinoma at Royal Prince Alfred Medical Centre, Sydney

	Years post-treatment					
	1	2	3	4	5	>5
Office visit[a]	4	4	2	1	1	1
Serum AFP level	4	4	4	4	4	2

The number in each cell indicates the number of times a particular modality is recommended in a particular post-treatment year.
AFP alpha fetoprotein.
[a]Imaging studies are ordered according to clinical findings or serum AFP (alpha fetoprotein) level evidence of disease recurrence.
Imaging is often performed for reasons not related to the index cancer (such as complications related to immunosuppression).

Table 29.2 Surveillance after curative-intent hepatic resection for hepatocellular carcinoma at Royal Prince Alfred Medical Centre, Sydney

	Years post-treatment					
	1	2	3	4	5	>5
Office visit with imaging[a]	2–4	2–4	2	2	2	2
Serum AFP level	4	4	4	4	4	4

The number in each cell indicates the number of times a particular modality is recommended in a particular post-treatment year.
AFP: alpha fetoprotein.
[a]Imaging includes ultrasound alternating with triple-phase CT.
Serum AFP (alpha fetoprotein) levels are followed in all patients irrespective of the initial level.

There are a small number of patients with high risk for recurrence where the yield from surveillance might be higher (those with tumours with vascular invasion, high mitotic rates or outside criteria [1, 2] on explant pathologic examination). However, these recurrences are usually multifocal and incurable, again making aggressive screening hard to justify.

Why then are AFP levels measured at all? There is no good oncological reason, since a rising AFP after liver transplant usually represents incurable recurrence. The test is performed because both the patient and medical staff find it reassuring when normal and because it is inexpensive, added to blood tests already being performed, and does not harm the patient.

Surveillance after curative-intent resection for HCC is also rather simple (Table 29.2). Most (>70%) patients who undergo resection for HCC develop recurrence. Some are true recurrences (local or metastatic), whereas some are new primary cancers occurring in a "field effect" due to the underlying liver disease. Recurrent HCC outside of the liver is evidence of systemic metastasis and is generally considered incurable. Recurrent disease within the liver represents either loco-regional recurrence or a new primary. When HCC recurs within the liver, an assessment is made about curability. This depends on the number of lesions and their size, location and evidence of vascular invasion or distant metastasis. The options for cure of intra-hepatic recurrence following resection are essentially the same as for the initial primary tumour: re-resection, liver transplant (sometimes called "salvage transplant" in this setting) and to a lesser degree ablative techniques. Non-curative life-extending options include TACE and systemic chemotherapy. The case for surveillance after liver resection is weaker than that after transplant.

There are no identified guidelines that are specifically designed to address follow-up after curative surgery for HCC. This is addressed in the NCCN practise guidelines [4], and a version of the recommended schedule is given in the first part of this chapter. European Society for Medical Oncology (ESMO) guidelines [5] recommend 3–6 monthly serum AFP level determination and liver imaging for 2 years. Most other guidelines addressing issues related to HCC do not comment on follow-up after surgery. There is a protocol for a systematic review of the surgical treatment of HCC published in the Cochrane library but it does not seem that there will be any assessment of the type or schedule of surveillance once that review is complete [6]. Most large studies reporting outcomes following hepatectomy for HCC come from Asia (often Japan) and cite-intensive schedules. One review article (English abstract) was identified that attempted to address the issue of surveillance after hepatectomy for HCC and recommended an intensive approach, while admitting a lack of evidence for it [7].

In the authors' practise, resection is followed in non-trial patients by therapeutic adjuvant intra-arterial 131-Iodine lipiodol therapy at around 6 weeks post-operatively. One month later a CT scan is performed, looking particularly for intra-hepatic lipiodol retention. A triple-phase CT is performed 6 months after surgery, and then 6 months later. Following this first 12-month period, a liver CT is performed yearly. An ultrasound is performed every 6 months for 5 years. Clinical examination takes place each time imaging is performed. Serum AFP levels are measured every 3 months (see Table 29.2). After 5 years, cirrhotic patients are returned to pre-hepatectomy surveillance schedules with serum AFP levels and US every 6 months.

This approach is more intensive than that given in the first part of this chapter. It is justified by the high probability of recurrence, the improved chances of salvage when recurrence is discovered early and the relatively low cost involved. It is similar to the surveillance strategy recommended for patients with hepatitis B-related cirrhosis who are not known to have a tumour (AFP and US every 6 months). Patients with cirrhosis are also followed for potential complications of their underlying liver disease including biochemical markers and endoscopy for the assessment and management of varices.

One could argue that the improved probability of survival in patients with recurrence detected by surveillance is only the result of lead-time bias. There is no randomised controlled study to prove that it is helpful. It does, however, make sense that the detection of recurrence (or new primary) while they are still suitable for curative therapy would be a good thing, and it is unlikely that a randomised trial will ever be conducted. Overall, doctors and patients expect some form of cancer surveillance and find this schedule to be appropriate.

Cholangiocarcinoma (cancer of the biliary epithelium) is a rarer form of primary hepatobiliary cancer. There are widespread geographic variations, reflecting differences in the incidence of pre-disposing factors. The well-established pre-disposing factors for the development of cholangiocarcinoma are primary sclerosing cholangitis, intra-hepatic cholelithiasis (particularly oriental cholangiohepatitis), choledochal cysts and other rare factors. Obesity, alcohol abuse and gallstone disease have also been implicated in large case–control studies, but even with these factors, cholangiocarcinoma is rare. In the western world, the majority of cholangiocarcinomas arise without any clear pre-disposing factors.

The treatment and prognosis depend not only on the tumour stage and histological differentiation but also on the location of the tumour. Essentially, cholangiocarcinoma can be divided into three types according to location. First is the peripheral or intra-hepatic type, which is usually diagnosed late or as an incidental finding on liver function tests or imaging where it may appear as a mass with or without bile duct dilation. Second is the hilar type (Klatskin tumour) that arises at or near the confluence of the hepatic ducts and usually presents with jaundice or abnormalities in liver function tests with intra-hepatic duct dilation on imaging. A well-defined mass on imaging studies is often a late event. Third is distal cholangiocarcinoma which arises in the extrahepatic biliary tree, including those that arise in the intra-pancreatic bile duct, which usually presents with painless jaundice. Peri-ampullary carcinoma is not considered in this chapter.

The only option for cure is aggressive surgical resection. For intra-hepatic cholangiocarcinoma, an anatomical liver resection ± portal node dissection is routine. For Klatskin tumours, an extended (left or right) hemi-hepatectomy and caudate resection with extrahepatic bile duct resection and portal node clearance is recommended. There are a small number of centres performing liver transplantation following aggressive chemo-radiotherapy for Klatskin tumours (Mayo protocol) [8], but this protocol is not universally accepted or applied. For extrahepatic cholangiocarcinoma, a radical bile duct resection including regional lymph nodes with (or without) a pancreaticoduodenectomy is performed.

The reported 5-year overall survival probability after curative-intent resection for cholangiocarcinoma is poor and varies with different series, ranging from around 10 to 30% after resection for Klatskin tumours to around 30–40% for distal bile duct carcinoma and peripheral (intra-hepatic) cholangiocarcinoma [9]. The chance of cure is dependent on the tumour stage and the resection margin. There is no convincing evidence for the role of neoadjuvant chemotherapy, radiotherapy or photodynamic therapy. However, this is an area of interest to experts and is continuously under review. Post-operative adjuvant therapy is not routinely recommended, although there is a theoretical advantage for radiotherapy following an R1 resection (macroscopically clear, but microscopically involved margin). The role for post-operative adjuvant chemotherapy has not been established.

Table 29.3 Surveillance following curative-intent resection for cholangiocarcinoma and gallbladder cancer at Royal Prince Alfred Medical Centre, Sydney

	Years post-treatment					
	1	2	3	4	5	>5
Office visit with imaging[a]	2–4	2–4	2	2	2	0
Serum tumour marker levels[b]	4	4	4	4	4	0

The number in each cell indicates the number of times a particular modality is recommended in a particular post-treatment year.
[a]Imaging consists of CT scan of abdomen and pelvis.
[b]CA 19-9 ± CEA if elevated pre-operatively.

Surveillance after curative-intent resection for cholangiocarcinoma is not complex. The tools available for the detection of tumour recurrence include office visit, serum tumour marker levels and imaging tests. The NCCN clinical practise guidelines [4] are the only guidelines identified that suggest a schedule, given in the first part of this chapter. Recurrence following resection of Klatskin or distal bile duct carcinomas is almost always incurable. The pattern of recurrence is often peritoneal, followed by systemic metastases. Surveillance is warranted to assess for wound or drain site recurrence that would be amenable to resection or local radiotherapy which, in rare circumstances, might be curative but is usually palliative. The detection of clinically occult recurrent disease is unlikely to lead to cure or extension of life and cannot be defended by the available literature. Rare cases of local recurrence or intra-hepatic disease after hepatectomy for peripheral cholangiocarcinoma may be cured by re-resection.

The author obtains serum CA 19-9 and CEA levels (when initially elevated) and liver function tests every 3 months. CT imaging and clinical examination are obtained every 6 months for 2 years and then yearly for at least a further 3 years (Table 29.3). The author is at variance with the NCCN guidelines beyond 2 years post resection. NCCN guidelines recommend no further surveillance [4] but patients who develop recurrence beyond 2 years are selected to have slow-growing tumours and more aggressive therapies such as further resection or ablation might be appropriate in such selected cases. Again, there is minimal evidence for surveillance and it is largely performed because of patient expectations. If recurrence is identified, a referral for palliative care, and (when suitable) palliative chemotherapy or radiotherapy is made. There is no evidence that early detection has an impact on quality of life or survival duration in the long run. In the event of actual or impending biliary obstruction, percutaneous or endoscopic cholangiography and metallic stent placement (with or without brachytherapy) are usually recommended, particularly when there is a high suspicion of a malignant stricture.

Gallbladder cancer is the most common malignancy of the biliary tract. It tends to occur in later life. It is more common in women than men and usually associated with gallstone disease. There is wide geographic variability with high rates in Native Americans, South Americans and Northern Indians [10]. Gallbladder cancer can present with pain, jaundice, palpable mass, cholecystitis, metastatic disease or as an incidental finding at the time of imaging. It may be discovered at the time of cholecystectomy for benign biliary disease. Not surprisingly, patients with incidentally diagnosed gallbladder carcinoma tend to have a better prognosis than those diagnosed with symptoms.

Surgery is the mainstay of curative therapy. The extent of surgery depends on the stage of the tumour, the mode of presentation and the surgeon's experience. Following an unanticipated histological finding of cancer after cholecystectomy, second stage radical clearance is often recommended depending on tumour stage. The prognosis after surgery is heavily influenced by the stage of the cancer and whether the margins are clear. Resection of early [Tis or T1N0M0 (Stage 0 or IA)] disease has good results even with standard cholecystectomy. Radical resection of T2N0M0 (Stage IB) tumours gives good results also. The role of surgery for more advanced lesions (T3 or T4N0M0) and for those with positive lymph nodes remains somewhat controversial, but there is a trend towards aggressive surgery with curative intent, and some studies showing reasonable long-term outcomes (particularly in Japanese series). Radical surgery includes resection of port sites for tumours diagnosed after laparoscopic cholecystectomy.

Surveillance after curative-intent resection for gallbladder carcinoma rarely, if ever, identifies curable tumour recurrence. Patients with early tumours are usually cured and those with late tumours usually die of their disease despite surveillance. Strategies include office visit, serum tumour marker level (particularly CA 19-9) and imaging. Occasional implantation metastases (wound or drain site) may be identified and removed but they commonly reflect underlying peritoneal disease even when the imaging is otherwise negative. Isolated ovarian metastases are occasionally seen but there is no evidence that resection of these contributes to survival. The author follows patients with T2 or more invasive tumours with serum CA 19-9 levels every 3 months and clinical examination with CT scan imaging (abdomen and pelvis) every 6 months for 2 years and then yearly until 5 years (Table 29.3). Medical staff and patients seem happy with this surveillance regimen.

There is no compelling data to support surveillance after curative therapy for patients with liver or biliary tract carcinoma. However, there is a reasonable case for doing so, particularly in those who would be fit enough to undergo further procedures aimed at cure in the event of discovery of early recurrence. Furthermore, it is an expectation of most patients (and their doctors) that such a strategy be employed.

References

1. Mazzaferro V, Regalia E, Doci R, et al. Liver transplantation for the treatment of small hepatocellular carcinomas in patients with cirrhosis. N Engl J Med. 1996;334:693–9.
2. Yao FY, Ferrell L, Bass NM, Bacchetti P, Ascher NL, Roberts JP. Liver transplantation for hepatocellular carcinoma: comparison of the proposed UCSF criteria with the Milan criteria and the Pittsburgh modified TNM criteria. Liver Transplant. 2002;8(9):765–74.
3. Duffy JP, Vardanian A, Benjamin E, Watson M, Farmer DG, Ghobrial RM, Lipshutz G, Yersiz H, Lu DS, Lassman C, Tong MJ, Hiatt JR, Busuttil RW. Liver transplantation criteria for hepatocellular carcinoma should be expanded: a 22-year experience with 467 patients at UCLA. Ann Surg. 2007;246(3):502–9.
4. NCCN. National Comprehensive Cancer Network. Clinical practice guidelines in oncology. Hepatobiliary Cancers. v.2.2008 (http://www.nccn.org).
5. Parikh P, Malhotra H, Jelic S. (ESMO Guidelines Working Group). Hepatocellular carcinoma: ESMO Clinical Recommendations for diagnosis, treatment and follow-up. Ann Oncol. 2008;19(S2):ii27–8.
6. Abrishami A, Nasseri-Moghaddam S, Eghtesad B, Sherman M. Surgical resection for hepatocellular carcinoma. (Protocol) Cochrane Database Syst Rev. 2008. (http://www.mrw.interscience.wiley.com/cochrane).
7. Kokudo N, Makuuchi M. Surveillance after curative resection of hepatocellular carcinoma (*Japanese*). J Japan Surg Soc. 2007;108(3):131–6.
8. Rea DJ, Heimbach JK, Rosen CB, Haddock MG, Alberts SR, Kremers WK, et al. Liver transplantation with neoadjuvant chemoradiation is more effective than resection for hilar cholangiocarcinoma. Ann Surg. 2005;242:451–8.
9. Malhi H, Gores G. Review Article: the modern diagnosis and therapy of cholangiocarcinoma. Aliment Pharmacol Ther. 2006;23:1287–96.
10. Misra S, Chatyrvedi A, Misra N, Sharma I. Carcinoma of the gallbladder. Lancet Oncol. 2003;4:167–76.

30 Liver and Biliary Tract Carcinoma Surveillance Counterpoint: Japan

Akinobu Taketomi and Yoshihiko Maehara

Keywords
Postoperative • Japan • Resection • Intrahepatic recurrence • Cholangiocarcinoma

A number of factors determine the optimal strategy for postoperative follow-up patients who have had surgical resection of primary liver cancer. Our recommendations are described here, based on our experience at Kyushu University in Fukuoka, Japan.

Hepatocellular carcinoma is common in Japan as well as in other East Asian countries. However, the proportion of hepatitis B and hepatitis C infections differs considerably from country to country. In Japan, more than 70% of patients with hepatocellular carcinoma are positive for hepatitis C viral antibody [1]. Briefly, the clinical follow-up of patients after resection of hepatocellular carcinoma follows a strict protocol. Patients are seen biweekly for the first month and then every 3–4 months. We obtain ultrasound scans and enhanced CT scans at every visit. Hepatic angiography, bone scintigraphy, or a thoracic CT scan is also performed if recurrence is suspected or if a rise in the serum alpha-fetoprotein (AFP) level or des-gamma-carboxy prothrombin (DCP) level is noted (Table 30.1).

Hepatocellular carcinoma recurs in up to 90% of patients after resection [2], often in the remnant liver, but long-term survival is possible when the recurrence is appropriately treated on a timely basis [3]. Early recurrence (<1 year after initial resection) is one of the most important prognostic indicators. Therefore, we use a rigorous follow-up program during the first year after initial hepatectomy. Resection of intrahepatic recurrence is safe and clearly improves survival, with 5-year survival rates of up to 50% [3]. Frequent and intensive surveillance is necessary to provide early diagnosis since recurrent carcinoma can be very aggressive. We perform blood tests and measure tumor markers every 3 months until 2 years after the initial hepatectomy and every 4 months thereafter. Tumor markers, particularly AFP and des-gamma carboxyprothrombin (DCP), are sensitive and specific in patients with HCC for differentiating recurrence from nonmalignant chronic liver disease [4]. The serum des-gamma carboxyprothrombin level is significantly correlated with the risk of portal venous invasion, which is known to be a major prognostic factor after hepatectomy [5]. For patients receiving liver transplant, the pretransplant DCP level is also significantly correlated with macroscopic portal invasion and intrahepatic metastasis in the explanted liver [6]. Our experience confirms that the serum DCP level is a reliable marker.

Ultrasound is a noninvasive and simple tool to detect recurrence after hepatic resection. The limits of ultrasound in screening for HCC are well known. In particular, its reliability depends on the examiner's technique and experience. Indeed, the high rate of early recurrence of HCC after percutaneous ethanol injection (PEI) or surgery in patients with a single nodule detected by ultrasound is felt to be due to the low sensitivity of ultrasound in staging of HCC. Some authors argue that ultrasound has no substantial impact on the overall survival of cirrhotic patients with hepatocellular carcinoma [7, 8]. However, all liver surgeons should be familiar with ultrasound, since it is essential for modern hepatic surgery.

Spiral-computed tomography is very accurate in the diagnosis of hepatocellular carcinoma, since it recognizes the development of the new, pathological arterial vascularization. It has been reported that CT arterial portography (CTAP) combined with CT hepatic angiography (CTHA) improves

A. Taketomi, M.D., Ph.D., F.A.C.S (✉) • Y. Maehara, M.D., Ph.D., F.A.C.S.
Department of Surgery and Science, Graduate School of Medicine, Kyushu University, 3-1-1 Maidashi, Higashi-ku, Fukuoka 812-8582, Japan
e-mail: taketomi@surg2.med.kyushu-u.ac.jp; maehara@surg2.med.kyushu-u.ac.jp

F.E. Johnson et al. (eds.), *Patient Surveillance After Cancer Treatment*, Current Clinical Oncology, DOI 10.1007/978-1-60327-969-7_30,

Table 30.1 Follow-up of patients with hepatocellular carcinoma: Kyushu University, Japan

	Years posttreatment					
	1	2	3	4	5	>5
Office visit	4	4	3	3	3	2
CBC	4	4	3	3	3	2
LFTs	4	4	3	3	3	2
Serum electrolyte levels	4	4	3	3	3	2
Serum AFP level	4	4	3	3	3	2
Serum AFP-L3 level[a]	4	4	3	3	3	2
Serum DCP level	4	4	3	3	3	2
Abdominal ultrasound	4	4	3	3	3	2
Abdominal CT	4	4	3	3	3	2
MRI	b	b	b	b	b	b

The same follow-up regimen is recommended for patients receiving transplant and nontransplant resection
The numbers in each cell indicate the number of times a particular modality is recommended during a particular posttreatment year
CBC complete blood count; *DCP* des-gamma-carboxyl prothrombin; *LFTs* liver function tests
[a]AFP-L3: an isoform of alpha-fetoprotein
[b]Performed only if clinically indicated

Table 30.2 Gallbladder cancer and extrahepatic or intrahepatic cholangiocarcinoma: Kyushu University, Japan

	Years posttreatment					
	1	2	3	4	5	>5
Office visit	4	4	3	3	3	2
CBC	4	4	3	3	3	2
LFTs	4	4	3	3	3	2
Serum electrolyte levels	4	4	3	3	3	2
Serum CEA level	4	4	3	3	3	2
Serum CA19-9 level[a]	4	4	3	3	3	2
Abdominal US	4	4	3	3	3	2
Thoracic CT	4	4	3	3	3	2
Abdominal CT	4	4	3	3	3	2
PET-CT	a	a	a	a	a	a

The numbers in each cell indicate the number of times a particular modality is recommended during a particular posttreatment year
CEA carcinoembryonic antigen; *CA19-9* carbohydrate antigen 19-9; *CT* computed tomography; *PET* positron emission tomography; *US* ultrasonogram; *CBC* complete blood count; *LFTs* liver function tests
[a]Performed only if clinically indicated

the detection of hypervascular HCCs compared with either CTAP or CTHA alone because the enhancement characteristics of CTHA help to characterize the perfusion abnormalities seen during CTAP. Superparamagnetic iron oxide (SPIO)-enhanced magnetic resonance (MR) imaging scan is also performed if there are any equivocal lesions in the liver.

Although the continued improvement in imaging techniques may decrease the gap between the imaging and the pathology of hepatocellular carcinoma, some discrepancy will certainly continue to exist. Consequently, we believe that the combination of tumor markers and imaging should be utilized routinely in patient surveillance after resection.

It has been reported that hepatitis viral type is an independent factor for recurrence [9]. Some authors contend that intrahepatic metastasis is the main type of recurrence in patients with advanced-stage HCC after curative-intent surgery. Therefore, for advanced-stage HCC, regardless of the type of hepatitis virus, we are alert to the possibility of intrahepatic metastasis in the early follow-up years after surgery, and adjuvant chemotherapy may be recommended. Our surveillance for hepatitis C virus-related HCC (stages I or II) emphasizes close follow-up to check for intrahepatic recurrence for greater than 2 years after surgery or later. Some experts believe that antiviral treatment such as interferon, with or without ribavirin, might be useful in preventing a second primary HCC [9].

Cholangiocarcinoma is the second most common primary hepatic malignant disease after hepatocellular carcinoma. Several studies have shown that the incidence and mortality rates are rising worldwide. Biliary tract cancer accounts for 2% of all human malignancies and has a poor prognosis. A 5-year survival rate of 9–18% is reported for proximal bile duct cancer and 20–30% for distal bile duct cancer. Prognostic factors for survival after surgical resection include the stage of disease, grade, adequacy of resection margins, depth of invasion, and presence or absence of perineural invasion (Table 30.2).

Recurrent biliary cancer is usually fatal. If relapse could be detected earlier, the appropriate anticancer treatment might improve the prognosis. Long-term follow-up is needed because late recurrence (greater than 5 years) has been reported. We recommend serum carcinoembryonic antigen (CEA) and carbohydrate antigen 19-9 (CA19-9) levels every 3 months until 2 years after the initial surgery and every 4 months thereafter. The sensitivity and the specificity of serum CEA levels are 63–69% and 78–81%, respectively. The sensitivity and the specificity of serum CA19-9 levels are 77–78% and 81–85%, respectively. Qin et al. reported the results of a clinical study in which serum CA19-9 and CEA concentrations were measured in 15 of 35 patients with cholangiocarcinoma after curative resection [10]. The sensitivity of serum CA19-9 was higher than that of serum CEA in detecting recurrence, but the sensitivity and specificity improved by combining them. Mataki et al. reported the usefulness of CEA messenger RNA expression in the peripheral blood during follow-up periods of patients who underwent curative surgery for biliary-pancreatic cancer [11].

CT scan is a useful tool for detecting intrahepatic or pulmonary recurrence of biliary cancer after curative-intent surgery. However, its accuracy in detecting lymph node metastasis is poor. Noji et al. recently addressed this point [12]. They compared the CT scans and pathological results from 146 patients who had undergone regional lymphadenectomy for biliary carcinoma and concluded that CT is not useful for predicting regional lymph nodal metastases smaller than 18 mm in size. In our experience, multimodality imaging to detect the recurrence is required.

Several investigators have reported on the usefulness of conventional positron emission tomography (PET) or integrated PET-CT in the diagnosis and staging of cholangiocarcinoma. It has been reported that the diagnostic accuracies of FDG-PET, CT, and MRI for detection of lymph node metastasis are 86%, 68%, and 57%, the sensitivities are 43%, 43% and 43%, and the specificities were 100%, 76%, and 64%, respectively [13]. PET-CT now has an established role in surveillance.

References

1. The Liver Cancer Study Group of Japan. Primary liver cancer in Japan: clinicopathological features and results of surgical treatment. Ann Surg. 1990;211:277–87.
2. Kanematsu T, Furui J, Yanaga K, Okudaira S, Shimada M, Shirabe K. A 16-year experience in performing hepatic resection in 303 patients with hepatocellular carcinoma: 1985-2000. Surgery. 2002;131(1 Suppl):S153–8.
3. Shimada M, Takenaka K, Taguchi K, et al. Prognostic factors after repeat hepatectomy for recurrent hepatocellular carcinoma. Ann Surg. 1998;227:80–5.
4. Marrero JA, Su GL, Wei W, Emick D, Conjeevaram HS, Fontana RJ, et al. Des-gamma carboxyprothrombin can differentiate hepatocellular carcinoma from nonmalignant chronic liver disease in American patients. Hepatology. 2003;37:1114–21.
5. Hagiwara S, Kudo M, Kawasaki T, et al. Prognostic factors for portal venous invasion in patients with hepatocellular carcinoma. J Gastroenterol. 2006;41:1214–9.
6. Taketomi A, Sanefuji K, Soejima Y, et al. The impact of des-gamma carboxyprothrombin and tumor size on the recurrence of hepatocellular carcinoma after living donor liver transplantation. Transplantation. 2009;87:531–7.
7. Craig JR, Klatt EC, Yu M. Role of cirrhosis and development of HCC: evidence from histologic studies and large population studies. In: Tabor E, Di Bisceglie AM, Purcell RH, editors. Etiology, pathology, and treatment of hepatocellular carcinoma in North America. Houston, TX: Portfolio Publishing; 1991. p. 177–90.
8. Dodd GD, Miller WJ, Baron RL. Detection of malignant tumors in end stage cirrhotic livers: efficacy of sonography as a screening technique. Am J Roentgenol. 1992;159:727–33.
9. Sasaki Y, Yamada T, Tanaka H, et al. Risk of recurrence in a long-term follow-up after surgery in 417 patients with hepatitis B- or hepatitis C-related hepatocellular carcinoma. Ann Surg. 2006;244:771–80.
10. Qin XL, Wang ZR, Shi JS, Lu M, Wang L, He QR. Utility of serum CA19-9 in diagnosis of cholangiocarcinoma: in comparison with CEA. World J Gastroenterol. 2004;10:427–32.
11. Mataki Y, Takao S, Maemura K, et al. Carcinoembryonic antigen messenger RNA expression using nested reverse transcription-PCR in the peripheral blood during follow-up period of patients who underwent curative surgery for biliary-pancreatic cancer: longitudinal analyses. Clin Cancer Res. 2004;10:3807–14.
12. Noji T, Kondo S, Hirano S, Tanaka E, Suzuki O, Shichinohe T. Computed tomography evaluation of regional lymph node metastases in patients with biliary cancer. Br J Surg. 2008;95:92–6.
13. Seo S, Hatano E, Higashi T, et al. Fluorine-18 fluorodeoxyglucose positron emission tomography predicts lymph node metastasis, P-glycoprotein expression, and recurrence after resection in mass-forming intrahepatic cholangiocarcinoma. Surgery. 2008;143:769–77. Epub 2008 Apr 11.

Liver and Biliary Tract Carcinoma Surveillance Counterpoint: Canada

31

Oliver F. Bathe and Kelly Warren Burak

Keywords
Cancer-related mortality • Canada • Bile duct cancer • Tests • mTOR

The Tom Baker Cancer Centre and the University of Calgary serve as a tertiary referral resource for about 1.5 million people. Virtually all hepatobiliary tumors from Southern Alberta are seen by our group, which consists of surgeons, hepatologists, gastroenterologists, interventional and diagnostic radiologists, and medical oncologists. The centralized referral pattern and weekly multidisciplinary meetings provide the group with a large experience in treating patients with these tumors.

On a provincial level, members of the Alberta Gastrointestinal Tumor Group meet on a biannual basis in an attempt to devise provincial standards of care, based on recent evidence from the medical literature. The majority of these efforts are focused on the development of treatment algorithms. These discussions seldom focus on the optimal way to survey patients after potentially curative treatments. Therefore, no provincial standards have so far been devised on posttherapeutic surveillance. Similarly, at an institutional level, we have not devised a standard approach to following patients after definitive treatment. On the other hand, the dialogue derived from weekly multidisciplinary hepatobiliary tumor rounds has resulted in some degree of uniformity in the management of hepatobiliary tumors, and an institutional philosophy has emerged.

O.F. Bathe, M.D., M.Sc., F.R.C.S.C., F.A.C.S. (✉)
Division of Surgical Oncology, Tom Baker Cancer Centre, 1331—29th Street NW, Calgary, AB, Canada T2N 4N2
e-mail: bathe@ucalgary.ca

K.W. Burak, M.D., F.R.C.P.C., M.Sc. (Epid)
Southern Alberta Liver Transplant Clinic, University of Calgary Liver Unit, Room 6D35 TRW Bldg, 3280 Hospital Drive NW, Calgary, AB, Canada, T2N 4N1

Any surveillance strategy depends on a number of factors. Most importantly, the likelihood that a recurrence can be successfully treated must be considered. If a therapeutic strategy exists that can salvage a patient if a recurrence is identified early, then a more intensive follow-up program is justifiable. Historical data about the timing of recurrence influences the frequency of follow-up testing. That is, diagnostic tests intended to identify recurrences will be most frequent when the majority of recurrences are expected. A less intensive follow-up regimen would be appropriate when recurrence is less common. The sites at risk for recurrence dictate the types of tests utilized on follow-up. These factors can each be assessed using available evidence, enabling one to devise a justifiable follow-up strategy. Another factor that affects any follow-up strategy is the psychological needs of the patient. Specifically, if a patient expresses a need to know if there is a recurrence (for example, for the purposes of prognostication), then a closer surveillance strategy may be indicated, even if there is little objective evidence of benefit. This is an important factor to consider in patients who have undergone surgery with curative intent for tumors for which there are few (if any) opportunities for salvage therapy.

Hepatocellular Carcinoma

There are approximately 600,000 new cases of hepatocellular carcinoma worldwide, making it the sixth most common cancer and the third leading cause of cancer-related mortality globally [1]. Approximately 80% occur in the developing world [1]. However, data from the SEER registry in the USA have shown that hepatocellular carcinoma is one of the only four cancers increasing in incidence during 2000–2004 and is the only cancer in North America with an

F.E. Johnson et al. (eds.), *Patient Surveillance After Cancer Treatment*, Current Clinical Oncology,
DOI 10.1007/978-1-60327-969-7_31, © Springer Science+Business Media New York 2013

increased mortality rate over the same time period [2]. Locally, we have seen a dramatic increase in the number of liver resections for hepatocellular carcinoma in recent years [3]. Between 2002 and 2007, 17–34% of adult liver transplants in Alberta were performed for hepatocellular carcinoma. The vast majority in North America develop in the setting of cirrhosis [4]. It is therefore important to consider that two diseases must typically be managed concomitantly, namely the carcinoma and the underlying cirrhosis. Worldwide, hepatitis B virus is the most common cause of liver disease leading to hepatocellular carcinoma [1]. In North America, hepatitis C virus is the most important cause of cirrhosis leading to hepatocellular carcinoma [5].

Data derived from studies on screening for hepatocellular carcinoma in patients at risk are valuable when devising a surveillance strategy following curative therapy for hepatocellular carcinoma. Biannual screening ultrasounds have been recommended in all cirrhotic patients and noncirrhotic hepatitis B virus carriers beyond middle age [4]. This screening interval is based on natural history studies of hepatocellular carcinoma which demonstrate a median doubling time of approximately 4 months [6]. As the serum alpha-fetoprotein level lacks sensitivity and specificity, it is no longer endorsed as a screening tool on its own, although it is still often combined with ultrasound examination at the same intervals [4]. If suspicious findings are encountered on ultrasonography, further imaging is indicated. The characteristic finding of hepatocellular carcinoma on computerized tomography, magnetic resonance imaging, and contrast enhanced ultrasound is arterial phase enhancement and portal venous washout [4]. Nodules that are 1–2 cm should have concordant findings on two contrast enhanced studies, but nodules which are >2 cm require only one imaging study with typical findings (or atypical radiologic findings with a serum AFP level >200 mg/dL) to establish the diagnosis of hepatocellular carcinoma. A biopsy is needed to establish the diagnosis only in a minority of cases, where the imaging is discordant and the AFP is not elevated [4]. This diagnostic algorithm has been prospectively validated in a recent study from Barcelona [7].

The management of hepatocellular carcinoma is complex and is best done in a multidisciplinary manner [4]. Our multidisciplinary Hepatopancrea to biliavy Neoplasia Group uses the Barcelona Clinic Liver Cancer staging system for determining the most appropriate therapy for patients with hepatocellular carcinoma. The Barcelona Clinic Liver Cancer staging system is now endorsed by the American Association for the Study of Liver Diseases as the best staging system for hepatocellular carcinoma because it takes into consideration the patient's liver function (Child-Turcotte-Pugh classification), performance status (Eastern Cooperative Oncology Group status), as well as specific tumor characteristics [4]. The Barcelona Clinic Liver Cancer staging system links the patient and tumor characteristics with therapy and prognosis (Fig. 31.1) [8]. Unfortunately, only 30% of patients present at a sufficiently early stage (BCLC Stage 0 or A) where potentially curative therapies can be offered.

After curative-intent resection, liver transplantation, or radiofrequency ablation, patients have 5-year survival rates approaching 70%, although tumor recurrence remains common [4]. Liver failure following surgical resection in a cirrhotic patient is often fatal and therefore surgery is an option only for patients with well-compensated liver disease. Child-Turcotte-Pugh class A cirrhotic patients may be candidates for nontransplant resections, although an elevated serum bilirubin level or evidence of portal hypertension (varices, ascites, splenomegaly, or a platelet count $<100 \times 10^9$/L) predict an increased risk of liver failure and decreased survival rate following resection [9]. Liver transplantation has the advantage of treating the underlying cirrhosis, liver failure, and the carcinoma. Transplantation is therefore the preferred strategy in patients with advanced liver disease and portal hypertension. While lifelong immunosuppression is required following liver transplantation, the risk of recurrence is low if patients are carefully selected according to the Milan criteria (one tumor <5 cm or up to three tumors each <3 cm) [10]. Radiofrequency ablation is typically offered to patients who are not candidates for surgical resection because of liver failure or portal hypertension and who are not candidates for liver transplantation because of age or comorbid conditions. Radiofrequency ablation can also be used as a temporizing measure to prevent tumor growth beyond acceptable limits for liver transplantation [11]. Radiofrequency ablation is preferred to percutaneous ethanol injection because it requires fewer sessions; it results in better local control and has been shown to result in improved recurrence-free survival in randomized controlled trials [4]. Due to the complexity of this management algorithm, the decision to perform surgery, liver transplantation, or radiofrequency ablation is best done on a case-by-case basis by a multidisciplinary group [4].

The majority of recurrences following curative-intent nontransplant surgery present within the remnant liver, either due to intrahepatic metastases or because of the development of new tumors in the cirrhotic liver. If recurrence is detected at an early stage, it may be possible to offer further therapy with curative intent. In a patient with cirrhotic liver, a second surgical resection is seldom an option, although it is the preferred treatment option in a noncirrhotic patient [12]. Salvage liver transplantation can be offered [13, 14]. However, tumors which are large, high-grade, or with microvascular invasion are at high risk for recurrence following salvage transplant [15]. Radiofrequency ablation remains a good option for patients with recurrent hepatocellular carcinoma but it is most successful for tumors <2 cm [16, 17]. If there is progression to an intermediate stage (Barcelona Clinic Liver Cancer Stage B) without portal vein thrombosis, transarterial

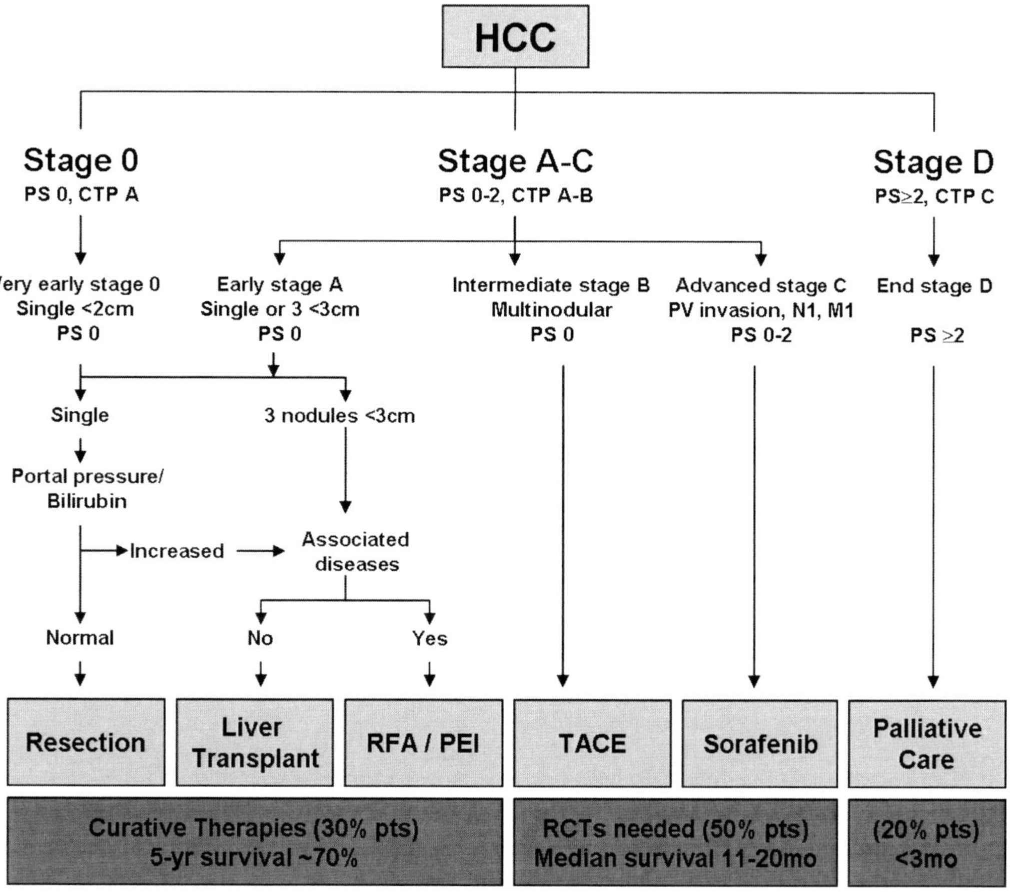

HCC

Stage 0
PS 0, CTP A

Stage A-C
PS 0-2, CTP A-B

Stage D
PS≥2, CTP C

Very early stage 0
Single <2cm
PS 0

Early stage A
Single or 3 <3cm
PS 0

Intermediate stage B
Multinodular
PS 0

Advanced stage C
PV invasion, N1, M1
PS 0-2

End stage D
PS ≥2

Single

3 nodules <3cm

Portal pressure/
Bilirubin

Increased

Associated diseases

Normal

No

Yes

Resection | Liver Transplant | RFA / PEI | TACE | Sorafenib | Palliative Care

Curative Therapies (30% pts)
5-yr survival ~70%

RCTs needed (50% pts)
Median survival 11-20mo

(20% pts)
<3mo

Fig. 31.1 Barcelona clinic liver cancer (BCLC) staging system for hepatocellular carcinoma (adapted from Reference [8]). *HCC* hepatocellular carcinoma; *PS* performance status; *CTP* Child-Turcotte-Pugh classification; *RFA* radiofrequency ablation; *PEI* percutaneous ethanol injection; *TACE* transarterial chemoembolization; *RCT* randomized clinical trials; *PV* portal vein; *pts* patients

chemoembolization is an option. A recent meta-analysis of randomized studies has shown that transarterial chemoembolization provides a survival benefit in carefully selected patients, with median survival duration increasing from about 16 months in patients managed with best supportive care to about 20 months in patients treated with transarterial chemoembolization [18]. If there is a recurrence with unfavorable tumor characteristics (e.g., portal vein invasion, metastasis, or lymph node involvement), palliative sorafenib can be offered for Barcelona Clinic Liver Cancer Stage C disease (Fig. 31.1). In a multicenter, randomized, controlled trial, which included many patients who had failed previous curative-intent therapies, this new drug was recently shown to improve median survival duration from 7.9 months (placebo arm) to 10.7 months (sorafenib arm) [19].

The patient who has undergone surgical resection requires close follow-up, not only to watch for recurrence, but also to monitor for development of other complications of cirrhosis (Table 31.1). It is our practice to perform laboratory tests including a complete blood count, liver function tests (serum alanine aminotransferase, aspartate aminotransferase, and alkaline leukocyte phosphatase, bilirubin, and albumin levels, prothrombin time international normalized ratio) plus serum electrolyte and creatinine levels at least monthly for the first 3 months, then every 3 months for the first year and every 6 months thereafter. Patients who require diuretics should have monthly monitoring of serum electrolyte and creatinine levels. The serum alpha-fetoprotein level is followed every 3 months for 3 years and then every 6 months thereafter, although this has been shown to be most useful if the alpha fetoprotein level was elevated preoperatively [20]. Patients are more likely to have an early recurrence within 1 year of surgery if the serum alpha fetoprotein level was elevated prior to surgery (>100 ng/mL) and if it does not normalize following resection [21]. At our institution, patients have regular follow-up visits not only with a hepatobiliary surgeon but also with a hepatologist to address other problems related to their liver disease, including screening for varices and, in patients infected with hepatitis B virus or hepatitis C virus, regular monitoring of viral load and supervision of antiviral therapy [22, 23].

Recurrence of hepatocellular carcinoma occurs in approximately 70% of patients within 5 years of surgical resection [4]. Since more than half of patients experience

Table 31.1 Surveillance of patients with hepatocellular carcinoma following liver resection: University of Calgary, Calgary, Alberta, Canada

	Year					
Modality	1	2	3	4	5	>5
Office visit	4	4	2	2	2	2
CBC, LFTs[a]	6	4	2	2	2	2
Serum alpha-fetoprotein level	4	4	2	2	2	2
US/CEUS	2	2	2	1	1	1
Abdominal CT or MRI	2	2	2	1	1	1

The serum alpha-fetoprotein level is most useful if it was elevated before surgery

The number in each cell indicates the number of times a particular modality is recommended during a particular posttreatment year

CBC complete blood count; *LFTs* liver function tests; *US* ultrasound examination; *CEUS* contrast enhanced ultrasound examination; *CT* computerized tomography; *MRI* magnetic resonance imaging

[a]LFTs = serum alanine aminotransferase, aspartate aminotransferase, and alkaline leukocyte phosphatase levels; serum Na, K, Cl, CO_2, creatinine levels

recurrence within 3 years of surgery [9], we feel that it makes sense to perform surveillance tests often for 3 years after surgical resection in an effort to detect recurrence at an early and potentially more treatable stage. As all cirrhotic patients require an ultrasound examination every 6 months (as surveillance for hepatocellular carcinoma), we recommend enhanced surveillance in patients treated with curative-intent resection of any sort. This involves both cross-sectional imaging (either CT or MRI) alternating with abdominal ultrasound examination every 3 months during the first three postoperative years. Thereafter, we recommend alternating imaging modalities every 6 months. After 5 years, patients may return to regular surveillance with abdominal ultrasound examinations every 6 months. At our institution, ultrasonographers have the ability to perform a contrast-enhanced ultrasound scan if a suspicious nodule is found on the non-enhanced scan of the liver. This improves the diagnostic accuracy of ultrasound and improves efficiency because the patient does not need to return for a contrast study at a later date [24]. Unfortunately, contrast-enhanced ultrasound in Canada is currently available in only two centers, Calgary and Toronto.

Fibrolamellar hepatocellular carcinoma, which typically occurs in young patients with noncirrhotic livers, represents a special situation. Because lymph nodes are more frequently involved in this subtype of hepatocellular carcinoma [25], it may be argued that a lymph node dissection should accompany a liver resection. Unlike other variants of hepatocellular carcinoma, because of the absence of cirrhosis, the remainder of the liver is not at as high a risk of *de novo* tumor formation. Moreover, the natural history of these tumors is more protracted, with recurrences often occurring years after resection [25]. Therefore, if a patient is encountered with a fibrolamellar variant of hepatocellular carcinoma, the more frequent and intensive follow-up testing that is typical in the first 3 years after resection for other variants of hepatocellular carcinoma is less important. On the other hand, we feel that surveillance should continue for up to 10 years after resection, due to the propensity for late recurrence.

Although curative-intent percutaneous radiofrequency ablation can be offered to patients with hepatocellular carcinoma up to 5 cm in size, it is most effective for smaller tumors. A recent study of radiofrequency ablation demonstrated complete response in 97% of lesions ≤2 cm with a median follow-up duration of 31 months, and a 5-year survival rate of 68.5% in 100 patients who would have been surgical resection candidates [17]. A randomized controlled trial from China of radiofrequency ablation vs. surgery for single tumors <5 cm demonstrated comparable 4-year survival in the two groups (67% vs. 64%) [26]. Other data suggest that recurrence rates are higher following radiofrequency ablation than resection. A recent review of the Japanese nationwide hepatocellular carcinoma database of 17,149 patients found that 2-year recurrence rates were lower after surgery (35.5%) than after radiofrequency ablation (55.4%) and percutaneous ethanol injection (73.3%), although overall survival duration was not different among these groups [27]. A recent analysis confirmed that tumor size was the only independent risk factor for recurrence following radiofrequency ablation, with decreased efficacy and higher local recurrence rates for tumors >2.5 cm [16]. In addition to recurrence at the ablation site and elsewhere within the cirrhotic liver, patients have about a 1% chance of tumor seeding in the peritoneum or abdominal wall. This is felt to be related to the procedure itself [28]. Therefore, it is our practice to burn the needle-tract at the liver capsule while withdrawing the probe, to prevent bleeding and tumor seeding.

We recommend a contrast-enhanced study (magnetic resonance imaging, computed tomography, or contrast-enhanced ultrasonography) 1 month following radiofrequency ablation to assess response to the procedure and to confirm eradication of the tumor. We find MRI with subtraction images to be particularly useful to confirm complete ablation or to monitor for local recurrence of hepatocellular carcinoma at the site of thermal injury. Specifically, subtraction images in which precontrast images are subtracted from postcontrast (enhanced) images can better demonstrate areas of enhancement. Such images have been shown to be useful in assessing hepatic lesions [29]. In our experience, subtraction images greatly improve the ability to determine the extent of thermal injury and the characteristics of enhancement around ablation beds. Therefore, magnetic resonance imaging clearly defines the completeness of necrosis and the extent of the necrotic injury. At our center, patients then undergo surveillance

Table 31.2 Surveillance of patients with hepatocellular carcinoma following curative-intent radiofrequency ablation: University of Calgary, Calgary, Alberta, Canada

	Year					
Modality	1	2	3	4	5	>5
Office visit	4	4	2	2	2	2
CBC, LFTs*	6	4	2	2	2	2
Serum alpha-fetoprotein level	4	4	2	2	2	2
US/CEUS*	2	2	2	1	1	1
CT/MRI*	2	2	2	1	1	1

The serum alpha-fetoprotein level is most useful if it was elevated before radiofrequency ablation

The number in each cell indicates the number of times a particular modality is recommended during a particular posttreatment year

CBC complete blood count; *LFTs* liver function tests; *US* ultrasound examination; *CEUS* contrast enhanced ultrasound examination; *CT* computerized tomography; *MRI* magnetic resonance imaging

*Following radiofrequency ablation, we also obtain a CEUS, MRI, or CT 1 month after the ablation to confirm eradication of the hepatocellular carcinoma. Thereafter, with radiofrequency ablation, and following surgery, patients undergo enhanced surveillance for the first 3 years with cross-sectional imaging (CT or MRI), alternating with US/CEUS every 3 months. Thereafter, if there is no evident tumor, patients return to surveillance every 6 months with alternating CT or MRI and US/CEUS. MRI is our preferred cross-sectional imaging modality after radiofrequency ablation

*LFTs=serum alanine aminotransferase, aspartate aminotransferase, and alkaline leukocyte phosphatase levels; serum Na, K, Cl, CO_2, creatinine levels

testing much like patients who have received conventional surgical resection (Table 31.2), except that magnetic resonance imaging is the main cross-sectional imaging modality used.

Recurrence following radiofrequency ablation can often be managed with a repeat radiofrequency ablation procedure. At our center, percutaneous ethanol injection is reserved for patients with hepatocellular carcinoma near major blood vessels, where the tumor cannot be completely ablated by radiofrequency ablation due to a "heat-sink" effect (heat dissipation secondary to the flow of cooler blood in adjacent major vessels). Patients with multifocal recurrence may be candidates for transarterial chemoembolization. There is emerging evidence that transarterial chemoembolization can be combined with radiofrequency ablation to improve the efficacy of the ablation and to decrease recurrence rates [30]. Patients who fail radiofrequency ablation and develop portal vein invasion or distant metastases can be offered sorafenib as a palliative treatment. Sorafenib is now also being evaluated as adjuvant therapy in a placebo-controlled trial of patients at high risk of recurrence following radiofrequency ablation or surgical resection (sponsored by Bayer Pharmaceutical; clinicaltrials.gov NCT00692770).

Outcomes of liver transplantation were greatly improved when programs began adhering to the Milan criteria (1 tumor <5 cm or 3 tumors <3 cm each), with recurrence rates of approximately 25% and 5-year survival rates exceeding 70% [15]. The total number and size of lesions prior to liver transplantation are surrogate markers for microvascular invasion, which is one of the most important predictors of recurrence following liver transplantation [15]. Since the original publication of the Milan criteria [10], other groups have attempted to expand these criteria in an attempt to offer liver transplantation to more patients with hepatocellular carcinoma. The University of California San Francisco has reported excellent outcomes after transplanting patients with a single tumor nodule up to 6.5 cm, or up to three tumors (largest <4.5 cm), with the sum of the total tumor diameters <8 cm [31]. In Alberta, we have transplanted many patients beyond the Milan criteria and have documented excellent outcomes in these patients using sirolimus-based immunosuppression following liver transplantation [32]. We noted recurrence in 2 of 34 transplanted patients when the Milan criteria were respected (6%) and 6 of 36 who were beyond the Milan criteria (17%), and the 4-year tumor-free survival duration was the same in the two groups (73% vs. 75%) [32]. A recent analysis from the University of Alberta has shown that a total tumor volume of >115 cm^3 is more predictive of recurrence than the Milan and UCSF criteria [33]. It is now recognized that mTOR inhibitors, like sirolimus, may be effective in the management of hepatocellular carcinoma [34]. Whether immunosuppression based on an mTOR inhibitor (sirolimus) is better than immunosuppression based on a calcineurin inhibitor (cyclosporine or tacrolimus) for decreasing the risk of recurrence following liver transplantation is now the subject of a multicenter international randomized clinical trial (clinicaltrials.gov NCT00355862). A recent analysis of 6,478 adult liver transplantation recipients registered in the Scientific Registry of Transplant Recipients Database determined that both a total tumor volume >115 cm^3 and serum alpha-fetoprotein level >400 ng/mL were most predictive of tumor recurrence following liver transplantation [35]. Therefore, in Alberta, patients must now have a total tumor volume <115 cm^3 and an AFP <400 ng/mL to be eligible for liver transplantation.

Monitoring for recurrence following liver transplantation is influenced by the fact that recurrences tend to occur at distant sites with disseminated disease, which is believed to be related to the patient's immunosuppressed state. In general, survival duration following recurrence of hepatocellular carcinoma after liver transplantation is poor, with median survival duration of 23 months in Alberta [32]. Following transplantation, patients have frequent blood tests and clinic appointments to monitor their liver allograft function and to monitor for complications of immunosuppression (Table 31.3). It is our practice to survey for recurrence following liver transplantation with alpha-fetoprotein levels and abdominal ultrasonography every 3 months for

Table 31.3 Surveillance of patients with hepatocellular carcinoma following liver transplantation: University of Calgary, Calgary, Alberta, Canada

	Year					
Modality	1	2	3	4	5	>5
Office visit	≥6	4	2	2	2	1
CBC, LFTs	≥24	12	12	12	12	6
Serum alpha-fetoprotein level	4	4	4	4	4	2
US/CEUS	4	4	2	2	2	2

The serum alpha-fetoprotein level is most useful if it was elevated before liver transplantation

The number in each cell indicates the number of times a particular modality is recommended during a particular posttreatment year

CBC complete blood count; *LFTs* liver function tests; *US* ultrasound examination; *CEUS* contrast enhanced ultrasound examination; *CT* computerized tomography; *MRI* magnetic resonance imaging

[a]Following liver transplantation, other imaging tests are performed only if there is a clinical suspicion of intrahepatic recurrence or distant metastasis

[b]LFTs = serum alanine aminotransferase, aspartate aminotransferase, and alkaline leukocyte phosphatase levels; serum Na, K, Cl, CO_2, creatinine levels

Table 31.4 Surveillance of patients with extrahepatic cholangiocarcinoma following resection: University of Calgary, Calgary, Alberta, Canada

	Year					
Modality	1	2	3	4	5	>5
Office visit	4	4	4	2	2	2
CBC, LFTs[*]	4	4	4	2	2	2
Serum CA19-9 and CEA levels	4	4	2	2	2	2

The number in each cell indicates the number of times a particular modality is recommended during a particular posttreatment year

CBC complete blood count; *LFTs* liver function tests; *CA19-9* carbohydrate antigen 19-9; *CEA* carcinoembryonic antigen; *CT* computerized tomography

[*]For extrahepatic cholangiocarcinoma, CT scans are done to investigate changes in tumor markers or LFTs, or if a patient requests a more intensive follow-up. In the latter instance, the schedule for CT examinations is similar to that for intrahepatic cholangiocarcinoma.

[*]LFTs = serum alanine aminotransferase, aspartate aminotransferase, and alkaline leukocyte phosphatase levels; serum Na, K, Cl, CO_2, creatinine levels

the first 2 years, and then every 6 months thereafter. If patients have unexplained weight loss, fever, dyspnea, or bone pain, these symptoms are investigated with conventional imaging modalities to look for evidence of metastatic recurrent hepatocellular carcinoma. Treatment options for patients with recurrent hepatocellular carcinoma after liver transplantation are limited. If the patient is not already taking sirolimus, switch to an mTOR inhibitor may theoretically be helpful [34]. The role of sorafenib following transplantation has not been clearly defined, but a recent multicenter experience from liver transplantation programs in France suggests there may be a role for this drug in patients with recurrent hepatocellular carcinoma after transplantation [36].

Bile Duct Cancer

Cholangiocarcinoma arises from the biliary ductal epithelium. There are two main variants: intrahepatic cholangiocarcinoma, which occurs within the liver, and extrahepatic cholangiocarcinoma, the more common variant, which arises in the extrahepatic biliary tree. Distal (extrahepatic) cholangiocarcinoma is not included in this discussion, as the postresection surveillance is more consistent with the principles of care for other periampullary lesions. The clinical behavior and the treatments of intrahepatic cholangiocarcinoma and extrahepatic cholangiocarcinoma vary. Therefore, the considerations for postoperative surveillance also differ.

At our institution, the treatment of choice for extrahepatic cholangiocarcinoma is resection alone. This involves a resection of the involved bile ducts and all periportal lymph nodes [37, 38]. Construction of a subfascial jejunostomy for future retrograde access of the biliary tree [39] is also frequently performed. Negative margins have been reported to confer an improved survival [38, 40]. Intraoperative frozen sections of margins are therefore important. If necessary, a liver resection (frequently including the caudate lobe) is done to ensure an R0 resection. This aggressive approach has been reported to enhance the likelihood of long-term disease control [38]. We do not routinely administer adjuvant chemotherapy because there is no convincing data that it is advantageous. The propensity for tumors to recur locally provides some rationale for adjuvant radiation [41]. However, patient survival does not seem to be improved in those who receive adjuvant chemotherapy plus radiation [42]. Therefore, we do not typically offer radiation to our patients. Recently, it has been reported that tumors at higher risk for recurrence can benefit from adjuvant chemotherapy plus radiation [43], which may prompt reconsideration of this practice.

Our surveillance strategy for resected extrahepatic cholangiocarcinoma was devised based on patterns of recurrence and the likelihood of salvage following recurrence (Table 31.4). It is known that the majority of recurrences appear at the resection line, in the liver, and in periportal lymph nodes, although up to 25–40% appear in extrahepatic sites such as the peritoneum, lungs, and bone [38, 44, 45]. The median time to recurrence is 13–31 months. Most recurrences appear in the first 3 years. At 5 years, 29–38% are still alive, but recurrences still appear at a high rate even after 5 years [38, 40, 41, 45–48]. If the cancer recurs, it is very unlikely that re-resection will be possible, although this has been reported for isolated hepatic recurrences remote from the hilum [45] and for recurrent mid-duct tumors [48]. If the recurrence is unresectable, palliative chemotherapy (including various combinations of gemcitabine, cisplatin, and capecitabine) has been used, with response rates in phase II trials ranging from 25 to 34% [49, 50]. While reported survival rates in these patients are encouraging, there is no evidence that earlier identification of recurrent disease and administration of chemotherapy is associated with a survival advantage.

Based on the above observations on extrahepatic cholangiocarcinoma, close surveillance is not likely to alter outcomes. On the other hand, any patient who has undergone resection and biliary reconstruction is susceptible to biliary complications, including biliary strictures and ascending cholangitis. Therefore, patients are followed for signs of obstructive cholestasis and/or cholangitis, so that timely biliary decompression may be achieved should a stricture (benign or malignant) appear. Liver enzymes and bilirubin are followed closely. Alkaline phosphatase levels are almost always elevated after biliary reconstruction, but sudden increases may signal the development of a stricture. Serum CA19-9 and carcinoembryonic antigen levels complement liver function tests, since abrupt elevations help to distinguish benign from malignant causes of new onset biliary obstruction. Surveillance is most intensive in the first 3 years, but should continue indefinitely. Further investigations are done as clinically indicated.

Radiologic surveillance for resected extrahepatic cholangiocarcinoma is not well standardized at our institution. There is little rationale to do routine computed tomography, since early (local) recurrence is not easily seen and since the probability of salvage is low. Moreover, in the case of local recurrence, we have found that changes in liver function tests or serum tumor marker levels almost always precede anatomical changes. On the other hand, patients who have undergone resection of a bile duct cancer are anxious about recurrence and desire early diagnosis for the purpose of prognostication. This spurs the clinician to follow up with radiologic investigations. If radiologic surveillance is used for this reason, we usually recommend an abdominal computed tomography alone. It may be argued that a more comprehensive evaluation for recurrent disease would involve a chest computed tomography or bone scans, but such testing can become prohibitively expensive with little evidence of benefit.

In Alberta, intrahepatic cholangiocarcinoma is very rare; only two to four cases are encountered annually by our group. As with extrahepatic cholangiocarcinoma, resection is the only potentially curative treatment. This involves liver resection, although bile duct resection is also performed if the tumor encroaches on the main bile ducts. The role of lymph node dissection is not well defined. In several series, a negative margin has been shown to impart a better prognosis [51, 52]. However, in a recent series, outcomes were not found to be adversely affected by positive margins [53]. This may be due to an underlying multicentric defect in the bile ducts such as biliary papillomatosis [54], leading to a high risk of recurrence in the remnant liver. Despite this controversy, our practice is to resect in an effort to obtain a negative margin (R0 status). Neither adjuvant chemotherapy nor radiation is routinely offered.

Table 31.5 Surveillance of patients with intrahepatic cholangiocarcinoma following resection: University of Calgary, Calgary, Alberta, Canada

	Year					
Modality	1	2	3	4	5	>5
Office visit	4	4	4	2	2	2
CBC, LFTs[a]	4	4	4	2	2	2
Serum CA19-9 and CEA levels	4	4	2	2	2	2
Abdominal CT/MRI	2	2	2	1	1	1

The number in each cell indicates the number of times a particular modality is recommended during a particular posttreatment year

CBC complete blood count; *LFTs* liver function tests; *US* ultrasound examination; *CT* computerized tomography; *MRI* magnetic resonance imaging

[a]LFTs = serum alanine aminotransferase, aspartate aminotransferase, and alkaline leukocyte phosphatase levels; serum Na, K, Cl, CO_2, creatinine levels

It has been suggested that, because of a more favorable tumor location, the prognosis for intrahepatic cholangiocarcinoma is better than for extrahepatic cholangiocarcinoma [46, 53]. While the more favorable tumor location does enhance the likelihood of successful resection, the prognosis is still dismal for patients with intrahepatic cholangiocarcinoma even after curative-intent resection. Aggregate numbers do not suggest that survival is much better than for extrahepatic cholangiocarcinoma. The median disease-free survival duration is 10–12 months [52, 53]. Most recurrences appear in the liver, and the remainder appears at distant sites such as peritoneum, bone, and lung [51–53, 55]. The survival rates at 5 years are 23–29% and the median survival duration is 31–37 months [52, 53, 55].

Postresection surveillance differs significantly from that of intrahepatic cholangiocarcinoma because salvage hepatectomy may be possible after resection of an intrahepatic cholangiocarcinoma [56]. Therefore, there is a better rationale for radiologic surveillance (Table 31.5). This is accomplished most cost-effectively with abdominal computed tomography scans. Only if a resectable recurrence is seen or if symptoms arise would more intensive radiologic testing (e.g., chest computed tomography, bone scan) be indicated. Serum CA19-9 and carcinoembryonic antigen levels, as well as liver function tests, are done during intervals between computed tomography scans and in parallel with computed tomography scans. Because a bile duct reconstruction is often not required to resect intrahepatic cholangiocarcinoma, it is not as critical to evaluate for obstructive cholestasis, although this still remains part of our routine evaluation. As with extrahepatic cholangiocarcinoma, most recurrences appear in the first 3 years after initial resection, but some still appear after 5 years. Therefore, surveillance should be most intensive in the first 3 years, but should continue indefinitely.

Transplantation for Cholangiocarcinoma

Liver transplantation for cholangiocarcinoma is generally avoided, as the recurrence rate is very high. However, in recent years, some centers have reported series of highly selected patients who have received neoadjuvant radiation and chemotherapy, followed by liver transplantation. These highly selected patients have 5-year survival rates of 31–76% [44, 57]. Patients with recurrent cholangiocarcinoma are not frequently included in reported transplantation series. Therefore, transplantation cannot be considered a viable salvage strategy for recurrent bile duct cancer at this time. Since liver transplantation is not offered to patients with cholangiocarcinoma in Alberta, we have not devised a surveillance strategy for transplant patients in this context. Rather, if an individual does pursue a liver transplantation at another center, we defer to the follow-up strategies employed by that center.

Gallbladder Carcinoma

In Southern Alberta, about 60 cases of gallbladder cancer are encountered annually. Resection is possible only in a minority. The greatest potential for cure is when early stage disease is diagnosed incidentally following a cholecystectomy for presumed benign disease. The standard resection consists of a resection of the gallbladder (if still present), segments IV and V of the liver, and periportal lymph nodes. If the cystic duct margin is positive, the bile duct is resected [58]. More extensive liver resections are indicated when disease extends further into the liver substance [59]. For gallbladder cancer, positive margins portend a recurrence. Therefore, our group very aggressively strives to achieve a negative margin. If the gallbladder cancer was discovered incidentally following a laparoscopic cholecystectomy and further surgery is warranted, we routinely excise port sites, due to the high incidence of recurrence at port sites [60]. While there are cytotoxic agents with some activity against gallbladder carcinoma [49], there are no convincing data that demonstrate a survival advantage with adjuvant chemotherapy. Therefore, this is not routinely offered following resection. Given the propensity of gallbladder cancer to recur at distant sites [41, 61], we feel that there is no rationale to administer adjuvant radiation.

The tumor biology of gallbladder carcinoma (and its attendant clinical behavior) contrasts starkly with that of bile duct cancer. The median survival duration is 17–34 months and the 5-year survival rate after aggressive surgery is 35–42% [59, 61, 62]. The recurrence rate increases dramatically with more advanced disease, and the survival rate drops proportionately. Overall, the median time to recurrence is 10–18 months [41, 62–64]. Only about 15–35% recur locoregionally; most recur at distant sites or at multiple sites [41, 61]. Therefore, re-resection to salvage a recurrence is virtually impossible, although there have been reports of salvage surgery after a simple cholecystectomy [65].

Given that the possibility of performing repeat surgery for potential cure is remote, radiologic surveillance is of secondary importance. Rather, the priority is to follow the patient clinically, watching for new constitutional symptoms, changes in performance status, and signs of biliary obstruction. Therefore, the standard follow-up would consist of periodic office visits and liver function tests, as well as serum tumor marker levels (Table 31.6). Worrisome findings would prompt further investigation to more definitively identify recurrent disease and initiate palliative treatment. Of course, as in bile duct cancer, many patients desire more detailed follow-up, for reassurance or prognostication. If that is the case, then an abdominal CT may be beneficial.

Table 31.6 Surveillance of patients with gallbladder carcinoma following resection: University of Calgary, Calgary, Alberta, Canada

	Year					
	1	2	3	4	5	>5
Office visit	4	4	4	2	2	2
CBC, LFTs[a]	4	4	4	2	2	2
Serum CA19-9 and CEA levels	4	4	4	2	2	2

The number in each cell indicates the number of times a particular modality is recommended during a particular posttreatment year

CBC complete blood count; *LFTs* liver function tests; *CA19-9* carbohydrate antigen 19-9; *CEA* carcinoembryonic antigen; *CT* computerized tomography; *MRI* magnetic resonance imaging

[a]LFTs = serum alanine aminotransferase, aspartate aminotransferase, and alkaline leukocyte phosphatase levels; serum Na, K, Cl, CO_2, creatinine levels

References

1. Parkin DM, Bray F, Ferlay J, Pisani P. Global cancer statistics, 2002. CA Cancer J Clin. 2005;55:74–108.
2. Ries L, Melbert D, Krapcho M, et al. SEER Cancer Statistics Review, 1975–2005, National Cancer Institute. 2008; http://seer.cancer.gov/csr/1975_2005, based on November 2007 SEER data submission, posted to the SEER web site; 2008.
3. Dixon E, Bathe O, McKay A, et al. A population based review of the outcomes following hepatic resection in a Canadian health region. Can J Surg. 2009;52:12–7.
4. Bruix J, Sherman M. Practice Guidelines Committee AAftSoLD. Management of hepatocellular carcinoma. Hepatology. 2005;42:1208–36.
5. DiBisceglie A, Lyra A, Schwartz M, et al. Hepatitis C-related hepatocellular carcinoma in the United States: influence of ethnic status. Am J Gastroenterol. 2003;98:2060–3.

6. Okuda K, Ohtsuki T, Obata H, et al. Natural history of hepatocellular carcinoma and prognosis in relation to treatment. Cancer. 1985;56:918–28.
7. Forner A, Vilana R, Ayuso C, et al. Diagnosis of hepatic nodules 20 mm or smaller in cirrhosis: prospective validation of the noninvasive diagnostic criteria for hepatocellular carcinoma. Hepatology. 2008;47:97–104.
8. Llovet J, DiBisceglie A, Bruix J, et al. Design and endpoints of clinical trials in hepatocellular carcinoma. J Natl Cancer Inst. 2008;100:698–711.
9. Llovet J, Fuster J, Bruix J. Intention-to-treat analysis of surgical treatment for early hepatocellular carcinoma: resection versus transplantation. Hepatology. 1999;30:1434–40.
10. Mazzaferro V, Regalia E, Montalto F, et al. Liver transplantation for the treatment of small hepatocellular carcinomas in patients with cirrhosis. N Engl J Med. 1996;334:693–9.
11. Heckman JT, Devera MB, Marsh JW, et al. Bridging locoregional therapy for hepatocellular carcinoma prior to liver transplantation. Ann Surg Oncol. 2008;15:3169–77.
12. Nakajima Y, Ko S, Kanamura T, et al. Repeat liver resection for hepatocellular carcinoma. J Am Coll Surg. 2001;192:339–44.
13. Vennarecci G, Ettorre G, Antonini M, et al. First-line liver resection and salvage liver transplantation are increasing therapeutic strategies for patients with hepatocellular carcinoma and child a cirrhosis. Transplant Proc. 2007;39:1857–60.
14. Ng K, Lo C, Liu C, Poon R, Chan S, Fan S. Survival analysis of patients with transplantable recurrent hepatocellular carcinoma: implications for salvage liver transplant. Arch Surg. 2008;143: 68–74.
15. Mazzaferro V. Results of liver transplantation: with or without Milan criteria? Liver Transpl. 2007;13(11Suppl 2):S44–7.
16. Lam V, Ng K, Chok K, et al. Risk factors and prognostic factors of local recurrence after radiofrequency ablation of hepatocellular carcinoma. J Am Coll Surg. 2008;207:20–9.
17. Livraghi T, Meloni F, DiStasi M, et al. Sustained complete response and complications rates after radiofrequency ablation of very early hepatocellular carcinoma in cirrhosis: is resection still the treatment of choice? Hepatology. 2008;47:82–9.
18. Marelli L, Stigliano R, Triantos C, et al. Transarterial therapy for hepatocellular carcinoma: which technique is more effective? A systematic review of cohort and randomized studies. Cardiovasc Intervent Radiol. 2007;30:6–25.
19. Llovet J, Ricci S, Mazzaferro V, et al. Sorafenib in advanced hepatocellular carcinoma. N Engl J Med. 2008;359:378–90.
20. Koh T, Taniguchi H, Katoh H, Kunishima S, Yamaguchi A, Yamagishi H. Are both PIVKA-II and alpha-fetoprotein necessary in follow-up management after hepatic resection for hepatocellular carcinoma? Hepatogastroenterology. 2002;49:1615–8.
21. Shirabe K, Takenaka K, Gion T, Shimada M, Fujiwara Y, Sugimachi K. Significance of alpha-fetoprotein levels for detection of early recurrence of hepatocellular carcinoma after hepatic resection. J Surg Oncol. 1997;64:143–6.
22. Sherman M, Shafran S, Burak K, et al. Management of chronic hepatitis B: consensus guidelines. Can J Gastroenterol. 2007; 21(Suppl C):5C–24C.
23. Sherman M, Shafran S, Burak K, et al. Management of chronic hepatitis C: consensus guidelines. Can J Gastroenterol. 2007;21 (Suppl C):25C–34C.
24. Wilson S, Jang H, Kim T, Burns P. Diagnosis of focal liver masses on ultrasonography: comparison of unenhanced and contrast-enhanced scans. J Ultrasound Med. 2007;26:775–87.
25. Kakar S, Burgart LJ, Batts KP, Garcia J, Jain D, Ferrell LD. Clinicopathologic features and survival in fibrolamellar carcinoma: comparison with conventional hepatocellular carcinoma with and without cirrhosis. Mod Pathol. 2005;18:1417–23.
26. Chen M, Li J, Zheng Y, et al. A prospective randomized trial comparing percutaneous local ablative therapy and partial hepatectomy for small hepatocellular carcinoma. Ann Surg. 2006; 243:321–8.
27. Hasegawa K, Makuuchi M, Takayama T, et al. Surgical resection vs. percutaneous ablation for hepatocellular carcinoma: a preliminary report of the Japanese nationwide survey. J Hepatol. 2008;49:589–94.
28. Stigliano R, Marelli L, Yu D, Davies N, Patch D, Burroughs A. Seeding following percutaneous diagnostic and therapeutic approaches for hepatocellular carcinoma. What is the risk and the outcome? Seeding risk for percutaneous approach of HCC. Cancer Treat Rev. 2007;33:437–47.
29. Yu H, Cheng J, Lai K, et al. Factors for early tumor recurrence of single small hepatocellular carcinoma after percutaneous radiofrequency ablation therapy. World J Gastroenterol. 2005;11:1439–44.
30. Yang P, Liang M, Zhang Y, Shen B. Clinical application of a combination therapy of lentinan, multi-electrode RFA and TACE in HCC. Adv Ther. 2008;25:787–94.
31. Yao F, Ferrell L, Bass N, et al. Liver transplantation for hepatocellular carcinoma: expansion of the tumor size limits does not adversely impact survival. Hepatology. 2001;33:1394–403.
32. Toso C, Meeberg G, Bigam D, et al. De novo sirolimus-based immunosuppression after liver transplantation for hepatocellular carcinoma: long-term outcomes and side effects. Transplantation. 2007;83:1162–8.
33. Toso C, Trotter J, Wei A, et al. Total tumor volume predicts risk of recurrence following liver transplantation in patients with hepatocellular carcinoma. Liver Transpl. 2008;14:1107–15.
34. Villanueva A, Chiang D, Newell P, et al. Pivotal role of mTOR signaling in hepatocellular carcinoma. Gastroenterology. 2008;135(6):1972–83. Epub 2008 Aug 20, e1-e11, ahead of print.
35. Toso C, Asthana S, Bigam D, Shapiro A, Kneteman N. Reassessing selection criteria prior to liver transplantation for hepatocellular carcinoma with the scientific registry of transplant recipients database. Hepatology. 2009;49:832–8.
36. Dharancy S, Romano O, Lorho R, et al. Tolerability and efficacy of sorafenib in recurrent hepatocellular carcinoma after liver transplantation: a case-control study. Hepatology. 2008;48(4 Suppl):310A.
37. Kitagawa Y, Nagino M, Kamiya J, et al. Lymph node metastasis from hilar cholangiocarcinoma: audit of 110 patients who underwent regional and paraaortic node dissection. Ann Surg. 2001;233:385–92.
38. Ito F, Agni R, Rettammel RJ, et al. Resection of hilar cholangiocarcinoma: concomitant liver resection decreases hepatic recurrence. Ann Surg. 2008;248:273–9.
39. Bathe OF, Pacheco JT, Ossi PB, et al. A subcutaneous or subfascial jejunostomy is beneficial in the surgical management of extrahepatic bile duct cancers. Surgery. 2000;127:506–11.
40. Endo I, House MG, Klimstra DS, et al. Clinical significance of intraoperative bile duct margin assessment for hilar cholangiocarcinoma. Ann Surg Oncol. 2008;15:2104–12.
41. Jarnagin WR, Ruo L, Little SA, et al. Patterns of initial disease recurrence after resection of gallbladder carcinoma and hilar cholangiocarcinoma: implications for adjuvant therapeutic strategies. Cancer. 2003;98:1689–700.
42. Bathe OF, Pacheco JT, Ossi PB, et al. Management of hilar bile duct carcinoma. Hepatogastroenterology. 2001;48:1289–94.
43. Borghero Y, Crane CH, Szklaruk J, et al. Extrahepatic bile duct adenocarcinoma: patients at high-risk for local recurrence treated with surgery and adjuvant chemoradiation have an equivalent overall survival to patients with standard-risk treated with surgery alone. Ann Surg Oncol. 2008;15:3147–56.
44. Thelen A, Neuhaus P. Liver transplantation for hilar cholangiocarcinoma. J Hepatobiliary Pancreat Surg. 2007;14:469–75.
45. Huang JL, Biehl TR, Lee FT, Zimmer PW, Ryan Jr JA. Outcomes after resection of cholangiocellular carcinoma. Am J Surg. 2004;187:612–7.
46. Sano T, Shimada K, Sakamoto Y, Ojima H, Esaki M, Kosuge T. Prognosis of perihilar cholangiocarcinoma: hilar bile duct cancer

versus intrahepatic cholangiocarcinoma involving the hepatic hilus. Ann Surg Oncol. 2008;15:590–9.
47. Allen PJ, Reiner AS, Gonen M, et al. Extrahepatic cholangiocarcinoma: a comparison of patients with resected proximal and distal lesions. HPB (Oxford). 2008;10:341–6.
48. Thomas H, Heaton ND. Late recurrence after surgery for cholangiocarcinoma: implications for follow-up? Hepatobiliary Pancreat Dis Int. 2008;7:544–6.
49. Knox JJ, Hedley D, Oza A, et al. Combining gemcitabine and capecitabine in patients with advanced biliary cancer: a phase II trial. J Clin Oncol. 2005;23:2332–8.
50. Verslype C, Prenen H, Van Cutsem E. The role of chemotherapy in biliary tract carcinoma. HPB (Oxford). 2008;10:164–7.
51. Ohtsuka M, Ito H, Kimura F, et al. Results of surgical treatment for intrahepatic cholangiocarcinoma and clinicopathological factors influencing survival. Br J Surg. 2002;89:1525–31.
52. Weber SM, Jarnagin WR, Klimstra D, DeMatteo RP, Fong Y, Blumgart LH. Intrahepatic cholangiocarcinoma: resectability, recurrence pattern, and outcomes. J Am Coll Surg. 2001;193: 384–91.
53. Tamandl D, Herberger B, Gruenberger B, Puhalla H, Klinger M, Gruenberger T. Influence of hepatic resection margin on recurrence and survival in intrahepatic cholangiocarcinoma. Ann Surg Oncol. 2008; 15:2787–94.
54. Cox H, Ma M, Bridges R, et al. Well differentiated intrahepatic cholangiocarcinoma in the setting of biliary papillomatosis: a case report and review of the literature. Can J Gastroenterol. 2005; 19:731–3.
55. Miwa S, Miyagawa S, Kobayashi A, et al. Predictive factors for intrahepatic cholangiocarcinoma recurrence in the liver following surgery. J Gastroenterol. 2006;41:893–900.
56. Kurosaki I, Hatakeyama K. Repeated hepatectomy for recurrent intrahepatic cholangiocarcinoma: report of two cases. Eur J Gastroenterol Hepatol. 2005;17:125–30.
57. Heimbach JK, Gores GJ, Haddock MG, et al. Predictors of disease recurrence following neoadjuvant chemoradiotherapy and liver transplantation for unresectable perihilar cholangiocarcinoma. Transplantation. 2006;82:1703–7.
58. Nakata T, Kobayashi A, Miwa S, Soeda J, Miyagawa S. Impact of tumor spread to the cystic duct on the prognosis of patients with gallbladder carcinoma. World J Surg. 2007;31:155–61; discussion 162–53.
59. Dixon E, Vollmer Jr CM, Sahajpal A, et al. An aggressive surgical approach leads to improved survival in patients with gallbladder cancer: a 12-year study at a North American Center. Ann Surg. 2005;241:385–94.
60. Giuliante F, Ardito F, Vellone M, Clemente G, Nuzzo G. Port-sites excision for gallbladder cancer incidentally found after laparoscopic cholecystectomy. Am J Surg. 2006;191:114–6.
61. Park JS, Yoon DS, Kim KS, et al. Actual recurrence patterns and risk factors influencing recurrence after curative resection with stage II gallbladder carcinoma. J Gastrointest Surg. 2007;11: 631–7.
62. D'Angelica M, Dalal KM, Dematteo RP, Fong Y, Blumgart LH, Jarnagin WR. Analysis of the extent of resection for adenocarcinoma of the gallbladder. Ann Surg Oncol. 2008;16:806–16.
63. Duffy A, Capanu M, Abou-Alfa GK, et al. Gallbladder cancer (GBC): 10-year experience at Memorial Sloan-Kettering Cancer Centre (MSKCC). J Surg Oncol. 2008;98:485–9.
64. Chan SY, Poon RT, Lo CM, Ng KK, Fan ST. Management of carcinoma of the gallbladder: a single-institution experience in 16 years. J Surg Oncol. 2008;97:156–64.
65. Tasaki K, Yamamoto H, Watanabe K, et al. Successful treatment of lymph node metastases recurring from gallbladder cancer. J Hepatobiliary Pancreat Surg. 2003;10:113–7.

32 Colon and Rectum Carcinoma

David Y. Johnson, Shilpi Wadhwa, and Frank E. Johnson

Keywords
Colorectal cancers • Risk factors • Common • Incidence • Variability

The International Agency for Research on Cancer (IARC), a component of the World Health Organization (WHO), estimated that there were 1,023,152 new cases of colorectal cancers worldwide in 2002 [1]. The IARC also estimated that there were 528,978 deaths due to this cause in 2002 [1].

The American Cancer Society estimated that there were 153,760 new cases and 52,180 deaths due to this cause in the USA in 2007 [2]. The estimated 5-year survival rate (all races) in the USA in 2007 was 65 % for colon cancer and 66 % for rectal cancer [2]. Survival rates were adjusted for normal life expectancies and were based on cases diagnosed from 1996 to 2002 and followed through 2003.

Risk factors for this cancer include age, colorectal polyps, various known genetic syndromes (such as familial adenomatous polyposis and Lynch syndromes I and II), inflammatory bowel disease, and hamartoma syndromes (such as Peutz-Jeghers syndrome). Other risk factors include smoking, obesity, and high-fat, high-calorie, and low-fiber diets [3, 4].

D.Y. Johnson • S. Wadhwa
Department of Internal Medicine, Saint Louis University Medical Center, Saint Louis, MO, USA

F.E. Johnson (✉)
Saint Louis University Medical Center and Saint Louis Veterans Affairs Medical Center, Saint Louis, MO, USA
e-mail: frank.johnson1@va.gov

Geographic Variation Worldwide

Colorectal cancer is one of the most common cancers worldwide [5]. The majority of colorectal cancers arise in industrialized countries with more variation in incidence for colon cancer than rectal cancer worldwide. High colorectal cancer rates are found in the USA, Canada, Japan, and New Zealand; rates are low in Algeria and India. In most countries, men are more likely to develop rectal cancer than women [3]. Geographic variation in the USA is also pronounced [6].

Surveillance Strategies Proposed by Professional Organizations or National Government Agencies and Available on the Internet

National Comprehensive Cancer Network (www.nccn.org)

National Comprehensive Cancer Network (NCCN) guidelines were accessed on 1/28/12 (Tables 32.1 and 32.2). There were minor quantitative and qualitative changes compared to the guidelines accessed on 4/10/07.

American Society of Clinical Oncology (www.asco.org)

American Society of Clinical Oncology (ASCO) guidelines were accessed on 1/28/12 (Table 32.3). There were no significant changes compared to the guidelines accessed on 10/31/07.

F.E. Johnson et al. (eds.), *Patient Surveillance After Cancer Treatment*, Current Clinical Oncology,
DOI 10.1007/978-1-60327-969-7_32, © Springer Science+Business Media New York 2013

Table 32.1 Colon cancer

	Years posttreatment[a]					
	1	2	3	4	5	>5
Office visit	2–4	2–4	2	2	2	0
Serum CEA level[b]	2–4	2–4	2	2	2	0
Chest/abdominal/pelvic CT[c]	1	1	1	0–1	0–1	0
Colonoscopy[d, e]	1	0–1	0–1	0	0–1	0–1

• PET-CT scan is not routinely recommended

Obtained from NCCN (www.nccn.org) on 1/28/12
NCCN guidelines were accessed on 1/28/12. There were minor quantitative and qualitative changes compared to the guidelines accessed on 4/10/07
[a]The numbers in the table indicate the number of times the modality is recommended during the indicated year posttreatment
[b]For T2 or greater lesions, if patient is a potential candidate for further intervention
[c]For patients at high risk for recurrence (e.g., lymphatic or venous invasion by tumor, or poorly differentiated tumors)
[d]All patients with colon cancer should be counseled for family history and considered for risk assessment. Patients with suspected hereditary non-polyposis colon cancer (HNPCC), familial adenomatous polyposis (FAP), and attenuated FAP: see the NCCN Colorectal Cancer Screening Guidelines
[e]Colonoscopy in 1 year except if no preoperative colonoscopy due to obstructing lesion, colonoscopy in 3–6 months. If advanced adenoma (villous polyp, polyp >1 cm, or high grade dysplasia), repeat in 1 year. If no advanced adenoma, repeat in 3 years, then every 5 years

Table 32.2 Rectal cancer

	Years posttreatment[a]					
	1	2	3	4	5	>5
Office visit	2–4	2–4	2	2	2	0
Serum CEA level[b, c]	2–4	2–4	2	2	2	0
Chest/abdomen/pelvis CT[d]	1	1	1	0–1	0–1	0
Colonoscopy[e]	1	0–1	0–1	0	0–1	0–1
Proctoscopy[f, g]	2	2	2	2	2	0

• PET-CT scan is not routinely recommended

Obtained from NCCN (www.nccn.org) on 1/28/12
NCCN guidelines were accessed on 1/28/12. There were minor quantitative and qualitative changes compared to the guidelines accessed on 4/10/07
[a]The numbers in the table indicate the number of times the modality is recommended during the indicated year posttreatment
[b]For T2 or greater lesions
[c]If patient is a potential candidate for resection of isolated metastasis
[d]For patients at high risk for recurrence (e.g., lymphatic or venous invasion by tumor, or poorly differentiated tumors)
[e]Colonoscopy in 1 year except if no preoperative colonoscopy due to obstructing lesion, colonoscopy in 3–6 months. If advanced adenoma (villous polyp, polyp >1 cm, or high grade dysplasia), repeat in 1 year. If no advanced adenoma, repeat in 3 years, then every 5 years
[f]For patients status post low anterior resection of the rectum
[g]Patients with rectal cancer should also undergo limited endoscopic evaluation of the rectal anastomosis to identify local recurrence. Optimal timing for surveillance in not known. No specific data clearly support rigid vs. flexible proctoscopy. The utility of routine endoscopic ultrasound for early surveillance is not defined

The Society of Surgical Oncology (www.surgonc.org)

The Society of Surgical Oncology (SSO) guidelines were accessed on 1/28/12. No quantitative guidelines exist for colorectal cancer surveillance, including when first accessed on 10/31/07.

Table 32.3 Colorectal cancer

	Years posttreatment[a]					
	1	2	3	4	5	>5
Office visit	2–4	2–4	2–4	2	2	0[b]
Serum CEA level[c, d]	4	4	4	0	0	0
Chest/abdomen CT[e]	1	1	1	0	0	0
Colonoscopy[f, g]	1	0	1	0	1	0–1
Flexible proctosigmoidoscopy[h]	2	2	2	2	2	0

• Routine blood tests (i.e., CBC, LFTs), fecal occult blood testing, yearly chest X-rays are not recommended
• Use of molecular or cellular markers should not influence the surveillance strategy

Obtained from ASCO (www.asco.org) on 1/28/12
ASCO guidelines were accessed on 1/28/12. There were no significant changes compared to the guidelines accessed on 10/31/07
[a]The numbers in the table indicate the number of times the modality is recommended during the indicated year posttreatment
[b]Physician visit after 5 years at the discretion of the physician
[c]For patients with stage II or III disease if the patient is a candidate for surgery or systemic therapy
[d]Since fluorouracil-based therapy may falsely elevate CEA values, waiting until adjuvant treatment is finished to initiate surveillance is advised
[e]For patients who are at a higher risk or recurrence, and who could be candidates for curative-intent surgery. A pelvic CT scan should be considered for rectal cancer surveillance, especially for patients who have not been treated with radiotherapy
[f]All patients with colon and rectal cancer should have a colonoscopy for pre- and perioperative documentation of a cancer- and polyp-free colon. If normal at 3 years, once every 5 years thereafter
[g]For colorectal cancer patients with high-risk genetic syndromes, the physician should consider the guideline published by the American Gastroenterology Association
[h]For rectal cancer patients who have not received pelvic radiation

European Society for Medical Oncology (www.esmo.org)

European Society for Medical Oncology (ESMO) guidelines were accessed on 1/28/12 (Tables 32.4, 32.5, 32.6, and 32.7). There were minor quantitative and qualitative changes and new quantitative guidelines compared to the guidelines accessed on 10/31/07.

European Society of Surgical Oncology (www.esso-surgeonline.org)

European Society of Surgical Oncology (ESSO) guidelines were accessed on 1/28/12. No quantitative guidelines exist for colorectal cancer surveillance, including when first accessed on 10/31/07.

Table 32.4 Primary colon cancer

	Years posttreatment[a]					
	1	2	3	4	5	>5
Office visit	2–4	2–4	2–4	1–2	1–2	0
Serum CEA level	2–4	2–4	2–4	1–2	1–2	0
Colonoscopy[b]	1	0	0	0–1	0–1	0–1
CT scan of chest and abdomen[c]	1–2	1–2	1–2	0	0	0

- Contrast-enhanced ultrasound could substitute for abdominal CT scan
- Other laboratory and radiological examinations are of unproven benefit and must be restricted to patients with suspicious symptoms

Obtained from ESMO (www.esmo.org) on 1/28/12
ESMO guidelines were accessed on 1/28/12. There were minor quantitative and qualitative changes compared to the guidelines accessed on 10/31/07
[a]The numbers in the table indicate the number of times the modality is recommended during the indicated year posttreatment
[b]Colonoscopy must be performed at year 1 and thereafter every 3–5 years, looking for metachronous adenomas and cancers
[c]For patients who are at higher risk for recurrence

Table 32.5 Familial colorectal cancer: familial adenomatous polyposis

	Years posttreatment[a]					
	1	2	3	4	5	>5
Office visit[b]	0.5–2	0.5–2	0.5–2	0.5–2	0.5–2	0.5–2
Endoscopy[c]	0.5–2	0.5–2	0.5–2	0.5–2	0.5–2	0.5–2

Obtained from ESMO (www.esmo.org) on 1/28/12
ESMO guidelines were accessed on 1/28/12. These are new quantitative guidelines compared to no guidelines found on 10/31/07
[a]The numbers in the table indicate the number of times the modality is recommended during the indicated year posttreatment
[b]Endoscopy was the only quantitative recommendation given. We inferred that office visit would be recommended as frequently as this
[c]When proctocolectomy is performed, surveillance of the pouch can be repeated every 1–2 years, but if the rectum is in place the interval between examinations should be reduced to 6–12 months. In patients with attenuated FAP conservatively managed with endoscopic polypectomy, examination of the entire colon and rectum should be performed annually. Surveillance of duodenal manifestations will depend on it extension. When it corresponds to Spigelman stage I or II, upper endoscopy can be performed every 5—3 years, respectively, whereas in more advanced forms intervals between examinations should be shortened to 1–2 years (Spigelman stage III) or 6 months (Spigelman IV)

Cancer Care Ontario (www.cancercare.on.ca)

Cancer Care Ontario (CCO) guidelines were accessed on 1/28/12 (Table 32.8). There were major quantitative and qualitative changes compared to the guidelines accessed on 10/31/07.

National Institute for Clinical Excellence (www.nice.org.uk)

National Institute for Clinical Excellence (NICE) guidelines were accessed on 1/28/12 (Table 32.9). There were major quantitative and qualitative changes compared to the guidelines accessed on 10/31/07.

Table 32.6 Familal colorectal cancer: MUTYH-associated polyposis

	Years posttreatment[a]					
	1	2	3	4	5	>5
Office visit[b]	1–2	1–2	1–2	1–2	1–2	1–2
Endoscopy[c]	1–2	1–2	1–2	1–2	1–2	1–2

Obtained from ESMO (www.esmo.org) on 1/28/12
ESMO guidelines were accessed on 1/28/12. These are new quantitative guidelines compared to no guidelines found on 10/31/07
[a]The numbers in the table indicate the number of times the modality is recommended during the indicated year posttreatment
[b]Endoscopy was the only quantitative recommendation given. We inferred that office visit would be recommended as frequently as this
[c]After total colectomy, regular endoscopic surveillance of the rectum every 6–12 months is recommended. In patients conservatively managed with endoscopic polypectomy, examination of the entire colon and rectum should be performed annually. Surveillance of duodenal manifestations will depend on its extension. When disease corresponds to Spigelman stage I or II, upper endoscopy can be performed every 5 or 3 years, respectively, whereas in more advanced forms intervals between examinations should be shortened to 1–2 year (Spigelman stage III) or 6 months (Spigelman IV)

Table 32.7 Rectal cancer

	Years posttreatment[a]					
	1	2	3	4	5	>5
Office visit	2	2	0	0	1	0–1
Rectosigmoidoscopy	2	2	0	0	0	0
Colonoscopy[b]	1	0	0	0	1	0–1
Imaging of liver, lungs	1	0	1	0	0	0

- The value of regular clinical, laboratory, and radiological examinations are not known

Obtained from ESMO (www.esmo.org) on 1/28/12
ESMO guidelines were accessed on 1/28/12. There were minor quantitative and qualitative changes compared to the guidelines accessed on 10/31/07
[a]The numbers in the table indicate the number of times the modality is recommended during the indicated year posttreatment
[b]A completion colonoscopy, if not done at the time of diagnostic work-up (e.g., if obstruction was present), should be performed within the first year. History and colonoscopy with resection of colonic polyps every 5 years

The Cochrane Collaboration (CC, www.cochrane.org)

CC guidelines were accessed on 1/28/12. No quantitative guidelines exist for colorectal cancer surveillance, including when first accessed on 10/31/07.

The American Society of Colon and Rectal Surgeons (www.fascrs.org)

The American Society of Colon and Rectal Surgeons (ASCRS) guidelines were accessed on 1/28/12 (Table 32.10).

Table 32.8 Colorectal cancer

	Years posttreatment[a]					
	1	2	3	4	5	>5
Office visit[b]	1–2	1–2	1–2	1	1	1
Serum CEA level	1–2	1–2	1–2	1	1	1
Chest X-ray	1–2	1–2	1–2	1	1	1
Liver ultrasound	1–2	1–2	1–2	1	1	1
Colonoscopy[c]	1	0–1	1	0–1	1	0–1

- When recurrences of disease are detected, patients should be assessed by a multidisciplinary oncology team including surgical, radiation, and medical oncologists to determine the best treatment options
- Patients should be encouraged to participate in clinical trials investigating screening tests added on to their clinical assessment

Obtained from CCO (www.cancercare.on.ca) on 1/28/12
CCO guidelines were accessed on 1/28/12. There were major quantitative and qualitative changes compared to the guidelines accessed on 10/31/07
[a]The numbers in the table indicate the number of times the modality is recommended during the indicated year posttreatment
[b]For patients at high risk of recurrence (stages IIb and III). In patients at high risk of relapse but who have comorbidities that may interfere with prescribed tests or potential treatment for recurrence, or who are unwilling to undergo prescribed tests or potential treatment for recurrence, clinical assessments yearly or for suggestive symptoms of relapse. For patients at lower risk of recurrence (stages I and Ia) or those with comorbidities impairing future surgery, only visits yearly or when symptoms occur are recommended
[c]Colonoscopy postoperatively if not yet done. If polyps present, excise as they are potential precursors of colorectal cancer; repeat colonoscopy yearly as long as polyps are found. If there are no polyps, repeat colonoscopy in 3–8 years. All patients should have a colonoscopy before or within 6 months of initial surgery, repeated yearly if villous or tubular adenomas >1 cm are found; otherwise, repeat every 3–5 years

Table 32.9 Colorectal cancer

	Years posttreatment[a]					
	1	2	3	4	5	>5
Office visit[b, c]	≥2	≥2	≥2	0	1	0
Serum CEA level	≥2	≥2	≥2	0	0	0
CT scan of chest, abdomen, pelvis[d]	≤1	≤1	≤1	0	0	0
Colonoscopy[e]	1	0	0	0	1	0

- Start reinvestigation if there is any clinical, radiological, or biochemical suspicion of recurrent disease
- Stop regular follow-up when the patient and healthcare professional have discussed and agreed that the likely benefits no longer outweigh the risks of further tests or when the patient cannot tolerate further treatments

Obtained from NICE (www.nice.org.uk) on 1/28/12
NICE guidelines were accessed on 1/28/12. There were major quantitative and qualitative changes compared to the guidelines accessed on 10/31/07
[a]The numbers in the table indicate the number of times the modality is recommended during the indicated year posttreatment
[b]Start follow-up at a clinic visit 4–6 weeks after potentially curative treatment
[c]CEA, CT, and colonoscopy were the only quantitative recommendations given. We inferred that office visit would be recommended as frequently as these
[d]A minimum of two CTs of the chest, abdomen, and pelvis in the first 3 years
[e]Surveillance colonoscopy at 1 year after initial treatment. If this investigation is normal, consider further colonoscopic follow-up after 5 years, and thereafter as determined by cancer networks. The timing of surveillance for patients with subsequent adenomas should be determined by the risk status of the adenoma

Table 32.10 Colon and rectal cancer

	Years posttreatment[a]					
	1	2	3	4	5	>5
Office visit[b]	3	3	0	0	0	0
Serum CEA level	3	3	0	0	0	0
Colonoscopy[c]	1	0	0	1	0	0–1

- Periodic anastomotic evaluation is recommended for patients who have undergone resection/anastomosis or local excision of rectal cancer
- There is insufficient data to recommend for or against chest X-ray as part of routine colorectal cancer follow-up
- Serum hemoglobin, hemoccult II, and liver function tests (hepatic enzymes tests) should not be routine components of a follow-up program
- Routine use of hepatic imaging studies in the follow-up of colorectal cancer should not be performed

Obtained from ASCRS (www.fascrs.org) on 1/28/12
ASCRS guidelines were accessed on 1/28/12. These are new quantitative guidelines compared to the qualitative guidelines accessed on 12/13/07
[a]The numbers in the table indicate the number of times the modality is recommended during the indicated year posttreatment
[b]Data concerning proper timing of office visits, CEA, and CXR is insufficient to recommend one particular schedule of follow-up over another; however, office visits and CEA evaluations should be performed at a minimum of three times per year for the first 2 years of follow-up
[c]Complete visualization of the colon should be performed if practical in all patients being considered for colon or rectal cancer resection; posttreatment colonoscopy should be performed at 3-year intervals

Table 32.11 Cancer of colon or rectum

	Years posttreatment[a]					
	1	2	3	4	5	>5
Office visit[b]	2–4	2–4	2–4	1	0	0–1
Serum CEA level	2–4	2–4	2–4	0	0	0
Colonoscopy[c]	1	0	0	1	0	0–1

- Based on clinical indications, radiographic imaging such as chest X-ray, ultrasound, CT and/or MRI scan may also be indicated to evaluate for regional recurrence or metastatic disease
- Whole body FDG-PET scanning is a new modality that may be useful in selected circumstances for identifying metastatic disease
- Patients with recurrent colon or rectal cancer who do not have evidence of distant disease may be candidates for surgical resection with or without adjuvant radiation therapy
- Localized hepatic or pulmonary metastases detected during surveillance should be evaluated for possible resection. If one or a few lesions can be completely resected, survival is significantly prolonged

Obtained from SSAT (www.ssat.com) on 1/28/12
SSAT guidelines were accessed on 1/28/12. These are new quantitative guidelines compared to the qualitative guidelines accessed on 12/18/07
[a]The numbers in the table indicate the number of times the modality is recommended during the indicated year posttreatment
[b]Serum CEA level and colonoscopy were the only quantitative recommendations given. We inferred that office visit would be recommended as frequently as these
[c]Colonoscopy 1 year after surgery and then every 3 years

There are new quantitative guidelines compared to the qualitative guidelines accessed on 12/13/07.

Society for Surgery of the Alimentary Tract (www.ssat.com)

Society for Surgery of the Alimentary Tract (SSAT) guidelines were accessed on 1/28/12 (Table 32.11). There were no significant changes compared to the guidelines accessed on 12/18/07.

The M.D. Anderson Surgical Oncology Handbook also has follow-up guidelines, proposed by authors from a single National Cancer Institute-designated Comprehensive Cancer Center, for many types of cancer [7]. Some are detailed and quantitative, others are qualitative.

Summary

This is a common cancer with significant variability in incidence worldwide. We found guidelines based on consensus as well as evidence, but the evidence currently available is derived from multiple trials that are all underpowered.

References

1. Parkin DM, Whelan SL, Ferlay J, Teppo L, Thomas DB. Cancer incidence in five continents, Vol. VIII, International Agency for Research on Cancer. (IARC Scientific Publication 155). Lyon, France: IARC Press; 2002. ISBN 92-832-2155-9.
2. Jemal A, Seigel R, Ward E, Murray T, Xu J, Thun MJ. Cancer statistics, 2007. CA Cancer J Clin. 2007;57:43–66.
3. Schottenfeld D, Fraumeni JG. Cancer epidemiology and prevention. 3rd ed. New York, NY: Oxford University Press; 2006. ISBN 13:978-0-19-514961-6.
4. DeVita VT, Hellman S, Rosenberg SA. Cancer. 7th ed. Philadelphia, PA: Lippincott Williams & Wilkins; 2005. ISBN 0-781-74450-4.
5. Mackay J, Jemal A, Lee NC, Parkin M. The Cancer Atlas. 2006 American Cancer Society 1599 Clifton Road NE, Atlanta, Georgia 30329, USA; 2006. Can also be accessed at www.cancer.org. ISBN 0-944235-62-X.
6. Devesa SS, Grauman DJ, Blot WJ, Pennello GA, Hoover RN, Fraumeni JF Jr. Atlas of Cancer Mortality in the United States. National Institutes of Health, National Cancer Institute. NIH Publication No. 99-4564; Sep 1999.
7. Feig BW, Berger DH, Fuhrman GM. The M.D. Anderson surgical oncology handbook. 4th ed. Philadelphia, PA: Lippincott Williams & Wilkins; 2006. ISBN 0-7817-5643-X (paperback).

33 Colon and Rectum Carcinoma Surveillance Counterpoint: USA

Mohamedtaki A. Tejani and Steven J. Cohen

Keywords
Colonoscopy • Detection strategies • US

Colorectal adenocarcinoma is a leading cause of cancer-related death in the United States, accounting for more than estimated 50,000 deaths in each year [1]. Approximately two thirds of patients present with potentially curable disease. This group of patients undergoes surgical resection with or without adjuvant treatment (chemotherapy with or without radiation).

After a patient's definitive care is completed, follow-up care is established with three primary goals. The first is to help address treatment complications such as post-chemotherapy residual neuropathy or postsurgical bowel issues. Patients and their oncologists develop relationships of trust during treatment and follow-up care gives an opportunity to provide reassurance and support. A second goal is to detect tumor recurrence at an early time point to pursue additional curative-intent therapy. There is increasing evidence of true cures in patients who undergo resection of limited distant (liver or lung) recurrences [2, 3]. This is a major rationale for intensive surveillance in patients who are medically fit and potentially able to tolerate salvage surgery. For medically unfit patients who would not be able to tolerate liver or lung metastasectomy, the benefit of intense surveillance is unclear.

A third goal of posttreatment follow-up is to identify and optimally manage early-stage metachronous colorectal cancers and pre-cancerous polyps. Patients can be reminded of the importance of colonoscopy and other cancer detection strategies such as mammograms and pap smears. The field of cancer survivorship is attracting increasing interest to better coordinate routine health maintenance for a growing number of survivors, including those with a history of colorectal cancer. Another goal is identification of patients with genetic syndromes such as familial adenomatous polyposis or hereditary nonpolyposis colon cancer who require heightened surveillance. Their specific management will not be discussed further.

There have been a number of small randomized controlled trials that have high-intensity to low-intensity surveillance [4–11]. The studies, ranging in sample size from 100 to 600, were heterogeneous in their patient populations and surveillance strategies. Overall, the recurrence rates were similar in the two groups, but recurrences were found earlier and more commonly in asymptomatic patients in the group receiving intensive surveillance. Most importantly, surgery with curative intent was reported more frequently in the intensive surveillance groups. However, a statistically significant improvement in overall survival was noted in only two out of six studies. Three independent meta-analyses [12–14] of these trials have been reported and found reduction in death from all causes and associated overall survival benefit in the intensive surveillance group. Particular aspects of surveillance that may account for this apparent reduction in death rate are mentioned below.

New symptoms reported by a patient may provide the first indication of recurrence. Thus, periodic patient assessment with history and physical examination is important. Inquiry about general well-being, fatigue, anorexia, weight loss, rectal bleeding, and pain should be included. Physical examination consists of evaluating for weight loss, jaundice, adenopathy, abdominal distension, and hepatosplenomegaly.

A follow-up office visit is usually performed at our institution every 3 months for the first 2 years and every 4–6 months in the ensuing 3 years as per National Comprehensive Cancer Network guidelines [15]. At the 5-year mark, the

M.A. Tejani, M.D (✉) • S.J. Cohen, M.D.
Fox Chase Cancer Center, 333 Cottman Avenue, Philadelphia, PA 19111, USA
e-mail: Mohamed.Tejani@fccc.edu; Steven.Cohen@fccc.edu

F.E. Johnson et al. (eds.), *Patient Surveillance After Cancer Treatment*, Current Clinical Oncology,
DOI 10.1007/978-1-60327-969-7_33, © Springer Science+Business Media New York 2013

patients are discharged to their primary care physicians for routine care. This pattern reflects the fact that the vast majority of colorectal cancer recurrences occur within the first 5 years after diagnosis and most of these are in the first 2 years [16, 17]. It is possible that, with improved adjuvant chemotherapy, more late recurrences may be noted.

Carcinoembryonic antigen (CEA) was first identified in colorectal cancer tissue in 1965 by Gold and Freedman [18]. It is elevated in about 50% of patients with colorectal cancer before surgery. After curative resection, the serum CEA level should fall to normal levels in 4–8 weeks. The sensitivity and specificity of CEA levels in detecting recurrent colorectal cancer are approximately 80% and 70%, respectively [19]. It is frequently the first test to identify relapse and typically increases before the onset of physical symptoms. While there is no absolute serum CEA level that distinguishes recurrence from nonrecurrence, serial increases strongly suggest recurrent disease. In our practice, we typically check CEA levels with each office visit. We usually repeat the measurement in 1 month after a modest elevation is noted. A large rise or serial rise in CEA level should trigger radiographic evaluation. CT scans are often the first test ordered, although use of PET/CT is increasing. Blood tests other than CEA (complete blood count, liver function tests) are neither sensitive nor specific in detecting colorectal cancer recurrence.

The role of routine surveillance imaging in patients after curative-intent initial therapy in colorectal cancer remains controversial. A Cochrane meta-analysis suggested a survival benefit with periodic CT scans while others did not. Specifically, there was reported survival benefit with liver imaging [14]. Current approaches to surveillance imaging range from no imaging at all to periodic abdominal ultrasound or CT. At Fox Chase Cancer Center, the general consensus of our group is to follow National Comprehensive Cancer Network guidelines and obtain yearly CT scans for 3 years for patients with high-risk disease. We have typically interpreted that term to include patients who were eligible to receive adjuvant therapy based on risk analysis. At the current time, we do not utilize routine PET/CT imaging in the average-risk surveillance setting. However, in the setting of a rising CEA, PET/CT likely has utility in detecting recurrence and is frequently ordered [20].

Colonoscopy is also included in routine surveillance following potentially curative treatment. Although colonoscopy may detect early anastomotic or perianastomotic recurrence, such events are uncommon [21]. Local recurrence of rectal cancer is also becoming increasingly rare in the era of more effective preoperative radiotherapy and better quality surgery. However, an important role of colonoscopy remains the detection of metachronous cancers and pre-cancerous adenomatous polyps. Patients with prior colorectal cancers have a risk of second primary tumors that is increased by a factor of 1.5–3.0 compared to the population at large [22].

Table 33.1 Surveillance for colorectal cancer patients after curative-intent initial treatment at the Fox Chase Cancer Center

	Year				
Modality	1	2	3	4	5
Office visit	4	4	2–3	2–3	2–3
Serum CEA level	4	4	2–3	2–3	2–3
Colonoscopy	1	[a]	[a]	[a]	[a]
CT abdomen/pelvis	1	1	1	[a]	[a]

After 5 years of surveillance, a patient who is clinically well is discharged to the primary care physician

The number in each cell indicates the number of times a particular modality is recommended during a particular posttreatment year

CEA carcinoembryonic antigen

[a]Dictated by findings at previous colonoscopy and serum CEA level

All patients should undergo a full colonoscopy prior to colorectal resection since 3–7% of patients have a synchronous tumor [23]. If patients with obstruction or perforation do not have colonoscopy preoperatively, it should be done within 3–6 months of primary surgery. Even if the initial examination does not reveal any polyps, it should be repeated 1 year postoperatively. The frequency of subsequent colonoscopies depends on endoscopic findings.

Table 33.1 presents a consensus summary of surveillance for patients with colorectal cancer at Fox Chase Cancer Center. As a founding member of the National Comprehensive Cancer Network, our surveillance strategies mirror their recommendations.

Further prospective studies are needed to compare high-intensity vs. low-intensity surveillance strategies. It would be helpful for these studies to make a special effort to elucidate differences in follow-up for high-risk vs. low-risk patients, the role of surveillance beyond 5 years in this era of adjuvant treatment, and the addition of newer imaging techniques such as PET-CT and virtual colonoscopy to our clinical toolkit.

References

1. Jemal A, Siegel R, Xu J, Ward E. Cancer statistics. CA Cancer J Clin. 2010;60:277–300.
2. Guyot F, Faivre J, Manfredi S, et al. Time trends in the treatment and survival of recurrences from colorectal cancer. Ann Oncol. 2005;16:756–61.
3. Tomlinson JS, Jarnagin WR, DeMatteo RP, et al. Actual 10-year survival after resection of colorectal liver metastases defines cure. J Clin Oncol. 2007;25:4575–80.
4. Schoemaker D, Black R, Giles L, Toouli J. Yearly colonoscopy, liver CT and chest radiography do not influence 5-year survical of colorectal cancer patients. Gastroenterology. 1998;114:7–14.
5. Pietra N, Sarli L, Costi R, Ouchemi C, Grattarola M, Peracchia A. Role of follow-up in management of local recurrences of colorectal cancer: a prospective, randomized trial. Dis Colon Rectum. 1998;41:1127–33.
6. Kjeldsen BJ, Kronborg O, Fenger C, Jorgensen OD. A prospective randomized study of follow-up after radical surgery for colorectal cancer. Br J Surg. 1997;84:666–9.

7. Ohlsson B, Breland U, Ekberg H, et al. Follow-up after curative surgery for colorectal carcinoma: randomized comparison with no follow-up. Dis Colon Rectum. 1995;38:619–26.
8. Makela JT, Laitinen SO, Kairaluoma MI. Five-year follow-up after radical surgery for colorectal cancer: results of a prospective randomized trial. Arch Surg. 1995;130:1062–7.
9. Secco GB, Fardelli R, Gianquinto D, et al. Efficacy and cost of risk-adapted follow-up in patients after colorectal cancer surgery: a prospective, randomized and controlled trial. Eur J Surg Oncol. 2002;28:418–23.
10. Ovaska J, Jarvinen H, Kujari H, Pertilla I, Mecklin JP. Follow-up of patients operated on for colorectal carcinoma. Am J Surg. 1990;159:593–6.
11. Rodriguez-Moranta F, Salo J, Arcusa A, et al. Postoperative surveillance in patients with colorectal cancer who have undergone curative resection: a prospective, multicenter, randomized, controlled trial. J Clin Oncol. 2006;24:386–93.
12. Figueredo A, Rumble RB, Maroun J, et al. Follow-up of patients with curatively resected colorectal cancer: a practice guideline. BMC Cancer. 2003;3:26.
13. Renehan AG, Egger M, Saunders MP, et al. Impact on survival of intense follow up after curative resection for colorectal cancer: systematic review and meta-analysis of randomized trials. BMJ. 2002;324:813.
14. Jeffery GM, Hickey BE, Hider P. Follow-up strategies for patients treated for non-metastatic colorectal cancer. Cochrane Database Syst Rev. 2002;1:CD002200.
15. NCCN colon cancer clinical practice guidelines in oncology. J Natl Compr Cancer Network. 2008;1:1–18.
16. Kjeldsen BJ, Kronborg O, Fenger C, Jorgensen OD. The pattern of recurrent colorectal cancer in a prospective randomized study and the characteristics of diagnostic tests. Int J Colorectal Dis. 1997;12:329–34.
17. Sargent D, Sobrero A, Grothey A, et al. Evidence for cure by adjuvant therapy in Colon Cancer: observations based on individual patient data from 20, 898 patients on 18 randomized trials. J Clin Oncol. 2009;6:872–7.
18. Gold P, Freedman SO. Demonstration of tumor-specific antigens in colonic carcinomata by immunological tolerance and absorption techniques. J Exp Med. 1965;121:439–62.
19. Arnaud JP, Koehl C, Adloff M. Carcinoembryonic antigen (CEA) in the diagnosis and prognosis of colorectal carcinoma. Dis Colon Rectum. 1980;23:141–4.
20. Libutti SK, Alexander HR, Choyke P, et al. A prospective study of 2-[18F] fluoro-2-deoxy-D-glucose/positron emission tomography scan, 99 m Tc-labeled arcitumomab (CEA-scan), and blind second-look laparotomy for detecting colon cancer recurrence in patients with increasing CEA levels. Ann Surg Oncol. 2001;8:779–86.
21. Tsikitis VL, Malireddy K, Green EA, et al. Postoperative recommendations for early stage colon cancer based on results from the clinical outcomes of surgical therapy trial. J Clin Oncol. 2009;22:3671–6.
22. Green RJ, Metlay JP, Propert K, et al. Surveillance for second primary colorectal cancer after adjuvant chemotherapy: an analysis of Intergroup 0089. Ann Intern Med. 2002;136:261–9.
23. Graffner H, Hultberg B, Johansson B, Moller T, Petersson BG. Detection of recurrent cancer of the colon and rectum. J Surg Oncol. 1985;28:156–9.

Colon and Rectum Carcinoma Surveillance Counterpoint: Australia

34

Toufic El-Khoury, Michael Solomon, and Jane Young

Keywords
Australia • Postoperative • Recurrence • Surveillance • Therapy

Surveillance for colorectal cancer should aim to identify recurrence at a point when therapy, in the form of surgery and/or adjuvant therapy, could impact survival duration and/or quality of life (QOL). The identification of metachronous neoplasms and early diagnosis of other conditions also improves overall survival duration [1]. Standardized surveillance strategies are also important to provide information to drive quality improvement through audit of outcomes against professional and national standards.

Meta-analysis provides the best available evidence thus far in support of intensive surveillance. Published randomized controlled trials are fraught with power and sample size issues. Meta-analyses have methodological problems such as dissimilar follow-up pathways in the published trials. They are unable to answer the question: What *types* and *timing* of tests are useful? Some randomized trials showed that increasing the number of surveillance modalities had no impact on overall survival but increasing the frequency of testing did. The meta-analyses have suggested a small but statistically significant survival advantage in support of intensive follow-up (www.cancer.org.au/aboutcancer/cancertypes/colorectal-cancer.htm; www.aihw.gov.au) [2], most recently by Tjandra et al. [1]. The heterogeneity among the different regimens makes it difficult to recommend a particular pathway. The most recent meta-analysis of eight randomized trials [1] supports the findings of previous meta-analyses; intensive surveillance seems to reduce mortality and leads to more curative reoperations. Intensive monitoring using serum carcinoembryonic antigen (CEA) level was the only test associated with improved overall survival duration, higher detection rate of asymptomatic recurrence, and higher curative-intent reoperation rate.

Generally, our strategy relies on four routine components: office visit, CEA, CT, and colonoscopy. Other diagnostic tests are used selectively. Office visits aim to detect symptomatic disease, whether recurrent or metachronous, colorectal or noncolorectal, oncological or nononcological. CEA, CT, and colonoscopy, on the other hand, specifically target the asymptomatic recurrence.

After the early postoperative office visit, surveillance is frequent for 2 years and less frequent thereafter. It consists of history and physical examination, including frequent digital rectal examination and rigid sigmoidoscopy in those with rectal cancer. CEA level is obtained at each visit and colonoscopy is carried out every 3 years. CT scan is performed after the completion of adjuvant treatment. Other tests are used selectively when the above regimens raise suspicion of recurrence (Table 34.1).

In Australia, colorectal cancer is the second most common cancer in both men and women following prostate and breast cancer. There are more than 12,500 new cases and 4,372 deaths from colorectal cancer each year [3]. The Australian Institute of Health and Welfare reported 8,546 new cases of colon cancer in 2004 and 4,431 rectal and rectosigmoid cancers [4]. One in ten men and one in fifteen women develop colorectal cancer by the age of 85. When stratified by age, colorectal cancer is the third most common cancer for those aged 15–44, the second most common cancer for those aged 45–64, and the most common cancer for

T. El-Khoury, MBBS, FRACS, (✉) • M. Solomon, MB BCh(Hons) MSc (Clin Epidemiol) FRACS • J. Young, MBBS, MPH, PhD, FAFPHM
Surgical Outcome Research Centre (SOuRCe), Royal Prince Alfred Hospital Sydney and University of Sydney, Level 9, Building 50, Camperdown, NSW 2050, Australia

F.E. Johnson et al. (eds.), *Patient Surveillance After Cancer Treatment*, Current Clinical Oncology,
DOI 10.1007/978-1-60327-969-7_34,

Table 34.1 Surveillance of patients with colorectal cancer after curative-intent primary therapy at the Royal Prince Alfred Hospital, Sydney

	Years posttreatment				
Modality	1	2	3	4	5
Office visit	2–4	2–4	1–2	1–2	1–2
DRE and sigmoidoscopy*	2–4	2–4	1–2	1–2	1–2
Serum CEA level	2–4	2–4	1–2	1–2	1–2
Colonoscopy	1**	0	1	0	0
CT scan abdomen/pelvis	1	0	0	0	0
EAUS***	2	2	2	2	2

The number in each cell indicates the number of times a particular modality is recommended during a particular posttreatment year

DRE digital rectal examination, *EAUS* endoanal ultrasonography

*Digital Rectal Examination and sigmoidoscopy for patients after anterior resection

**Early postoperative colonoscopy is indicated if the proximal part of the colon was not examined preoperatively

***For patients after local excision of rectal cancer

people aged over 65. It is the third most common cause of cancer deaths in both men and women [5].

Thirty to fifty percent of patients treated for colorectal cancer with curative intent develop recurrent disease [1]. Eighty percent of the recurrences occur in the first 3 years [6] and 90 % by 5 years [1]. Approximately 7.7 % of patients develop a metachronous colorectal cancer.

Colorectal cancer is the second most expensive cancer in Australia; the burden is estimated at 10.8 % of the total cost of cancer care [2]. Costs of surveillance regimens are substantial and not proven to be cost-effective in the Australian setting.

Different follow-up regimens have different cost-effectiveness profiles. Worthington et al. [7] compared the Norwegian surveillance protocol to the Australian one and found marked differences in cost per patient with a resectable recurrence of colorectal cancer.

At our institution, we follow the clinical practice guidelines made by the working party of the Australian Cancer Network, with support from the Cancer Council Australia and the Clinical Oncological Society of Australia, and approved by the National Health and Medical Research Council [2], as well as the Practice Parameters for the *Surveillance and Follow-Up of Patients with Colon and Rectal Cancer* published in Diseases of the Colon and Rectum [8], the official journal of the colorectal surgical society of Australia and New Zealand (CSSANZ).

- The National Health and Medical Research Council guidelines are updated every 5 years and were last reviewed in 2005. They can be accessed electronically on the following websites: www.cancer.org.au/Healthprofessionals/clinicalguidelines/colorectalcancer.htm and www.nhmrc.gov.au/publications/synopses/cp106/cp106syn.htm
- The CSSANZ practice guidelines can be accessed by members at www.cssa.org.au.htm.

When compared to surveillance strategies proposed by other professional organizations, the National Health and Medical Research Council guidelines have not developed pathways as detailed as those of the National Comprehensive Cancer Network or the American Society of clinical Oncology, nor as complex as those of Cancer Care Ontario. It does not stratify surveillance according to the risk of recurrence nor does it differentiate the follow-up of colon from rectal cancer.

National Health and Medical Research Council practice recommendations are that: *intensive follow-up for colorectal cancer should be considered for patients who have potentially curable disease*. The benefit from increased intensity is supported only by meta-analysis of published randomized trials. The overall benefit seen is small but significant and is not evident in the individual studies themselves. The definition of *intensive* is not specified, however. The intensity can be increased by increasing the frequency of tests, increasing the number of investigations performed at each office visit, or by increasing both. For example, the median number of office visits in year 5 ranges from 4 to 14 for nonintensive and intensive regimens, respectively, and the median number of different investigations are 5 and 7 for nonintensive and intensive regimens, respectively [9]. One can argue that our regimen is intensive, given the frequency of office visits (7–14 visits in 5 years), but others may consider it nonintensive as we only use three investigations (CEA, CT, and colonoscopy).

The role of monoclonal antibodies, although expanding in the area of adjuvant treatment, is still experimental in surveillance. We do not use anti-CEA or anti-TAG-72 labeled antibodies in follow-up or in a trial setting.

In our institution, surveillance, like the management of the primary cancer, is of a multidisciplinary nature. There seems to be agreement on regimens among different care providers, with rectal cancer followed up by surgeons, while colon cancer patients are followed up primarily by surgeons once the chemotherapy has concluded. There is a consensus on who should carry out the surveillance; it is the responsibility of the specialist clinician and not of the general practitioner (GP) [2].

Wattchow and colleagues [10] conducted a multicenter randomized controlled trial from hospitals across four states in Australia, comparing outcomes between GP-led and surgeon-led follow-up regimens. The trial that recruited from 1998 till 2001 was powered for QOL measured at 12 and 24 months. Survival duration, time to recurrence, number, and type of investigations were secondary outcomes. The trial found no significant difference in QOL recurrence rate or survival duration between patients followed by surgeons or GPs. The type of investigations varied, with GPs ordering more fecal occult blood tests and surgeons ordering more colonoscopies and ultrasounds. The findings of this study might cause a change in National Health and Medical Research Council recommendations.

Although there is a consensus among practitioners in our institution, there has been no survey among members of the CSSANZ who measured actual practice patterns. In addition, a significant number of colorectal malignancies are managed by non-colorectal surgeons, some outside tertiary centers and in rural settings with a wide range of protocols. Pathways for surveillance after surgery for colon cancer do not differ greatly from rectal cancer in our institution.

Rectal cancer treatment is associated with a higher rate of local recurrence than colon cancer treatment and an equal rate of liver and lung metastasis compared with recurrence of colon cancer which affects mostly the liver, with low risk of local or pulmonary metastasis.

There are insufficient data to recommend for or against the use of chest X-ray, and we do not routinely use it for follow-up of patients with rectal cancer. Although studies [11–13] have shown that resectable lung disease can be identified in 1.8–12 % of patients, the effect on survival is not clear.

Local excision of rectal cancer may be used in selected cancer patients, according to National Health and Medical Research Council guidelines: T1 on endorectal ultrasound, mobile tumor <3 cm and not poorly differentiated. It is also a surgical option for those who refuse or are unfit for major surgery. The follow-up of patients following local excision differs slightly from those following conventional excision. The recurrence rate following local resection of rectal cancer is 12 % and 24 % for T1 and T2, respectively.

Following local excision for rectal cancer, most local recurrences occur within the undissected intact mesorectum. Endoanal ultrasound and serum CEA measurements may lead to detection of the more common extraluminal recurrence and should complement tests of intraluminal evaluation such as endoscopy and fecal occult blood tests.

At each office visit for a rectal cancer patient we perform a digital rectal examination and a rigid sigmoidoscopy. We perform six-monthly endoanal ultrasounds for locally excised rectal cancer while the other investigations are used for colon cancer.

We do not tailor the surveillance program risk groups. The main reason is that calculation of risk of recurrence is complicated with other factors such as the patient's overall medical and psychological well being as well as geographical remoteness. We adhere to one regimen for all patients (Table 34.1).

Intensifying surveillance for those at greater risk does not guarantee a greater benefit. Although the incidence of recurrence depends largely on the stage of the primary tumor, the study by Rodriguez-Moranta and colleagues [14] showed that patients with stage II benefited more from intensive follow-up than those with stage III. Intensive follow-up led to the detection of double the number of metachronous lesions than the standard follow-up in stage II cancers but there was no observed difference for those with stage III cancers. In addition, the wide range of factors, in addition to stage, which influence recurrence, makes calculation of risk difficult. Factors, such as grade, lymphovascular invasion, perineural invasion, CEA level, perforation, and the level of the anastomosis from the anal verge [3], all have to be considered along with the adequacy in the surgical and adjuvant treatment.

The effect of adjuvant therapy in prolonging time to recurrence is documented for both colon and rectal cancers. Some have suggested a longer surveillance period for those who have received adjuvant therapy. As an example, the six-year follow-up report from the Dutch trial [15] shows that preoperative radiotherapy postpones local recurrence of rectal cancer. In patients assigned to total mesorectal excision alone, 10 % of local recurrences appeared after 3 years, compared with 31 % of local recurrence when preoperative radiotherapy preceded total mesorectal excision.

One of the purposes of an office visit is the detection of symptomatic recurrences and other secondary neoplasms to which colorectal cancer survivors are susceptible (for example, breast, prostate, and thyroid cancers). The finding by Tjandra and colleagues [1] in the most recent meta-analysis of an overall survival benefits from intensive surveillance, despite no improvement in cancer-specific mortality, suggests that regular surveillance may be identifying nononcological factors which could be implicated in the overall survival advantage.

We believe that there is no modality more useful than CEA. Variable reports exist on its sensitivity, specificity, and accuracy, all of which depend on the chosen cut-off levels as well as the site of recurrence. The serum CEA level has been shown to be the first indicator of disease recurrence [11] leading the other tests by 3 months. It is also the most cost-effective and most widely used test [16]. All patients with recurrence detected by the serum CEA level monitoring in a French series [16] who had a radical resection were alive 5 years after the diagnosis of recurrence.

What has been debatable is the usefulness of the serum CEA level in patients with a normal preoperative CEA level. A recent study [17] calculating posttest probability of recurrence found that postoperative CEA elevation indicates recurrence with high probability; a normal postoperative CEA level is not useful for excluding the probability of recurrence, which is common in patients without preoperative CEA elevation. The analysis went further in defining the usefulness of CEA as a site-specific detector of recurrence. Postoperative CEA elevation predicted liver metastasis with high reliability in both those with normal or high preoperative serum CEA levels. It had a lower positive predictive value for lung metastases especially in those with normal preoperative CEA. The sample of population in this study was comprised of patients with Dukes C, and whether these findings apply to the earlier stages of cancer is difficult to say.

The second most effective indicator of recurrence is the presence of symptoms. For this reason, our policy is to intensify both office visits and CEA in the early years of follow-up, with less intense and more selective use of other diagnostic tests such as colonoscopy, liver ultrasound, and liver chemistry.

Some argue that performing a colonoscopy in the first 5 years posttreatment of the primary is unlikely to detect recurrent or metachronous lesions in the absence of clinical or screening abnormalities. In the study by Shoemaker et al. [13], all but 1 of 23 lesions identified endoscopically were associated with clinical and/or screening abnormalities. They argued that colonoscopy is not justified in the first 5 years in asymptomatic patients.

Our practice differs from this as we perform colonoscopy every 3–5 years for two reasons. In order to detect asymptomatic recurrence, Shoemaker et al. [13] used fecal occult blood tests, liver function tests, and CEA levels as screening investigations at each follow-up visit; we regularly use CEA alone. The second reason is that the benefit of colonoscopy lies in the identification of metachronous adenomas, and this has been proven within the average risk population. When using colonoscopy to screen the general population, an interval of 5 years or longer is recommended. For patients after treatment of colorectal cancer, a shorter interval seems warranted.

In our practice, colonoscopy is carried out every 3 years after the initial operation. The aim of colonoscopy is the detection of metachronous and luminal recurrence. If a preoperative colonoscopy was not performed, it should be carried out 3–6 months from surgery. When technically difficult, CT colonography can replace colonoscopy.

The use of CT scan is supported neither by prospective trials nor by a recent meta-analysis. A prospective study by Howell et al. [18] found that annual CT scan leads to resection of liver metastasis in 2 of 157 (1.3 %). Makela et al. [12] found that routine abdominal CT scan leads to an increase in the detection rate of asymptomatic recurrence but, despite that, there was no difference in the attempted resection rate. The meta-analysis by Tjandra [1] and colleagues found that the use of CT scan leads to an insignificant improvement in overall mortality despite the fact that there was an increase in detection of asymptomatic tumor recurrence and in curative reoperation rate. Similarly, a study from South Australia [13] showed that yearly liver CT was able to detect more hepatic metastases while patients were asymptomatic, but this did not translate into a higher curative resection rate compared with patients who did not undergo no CT scanning. We routinely use CT scan once in the follow-up of patients, usually after the completion of chemotherapy, or at one year. CT of the chest and abdomen is used to investigate a raised CEA level.

In the South Australian study [13], 6 % of the patients in the standard surveillance group and 5 % in the intensive surveillance group developed lung metastasis. In the intensive group, a yearly chest X-ray was performed, with a total of 750 chest X-rays performed. Only one patient with lung recurrence was alive at 4 years follow-up.

Surveillance strategies proposed by National Comprehensive Cancer Network, American Society of Clinical Oncology, European Society for Medical Oncology, Cancer Care Ontario, and National Institute for Health and Clinical Excellence do not routinely use chest X-ray. National Comprehensive Cancer Network recommends CT chest for rectal and advanced colon cancer, while American Society of Clinical Oncology recommends CT chest for 3 years for colon and rectal cancer follow-up. In our practice and according to the National Health and Medical Research Council [2] and the Practice Parameters of the American Society of Colon and Rectal Surgeons [5], there are insufficient data to recommend for or against chest X-ray as part of routine colorectal cancer follow-up.

There are insufficient data to recommend the use of other colorectal tumor markers such as CA 19–9, or markers of inflammation such as C-reactive protein.

Serum hemoglobin level, Hemoccult II, and liver function tests are not part of routine follow-up [5]. In Australia, the role of fecal occult blood test in screening for colorectal cancer has been clarified, but its use in follow-up remains controversial. We believe that patients cured from colorectal cancer remain in the high-risk category for life, and general population screening tests should not target them.

There are no data to support the use of PET scan as a primary follow-up tool. We limit its use to those with raised CEA levels. In patients with pulmonary or hepatic metastasis, PET scan is used prior to embarking on a major operation. A recent published Australian study showed that PET scan changed the management plan in 49 % of patients with recurrent disease [19].

Surgery offers the only chance of cure after colorectal recurrences whether it is local, hepatic, or pulmonary. Recurrence tends to be multifocal in the majority of cases, and thus incurable. Chemotherapy may improve survival and QOL.

Liver and lung metastases are sites amenable to curative-intent surgery. The refinement in patient selection, along with advances in perioperative care and chemotherapy, has led to a recent improvement in survival. An overall five-year survival of 37 % [20] has been reported following hepatic resection and up to 60 % [21] following pulmonary resection for colorectal cancer.

Our institution published the outcome of 160 patients with locally recurrent rectal cancer. Salvage treatment was possible in 95 % of them (39 % underwent radical resection, 56 % underwent extended radical resection). We achieved a negative resection margin in 61 %. The five-year cancer-specific and overall survival probability was 41.5 % and 36.6 %, respectively [22].

New primary neoplasms are divided into colorectal (or metachronous) and noncolorectal primary.

Patients treated for colorectal cancer have a 7.7 % lifetime risk of developing a new primary colorectal cancer and 62 % risk of developing an adenoma. Detection and removal of colorectal adenomas reduces the incidence of subsequent new primary cancers. The detection of a new primary cancer has a negative impact on survival, in particular if it is detected during the period of adjuvant treatment.

Patients treated for colorectal cancer are also at risk of developing a new primary noncolorectal cancer, and we rely on a multidisciplinary approach to patients with familial adenomatous polyposis, hereditary nonpolyposis colorectal cancer, and other familial colorectal carcinomas, and on office visits to diagnose symptomatic new primary cancers. We emphasize the importance of screening for prostate and breast cancer, the two commonest cancers in men and women in Australia.

Future trials could address three aspects of posttreatment surveillance: the impact of different follow-up strategies on patient survival duration, the impact on QOL, and the relative cost-effectiveness of different strategies.

There are no randomized trials addressing the issue of cost-effectiveness of different surveillance regimens in the Australian setting. Most Australian authors publishing on this topic convert other reported costs to the Australian dollar. Large trials comparing different pathways for different risk groups are needed to prove their cost-effectiveness. Our medical resources differ from that of the European and American counterparts and are mostly publicly funded. An investigation into cost-effectiveness of follow-up programs in the Australian setting is greatly needed.

On an international basis we need to await the GILDA trial [23] to complete recruitment of 1,500 patients in order to become adequately powered to detect a hazard-rate reduction of 24 %. The FACS trial will also continue to recruit until December 2008. Until then we have to accept the conclusion of the meta-analysis of randomized clinical trials [1, 9] as best available evidence. The GILDA and the FACS do not address the use of PET scan and fecal occult blood test for colorectal cancer or the use of endoanal ultrasound for rectal cancer [24].

It would be feasible to carry a multicenter randomized controlled trial in Australia, similar to these international trials, to determine the surveillance regimen which best improves QOL and increases the length of life without overusing our limited medical resources.

Studying the prognostic significance of cancer biology such as the overexpression of p53 or the mutation of Ki-ras may aid in stratifying patients into risk of recurrence, but gene expression profiling seems to be a long way away from altering surveillance strategies. Yang and colleagues [25] studied a set of 20 genes; they have shown promising results in predicting the behavior of colonic cancer. Monoclonal antibody-guided diagnostic approaches are still experimental.

References

1. Tjandra J, Chan M. Follow-up after curative resection of colorectal cancer: a meta-analysis. Dis Colon Rectum. 2007;50:1783–99.
2. National Health and Medical Research Council (NHMRC). Clinical practice guidelines for the Prevention, early detection and management of colorectal cancer. The Cancer Council Australia, Australian Cancer Network, The Commonwealth of Australia, Canberra 2005.
3. Yun H, Lee L, Park J, et al. Local recurrence after curative resection in patients with colon and rectal cancers. Int J Colorectal Dis. 2008;23:1081–7.
4. Worthington T, Wilson T, Padbury R. Case for postoperative surveillance following colorectal cancer resection. ANZ J Surg. 2004;74:43–5.
5. Anthony T, Simmang C, Hyman N, et al. Practice parameters for the surveillance and follow-up of patients with colon and rectal cancer. Dis Colon Rectum. 2004;47:807–17.
6. Raptis DA, Gore DM, Boulos PB. The value of CEA and CT in early diagnosis of colorectal cancer recurrence. American Society of Colon and Rectal Surgeons Tripartite Meeting 2008. Oral presentation. Boston 2008.
7. Bruinvells D, Stiggerbart A, Kievet J, Van de Velde J. Follow-up of patients with colorectal cancer: a meta-analysis. Ann Surg. 1994;219:174–82.
8. Rosen M, Chan L, Beart R, Valksoin P, Anthone G. Follow-up of colorectal cancer: a meta analysis. Dis Colon Rectum. 1998;41:1116–25.
9. Renehan A, Egger M, O'Dwyer S. Impact on survival of intensive follow-up after curative resection for colorectal cancer: systemic review and meta-analysis of randomised trials. Br Med J. 2002;324:813–30.
10. Wattchow DA, Weller DP, Esterman A, Pilotto LS, McGorm K, Hammett Z, Platell C, Silagy C. General practice vs. surgical-based follow-up for patients with colon cancer: randomised controlled trial. Br J Cancer. 2006;94:116–21.
11. Ohlesson B, Breland U, Ekberg H, Graffner H, Tranberg KG. Follow-up after curative surgery for colorectal carcinoma. Dis Colon Rectum. 1995;38:619–26.
12. Makela J, Laitnen S, Kairaluoma M. Five-year follow-up after radical surgery for colorectal cancer. Results of a prospective randomised trial. Arch Surg. 1995;130:1062–7.
13. Schoemaker D, Black R, Giles L, Toouli J. Yearly colonoscopy, liver CT and chest radiography do not influence 5-year survival of colorectal cancer patients. Gastroenterology. 1998;114:7–14.
14. Rodriguez-Moranta F, Salo J, Arcusa A. Postoperative surveillance in patients with colorectal cancer who have undergone curative resection: a prospective multicenter, randomised, controlled trial. J Clin Oncol. 2006;24:386–93.
15. Peeters K, Marijnen C, Nagtegaal I, et al. The TME trial after a median follow up of 6 years. Ann Surg. 2007;246:693–701.
16. Borie F, Daures JP, Millat B, Tretarre B. Cost and effectiveness of follow-up examinations in patients with colorectal cancer resected for cure in a French population-based study. J Gastrointest Surg. 2004;8:552–8.
17. Hara M, Kanemitsu Y, Hirai T, Komori K, Kato T. Negative Serum CEA has insufficient accuracy for excluding recurrence from patients with Dukes C colorectal cancer: analysis with likelihood ratio and post test probability in a follow-up study. Dis Colon Rectum. 2008;51:1675–80.

18. Howell J, Wotherspoon H, Leen E, coke T, McArdle C. Evaluation of a follow-up program after curative resection fro colorectal cancer. Br J Cancer. 1999;79:308–10.
19. Scott A, Gunawardana D, Kelley B, Stuckey J, Byrne A, Ramshaw J, Fulham M. PET Changes Management and Improves Prognostic Stratification in Patients with Recurrent Colorectal Cancer: Results of a Multicenter Prospective Study. J Nucl Med. 2008;49:1451–7.
20. Zakaria S, Donohue JH, Florenia G, Farnell MB, et al. Hepatic resection for colorectal metastases, value for risk scoring systems? Ann Surg. 2007;246:183–91.
21. Hideyuki I, Shimada H, Ohki S, Togo S, Yamaguchi S, Ichikawa Y. Results of aggressive resection of lung metastases from colorectal carcinoma detected by intensive follow-up. Dis Colon Rectum. 2002;45:468–75.
22. Heriot A, Byrne C, Lee P, Dobbs B, Tilney H, Solomon M, Mackay J, Frizelle F. Extended radical resection: the choice for locally recurrent rectal cancer. Dis Colon Rectum. 2008;51:284–91.
23. Grossman EM, Johnson FE, Vigro KS, Longo WE, Fossati R. Follow-up of colorectal cancer patients after resection with curative intent: the GILDA trial. Surg Oncol. 2004;13:119–24.
24. Primrose J, Mant D. A randomised controlled trial to assess the cost-effectiveness of intensive versus no scheduled follow-up in patient who have undergone resection for colorectal cancer with curative intent. A protocol. Website -http://www.controlled-trials.com/isrctn/pf/61091474.
25. Yang I, Eschrich S, Bloom G, Quackenbush J, Yeatman T. Molecular profiling predicts colon cancer survival better than Dukes staging. Ann Surg Oncol. 2004;1 Suppl 2:S54.

Colon and Rectum Carcinoma Surveillance Counterpoint: Japan

35

Yasushi Toh and Yoshihisa Sakaguchi

The primary aim of surveillance after curative resection of colorectal cancer is to detect metastasis, local recurrence, or metachronous primary cancers at an early stage when curative reoperations are possible, leading to improvement of the prognosis. Recent meta-analyses show that more intensive postoperative surveillance results in a reduction of mortality and an improvement in the curative reoperation rate in comparison to minimal surveillance [1-6]. Furthermore, the early detection of recurrence of colorectal cancer also results in prolongation of life by chemotherapy and/or radiotherapy, even in patients with unresectable disease [7]. While several recommendations are now available from the American Society of Clinical Oncology (ASCO), the European Society for Medical Oncology (ESMO) and so on [8,9], the best strategy for the surveillance still remains controversial.

Surveillance seems more intensive in Japan than in Western countries. However, the most reliable method of surveillance has not yet been established in Japan because of lack of data. Therefore, the Japanese Society for Cancer of the Colon and Rectum (JSCCR) carried out a retrospective multicenter study to clarify the characteristics of recurrence and the effectiveness of surveillance after curative-intent resection of colorectal cancer in Japan [10]. Based on the results of this study, standard surveillance schedules have been published [11].

In determining the best surveillance strategy after curative-intent resection of colorectal cancer in Japan, it is necessary to consider certain aspects of treatments and outcomes in this country: (1) The five-year survival rates after resection seem to be higher in Japan than in Western countries, possibly because of a more extensive lymph node dissection; (2) The method for pathological detection of lymph node metastases is different and more extensive, thus resulting in more accurate pathological staging in Japan [12]; (3) Neoadjuvant chemoradiotherapy is not popular for rectal cancer in Japan; and (4) Strategies for adjuvant chemotherapy are different in Japan where oral anticancer drugs are used for many of the patients with high-risk stage II and stage III cancers.

The study by the JSCCR showed the characteristics of recurrence and surveillance tools after a curative resection for colorectal cancer in Japan [10]. They enrolled 5,230 consecutive patients (stage I = 1367; stage II = 1912; stage III = 1951) who underwent curative-intent resections at 14 hospitals from 1991 to 1996. The median follow-up periods were 3.5 ± 2.9 years for the patients with recurrence and 7.1 ± 3.1 years for those without.

Of the 5,230 patients, 906 (17.3%) developed recurrence. The recurrences occurred in 3.7%, 14%, and 31% of patients with stages I, II, and III disease, respectively. In each stage, the rate of recurrence was higher in patients with rectal cancer than in those with colon cancer. The sites of recurrence in patients with colon cancer were liver (7.9%), lung (3.5%), local recurrence (1.8%), anastomotic recurrence (0.3%), and other (1.8%). The rates for rectal cancer were liver (7.3%), lung (7.5%), local recurrence (8.8%), anastomotic recurrence (0.8%), and other (4.2%), respectively. The median time to recurrence was 1.4 ± 1.4 years. Approximately 80% and 95% of all recurrences occurred within three and five years after the initial operation, respectively. About 95% of anastomotic recurrences occurred within three years. The recurrence rates one year after resection were 22% for stage I, 31% for stage II, and 45% for stage III in patients. The rates at three years were 69%, 77%, and 87%, and those at five years were 96%, 93%, and 98%, respectively. Therefore, the recurrence rate in patients with stages II and III disease increased rapidly for the first three years, while those with stage I showed a gradual and constant increase for five years. Recurrences later than five years after the initial resection were extremely rare (0.14%, 0.94%, and 0.67% in stages I, II, and III, respectively).

Y. Toh, MD, PhD, FACS (✉) • Y. Sakaguchi, MD, PhD, FACS
Department of Gastroenterological Surgery, National Kyushu Cancer Center, 3-1-1 Notame, Minami-ku, Fukuoka 811-1395, Japan
e-mail: ytoh@nk-cc.go.jp; ysakaguchi@nk-cc.go.jp

F.E. Johnson et al. (eds.), *Patient Surveillance After Cancer Treatment*, Current Clinical Oncology,
DOI 10.1007/978-1-60327-969-7_35, © Springer Science+Business Media New York 2013

Of the 906 patients with recurrence, 379 (42%) underwent a resection with curative intent. The resection rates for liver metastasis, lung metastasis, local recurrence, and anastomotic recurrence were 46%, 38%, 34%, and 68%, respectively. The five-year survival rates after a resection of the liver, lung, local and anastomotic recurrence were 45%, 48%, 27%, and 33%, respectively, and the prognosis of patients who underwent a resection for any recurrence was better than that of patients who did not. Among the patients with resection of a recurrence, 37% developed no re-recurrence during a median follow-up of 6.0 ± 2.8 years.

The study group of the JSCCR also investigated surveillance tools that first indicated a suspicion of recurrence (first indicator). When the first indicator was a symptom or physical finding, the curative-intent resection rate was low in patients with hepatic and pulmonary recurrence but high in local and anastomotic recurrence. The detection rates of recurrence by a combination of clinical visits and the measurement of serum carcinoembryonic antigen (CEA) levels were 52%, 35%, 71%, and 68% in hepatic, pulmonary, local and anastomotic recurrences, respectively. Therefore, a considerable number of recurrences could be detected by clinical visits plus CEA monitoring alone, except for lung metastasis. For liver metastasis, the addition of liver imaging to clinical visits and CEA measurement increased the detection rate to 95%. The resection rate for lung metastasis was high when a chest X-ray was the first indicator; 80% of lung metastasis could be detected with chest X-ray combined with clinical visits and CEA measurement. More than 80% of recurrences (other than liver and lung) could be detected by computed tomography (CT) combined with clinical visits and CEA measurement. The first indicator for anastomotic recurrence was usually physical examination. A digital rectal examination was the most important way to detect local recurrence of rectal cancer.

In the most recent JSCCR guidelines for the treatment of colorectal cancer in Japan [11], examples of surveillance protocols after curative resection are presented separately for patients with colon cancer and rectal cancer of stages I, II, and III, taking the present status of surveillance in Japan and the data mentioned above into consideration. These guidelines suggest that surveillance for patients with a mucosal colorectal cancer with cancer-free resection margin might be omitted due to the extremely low recurrence rate. Although not yet been validated, our institute follows this recommendation.

The duration of surveillance is five years because rate of recurrence greater than five years after the initial operation is extremely low. Considering the rate and timing of recurrence, surveillance should be more intensive for the first three years and less intensive for the following two years.

According to the JSCCR guidelines [11], patients with stages I, II, and III colorectal cancers should be seen in the office every three months for the first three years and every six months thereafter until five years after the initial operation. About half of the local or anastomotic recurrences are found by history and/or physical examination during a clinical visit [10]. For patients with rectal cancer, a digital rectal examination should be performed every six months for the first three years after the operation, irrespective of stage.

An increase in the serum CEA level is the first indicator of recurrence in 40–89% of recurrences [13]. Recent meta-analyses indicate that more intensive monitoring of CEA has a significant impact on the mortality rate and the curative-intent resection rate [2,6]. ASCO guidelines recommend measurement of CEA levels for patients with stage II–III disease every three months for at least three years after the initial treatment provided that the patient is a candidate for surgery or systemic therapy [8]. The recommendation by The European Society of Medical Oncology (ESMO) is similar: CEA measurement every three to six months for the first three years and every six to twelve months in the following two years after surgery if initially elevated [9]. In JSCCR guidelines [11], measurement of the CEA level is recommended on every clinic visit for all patients with stages I, II, and III colorectal cancers: every three months for the first three years and every six months thereafter until five years after initial operation. The measurement of CA19-9 is also recommended in the surveillance of patients following a curative resection of colorectal cancer in Japan. However, the significance of CA19-9 monitoring in surveillance of patients following a curative resection of colorectal cancers remains controversial.

Kobayashi et al. reported that curative-intent resection rate of lung metastasis was 50%, when it was found by chest X-ray [10]. A meta-analysis by Tjandra et al. showed a significantly lower mortality with the use of chest X-ray, in comparison with the control in which no chest X-ray was performed [6]. Furthermore, more frequent use of chest X-ray was shown to have a significant impact on the curative operation rate of recurrence in comparison to less frequent use in this study. ASCO does not recommend routine chest X-rays and ESMO recommends the annual use of chest X-ray for five years [8,9]. Routine chest X-ray is not recommended (but is permitted) in JSCCR guidelines (Tables 35.1 and 35.2).

Few reports have shown the superiority of chest CT to chest X-ray as a routine imaging modality. JSCCR guidelines recommend a chest CT for patients with stages I, II, and III colorectal cancers every six months for five years. For patients with stages I or II, a chest CT can be done once a year in years 4 and 5 after initial operation in JSCCR guidelines. ASCO and ESMO recommend annual chest CT for three years for patients who are at high risk of recurrence and who could be candidates for curative-intent surgery [8,9].

The liver is the most common site of distant recurrence of colorectal cancer. However, the data available is inconclusive

Table 35.1 Surveillance for patients with stage I, II, and III colon cancer. National Kyushu Cancer Center, Japan

	Year Posttreatment#					
	1	2	3	4	5	>5
Office visit	4	4	4	2	2	0
Serum CEA and CA19-9 levels	4	4	4	2	2	0
Chest-/abdomen-computed tomography	2	2	2	2†	2†	0
Colonoscopy‡	1	0	1	0	0	‡

CEA: carcinoembryonic antigen
#Surveillance for only five years is recommended. Thereafter, the patient is returned to the primary care doctor.
†For patients with stage I or stage II disease, chest/abdomen CT can be once a year in years 4 and 5.
‡The recommended frequency of colonoscopy after five years is not determined.
For chest imaging, chest CT is more desirable, although chest X-ray is permitted instead.
For abdominal imaging, abdominal CT is more desirable, although abdominal ultrasonography is permitted instead.
The number in each cell indicates the number of times a particular modality is recommended during a particular posttreatment year.

Table 35.2 Surveillance for patients with stages I, II and III rectal cancer after curative-intent initial treatment National Kyushu Cancer Center, Japan

	Year Posttreatment#				
	1	2	3	4	5
Office visit	4	4	4	2	2
Digital rectal examination	2	2	2	0	0
Serum CEA and CA19-9 levels	4	4	4	2	2
Chest-/abdomen-/pelvis-computed tomography	2	2	2	2+	2+
Colonoscopy‡	1	1	1	0	0

CEA: carcinoembryonic antigen
#Surveillance for only five years is recommended. Thereafter, the patient is returned to the primary care doctor.
†For patients with stage I or stage II disease, chest/abdomen/pelvis CT can be once a year in years 4 and 5.
‡The recommended frequency of colonoscopy after five years is not determined.
For chest imaging, chest CT is more desirable, although chest X-ray is permitted instead.
For abdominal imaging, abdominal CT is more desirable, although abdominal ultrasonography is permitted instead.
The number in each cell indicates the number of times a particular modality is recommended during a particular posttreatment year.

with regard to the timing and frequency of imaging as well as to the modalities to detect liver metastasis. In several meta-analyses, a survival benefit of liver imaging has been shown [2-4]. The most recent meta-analysis showed that abdominal ultrasonography (US) significantly reduces the overall mortality rate and increases the curative-intent reoperation rate for liver metastasis [6]. Although the sensitivity of abdominal US to detect liver metastasis is inferior to that of abdominal CT [14], ESMO recommends US for liver imaging every six months for three years and then yearly for two years. An abdominal CT is recommended in ESMO guidelines only for patients with suspicion of recurrence. ASCO guidelines recommend annual abdominal CT instead of abdominal US for three years for such patients. An abdominal US is not recommended (but is permitted) for surveillance of liver metastasis in the JSCCR guidelines. In these guidelines, abdominal CT is recommended for liver imaging [11].

A pelvic CT is the most effective modality for detecting pelvic recurrence after a curative resection of rectal cancer and, therefore, the use of pelvic CT is considered to be appropriate for postoperative surveillance. Whether pelvic CT is superior to CEA level in detecting asymptomatic local recurrence is questionable [15]. Since local recurrences are frequently inoperable even if they are found at an early stage, the significance of pelvic CT in postoperative surveillance remains controversial. Furthermore, the specificity of pelvic CT to detect local recurrence is low (52%) reflecting the difficulty in distinguishing recurrent cancer from postoperative fibrosis in spite of its high sensitivity (82%) [16]. In Japan, pelvic CT is recommended every six months for five years for patients with rectal cancer. For those with stage I or II disease, it can be once a year in years 4 and 5. According to ASCO guidelines, pelvic CT is also considered for rectal cancer surveillance, especially for patients who have not been treated with radiotherapy [8].

Magnetic resonance imaging (MRI) has a higher sensitivity than CT for detection of liver metastasis, especially in combination with superparamagnetic iron oxide (SPIO). It is also more sensitive than CT for detecting pelvic local recurrence [14]. Because of its low cost-effectiveness, MRI is reserved for a more accurate diagnosis of hepatic or pelvic local recurrence for which a curative resection is indicated. Therefore, MRI is not recommended for surveillance in Japan.

Fluorodeoxyglucose (FDG)-PET is significantly more sensitive than CT or MRI for detecting liver metastasis [14], but it is inappropriate for surveillance due to its high cost and limited availability. The role of FDG-PET is to confirm operability by excluding unexpected additional metastases. FDG-PET is also valuable in the investigation of patients with increased tumor marker levels and negative conventional imaging.

The aim of colonoscopy is to identify either anastomotic recurrence or metachronous primary cancer. There is, however, no conclusive evidence of a survival benefit for the detection of intraluminal recurrence [13], although one meta-analysis demonstrated that colonoscopy had a significant impact on the overall mortality rate and curative-intent operation rate after detection of recurrence [6]. Since it is reported that metachronous primary colorectal cancer usually occurs in the first two years after the initial operation, the first postoperative colonoscopy is recommended at year 1 after the initial operation [13]. ASCO guidelines recommend the first colonoscopy at year 3 and then, if normal, once every five years thereafter, while ESMO guidelines call for the first colonoscopy at year 1 and every three years thereafter [8,9]. In Japan, colonoscopy is recommended at years 1 and 3 for colon cancer patients and annually for the first three years for those with rectal cancer. The optimal frequency of colonoscopic surveillance after three years is not addressed in the JSCCR recommendation.

There is no evidence that patients with colorectal cancer have a higher risk of developing second cancers in other organs or that surveillance for such cancers is valuable.

In Japan, standard surveillance schedules after a curative resection of colorectal cancer were published in 2010 [11]. Most institutes in Japan follow these recommendations. They are more intensive than those in the Western countries. Taking into account the peculiar situation of the treatment strategies and outcomes for colorectal cancers in Japan, the JSCCR recommendations, therefore, need to be validated in order to establish the optimal surveillance methods in Japan. Cost-effectiveness also needs to be considered. Moreover, it must always be kept in mind that the surveillance strategies might need to be changed if new effective diagnostic modalities or treatments are developed.

References

1. Rosen M, Chan L, Beart Jr RW, et al. Follow-up of colorectal cancer: a meta-analysis. Dis Colon Rectum. 1998;41:1116–26.
2. Figueredo A, Rumble RB, Maroun J, et al. Follow-up of patients with curatively resected colorectal cancer: a practice guideline. BMC Cancer. 2003;3:26.
3. Jeffery GM, Hickey BE, Hider P. Follow-up strategies for patients treated for non-metastatic colorectal cancer. Cochrane Database Syst Rev. 2002:CD002200.
4. Renehan AG, Egger M, Saunders MP, O'Dwyer ST. Impact on survival of intensive follow-up after curative resection for colorectal cancer: systematic review and meta-analysis of randomised trials. Br Med J. 2002;324:813–6.
5. Renehan AG, O'Dwyer ST, Whynes DK. Cost effectiveness analysis of intensive versus conventional follow up after curative resection for colorectal cancer. Br Med J. 2004;328:81–4.
6. Tjandra JJ, Chan MK. Follow-up after curative resection of colorectal cancer: a meta-analysis. Dis Colon Rectum. 2007;50: 1783–99.
7. McArdle C. ABC of colorectal cancer: effectiveness of follow up. Br Med J. 2000;21:1332–5.
8. Desch CE, Benson III AB, Somerfield MR, et al. Colorectal cancer surveillance: 2005 update of an American Society of Clinical Oncology practice guideline. J Clin Oncol. 2005;23:8512–9.
9. Van Cutsem EJ. Colon cancer: ESMO clinical recommendations for diagnosis, adjuvant treatment and follow-up. Ann Oncol. 2007; 18 Suppl 2:ii21-2.
10. Kobayashi H, Mochizuki H, Sugihara K, et al. Characteristics of recurrence and surveillance tools after curative resection for colorectal cancer: a multicenter study. Surgery. 2007;141:67–75.
11. The Japanese Society for Cancer of the Colon and Rectum. JSCCR guidelines 2010 for the treatment of colorectal cancer. (In Japanese) Tokyo, Kanehara; 2010; 36.
12. Ratto C, Sofo L, Ippoliti M, et al. Accurate lymph-node detection in colorectal specimens resected for cancer is of prognostic significance. Dis Colon Rectum. 1999;42:143–54.
13. Gan S, Wilson K, Hollington P. Surveillance of patients following surgery with curative intent for colorectal cancer. World J Gastroenterol. 2007;13:3816–23.
14. Miles K, Burkill G. Colorectal cancer: imaging surveillance following resection of primary tumour. Cancer Imaging. 2007;7:S143–149.
15. Pietra N, Sarli L, Costi R, et al. Role of follow-up in management of local recurrences of colorectal cancer: a prospective, randomized study. Dis Colon Rectum. 1998;41:1127–33.
16. Schaefer O, Langer M. Detection of recurrent rectal cancer with CT, MRI and PET/CT. Eur Radiol. 2007;17:2044–54.

Colon and Rectum Carcinoma Surveillance Counterpoint: Canada

36

Marko Simunovic

Keywords
Cancer Care Ontario • Computed tomography • Carcinoembryonic antigen • Magnetic resonance imaging • Position emissions tomography • Program in Evidence Based Care

In Canada, approximately 20,000 people are diagnosed annually with colon or rectal cancer, and cancer in these two related sites is the second leading cause of cancer deaths [1]. A similar pattern is present in other jurisdictions around the world [2, 3]. Surgical removal of the appropriate bowel segment and attached lymphatic basin is the cornerstone of curative therapy. Unfortunately, many patients do not undergo such resections due to the presence of advanced unresectable disease or underlying patient comorbidities. Population-based data from Ontario, Canada (population 13 million) show that 18% and 24% of patients with colon and rectal cancer, respectively, do not undergo a resection of their tumor [4]. Other data, also from Ontario, suggest that 10% of patients undergoing resection of their primary colon or rectal tumor have stage IV or metastatic disease [5] (see Table 36.1). Rarely is stage IV disease curable. Patients who present with metastatic disease do not enter surveillance regimens, but may enter testing regimens that monitor response to therapy. One may estimate then that, in Ontario and likely in many other large populations, approximately 70% of patients with colon or rectal cancer undergo resective surgery for cure. This chapter addresses surveillance for these patients.

Following curative-intent surgery, a patient may develop a second primary colorectal cancer—a metachronous lesion—or have the original tumor recur. Recurrent disease may recur locally—in the anatomic site of the previous relevant surgery—or in distant sites such as the liver, lung, or bone. The purpose of surveillance in colon and rectal cancer is threefold: to detect a new asymptomatic primary cancer; to prevent a new primary cancer; or to identify asymptomatic recurrent disease.

Asymptomatic metachronous colon or rectal cancer is estimated to occur in 5% of patients [6, 7]. Such lesions, when detected, are often resectable and curable. The removal of adenomas from the colon or rectum may prevent the development of a new cancer [8]. Such polypectomies are usually performed through an endoscope. The risk of asymptomatic recurrent disease after initial therapy influences the utility of surveillance tests, especially cross-sectional imaging tests. The risk of recurrent disease for patients with Stage II or III colon or rectal cancer ranges from 30 to 50% [9]. The risk of recurrent disease for patients with Stage I disease is low (10% or less).

Treatments following the discovery of asymptomatic recurrent disease can include surgery, chemotherapy, or radiation therapy. Radiation treatments are used as an adjunct to surgery or to palliate symptoms. Randomized trials demonstrate that chemotherapy can extend the survival duration of patients who present with stage IV disease or who develop distant recurrent disease. Such trials have not assessed the value of surveillance regimens to identify patients with recurrent disease in an effort to expedite treatment with chemotherapy or to lengthen the lives of such patients. The main purpose of surveillance is to identify asymptomatic metachronous or recurrent disease that can be surgically removed with a curative intent. For an individual patient, if surgery is not possible due to comorbid conditions or patient choice, then the use of surveillance tests should be discouraged—unless there are other reasons such as participation in a research study.

M. Simunovic, M.D., M.P.H., F.R.C.S.(C) (✉)
Department of Surgery, McMaster University,
1280 Main Street West, Hamilton, ON L8S 4L8, Canada

Surgical Oncologist, Juravinski Cancer Centre, Hamilton Health Sciences, 699 Concession Street, Hamilton, ON, Canada L8V 5C2
e-mail: marko.simunovic@jcc.hhsc.ca

F.E. Johnson et al. (eds.), *Patient Surveillance After Cancer Treatment*, Current Clinical Oncology,
DOI 10.1007/978-1-60327-969-7_36,

Table 36.1 TNM staging for colorectal cancer

	T category	*N* category	*M* category
Stage I	T1 into submucosa	Negative	Negative
	T2 into muscularis propria		
Stage II	T3 into surrounding mesenteric fat	Negative	Negative
	T4 involving visceral peritoneum or adjacent organ		
Stage III	Not relevant	Positive	Negative
Stage IV	Not relevant	Not relevant	Positive

Adapted from Greene FL, Page DL, Fleming ID, et al. AJCC Cancer Staging Manual, 7th ed. New York: Springer, 2002.
T—depth of penetration of primary tumor.
N—involvement of regional lymph nodes.
M—presence of metastatic disease.

Rarely is locally recurrent colon or rectal cancer resectable since such lesions often invade unresectable structures (e.g., pelvic side wall) or occur in concert with metastatic deposits [10, 11]. Only a small percentage of local recurrences undergo potentially curative resection and the prognosis for patients following surgical removal is poor. For patients with locally recurrent rectal cancer, who have had a resection with negative postoperative pathologic margins, the chance of long-term cure is approximately 20%. Regardless, surgeons are increasingly aggressive with recommendations for the resection of local recurrences—with or without the resection of metastatic deposits. For the appropriate patient, even if cure is not possible, local resection can still lead to local disease control and an ensuing important palliative benefit (e.g., the avoidance of disabling pain).

The liver is the most common of distant metastases following potentially curative colorectal cancer surgery. Liver metastases develop in approximately 30% of patients with stage II or III colorectal cancer [9, 12]. At the population level, a minority of such patients undergo resection of their liver metastases, though such resections are the most common type of surgery for distant recurrent disease [12]. Most case series reporting on the successful resection of liver metastases quote 5-year survival rates among patients of approximately 40% [13, 14]. There is much less data on the resection of metastatic disease in other organs or sites but, as with local surgery for local recurrence, clinicians are increasingly likely to recommend the resection of metastatic disease, especially if all evident disease can be resected.

In summary, surveillance regimens are used among patients who have undergone potentially curative surgery, who are at high risk for developing recurrent disease, and who are candidates for subsequent surgical treatments such as bowel or liver resection.

There are three forms of surveillance testing in colon and rectal cancer. The first is blood tests. Routine blood counts may demonstrate perturbations in the loss or production of red cells or platelets, while elevated liver function tests may indicate obstruction of the biliary system due to lymph node enlargement in the portal triad area or metastatic deposits in the liver. Serum carcinoembryonic antigen (CEA) levels are elevated in approximately 15% of patients with primary colon or rectal cancer, and an elevated CEA level is a poor prognostic factor [15, 16]. This antigen is located on the surface of colorectal adenocarcinoma cells and, if elevated, should drop to normal levels following curative surgery. A persistent elevation in CEA levels postsurgery usually indicates persistent cancer while a later rise may indicate metachronous or recurrent disease.

The second form of surveillance testing is endoscopic examination of the lower gastrointestinal tract. Endoscopy can identify metachronous disease or locally recurrent disease. The endoscopic removal of adenomas in a given patient may also prevent the development of metachronous colorectal cancer [8]. The time needed for transformation of a benign polyp to carcinoma is 5–10 years [17].

The third form of surveillance testing is imaging of the chest, abdomen, and pelvis [18]. The chest can be assessed using chest X-rays or cross-sectional imaging with computed tomography (CT), magnetic resonance imaging (MRI), or positron emissions tomography scans (PET). MRI scans are more likely to be used to assess the resectability of recurrent disease, while PET scans are best used to identify inconspicuous deposits of tumor outside an area of suspected recurrence. Similarly, the abdomen and pelvis can be assessed using CT scans, with MRI or PET scans ordered when there is a suspicion of recurrent disease. Ultrasound can also be used to detect metastatic disease in the liver, though it is of little use to detect recurrent disease in other parts of the abdomen and pelvis.

There are other tests available to detect recurrent colorectal cancer such as bone scan or cross-sectional imaging of the head. However, it is unlikely that asymptomatic recurrent colorectal cancer will appear in the bone or brain of a patient, prior to the development of liver or lung metastases. Thus, such tests are not used in routine care. These tests should be considered as resulting from a surveillance regimen when such tests were precipitated by a relevant symptom or sign that was elicited or observed, respectively, during a routine follow-up clinic visit.

High-quality evidence on surveillance in colon and rectal cancer is available from studies that have randomized patients to intense vs. less intense strategies. These will be discussed below. There is little evidence supporting individual surveillance tests or visits, or varying intervals for such interventions. Lennon et al. assessed the survival benefit of CEA monitoring [19]. Patients with an elevated CEA were randomized to aggressive investigation for recurrent disease, including a second-look laparotomy, vs. a conventional approach. Survival was similar in both arms of the trial suggesting little utility for

Table 36.2 Summary of intense vs. less intense randomized trials for colorectal cancer surveillance

Study, year	References	Surveillance intensity	Number of patients randomized	Median observation time (months)	Overall recurrence rate (%)	Number of second bowel cancers	Radical reoperation rate (%)	5-Year survival rate (%)
Ohlsson 1995	21	Less	54	82	33	NR	17	67
		More	53		32		29	75
Makela 1995	22	Less	54	>60	39	NR	14	54
		More	52		42		23	59
Schoemaker 1998	23	Less	158	>60	NR	5	NR	70
		More	167			3		76
Kjeldsen 1997	24	Less	307	>60	26	3	NR	68
		More	290		26	7		70
Pietra 1998	25	Less	103	>60	19	1	10	58
		More	104		25[a]	0	65	73[b]
Secco 2002	26	Less	145	>60	53	NR	16	48
		More	192		57		31	63

Reproduced from Figueredo A, Rumble R, Maroun J, Earle C, Cummings B, McLeod R, Zuraw L, Zwall C, and the members of the Gastrointestinal Cancer Disease Site Group of Cancer Care Ontario's Program in Evidence Based Care. Follow-up of patients with curatively resected colorectal cancer: a practice guideline. BMC Cancer. 2003 Oct;3(26): 1–13. http://www.biomedcentral.com/content/pdf/1471-2407-3-26.pdf
Note: *NR* Not reported
[a]$p<0.01$
[b]$p<0.05$

isolated CEA monitoring. Recommendations on the role of surveillance bowel imaging following colon or rectal cancer surgery are often extrapolated from cohort or case series studies, and observations that patients with a history of colorectal cancer are at greater risk over the normal population of developing a synchronous or metachronous bowel cancer [8]. We are unaware of randomized studies that have tested the efficacy of isolated surveillance imaging tests.

Cancer Care Ontario is mandated to oversee cancer control in the province of Ontario (population 13 million), Canada. The Program in Evidence Based Care at Cancer Care Ontario produces evidence-based standards, documents, and guidelines related to the diagnosis, treatment, and surveillance of patients with cancer. Such a document—a systematic review of the literature—has been produced on surveillance regimens among patients who have undergone potentially curative colorectal cancer surgery [12]. The review identified six high-quality trials that randomized patients with stage II or III colorectal cancer to a more vs. less intense surveillance strategy [20–25]. Recurrence and 5-year survival rates were calculated for over 1,150 patients. Details of the individual trial are summarized in Table 36.2.

In some of the studies, tests such as CEA testing, endoscopy, or imaging of the liver were used in both arms of the trial. Only one of the trials detected a statistically significant survival benefit favoring the more intense follow-up program [24]. However, when the data were pooled, a significant improvement was demonstrated in overall survival favoring the more intense follow-up program (relative risk ratio = 0.80, 95% CI, 0.70–0.91; $p=0.0008$) [12]. Of note, while rates of recurrence were similar in both surveillance schedules, asymptomatic recurrences and reoperations were more common in patients randomized to more intense schedules. This provides clinical plausibility for a more intense surveillance regimen. The review also discussed two meta-analyses which corroborated the Ontario guideline results [26, 27]. The authors of the Ontario practice guideline concluded that, while there is insufficient evidence to recommend specific surveillance tests, a more intense regimen results in a survival advantage.

Following the combining of current standards of care, expert opinion, and the results of the meta-analysis discussed above, stakeholders in Ontario made recommendations about a surveillance strategy [12]. These recommendations were modified slightly following the production of an Ontario guideline on cross-sectional imaging in colorectal cancer [18]. This latter guideline highlighted evidence demonstrating that CT identifies local recurrences and liver metastases better than ultrasound. Resection of liver metastases is likely the major driver of improved survival duration among patients enrolled in more intense surveillance strategies. Current recommendations in Ontario based on these two guidelines are summarized in table 36.3. The following post-surgery interventions are recommended for asymptomatic patients with stage II or III cancer: clinic visits every 6 months for 3 years and yearly thereafter for 2 years; during each visit serum CEA level and liver function tests are obtained; annual chest X-ray; annual cross-sectional imaging of the abdomen and pelvis with CT or MRI scanning; ultrasound of the abdomen at months 6, 18, and 30; and, colonoscopy within 1 year

Table 36.3 Current recommendations for stage II and III disease

	Time after primary treatment				
Category	Year 1	Year 2	Year 3	Year 4	Year 5
Clinic visits	2	2	2	1	1
Blood tests (CEA, liver)	2	2	2	1	1
Chest X-ray	1	1	1	1	1
CT or MRI abdomen and pelvis[a]	1	1	1	1	1
US abdomen[b]	1	1	1	–	–
Colonoscopy[c]	1	–	–	–	–

Adapted from guideline I and II
[a]Recommended end of the year
[b]Recommended mid-year
[c]3–5 years later if first scope is normal

Table 36.4 Current recommendations for stage I disease

	Time after primary treatment				
Category	Year 1	Year 2	Year 3	Year 4	Year 5
Clinic visits	2	2	2	1	1
Blood tests (CEA, liver)	2	2	2	1	1
Chest X-ray	1	1	1	1	1
CT abdomen and pelvis	1	1	1	–	–
Colonoscopy[a]	1	–	–	–	–

[a]3–5 years later if first scope is normal

of surgery and repeated annually if clinically significant polyps are removed, or repeated in 3–5 years if no clinically significant polyps are detected. Early postoperative colonoscopy is recommended if it was not done prior to surgery. There is no evidence of a difference between CT and MRI for diagnosing recurrence even among patients with a clinical suspicion of disease recurrence, though it is likely that MRI is more accurate in differentiating scar tissue from recurrence [28]. Thus a practical approach to abdominal and pelvic imaging is initial use of CT scans followed by MRI if local recurrence is suspected. The Ontario guidelines do not advocate the use of routine chest CT to detect lung recurrences. This is due to the high rate of identifying false positive lesions and the attendant risks of investigating or removing such lesions.

It is important to recognize that the Ontario guidelines make no comment on surveillance among patients with Stage I colorectal cancer, since such patients were not included in the randomized trials assessed in the relevant systematic review, outlined above [12]. Such patients were likely not included in trials since their risk of recurrent disease is low. As well, if comorbidities or patient choice preclude future surgery, only annual visits or testing when symptoms occur are recommended.

The author follows the Cancer Care Ontario guidelines for surveillance among patients with stages II and III disease (Table 36.3). Surveillance regimens are similar for patients with rectal and colon cancer, with the exception of a rigid sigmoidoscopy provided at each office visit for patients treated for rectal cancer. Of importance, rectal cancer patients, and a small number of colon cancer patients, treated with neoadjuvant therapy for locally advanced disease can have tumor downsizing, and postoperative pathological examination is not always predictive of the presenting tumor stage. Thus, I assume all patients who receive neoadjuvant therapy were originally stages II or III, regardless of pathology, and such patients enter the surveillance regimen outlined in Table 36.3.

The Ontario guidelines do not deal with patients with stage I disease. For such patients I follow the office visit, blood work, chest X-ray, and endoscopy surveillance schedule outlined in Table 36.3, but will modify cross-sectional imaging of the abdomen and pelvis. Generally, I recommend CT scans annually for 2–3 years only (Table 36.4).

Surgical cancer care in Ontario is relatively centralized. For example, the median distance traveled by patients to receive colon cancer surgery is only 5 km [29]. As well, in most regions of the country, the Canadian Cancer Society organizes fleets of volunteers—often former patients treated for cancer—to drive cancer patients to tests or office visits. Thus, in this practice, it is not an undue burden for most patients to travel to the clinic for follow-up visits and tests. For the small number of patients referred by surgeons from parts of the province where the patient must travel a long distance for care, surveillance recommendations are summarized in a letter which requests that the referring surgeon oversee such tests and visits. Rarely do patients object to follow-up endoscopy, blood tests, or imaging. Primary care physicians are the backbone of the medical system in Ontario. Nearly every patient diagnosed with colorectal cancer is initially referred to an appropriate specialist for investigation or treatment from their family physician. Despite this, family physicians do not play a role in routine surveillance of my patients for two main reasons. Subtle signs or symptoms related to recurrent disease may not be noted on testing or during office visits by the family physician, a physician who must deal with a myriad of unrelatd issues for an individual patient. As well, I believe that an expectation of routine visits and tests ensures greater completeness of surveillance and more accurate measurement of overall outcomes for patients I treat. Medical and radiation oncologists play little role in the routine surveillance of my patients treated with stage I–III colorectal cancer. The development of recurrent disease in a patient will trigger the appropriate involvement or reinvolvement of other oncologists in the care of patients.

There are variations on recommendations for colorectal cancer surveillance regimens from different organizations around the world. The American Society of Clinical Oncology suggests that, for patients with stage II or III disease, CEA testing should be done every 3 months for at least

3 years, along with annual CT scans of the chest and abdomen, and colonoscopy according to intervals similar to the Ontario schedule outlined above [30]. The American Society of Gastrointestinal Endoscopy surveillance guideline comments only on colonscopy. The colonoscopy recommendations are similar to those in Ontario [31]. The American Society of Colon and Rectal Surgeons suggests that, for patients with completely resected colorectal cancer, routine imaging of the liver should not be performed, while clinic visits and CEA testing should occur at least three times per year for the first 2 years of follow-up [32]. The Association of Coloproctology of Great Britain and Ireland recommends that a colon cleared of polyps or cancer be colonoscoped every 5 years, and that a single CT scan of the chest and abdomen be performed at some point in the 2 years following surgery with the intent of discovering asymptomatic resectable liver metastases [33]. The Scottish Intercollegiate Guidelines Network simply recommends that "patients who have undergone curative resection for colorectal cancer should undergo formal follow up in order to facilitate the early detection of metastatic disease [34]." The New Zealand Guidelines Group provides little detail on specific recommended surveillance interventions except that colonoscopy should be performed at 3- to 5-year intervals [35]. Of interest, it is also suggested that patients "should be informed of the uncertain efficacy of follow-up with regard to survival benefit."

In summary, a meta-analysis of six well-designed randomized trials demonstrated a survival benefit for an intense vs. less intense surveillance regimen among patients who have undergone curative resection for colorectal cancer [12]. There was a 20% drop in the risk of death among patients enrolled in intense surveillance (relative risk ratio=0.80, 95% CI, 0.70–0.91; $p=0.0008$). These results were the basis of the Ontario surveillance recommendations outlined in Table 36.3, and the basis of my surveillance recommendations to patients. The benefit of intense surveillance is likely due to increased rates of identification and resection of asymptomatic liver metastases. It follows that surveillance tests are of less benefit if the risk of recurrent disease is very low (e.g., patients with stage I disease) and of no benefit among patients who will be unable to undergo subsequent surgery due to comorbidities. Surveillance recommendations around the world are fairly consistent for colonoscopy. It is generally agreed that the large bowel should be cleared of synchronous disease and adenomatous polyps in the perioperative period, and that a repeat colonoscopy be repeated within 1 year of surgery. If the bowel is clear at this point, then colonoscopy should be repeated every 3–5 years. There is more variability for blood testing, especially for CEA monitoring, and for cross-sectional imaging of the chest, abdomen, and pelvis. It must be emphasized that surveillance recommendations apply to the postoperative patient who is asymptomatic and apparently cancer-free. A new worrisome sign or symptom brought to the attention of the attendant physician should be appropriately investigated, regardless of the time since surgery or, within reason, results of recent tests. Surveillance recommendations in colorectal cancer complement, rather than replace, clinical judgment.

References

1. Canadian Cancer Society/National Cancer Institute of Canada: Canadian Cancer Statistics 2008, Toronto, Canada, 2008. ISSN 0835-2976. http://www.cancer.ca/canada-wide/about%20cancer/cancer%20statistics/~/media/CCS/Canada%20wide/Files%20List/English%20files%20heading/pdf%20not%20in%20publications%20section/Canadian%20Cancer%20Society%20Statistics%20PDF%202008_614137951.ashx (Accessed November 19, 2009).
2. Boyle P, Ferlay J. Cancer incidence and mortality in Europe, 2004. Ann Oncol. 2005;16:481–8. http://coloncancer.about.com/gi/dynamic/offsite.htm?zi=1/XJ&sdn=coloncancer&cdn=health&tm=12&gps=86_189_931_562&f=10&su=p284.9.336.ip_p736.8.336.ip_&tt=2&bt=0&bts=0&zu=http%3A//dx.doi.org/10.1093/annonc/mdi098.
3. Horner MJ, Ries LAG, Krapcho M, Neyman N, Aminou R, Howlader N, et al., editors. SEER cancer statistics review, 1975–2006. Bethesda, MD: National Cancer Institute; 200. http://seer.cancer.gov/csr/1975_2006/, based on November 2008 SEER data submission, posted to the SEER web site.
4. Nenshi R, Baxter N, Kennedy E, Schultz SE, Gunraj N, Wilton AS, et al. Cancer surgery in Ontario: surgery for colorectal cancer; ICES atlas. Toronto: Institute for Clinical Evaluative Sciences; 2008. Chapter 4, p. 53–96.
5. Simunovic M, Coates A, Goldsmith C, Thabane L, Reeson D, Smith A, et al. The cluster-randomized Quality Initiative in Rectal Cancer (QIRC) trial: evaluating a quality improvement strategy in surgery. CMAJ. 2010;182(12):1301–1306 [ISRCTN 78363167].
6. Enblad P, Adami HO, Glimelius B, Krusemo U, Påhlman L. The risk of subsequent primary malignant diseases after cancers of the colon and rectum. A nationwide cohort study. Cancer. 1990;65:2091–100.
7. Bülow S, Svendsen LB, Mellemgaard A. Metachronous colorectal carcinoma. Br J Surg. 1990;77:502–5.
8. Winawer S, Zauber A, Ho M, O'Brien M, Gottlieb L, Sternberg S, et al. The National Polyp Study Workgroup. Prevention of colorectal cancer by colonscopic polypectomy. N Engl J Med. 1993;329:1977–81.
9. O'Connell MJ, Campbell ME, Goldberg RM, Grothey A, Seitz JF, Benedetti JK, et al. Survival following recurrence in stage II and III colon cancer: findings from the ACCENT data set. J Clin Oncol. 2008;26:2336–41.
10. Heriot AG, Tekkis PP, Darzi A, Mackay J. Surgery for local recurrence of rectal cancer. Colorectal Dis. 2006;8:733–47.
11. Moriya Y. Treatment strategy for locally recurrent rectal cancer. Jpn J Clin Oncol. 2006;36:127–31.
12. Gastrointestinal Cancer Disease Site Group. Figueredo A, Rumble RB, Maroun J, Earle CC, Cummings B, McLeod R, Zuraw L, Zwaal C. Follow-up of patients with curatively resected colorectal cancer [full report]. Toronto (ON): Cancer Care Ontario (CCO); 2004 [online update]. 30 p. (Practice guideline report; no. 2–9).
13. Shah SA, Bromberg R, Coates A, Rempel R, Simunovic M, Gallinger S. Survival after liver resection for metastatic colorectal carcinoma in a large population. J Am Coll Surg. 2007;205:676–83.

14. Cummings LC, Payes JD, Cooper GS. Survival after hepatic resection in metastatic colorectal cancer: a population-based study. Cancer. 2007;109:718–26.
15. Takagawa R, Fujii S, Ohta M, et al. Preoperative serum carcinoembryonic antigen level as a predictive factor of recurrence after curative resection of colorectal cancer. Ann Surg Oncol. 2008;15:3433–9.
16. Goldstein MJ, Mitchell EP. Carcinoembryonic antigen in the staging and follow-up of patients with colorectal cancer. Cancer Invest. 2005;23:338–51.
17. Imperiale TF, Glowinski EA, Lin-Cooper C, Larkin GN, Rogge JD, Ransohoff DF. Five-year risk of colorectal neoplasia after negative screening colonoscopy. N Engl J Med. 2008;359:1218–24.
18. Simunovic M, Stewart L, Zwaal C, Johnston M. Diagnostic Imaging Guidelines Panel. Cross-sectional imaging in colorectal cancer: recommendations report. Toronto, ON: Cancer Care Ontario (CCO); 2006. p.20.
19. Lennon T, Houghton J, Northover J. What is the value of clinical follow-up for colorectal cancer patients? The experience of the CRC/NIH CEA second-look trial. In the proceedings of the Nottingham International Colorectal Cancer Symposium, Nottingham; 1995.
20. Ohlsson B, Breland U, Ekberg H, Graffner H, Tranberg KG. Follow-up after curative surgery for colorectal carcinoma. Randomized comparison with no follow-up. Dis Colon Rectum. 1995;38:619–26.
21. Mäkelä JT, Laitinen SO, Kairaluoma MI. Five-year follow-up after radical surgery for colorectal cancer. Results of a prospective randomized trial. Arch Surg. 1995;130:1062–7.
22. Schoemaker D, Black R, Giles L, Toouli J. Yearly colonoscopy, liver CT, and chest radiography do not influence 5-year survival of colorectal cancer patients. Gastroenterology. 1998;114:7–14.
23. Kjeldsen BJ, Kronborg O, Fenger C, Jørgensen OD. A prospective randomized study of follow-up after radical surgery for colorectal cancer. Br J Surg. 1997;84:666–9.
24. Pietra N, Sarli L, Costi R, Ouchemi C, Grattarola M, Peracchia A. Role of follow-up in management of local recurrences of colorectal cancer: a prospective, randomized study. Dis Colon Rectum. 1998;41:1127–33.
25. Secco GB, Fardelli R, Gianquinto D, et al. Efficacy and cost of risk-adapted follow-up in patients after colorectal cancer surgery: a prospective, randomized and controlled trial. Eur J Surg Oncol. 2002;28:418–23.
26. Rosen M, Chan L, Beart Jr RW, Vucasin P, Anthone G. Follow-up of colorectal cancer. A meta-analysis. Dis Colon Rectum. 1998;41:1116–26.
27. Bruinvels DJ, Stiggelbout AM, Kievit J, van Houwelingen HC, Habbema DF, van de Velde CJ. Follow-up of patients with colorectal cancer. A meta-analysis. Ann Surg. 1994;219:174–82.
28. Blomqvist L, Holm T, Göranson H, Jacobsson H, Ohlsén H, Larsson SA. MR imaging, CT and CEA scintigraphy in the diagnosis of local recurrence or rectal carcinoma. Acta Radiol. 1996;37:779–84.
29. Simunovic M, Rempel E, Thériault ME, et al. Influence of hospital characteristics on operative death and survival of patients after major cancer surgery in Ontario. Can J Surg. 2006;49:251–8.
30. Desch CE, Benson 3rd AB, Somerfield MR, et al. Colorectal cancer surveillance: 2005 update of an American Society of Clinical Oncology practice guideline. J Clin Oncol. 2005;20(23):8512–9.
31. Rex DK, Kahi CJ, Levin B, et al. Guidelines for colonoscopy surveillance after cancer resection: a consensus update by the American Cancer Society and US Multi-Society Task Force on Colorectal Cancer. CA Cancer J Clin. 2006;56:160–7.
32. Anthony T, Simmang C, Hyman N, et al. American Society of Colon and Rectal Surgeons Practice parameters for the surveillance and follow-up of patients with colon and rectal cancer. Dis Colon Rectum. 2004;47:807–17.
33. Association of Coloproctology of Great Britain and Ireland. Guidelines for the management of colorectal cancer. London, UK: Association of Coloproctology of Great Britain and Ireland; 2007. 117 p.
34. Scottish Intercollegiate Guidelines Network (SIGN). Management of colorectal cancer. A national clinical guideline. Edinburgh, Scotland: Scottish Intercollegiate Guidelines Network (SIGN); 2003. 47 p. (SIGN publication; No. 67).
35. New Zealand Guidelines Group (NZGG). Surveillance and management of groups at increased risk of colorectal cancer. Wellington, NZ: New Zealand Guidelines Group (NZGG); 2004. 84 p.

Anal Carcinoma

37

David Y. Johnson, Shilpi Wadhwa, and Frank E. Johnson

Keywords
Anal carcinoma • Common • Incidence • Risk factors • Variability

The data for the estimated new cases and deaths worldwide in 2002 for anal carcinoma was not available through the international agency for research on cancer (IARC), a component of the world health organization (WHO) [1].

The American Cancer Society estimated that there were 4,650 new cases and 690 deaths due to anal carcinoma in the USA in 2007 [2]. The cases included carcinoma of the anus, anal canal, and anorectum. The data for the estimated five-year survival rate (all races) in the USA in 2007 was not available for this type of cancer [2].

The incidence of anal cancer is approximately 10 % the incidence of rectal cancer. There is considerable geographic variation in histology (squamous cell carcinoma versus adenocarcinoma). Risk factors include human papilloma virus infection, immunosuppression, history of a prior sexually transmitted disease, and tobacco smoking [3, 4].

Geographic Variation Worldwide

The incidence of anal cancer is higher among women than men in Switzerland, Western Europe, and Central and South America. In North America, Middle and Far East, and Oceania, the differences in incidence between the sexes are generally small. The incidence is low in Israel and Japan [3]. Within the USA, the incidence of anal cancer is high among black and white men in California [3].

Surveillance Strategies Proposed By Professional Organizations or National Government Agencies and Available on the Internet.

National Comprehensive Cancer Network (NCCN, www.nccn.org)—NCCN guidelines were accessed on 1/28/12 (Table 37.1). There were no significant changes compared to the guidelines accessed on 4/10/07.

American Society of Clinical Oncology (ASCO, www.asco.org)—ASCO guidelines were accessed on 1/28/12. No quantitative guidelines exist for anal cancer surveillance, including when first accessed on 10/31/07.

The Society of Surgical Oncology (SSO, www.surgonc.org)—SSO guidelines were accessed on 1/28/12. No quantitative guidelines exist for anal cancer surveillance, including when first accessed on 10/31/07.

European Society for Medical Oncology (ESMO, www.esmo.org)—ESMO guidelines were accessed on 1/28/12 (Table 37.2). There are new quantitative guidelines compared to the guidelines accessed on 10/31/07.

European Society of Surgical Oncology (ESSO, www.esso-surgeonline.org)—ESSO guidelines were accessed on 1/28/12. No quantitative guidelines exist for anal cancer surveillance, including when first accessed on 10/31/07.

Cancer Care Ontario (CCO, www.cancercare.on.ca)—CCO guidelines were accessed on 1/28/12. No quantitative guidelines exist for anal cancer surveillance, including when first accessed on 10/31/07.

National Institute for Clinical Excellence (NICE, www.nice.org.uk)—NICE guidelines were accessed on 1/28/12. No quantitative guidelines exist for anal cancer surveillance, including when first accessed on 10/31/07.

D.Y. Johnson (✉) • S. Wadhwa
Department of Internal Medicine, Saint Louis University Medical Center, Saint Louis, MO, USA
e-mail: dyjohnson@gmail.com

F.E. Johnson, M.D., FACS (✉)
Saint Louis University Medical Center and Saint Louis Veterans Affairs Medical Center, Saint Louis, MO, USA
e-mail: frank.johnson1@va.gov

F.E. Johnson et al. (eds.), *Patient Surveillance After Cancer Treatment*, Current Clinical Oncology,
DOI 10.1007/978-1-60327-969-7_37,

Table 37.1 Obtained from NCCN (www.nccn.org) on 1-28-12 Anal Carcinoma

	Years posttreatment[a]					
	1	2	3	4	5	>5
Office visit[b]	2–4	2–4	2–4	2–4	2–4	0
Anoscopy[c]	2–4	2–4	2–4	2–4	2–4	0
Chest/abdomen/ pelvic imaging[d]	1	1	1	0	0	0

NCCN guidelines were accessed on 1/28/12. There were no significant changes compared to the guidelines accessed on 4/10/07
[a]The numbers in the table indicate the number of times the modality is recommended during the indicated year posttreatment
[b]Includes digital rectal examination and inguinal node palpation
[c]Does not apply to patients status post abdominoperineal resection
[d]For T3-T4 or inguinal node positive disease

Table 37.2 Obtained from ESMO (www.esmo.org) on 1-28-12 Anal Cancer

	Years posttreatmenta					
	1	2	3	4	5	>5
Office visit[b]	2–4	2–4	1–2	1–2	1–2	0

- Regular CT scans for metastatic surveillance outside trials remains controversial, as there is no evidence for benefit of resection of metastases as in colorectal cancer

ESMO guidelines were accessed on 1/28/12. These are new quantitative guidelines compared to the guidelines accessed on 10/31/07
[a]The numbers in the table indicate the number of times the modality is recommended during the indicated year posttreatment
[b]Includes digital rectal examination and palpation of the inguinal lymph nodes

Table 37.3 Obtained from ASCRS (www.fascrs.org) on 1-28-12 Anal Canal Squamous-Cell Carcinoma

	Years Posttreatment[a]					
	1	2	3	4	5	>5
Office visit[b]	2–4	2–4	2–4	2–4	2–4	2–4
Anoscopy with biopsy[c]	2–4	2–4	2–4	2–4	2–4	2–4
CT scan[d]	2–4	2–4	2–4	2–4	2–4	2–4

- Endorectal ultrasound (ERUS) may help in early detection of recurrence[e]

ASCRS guidelines were accessed on 1/28/12. These are new quantitative guidelines compared to no guidelines found on 12/13/07
[a]The numbers in the table indicate the number of times the modality is recommended during the indicated year posttreatment
[b]Includes digital rectal examination and inguinal palpation
[c]Controversy exists about the need for multiple random biopsies vs. biopsy of suspicious lesions only
[d]For more advanced disease
[e]Three dimensional ERUS in conjunction with digital rectal examination and anoscopy can improve detection rates compared with two-dimensional ERUS and three-dimensional ERUS alone

The Cochrane Collaboration (CC, www.cochrane.org)—CC guidelines were accessed on 1/28/12. No quantitative guidelines exist for anal cancer surveillance, including when first accessed on 11/24/07.

The American Society of Colon and Rectal Surgeons (ASCRS, www.fascrs.org)—ASCRS guidelines were accessed on 1/28/12 (Table 37.3). There are new quantitative guidelines compared to no guidelines found on 12/13/07.

Society for Surgery of the Alimentary Tract (SSAT, www.ssat.com)—SSAT guidelines were accessed on 1/28/12. No quantitative guidelines exist for anal cancer surveillance, including when first accessed on 12/18/07.

The M.D. Anderson Surgical Oncology Handbook also has follow-up guidelines, proposed by authors from a single National Cancer Institute-designated Comprehensive Cancer Center, for many types of cancer [5]. Some are detailed and quantitative, others are qualitative.

Summary

This is a relatively uncommon cancer with significant variability in incidence worldwide. We found consensus-based guidelines but none based on high-quality evidence.

References

1. Parkin DM, Whelan SL, Ferlay J, Teppo L, Thomas DB. Cancer incidence in five continents, vol. VIII, international agency for research on cancer (IARC Scientific Publication 155). Lyon: IARC Press; 2002. ISBN 92-832-2155-9.
2. Jemal A, Seigel R, Ward E, Murray T, Xu J, Thun MJ. Cancer Statistics, 2007. CA Cancer J Clin. 2007;57:43–66.
3. Schottenfeld D, Fraumeni JG. Cancer epidemiology and prevention. 3rd ed. New York, NY: Oxford University Press; 2006. ISBN ISBN 13:978-0-19-514961-6.
4. DeVita VT, Hellman S, Rosenberg SA. Cancer. 7th ed. Philadelphia, PA: Lippincott Williams & Wilkins; 2005. ISBN ISBN 0-781-74450-4.
5. Feig BW, Berger DH, Fuhrman GM. The M.D. Anderson Surgical Oncology Handbook. 4th ed. Philadelphia, PA: Lippincott Williams & Wilkins; 2006. paperback. ISBN ISBN 0-7817-5643-X.

Anal Carcinoma Surveillance Counterpoint: USA

38

Jonathan M. Hernandez, Erin M. Siegel, Abby Koch, and David Shibata

Keywords
Human papillomavirus • Human immunodeficiency virus • Anal canal • Anal margin • Surveillance after therapy • Anal cancer in special populations • Anal adenocarcinoma

Anal cancer accounts for 4% of all lower gastrointestinal tract malignancies in the United States [1]. The incidence of anal cancer appears to be on the rise, with increases in incidence rates of 2.6% per year reported between 1992 and 2000 [2]. Over 5,000 new cases of anal cancer are diagnosed in the U.S. annually [3]. The overall 5-year survival rate is 66.5% [4]. This varies by stage at diagnosis (82% for local disease; 59% for regional disease and 19% for distant disease) [3]. The vast majority (65–85%) of anal malignancies are squamous cell carcinomas, which include various histological subtypes such as cloacogenic, basaloid, and transitional cell cancers [2]. Cancers of the anus have been categorized as those arising in the anal canal, or intraanal, and those arising at the anal margin, or perianal region [5].

J.M. Hernandez, M.D.
Department of Surgery, University of South Florida, Tampa, FL, USA

Department of Gastrointestinal Oncology, H. Lee Moffitt Cancer Center and Research Institute, Tampa, FL, USA
e-mail: Jonathan.hernandez@moffitt.org

E.M. Siegel, Ph.D. • A. Koch, B.S.
Department of Cancer Epidemiology and Genetics, Risk Assessment, Detection & Intervention Program, H. Lee Moffitt Cancer Center and Research Institute, 12902 Magnolia Drive, MRC-2, Tampa, FL 33612, USA
e-mail: Erin.siegel@moffitt.org; Abby.koch@moffitt.org

D. Shibata, M.D., F.A.C.S., F.A.S.C.R.S (✉)
Department of Gastrointestinal Oncology, H. Lee Moffitt Cancer Center and Research Institute, 12902 Magnolia Drive, SRB-2, Tampa, FL 33612, USA
e-mail: David.shibata@moffitt.org

Anal squamous cell carcinoma is highly associated with the presence of human papillomavirus (HPV), a sexually acquired virus with >50 different genotypes that infect the anogenital region [6, 7]. HPV DNA has been identified in over 85% of anal tumors. The HPV prevalence rate in cancer of the anal canal is similar to that found in cervical cancer, reflecting similar anatomy and presence of a transformation zone, which is the preferential site of HPV infection. Its prevalence in anal margin cancer is similar to that of vulvar or penile cancer, and lower than cancers of the anal canal [7]. Risk factors for anal cancer include those associated with exposure to HPV, such as sexual promiscuity, anal receptive anal intercourse, and homosexuality (specifically for males), as well as conditions affecting immune status such as human immunodeficiency virus (HIV) infection and use of immunosuppressant medication [8]. Additional risk factors for anal cancer include age, gender, smoking history, and history of cervical dysplasia or cancer [5, 8].

Despite the growing incidence of anal squamous cell carcinoma and increasing knowledge regarding a viral etiology, there has been minimal progress toward improving the overall clinical outcomes of this disease since the establishment of definitive chemoradiation as standard first-line treatment by Nigro et al. in the 1970s [9]. However, given the treatment-associated toxicities of 5-fluorouracil and mitomycin C and concomitant external beam radiotherapy, many investigators have attempted to identify equally efficacious regimens with improved patient tolerance. Most recently, the Radiation Therapy Oncology Group randomized 644 patients to either two cycles of 5-fluorouracil and cisplatin followed by concurrent chemotherapy plus radiotherapy with 5-fluorouracil and cisplatin or concurrent chemotherapy plus radiotherapy with 5-fluorouracil and mitomycin C [10]. Although there were no

F.E. Johnson et al. (eds.), *Patient Surveillance After Cancer Treatment*, Current Clinical Oncology,
DOI 10.1007/978-1-60327-969-7_38,

differences in disease-free or overall survival, the colostomy rate was significantly higher in patients receiving cisplatin, demonstrating a lack of superiority as compared to combination chemoradiotherapy using 5-fluorouracil and mitomycin C. With the overall success rate of chemotherapy plus radiation in the range of 60–80%, appropriate surveillance of patients with squamous cell carcinoma remains critical and personalized surveillance regimens may need to be considered for unique patient populations, such as HPV- and HIV-positive patients or those who are immunosuppressed [10–15].

Accumulating evidence supporting HPV as an etiological cause of anal cancers [7] and the differential treatment response by HPV status of other HPV-associated cancers, such as oropharyngeal cancer [16, 17], suggests that HPV infection may be an important factor influencing treatment response among anal squamous cell carcinoma patients. Currently, the routine assessment of the HPV status of tumors has not been a part of treatment trials and consequently, evaluation of response by HPV status or HPV type has not been feasible. Thus, clinical guidelines currently do not support HPV testing in the management of anal cancer [18]. A better understanding of the treatment response and patient outcomes according to HPV status has the potential to influence treatment and surveillance regimens.

Patterns of Treatment Failure

The initial success rate of chemoradiation is reported to be as high as 86%, although persistent disease may be present in up to 15% of patients [12, 19]. Even among patients with complete pathologic responses, as many as 30% sustain disease recurrence [19–21]. Recurrent disease occurs locally in the anal margin or canal, regionally in the pelvis including inguinal lymph nodes, and/or systemically outside the pelvis. Knowledge of the patterns of failure and patient predisposition to failure for both cancers of the anal canal and anal margin can contribute to the development of rational patient surveillance regimens.

Squamous Cell Carcinoma of the Anal Canal

Failure following definitive chemotherapy plus radiation for squamous cell carcinoma of the anal canal is primarily local and occurs in approximately 11–30% of patients [19–21]. Local recurrence is defined as a recurrence of disease in the anal canal or rectum after a disease-free interval of at least 6 months following completion of chemoradiation, thus distinguishing recurrence from disease persistence [1]. Both tumor-specific factors and treatment compliance are known to impact local recurrence rates. Das et al., in a multivariable analysis of 167 patients treated at M.D. Anderson Cancer Center, found that both T and N stages predicted an increased risk for treatment failure at the primary site [12]. Specifically, 3-year local control rates were 90% for T1 tumors and 63% for T4 tumors, and 85% and 39% for N0 tumors and tumors with extensive nodal metastases, respectively. Similarly, Peiffert et al., in a review of 106 patients, found that patients with tumors larger than 4 cm had increased rates of local recurrence compared to those having smaller tumors [22]. Nodal status was found to be a significant predictor of local control in the European Organization for Research and Treatment of Cancer phase III trial [23]. Roohipour et al. reported the Memorial Sloan-Kettering experience with 131 patients, demonstrating again that overall stage had a significant impact upon local recurrence rate [14]. In addition, the total dose of radiation received and duration of radiation treatment were identified as strong independent predictors of local treatment failure. In the Radiation Therapy Oncology Group 92-08 trial, planned 2-week treatment breaks were associated with increased local failure rate [24]. Of note, the majority of patients with local recurrences present within the first 12 months following completion of therapy, and nearly all are identified by the end of the second year [1, 22, 25, 26].

Regional failures, defined as recurrences in the pelvis but outside the anal canal and rectum, occur in isolation far less frequently than local recurrences. Regional failure sites include perirectal, iliac, and inguinal lymph nodes, vagina, prostate, and urinary bladder. Generally, tumor-specific factors affecting local control also impact regional control (i.e., T stage, N stage, and overall stage). The absence of nodal disease at presentation does not obviate the need for nodal surveillance. Peiffert et al. reported a large series of regional recurrences with or without concomitant local recurrence [22]. Fifteen patients (14%) experienced regional recurrence in inguinal lymph nodes (5%), perirectal lymph nodes (2%), iliac lymph nodes (5%), and other pelvic sites (3%). Only 4 of the 12 patients with lymph node recurrence had evident lymphatic involvement at the time of initial presentation. This phenomenon may be secondary to the inability to accurately identify lymphatic disease by computed tomography alone. Using positron emission tomography, Trautmann et al. demonstrated nodal disease in 24% of patients studied who were initially thought to be node-negative by computed tomography [27]. In support of this concept of subclinical lymphatic disease are the recommendations for the inclusion of inguinal nodes in the radiotherapy fields in any patient estimated to be at increased risk [18]. The vast majority of isolated regional nodal recurrences present within 2 years following completion of chemotherapy plus radiation [22, 25, 26].

Distant failure, defined as cancer recurrence outside the pelvis, most commonly affects liver, lung, bone, and extrapelvic lymph nodes [28, 29]. Distant recurrences are frequently reported as occurring either simultaneously with or following local/regional failure [12, 22]. Local and/or regional failure is a predictive factor for the development of distant metastatic disease. In addition, the presence of nodal disease at presentation is associated with recurrent disease at distant sites. For example, Das et al. reported a 94% 3-year distant control rate for patients with N0 tumors vs. 79% for those with nodal disease [12]. Higher N stage independently predicted increased rates of distant metastasis. Additionally, Peiffert reported nine distant failures among 106 patients, five of whom had lymphatic disease at initial presentation. Time to distant failure ranged from three to 41 months, with a median of 18 months [22]. Similarly, Toboul et al. reported that over 90% of distant metastases were recognized within 38 months following initial irradiation [26].

Squamous Cell Carcinoma of the Anal Margin

Local recurrence in patients with carcinoma of the anal margin is less frequent than in patients with carcinoma of the anal canal but is nonetheless the most frequent location of treatment failure [13]. Data concerning predisposition to local recurrence is limited. No series in the literature is larger than 60 patients and many have reported on less than half this number [11, 13, 30–35]. Consequently, it is difficult to correlate tumor-associated factors and/or treatment variables with recurrence. For example, in a study of 45 patients, Khanfir et al. found no correlation between local control and T stage, N stage, or tumor grade [13]. However, others have reported that lymph nodes metastasis at presentation has a significant impact on the rate of local control. A review of 32 patients treated in France demonstrated lymph node status to be the only significant factor affecting local and regional recurrence [31]. In another small series, Bieri et al. reported nodal disease at presentation in 4 of 24 patients with anal margin cancer, 3 of whom went on to suffer local recurrences [33].

Regional nodal recurrence is common in patients with squamous cell carcinoma of the anal canal as well as squamous cell carcinoma of the anal margin, but the nodes involved with the metastases in carcinoma of the anal margin are almost solely the inguinal lymph nodes [11]. Not surprisingly, the presence of nodal metastasis at presentation predisposes patients to recurrence in the involved nodal site [11]. Another strong predictor of nodal recurrence is failure to include the inguinal lymph nodes in the radiation field. Papillon et al. documented nodal recurrence in 6 of 42 patients with N0 disease without inguinal lymph node irradiation and 3 of 15 patients with N1 disease without inguinal lymph node irradiation [35]. Cutili et al. observed nodal recurrence in 3 of 18 patients with anal margin carcinoma in whom inguinal nodal irradiation was omitted [34]. In addition, Newlin et al. reported a single inguinal nodal recurrence in 19 patients, which occurred in the only patient who did not receive inguinal nodal radiation [30].

As with squamous cell carcinoma of the anal canal, distant recurrences in patients with carcinoma of the anal margin occur most commonly in patients with high T stage and/or N stage, and after local/regional recurrence. Given the paucity of patients with distant recurrence after treatment of anal margin cancer, no other predisposing tumor-specific factors or treatment variables have been identified.

Surveillance

Definitive chemoradiation has been firmly established as the preferred initial treatment for all patients with anal squamous cell carcinoma with the possible exception of T1 anal margin carcinoma [18]. Close surveillance is important following completion of chemotherapy plus radiation. At Moffitt Cancer Center, initial pretreatment assessment and patient surveillance are carried out by a multidisciplinary team of clinicians. Colorectal surgical oncologists play a central role in patient surveillance regardless of whether an operation was required as part of the initial treatment. This is mainly due to their expertise in anorectal anatomy, physical examination, endoscopy, biopsy, and surgery. Cancers can recur locally, regionally, and/or systemically, and therefore posttreatment surveillance must address each potential site of failure.

For patients with low-risk tumors (T1 or T2, N0), follow-up visits should occur every 3 months for the first 2 years and then every 6 months for 3 years (follow-up visits are generally not mandated after a disease-free interval of 5 years). They should include digital rectal examination, anoscopy/proctoscopy, and inguinal lymph node palpation at each visit (Table 38.1). Given that regional and distant recurrences are generally uncommon for patients with low-risk tumors (less than 5%), routine computed tomography scan surveillance is generally not performed [26].

For patients with high-risk tumors (T3, T4, or N+), follow-up visits should occur every 3 months for 2 years and every 6 months for 3 years. They should include digital rectal examination, anoscopy/proctoscopy, and inguinal lymph node palpation at each visit. Due to the substantial risk of both regional and distant recurrences for patients with high-risk tumors, we obtain a computed tomography scan of the chest, abdomen, and pelvis annually for 3 years (Table 38.2). Given our practice of using positron emission tomography scan for pretreatment planning and the incidence of false negative computed tomography scans in regional disease [27], we also obtain a concomitant positron emission tomography scan in these high-risk individuals. For the most part, we adhere to the surveillance guidelines published by the National Comprehensive Cancer Network but differ slightly in this regard [18].

Table 38.1 Follow-up schedule for patients with anal squamous cell carcinoma at low risk (T1/T2 and N0) for recurrence after chemotherapy plus radiation at Moffitt Cancer Center

	Year 1	Year 2	Year 3	Year 4	Year 5
Office visit[a]	4	4	2	2	2

[a]Includes digital rectal examination, anoscopy/proctoscopy, and inguinal node palpation
The numbers in each cell indicate the number of times in a particular year that the surveillance modality is recommended

Table 38.2 Follow-up schedule for patients with anal squamous cell carcinoma at high risk (T3/T4 and/or N+) for recurrence after chemotherapy plus radiation at Moffitt Cancer Center

	Year 1	Year 2	Year 3	Year 4	Year 5
Office visit[a]	4	4	2	2	2
CT	1	1	1	–	–
Positron emission tomography	1	1	1	–	–

[a]Includes digital rectal examination, anoscopy/proctoscopy, and inguinal node palpation
The numbers in each cell indicate the number of times in a particular year that the surveillance modality is recommended

At our institution, both providers and patients have been generally compliant with our surveillance strategy for squamous cell carcinoma of the anus. The frequent visits over the initial 2 years, in addition to oncologic surveillance, also allow patients to seek care and advice regarding treatment side effects such as proctitis, cystitis, and vaginal stenosis. Cost-related issues with respect to anal cancer surveillance require further study.

Physical examination is one of the most critical components of the surveillance regimen, particularly for the assessment of local disease status. We generally perform an examination at approximately 10–12 weeks following the completion of treatment. This allows enough time for healing of any perianal inflammation or desquamation such that digital rectal examination and anoscopy/sigmoidoscopy will be well tolerated by the patient. At this point a baseline response of the primary tumor mass is assessed along with the status of any clinical inguinal lymphadenopathy. The treated area is visualized by anoscopy and any baseline proctitis is also evaluated. Occasionally, significant posttreatment distortion of the anorectal anatomy, such as induration, inflammation, ulceration, or tissue loss, can be present and such changes should be meticulously documented for future follow-up. The majority of patients experience complete clinical response with either absence of any disease or the presence of a small scar or cicatrix. In the presence of any residual mass or suspicious abnormality, observation is carried out for an additional 4 weeks. Any persistent lesion is then biopsied. In the absence of any abnormality, we do not perform random blind biopsies. It is our experience that the majority of locoregional recurrences occur in the first 2 years and, as such, patients are scheduled for office visits every 3 months for the first 2 years. Continuity of care with the same clinician is highly desirable. The use of serum markers such as SCCAg has been described but we have not found that it adds value to our standard surveillance methods. Although this and other serological tests are of potential interest, we do not routinely use them [36].

The role of transrectal endoscopic ultrasound in pretreatment evaluation and surveillance remains somewhat controversial [25]. It is our opinion that comprehensive anoscopy and digital rectal examination yield equivalent if not greater information in the posttreatment setting. Evaluation with transrectal ultrasound examination may be confounded by postradiation inflammation with frequent fusion of the anatomic layers of the rectal wall. Therefore, we do not use transrectal ultrasound examination routinely in the follow-up of patients with anal cancer. As noted previously, stage at diagnosis is the most reliable determinant of treatment response and therefore accurate staging is of utmost importance. Although it has been suggested that transrectal ultrasound may provide improved accuracy of pretreatment staging, high quality evidence to support this contention is lacking [37, 38].

The most common sites of distant metastases from anal squamous cell carcinoma are extrapelvic lymph nodes, liver, lung, and bone [28, 29]. Rather than relying on a combination of different modalities such as chest X-ray, liver ultrasound, and pelvic computed tomography for site-directed imaging, we prefer to use computed tomography scan of the chest, abdomen, and pelvis for both pretreatment staging and subsequent assessments. This also provides additional assessment of inguinal node status and is particularly helpful for patients in whom physical examination is suboptimal (e.g., due to obesity, postradiation induration, etc.). For high-risk patients (T3/T4 and/or node positive), we obtain an annual computed tomography scan for a total of 3 years in accordance with National Comprehensive Cancer Network guidelines [18].

At our institution, the use of pretreatment positron emission tomography scans for anal squamous cell carcinoma serves a dual purpose. As endorsed by the National Comprehensive Cancer Network, we utilize positron emission tomography scan for preoperative staging purposes [18]. With the addition of positron emission tomography scanning, additional occult nodal disease can be detected in a significant number of patients initially thought to be node-negative by computed tomography [27]. Additionally, our radiation oncologists prefer the use of intensity-modulated radiation therapy techniques for the delivery of external beam radiation for anal squamous cell carcinoma, and positron emission tomography scan is routinely used as part of the target contouring process [39–41]. Consequently, positron emission tomography scans for anal squamous cell carcinoma are scheduled, observed, and integrated into the treatment plan by the radiation oncology team. The post-treatment positron emission tomography scan is usually obtained 12–16 weeks after completion of therapy. Schwartz et al. have demonstrated that a favorable metabolic response to chemotherapy and radiation after completion of therapy is strongly predictive of progression-free survival and cause-specific survival [42]. For high-risk patients, we obtain an annual positron emission tomography scan for 3 years in conjunction with annual computed tomography scanning. The utility of positron emission tomography scan in longer term surveillance and for lower risk patients requires additional study.

Management and Surveillance in the Setting of Recurrence

Treatment failure following chemoradiation includes those with persistent disease and those with recurrence following apparent complete response. Upon identification and biopsy confirmation of persistent or recurrent disease, we recommend restaging with computed tomography scan and positron emission tomography scan.

In the setting of locoregional treatment failure, the extent of local contiguous involvement (e.g., anus, vagina, prostate, bladder) and perirectal/pelvic lymph node disease must be ascertained. With disease confined to the pelvis and with exclusion of distant metastases, we generally recommend surgical resection by abdominoperineal resection or pelvic exenteration as indicated. Due to the often wide perineal excision and impaired wound healing secondary to radiation treatment, muscle flap reconstruction of the perineum is often employed. As an alternative to surgery, additional treatment with 5-fluorouracil and cisplatin and reirradiation may also be considered. However, our experience suggests that the likelihood of success with this approach is very low. If isolated inguinal lymph node recurrence is identified, groin dissection should be undertaken, assuming inguinal regions were included in the original radiation fields. If no prior inguinal radiation was administered, we prefer irradiation over groin dissection, given the morbidity associated with the latter. Local and regional control for palliative purposes remains a meaningful goal in patients with distant metastatic disease. Patients with local and locoregional recurrence who are treated with curative intent are at high risk for additional recurrences [43]. For surveillance of patients with locoregional treatment failure, we apply our regimen for high-risk patients, as outlined in Table 38.2, with few exceptions. We follow these patients with computed tomography scan every 6 months for 2 years. In patients treated by abdominoperineal resection or exenteration, digital rectal exam is no longer possible. Similarly, inguinal node examination can be difficult in patients previously treated by both radiation and inguinal node dissection. Consequently, we use serial positron emission tomography scans along with computed tomography scan surveillance for these patients.

The development of distant metastatic and/or unresectable locoregionally recurrent disease should prompt enrollment, when possible, in a clinical trial, given the modest survival benefit, imparted by standard palliative 5-fluorouracil and cisplatin chemotherapy. Anecdotally, although most often unsuccessful, metastasectomy can be considered if a single focus of distant metastatic disease is identified in a patient with both local/regional control and a long disease-free interval [22]. There is no strong evidence to support the resection of distant metastatic disease in the setting of anal cancer.

Anal Cancer in Special Populations

Although we have outlined the care and management of patients with anal squamous cell carcinoma in our institution, it is imperative that the practicing clinician realize that guidelines are meant for all patients in general, not necessarily any one individual patient. There are subpopulations of patients with anal squamous cell carcinoma which deserve further mention. Immunosuppressed patients, particularly those who are HIV-positive or those who have solid organ and bone marrow transplants, account for approximately 20–35% of patients diagnosed with anal squamous cell carcinoma. In the era of highly active antiretroviral therapy, HIV-positive patients are at increased risk for anal squamous cell carcinoma as their first manifestation of HIV/AIDS, due to high-risk behaviors (e.g., HPV infection and anal intercourse). The disease-free survival duration in this subgroup of patients is equivalent to that of other similarly staged patients, assuming treatment compliance [44]. HIV-positive squamous cell carcinoma patients with other HIV/AIDS-associated conditions are less likely to tolerate chemoradiation and may require treatment modifications [18, 45]. We have found that a large percentage of immunosuppressed individuals (predominantly from chemotherapy) treated at our institution require dose adjustments and treatment breaks, placing them at higher risk for treatment failure. Similarly, immunosuppressed patients with solid organ or bone marrow transplants appear particularly susceptible to aggressive disease progression and/or recurrence. Standard surveillance regimens may require individualized alterations for such patients.

Adenocarcinoma of the Anus

Adenocarcinoma of the anus is a rare diagnosis accounting for approximately 5% of anal cancers. It is thought to arise from the mucin-secreting stratified columnar epithelium of the anal glands and is generally believed to behave more aggressively than squamous cell carcinoma and therefore carries a worse prognosis [46]. Abdominoperineal resection has been advocated as primary treatment for adenocarcinoma of the anus, although chemoradiation may be equally efficacious [47–52]. We recommend that chemoradiation be reserved for patients unwilling or unable to undergo an abdominoperineal resection. If chemoradiation is chosen as a primary treatment modality, we recommend that these patients be considered at high risk for recurrence and followed accordingly (See Table 38.1). Consequently, the recommended schedule of follow-up for patients with adenocarcinoma of the anus is the same as that for high-risk squamous cell carcinoma.

Summary

Anal squamous cell carcinoma is an uncommon cancer accounting for approximately 5% of gastrointestinal tract malignancies, although the prevalence has been steadily increasing over the last several decades. Primary treatment emphasizes sphincter preservation using combination chemotherapy with 5-fluorouracil and mitomycin C and concomitant radiotherapy. Such an approach is curative for 60–70% of patients, although many patients experience significant treatment-associated toxicity, leading to noncompliance and/or unplanned treatment breaks. At present, the subpopulation of patients that fail chemotherapy plus radiation cannot be identified with certainty; therefore, careful surveillance is mandatory, particularly given the viability of salvage resection for cure. With the development of an efficacious vaccine against HPV, it is distinctly possible that the epidemiology and pathophysiology of anal squamous cell carcinoma will be altered [17]. Furthermore, there is growing interest in the identification of molecular signatures to predict the response of individual cancers to treatment regimens. In the future, such discoveries are likely to enhance our ability to predict the outcome of patients with anal squamous cell carcinoma [53–58]. In the meantime, knowledge of the patterns of recurrence as well as of tumor- and patient-associated factors which predispose to failure, allows for the development of guidelines to aid the clinician in surveillance after treatment of anal carcinoma.

References

1. Eng C. Anal cancer: current and future methodology. Cancer Invest. 2006;24(5):535–44.
2. Joseph DA, Miller JW, Wu X, et al. Understanding the burden of human papillomavirus-associated anal cancers in the US. Cancer. 2008;113(10 Suppl):2892–900.
3. American Cancer Society. Cancer facts & figures 2008. Atlanta: American Cancer Society, Inc; 2008.
4. SEER Cancer Statistics Review, 1975–2005. 2007 [cited 22 Sept 20008]; Available from: http://seer.cancer.gov/csr/1975_2005
5. Welton ML, Sharkey FE, Kahlenberg MS. The etiology and epidemiology of anal cancer. Surg Oncol Clin N Am. 2004;13(2):263–75.
6. Giuliano AR, Tortolero-Luna G, Ferrer E, et al. Epidemiology of human papillomavirus infection in men, cancers other than cervical and benign conditions. Vaccine. 2008;26 Suppl 10:K17–28.
7. IARC. IARC monographs on the evaluation of carcinogenic risks to humans. Human Papillomaviruses. 2007;90:1–670.
8. Daling JR, Madeleine MM, Johnson LG, et al. Human papillomavirus, smoking, and sexual practices in the etiology of anal cancer. Cancer. 2004;101(2):270–80.
9. Nigro ND, Vaitkevicius VK, Considine Jr B. Combined therapy for cancer of the anal canal: a preliminary report. Dis Colon Rectum. 1974;17(3):354–6.
10. Ajani JA, Winter KA, Gunderson LL, et al. Fluorouracil, mitomycin, and radiotherapy vs fluorouracil, cisplatin, and radiotherapy for carcinoma of the anal canal: a randomized controlled trial. JAMA. 2008;299(16):1914–21.
11. Chapet O, Gerard JP, Mornex F, et al. Prognostic factors of squamous cell carcinoma of the anal margin treated by radiotherapy: the Lyon experience. Int J Colorectal Dis. 2007;22(2):191–9.
12. Das P, Bhatia S, Eng C, et al. Predictors and patterns of recurrence after definitive chemoradiation for anal cancer. Int J Radiat Oncol Biol Phys. 2007;68(3):794–800.
13. Khanfir K, Ozsahin M, Bieri S, Cavuto C, René O, Mirimanoff RO, et al. Patterns of failure and outcome in patients with carcinoma of the anal margin. Ann Surg Oncol. 2008;15(4):1092–8.
14. Roohipour R, Patil S, Goodman KA, et al. Squamous-cell carcinoma of the anal canal: predictors of treatment outcome. Dis Colon Rectum. 2008;51(2):147–53.
15. Flam M, John M, Pajak TF, et al. Role of mitomycin in combination with fluorouracil and radiotherapy, and of salvage chemoradiation in the definitive nonsurgical treatment of epidermoid carcinoma of the anal canal: results of a phase III randomized intergroup study. J Clin Oncol. 1996;14(9):2527–39.
16. Fakhry C, Westra WH, Li S, et al. Improved survival of patients with human papillomavirus-positive head and neck squamous cell carcinoma in a prospective clinical trial. J Natl Cancer Inst. 2008;100(4):261–9.
17. Gillison ML, Chaturvedi AK, Lowy DR. HPV prophylactic vaccines and the potential prevention of noncervical cancers in both men and women. Cancer. 2008;113 Suppl 10:3036–46.
18. Engstrom PF, Benson III AB, Chen YJ, et al. Anal canal cancer clinical practice guidelines in oncology. J Natl Compr Canc Netw. 2005;3(4):510–5.
19. Akbari RP, Paty PB, Guillem JG, et al. Oncologic outcomes of salvage surgery for epidermoid carcinoma of the anus initially managed with combined modality therapy. Dis Colon Rectum. 2004;47(7):1136–44.
20. Ellenhorn JD, Enker WE, Quan SH. Salvage abdominoperineal resection following combined chemotherapy and radiotherapy for epidermoid carcinoma of the anus. Ann Surg Oncol. 1994;1(2):105–10.
21. Longo WE, Vernava 3rd AM, Wade TP, Coplin MA, Virgo KS, Johnson FE. Recurrent squamous cell carcinoma of the anal canal. Predictors of initial treatment failure and results of salvage therapy. Ann Surg. 1994;220(1):40–9.
22. Peiffert D, Bey P, Pernot M, et al. Conservative treatment by irradiation of epidermoid cancers of the anal canal: prognostic factors of tumoral control and complications. Int J Radiat Oncol Biol Phys. 1997;37(2):313–24.
23. Epidermoid anal cancer: results from the UKCCCR randomised trial of radiotherapy alone versus radiotherapy, 5-fluorouracil, and mitomycin. UKCCCR Anal Cancer Trial Working Party. UK Co-ordinating Committee on Cancer Research. Lancet. 1996;348(9034):1049–1054.

24. Konski A, Garcia Jr M, Madhu J, et al. Evaluation of planned treatment breaks during radiation therapy for anal cancer: update of RTOG 92-08. Int J Radiat Oncol Biol Phys. 2008;72(1):114–8.
25. Faynsod M, Vargas HI, Tolmos J, et al. Patterns of recurrence in anal canal carcinoma. Arch Surg. 2000;135(9):1090–3. discussion 1094–1095.
26. Touboul E, Schlienger M, Buffat L, et al. Epidermoid carcinoma of the anal canal. Results of curative-intent radiation therapy in a series of 270 patients. Cancer. 1994;73(6):1569–79.
27. Trautmann TG, Zuger JH. Positron Emission Tomography for pretreatment staging and posttreatment evaluation in cancer of the anal canal. Mol Imaging Biol. 2005;7(4):309–13.
28. Johnson LG, Madeleine MM, Newcomer LM, et al. Anal cancer incidence and survival: the surveillance, epidemiology, and end results experience, 1973–2000. Cancer. 2004;101(2):281–8.
29. Myerson RJ, Karnell LH, Menck HR. The National Cancer Data Base report on carcinoma of the anus. Cancer. 1997;80(4):805–15.
30. Heather B, Newlin HE, Zlotecki RA, et al. Squamous cell carcinoma of the anal margin. J Surg Oncol. 2004;86(2):55–62. discussion 63.
31. Peiffert D, Bey P, Pernot M, et al. Conservative treatment by irradiation of epidermoid carcinomas of the anal margin. Int J Radiat Oncol Biol Phys. 1997;39(1):57–66.
32. Touboul E, Schlienger M, Buffat L, et al. Epidermoid carcinoma of the anal margin: 17 cases treated with curative-intent radiation therapy. Radiother Oncol. 1995;34(3):195–202.
33. Bieri S, Allal AS, Kurtz JM. Sphincter-conserving treatment of carcinomas of the anal margin. Acta Oncol. 2001;40(1):29–33.
34. Cutuli B, Fenton J, Labib A, Bataini JP, Mathieu G, et al. Anal margin carcinoma: 21 cases treated at the Institut Curie by exclusive conservative radiotherapy. Radiother Oncol. 1988;11(1):1–6.
35. Papillon J, Chassard JL. Respective roles of radiotherapy and surgery in the management of epidermoid carcinoma of the anal margin. Series of 57 patients. Dis Colon Rectum. 1992;35(5):422–9.
36. Goldman S, Svensson C, Brönnergård M, Glimelius B, Wallin G. Prognostic significance of serum concentration of squamous cell carcinoma antigen in anal epidermoid carcinoma. Int J Colorectal Dis. 1993;8(2):98–102.
37. Martellucci J, Naldini G, Colosimo C, Cionini L, Rossi M. Accuracy of endoanal ultrasound in the follow-up assessment for squamous cell carcinoma of the anal canal treated with radiochemotherapy. Surg Endosc. 2009;23:1054–7.
38. Saranovic D, Saranovic D, Barisic G, Krivokapic Z, Masulovic D, Djuric-Stefanovic A. Endoanal ultrasound evaluation of anorectal diseases and disorders: technique, indications, results and limitations. Eur J Radiol. 2007;61(3):480–9.
39. Milano MT, Jani AB, Farrey KJ, Rash C, Heimann R, Chmura SJ. Intensity-modulated radiation therapy (IMRT) in the treatment of anal cancer: toxicity and clinical outcome. Int J Radiat Oncol Biol Phys. 2005;63(2):354–61.
40. Chen YJ, Liu A, Tsai PT. Organ sparing by conformal avoidance intensity-modulated radiation therapy for anal cancer: dosimetric evaluation of coverage of pelvis and inguinal/femoral nodes. Int J Radiat Oncol Biol Phys. 2005;63(1):274–81.
41. Cotter SE, Grigsby PW, Siegel BA. FDG-PET/CT in the evaluation of anal carcinoma. Int J Radiat Oncol Biol Phys. 2006;65(3):720–5.
42. Schwarz JK, Siegel BA, Dehdashti F, Myerson RJ, Fleshman JW, Grigsby PW. Tumor response and survival predicted by post-therapy FDG-PET/CT in anal cancer. Int J Radiat Oncol Biol Phys. 2008;71(1):180–6.
43. Stewart D, Yan Y, Kodner IJ, et al. Salvage surgery after failed chemoradiation for anal canal cancer: should the paradigm be changed for high-risk tumors? J Gastrointest Surg. 2007;11(12):1744–51.
44. Wexler A, Bersom AM, Goldstone SE. Invasive anal squamous-cell carcinoma in the HIV-positive patient: outcome in the era of highly active antiretroviral therapy. Dis Colon Rectum. 2008;51(1):73–81.
45. Uronis HE, Bendell JC. Anal cancer: an overview. Oncologist. 2007;12(5):524–34.
46. Gaertner WB, Hagerman GF, Finne CO. Fistula-associated anal adenocarcinoma: good results with aggressive therapy. Dis Colon Rectum. 2008;51(7):1061–7.
47. Lee J, Corman M. Recurrence of anal adenocarcinoma after local excision and adjuvant chemoradiation therapy: report of a case and review of the literature. J Gastrointest Surg. 2009;13(1):150–4.
48. Belkacemi Y, Berger C, Poortmans P, et al. Management of primary anal canal adenocarcinoma: a large retrospective study from the Rare Cancer Network. Int J Radiat Oncol Biol Phys. 2003;56(5):1274–83.
49. Joon DL, Chao MW, Ngan SY, Joon ML, Guiney MJ. Primary adenocarcinoma of the anus: a retrospective analysis. Int J Radiat Oncol Biol Phys. 1999;45(5):1199–205.
50. Papagikos M, Crane CH, Skibber J. Chemoradiation for adenocarcinoma of the anus. Int J Radiat Oncol Biol Phys. 2003;55(3):669–78.
51. Li LR, Wan DS, Pan ZZ, et al. Clinical features and treatment of 49 patients with anal canal adenocarcinoma. Zhonghua Wei Chang Wai Ke Za Zhi. 2006;9(5):402–4.
52. Beal KP, Wong D, Guillem JG, et al. Primary adenocarcinoma of the anus treated with combined modality therapy. Dis Colon Rectum. 2003;46(10):1320–4.
53. Brabender J, Vallböhmer D, Grimminger P, et al. ERCC1 RNA expression in peripheral blood predicts minor histopathological response to neoadjuvant radio-chemotherapy in patients with locally advanced cancer of the esophagus. J Gastrointest Surg. 2008;12(11):1815–21.
54. Paré L, Marcuello E, Altés A, et al. Pharmacogenetic prediction of clinical outcome in advanced colorectal cancer patients receiving oxaliplatin/5-fluorouracil as first-line chemotherapy. Br J Cancer. 2008;99(7):1050–5.
55. Pentheroudakis G, Kalogeras KT, Wirtz RM, et al. Gene expression of estrogen receptor, progesterone receptor and microtubule-associated protein Tau in high-risk early breast cancer: a quest for molecular predictors of treatment benefit in the context of a Hellenic Cooperative Oncology Group trial. Breast Cancer Res Treat. 2009;116(1):131–43.
56. Razis E, Briasoulis E, Vrettou E, et al. Potential value of PTEN in predicting cetuximab response in colorectal cancer: an exploratory study. BMC Cancer. 2008;8:234.
57. Takahari D, Yamada Y, Okita N, et al. Relationships of insulin-like growth factor-1 receptor and epidermal growth factor receptor expression to clinical outcomes in patients with colorectal cancer. Oncology. 2009;76(1):42–8.
58. Zhang X, Chang A. Molecular predictors of EGFR-TKI sensitivity in advanced non-small cell lung cancer. Int J Med Sci. 2008;5(4):209–17.

Anal Carcinoma Surveillance Counterpoint: Australia

39

Toufic El-Khoury, Michael Solomon, and Jane Young

Surveillance after treatment of anal carcinoma is not as firmly established as surveillance for colorectal cancer. The rarity of the disease means that there is a paucity of data or clinical trials comparing different regimens. The current standard of care for squamous cell carcinoma of the anus consists of combined modality treatment, with a surveillance regimen that aims at detecting recurrent or persistent disease, assessing treatment tolerance and related complications, with salvage surgery being reserved for locoregional failures.

Several risk factors are known. Human Papilloma Virus (HPV), Human Immune-Deficiency Virus (HIV), a compromised immune system, and anal intercourse are interrelated factors in the causation of anal cancer. In Australia there were 265 new cases (137 females and 128 males) in 2004 reported by the Australian Institute of Health and Welfare [1]. The rate of newly diagnosed anal cancer has been on the increase, with 120 and 184 new cases per year reported in 1984 and 1994, respectively.

The recent observed shift in demographics of homosexual men in Australia may alter the demographics of anal carcinoma in the future. Currently, a larger proportion of homosexual men reside in New South Wales than in the other Australian states. At the end of 2006, 68% of all HIV infections among homosexual men in Australia had occurred in New South Wales [2] despite the fact that New South Wales accounts for only 32.9% of the national population. There may be a shift in the population of homosexual and bisexual men, including those with HIV, away from New South Wales and into Queensland [2]. Together with the HPV Vaccination Program introduced by the Australian Government in 2006, this will have an unpredictable effect on the demographics of anal cancer in Australia. On the other hand, we may see a rise in the overall rate of anal cancer as the rate of HIV and HPV infection rises and as effective treatment of HIV prolongs the lives of HIV-positive patients. Surveillance of patients with rare diseases such as anal cancer may not have great overall cost implications and cost-effectiveness may be difficult to prove. Another challenge in comparing surveillance protocols is variability among institutions.

There are no clinical practice guidelines for surveillance approved by the National Health and Medical Research Council [3]. Diseases of the Colon and Rectum, the official journal of the Colorectal Surgical Society of Australia and New Zealand, has published Practice Parameters for Anal Squamous Neoplasms in 2008 [4]. These can be accessed only by members on (www.cssa.org.au.htm). Some of our practice is based on these recommendations. These parameters are not as detailed as those of the National Comprehensive Cancer Network.

Although the treatment of patients with anal margin and anal canal carcinoma differ slightly, their follow-up regimens are the same. However, both treatment and follow-up of squamous cell carcinoma and adenocarcinoma differ, with adenocarcinoma treated and followed as per rectal cancer (see our counterpoint, Chapter 32). Cancer of the anal margin is treated with local excision for T1N0 and for the more advanced stages the treatment is similar to that for cancer of the anal canal. The success rate of treating small anal cancers (<2 cm) with local excision is well documented. However, in our reported series of 120 anal cancers, the local recurrence of small anal cancers treated with local excision was four out of nine [5].

After completion of primary treatment, surveillance begins at 12 weeks. The aim is to classify patients into complete responders or locoregional failures; these latter are classified as having persistent or recurrent disease. The other aim is to detect radiotherapy-related complications such as anal stenosis, nonhealing ulcers, or incontinence, and to assess patient tolerance to treatment, particularly in those who are immunosuppressed.

T. El-Khoury, M.B.B.S., F.R.A.C.S. (✉) • M. Solomon, M.B., B.Ch. (Hons) M.Sc. (Clin Epidemiol) F.R.A.C.S. • J. Young, M.B.B.S., M.P.H., Ph.D., F.A.F.P.H.M.
Surgical Outcome Research Centre (SOuRCe), Royal Prince Alfred Hospital Sydney and the University of Sydney, Level 9, Building 50, Camperdown, NSW 2050, Australia
e-mail: toufic.el-khoury@email.cs.nsw.gov.au

F.E. Johnson et al. (eds.), *Patient Surveillance After Cancer Treatment*, Current Clinical Oncology,
DOI 10.1007/978-1-60327-969-7_39, © Springer Science+Business Media New York 2013

At our institution patients are managed in a multidisciplinary setting with an aim of preserving the sphincter and avoiding colostomy [5]. There seems to be a consensus among varying specialists in our center but a lack of agreement among different institutions. This is mostly due to shortage of data and the lack of evidence supporting one practice over another.

We usually use physical examination and endoanal ultrasonography to determine the T-stage, physical examination alone without biopsy to determine the status of inguinal nodes, and CT scan of the chest, abdomen, pelvis, and groins for determining N and M stages.

Physical examination has a critical role in both treatment and follow-up because of the accessibility of the anal canal and regional lymph nodes. Each office visit includes visual assessment of the anal margin, digital anorectal examination, palpation of inguinal regions, and rigid sigmoidoscopy, or inspection of the gluteal cleft in those who had an abdominoperineal resection. Flexible sigmoidoscopy, with a retroflexed view, is not routinely used because rigid sigmoidoscopy is easily performed in the office without the use of anesthesia and we consider direct visualization to be of superior quality. Office visits are carried out every 3–6 months for the first 2 years, starting 3 months after the completion of treatment. The follow-up period continues for 5 years, with two office visits per year in years 3–5 (Table 39.1).

Endoanal ultrasound and CT scans are of value in both anal cancer workup and surveillance. We rely on digital anorectal examination to assess the size of the primary tumor and endoanal ultrasound to assess the involvement of the anal sphincters, adjacent organs, and perirectal lymph nodes. CTs of the chest, abdomen and pelvis, and endoanal ultrasound are used as needed. The 3-D endoanal ultrasound is not currently available. Its superiority to the 2-D endoanal ultrasound has been shown in a study from the Denmark [6]. It showed that 3-D endoanal ultrasound, in combination with digital anorectal examination and anoscopy, had sensitivity of 100% at detecting recurrence; it surpasses 2-D ultrasound in the evaluation of local recurrence, especially in combination with anoscopy and digital anorectal examination. Currently we use 2-D digital anorectal examination at alternate office visits (Table 39.1).

There seems to be some variation among surgeons in the use of routine biopsies. We do not routinely biopsy unless a suspicious lesion is seen. Colonoscopy is not used in our follow-up regimen. Patients with anal carcinoma are in the same risk category as the general population for developing colorectal malignancy.

Cytology has an important role in the management of anal intraepithelial neoplasia but no identified role in surveillance [4]. Pap cytology is an integral part of follow-up in those with associated cervical HPV.

In our institution tumor markers are not used. Some studies have advocated the use of pretreatment serum squamous cell cancer antigen (SCCAg) level as a prognostic marker [7] and posttreatment SCCAg levels as a marker of recurrence [8]. The role of serum CEA level is clear when dealing with colorectal malignancy but has a doubtful role in anal cancer. The serum Ca-19.9 level has no role in surveillance of anal cancer.

Table 39.1 Surveillance of patients with anal cancer after curative-intent initial treatment. Royal Prince Alfred Hospital, Sydney

	Posttreatment year				
	1	2	3	4	5
Office visit[a]	2–4	2–4	2	2	2
Anoscopy[b]	2–4	2–4	2	2	2
EAUS[c]	1–2	1–2	1	1	1
CT scan[d]	1	1	1	1	1
CT scan[e]	2	2	1	1	1

[a]Includes digital rectal examination and inguinal palpation
[b]Anoscopy is accompanied by biopsy if a suspicious lesion is identified
[c]EAUS (endoanal ultrasound) is carried out at alternate office visits
[d]For low-stage disease, CT of the abdomen and pelvis
[e]For high-stage disease, CT of the chest, abdomen and pelvis
The number in each cell indicates the number of times a particular modality is recommended in a particular posttreatment year

PET technology continues to progress with the development of PET-CT and changes in the tracers used. PET scans have been shown to improve staging of nodal disease in anal cancer. It influences management decisions in a proportion of patients [9]. In the future PET scanning may find a role in surveillance in anal cancer patients. For the time being, however, there is a limited role for PET in Australia.

As mentioned above, the other aims of follow-up include assessing treatment tolerance and treatment-related complications. Tolerance to treatment has been shown to be an important predictor of treatment success [10]. The most common late radiotherapy toxicities in our series of 80 patients [5] who received radiotherapy were fecal incontinence, bleeding, and telangiectasia. Less common toxicities were anal pain, chronic diarrhea, and stenosis.

Anal intercourse, immune suppression, and HPV infection tend to coexist with HIV infection. Although HPV has been directly linked to the development of anal intraepithelial neoplasia and anal cancer, the role of HIV as an independent causative virus is not clear. The majority of high-risk HPV (16 and 18)-positive patients do not develop anal cancer as the noncompromised immune system is able to clear infected cells. HIV infection appears to play an important role in the development of anal cancer as it allows the HPV infection to persist. HIV-positive patients have evidence of persistent HPV infection in the anal canal [1]. In the immunocompromised patient, HPV infection can lead to malignant transformation. Anal intraepithelial neoplasia seems to progress at a faster rate to squamous cell carcinoma in HIV-positive patients than in patients without HIV infection and cancer develops at a much younger age [11].

The main aim of treatment of HPV lies in the prevention of anal intraepithelial neoplasia and subsequent prevention of anal cancer. Increasing the CD4 count in HIV-positive patients aims to improve tolerance to adjuvant treatment for anal cancer. Associations between HPV infection, intraepithelial neoplasia, and anal cancer have been demonstrated. In our series of 120 patients with anal cancer, 26% of female patients had associated cervical, vulvar, or vaginal malignancies [5], indicating an association between HPV and anal cancer. Varying recommendations for the screening and prevention of anal cancer abound, including use of 5% imiquimod cream, topical 5% 5-FU cream, photodynamic therapy, and infrared coagulation [4]. Follow-up and treatment of anal intraepithelial neoplasia at 6-month intervals for as long as dysplasia is present may prevent anal cancer.

It is important to determine the CD4 count in patients with HIV and anal cancer as it affects their management. Patients with CD4 counts <200 do not tolerate chemoradiotherapy as well as those with higher CD4 count. This has led to substandard treatment of anal cancer in many cases. By using highly active antiviral therapy to increase the CD4 count, both tolerance and outcome may improve [12] and there is no need to compromise the treatment of anal cancer because of the potential toxicity of the chemotherapy. Even though highly active antiviral therapy has been shown to improve immune function and reduce the rate of neoplasms, it has not been shown to cause anal intraepithelial neoplasia to regress [13]. The benefit of highly active antiviral therapy seems to be solely in improving tolerance to treatment. The CD4 count also affects the response rate to chemoradiotherapy [14].

At the Royal Prince Albert Hospital, surveillance intensity for patients with anal cancer depends on T-and N-stage, histology, and the completion of treatment. There are conflicting findings with regard to predictors of local failure. T-stage, overall stage, and gender have been reported by some authors to be associated with local failure [15], while others disagree [1]. Completion of radiotherapy and total radiotherapy dose are predictors of disease-free survival [1, 16]. The recently published US Gastrointestinal Intergroup RTOG 98-11 randomized controlled trial [1] showed that male sex, clinically positive nodes, and tumor size greater than 5 cm were independent prognosticators for worse disease-free survival.

At our institution, the treatment of T3, T4, or any T with node-positive anal cancer is different than the treatment of early T-stage anal cancer in two respects. First, the total radiotherapy dosage is increased and the field covered is widened to include both inguinal and low pelvic basins. Second, surveillance differs in that patients in this higher risk group undergo a CT more frequently (Table 39.1). Tumor location has not been shown to predict disease recurrence [15], and the subtypes of anal cancer described by the World Health Organization do not affect follow-up practices at our hospital.

Locoregional failure occurs in up to 30% of patients treated with sphincter-preserving nonsurgical treatment using combined modality treatment. Half of those locoregional failures are local recurrences and the other half are due to persistent disease. Abdominoperineal resection is an effective salvage therapy for persistent or recurrent disease (level III evidence), offering a better overall survival advantage for recurrent disease than for persistent disease [4].

Persistent disease can be classified as either stable or progressive. For those who show disease progression, salvage treatment in the form of abdominoperineal resection is usually recommended, and this offers a 30–56% overall 5-year survival rate [17–19]. Recent studies have demonstrated survival rates at the higher end of this range compared with older studies. There is also a group of patients who, on serial observation, do not show regression or progression. We continue to evaluate this group on a monthly basis for 3 months; stable disease by 6 months is considered persistent and salvage treatment is offered.

When considering salvage surgery following a local failure in a patient with a previously irradiated perineum, prevention of wound failure and achieving a negative resection margin are the two priorities of management of distant metastasis-free local failure. Salvage surgery often requires a multimodality approach with colorectal surgeons performing the abdominoperineal resection and plastic surgeons performing a myocutaneous flap [19, 20]. Primary closure, omentoplasty, and various packing techniques for healing with secondary intention are less desirable options. A multimodality surgical approach is also needed to obtain negative resection margins. Microscopically and macroscopically involved margins strongly predict an adverse outcome [19].

Recurrences following salvage abdominoperineal resection are referred for chemotherapy. The survival rate is dismal and resection for metastatic disease is not supported by the literature. The common sites of metastasis are liver, lung, and extrapelvic lymph nodes, and investigations to detect metastasis in these regions are only used in high-risk groups. The risk factors for recurrence following salvage surgery include poorly differentiated cancers, positive resection margins, and a short-time interval between treatment and failure [1].

There are no data available comparing the prognosis of those with recurrent anal cancer vs. a new primary anal cancer. In our practice, salvage surgery in the form of abdominoperineal resection is the treatment of choice for a new primary anal canal cancer.

There are similarities in the histology of both the cervical and anal canal and a similarity between the risk factors of their cancers. In particular, an infectious etiology is implicated in both. The persistent nature of these risk factors causes a continuous exposure of these canals to the carcinogenic effect of HPV [1], warranting a careful monitoring of the cervix for the development of primary cervical cancer.

The different outcomes in subgroups of patients based on risk factors, as well as the rarity of the disease, make comparative trials unfeasible. Australian national guidelines need to be established first to standardize the treatment of anal cancer in order to give future trials sufficient power (sample size). Cost-effectiveness analysis can then follow. Before preventive measures for anal cancer can be established, we need to concentrate on understanding the natural history of anal intraepithelial neoplasia and to standardize an effective way of treating anal intraepithelial neoplasia.

Risk factors for anal cancer are known but the natural history of the development of anal cancer is not clear, making screening difficult. In Australia, women are now offered HPV immunization and cervical cancer screening. The immunization is delivered to females at age 12 through community-based or school-based programs, while Pap smear is used for screening for cervical cancer. The available data does support neither the implementation of the immunization nor the screening programs in the high-risk male population.

References

1. www.aihw.gov.au
2. Prestage G, Ferris J, Grierson J, et al. Homosexual men in Australia: population, distribution and HTV prevalence. Sex Health. 2008;5:97–102.
3. National Health and Medical Research Council (NHMRC). Clinical practice guidelines for the prevention, early detection and management of colorectal cancer. The Cancer Council Australia, Australian Cancer Network, The Commonwealth of Australia, Canberra; 2005.
4. Fleshner P, Chalasani S, Chang G, et al. Practice parameters for anal squamous neoplasms. Dis Colon Rectum. 2008;51:2–9.
5. Young SC, Solomon MJ, Hruby G, Frizelle FA. Review of 120 anal cancer patients. Colorectal Dis. 2009;11:909–14. Epub 2008 Oct 25.
6. Christensen A, Nielsen M, Svendsen L, Engelholm S. Three-dimensional anal endosonography may improve detection of recurrent anal cancer. Dis Colon Rectum. 2006;49:1527–32.
7. Goldman S, Svensson C, Bronnergard M, Glimelius B, Wallin G. Prognostic significance of serum concentration of squamous cell carcinoma antigen in anal epidermal carcinoma. Ing J Colorectal Dis. 1993;8:98–102.
8. Petrelli NJ, Palmer M, Herrera L, Bhargava A. The utility of squamous cell carcinoma antigen for the follow-up of patients with squamous cell carcinoma of the anal canal. Cancer. 1992;70:35–9.
9. Tasevski R, De Winton E, Ngan S, Mackay J, Hicks R, Heriot A. CR13 utility of 18- fluorodeoxyglucose PET in the staging and management of anal cancer. ANZ J Surg. 2007;77(Suppl sl):A17.
10. Roohipour R, Patil S, Goodman K, et al. Squamous-cell carcinoma of the anal canal:·predictors of treatment outcome. Dis Colon Rectum. 2008;51:147–53.
11. Gervaz P, Hirschel B, Morel P. Molecular biology of squamous cell carcinoma of the anus. Br J Surg. 2006;93:531–8.
12. Place R, Gregorcyk S, Huber P, Simmang C. Outcome analysis of HIV-positive patients with anal squamous cell carcinoma. Dis Colon Rectum. 2001;44:506–12.
13. Martin F, Bower M. Anal intraepithelial neoplasia in HIV positive people. Sex Transm Infect. 2001;5:327–31.
14. Hoffinan R, Welton M, Klencke B, Weinberg V, Krieg R. The significance of pretreatment CD4 count on the outcome and treatment tolerance of HIV-positive patients with anal cancer. Int J Radiat Oncol Biol Phys. 1999;44:127–31.
15. Ajani J, Winter K, Gunderson L, et al. Fluorouracil, mitomycin and radiotherapy vs fluorouracil, cisplatin and radiotherapy for carcinoma of the anal canal. JAMA. 2008;299:1914–21.
16. Renehan A, Saunders M, Schofield P, O'Dwyer S. Patterns of local disease failure and outcome after salvage surgery in patients with anal cancer. Br J Surg. 2005;92:605–14.
17. Mariani P, Ghanneme A, De la Rochefordiere A, Girodet J, Falcou M, Salmon R. Abdominoperineal resection for anal cancer. Dis Colon Rectum. 2008;51:1495–501.
18. Nilsson PJ, Svenson C, Goldman S, Glimelius B. Salvage abdominoperineal resection in anal epidermoid cancer. Br J Surg. 2002; 89:1425–9.
19. Ferenschild F, Vermaas M, Hofer SO, Verhoef C, Eggermont A, de Witt JHW. Salvage abdominoperineal resection and perineal wound healing in local recurrent or persistent anal cancer. World J Surg. 2005;29:1452–7.
20. Sunesen KG, Buntzen T, Lindegaard J, Norgaard M, Laurberg S. Perineal healing and survival after anal cancer salvage surgery: 10-year experience with primary perineal reconstruction using the vertical rectus abdominis myocutaneous flap. Ann Surg Oncol. 2009;16:68–77. Epub 2008 Nov 5.

Anal Carcinoma Surveillance Counterpoint: Japan

40

Yoshihisa Sakaguchi and Yasushi Toh

There is no evidence-based, established surveillance strategy for anal carcinoma. Neither the American Society of Clinical Oncology (ASCO) nor the European Society of Medical Oncology (ESMO) has so far established any guidelines for the follow-up after initial treatment. Characteristics of anal carcinoma, such as its rarity, diverse histological types, and the various treatment modalities, make it difficult to standardize the protocol.

Anal carcinoma is an uncommon malignancy of the gastrointestinal tract and represents only 10% of anorectal malignancies [1]. Moreover, the incidence is lower in Japan in comparison to Western countries. Only 20 patients with primary anal carcinoma have undergone treatment in the last decade at the National Kyushu Cancer Center in Fukuoka. This disease represents 2.9% of all patients treated for large bowel cancer. Because of the variety of the epithelium within the anal mucosa, anal carcinomas have different histological appearance and there is considerable geographic difference in the histological types. In the United States, nearly 80% of anal carcinomas are squamous cell carcinomas and about 10% are adenocarcinomas [2]. In Japan, adenocarcinoma accounts for 70% of anal carcinomas and squamous cell carcinomas comprise only 20%. These different types of anal carcinomas are treated initially by different modalities. Adenocarcinomas are treated by surgery and squamous cell carcinomas are usually treated by chemoradiotherapy, except for the local excision of small cancers without sphincter invasion. These characteristics require separate surveillance strategies for adenocarcinomas and squamous cell carcinomas of the anal canal (Tables 40.1 and 40.2).

Anal canal adenocarcinoma originating from the anal canal glands is very rare. It is likely that most cases represent lower rectal cancers extending into the anal canal. The true incidence of anal canal adenocarcinoma is probably significantly smaller [1]. However, in all cases, adenocarcinomas are usually managed by surgery, as low rectal cancers, because radiotherapy and chemotherapy are considered less effective. Early cancers are treated by a local excision and advanced cancers are managed by an abdominoperineal resection. In advanced cases, adjuvant therapies of radiotherapy and/or chemotherapy are combined with surgery, resulting in some benefit for pelvic disease control.

In Japan, the surveillance strategy for patients with adenocarcinoma after a curative resection is the same as that of patients with lower rectal cancers. The schedules were recommended in the first guideline for the treatment of colorectal cancers published in 2005, by the Japanese Society for Cancer of the Colon and Rectum (JSCCR) [3]. In cases of early cancers which are successfully resected, a digital rectal examination is performed to detect local recurrence every 6 months for 2 years. If necessary, anoscopy and/or biopsy should be carried out. Other imaging examinations may be omitted.

The surveillance protocol for the patients with advanced adenocarcinomas at National Kyushu Cancer Center is shown in Table 40.1. A careful physical examination of the perineal wound and inguinal lymph nodes is performed at every office visit after a curative surgery, and the serum levels of CEA and CA19-9 are measured every 3 months for 3 years and every 6 months for the next 2 years. Computed tomography (CT) of the abdomen, including the pelvis, is evaluated every 6 months for 2 ears and once a year for the next 3 years. Chest CT is evaluated annually for 5 years. Abdominal ultrasonography is not performed routinely but is useful when liver metastasis is suspected. Magnetic resonance imaging (MRI) and positron emission tomography (PET) are not included in the basic schedule but are used to obtain more information of metastasis and to decide the indications for treatment when recurrence is suspected. In the case of recurrence, the options of salvage surgery, chemotherapy, and radiotherapy are evaluated.

Squamous cell carcinoma of the anal canal was treated with abdominoperineal resection, prior to the pioneering

Y. Sakaguchi (✉) • Y. Toh
Department of Gastroenterological Surgery, National Kyushu Cancer Center, 3-1-1 Notame, Minami-ku, Fukuoka 811-1395, Japan
e-mail: ysakaguchi@nk-cc.go.jp; ytoh@nk-cc.go.jp

F.E. Johnson et al. (eds.), *Patient Surveillance After Cancer Treatment*, Current Clinical Oncology,
DOI 10.1007/978-1-60327-969-7_40, © Springer Science+Business Media New York 2013

Table 40.1 Surveillance after curative-intent treatment for advanced adenocarcinoma of the anal canal at National Kyushu Cancer Center, Japan

	Year				
	1	2	3	4	5
Office visit[a]	4	4	4	2	2
CEA,CA19-9	4	4	4	2	2
Abdominal and pelvic CT	2	2	1	1	1
Chest CT	1	1	1	1	1

[a]Includes digital rectal examination
CT computed tomography
The numbers in each cell indicate the number of times a particular modality is recommended during a particular posttreatment year

Table 40.2 Surveillance after curative-intent treatment for squamous cell carcinoma of the anal canal at National Kyushu Cancer Center, Japan

	Year				
	1	2	3	4	5
Office visit[a]	4	4	2	2	2
Abdominal and pelvic CT	2	2	1	1	1
Chest CT	1	1	1	1	1

CT computed tomography
[a]Includes digital rectal examination
The numbers in each cell indicate the number of times a particular modality is recommended during a particular posttreatment year

work of Nigro et al. in 1974 [4], which demonstrated that chemoradiotherapy offers survival and recurrence rates equivalent to sphincter-removing surgery while preserving the sphincter function. Many investigators have confirmed those results and chemoradiotherapy has gained general acceptance as the standard treatment for squamous cell carcinoma [5]. Exceptionally, radiotherapy alone or local excision can provide excellent survival and local control for highly selected patients who have early-stage lesions [2]. Abdominoperineal resection is reserved as a salvage treatment in radioresistant cases.

In Japan, squamous cell carcinoma was traditionally treated by an abdominoperineal resection, even after Nigro et al. [4] demonstrated the efficacy of chemoradiotherapy. However, based on accumulating evidence, the Japanese Collage of Radiology recommended in 2004 that squamous cell carcinomas should be treated by radiotherapy with or without chemotherapy. Therefore, chemoradiotherapy has become the new standard treatment.

Carcinoma of the anal canal is primarily a locoregional disease which rarely (in less than 10% of cases) metastasizes [2], and optimizing local control is critical. Although chemoradiotherapy provides improved local control, there are concerns that the local disease failure rate remains high. Failure to achieve a complete response to chemoradiotherapy occurs in 10–15% of patients treated, and 10–30% of patients experience recurrence after an initial complete response to chemoradiotherapy [6]. Salvage surgery may be appropriate in some patients with durable local control. There is a chance of a potential cure only for the cases in which salvage surgery achieves a negative resection margin. Salvage treatment usually requires an abdominoperineal resection with a permanent colostomy, but there are some cases in which more radical procedures, such as pelvic exenterations, are necessary to obtain a negative surgical margin. A delayed recognition of persistent or recurrent disease may contribute to the low resection rate. Moreover, a positive margin is a highly significant negative prognostic factor, yielding an equivalent survival rate to that with no salvage therapy [5]. Therefore, to pursue cure and avoid the major surgery resulting in poor quality of life, careful follow-up after the initial treatment is very important to define persistent tumors as well as to detect local or regional recurrence as early as possible. Local failure is common, even within months of initial treatment, and the majority occurs in the first 3 years [5]. In addition, after completion of chemoradiotherapy, the anal tumor can continue to respond for 6–9 months [7].

There is no consensus about the optimal posttreatment surveillance strategy for patients with squamous cell carcinoma of the anal canal in Japan because of the low incidence. The National Kyushu Cancer Center uses an original protocol for the patients with squamous cell carcinoma, shown in Table 40.2. A physical examination, including digital rectal, is performed every 3 months for 2 years and every 6 months for the next 3 years. A digital rectal examination is the most convenient and the most effective procedure of the routine follow-up. Anoscopy, with or without biopsy, should be performed if disease persistence or recurrence is suspected. Imaging examinations are useful for detecting local recurrence, lymph node metastasis, and distant metastasis, which most commonly occur in the liver and lung. CT of the abdomen and pelvis is recommended every 6 months for 2 years, then once a year for the next 3 years. Chest CT is evaluated annually for 5 years. When persistent or recurrent tumors are detected, it is important to assess the extent of disease to determine the indications for treatment. Preoperative surgical planning is important before proposing salvage surgery to evaluate the curability and the extent of resection required to achieve negative margins [1]. CT and MRI have proved useful in evaluating adjacent organ involvement. Endorectal ultrasonography can also be useful to determine the extent of invasion and involvement of adjacent organs. Patients with distant metastatic disease have a poor prognosis and are not considered candidates for salvage resection of locally persistent or recurrent disease. When careful preoperative planning and patient selection are combined with an aggressive surgical resection, it is possible to achieve long-term survival [6].

No standard surveillance strategy of anal carcinoma has yet been established in Japan. It might be important to centralize patients with this uncommon cancer to the institutions which have a follow-up protocol and all modalities required for diagnosis and treatment.

References

1. Rousseau Jr DL, Petrelli NJ, Kahlenberg MS. Overview of anal cancer for the surgeon. Surg Oncol Clin N Am. 2004;13:249–62.
2. Klas JV, Rothenberger DA, Wong WD, Madoff RD. Malignant tumors of the anal canal. Cancer. 1999;85:1686–93.
3. The Japanese Society for Cancer of the Colon and Rectum. JSCCR guidelines 2005 for the treatment of colorectal cancer. Tokyo, Japan: Kanehara & Co., Ltd.; 2005.
4. Nigro ND, Vaitkevicius VK, Considine Jr B. Combined therapy for cancer of the anal canal: a preliminary report. Dis Colon Rectum. 1974;17:354–6.
5. Renehan AG, Saunders MP, Schofield PF, O'Dwyer ST. Patterns of local disease failure and outcome after salvage surgery in patients with anal cancer. Br J Surg. 2005;92:605–14.
6. Schiller DE, Cummings BJ, Rai S, et al. Outcomes of salvage surgery for squamous carcinoma of the anal canal. Ann Surg Oncol. 2007;14:2780–9.
7. Cummings BJ, Keane TJ, O'Sullivian B, Wong CS, Catton CN. Epidermoid anal cancer: treatment by radiation alone or by radiation and 5-fluorouracil with and without mitomycin C. Int J Radiat Oncol Biol Phys. 1991;21:111–25.

41 Anal Carcinoma Surveillance Counterpoint: Canada

Natasha Press and John Hay

Keywords
Squamous cell carcinoma • High-resolution Anoscopy • Radiation therapy • Chemotherapy • Survival duration

Anal dysplasia and intraepithelial neoplasia are part of a continuum of anal cancer that is typically treated with curative intent. Surveillance after treatment in our practice includes high-resolution anoscopy. This is similar to colposcopy in cervical cancer screening and treatment programs. It allows for the visualization of the anal canal, with biopsy of suspicious looking lesions [1]. In Canada, high-resolution anoscopy is performed in a few outpatient settings, and constitutes part of a screening program for individuals who are at high risk for anal dysplasia due to human papillomavirus (e.g., men who have sex with men and HIV-positive individuals). These high-risk individuals are usually screened with anal cytology, and referred for high-resolution anoscopy if the cytology result is abnormal. Following high-resolution anoscopy, biopsy may be indicated. If the biopsy shows high-grade dysplasia (anal intraepithelial neoplasia II/III, carcinoma in situ), lesions are treated with either 80% trichloroacetic acid or infrared coagulation. Recent data on infrared coagulation show that it is a safe and effective office-based procedure, and that repeated treatments lead to resolution of the high-grade dysplasia [2].

Once patients have been identified and treated for high-grade dysplasia, they continue to follow-up in the anal dysplasia clinic for ongoing surveillance using anal cytology, digital rectal examination, and high-resolution anoscopy with biopsies as needed. One study reported 10 years of experience with targeted surgical treatment using high-resolution anoscopy combined with office-based ablation of recurrences. It suggests that control of high-grade dysplasia with high-resolution anoscopy is effective in decreasing the risk of progression to anal cancer [3].

Some patients with previously excised anal cancer are referred to the Vancouver high-resolution anoscopy clinic for ongoing surveillance for recurrence. There have been no studies looking at high-resolution anoscopy follow-up in this population, and no guidelines exist regarding frequency of visits or utility of biopsies.

Patients are usually seen every 6 months for the first 2 years and then seen annually. If recurrent dysplasia is found, then the follow-up schedule is revised.

Invasive squamous cell cancer of the perianal skin and anal canal has the potential to be lethal.

Tumors that are ≤2 cm can usually be resected with clear margins without the need for prophylactic surgical treatment of the groins or any radiation therapy. The patient is seen at four to six weekly intervals until the incision has healed, then at three monthly intervals for 2 years, then at six monthly intervals for 5 years. At this point the patient is discharged back to the care of the family doctor. Late recurrence is unusual, but patients with invasive carcinoma on a background of widespread in situ disease, which is usually related to human papillomavirus, are at risk of developing a second primary and should therefore be followed indefinitely. Careful clinical examination of the perineum, anal canal, and groins is made at each visit. Biopsy is only performed to characterize an abnormality that is detected clinically. Routine anoscopy is not considered necessary unless the

N. Press, M.D., F.R.C.P.C.
Division of Infectious Diseases, University of British Columbia, St. Paul's Hospital, 667-1081 Burrard Street, Vancouver, BC, Canada V6Z 1Y6

J. Hay, M.B., B.Chir., F.R.C.P.C., F.R.C.R. (✉)
Radiation Oncologist, British Columbia Cancer Agency, Vancouver Cancer Centre, University of British Columbia, 600 West 10th Avenue, Vancouver, BC V5Z 4E6, Canada
e-mail: jhay@bccancer.bc.ca

F.E. Johnson et al. (eds.), *Patient Surveillance After Cancer Treatment*, Current Clinical Oncology,
DOI 10.1007/978-1-60327-969-7_41,

Table 41.1 Surveillance after curative-intent treatment for anal dysplasia and intraepithelial neoplasia

	Posttreatment year				
Modality	1	2	3	4	≥5
Office visit, including digital rectal examination and pap smear	2	2	1	1	1

High resolution anoscopy is utilized as indicated by clinical findings

Table 41.2 Surveillance after curative-intent treatment for perianal squamous cell carcinoma

	Posttreatment year					
Modality	1	2	3	4	5	≥5
Office visit, including digital rectal examination and groin node palpation	4–6	4	2	2	2	1

The number in each cell indicates the number of times a particular modality is recommended during a particular posttreatment year

Table 41.3 Surveillance after curative-intent treatment for anal canal squamous cell carcinoma

	Posttreatment year					
Modality	1	2	3	4	5	≥5
Office visit, including digital rectal examination and groin node palpation	6	4	2	2	2	1

Patients with cancer that could not be adequately palpated at the time of diagnosis and required CT or MRI imaging generally have the same imaging study every 3 months in the first year and then prior to each office visit thereafter. The number in each cell indicates the number of times a particular modality is recommended during a particular posttreatment year

Table 41.4 Surveillance after curative-intent treatment for adenocarcinoma of the anal canal

	Posttreatment year					
Modality	1	2	3	4	5	≥5
Office visit, including digital rectal examination and groin node palpation	4	4	2	2	2	1

The number in each cell indicates the number of times a particular modality is recommended during a particular posttreatment year

patient fits the criteria for high-resolution anoscopy. No routine imaging is performed.

Larger tumors of the perianal skin and anal canal are not uncommon. The vast majority of these patients are treated with definitive radiation therapy and concurrent chemotherapy with 5-fluorouracil and mitomycin C with the goal of preserving anal sphincter function as well as eradicating the cancer. Patients who are medically unfit for concurrent chemotherapy are treated with radiation alone. Patients with very advanced tumors that have already significantly damaged the sphincter are offered a defunctioning colostomy followed by radiation and chemotherapy. Even if these very large tumours regress completely, most of these patients require a permanent colostomy, although some regain sufficient sphincter function to have their colostomy closed.

At each surveillance visit attention is paid to managing treatment sequelae and detecting residual or recurrent disease. We recently reviewed the outcome of 85 patients with anal carcinoma, treated in British Columbia between January 2000 and December 2005, who subsequently developed locoregional recurrence or systemic metastases [4]. Sites of failure were anorectal in 54 (64%), regional nodal in 13 (15%), and distant in 26 (31%). Of the anorectal failures, 45/54 were confined to the anorectum, 4/54 also had regional nodal disease, 4/54 also had distant metastases, and 1/54 had nodal and distant disease. Of the distant failures, 16 had soft-tissue/visceral metastases, 5 had extrapelvic nodal involvement, and 5 had a combination of both. The median times to anorectal, regional nodal, and distant failure were 8, 6, and 10 months, respectively. The only long-term survivors were those who could be treated surgically but, for a variety of reasons, including extent of disease and coexisting medical problems, only 37 of the 54 patients with anorectal recurrence had abdominoperineal resections.

In a separate report, 57 patients treated in British Columbia between 1998 and 2006 with potentially curative surgery for recurrent anal carcinoma were reviewed [5]. This group included all the patients in the previous cohort. Fifty-one patients underwent salvage abdominoperineal resection and six patients had node dissections for inguinal recurrence. The 5-year overall survival probability after abdominoperineal resection was 29% (median survival duration, 22 months). Age, gender, human immunodeficiency virus status, TNM stage at presentation, node status, and failure type did not predict survival. A negative resection margin was strongly associated with improved overall and disease-free survival duration ($p = 0.03$ and $p < 0.0001$, respectively). The median survival duration for the six patients undergoing inguinal lymph node dissection for regional recurrence was 11 months, with freedom from recurrence achieved in two of them; the other four succumbed to their disease.

Thus, the focus of surveillance is on the detection of potentially curable locoregional failure which is most likely to occur in the first year after treatment. Patients are followed more closely until acute treatment sequelae—such as urgency and frequent defecation—have settled, with or without treatment, such as anti-inflammatory suppositories, until there has been complete clinical eradication of their cancer. Our experience [4, 6] is similar to that of Cummings [7] in that the majority of local failures have incomplete regression of their disease rather than recurrence after an apparently complete response, although a few relapses occur several years after treatment [8]. Surveillance usually entails visits at 6-week intervals for 6 months and then 2-month intervals up to 1 year. If there is no cause for concern, patients are then seen at 3-month intervals for 2 years and then every 6 months for up to 5 years after treatment. In our experience, careful clinical examination is the most useful investigation. Routine biopsies are not used unless a clinical abnormality is detected. Anoscopy is not routinely used in the asymptomatic patient.

There is increasing evidence that FDG-PET scanning can be very useful in the post treatment assessment of patients who have been treated for anal cancer. Disease free survival rates of approximately 95% have been reported in patients who experience a complete metabolic response [8, 9]. When available, a PET scan done between 10 and 16 weeks post treatment appears to be the imaging modality of choice for the assessment of these patients. This is particularly relevant for patients with T3 and T4 tumours which have the highest rates of loco-regional recurrence.

When PET is not available, the use of other imaging modalities depends on the pretreatment findings. Unless large, the primary tumor is often poorly defined by either CT or MRI. However, both these modalities may show inguinal and pelvic lymphadenopathy and more distant disease. If the pretreatment scan did not show the primary lesion well, and there was no adenopathy, then one scan is usually performed 3 months after treatment to ensure that no new abnormality has arisen. The vast majority of these scans are negative, although occasionally metastases are detected in the regional nodes or elsewhere. If the follow-up scan is negative, it is not repeated in the absence of new symptoms or clinical findings.

If the pretreatment scan shows an abnormality at the primary site or significant lymphadenopathy, then a follow-up scan is performed 3 months after treatment. If there is a residual abnormality, then a biopsy is considered. If the scan is negative, it is repeated once more at 1 year. If the second scan is negative, then no further scans are performed unless the original abnormality was in an area that is not palpable—such as a high pelvic node. In this case, the scans are repeated prior to each clinic visit.

Primary adenocarcinoma of the anal canal is a rare tumor thought to originate in the anal glands. In our experience and that of others [10], these have not responded well to primary radiation with or without chemotherapy and, unless medically unfit, the patients have required an abdominoperineal resection. The prognosis is not as good as for patients with squamous cell carcinoma with 5-year survival rates of 50% or less [11]. Postoperative follow-up is primarily clinical; three monthly visits to 2 years with six monthly visits to 5 years is our typical practice.

References

1. Jay N, Berry JM, Hogeboom CJ, et al. Colposcopic appearance of anal squamous intraepithelial lesions: relationship to histopathology. Dis Colon Rectum. 1997;40:919–28.
2. Goldstone SE, Hundert JS, Huyett JW. Infrared coagulator ablation of high-grade anal squamous intraepithelial lesions in HIV-negative males who have sex with males. Dis Colon Rectum. 2007;50:565–75.
3. Pineda CE, Berry JM, Jay N, et al. High-resolution anoscopy targeted surgical destruction of anal high-grade squamous intraepithelial lesions: a ten-year experience. Dis Colon Rectum. 2008;51:829–37.
4. Foo M, Harrow S, Ma R, et al. Outcomes and treatment following recurrence of anal carcinoma after radical radiotherapy: the British Columbia experience. Radiother Oncol. 2010;96 Suppl 2:S44 (Abstr. 133).
5. Eeson G, Foo M, Harrow S, et al. Outcomes of salvage surgery for epidermoid carcinoma of the anus following failed combined modality treatment. Am J Surg. 2011;201:624–9.
6. Newman G, Calverly DC, Acker BD, et al. The management of carcinoma of the anal canal by external beam radiotherapy, experience in Vancouver 1971–1988. Radiother Oncol. 1992;25:196–202.
7. Cummings BJ, Keane TJ, O'Sullivan B, et al. Epidermoid anal cancer: treatment by radiation alone or radiation and 5-Fluorouracil with and without Mitomycin C. Int J Radiat Oncol Biol Phys. 1991;21:1115–25.
8. Schwarz JK. Siegel BA. Dehdashti F. et al.Tumor response and survival predicted by post-therapy FDG-PET/CT in anal cancer. Int J Radiat Oncol Biol Phys. 2008;71(1):180–86.
9. Day FL, Link E, Ngan S et al. FDG-PET metabolic response predicts outcomes in anal cancer managed with chemoradiotherapy. Br J Cancer. 2011;105:498–504.
10. Ajani AJ, Winter KA, Gunderson L, et al. Fluorouracil, Mitomycin and radiotherapy vs Fluorouracil, Cisplatin and radiotherapy for carcinoma of the anal canal. A randomized controlled trial. JAMA. 2008;299:1914–21.
11. Belkacemi Y, Berger C, Poortmans P, et al. Management of primary anal canal adenocarcinoma: a large retrospective study from the Rare Cancer Network. Int J Radiat Oncol Biol Phys. 2003;56:1274–83.

Soft Tissue Sarcoma

42

David Y. Johnson, Shilpi Wadhwa, and Frank E. Johnson

Data concerning the estimated new cases and deaths worldwide in 2002 for soft tissue sarcoma were not available through the International Agency for Research on Cancer (IARC), a component of the World Health Organization (WHO) [1].

The American Cancer Society estimated that there were 9,220 new cases and 3,560 deaths due to this cause in the USA in 2007 [2]. The data for the estimated 5-year survival rate (all races) in the USA in 2007 were not available for this type of cancer [2].

The best-established risk factor is ionizing radiation. Genetic factors predisposing to soft tissue sarcomas include Li-Fraumeni syndrome (p53 mutations), retinoblastoma gene (Rb-1) mutations, KIT mutations, neurofibromatosis type I; others have been reported. Certain occupations, particularly those involving toxic organic chemicals such as herbicides, are associated with sarcoma development. Immunosuppression is also a risk factor [3–8].

Geographic Variation Worldwide

The highest rates for connective tissue tumors in the world are in South African white males and females, with Ugandan females a close second. The incidence of Kaposi sarcoma is very high in Uganda, with the USA as a distant second. It is possible that lower rates in other countries may be a function of incomplete ascertainment rather than a true reflection of incidence [3]. There is considerable variation in the incidence among races in the USA [3].

D.Y. Johnson • S. Wadhwa
Department of Internal Medicine, Saint Louis University Medical Center, Saint Louis, MO, USA

F.E. Johnson (✉)
Saint Louis University Medical Center and Saint Louis Veterans Affairs Medical Center, Saint Louis, MO, USA
e-mail: frank.johnson1@va.gov

Surveillance Strategies Proposed by Professional Organizations or National Government Agencies and Available on the Internet

National Comprehensive Cancer Network (NCCN, www.nccn.org)

NCCN guidelines were accessed on 1/28/12 (Tables 42.1–42.8). There were major quantitative changes and new quantitative guidelines compared to the guidelines accessed on 4/10/07.

American Society of Clinical Oncology (ASCO, www.asco.org)

ASCO guidelines were accessed on 1/28/12. No quantitative guidelines exist for sarcoma surveillance, including when first accessed on 10/31/07.

The Society of Surgical Oncology (SSO, www.surgonc.org)

SSO guidelines were accessed on 1/28/12. No quantitative guidelines exist for sarcoma surveillance, including when first accessed on 10/31/07.

European Society for Medical Oncology (ESMO, www.esmo.org)

ESMO guidelines were accessed on 1/28/12 (Tables 42.9–42.12). There were major quantitative and qualitative changes compared to the guidelines accessed on 10/31/07.

F.E. Johnson et al. (eds.), *Patient Surveillance After Cancer Treatment*, Current Clinical Oncology, DOI 10.1007/978-1-60327-969-7_42,

Table 42.1 Soft tissue sarcoma: extremity/trunk (stage I)

	Years posttreatment[a]					
	1	2	3	4	5	>5
Office visit	2–4	2–4	1–4	1	1	1
Chest imaging[b]	1–2	1–2	1–2	1–2	1–2	1–2

[a]The numbers in the table indicate the number of times the modality is recommended during the indicated year posttreatment
[b]Consider obtaining postoperative baseline and periodic imaging of primary site based on estimated risk of locoregional recurrence (MRI, CT, consider ultrasound). In situations where the area is easily followed by physical examination, imaging may not be required. After 10 years, the likelihood of developing a recurrence is small and follow-up should be individualized
Evaluation for rehabilitation (occupational therapy, physical therapy), continue until maximal function is achieved
Obtained from NCCN (www.nccn.org) on 1-28-12
NCCN guidelines were accessed on 1/28/12. There were no significant changes compared to the guidelines accessed on 4/10/07

Table 42.2 Soft tissue sarcoma: extremity/trunk (stage II–III)

	Years posttreatment[a]					
	1	2	3	4	5	>5
Office visit	2–4	2–4	2–4	2	1–2	1
Chest imaging[b,c]	2–4	2–4	2–4	2	1–2	1

[a]The numbers in the table indicate the number of times the modality is recommended during the indicated year posttreatment
[b]Plain radiograph or chest CT
[c]Consider obtaining postoperative baseline and periodic imaging of primary site based on estimated risk of locoregional recurrence (MRI, CT, consider ultrasound). In situations where the area is easily followed by physical examination, imaging may not be required. After 10 years, the likelihood of developing a recurrence is small and follow-up should be individualized
Evaluation for rehabilitation (occupational therapy, physical therapy), continue until maximal function is achieved
Obtained from NCCN (www.nccn.org) on 1-28-12
NCCN guidelines were accessed on 1/28/12. There were no significant changes compared to the guidelines accessed on 4/10/07

Table 42.3 Soft Tissue Sarcoma: Retroperitoneal/Intra Abdominal, R0 Resection

	Years Posttreatment[a]					
	1	2	3	4	5	>5
Office visit	2–4	2–4	1–4	1	1	1
Abdominal/pelvic CT	2–4	2–4	1–4	1	1	1

[a]The numbers in the table indicate the number of times the modality is recommended during the indicated year posttreatment
Consider chest imaging
Obtained from NCCN (www.nccn.org) on 1-28-12
NCCN guidelines were accessed on 1/28/12. There were no significant changes compared to the guidelines accessed on 4/10/07

Table 42.4 Soft tissue sarcoma: retroperitoneal/intra abdominal, R1 resection

	Years posttreatment[a]					
	1	2	3	4	5	>5
Office visit	2–4	2–4	2–4	2	1–2	1
Abdominal/pelvic CT	2–4	2–4	2–4	2	1–2	1

[a]The numbers in the table indicate the number of times the modality is recommended during the indicated year posttreatment
Consider chest imaging
Obtained from NCCN (www.nccn.org) on 1-28-12
NCCN guidelines were accessed on 1/28/12. There were no significant changes compared to the guidelines accessed on 4/10/07

Table 42.5 Soft tissue sarcoma: gastrointestinal stromal tumors (GIST), very small gastric GISTs[a]

	Years posttreatment[b]					
	1	2	3	4	5	>5
Office visit[c]	2–4	2–4	2–4	1–4	1–4	1
Abdominal/pelvic CT with contrast	2–4	2–4	2–4	1–4	1–4	1

[a]<2 cm
[b]The numbers in the table indicate the number of times the modality is recommended during the indicated year posttreatment
[c]Abdominal/pelvic CT was the only quantitative recommendation given. We inferred that office visit would be recommended as frequently as this
Obtained from NCCN (www.nccn.org) on 1-28-12
NCCN guidelines were accessed on 1/28/12. There were major quantitative changes compared to the guidelines accessed on 4/10/07

Table 42.6 Soft tissue sarcoma: gastrointestinal stromal tumors (GIST) without preoperative imatinib

	Years posttreatment[a]					
	1	2	3	4	5	>5
Office visit[b]	2–4	2–4	2–4	2–4	2–4	1
Abdominal/pelvic CT[c]	2–4	2–4	2–4	1–4	1–4	1

[a]The numbers in the table indicate the number of times the modality is recommended during the indicated year posttreatment
[b]Less frequent surveillance may be acceptable for very small tumors (<2 cm)
[c]Abdominal/pelvic CT was the only quantitative recommendation given. We inferred that office visit would be recommended as frequently as this
Obtained from NCCN (www.nccn.org) on 1-28-12
NCCN guidelines were accessed on 1/28/12. There were no significant changes compared to the guidelines accessed on 4/10/07

Table 42.7 Soft tissue sarcoma: gastrointestinal stromal tumors (GIST) with preoperative imatinib

	Years posttreatment[a]					
	1	2	3	4	5	>5
Office visit[b]	2–4	2–4	2–4	2–4	2–4	2–4
Abdominal/pelvic CT[10]	2–4	2–4	2–4	2–4	2–4	2–4

[a]The numbers in the table indicate the number of times the modality is recommended during the indicated year posttreatment
[b]Less frequent surveillance may be acceptable for very small tumors (<2 cm)
Obtained from NCCN (www.nccn.org) on 1-28-12
NCCN guidelines were accessed on 1/28/12. There were minor quantitative changes compared to the guidelines accessed on 4/10/07

Table 42.8 Soft Tissue Sarcoma: Desmoid Tumors (Fibromatosis)

	Years posttreatmenta					
	1	2	3	4	5	>5
Office visit	2–4	2–4	1–4	1	1	1
Appropriate imaging	2–4	2–4	1–4	1	1	1

[a]The numbers in the table indicate the number of times the modality is recommended during the indicated year posttreatment
Evaluation for rehabilitation (occupational therapy, physical therapy), continue until maximal function is achieved
Obtained from NCCN (www.nccn.org) on 1-28-12
NCCN guidelines were accessed on 1/28/12. These new quantitative guidelines compared to no guidelines found on 4/10/07

Table 42.9 Soft tissue sarcomas: low-grade sarcoma

	Years posttreatment[a]					
	1	2	3	4	5	>5
Office visit	2–3	2–3	2–3	2–3	2–3	2–3
Chest x-ray or CT scan[b]	2–3	2–3	2–3	1–3	1–3	1

[a]The numbers in the table indicate the number of times the modality is recommended during the indicated year posttreatment
[b]Chest x-ray or CT scan should be obtained at more relaxed intervals than office visits in the first 3–5 years, then yearly
Obtained from ESMO (www.esmo.org) on 1-28-12
ESMO guidelines were accessed on 1/28/12. There were major quantitative and qualitative changes compared to the guidelines accessed on 10/31/07

Table 42.10 Soft tissue sarcomas: intermediate-/high-grade sarcoma

	Years posttreatment[a]					
	1	2	3	4	5	>5
Office visit	3–4	3–4	2–4	2	2	1
Chest x-ray or CT scan[b,c]	3–4	3–4	2–4	1–2	1–2	1

[a]The numbers in the table indicate the number of times the modality is recommended during the indicated year posttreatment
[b]ESMO guidelines do not directly mention imaging for intermediate-/high-grade sarcoma surveillance. However, chest x-ray or CT scan is directly recommended for low-grade sarcoma in relation to office visit frequency. We inferred that imaging should be pursued in a similar fashion for intermediate-/high-grade sarcoma
[c]Chest x-ray or CT scan should be obtained at more relaxed intervals than office visits in the first 3–5 years, then yearly
Obtained from ESMO (www.esmo.org) on 1-28-12
ESMO guidelines were accessed on 1/28/12. There were major quantitative and qualitative changes compared to the guidelines accessed on 10/31/07

European Society of Surgical Oncology (ESSO, www.essoweb.org)

ESSO guidelines were accessed on 1/28/12. No quantitative guidelines exist for sarcoma surveillance, including when first accessed on 10/31/07.

Table 42.11 Soft tissue sarcomas: gastrointestinal stromal tumors (GIST), low-risk tumors

	Years posttreatment[a]					
	1	2	3	4	5	>5
Office visit[b]	2	2	2	2	2	0
CT scan	2	2	2	2	2	0

[a]The numbers in the table indicate the number of times the modality is recommended during the indicated year posttreatment
[b]Very low-risk GIST probably do not deserve routine follow-up, although one must be aware that the risk is not nil
Obtained from ESMO (www.esmo.org) on 1-28-12
ESMO guidelines were accessed on 1/28/12. There were no significant changes compared to the guidelines accessed on 10/31/07

Table 42.12 Soft tissue sarcomas: gastrointestinal stromal tumors (GIST), intermediate-/high-risk tumors

	Years posttreatment[a]					
	1	2	3	4	5	>5
Office visit	3–4	3–4	3–4	2	2	0
CT scan	3–4	3–4	3–4	2	2	0

[a]The numbers in the table indicate the number of times the modality is recommended during the indicated year posttreatment
Obtained from ESMO (www.esmo.org) on 1-28-12
ESMO guidelines were accessed on 1/28/12. There were no significant changes compared to the guidelines accessed on 10/31/07

Cancer Care Ontario (CCO, www.cancercare.on.ca)

CCO guidelines were accessed on 1/28/12. No quantitative guidelines exist for sarcoma surveillance, including when first accessed on 10/31/07.

National Institute for Clinical Excellence (NICE, www.nice.org.uk)

NICE guidelines were accessed on 1/28/12. No quantitative guidelines exist for sarcoma surveillance, including when first accessed on 10/31/07.

The Cochrane Collaboration (CC, www.cochrane.org)

CC guidelines were accessed on 1/28/12. No quantitative guidelines exist for sarcoma surveillance, including when first accessed on 10/31/07.

The M.D. Anderson Surgical Oncology Handbook also has follow-up guidelines, proposed by authors from a single National Cancer Institute-designated Comprehensive Cancer Center, for many types of cancer [8]. Some are detailed and quantitative, others are qualitative.

Summary

This is a rare cancer with high incidence in South Africa and Uganda. We found consensus-based guidelines but none based on high-quality evidence.

References

1. Parkin DM, Whelan SL, Ferlay J, Teppo L, Thomas DB. Cancer incidence in five continents, Vol. VIII. Lyon, France: International Agency for Research on Cancer; 2002 (IARC Scientific Publication 155). ISBN 92-832-2155-9.
2. Jemal A, Seigel R, Ward E, Murray T, Xu J, Thun MJ. Cancer Statistics, 2007. CA Cancer J Clin. 2007;57:43–66.
3. Schottenfeld D, Fraumeni JG. Cancer epidemiology and prevention. 3rd ed. New York, NY: Oxford University Press; 2006. ISBN 13:978-0-19-514961-6.
4. DeVita VT, Hellman S, Rosenberg SA. Cancer. 7th ed. Philadelphia, PA: Lippincott Williams & Wilkins; 2005. ISBN 0-781-74450-4.
5. CDC: National Center for Chronic Disease Prevention and Health Promotion Oral Health Resources. Resource Library Fact Sheet. Oral cancer: deadly to ignore. February 2002. Available online at http://www.cdc.gov/OralHealth/factsheets/oc-facts.htm.
6. International Agency for Research on Cancer IARC Screening Group. Lancet 2005: 365:1927-33. Available online at http://www.screening.iarc.fr/oralindex.php.
7. Devesa SS, Grauman DJ, Blot WJ, Pennello GA, Hoover RN, Fraumeni JF Jr. Atlas of Cancer Mortality in the United States. National Institutes of Health, National Cancer Institute; September 1999 (NIH Publication No. 99-4564).
8. Feig BW, Berger DH, Fuhrman GM. The M.D. Anderson surgical oncology handbook. 4th ed. Philadelphia, PA: Lippincott Williams & Wilkins; 2006 (paperback). ISBN 0-7817-5643-X.

43 Soft Tissue Sarcoma Surveillance Counterpoint: USA

Valeriy Sedov and Janice M. Mehnert

Keywords

Sarcoma: soft tissue, retroperitoneal, extremity, uterine • Surveillance of • Adjuvant radiation therapy of • Adjuvant chemotherapy forIntroduction

Sarcomas are malignant tumors originating from mesenchymal tissue. They are quite rare, accounting for approximately 1% of all newly diagnosed malignancies. The estimated number of new soft tissue cancers in the United States is >10,000 per year with >3,000 deaths [1]. The incidence is thought to be underestimated [2], but these cancers represent a significant clinical and financial burden [3].

Surgical resection is the only potentially curative therapy. Adjuvant radiation therapy is commonly recommended for patients with high-grade resected sarcomas involving the extremities, retroperitoneum, trunk, or head and neck region. The main benefit of radiation is improved local control, and no meaningful impact on survival has been shown. The role of adjuvant chemotherapy remains controversial. With the exception of childhood soft tissue sarcomas such as rhabdomyosarcoma and extraskeletal Ewing's sarcoma, the benefit of adjuvant chemotherapy for other histologic subtypes of soft tissue sarcoma is still a subject of a debate. No clear benefit has been shown for adjuvant chemotherapy in patients with retroperitoneal or uterine sarcomas A survival benefit for adjuvant doxorubicin and ifosfamide-based regimens has been suggested in some trials and a recent meta-analysis involving patients with extremity soft tissue sarcomas [4, 5] but has not been seen in other trials [6–8], making it difficult to adopt this approach as standard therapy. Preoperative radiation therapy and/or systemic chemotherapy are often used in neo-adjuvant settings to improve resectability depending on site, stage, histologic grade, feasibility of primary resection, or clinician/institutional experience. Unfortunately, however, soft tissue sarcomas have a high potential for recurrence, particularly those that are large (> 5 cm) and exhibit high-grade pathology. After primary treatment, 40–60% of all patients develop local or distant recurrence, most occurring within 2 years of primary treatment [9]. Many experts agree that sarcoma patients benefit from a team approach of a multidisciplinary sarcoma program.

According to the American Joint Committee on Cancer, the overall 5-year survival rate for soft tissue sarcoma of the extremities is 50–60% in the United States [2] with 90% survival for stage 1 and less than 5% for stage IV lesions. Patients with retroperitoneal tumors have poorer survival rates. Over 50% of patients die each year of metastatic disease, due to development of distant metastases. Some local recurrences or isolated metastases can be treated by repeat surgical resection with or without adjuvant chemotherapy or radiotherapy. Because early treatment of local recurrence or distant metastases may prolong survival and might be curative [9], development of an appropriate surveillance protocol is important.

There are no guidelines rooted in evidence based-data. This leaves much of the decision making to a practicing physician, sometimes subjecting patients to inappropriate diagnostic modalities or delaying timely diagnosis. Surveillance can be quite expensive. Studies have shown a significant difference between the least and the most expensive approaches: 7-to-20-fold in UK (£372–7,961 as of 2006 [10]), and more than 40-fold in the United States ($485–21,235 [3]). These estimates do not include cost of care after diagnosis of recurrence. Guidelines for surveillance after primary treatment have been proposed by several institutions, but there is no consensus [9, 11–13]. Some are mostly qualitative, emphasizing the importance of surveillance and stressing participation in clinical trials [11].

V. Sedov, M.D. • J.M. Mehnert, M.D. (✉)
Melanoma and Soft Tissue Oncology, The Cancer Institute of New Jersey, 195 Little Albany Street, Room 5543, New Brunswick, NJ 08903, USA
e-mail: sedovva@umdnj.edu; mehnerja@umdnj.edu

F.E. Johnson et al. (eds.), *Patient Surveillance After Cancer Treatment*, Current Clinical Oncology, DOI 10.1007/978-1-60327-969-7_43,

Tables 43.1 Surveillance after curative-intent therapy for patients with low-grade soft tissue sarcoma of the extremities at the Cancer Institute of New Jersey

	Year					
Modality	1	2	3	4	5	>5
Office visit	2–4	2–4	2–4	1	1	1
Chest X-ray	0–2	0–2	0–2	1	1	0–1
CT of chest, abdomen and pelvis	0–2	0–2	0–2	0	0	0
CT or MRI or extremity	0–1	0–1	0–1	0	0	0

The number in each cell indicates the number of times a particular modality is recommended during a particular posttreatment year

Tables 43.2 Surveillance after curative-intent therapy for patients with high-grade soft tissue sarcoma of the extremities at the Cancer Institute of New Jersey

	Year					
Modality	1	2	3	4	5	>5
Office visit	2–4	2–4	2–4	2	2	1
Chest X-ray	1–2	1–2	1–2	2	2	1
CT of chest, abdomen and pelvis	1–2	1–2	1–2	0–1	0–1	0
CT or MRI or extremity	1–2	0–1	0–1	0	0	0

The number in each cell indicates the number of times a particular modality is recommended during a particular posttreatment year

Tables 43.3 Surveillance after curative-intent therapy for patients with retroperitoneal soft tissue sarcoma at the Cancer Institute of New Jersey

	Year					
Modality	1	2	3	4	5	>5
Office visit	2–4	2–4	2–4	2	2	1
CT of chest,	2–4	2–4	2–4	1–2	1–2	0–1*
abdomen and pelvis	0–2	0–2	0–2	0–1	0–1	0**

* = high grade, ** = low grade

The number in each cell indicates the number of times a particular modality is recommended during a particular posttreatment year

Others are more specific, as outlined earlier in this chapter. The duration of follow-up varies from 5 to 10 years from the time of primary treatment. The backbone of each protocol is the understanding that sarcomas have a high potential for recurrence, which defines survival, and that patterns of recurrence depend on the grade and size of the tumor and primary anatomical site [12].

Tables 43.1, 43.2, and 43.3 summarize our practice at the Cancer Institute of New Jersey. They resemble NCCN and ESMO guidelines. For high-grade extremity sarcomas or for retroperitoneal sarcomas, given the high risk of recurrence within the first 2–3 years, CT scans are often employed rather than a chest X-ray. We obtain MRI scans of the primary site with extremity tumors after the initial 6 months, then yearly if physical examination is easy to perform (superficial location, small body habitus, etc.) for 3 years. If physical examination is problematic (deep location, woody edema from radiation, large body habitus), MRI is continued every 6 months for 3 years. This may vary given the age of the patient. For instance, for younger females of child-bearing age we may recommend alternating chest X-rays with CT scans to minimize repeated radiation exposure. These guidelines have been developed as a consensus within the Melanoma and Soft Tissue Oncology Group. The imaging studies have not appeared to be prohibitive in terms of cost to our patient population, although no formal analysis of this issue has been completed. We recognize that some flexibility is needed, usually driven by factors such as availability of resources, the patient's ability to comply, and his/her level of anxiety (which sometimes results in higher costs).

References

1. Jemal A, Siegel R, Ward E, et al. Cancer Statistics, 2008. CA Cancer J Clin. 2008;58:71–96.
2. The NCCN Clinical Practice Guidelines in Oncology™ GUIDELINE NAME (Version 2.2008). © 2009 National Comprehensive Cancer Network, Inc. http://www.nccn.org/. Accessed March 2009.
3. Goel A, Christy ME, Virgo KS, Kraybill WG, Johnson FE. Costs of follow-up after potentially curative treatment for extremity soft-tissue sarcoma. Int J Oncol. 2004;25(2):429–35.
4. Adjuvant chemotherapy in soft tissue sarcoma (STS): a meta-analysis of published data. 2008 ASCO Annual Meeting. J Clin Oncol. 2008; (May 20 Suppl; Abstr 10526).
5. Pervaiz N, Colterjohn N, Farrokhyar F, et al. A systematic metaanalysis of randomized controlled trials of adjuvant chemotherapy for localized resectable soft-tissue sarcoma. Cancer 2008; 113:573.
6. Bramwell V, Rouesse J, Steward W, et al. Adjuvant CYVADIC chemotherapy for adult soft tissue sarcoma--reduced local recurrence but no improvement in survival: a study of the European Organization for Research and Treatment of Cancer Soft Tissue and Bone Sarcoma Group. J Clin Oncol 1994; 12:1137.
7. Le Cesne A, Van Glabbeke M, Woll PJ, et al. The end of adjuvant chemotherapy era with doxorubicin-based regimen in resected high-grade soft tissue sarcoma: Pooled analysis of the two STBSG-EORTC phase III clinical trials (abstract). J Clin Oncol 2008; 26:559s.
8. Woll PJ, Reichardt P, Le Cesne A, et al. Adjuvant chemotherapy with doxorubicin, ifosfamide, and lenograstim for resected soft-tissue sarcoma (EORTC 62931): a multicentre randomised controlled trial. Lancet Onco12012; 13:1045.
9. Whooley BP, Gibbs JF, Mooney MM, McGrath BE, Kraybill WG. Primary extremity sarcoma: what is the appropriate follow-up? Ann Surg Oncol. 2000;7:9–14.
10. Gerrand CH, Billingham LJ, Woll PJ, Grimer RJ. Follow up after primary treatment of soft tissue sarcoma: a survey of current practice in the United Kingdom. Sarcoma. 2007;2007:34128.
11. National Institute for Health and Clinical Excellence, Improving outcomes for people with sarcoma, the manual. http://www.nice.org.uk/nicemedia/pdf/SarcomaFullGuidance.pdf.
12. Whooley BP, Mooney MM, Gibbs JF, Kraybill WG. Effective follow-up strategies in soft tissue sarcoma. Semin Surg Oncol. 1999;17:83–7.
13. Casali PG, Jost L, Sleijfer S, Verweij J, Blay JY. ESMO Guidelines Working Group. Soft tissue sarcomas: ESMO clinical recommendations for diagnosis, treatment and follow-up. Ann Oncol. 2008;19 Suppl 2:ii89–93.

Soft-Tissue Sarcoma Surveillance Counterpoint: Japan

44

Shuichi Matsuda and Yukihide Iwamoto

Keywords
Soft-tissue sarcoma • CT scan • MRI • PET • Chemotherapy • Radiation • Liposarcoma

Soft-tissue sarcomas are rare malignant soft-tissue tumors that arise from mesodermal tissue, most commonly from the connective, muscle, adipose, neural, and vascular tissues. Approximately two new cases of soft-tissue sarcoma are diagnosed in Japan annually per 100,000 population. They are very heterogeneous, and more than 50 different types have been described. They can be managed through multidisciplinary care provided by surgeons, medical oncologists, and radiation oncologists.

The majority of patients with low-grade sarcoma require surgery alone, but those with a high-grade sarcoma typically require chemotherapy and radiation therapy also. The mainstay of local treatment is excision with wide surgical margins. Radiation has been shown to improve local control in the management of soft-tissue sarcomas with wide local excision [1, 2]. The decision to use chemotherapy is difficult because no consensus exists regarding indications.

After curative-intent primary therapy, patients with stage I tumors are followed up every 6 months with chest and tumor-site imaging during the first 3 years and once per year thereafter (Table 44.1) [3, 4]. This strategy is very similar to the guidelines from the National Comprehensive Cancer Network (NCCN).

The prognosis of patients with low-grade tumors is excellent, with a 90% 5-year survival rate; however, late recurrence and metastasis can occur. For stage II and III patients, follow-up should be performed every 3 months for 2 years because most patients who ever experience relapse have recurrence within this interval. After 2–3 years, follow-up frequency can be decreased to every 6 months and then once per year at year 5 (Table 44.2) [3, 4]. In addition to the strategy from the NCCN, we recommend imaging of the local site by magnetic resonance imaging (MRI) or computed tomography (CT) scan to identify local recurrence [5]. A marginally or incompletely excised soft-tissue sarcoma should be followed more carefully because the rate of local recurrence is increased in this situation, even if radiation therapy is given [6]. Clinicians should be aware that postradiation sarcoma could develop in irradiated tissues [7]. Serial chest CT scans are recommended because metastasis occurs predominantly by a hematogenous route to the lungs [8]. Lymphatic metastasis is uncommon, occurring in approximately 5% of cases [9]; however, certain histologic subtypes of sarcoma, such as epithelioid sarcoma, clear cell sarcoma, and synovial sarcoma, display a propensity to lymphatic spread. No specific tumor markers have been identified for soft-tissue sarcoma. Appropriate tests should be carried out to detect treatment-related toxicities. When a recurrent or metastatic lesion is found during follow-up, surgical resection is the first choice for treatment. Surgical treatment of known local recurrence improves survival and decreases morbidity. Therefore, early detection of recurrent or metastatic disease allows a greater chance for resection, leading to salvage in some patients. In our hospital, it is not difficult to obtain a CT scan every 3 months. Patients understand that it is difficult to find lung metastasis without serial CT scans. We believe that patients and doctors are satisfied with this strategy.

Since soft-tissue sarcoma is a rare cancer, it is very important to perform multicenter studies, especially for evaluating the effect of chemotherapy. In Japan, multi-institution prospective trials are in progress to evaluate the effect of pre- and postoperative chemotherapy for high-grade soft-tissue sarcoma.

Positron emission tomography (PET) is useful in monitoring for local tumor recurrence and metastasis, especially

S. Matsuda, M.D., Ph.D. (✉) • Y. Iwamoto, M.D., Ph.D.
Department of Orthopaedic Surgery, Kyushu University,
3-1-1 Maidashi, Higashiku, Fukuoka city 812-8582, Japan
e-mail: mazda@ortho.med.kyushu-u.ac.jp;
yiwamoto@ortho.med.kyushu-u.ac.jp

F.E. Johnson et al. (eds.), *Patient Surveillance After Cancer Treatment*, Current Clinical Oncology,
DOI 10.1007/978-1-60327-969-7_44, © Springer Science+Business Media New York 2013

Table 44.1 Patient surveillance after curative-intent initial therapy for soft-tissue sarcoma (stage I) at Kyushu University, Japan

	Years posttreatment					
	1	2	3	4	5	>5
Office visit	2	2	2	1	1	1
Chest X-ray	2	2	2	1	1	1

Consider baseline imaging after primary therapy
Consider periodic imaging of the primary site based on estimated risk of locoregional recurrence
The number in each cell indicates the number of times a particular modality is recommended in a particular posttreatment year

Table 44.2 Patient surveillance after curative-intent initial therapy for soft-tissue sarcoma (stages II-III) at Kyushu University, Japan

	Years posttreatment[#]					
	1	2	3	4	5	>5
Office visit	4	4	4	2	2	1
Chest CT	4	4	4	2	2	1
MRI or CT of primary site[a]	2	2	2	1	1	1

Testing to detect treatment toxicities is warranted, depending on clinical factors
The number in each cell indicates the number of times a particular modality is recommended in a particular posttreatment year
[a]Increased frequency of imaging of the primary site (based on the estimated risk of locoregional recurrence) may be advisable

for sarcomas such as myxoid/round cell liposarcoma, which metastasize to various organs in addition to lung. The main current limitation of PET scanning is its expense. Molecular biology approaches have not been established for surveillance of soft-tissue sarcoma patients.

References

1. Yang JC, Chang AE, Baker AR, et al. Randomized prospective study of the benefit of adjuvant radiation therapy in the treatment of soft tissue sarcomas of the extremity. J Clin Oncol. 1998;16:197–203.
2. Pisters PW, Harrison LB, Leung DH, Woodruff JM, Casper ES, Brennan MF. Long-term results of a prospective randomized trial of adjuvant brachytherapy in soft tissue sarcoma. J Clin Oncol. 1996;14:859–68.
3. Gilbert NF, Cannon CP, Lin PP, Lewis VO. Soft-tissue sarcoma. J Am Acad Orthop Surg. 2009;17:40–7.
4. Conrad III EU. Multimodality management of malignant soft-tissue tumors. In: Menedenz LR, editor. Orthopaedic knowledge update: musculoskeletal tumors. Rosemont, IL: American Academy of Orthopaedic Surgeons; 2002. p. 255–9.
5. Garner HW, Kransdorf MJ, Bancroft LW, Peterson JJ, Bequiest TH. Murphey M.D. Benign and malignant soft tissue tumors: posttreatment MR imaging. Radiographics. 2009;29:119–34.
6. Zagars GK, Ballo MT, Pisters PW, Pollock RE, Patek SR, Benjamin RS. Surgical margins and reresection in the management of patients with soft tissue sarcoma using conservative surgery and radiation therapy. Cancer. 2003;97:2544–53.
7. Davis AM, O'Sullivan B, Turcotte R, et al. Late radiation morbidity following randomization to preoperative versus postoperative radiotherapy in extremity soft tissue sarcoma. Radiother Oncol. 2005;75:48–53.
8. Billingsley KG, Burt ME, Jara E, et al. Pulmonary metastases from soft tissue sarcoma: Analysis of patterns of diseases and postmetastasis survival. Ann Surg. 1999;229:602–10.
9. Fong Y, Coit DG, Woodruff JM, Brennan MF. Lymph node metastasis from soft tissue sarcoma in adults: Analysis of data from a prospective database of 1772 sarcoma patients. Ann Surg. 1993;217:72–7.
10. van de Luijtgaarden AC, de Rooy JW, de Geus-Oei LF, van der Graaf WT, Oyen WJ. Promises and challenges of positron emission tomography for assessment of sarcoma in daily clinical practice. Cancer Imaging. 2008;8(Suppl A):S61–8.

Soft Tissue Sarcoma Surveillance Counterpoint: Canada

45

Lloyd A. Mack and Vivien H.C. Bramwell

Keywords
Surveillance • Canada • GIST • Childhood cancer survivors • Biopsy

Introduction

Soft tissue sarcomas are malignant tumors derived from mesenchymal tissue outside the skeleton. In addition to being comparatively rare (<1% of all cancers), many histological subtypes are recognized, and soft tissue sarcoma can arise in any anatomical location [1]. This heterogenity presents a challenge to the development of management and follow-up guidelines. This counterpoint will focus on adult soft tissue sarcomas, divided into extremity and non-extremity groupings. Also included are separate sections on gastrointestinal stromal tumors (GIST) focusing on their unique biology, treatment, and follow-up. The short- and long-term morbidities of treatment for cancers occurring in children are very different from those seen in adults and require different follow-up protocols. For this reason, pediatric rhabdomyosarcomas will not be covered in this counterpoint. Although nominally a sarcoma, Kaposi's sarcoma is a multifocal malignant spindle cell proliferation seen almost exclusively now in the setting of acquired immunodeficiency syndrome (AIDS) associated with human immunodeficiency virus (HIV) infection. These spindle cells express endothelial and macrophage markers and are thought to originate from circulating peripheral blood hematopoietic precursor cells [2]. In Chapter 42, Wadhwa and Johnson state that the highest rates of connective tissue tumors in the world are seen in South Africa and Uganda. However, these figures are certainly skewed by the inclusion of AIDS-related Kaposi sarcomas, whose incidence correlates with the prevalence of HIV infection in a given country. Given that Kaposi sarcomas have nothing in common with classic adult soft tissue sarcomas, they will not be considered further in this counterpoint.

Cancer statistics compiled by the Canadian Cancer Society (http://cancer.ca/statistics/Accessed 24 November 2010) document 1,050 (610 male/440 female) new soft tissue tumors (2006 figures) and 374 deaths annually (2005 figures), in an estimated Canadian population of around 32 million. For 2010, the total new cancer cases were 173,800 with 76,200 deaths. Thus, numerically, these tumors represent a tiny fraction of the overall cancer burden. Nevertheless, soft tissue sarcoma ranks as the eleventh commonest cancer (approximately 4%) occurring in young adults (ages 20–44 years) in Canada, and it ranks seventh in mortality [3], with a disproportionately high economic impact in the working population.

Although the framework for health care delivery is mandated through the Canada Health Act, service delivery is a provincial responsibility. Provincial cancer agencies exist in many of the provinces and have varying degrees of responsibility for organization and delivery of cancer services. Radiation treatment machines have generally been confined to a limited number of cancer centers or university teaching hospitals, and sarcoma expertise in medical and radiation oncology is usually concentrated at these

L.A. Mack, M.D., F.R.C.S.C., F.A.C.S. (✉)
Department of Surgical Oncology, Alberta Health Services—Cancer Care, Tom Baker Cancer Centre, University of Calgary, Surgical Oncologist, 1331 – 29 Street NW, Calgary, AB, Canada T2N 4N2
e-mail: Lloyd.Mack@albertahealthservices.ca

V.H. Bramwell, Ph.D., M.B.B.S., F.R.C.P.C.
Department of Medicine, Alberta Health Services—Cancer Care, Tom Baker Cancer Centre, University of Calgary, 1331 – 29 Street NW, Calgary, AB, Canada T2N 4N2

Division of Medical and Radiation Oncology, Alberta Health Services, Calgary Zone, 1331 – 29 Street NW, Calgary, AB, Canada T2N 4N2
e-mail: Vivien.Bramwell@albertahealthservices.ca

F.E. Johnson et al. (eds.), *Patient Surveillance After Cancer Treatment*, Current Clinical Oncology,
DOI 10.1007/978-1-60327-969-7_45,

sites. As sophisticated limb salvage techniques have been developed for patients with extremity sarcomas, increasingly these individuals are referred to provincial cancer centers to be seen by sarcoma multidisciplinary teams comprising surgical, radiation, and medical oncologists as well as specialized pathologists and radiologists. It is also common practice in Canada for patients with sarcoma to be followed in cancer centers (generally for 5 years) by one or more members of the multidisciplinary teams. Of interest, a Canadian study reviewing data of a population-based cohort of 1,467 cases of extremity soft tissue sarcoma treated in Ontario1987–1996 documented significant increases in the relative risk of amputation at any time and death from any cause, of 3.48 and 1.4, respectively, for those patients not seen in a multidisciplinary cancer center within 3 months following the diagnosis [4].

In Canada, there are few published guidelines for management of STS and/or GIST. The British Columbia Cancer Agency provides consensus guidelines for cancer including sarcomas, covering demographics, predisposing factors/prevention, screening/early detection, diagnosis, staging, and management, including follow-up (http://www.bccancer.bc.ca/HPI/cancermanagementguidelines/musculoskeletalandsarcoma Accessed 24 November 2010). In contrast, Cancer Care Ontario (CCO), through its Program in Evidence Based Care, produces evidence-based guidelines for a range of cancers, including sarcoma (http://www.cancercare.on.ca/english/home/toolbox/qualityguidelines/diseasesite/sarcoma-ebs Accessed 10 December 2008). To date, these have been limited to systemic treatments for soft tissue sarcoma and GIST, and follow-up guidelines are not available. A recently published guideline (11.9: May 12, 2010) makes recommendations for "Multidisciplinary Specialist Care for Sarcoma" but does not cover follow-up care.

The rationale behind follow-up recommendations can only be appreciated based on a clear understanding of current assessment and treatment of soft tissue sarcoma, as described here.

Table 45.1 AJCC stage grouping for soft tissue sarcoma

Histological grade				
GX	Grade cannot be assessed			
G_1	Well-differentiated			
G_2	Moderately differentiated			
G_3	Poorly differentiated			
G_4	Undifferentiated			
TNM				
Primary tumor (T)				
TX	Primary tumor cannot be assessed			
T_0	No evidence of primary tumor			
T_1	Tumor 5 cm or less in greatest dimension			
T_2	Tumor more than 5 cm in greatest dimension			
Depth				
a	Superficial to muscular fascia			
b	Is deep to or involves muscular fascia			
Regional lymph nodes (N)				
NX	Regional lymph nodes cannot be assessed			
N_0	No regional lymph node metastasis			
N_1	Regional lymph node metastasis			
Distant metastasis (M)				
Mx	Presence of distant metastasis cannot be assessed			
M_0	No distant metastasis			
M_1	Distant metastasis			
Stage grouping				
Stage I	G_1	T_{1a}, 1b, 2a, 2b	N_0	M_0
Stage II	G_{2-3}	T_{1a}, 1b, 2a	N_0	M_0
Stage III	G_{2-3}	T_{2b}	N_0	M_0
Stage IV	Any G	Any T	N_1	M_0
	Any G	Any T	N_0	M_1

Initial Assessment

At our center, initial assessment of a patient with suspected soft tissue sarcoma includes a full history and examination, concentrating on presenting symptoms and signs, including lump or swelling, pain, and neurovascular deficits, as well as constitutional symptoms or signs that could indicate metastatic disease. Most extremity and nonextremity tumors of the head and neck and superficial trunk are evaluated similarly. For suspected soft tissue sarcoma of the retroperitoneum or primary GIST, attention is directed to complaints associated with an abdominal mass—early satiety, back pain, and the development of lymphedema or leg discomfort as well as symptoms of bowel or urinary obstruction. Clinical evaluation includes assessment of the size of the mass, determination of whether a mass is mobile and superficial vs. fixed and deep to muscular fascia as well as an appropriate neurovascular assessment, including documentation of limb function with the Musculoskeletal Tumor Society Rating Scale (MSTS) [5] and the Toronto Extremity Salvage Score (TESS) [6] Tumor size and grade, as well as depth related to muscular fascia, are important prognostic features for soft tissue sarcoma [7, 8] and are components of the American Joint Committee on Cancer (AJCC) staging system for soft tissue sarcoma (Table 45.1).

Initial imaging includes plain radiographs of the affected area, chest radiograph (CXR), and assessment of the mass lesion with cross-sectional imaging, including computer tomography (CT) scan or magnetic resonance imaging (MRI) or both. MRI gives the most information regarding invasion of important neurovascular structures in STS of the extremity [9]. CT is often quite comparable and can also assess potential periosteal or bony invasion, although this is uncommon. CT scan of the chest, abdomen, and pelvis is required for appropriate initial evaluation of retroperitoneal tumors and GISTs.

The role of positron emission tomography (PET) in the management of soft tissue sarcoma is evolving [10, 11]. It has been suggested that ancillary information provided by PET (1) may assist in the prediction of grade, based on imaging alone, (2) differentiate benign vs. malignant lesions, (3) guide biopsy to areas with higher metabolic activity, and (4) help assess response to therapy [10, 11]. Further, PET/CT is increasingly used to exclude distant metastases and assist decision- making when particularly high-risk and morbid surgery, such as external hemipelvectomy, is being considered.

The use of image- or surgeon-directed core biopsy to obtain multiple samples is generally sufficient to make a diagnosis of soft tissue sarcoma in more than 90% of cases [12]. GISTs are usually biopsied via an endoscopic approach when in the stomach, duodenum, or rectum. The preference at our center is to employ image-directed core biopsy for suspected retroperitoneal soft tissue sarcoma to rule out other diagnoses, including benign tumors, lymphoma, and germ cell tumors. Further, a preoperative biopsy is required if neoadjuvant therapy is proposed. Tumor grading is often possible on core biopsy alone; in our center, the three-tiered system of the French Federation of Cancer Centers Sarcoma Group [13] is used. In cases where core biopsy is nondiagnostic, an incisional biopsy is needed and is performed by an experienced soft tissue oncology surgeon, ideally the same surgeon planning potential definitive surgical management. Small (≤3–5 cm, depending on site), superficial soft tissue masses can be removed by an excisional biopsy.

Pathologic assessment is performed by a pathologist experienced in the diagnosis and grading of soft tissue sarcomas, including standard microscopic evaluation, immunohistochemistry, and cytogenetic and molecular pathologic evaluation as appropriate. Most surgical procedures are planned after definitive pathological diagnosis. For GIST, CD117 (KIT) immunohistochemistry staining is positive in approximately 95% of cases, and important prognostic information includes tumor size, site, and mitotic rate.14

Current staging recommendations for exclusion of distant spread include CT chest for extremity soft tissue sarcoma and CT chest, abdomen, and pelvis for retroperitoneal and GIST subtypes. Evaluation of draining lymph nodes by sentinel lymph node biopsy may be performed in uncommon histological subtypes, including clear cell sarcoma or epithelioid sarcoma.

Local Treatment: Extremity/ Trunk/ Head and Neck

There is level 1 evidence showing that limb-sparing surgery and adjuvant irradiation can produce equivalent outcomes to amputation [15–17], but the ideal specific combinations and sequencing of surgery, radiotherapy ± chemotherapy remain controversial. Multidisciplinary discussion and planning are vital. The current surgical standard of care is limb-preserving, function-preserving, wide local excision (>1 cm), although narrower margins near critical neurovascular structures are acceptable when combined with irradiation. Our center uses a preoperative chemoradiation protocol with chemotherapy given primarily as a radiosensitizer [18], but most Canadian centers employ preoperative or postoperative external beam irradiation. The optimum timing of radiotherapy was evaluated in a Canadian randomized control trial [19], which showed no differences in local control, disease-free survival, or overall survival between the treatment arms. Wound complications were higher (35% vs. 17%; $p=0.01$) in the group treated with the preoperative irradiation and were most significant in the lower limb. Those treated with postoperative irradiation had better function at 6 weeks post-surgery but no significant differences at later time points [20]. However, there was more late radiation morbidity from fibrosis in the postoperative irradiation arm. Those with significant fibrosis had more joint stiffness and edema, which adversely affected patient function [21].

Table 45.2 Surveillance of patients with extremity/trunk/head and neck soft tissue sarcoma—low grade (Stage I) at Tom Baker Cancer Centre

	Years posttreatment				
	1	2	3	4	5
Office visit	2	2	2	1	1
CXR	2	2	2	1	1

Baseline imaging after primary therapy is usually obtained 3–4 months postoperatively

Local imaging (US/CT/MRI) repeated only if worrisome symptoms and/or signs are noted

The numbers in each cell indicate the number of times a particular modality is recommended during a particular posttreatment year

Retroperitoneal STS

Unlike extremity soft tissue sarcoma, where combined modality treatment is accepted and supported by level 1 evidence, the most appropriate treatment of retroperitoneal tumors is less clear. En bloc resection of the retroperitoneal soft tissue sarcoma, plus adjacent organs to obtain a histologically negative margin, is the mainstay of treatment [22]. Unfortunately, as many as 20% of tumors are deemed unresectable at presentation or gross residual disease remains after a resection attempt. Even among those completely resected, in approximately 25% of cases margins are microscopically positive. In their large series, 19% and 41% local recurrence rates at 2 and 5 years, respectively, were described for those undergoing a complete resection [22]. In retroperitoneal sarcomas, local recurrence without the development of systemic metastases is a leading cause of death. Therefore,

Table 45.3 Surveillance of patients with extremity/trunk/head and neck soft tissue sarcoma—high grade (Stages II/III) at Tom Baker Cancer Centre

	Years posttreatment				
	1	2	3	4	5
Office visit	3–4	3–4	2–3	2	2
CXR	3–4	3–4	2–3	2	2

Baseline imaging after primary therapy is usually obtained 3–4 months postoperatively
Local imaging (US/CT/MRI) is repeated only if worrisome symptoms and/or signs are noted
The numbers in each cell indicate the number of times a particular modality is recommended during a particular posttreatment year

Table 45.4 Surveillance of patients with retroperitoneal soft tissue sarcoma or GIST—all risk categories

	Years posttreatment				
	1	2	3	4	5
Office visit	2–3	2–3	2–3	2	2
CXR[a]	2	2	2	2	2
CT scan abdomen/pelvis[b]	2–3	2–3	2–3	2	2

Baseline imaging after primary therapy is usually obtained 3–4 months Postoperatively
[a]GIST rarely metastasize to lung, and annual CXR is adequate
[b]More frequent imaging (3×/year) is recommended for patients with large tumors (>5 cms) and/or high-grade (>mitoses/50 high power fields), and/or tumor spillage at surgery
The numbers in each cell indicate the number of times a particular modality is recommended during a particular posttreatment year

many centers have explored the use of various combinations of surgery and irradiation to reduce local recurrence rates [23], and follow-up guidelines reflect an emphasis on detecting local recurrence (Table 45.4).

GIST

For GIST, limited resectable disease should be completely excised (R0 resection) without dissection of clinically negative lymph nodes, taking care to avoid tumor rupture [24]. In cases of locally advanced disease, multidisciplinary consultation is essential and neoadjuvant imatinib should be considered with the intent of downstaging to limit surgical morbidity, particularly for rectal GIST [25]. Resecting the primary tumor in the setting of distant metastatic disease is appropriate, if feasible with low morbidity, to avoid treatment-related complications of tumor such as hemorrhage or perforation.

Adjacent Chemothereapy

We offer adjuvant chemotherapy to selected patients (stage III) with extremity and trunk soft tissue sarcoma, following a guideline (#11.2) developed by the Program in Evidence-Based Care of CCO (http://cancercare.on.ca/english/home/toolbox/qualityguidelines/diseasesite/sarcoma-ebs/ Accessed 24 November 2010). Six cycles of doxorubicin/ifosfamide is the most commonly recommended regimen and is accompanied by an extensive discussion of the potential benefit and risks. Adjuvant chemotherapy is rarely suggested for patients with STS of nonextremity sites.

For patients with GIST, imatinib is a highly active targeted therapy for patients with unresectable and/or metastatic disease [26, 27], producing objective response rates of 50–60%, with only 10–15% of tumors showing primary progression. However, treatment is not curative and the median duration of response is approximately 2 years. The American College of Surgeons Oncology Group (ACOSOG) performed a trial (Z9001) comparing 1 year of adjuvant imatinib with placebo, in patients who had complete resection of primary GIST and no evidence of metastases. Our center contributed patients to this trial, which closed in April 2007 after accrual of 756 patients, based on an interim analysis showing a highly significant difference in recurrence-free survival duration at 1 year, 97% for imatinib vs. 83% for placebo [48]. Patients still taking placebo were given 1 year of adjuvant imatinib. It was too early to demonstrate an overall survival benefit for adjuvant imatinib, and this may not be seen for many years, if ever, due to crossover of some patients. A similar European Organisation for Research and Treatment of Cancer (EORTC) open-label randomized trial, comparing 2 years of adjuvant imatinib with no further treatment and powered for an overall survival endpoint, has been completed, but results are not yet available. As imatinib is a highly active drug in GIST, timing of therapy (early or late) may not be critical. Thus, the use of adjuvant imatinib in all eligible patients can be questioned until an overall survival benefit is demonstrated in a randomized trial.

Currently, we discuss the results of this study with patients who have had resection of intermediate- or high-risk GIST [14]. Patients who choose to receive adjuvant imatinib are responsible for the cost of the medication personally or through private insurance. At present, there is variation in funding mechanisms for adjuvant imatinib across Canada. Patients at high risk for recurrence are followed closely so that imatinib can be initiated early for relapse (Table 45.4).

Surveillance

As stated in Chapter 42 by Wadhwa and Johnson, there are no evidence-based guidelines for follow-up of patients with STS. Thus, in their Tables 1–7, they provide consensus guidelines developed by the National Comprehensive Cancer Network (NCCN) (http://www.nccn.org/ Accessed 10 December 2008). The membership of the Sarcoma Panel comprises exclusively oncologists from the United States. Some sarcoma specialists in Canada have contributed to, and will follow, guidelines developed by CCO (http://www/cancercare.on.ca/english/home/toolbox/qualoityguidelines/diseasesite/sarcoma-ebs/ Accessed 24 November 2010), where these exist, or consensus-based guidelines developed locally. The only published follow-up guidelines in Canada are those of BCCA (http://www.bccancer.bc.ca/HPI/cancermanagementguidelines/musculoskeletalandsarcoma/ Accessed 24 November 2010).

In Calgary, surgical radiation and medical oncologists who are members of our multidisciplinary sarcoma team have developed consensus guidelines for follow-up of patients with soft tissue sarcoma (Tables 45.2 and 45.3), and these do not differ between patients treated by multimodality limb salvage techniques and those treated with radical surgery. In practice, our follow-up guidelines are not substantially different from those of NCCN, BCCA, and also the European Society for Medical Oncology [28].

In a large series of 1,224 patients treated with conservative surgery and radiation for localized soft tissue sarcoma, the risk of local or distant recurrence was highest in the first few years, with approximately two thirds of relapses occurring by 2 years and more than 90% by 5 years [29]. This pattern of relapse, together with information on initial stage, treatment, and prognostic factors, guides our follow-up practice. Important factors predictive of a higher risk of local recurrence include positive margins following resection, presentation with locally recurrent disease, and high-grade pathology [30, 31]. Prognostic factors predictive of systemic recurrence and death include older age at diagnosis, increasing tumor size (≤5, 5–10, or > 10 cm), higher tumor grade, depth (deep to muscular fascia), and site (head and neck, abdominal, retroperitoneal, and trunk worse than extremity) [8, 30–32], although not all of these factors influence our follow-up practice. Tumor grade probably influences rapidity of recurrence [33], and, thus, our follow-up protocol for patients with high/intermediate-grade soft tissue sarcoma differs slightly from that for patients with low-grade soft tissue sarcoma, in terms of frequency (Table 45.2 and 45.3). Clinic visits with attention to symptoms and clinical examination of the primary site is the core component of follow-up procedures. We perform baseline imaging with MRI of the primary site for extremity soft tissue sarcoma approximately 3–4 months postoperatively to allow sufficient time for recovery and resolution of postoperative changes. No further routine imaging of the primary site is performed unless symptoms or physical findings in follow-up are of concern. Soft tissue sarcoma of the head and neck, superficial trunk, and abdominal wall are managed similarly. For retroperitoneal sarcoma, or those in deep locations and not easily palpated, we perform CT scan imaging every 6 months posttreatment (Table 45.3). The role of PET scanning is even more uncertain in follow-up practice.

For patients with high-grade soft tissue sarcoma being considered for adjuvant chemotherapy, we obtain a CT scan of the chest in the postoperative period. Further follow-up imaging includes CXR, as described in Table 45.2. Concerning symptoms, physical findings, or radiologic abnormalities detected by CXR are further evaluated by chest CT scan when necessary. As there are no useful tumor markers for STS/GIST, routine blood work is not performed. Aspiration biopsy is used to evaluate suspicious local or distant lesions, as cytology is often adequate to establish recurrence.

In addition to oncologic outcomes, most patients are followed for wound complications and functional outcomes using a standardized wound complication scoring system, and the MSTS [5] and TESS [6] scoring systems. The best functional outcomes are among those in whom wound complications are avoided [20].

After appropriate combined modality treatment, local recurrence is uncommon (5–20%) in extremity soft tissue sarcoma but remains a significant problem for patients with retroperitoneal soft tissue sarcoma [22, 23]. Local recurrence is often a harbinger of systemic disease and repeat pretreatment staging, specifically CT scan of the chest for extremity soft tissue sarcoma, and CT scan of the chest, abdomen, and pelvis for retroperitoneal soft tissue sarcoma is necessary.

Generally, if concurrent distant metastases are discovered and are symptomatic, the most common treatment is palliative intent chemotherapy. If a local recurrence is likely to cause severe symptoms or local problems before patient deterioration related to metastases, further treatment is considered including reresection alone, palliative irradiation or amputation, generally accepting the least invasive technique. However, isolated local recurrence occurs in two-thirds of cases, and further combined modality treatment may produce long-term local control rates of approximately 45–50%[29]. Alternatively, a local recurrence may be treated with surgery alone including further wide local excision or amputation.

Unfortunately, local recurrence of retroperitoneal sarcoma is rarely completely resectable and is associated with poor overall survival [22]. True local recurrence of GIST is infrequent but may be resectable. Most cases present with metastatic regional disease in the peritoneum or liver metastases, but in selected cases, surgical resection is considered.

Surgery for Distant Metastases

Up to 40% of patients with soft tissue sarcoma develop distant metastases: lung is the most frequent initial site in extremity soft tissue sarcoma, with lung, liver, and widespread intra-abdominal sarcomatosis occurring in retroperitoneal soft tissue sarcoma [30]. Median survival duration is short following the development of distant metastases, in the range of 12–15 months [34]. Most patients are treated with palliative chemotherapy. However, close follow-up with regular CXR for the presence of lung metastases is justified in patients with intermediate-/high-grade sarcomas (Table 45.2), as distant metastases may be limited to the lungs in approximately 20% of cases [35, 36]. Such patients are referred for thoracic surgical evaluation. Resection of lung metastases in selected cases produces overall survival rates of 23–40% at 3 years and 15–30% at 5 years [35, 37].

Although less extensively studied, surgery is considered for isolated and technically resectable liver or intra-abdominal metastases [38], which together with the risk of local recurrence provide the rationale for regular CT scans of abdomen/pelvis in follow-up (Table 45.3). Particularly for GIST, surgery may be indicated if one or two metastases are growing in the setting of overall response on imatinib. Complete resection of residual metastatic disease appears to be associated with a better prognosis, although whether this is related to patient selection or surgery is uncertain [39].

New Primary Neoplasm

Childhood cancer survivors have approximately a ninefold increased risk (standardized incidence ratio) of developing secondary sarcomas, at a median of 11 years following their primary diagnosis of cancer [40]. The highest risks are associated with a young age at time of primary diagnosis, having a sarcoma as the primary diagnosis, and having a first-degree relative with cancer [40]. In multivariate analysis, increased risks were related to prior radiation therapy, a primary diagnosis of sarcoma, and treatment with higher doses of anthracyclines or alkylating agents. Patients with genetic predisposition such as Li-Fraumeni syndrome, neurofibromatosis type I, and retinoblastoma are also at a higher risk of developing a secondary sarcoma [41, 42]. GIST may occur synchronously or metachronously with other cancers in up to 10% of patients; however, soft tissue or bone sarcomas made up a minority (3%) of cases in one series [43]. However, for adults with soft tissue sarcoma, the risk of a second primary neoplasm is substantially lower than that of recurrent soft tissue sarcoma and thus does not influence follow-up practice.

Future Prespects

Although prospective randomized trials of follow-up practices in soft tissue sarcoma have the potential to rationalize use of limited resources (personnel, imaging tests), it is unlikely that such studies will be done, particularly in Canada. Their feasibility is limited by available patient numbers and the need to answer more critical questions about initial management.

Identification of chromosomal translocations [44] and gene microarray technology [45] are playing increasing roles in diagnosis of soft tissue sarcoma as well as identification of potential therapeutic targets. How this might affect our follow-up practices remains to be seen. However, recognition that progressive disease is often associated with new mutations in patients with GIST [46], which may be responsive to therapy with alternative tyrosine kinase inhibitors [47], would support a policy of more frequent biopsy and mutational analysis of recurrent tumors.

Active research continues exploring the role of PET in diagnosis, staging, and follow-up of soft tissue sarcoma [1, 10, 11]. New PET tracers including 18 F-fluorothymidine (18 F-FLT) and 18 F-misonidazole (18 F-MISO) are being investigated for their ability to reveal tumor growth rate, oxygen use, drug resistance properties, and blood supply of tumors [11].

References

1. Weiss SW, Goldblum JR. Enzinger and Weiss's soft tissue tumors. 4th ed. Marc Strauss editor. Mosby, Inc. 2001. p7–8.
2. Ambinder RF. Chapter 98 HIV associated malignancies, p2649. In: Abeloff JO, Niederhuber JE, Kastan MB, McKenna WG, editors. Clinical oncology. 3rd ed. Churchill, Livin`one: Elsevier; 2004.
3. Cancer care Ontario: cancer in young adults in Canada, Toronto, Canada 2006. ISBN 0-921325-10-X. Also available at htpp://www.cancercare.on.ca.
4. Paszat L, O'Sullivan B, Bell R, Bramwell V, Groome P, MacKillop W, et al. Processes and outcomes of care for soft tissue sarcoma of the extremities. Sarcoma. 2002;6:19–26.
5. Enneking W. Modification of the system for functional evaluation in the surgical management of musculoskeletal tumors. In: Enneking W, editor. Limb salvage in musculoskeletal oncology. New York, NY: Churchill, Livingstone; 1987. p. 627–39.
6. Davis AM, Wright JG, Williams JI, Bombardier C, Griffin A, Bell RS. Development of a measure of physical function for patients with bone and soft tissue sarcoma. Qual Life Res. 1996;5:508–16.
7. Soft tissue sarcoma. In: Greene FL, Page DL, Fleming ID, Fritz AG, Balch CM, Haller DG, Morrow M, editors. AJCC Cancer Staging Manual. 6th ed. New York: Springer, 2002. p. 193–197.
8. Kattan NW, Leung DH, Brennan MF. Postoperative nomogram for 12-year sarcoma-specific death. J Clin Oncol. 2002;20:791–6.
9. Heslin MJ, Smith JK. Imaging of soft tissue sarcomas. Surg Oncol Clin N Am. 1999;8:91–107.
10. Schuetze SM. Utility of positron emission tomography in sarcomas. Curr Opin Oncol. 2006;18:369–73.
11. Toner GC, Hicks RJ. PET for sarcomas other than gastrointestinal stromal tumors. Oncologist. 2008;13 Suppl 2:22–6.
12. Welker J, Henshaw RM, Jelinek J, Shmookler BM, Malawer MM. The percutaneous needle biopsy is safe and recommended in the diagnosis of musculoskeletal masses. Cancer. 2000;89:2677–86.
13. Coindre JM, Nguyen BB, Bonichon F, de Mascarel I, Trojani M. Histopathologic grading in spindle cell soft tissue sarcomas. Cancer. 1988;61:2305–9.
14. Fletcher CDM, Berman JJ, Corless C, Gorstein F, Lasota J, Longley BJ, et al. Diagnosis of gastrointestinal stromal tumors: a consensus approach. Human Pathol. 2002;33:459–65.
15. Rosenberg SA, Tepper J, Glatstein E, Costa J, Baker A, Brennan M, et al. The treatment of soft-tissue sarcomas of the extremities: prospective randomized evaluations of (1) limb-sparing surgery plus

radiation therapy compared with amputation and (2) the role of adjuvant chemotherapy. Ann Surg. 1982;196:305–15.

16. Yang JC, Chang AE, Baker AR, Sindelar WF, Danforth DN, Topalian SL, et al. Randomized prospective study of the benefit of adjuvant radiation therapy in the treatment of soft tissue sarcomas of the extremity. J Clin Oncol. 1998;16:197–203.
17. Pisters PW, Harrison LB, Woodruff JM, Gaynor JJ, Brennan MF. A prospective randomized trial of adjuvant brachytherapy in the management of low-grade soft tissue sarcomas of the extremity and superficial trunk. J Clin Oncol. 1994;12:1150–5.
18. Mack LA, Crowe PJ, Yang JL, Schachar NS, Morris DG, Kurien EC, et al. Preoperative chemoradiotherapy (modified Eilber protocol) provides maximum local control and minimal morbidity in patients with soft tissue sarcoma. Ann Surg Oncol. 2004;12:646–53.
19. O'Sullivan B, Davis AM, Turcotte R, Bell R, Catton C, Chabot P, et al. Preoperative versus postoperative radiotherapy in soft-tissue sarcoma of the limbs: a randomized trial. Lancet. 2002;359:2235–41.
20. Davis AM, O'Sullivan B, Bell RS, Turcotte R, Catton CN, Wunder JS, et al. Function and health status outcomes in a randomized trial comparing preoperative and postoperative radiotherapy in extremity soft tissue sarcoma. J Clin Oncol. 2002;20:4471–7.
21. Davis AM, O'Sullivan B, Turcotte R, Bell R, Catton C, Chabot P, et al. A Canadian Sarcoma Group and NCI Canada Clinical Trials Group Randomized Trial: late radiation therapy in extremity soft tissue sarcoma. Radiother Oncol. 2005;75:48–53.
22. Lewis JJ, Leung D, Woodruff JM, Brennan MF. Retroperitoneal soft-tissue sarcoma: analysis of 500 patients treated and followed at a single institution. Ann Surg. 1998;228:355–65.
23. Pawlik TM, Pisters PWT, Mikula L, Feig BW, Hunt KK, Cormier JN, et al. Long-term results of two prospective trials of preoperative external beam radiotherapy for localized intermediate- or high-grade retroperitoneal soft tissue sarcoma. Ann Surg Oncol. 2006;13: 508–17.
24. DeMatteo RP, Heinrich MC, El-rifai WM, Demetri G. Clinical Management of gastrointestinal stromal tumors: before and after STI-571. Human Pathol. 2002;33:466–77.
25. Eisenberg BL, Harris J, Blanke CD, Demetri GD, Heinrich MC, Watson JC, et al. Phase II trial of neoadjuvant/adjuvant imatinib mesylate (IM) for advanced primary and metastatic/recurrent operable gastrointestinal stromal tumor (GIST): early results of RTOG 0132/ACRIN 6665. J Surg Oncol. 2009;99:42–7.
26. Verweij J, Casali PG, Zalcberg J, LeCesne A, Reichardt P, Blay JY, et al. Judson I, for the EORTC soft Tissue and Bone Sarcoma Group, the Italian Sarcoma Group, and the Australasian Gastrointestinal Trials Group: progression-free survival in gastrointestinal stromal tumours with high-dose imatinib: randomized trial. Lancet. 2004;364:1127–34.
27. Blanke CD, Rankin C, Demetri GD, Ryan CS, von Mehren M, Benjamin RS, et al. Phase III randomized, intergroup trial assessing imatinib mesylate at two dose levels in patients with unresectable or metastatic gastrointestinal stromal tumors expressing the kit receptor tyrosine kinase: S0033. J Clin Oncol. 2008;26:626–32.
28. Casali PG, Jost L, Sleijfer S, Verweij J, Blay JY. ESMO Guidelines Working Group: soft tissue sarcomas: ESMO clinical recommendations for diagnosis, treatment and follow-up. Ann Oncol. 2008;19 (Suppl ii):89–93.
29. Zagars GK, Ballo MT, Pisters PWT, Pollock RE, Patel SR, Benjamin RS, et al. Prognostic factors for patients with localized soft-tissue sarcoma treated with conservation surgery and radiation therapy: an analysis of 1224 patients. Cancer. 2003;97:2530–43.
30. Pisters PWT, Leung DHY, Woodruff J, Shi W, Brennan MF. Analysis of prognostic factors in 1,041 patients with localized soft tissue sarcoma of the extremities. J Clin Oncol. 1996;14:1679–89.
31. Eilber FC, Rosen G, Nelson SD, Selch M, Dorey F, Eckardt J, Eilber FR. High-grade extremity soft tissue sarcomas: factors predictive of local recurrence and its effect on morbidity and mortality. Ann Surg. 2003;237(2):218–26.
32. Coindre JM, Terrier P, Guillou L, Doussal VL, Collin F, Ranchere D, et al. Predictive value of grade for metastasis development in the main histologic types of adult soft tissue sarcomas: a study of 1240 patients from the French Federation of Cancer Centers Sarcoma Group. Cancer. 2003;91:1914–26.
33. Stojadinovic A, Leung DHY, Allen P, Lewis JJ, Jaques DP, Brennan MF. Primary adult soft tissue sarcoma: time-dependent influence of prognostic variables. J Clin Oncol. 2002;20:4344–52.
34. Bramwell VH, Anderson D, Charette ML, Sarcoma Disease Site Group. Doxorubicin-based chemotherapy for the palliative treatment of adult patients with locally advanced or metastatic soft tissue sarcoma. Cochrane Database Syst Rev. 2003;(3): CD003293.
35. Gadd MA, Casper ES, Woodruff JM, McCormack PM, Brennan MF. Development and treatment of pulmonary metastases in adult patients with extremity soft tissue sarcoma. Ann Surg. 1993;218:705–12.
36. Potter DA, Glenn J, Kinsella T, Glatstein E, Lack EE, Restrepo C, et al. Patterns of recurrence in patients with high-grade soft-tissue sarcomas. J Clin Oncol. 1985;3:353–66.
37. Pastorino U, Buyse M, Frieel G, Ginsberg RJ, Girard P, Goldstraw P, et al. Long-term results of lung metastectomy: prognostic analyses based on 5206 cases. J Thorac Cardiovasc Surg. 1997;113:37–49.
38. DeMatteo RP, Shah A, Fong Y, Jarnagin WR, Blumgart LH, Brennan MF. Results of hepatic resection for sarcoma metastatic to liver. Ann Surg. 2001;234:540–7.
39. Andtbacka RH, Ng CS, Scaife CL, Cormier JN, Hunt KK, Pisters PW, et al. Surgical resection of gastrointestinal stromal tumors after treatment with imatinib. Ann Surg Oncol. 2007;14:14–24.
40. Henderson TO, Whitton J, Stovall M, Mertens AC, Mitby P, Friedman D, et al. Secondary sarcomas in childhood cancer survivors: a report from the childhood cancer survivor study. J Natl Cancer Inst. 2007;99:300–8.
41. Kingston JE, Hawkins MM, Draper GJ, Marsden HB, Kinnier Wilson LM. Patterns of multiple primary tumours in patients treated for cancer during childhood. Br J Cancer. 1987;56:331–8.
42. Krumerman MS, Stingle W. Synchronous malignant glandular schwannomas in congenital neurofibromatosis. Cancer. 1978;41: 2444–51.
43. Agaimy A, Wunsch PH, Sobin LH, Lasota J, Miettinen M. Occurrence of other malignancies in patients with gastrointestinal stromal tumors. Semin Diag Pathol. 2006;23:120–9.
44. Borden EC, Baker LH, Bell RS, Bramwell V, Demetri GD, Eisenberg BL, et al. Soft tissue sarcomas of adults: state of the translational science. Clin Cancer Res. 2003;9:1941–56.
45. Nielsen TO. Microarray analysis of sarcomas. Adv Anat Pathol. 2006;13(4):166–73.
46. Antonescu CR, Besmer P, Guo T, Arkun K, Hom G, Koryotowski B, et al. Acquired resistance to imatinib in gastrointestinal stromal tumor occurs through secondary gene mutation. Clin Cancer Res. 2005;11:4182–90.
47. Demetri GD, van Oosterom AT, Garrett CR, Blackstein ME, Shah MH, Verweij J, et al. Efficacy and safety of sunitinib in patients with advanced gastrointestinal stromal tumour after failure of imatinib: a randomized controlled trial. Nat Clin Pract Oncol. 2007; 4:342–3.
48. Dematteo RP, Ballman KV, Antonescu CR, Maki RG, Pisters PW, Demetri GD, et al. Adjuvant imatinib mesylate after resection of localized, primary gastrointestinal stromal tumour: a ranedomised, double-blind, placebo-controlled trial. Lancet. 2009;373: 1097–104.

Osteogenic Sarcoma and Dedifferentiated Chondrosarcoma

46

David Y. Johnson, Shilpi Wadhwa, and Frank E. Johnson

Keywords
Osteogenic sarcoma • Dedifferentiated chondrosarcoma • WHO • ASC • Surveillance

Data concerning estimated new cases and deaths worldwide in 2002 for osteogenic sarcoma and dedifferentiated chondrosarcoma were not available through the International Agency for Research on Cancer (IARC), a component of the World Health Organization (WHO) [1].

The American Cancer Society estimated that there were 2,370 new cases and 1,330 deaths due to cancers arising in bones and joints in the United States in 2007 [2]. The data for the estimated 5-year survival rate (all races) in the United States in 2007 were not available for these types of cancer [2].

Ionizing radiation causes osteogenic sarcoma and chondrosarcoma. Exposure to alkylating agents, particularly in childhood, appears to be a risk factor. Skeletal abnormalities such as Paget's disease, Ollier's syndrome (enchondromatosis), and Maffucci's syndrome (enchondromatosis and hemangiomatosis) are also risk factors. Li-Fraumeni syndrome (p53 mutation) is a rare but definite cause of these sarcomas [3, 4].

Geographic Variation Worldwide

Adequate data are not available to document worldwide variability in the incidence of this cancer.

D.Y. Johnson • S. Wadhwa
Department of Internal Medicine, Saint Louis University Medical Center, Saint Louis, MO, USA

F.E. Johnson (✉)
Saint Louis University Medical Center and Saint Louis Veterans Affairs Medical Center, Saint Louis, MO, USA
e-mail: frank.johnson1@va.gov

Surveillance Strategies Proposed By Professional Organizations or National Government Agencies and Available on the Internet

National Comprehensive Cancer Network (NCCN, www.nccn.org)

NCCN guidelines were accessed on January 28, 2012 (Tables 46.1–46.4). There were new quantitative guidelines in addition to quantitative guidelines with no significant changes compared to guidelines found on 4/10/07.

American Society of Clinical Oncology (ASCO, www.asco.org)

ASCO guidelines were accessed on January 28, 2012. No quantitative guidelines exist for bone cancer surveillance, including when first accessed on October 31, 2007.

The Society of Surgical Oncology (SSO, www.surgonc.org)

SSO guidelines were accessed on January 28, 2012. No quantitative guidelines exist for bone cancer surveillance, including when first accessed on October 31, 2007.

F.E. Johnson et al. (eds.), *Patient Surveillance After Cancer Treatment*, Current Clinical Oncology,
DOI 10.1007/978-1-60327-969-7_46, © Springer Science+Business Media New York 2013

Table 46.1 Bone cancer: chondrosarcoma, low grade and intracompartmental

	Years posttreatment[a]					
	1	2	3	4	5	>5
Office visit	1–2	1–2	1	1	1	1
Chest and lesion X-ray	1–2	1–2	1	1	1	1

Source: Obtained from NCCN (www.nccn.org) on January 28, 2012
NCCN guidelines were accessed on January 28, 2012. These were new quantitative guidelines compared to no guidelines found on April 10, 2007
[a]The numbers in the table indicate the number of times the modality is recommended during the indicated year posttreatment

Table 46.2 Bone cancer: chondrosarcoma, high grade (grade II, grade III) or clear cell or extracompartmental

	Years posttreatment[a]					
	1	2	3	4	5	>5
Office visit[b]	2–4	2–4	2–4	2–4	2–4	1[c]
Chest imaging	2–4	2–4	2–4	2–4	2–4	1[c]
Primary site radiographs and/or cross-sectional imaging as indicated						
Reassess function at every follow-up visit						

Source: Obtained from NCCN (www.nccn.org) on January 28, 2012
NCCN guidelines were accessed on January 28, 2012. These were new quantitative guidelines compared to no guidelines found on April 10, 2007
[a]The numbers in the table indicate the number of times the modality is recommended during the indicated year post-treatment
[b]Chest imaging was the only quantitative recommendation given. We inferred that office visit would be recommended as frequently as this
[c]After 5 years, yearly for a minimum of 10 years

Table 46.3 Bone cancer: Ewing's sarcoma

	Years posttreatment[a]					
	1	2	3	4	5	>5
Office visit[b]	4–6	4–6	4–6	4–6	4–6	1
Chest and local imaging[c,d]	4–6	4–6	4–6	4–6	4–6	1
CBC and other laboratory studies as indicated						

Source: Obtained from NCCN (www.nccn.org) on January 28, 2012
NCCN guidelines were accessed on January 28, 2012. These were new quantitative guidelines compared to no guidelines found on April 10, 2007
[a]The numbers in the table indicate the number of times the modality is recommended during the indicated year posttreatment
[b]Increase interval for physical examination after 24 months
[c]Increase interval for chest and local imaging after 24 months
[d]Consider PET scan or bone scan. Use the same imaging technique that was performed in the initial workup

European Society for Medical Oncology (ESMO, www.esmo.org)

ESMO guidelines were accessed on January 28, 2012 (Tables 46.5 and 46.6). There were significant quantitative and qualitative changes compared to the guidelines accessed on October 31, 2007.

Table 46.4 Bone cancer: osteosarcoma

	Years posttreatment[a]					
	1	2	3	4	5	>5
Office visit	4	4	3	2	2	1
Chest and local imaging[b]	4	4	3	2	2	1
CBC and other laboratory studies as indicated						
Reassess function every visit						

Source: Obtained from NCCN (www.nccn.org) on January 28, 2012
NCCN guidelines were accessed on January 28, 2012. There were no significant changes compared to the guidelines accessed on April 10, 2007
[a]The numbers in the table indicate the number of times the modality is recommended during the indicated year posttreatment
[b]Consider PET scan and/or bone scan. Use same imaging technique that was performed in the initial workup

Table 46.5 Bone sarcomas: low-grade tumors

	Years posttreatment[a]					
	1	2	3	4	5	>5
Office visit[b]	2	2	1	1	1	1
Local imaging, chest X-ray/CT[c]	2	2	1	1	1	1
Follow-up should include both a physical examination of the tumor site and assessment of the function and possible complications of any reconstruction						
In Ewing sarcoma, where osseous metastases are likely, isotope bone scanning can be used in addition						
It is important to evaluate the long-term toxicity effect of chemotherapy and radiotherapy if appropriate[d]						

Source: Obtained from ESMO (www.esmo.org) on January 28, 2012
ESMO guidelines were accessed on January 28, 2012. There were significant quantitative and qualitative changes compared to the guidelines accessed on October 31, 2007
[a]The numbers in the table indicate the number of times the modality is recommended during the indicated year posttreatment
[b]Late metastases as well as local recurrences and functional deficits may occur >10 years after diagnosis, and there is no universally accepted stopping point for tumor surveillance
[c]ESMO recommends that local imaging and chest X-ray/CT should be the norm. We inferred that ESMO recommends scheduled imaging as frequently as the office visit schedule
[d]Monitoring for late effects should be undertaken for >10 years after treatment, depending on the chemotherapy protocol and radiation used in conjunction with late-effects services when available. Secondary cancers may arise in survivors of bone sarcomas, either related to or independent of irradiation. Secondary leukemia, particularly acute myeloid leukemia, may rarely be observed following chemotherapy as early as 2–5 years after treatment

European Society of Surgical Oncology (ESSO, www.esso-surgeonline.org)

ESSO guidelines were accessed on January 28, 2012. No quantitative guidelines exist for bone cancer surveillance, including when first accessed on October 31, 2007.

Table 46.6 Bone sarcomas: high-grade tumors

	Years posttreatment[a]					
	1	2	3	4	5	>5
Office visit	4–9	4–9	3–6	3–6	2	1–2[b]
Local imaging, chest X-ray/CT[c]	4–9	4–9	3–6	3–6	2	1–2[b]
Follow-up should include both a physical examination of the tumor site and assessment of the function and possible complications of any reconstruction						
In Ewing sarcoma, where osseous metastases are likely, isotope bone scanning can be used in addition						
It is important to evaluate the long-term toxicity effect of chemotherapy and radiotherapy if appropriate[d]						

Source: Obtained from ESMO (www.esmo.org) on January 28, 2012

ESMO guidelines were accessed on January 28, 2012. There were significant quantitative and qualitative changes compared to the guidelines accessed on October 31, 2007

[a]The numbers in the table indicate the number of times the modality is recommended during the indicated year posttreatment

[b]Follow-up every 6 months for years 5–10 and thereafter every 6–12 months according to local practice

[c]ESMO recommends that local imaging and chest X-ray/CT should be the norm. We inferred that ESMO recommends scheduled imaging as frequently as the office visit schedule

[d]Monitoring for late effects should be undertaken for >10 years after treatment, depending on the chemotherapy protocol and radiation used in conjunction with late-effects services when available. Secondary cancers may arise in survivors of bone sarcomas, either related to or independent of irradiation. Secondary leukemia, particularly acute myeloid leukemia, may rarely be observed following chemotherapy as early as 2–5 years after treatment

Cancer Care Ontario (CCO, www.cancercare.on.ca)

CCO guidelines were accessed on January 28, 2012. No quantitative guidelines exist for bone cancer surveillance, including when first accessed on October 31, 2007.

National Institute for Clinical Excellence (NICE, www.nice.org.uk)

NICE guidelines were accessed on January 28, 2012. No quantitative guidelines exist for bone cancer surveillance, including when first accessed on October 31, 2007.

The Cochrane Collaboration (CC, www.cochrane.org)

CC guidelines were accessed on January 28, 2012. No quantitative guidelines exist for bone cancer surveillance, including when first accessed on November 24, 2007.

The M.D. Anderson Surgical Oncology Handbook also has follow-up guidelines, proposed by authors from a single National Cancer Institute-designated Comprehensive Cancer Center, for many types of cancer [5]. Some are detailed and quantitative, others are qualitative.

Summary

These are relatively uncommon cancers with little data available to document worldwide variation in incidence. We found consensus-based guidelines but none based on high-quality evidence.

References

1. Parkin DM, Whelan SL, Ferlay J, Teppo L, Thomas DB. Cancer incidence in five continents, Vol. VIII, International Agency for Research on Cancer, 2002. (IARC Scientific Publication 155). Lyon, France: IARC Press; 2002. ISBN 92-832-2155-9.
2. Jemal A, Seigel R, Ward E, Murray T, Xu J, Thun MJ. Cancer statistics, 2007. CA Cancer J Clin. 2007;57:43–66.
3. Schottenfeld D, Fraumeni JG. Cancer epidemiology and prevention. 3rd ed. New York, NY: Oxford University Press; 2006. ISBN 13:978-0-19-514961-6.
4. DeVita VT, Hellman S, Rosenberg SA. Cancer. 7th ed. Philadelphia, PA: Lippincott Williams & Wilkins; 2005. ISBN 0-781-74450-4.
5. Feig BW, Berger DH, Fuhrman GM. The M.D. Anderson surgical oncology handbook. 4th ed. Philadelphia, PA: Lippincott Williams & Wilkins; 2006. paperback. ISBN 0-7817-5643-X.

Osteogenic Sarcoma and Dedifferentiated Chondrosarcoma Surveillance Counterpoint: Japan

47

Shuichi Matsuda and Yukihide Iwamoto

Keywords
Osteosarcoma • Dedifferentiated chondrosarcoma • CT scan • MRI • PET • Chemotherapy • Radiation

Introduction

Osteosarcoma is a primary malignant tumor of the skeleton characterized by its production of osteoid matrix. The classic osteosarcoma is rare, with an estimated incidence of two cases/million population/year in Japan. It is most common in males and occurs primarily in the second decade of life. Years ago patients with osteosarcoma were treated with surgical resection only, with more than 80% of the patients ultimately dying of this disease. Today osteosarcoma is treated with pre- and postoperative chemotherapy plus surgery, and the percentage of patients cured varies between 60 and 70% [1, 2].

Dedifferentiated chondrosarcoma is a high-grade noncartilaginous sarcoma arising typically within a low-grade chondrosarcoma. Dedifferentiated chondrosarcoma is very rare. Only three to five new cases are registered annually in the bone tumor registry in Japan. It is highly malignant with a very poor prognosis with a reported 5-year survival rate of around 10% [3, 4].

Complete surgical resection is crucial for treatment of osteosarcoma. The outcome has dramatically improved with systemic chemotherapy. Therefore, pre- and postoperative chemotherapy with methotrexate, doxorubicin, cisplatin, and ifosfamide is currently a standard approach in most centers [5]. Controversy still exists about the efficacy and drawbacks of preoperative chemotherapy. Since the tumor is resistant to standard-dose radiotherapy, it is employed only when wide resection is not feasible.

Surveillance should be performed every 3 months during the first 3 years because most patients who experience relapse recur within this interval (Table 47.1). Our strategy is similar to that of the National Comprehensive Cancer Network (NCCN). If surgical margins are not adequate, the patients should be carefully followed because the rate of local recurrence is very high in such cases. The search for metastases should focus on lung and bone where the vast majority of all metastases appear [6]. Plain radiographs and computed tomography (CT) are useful to detect lung metastases, and 99 mTc-methylene diphosphonate (Tc-MDP) bone scan is useful for detecting bone metastasis. Since the prognosis of patients with primary metastatic lesions (stage IV) is still poor [2], such patients should be carefully followed. The amount of tumor necrosis following preoperative chemotherapy is another reliable prognostic factor [5]. The poor responders, whose tumor necrosis is less than 90%, should also be carefully observed. Although no specific tumor markers have been identified, a high level of serum alkaline phosphatase is frequently seen in recurrent disease. Appropriate tests should be carried out to detect treatment-related toxicities.

When a recurrent or metastatic lesion is found during follow-up, surgery is clearly the most important therapeutic method. Patients are rarely cured without complete resection of all lesions. Early detection of recurrent or metastatic disease allows a greater chance for complete resection, leading to salvage. In our department, we educate patients about this and our patients are generally satisfied with frequent imaging.

Surgical treatment should be prompt and aggressive for dedifferentiated chondrosarcoma. However, the local

S. Matsuda, M.D., Ph.D. (✉) • Y. Iwamoto, M.D., Ph.D.
Department of Orthopaedic Surgery, Kyushu University, 3-1-1 Maidashi, Higashiku, Fukuoka city 812-8582, Japan
e-mail: mazda@ortho.med.kyushu-u.ac.jp; yiwamoto@ortho.med.kyushu-u.ac.jp

F.E. Johnson et al. (eds.), *Patient Surveillance After Cancer Treatment*, Current Clinical Oncology,
DOI 10.1007/978-1-60327-969-7_47, © Springer Science+Business Media New York 2013

Table 47.1 Surveillance after curative-intent initial treatment for osteogenic sarcoma at Kyushu University, Japan

	Posttreatment year					
	1	2	3	4	5	>5
Office visit	4	4	4	2	2	1
CXR or chest CT	4	4	4	2	2	1
CBC	4	4	4	2	2	1

Reassess function at every office visit
Consider bone scan at every office visit
The number in each cell indicates the number of times a particular modality is recommended during the indicated posttreatment year

Table 47.2 Surveillance after curative-intent initial treatment for dedifferentiated chondrosarcoma at Kyushu University, Japan

	Posttreatment year					
	1	2	3	4	5	>5
Office visit	6	6	6	3	3	2
CXR or chest CT	6	6	6	3	3	2
CBC	3	3	3	3	3	2

Reassess function at every office visit
The number in each cell indicates the number of times a particular modality is recommended during the indicated posttreatment year

recurrence rate is very high even after wide resection [3, 4]. This suggests that occult local extension and metastases occur frequently. The role of adjuvant chemotherapy and radiotherapy in dedifferentiated chondrosarcoma remains unclear [7]. There is no guideline for surveillance for dedifferentiated chondrosarcoma from NCCN, but the patients with this disease should be followed every 2 months because of the poor prognosis, with most patients living less than 2 years (Table 47.2). Plain radiographs and CT scans are used to detect pulmonary metastasis and local recurrence, which occur with disappointingly high frequency. Metastasis at the time of presentation or a positive surgical margin is not prognostically very significant because the survival rates are so dismal. No specific tumor markers have been identified for dedifferentiated chondrosarcoma. Appropriate tests should be obtained to detect treatment-related toxicities. Although obtaining imaging tests every 2 months is a burden for patients, most understand the reason it is necessary. Surgery is the only way to treat recurrent or metastatic lesions with any expectation of success. Early detection of recurrent or metastatic disease allows greater chances for complete resection. However, no data are available regarding the effect of surgical resection of a recurrent lesion on overall prognosis.

Since osteosarcoma and dedifferentiated chondrosarcoma are rare, it is very important to perform multicenter studies, especially to evaluate the effect of chemotherapy. In Japan, multi-institution prospective trials will be started to evaluate the effect of pre- and postoperative chemotherapy for osteosarcoma.

Positron emission tomography (PET) is useful in monitoring for local tumor recurrence. For osteosarcoma, 18F-fludeoxyglucose PET is considered to be more accurate than CT or magnetic resonance imaging (MRI) to differentiate between local recurrence and benign mass lesions caused by postoperative tissue changes [8]. In addition, MRI is often hampered by image artifacts after implantation of metallic prostheses. The efficacy of MRI for detecting metastasis in patients with osteosarcoma has not been established.

Molecular biology approaches have not been established for surveillance of patients with osteosarcoma or dedifferentiated chondrosarcoma but are the subject of active research.

References

1. Picci P. Osteosarcoma (osteogenic sarcoma). Orphanet J Rare Dis. 2007;2:6.
2. Gebhardt MC, Hornicek FJ. Osteosarcoma. In: Menedenz LR, editor. Orthopaedic knowledge update: musculoskeletal tumors. Rosemont, IL: American Academy of Orthopaedic Surgeons; 2002. p. 175–86.
3. Dickey ID, Rose PS, Fuchs B, et al. Dedifferentiated chondrosarcoma: the role of chemotherapy with updated outcomes. J Bone Joint Surg Am. 2004;86:2412–8.
4. Mitchell AD, Ayoub K, Mangham DC, Grimer RJ, Carter SR, Tillman RM. Experience in the treatment of dedifferentiated chondrosarcoma. J Bone Joint Surg Br. 2000;82:55–61.
5. Sakamoto A, Iwamoto Y. Current status and perspectives regarding the treatment of osteosarcoma: chemotherapy. Rev Recent Clin Trials. 2008;3:228–31.
6. Bielack SS, Carrle D. State-of-the-art approach in selective curable tumors: bone sarcoma. Ann Oncol. 2008;19 Suppl 7:vii155–60.
7. Gelderblom H, Hogendoorn PC, Dijkstra SD, et al. The clinical approach towards chondrosarcoma. Oncologist. 2008;13:320–9.
8. Brenner W, Bohuslavizki KH, Eary JF. PET imaging of osteosarcoma. J Nucl Med. 2003;44:930–42.

Osteogenic Sarcoma and Dedifferentiated Chondrosarcoma Surveillance Counterpoint: Canada

48

Timothy R. Asmis, Joel Werier, and Shailendra Verma

Keywords
ESMO • Canada • Metastases • Osteosarcoma • Surveillance

Osteosarcomas are uncommon tumors that affect mainly children and adolescents. Statistics Canada estimates that 153 cases per year are diagnosed in Canadians 0–19 years old [1]. Survival has been dramatically improved through the routine use of neoadjuvant and adjuvant multidrug chemotherapy. Once multimodality therapy has been completed, surveillance commences. The goals of a surveillance program are multifactorial and include assessment of the primary tumor site for recurrence, assessment of functionality, especially when limb-sparing surgery has been employed, early detection of systemic (particularly pulmonary) metastases, and detection of treatment toxicities. Screening is defined by the National Cancer Institute as checking for disease when there are no symptoms. Since screening may find diseases at an early stage, it is hypothesized that this could improve chances for cure [2]. As a test for the presence or absence of a disease [3], screening can occur either prior to the detection of a disease (primary screening) or after a disease has been diagnosed and treated (secondary). A screening program should be effective in detecting potentially curable disease, be cost-effective, and available to patients.

Osteosarcoma patients should have secondary screening, as cure is possible in some cases if metastases are detected. In addition, patients are typically young and consequently must deal with multiple cancer survivor issues such as cardiac, endocrine, reproductive, renal, auditory problems, second malignancies, and psychological health.

T.R. Asmis, M.D., F.R.C.P.C. (✉)
• J. Werier, M.D., F.R.C.S.C. • S. Verma, M.D.
The Ottawa Hospital Regional Cancer Centre,
501 Smyth Road, Box 913, Ottawa, ON, Canada K1H 8L6
e-mail: tasmis@ottawahospital.on.ca; jwerier@toh.on.ca; sverma@toh.on.ca

It is therefore reasonable to expect that any surveillance strategy should have two main goals: to detect early, potentially curable, locally recurrent, or metastatic disease and to screen for complications of the disease and/or the consequences of therapy involving orthopedic, cardiac, endocrine, renal, and reproductive organs; labeling and other psychological/social effects; and secondary malignancies.

As osteogenic sarcoma is relatively rare, surveillance recommendations are based on expert opinion because of the difficulty of accumulating evidence [4]. There will likely never be a clinical trial to determine the relative benefits of different strategies that vary in intensity. This leaves oncologists to make clinical recommendations based on experience. Metastases most commonly occur in the lungs (85% of cases) and in many patients may be the sole site of involvement [5]. There have been multiple case series of long-term survivors of metastatic osteosarcoma following a complete resection of metastatic disease [6–12]. Hence, it is reasonable to conclude that detection of pulmonary metastases should be a goal of secondary screening. This is achieved by regular history and physical examinations as well as diagnostic imaging. The European Society of Medical Oncology (ESMO) has published recommended guidelines that we generally follow. The recommended interval between clinic visits is usually 3 months for the first 2 years following the diagnosis, and then every 4 months for years 3 and 4 and every 6 months in years 5–10 [13]. Each of these visits should consist of a history and physical examination as well as a chest X-ray. At our center, we perform thoracic CT scans every 6 months for the first 2 years. To limit radiation exposure, we suggest limiting imaging investigations to chest X-rays at all other interim visits within the first 2 years. Imaging by plain X-ray of the primary tumor site should be performed every 4 months until the end of year 4, with MRI scans recommended if there

F.E. Johnson et al. (eds.), *Patient Surveillance After Cancer Treatment*, Current Clinical Oncology,
DOI 10.1007/978-1-60327-969-7_48,

Table 48.1 Surveillance for patients after curative-intent initial therapy of osteogenic sarcoma at The Ottawa Hospital Regional Cancer Centre

	Year					
Modality	1	2	3	4	5	>5
Office visit	4	4	3	3	2	2
CXR	2	2	3	3	3	2
CT chest[a]	2	1	0	0	0	0
X-ray of tumor site	4	4	3	3	2	2
Echocardiogram[b]	2	1	0	0	0	0
Laboratory tests[c]	2	0	0	0	0	0

[a]Alternating with CXR
[b]For patients treated with doxorubicin
[c]Complete blood count, serum electrolyte levels, serum creatinine level
The number in each cell indicates the number of times a particular modality is recommended during a particular posttreatment year

are changes suspicious for recurrent disease. The majority of patients with osteosarcoma of the extremity have had a wide resection with a limb salvage procedure. X-rays of the operative site should be taken at surveillance visits, as recommended above, not only for potential recurrence but also to assess the integrity of the reconstruction and implant. If orthopedic reconstruction has been performed, this should be done in conjunction with the patient's orthopedic oncologist. Plain radiographs are generally adequate, with local CT/MRI imaging reserved for cases with special concern for recurrence on physical examination. For complex cases involving the pelvis and acetabulum, a baseline postoperative CT or MRI of the pelvis at 6–9 months may be useful as a reference for future comparative clinical evaluation. CT/MRI local imaging for these cases needs to be individualized depending on the type of resection, margins, and reconstruction performed. For patients in whom pulmonary metastases are detected and who are considered appropriate candidates for surgery (medically fit, disease-free survival >12 months), referral to a thoracic surgeon is required.

For patients treated with neoadjuvant chemotherapy that includes doxorubicin, annual monitoring of cardiac and renal function is recommended. All patients are counseled on the possible risks to reproductive health following systemic therapy and the possibility of second malignancies.

There has been dramatic progress in the treatment of this disease over the last few decades. We believe an important role of the multidisciplinary oncology team is to address the broad spectrum of health needs of osteosarcoma survivors.

References

1. Canada S: Canadian cancer statistics. 2008
2. National Cancer Institute, Dictionary of cancer terms, 2010
3. Oxford University Press. Oxford English dictionary. Oxford, England: Oxford University Press; 2003.
4. Hogendoorn PC, Athanasou N, Bielack S, et al. Bone sarcomas: ESMO Clinical Practice Guidelines for diagnosis, treatment and follow-up. Ann Oncol. 2010;21 Suppl 5:v204–13.
5. DeVita VT, Rosenberg SA, Hellman S. Cancer principles and practice of oncology, Books@Ovid. 7th ed. Lippincott, Williams & Wilkins: Philadelphia; 2005.
6. Telander RL, Pairolero PC, Pritchard DJ, et al. Resection of pulmonary metastatic osteogenic sarcoma in children. Surgery. 1978;84: 335–41.
7. Putnam Jr JB, Roth JA, Wesley MN, et al. Survival following aggressive resection of pulmonary metastases from osteogenic sarcoma: analysis of prognostic factors. Ann Thorac Surg. 1983;36: 516–23.
8. Goorin AM, Delorey MJ, Lack EE, et al. Prognostic significance of complete surgical resection of pulmonary metastases in patients with osteogenic sarcoma: analysis of 32 patients. J Clin Oncol. 1984;2:425–31.
9. Meyer WH, Schell MJ, Kumar AP, et al. Thoracotomy for pulmonary metastatic osteosarcoma. An analysis of prognostic indicators of survival. Cancer. 1987;59:374–9.
10. Han MT, Telander RL, Pairolero PC, et al. Aggressive thoracotomy for pulmonary metastatic osteogenic sarcoma in children and young adolescents. J Pediatr Surg. 1981;16:928–33.
11. Tronc F, Conter C, Marec-Berard P, et al. Prognostic factors and long-term results of pulmonary metastasectomy for pediatric histologies. Eur J Cardiothorac Surg. 2008;34:1240–6.
12. Harting MT, Blakely ML, Jaffe N, et al. Long-term survival after aggressive resection of pulmonary metastases among children and adolescents with osteosarcoma. J Pediatr Surg. 2006;41:194–9.
13. Bielack S, Carrle D, Jost L. Osteosarcoma: ESMO clinical recommendations for diagnosis, treatment and follow-up. Ann Oncol. 2008;19 Suppl 2:94–6.

Cutaneous Melanoma

49

David Y. Johnson, Shilpi Wadhwa, and Frank E. Johnson

Keywords
Cutaneous Melanoma • Xeroderma pigmentosum • Genetic factor • Immunosuppression • Transplantation

The International Agency for Research on Cancer (IARC), a component of the World Health Organization (WHO), estimated that there were 160,177 new cases of cutaneous melanoma worldwide in 2002 (1). The IARC also estimated that there were 40,781 deaths due to this cause in 2002 (1).

The American Cancer Society estimated that there were 59,940 new cases and 8,110 deaths due to this cause in the USA in 2007(2). The estimated 5-year survival rate (all races) in the USA in 2007 was 92% for this cancer (2). Survival rates were adjusted for normal life expectancies and were based on cases diagnosed from 1996 to 2002 and followed through 2003.

There is a marked effect of race. Whites, particularly fair-skinned individuals, are at much higher risk than darker-skinned people. There is a marked effect of age as well, although young people are affected. Exposure to ionizing radiation, particularly in the form of sunlight, is a major risk factor. Genetic factors have been known for decades and specific genes have been identified. Patients with xeroderma pigmentosum, a disorder of defective DNA repair, have a greatly increased risk (3, 4). Skin morphology, including the presence of many pigmented nevi and congenital nevi, appears to confer risk. Immunosuppression, such as in organ transplant patients, increases the risk of melanoma (3, 4).

D.Y. Johnson • S. Wadhwa
Department of Internal Medicine, Saint Louis University Medical Center, Saint Louis, MO, USA

F.E. Johnson (✉)
Saint Louis University Medical Center and Saint Louis Veterans Affairs Medical Center, Saint Louis, MO, USA
e-mail: frank.johnson1@va.gov

Geographic Variation Worldwide

The people of mainly non-European origin have much lower rates of melanoma than do people of mainly European origin. The highest incidence is found in Australia, New Zealand, Scandinavia, Switzerland, and white populations of the USA, including Hawaii. The populations with the lowest rates are those of Southern and Eastern Europe and South America (3). Within the USA, the incidence of this cancer is lower in northern regions than in southeastern and south-central regions (5).

Surveillance Strategies Proposed By Professional Organizations or National Government Agencies and Available on the Internet

National Comprehensive Cancer Network (NCCN, www.nccn.org)

NCCN guidelines were accessed on January 28, 2012 (Tables 49.1–49.3). There were major quantitative and qualitative changes compared to the guidelines accessed on April 10, 2007.

American Society of Clinical Oncology (ASCO, www.asco.org)

ASCO guidelines were accessed on January 28, 2012. No quantitative guidelines exist for melanoma surveillance, including when first accessed on October 31, 2007.

F.E. Johnson et al. (eds.), *Patient Surveillance After Cancer Treatment*, Current Clinical Oncology,
DOI 10.1007/978-1-60327-969-7_49, © Springer Science+Business Media New York 2013

Table 49.1 Melanoma: stage 0 in situ

	Years posttreatment[a]					
	1	2	3	4	5	>5
Office visit[b]	1	1	1	1	1	1
Educate patient in monthly self skin examination						
Routine blood tests are not recommended						
Radiologic imaging is indicated to investigate specific signs or symptoms						
Follow-up schedule influenced by risk or recurrence, prior primary melanoma, and family history of melanoma and includes other factors, such as atypical moles/dysplastic nevi, and patient anxiety						

Source: Obtained from NCCN (www.nccn.org) on January 28, 2012

NCCN guidelines were accessed on January 28, 2012. There were major qualitative changes compared to the guidelines accessed on April 10, 2007

[a]The numbers in the table indicate the number of times the modality is recommended during the indicated year posttreatment

[b]At least annual skin examination for life

Table 49.2 Melanoma: stage IA–IIA (no evidence of disease after treatment)

	Years posttreatment[a]					
	1	2	3	4	5	>5
Office visit[b,c]	1–4	1–4	1–4	1–4	1–4	1
Educate patient in monthly self skin examination						
Routine blood tests are not recommended						
Radiologic imaging is indicated to investigate specific signs or symptoms; routine radiologic imaging to screen for asymptomatic recurrent/metastatic disease is not recommended						
Follow-up schedule influenced by risk or recurrence, prior primary melanoma, and family history of melanoma and includes other factors, such as atypical moles/dysplastic nevi, and patient anxiety						

Source: Obtained from NCCN (www.nccn.org) on January 28, 2012

NCCN guidelines were accessed on January 28, 2012. There were major quantitative and qualitative changes compared to the guidelines accessed on April 10, 2007

[a]The numbers in the table indicate the number of times the modality is recommended during the indicated year posttreatment

[b]At least annual skin examination for life

[c]History and physical examination with emphasis on nodes and skin

The Society of Surgical Oncology (SSO, www.surgonc.org)

SSO guidelines were accessed on January 28, 2012. No quantitative guidelines exist for melanoma surveillance, including when first accessed on October 31, 2007.

European Society for Medical Oncology (ESMO, www.esmo.org)

ESMO guidelines were accessed on January 28, 2012. No quantitative guidelines currently exist for melanoma surveillance, compared to the quantitative guidelines accessed on October 31, 2007.

Table 49.3 Melanoma: stage IIB–IV (no evidence of disease after treatment)

	Years posttreatment[a]					
	1	2	3	4	5	>5
Office visit[b,c]	2–4	2–4	1–4	1	1	1
Chest x-ray, CT, and/or PET/CT scan	1–2	1–2	1–2	1–2	1–2	0
Brain MRI	1	1	1	1	1	0
Educate patient in monthly self skin examination						
Routine blood tests are not recommended						
Radiologic imaging is indicated to investigate specific signs or symptoms; routine radiologic imaging to screen for asymptomatic recurrent/metastatic disease is not recommended after 5 years						
Follow-up schedule influenced by risk or recurrence, prior primary melanoma, and family history of melanoma and includes other factors, such as atypical moles/dysplastic nevi, and patient anxiety						

Source: Obtained from NCCN (www.nccn.org) on January 28, 2012

NCCN guidelines were accessed on January 28, 2012. There were major quantitative and qualitative changes compared to the guidelines accessed on April 10, 2007

[a]The numbers in the table indicate the number of times the modality is recommended during the indicated year posttreatment

[b]At least annual skin examination for life

[c]History and physical examination with emphasis on nodes and skin

European Society of Surgical Oncology (ESSO, www.esso-surgeonline.org)

ESSO guidelines were accessed on January 28, 2012. No quantitative guidelines exist for melanoma surveillance, including when first accessed on October 31, 2007.

Cancer Care Ontario (CCO, www.cancercare.on.ca)

CCO guidelines were accessed on January 28, 2012. No quantitative guidelines exist for melanoma surveillance, including when first accessed on October 31, 2007.

National Institute for Clinical Excellence (NICE, www.nice.org.uk)

NICE guidelines were accessed on January 28, 2012. No quantitative guidelines currently exist for melanoma surveillance, compared to the quantitative guidelines accessed on October 31, 2007.

The Cochrane Collaboration (CC, www.cochrane.org)

CC guidelines were accessed on January 28, 2012. No quantitative guidelines exist for melanoma surveillance, including when first accessed on November 24, 2007.

Table 49.4 Primary cutaneous melanoma

	Years posttreatment[a]					
	1	2	3	4	5	>5
Office visit[b]	1	1	1	1	1	1
Baseline laboratory tests and imaging studies are generally not recommended in asymptomatic patients with newly diagnosed primary melanoma of any thickness						
Regular clinical follow-up and interval patient self-examination of skin and regional lymph nodes are most important means of detecting recurrent disease or new primary melanoma; findings from history and physical examination should direct need for further studies to detect local, regional, and distant metastasis						
Surveillance laboratory tests and imaging studies in asymptomatic patients with melanoma have low yield for detection of metastatic disease and are associated with relatively high false-positive rates						

Source: Obtained from AAD (www.aad.org) on January 28, 2012

AAD guidelines were accessed on January 28, 2012. These are new quantitative guidelines compared to the guidelines accessed on January 14, 2008

[a] The numbers in the table indicate the number of times the modality is recommended during the indicated year posttreatment

[b] No clear data regarding follow-up interval exist, but at least annual history and physical examination with attention to skin and lymph nodes are recommended

American Academy of Dermatology Association (AAD, www.aad.org)

AAD guidelines were accessed on January 28, 2012 (Table 49.4). There are new quantitative guidelines compared to the guidelines accessed on January 14, 2008.

The M.D. Anderson Surgical Oncology Handbook also has follow-up guidelines, proposed by authors from a single National Cancer Institute-designated Comprehensive Cancer Center, for many types of cancer (6). Some are detailed and quantitative, others are qualitative.

Summary

This is a common cancer with significant variability in incidence worldwide. We found consensus-based guidelines but none based on high-quality evidence.

References

1. Parkin DM, Whelan SL, Ferlay J, Teppo L, Thomas DB. Cancer incidence in five continents, Vol. VIII, International Agency for Research on Cancer, 2002. (IARC Scientific Publication 155). Lyon, France: IARC Press; 2002. ISBN 92-832-2155-9.
2. Jemal A, Seigel R, Ward E, Murray T, Xu J, Thun MJ. Cancer statistics, 2007. CA Cancer J Clin. 2007;57:43–66.
3. Schottenfeld D, Fraumeni JG. Cancer epidemiology and prevention. 3rd ed. New York, NY: Oxford University Press; 2006. ISBN 13:978-0-19-514961-6.
4. DeVita VT, Hellman S, Rosenberg SA. Cancer. 7th ed. Philadelphia, PA: Lippincott Williams & Wilkins; 2005. ISBN 0-781-74450-4.
5. Devesa SS, Grauman DJ, Blot WJ, Pennello GA, Hoover RN, Fraumeni JF Jr. Atlas of Cancer Mortality in the United States. National Institutes of Health, National Cancer Institute. NIH Publication No. 99-4564; 1999.
6. Feig BW, Berger DH, Fuhrman GM. The M.D. Anderson surgical oncology handbook. 4th ed. Philadelphia, PA: Lippincott Williams & Wilkins; 2006. paperback. ISBN 0-7817-5643-X.

Cutaneous Melanoma Surveillance Counterpoint: USA

50

Gerald Linette and Lynn A. Cornelius

Keywords
Skin Cancer • Nonmelanoma • Melanoma • UV • Metastases

Skin cancer represents the most common type of cancer diagnosed in the United States today, with rates of both nonmelanoma and melanoma skin cancers currently rising in young adults [1, 2]. Although melanoma accounts for less than 5% of all skin cancer cases, the majority of the skin cancer deaths are due to this disease. The American Cancer Society estimated that in 2009 there were over 68,000 new cases of melanoma diagnosed in the United States and over 8,600 deaths from melanoma. It is a disease primarily of the Caucasian population. Overall, the lifetime risk of getting melanoma is about 1 in 50 for whites, 1 in 1,000 for blacks, and 1 in 200 for Hispanics (www.cancer.org).

The annual percent change in melanoma incidence has increased significantly for both men and women between the time periods of 1975–1981 and 1981–2005 (http://seer.cancer.gov). Within these groups, however, certain subpopulations and trends deserve special mention: (1) Elderly white men (>65 years) are at the highest risk of developing and dying from the disease [3]. (2) Solid organ transplant [4] and bone marrow transplant [5] patients have increased incidence of melanoma, along with nonmelanoma skin cancer. (3) The incidence in young women (<40 years of age) is increasing for both thin (≤1 mm) and thicker (≥1 mm) melanoma tumors, with the increase in regional and distant disease (estimated annual percent change 9.2, Confidence Interval 3.8, 14.9) being greater than that of localized tumors (estimated annual percent change 1.9, Confidence Interval 1.6, 2.3) [2]. (4) White, Hispanic, and black patients with melanoma are significantly more likely to be diagnosed with higher stage of disease than non-Hispanics [6]. These findings may highlight those individuals and groups who could benefit from improved surveillance and education regarding melanoma.

Melanoma has a significant disease cost in the United States. One study estimated the direct annual cost of treating newly diagnosed melanoma over a decade ago (diagnosed in 1997) to be $563 million [7]. Given a 7.5% per year increase in health care costs [8], and a 2.6% per year increase in the incidence of melanoma, this extrapolates to a cost of $2.01 billion in today's health care dollars. As might be anticipated, approximately 90% of the cost incurred was from treatment of metastatic disease (Stage III and IV). In this analysis, assessments of cost included cost of physician visits, procedures, diagnostic tests (including pathologic diagnosis), and terminal care. This high cost of care for advanced, metastatic disease was later validated in 2001, with melanoma cost of care being among the highest for all malignancies [9].

As in most cancers, genes and environment interact to determine melanoma risk. Mutations in the CDKN2A gene, originally described in patients with familial melanoma [10], have also been detected in patients with a family history of melanoma and clinically atypical nevi [11–14]. In fact, patients with multiple clinically atypical nevi (formerly described as "dysplastic" nevi) and a strong family history of melanoma (approximately 10% of cases) are at significantly increased risk for disease [13, 15]. Mutations in this gene are found in ~40% of families that have at least three family members with melanoma [16]. Variant alleles in other genes, particularly those that determine skin pigmentation (phenotype) such as the Melanocortin 1 Receptor (MC1R) gene [17–19], have also been recognized to contribute to melanoma risk. Nonetheless, genetic screening is currently not recommended in melanoma, as DNA testing is not felt to

G. Linette, M.D., Ph.D. • L.A. Cornelius, M.D. (✉)
Department of Medical Oncology, Washington University School of Medicine, St. Louis, MO, USA
e-mail: cornelil@wustl.edu

F.E. Johnson et al. (eds.), *Patient Surveillance After Cancer Treatment*, Current Clinical Oncology,
DOI 10.1007/978-1-60327-969-7_50,

Table 50.1 Surveillance after curative-intent treatment for TNM stage 0 melanoma at Washington University Comprehensive Cancer Center

Modality	Year 1	2	3	4	5	>5
Office visit, including full skin and lymph node examination	1	1	1	1	1	1

The number in each cell indicates the number of times a particular modality is recommended during a particular posttreatment year

Table 50.2 Surveillance after curative-intent treatment for TNM stage IA–IIA melanoma at Washington University Comprehensive Cancer Center

Modality	Year 1	2	3	4	5	>5
Office visit, including full skin and lymph node examination	1–4	1–4	1–4	1–4	1–4	1
Chest X-ray	1[b]	1[b]	1[b]	1[b]	1[b]	1[b]
Serum LDH level	1–2	1–2	1–2	1–2	1–2	1–2

[a] Not recommended by NCCN guidelines but may be considered in men >65 who have the highest mortality in melanoma [68]
[b] CT and/or PET-CT and/or brain MRI only as indicated by clinical findings
The number in each cell indicates the number of times a particular modality is recommended during a particular posttreatment year

Table 50.3 Surveillance after curative-intent treatment for TNM stages IIB–IV melanoma at Washington University Comprehensive Cancer Center

Modality	Year 1	2	3	4	5	>5
Office visit, including full skin and lymph node examination	2–4	1–4	1–4	1–4	1–4	1–4
Chest X-ray	1[a]	1[a]	1[a]	1[a]	1[a]	1[a]
Serum LDH level	1–2	1–2	1–2	1–2	1–2	1–2

[a] Not recommended by NCCN guidelines but may be considered in men >65 who have the highest mortality in melanoma [68]
CT and/or PET-CT only as indicated by clinical findings
Brain MRI may be considered annually
The number in each cell indicates the number of times a particular modality is recommended during a particular posttreatment year

substitute for clinical examination and continued surveillance of patients with history of melanoma or other high-risk groups (i.e., individuals with a positive family history, fair skin, blue eyes, and significant ultraviolet exposure) [20].

Epidemiologic data support the role of ultraviolet light in cutaneous melanoma pathogenesis [21]. The World Health Organization has classified ultraviolet radiation (wavelengths between 100 and 400 nm: ultraviolet A, ultraviolet B, and ultraviolet C) as a Group 1 "known carcinogen," as is ionizing radiation. Tumor types linked to solar radiation include melanoma and nonmelanoma skin cancers (basal cell carcinoma and squamous cell carcinoma). Most recently, ultraviolet-emitting tanning devices have also been given a Group 1 "known carcinogen" classification based on evidence linking exposure to both cutaneous and ocular melanoma [22].

Quantifying absolute melanoma risk has proven somewhat difficult, with individual exposure type and frequency (solar vs. ultraviolet-emitting device; intermittent vs. chronic), genotype, and phenotype (fair skin, red hair) all affecting overall risk (reviewed in [23]). Recent insights into the molecular pathogenesis of melanoma have determined that specific gene mutations, such as BRAF, that contribute to its pathogenesis [24], stratify according to ultraviolet exposure type [25], supporting the pathogenic role of ultraviolet radiation in this disease. The alarming incidence in persons with fair complexion who reside in equatorial environments, such as Australia, also provides epidemiologic evidence for the role of ultraviolet radiation. In fact, the most recent clinical and practice guidelines for melanoma from New Zealand and Australia state that exposure to UV light from sunlight is the main known cause of melanoma (http://www.nhmrc.gov.au/publications/synopses/cp111syn.htm).

It is not surprising that patients with one primary melanoma are at high risk for the development of another primary melanoma, either synchronous or metachronous. In a large study of patients (>8,000) with thin to intermediate depth melanomas at John Wayne Cancer Institute, an incidence of 0.5% per year for a second primary melanoma was found in the first 5 years of patient follow-up with a 2.8% and 3.6% risk at 5 years and 10 years, respectively [26]. In a separate study of patients with primary melanomas followed for a median of 6.5 years, a 4.5 standardized incidence ratio of subsequent melanoma diagnosis was also documented (confidence interval 1.2–10.0) [27]. Finally, *SEER* data have shown that the rate of subsequent melanomas in patients with a primary diagnosis was greater than ten times the rate of melanoma in the general population, with the highest risk occurring in the 2 years following the original diagnosis [28]. Interestingly, in patients with multiple primary melanomas, the risk of carrying a *CDKN2A* mutation increases with the number of primary melanomas and a positive family history [29].

In patients who present with localized cutaneous melanoma, the primary mode of initial metastasis or recurrence in the majority (approximately two-thirds) of patients who develop metastases is locoregional (adjacent skin and regional lymph node basin) and significantly increases with tumor (Breslow) depth [30]. It is for this reason that in T1b–T4 melanomas (≤1 mm with ulceration or mitoses > 1/mm^3, or any melanoma > 1 mm), in which evidence of disease progression to the lymph nodes or other organs is not clinically evident, sentinel lymph node biopsy is performed. In this procedure, the first lymph node that drains the lymphatic basin of the primary tumor is identified by lymphoscintigraphy and evaluated for micrometastatic disease at the time of wide local excision of the tumor. The sentinel lymph node biopsy is predicated upon the belief that sentinel lymph nodes harboring tumor cells will ultimately progress to clinically significant nodal recurrence if not excised. Although the therapeutic benefit of sentinel lymph node biopsy has not yet been determined, sentinel lymph node status has prognostic significance [31].

In interim analysis of a large multi-institutional study (Melanoma Sentinel Lymph Node Trial-1: MSLT-1), this technique was reported to identify patients with nodal metastasis in whom subsequent removal of several lymph nodes in the draining nodal basin (lymphadenectomy) prolonged survival when compared to patients with similar melanomas who ultimately developed clinically evident nodal disease [32]. This study additionally claimed that if clinical evidence of metastasis developed, the number of involved nodes was significantly higher in those patients than in the patients who had micrometastasis determined by sentinel lymph node biopsy. It had previously been determined that melanoma patients who developed clinically evident nodal disease (detected by physical examination) had a worse prognosis than patients with micrometastatic disease (determined by sentinel lymph node biopsy) [33]. Questions had been raised regarding the conclusions reached in the MSLT-1 interim analysis, particularly the biologic significance of micrometastatic disease and the value of completion of lymph node dissections in patients who may never develop clinically significant disease. Concern regarding the appropriate comparison of study groups was also raised [34]. In the most recent analysis performed for the revised American Joint Committee on Cancer Staging system (7th Edition, 2010) [35, 36], Stage III patients with non-ulcerated primaries who had nodal micrometastases at the time of diagnosis did have a significantly improved survival rate at 15 years compared to patients who presented with clinically evident nodal disease, but their prognosis was not as favorable as patients with Stage II (localized) lesions. Therefore, sentinel lymph node dissection continues to be performed in patients with melanomas of Breslow thickness ≥ 1 mm and now, according to the revised staging guidelines, 1 mm with ulceration or mitoses $> 1/\text{mm}^3$ without clinically evident locoregional or distant metastatic disease at the time of diagnosis.

As in breast cancer, there has been some suggestion that nodal micrometastastic tumor volume may be of significance and that metastases below a certain size, or those detected only by immunohistochemistry [37], would have no impact on prognosis [38, 39]. (A term called prognostic false positivity has been applied by those investigators who subscribe to this belief [40]). This, in fact, had been incorporated into the previous 2002 American Joint Committee on Cancer Staging System, in which a 0.2 mm^3 tumor volume threshold was implied, and hematoxylin-eosin stain microscopic confirmation was required to establish micrometastatic node-positive status. The American Joint Committee on Cancer 2010 Staging System, however, has not incorporated a lower threshold for staging of node-positive disease and does allow immunohistochemical detection *only* of nodal micrometastases (without hematoxylin-eosin stain confirmation) as long as a melanoma-specific marker is used (HMB-45, Melan-A, MART-1) [35].

Melanoma recurrence was recently evaluated in a large cohort of localized American Joint Committee on Cancer Stage I and II melanoma patients (n=4,704) diagnosed between 1959 and 2002 in the Sydney Melanoma Unit [41]. The median follow-up time was 5.3 years. Eighteen percent of these patients had disease recurrence, with a median disease-free interval of 2.7 years (range, 0.37–27.6 years). Local recurrences (defined as ≤ 3 cm from the primary tumor) accounted for 10.9% of these recurrences; 9.9% were "in-transit" (defined as ≥ 3 cm from the primary tumor), 34.4% were regional lymph node metastases, and 44.9% were distant disease spread. Therefore, greater than 50% of the patients that recurred had locoregional recurrence, in accordance with other studies as reported here.

The presence of in-transit metastasis has now been incorporated into the American Joint Committee on Cancer staging system for melanoma (N2c, Stage IIIc). In-transit and clinical or microscopic "satellite" metastases are considered to be intralymphatic tumor spread where melanoma has spread into either the cutaneous or subcutaneous tissue located between the primary tumor and the draining lymphatics [42]. More specifically, satellite metastases have conventionally been described as clinically evident cutaneous or subcutaneous tumor deposits within 2 cm of the primary melanoma and in-transit metastasis as deposits located at sites >2 cm from the primary tumor. In patients with Stage I or II melanoma (localized tumor) at the time of original diagnosis, the development of intralymphatic tumor spread portends a poor prognosis (a 33–52% 10-year survival rate with the least favorable prognosis in patients having synchronous nodal involvement) [36]. Treatment of intralymphatic tumor spread is surgical excision of the persistent or metastatic cutaneous tumor with the goal of obtaining clear margins although, in the presence of multiple tumor deposits, this may not be possible. A sentinel lymph node biopsy may also be performed at the time of surgical excision if there is no current or previous evidence of nodal disease. When multiple satellite or in-transit metastases exist in an extremity without evidence of more distant metastases, systemic therapy (dependent upon clinical stage) and evaluation for enrollment into a clinical trial should be considered. Isolated limb perfusion of cytotoxic drugs (for deep and more numerous metastases) is a therapeutic option in select patients [43], but it should be reserved for appropriate patients and performed in large centers proficient in its use.

In addition, CO_2 laser ablation (for superficial metastases) may offer some palliation.

Melanoma has the propensity to spread to the brain, lung, liver, and gastrointestinal tract. The presence of systemic metastasis at the time of, or subsequent to, the initial diagnosis portends a poor prognosis (7–19% 5-year overall survival).

All patients with a recently diagnosed melanoma should have a complete history and physical examination performed with specific emphasis on the skin and lymph node examination. Ophthalmologic examination is not currently recommended.

In Stage IB–II patients, lymphoscintigraphy and sentinel lymph node biopsy are indicated in the staging workup. Chest X-ray examination is optional in patients with Stage IB and II melanoma as several studies have shown that chest X-ray is of limited benefit in identifying metastases [44]. According to the National Comprehensive Cancer Network melanoma guidelines (http://www.nccn.org), routine targeted imaging of either the regional tumor bed or the draining nodal basin for patients with Stage 0–II melanoma is only recommended to evaluate specific signs or symptoms. Studies have failed to demonstrate the benefit of routine imaging in detecting occult metastases in this patient population [45]. This is particularly relevant in light of recent reports about the ionizing radiation exposure risk imparted by routine imaging procedures such as CT [46].

Fluorine-18 deoxyglucose (FDG) positron emission tomography (FDG-PET), a metabolic imaging modality, is often employed in conjunction with low-resolution CT, to aid in the localization of FDG-avid metastatic lesions. PET-CT is of no benefit in the identification of micrometastatic nodal disease [47], and its sensitivity for the detection of occult disease smaller than 10 mm is not optimal [48]. Its use in the initial staging of Stage I and II patients in the absence of systemic symptoms is not indicated.

In patients with Stage IIIA disease (sentinel lymph node micrometastases), it is current practice to perform baseline imaging including CT ± PET-CT and magnetic resonance imaging for accurate staging and appropriate treatment stratification. In Stage III patients who present with clinically positive nodes, fine needle aspiration biopsy or conventional lymph node biopsy is indicated for diagnosis and staging, often with baseline imaging as described here. For positive inguinofemoral nodes, in particular, a pelvic CT is indicated. Fine needle aspiration or conventional biopsy is also indicated in Stage III patients who present with in-transit disease, together with these imaging recommendations. Finally, in patients who present with Stage IV disease, a biopsy is indicated to confirm the diagnosis. Initial staging workup of Stage IV melanoma patients typically includes brain magnetic resonance imaging and CT of chest, abdomen, and pelvis.

As outlined and referenced in the National Comprehensive Cancer Network guidelines for melanoma … "(a) structured follow-up program (in melanoma) could permit the earlier detection of recurrent disease at a time when it might be more amenable to potentially curative surgical resection. This follow-up would be particularly appropriate for patients at risk for regional nodal recurrence who have not undergone sentinel node biopsy or elective lymph node dissection. Several other reasons for a structured follow-up program include detection of a subsequent second primary melanoma, provision of ongoing psychosocial support, identification of familial kindreds, screening for second nonmelanoma primary malignancies, patient education, and documentation of the results of treatment…" [49–51]. The evidence for these guidelines is discussed later, and this consensus document forms the foundation of melanoma care by most physicians in the United States. Interestingly, they closely follow those outlined by Australia and New Zealand with few exceptions noted.

All patients with a previously diagnosed melanoma should have dermatologic surveillance throughout their lifetime. Not only are these patients at risk for recurrent disease, but they are also at increased risk to develop a second primary melanoma and/or nonmelanoma skin cancer. The surveillance schedule is dependent upon disease stage, patient risk factors, and the history or presence of nonmelanoma skin cancer. The National Comprehensive Cancer Network guidelines suggest that Stage 0 patients (melanoma in situ) receive annual complete skin and regional lymph node examination. Stage IA–IIA patients should be similarly followed up every 3–12 months for 5 years, then annually. Stage IIB–IV patients are at higher risk of melanoma recurrence, and examinations should be intensified (every 3–6 months) for the first 2 years, then every 3–12 months for 3 years, and then once per year as clinically indicated after 5 years.

Other groups have similarly attempted to develop a rational, evidenced-based approach to melanoma surveillance. The Scottish Melanoma Group evaluated 5-year surveillance in patients with cutaneous melanoma excised between 1979 and 1994. Close to half (47%) of the relapses that occurred in Stage I patients were detected by the patient, and 26% were initially detected on a follow-up visit [52] . This is consistent with a prospective Australian study in which the frequency and method of detection of first melanoma recurrence were determined in over 200 Stage I–III patients. These patients were advised to return for follow-up at least twice a year for the first 5 years after initial treatment [53]. One hundred sixty-eight patients were evaluable in this relatively small group and, consistent with other studies, the majority of patients with recurrence (76%) had locoregional recurrence only. In this patient cohort, over 70% of initial recurrences were detected by the patient. It has been suggested that surveillance regimens that are more rigorous (and may include

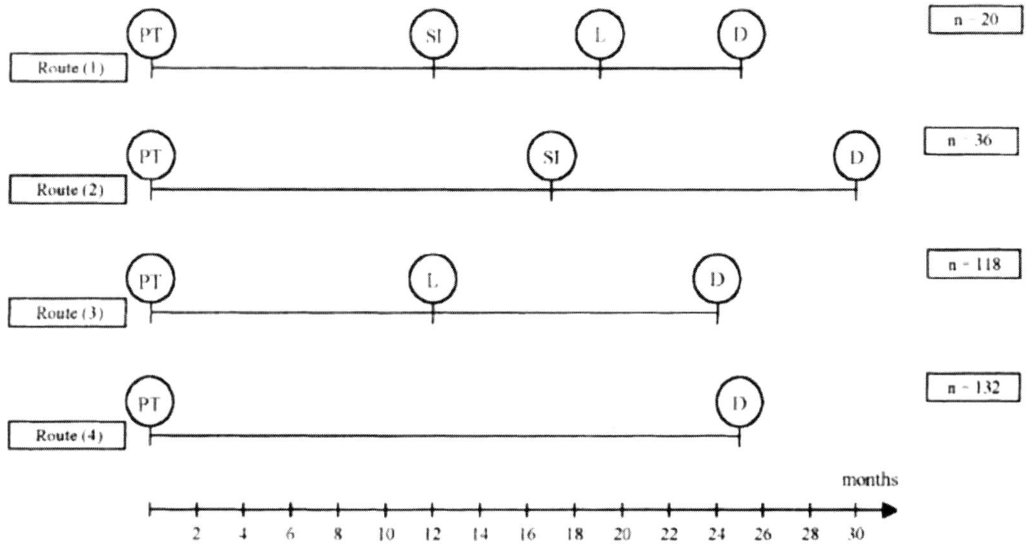

Fig. 50.1 Time course of the development of distant metastases and the routes to metastases. PT, primary tumor; SI, satellite/in-transit metastases; L, regional lymph node metastases; D, distant metastases. Reproduced with permission from Wiley-Blackwell 56

routine regional ultrasound examination) than those routinely employed in clinical practice may be of benefit in the detection of second primary tumors and early disease recurrence [44]. This group of investigators was able to translate early detection of recurrence (classified as organ or lymph node metastases of ≤2 cm in diameter, <10 individual nodes affected, and potential for surgery with intent to cure) to increased overall survival probability [44]. Consistent with this, studies have demonstrated that complete surgical removal of isolated distant metastases in certain cancers, including melanoma, may provide a survival benefit [54, 55]. These findings lend support to regimens that detect disease recurrence at an early stage and where surgical treatment is able to render the patient clinically cancer-free.

In all cases, follow-up strategies should be based upon the finding that patients are at highest risk of melanoma recurrence and second primaries within the first 2 years following their initial diagnosis. More specifically, one study examined the metastatic pathways and time course of progression of metastases in >3,000 patients with localized melanoma, among whom >400 patients developed disease recurrence (Fig. 50.1) [56]. In these patients, distant metastases developed after a median period of 25 months, regardless of whether distant disease was the initial presentation of melanoma progression or distant metastases followed satellite/in-transit metastases or regional nodal recurrence [56]. Direct regional lymph node recurrence and satellite/in-transit metastases (as detected by routine clinical examination) had median latency periods of 16 months and 17 months, respectively.

Yearly chest X-ray examinations to detect occult pulmonary involvement (National Comprehensive Cancer Network Guidelines, Melanoma, v.1, 2010) are optional in Stage IIB–IV NED patients, as they have been shown to be of questionable, if any, benefit [44]. (Elderly male patients with high-risk localized melanoma are one cohort at high risk for disease recurrence [57] and may represent an exception). Other imaging modalities such as CT are recommended in Stage IA–IIA disease only as directed by patient symptoms or physical examination. In practice, follow-up imaging strategies in asymptomatic patients at high risk of recurrence who have completed a course of interferon, enrolled in a clinical trial or have surgically resected Stage III disease, vary greatly by patient stage, individual practitioner, and institution. Recent guidelines do suggest that, in patients with Stage IIB–IV disease who are asymptomatic and clinically cancer-free, chest X-ray, CT, PET-CT, and brain MRI scans should be considered to screen for recurrent or metastatic disease. Routine imaging to screen for disease recurrence is not recommended in asymptomatic patients >5 years after initial treatment.

The disease-specific mortality rate increases significantly with increasing size and number of metastatic nodes [33]. Based upon these findings, as well as those described above, our colleagues in Australia and Europe have investigated the sensitivity of ultrasound examination in the detection of locoregional melanoma metastasis at an early stage and the outcome of interventions that were based on ultrasonography findings. One study evaluated the efficacy of ultrasound B-scan to detect nodal disease as compared to physical examination in the surveillance of melanoma patients [58]. Overall survival at 4 years was affected by the size of the nodal recurrence detected as well as the number of nodes involved (consistent with the current American Joint Committee on Cancer staging). The potential benefit of ultrasound examination of the draining nodal basin was illustrated by a prospective study in Stage I–III melanoma patients that employed a rigorous follow-up regimen including serial ultrasound examinations of the scar, lymphatic drainage area, and regional nodal basin. In this study, close surveillance resulted in early discovery of disease metastasis [44]. Seventy-six per cent of lymph node ultrasound examinations that were suspicious for metastases were confirmed as positive on further evaluation, and lymph node sonography detected 21% of all recurrences in the primary tumor stage. It has been documented that histologically proven melanoma metastasis of 4–4.5 mm can be detected by ultrasound, depending upon the nodal basin [59] as well as patient's body habitus, ultrasound Mhz resolution, and technical expertise.

Based on these findings, the use of serial ultrasound evaluation of the draining nodal basin (previously identified by lymphoscintigraphy) has been incorporated into the MSLT-2 multi-institutional melanoma trial (www.http://clinicaltrials.gov/show/NCT00297895). This trial was designed to determine the value of complete lymph node dissection in patients who have micrometastatic disease, since 70–80% of patients have no further nodal involvement upon completion of lymphadenectomy. MSLT-2 randomizes patients to completion lymphadenectomy vs. close clinical surveillance that includes ultrasound. To this point, ultrasound may be used in conjunction with clinical examination in the follow-up of patients with more advanced primary disease in Australia and New Zealand (http://www.nhmrc.gov.au/_files_nhmrc/file/publications/synopses/cp111.pdf.).

In Stage IV melanoma, the serum lactate dehydrogenase level (LDH) has been demonstrated to be an independent predictor of clinical outcome, although it is not a sensitive marker of metastatic disease [60]. Elevated serum LDH level has been incorporated into the 2010 American Joint Committee on Cancer staging system. It is therefore indicated in the staging work-up and should be considered in surveillance of Stage IV melanoma patients and patients with nodal recurrence. According to the National Comprehensive Cancer Network guidelines, LDH is optional, along with complete blood count, in patients with Stage IB–III disease (http://www.nccn.org). The use of other serum markers such as S100 to detect melanoma recurrence has also been investigated, although there are none routinely used in current clinical practice [61].

Patient education regarding ultraviolet protection and skin self-examination should be a routine part of patient follow-up in the melanoma population, as in the general population. As detailed earlier, patients with a prior melanoma diagnosis are at a higher risk for subsequent melanoma and nonmelanoma skin cancers. Population-based screening has not been shown to reduce melanoma mortality and is not currently recommended in Australia as the cost-effectiveness of such screenings has not been proven. Nonetheless, skin cancer screenings may facilitate early diagnosis of melanoma and nonmelanoma skin cancers in certain groups who would not otherwise have access to dermatologic care.

Educational campaigns by melanoma and skin cancer advocacy groups such as the American Academy of Dermatology, The Skin Cancer Foundation, American Skin Association, Melanoma Hope Network, and many others have certainly improved the general population's recognition of the signs of melanoma (asymmetry, border, color, diameter, evolution) and the importance of ultraviolet protection in melanoma and skin cancer prevention. Nation-wide efforts in countries such as Australia with campaigns regarding the use of sunscreens ("slip, slap, slop"), mandates regarding the availability of shade structures, and the use of sun protective clothing for school age children are particularly effective interventions. Currently, organizations such as the American Skin Association, as well as more localized groups (SPOTS, Sun Protection Outreach Taught by Students, www.SPOTS.wustl.edu), have formal educational programs reaching out to middle school and high school students. Although educational campaigns are effective in improving knowledge regarding UV risk and changing behavior [62], the effect of these campaigns on tumor incidence is not yet evident.

As outlined by the American Academy of Dermatology (http://www.aad.org/media/background/factsheets/fact_indoortanning.html), there is growing evidence that implicates indoor tanning as a risk factor in melanoma and skin cancer development. In particular, the overwhelming majority of indoor tanning patrons are girls and young women [63], and this behavior has not only been temporally linked to the increased melanoma incidence in this group [2], but recent findings have also documented a greater than fourfold increased risk of melanoma by the use of certain tanning bed devices [64]. As previously stated, the World Health Organization has recently classified ultraviolet-emitting tanning devices as a Group 1 "known carcinogen" because of evidence linking exposure to both cutaneous and ocular melanoma [22]. To date, 31 states in the United States have passed legislation to impose regulations on the tanning bed industry [65], with attempts to do so in many others.

Digital photography, or "mole mapping," may be employed in patients with multiple atypical nevi with or without a history of melanoma who are at high risk for the development of a primary, or subsequent, melanoma. Its use and efficacy in early detection of melanoma have been evaluated. Some studies have determined that serial photography can aid in the detection of melanomas at a relatively early stage based on subtle changes noted in photographic images [66]. Prospective case-controlled studies to determine the effect on overall survival comparing patients that have close physician follow-up with or without digital photography have not yet been performed. Cost-effectiveness has also not been determined, although American Medical Association Current Procedural Terminology category I status (96,904) (described as "whole body integumentary photography, for monitoring of high-risk patients with dysplastic nevus syndrome or a history of dysplastic nevi, or patients with a personal or familial history of melanoma") has been assigned. Dermoscopy, the use of skin surface microscopy using a handheld dermatoscope, improves clinical diagnosis of melanoma for those trained in its use. Newer noninvasive imaging technologies to aid in the earlier detection of melanoma including computer analysis of digital images and confocal microscopy are currently in the research and development stages (reviewed in [67]).

As in most cancers with a high risk of recurrence and metastases, the expertise of colleagues in dermatology, medical and surgical oncology, otolaryngology, radiology, and radiation oncology is key to the appropriate management of melanoma patients. In many large tertiary care centers, like ours, this is effectively accomplished through multidisciplinary clinics and conferences. In our practice, all Stage 0–III melanoma patients are routinely seen by the dermatologist, either for the initial consultation for their disease, or as a referral from the medical or surgical oncologist when treatment is instituted. The dermatologist is often, although not routinely, involved in the treatment and follow-up of patients who present with Stage IV disease.

Our practice functions as a "virtual" center, with patients seen in the different specialty clinics, often on the same day. For patients who either present with, or progress to, more advanced disease, their cases are presented in a multidisciplinary conference that is attended by the various specialties (including pathology) and treatment plans discussed. Our medical and surgical oncologists continue to follow patients with Stage III and IV disease through their treatment and postsurgical course at frequent intervals, as indicated by the specific therapy or intervention. For example, patients receiving interferon for Stage III disease are seen monthly by the medical oncologist and appropriate monitoring performed during their treatment course, as well as one to two times per year following completion of their therapy. Similarly, high-risk Stage II and Stage III patients who are status post wide local excision and/or lymph node dissection are evaluated frequently during the postoperative period as well as during the 1–2 years following treatment when recurrence is most likely. In patients who have no evidence of disease (NED) following treatment (either chemotherapy, surgery, or both), their visits to each specialist are often alternated so that they are seen at the appropriate intervals (for example, a patient with Stage IIB disease who is status post wide local excision and negative sentinel lymph node biopsy is seen at 3-month intervals—two visits per year with the surgical oncologist alternating with two visits per year with the dermatologist).

At this point in the care of melanoma patients with advanced disease, access to new immunologic and targeted therapies through clinical trials is important. We are all hopeful that effective therapies are on the horizon. Despite this, as discussed earlier, detection of locoregional or even systemic metastasis at the earliest stage where intervention with the intent to cure, when disease burden remains low, is challenging. Although national guidelines and consensus statements give us some guidance, much is left to the individual practitioner when decisions are required regarding the worth of radiologic or ultrasound imaging of melanoma patients who are without clinically detected evidence of disease, but yet at high risk for recurrence. Practices vary widely. One must weigh the cost of imaging procedures, the impact (both fiscal and psychological) of falsepositive studies, among other variables, with the overall sensitivity of detection of true disease amenable to effective treatment. The multi-institutional MSLT-2 trail will no doubt help us to better evaluate the use of ultrasound for surveillance of our high-risk melanoma patients. With this in mind, we are currently planning an institutional trial where we will follow our high-risk treated Stage IIB and III melanoma patients with a combination of ultrasound targeted at their primary tumor site as well at their draining lymph node basin and the use of surveillance PET-CT.

References

1. Christenson LJ, Borrowman TA, Vachon CM, et al. Incidence of basal cell and squamous cell carcinomas in a population younger than 40 years. JAMA. 2005;294:681–90.
2. Purdue MP, Freeman LE, Anderson WF, Tucker MA. Recent trends in incidence of cutaneous melanoma among US Caucasian young adults. www.jidonline.org. J Invest Dermatol. 2008;128:2905–8. Epub 2008 Jul 10.
3. Tsai S-H, Balch CM, Lange J. Epidemiology and treatment of melanoma in elderly patients. Nat Rev Clin Oncol. 2010;7:148–52.
4. Vajdic C, van Leewen M. Cancer incidence and risk factors after solid organ transplantation. Int J Cancer. 2009;125:1747–54.
5. Curtis RE, Rowlings PA, Deeg HJ, et al. Solid cancers after bone marrow transplantation. N Eng J Med. 1997;336:897–904.
6. Hu S, Parmet Y, Allen G, et al. Disparity in melanoma: a trend analysis of melnaoma incidence and stage at diagnosis among Whites, Hispanics and Blacks in Florida. Arch Dermatol. 2009; 145:1369–74.
7. Tsao H, Rogers GS, Sober A. An estimate of annual direct cost of treating cutaneous melanoma. J Am Acad Dermatol. 1998;38: 669–80.
8. Borger C, Smith S, Truffer C, et al. Health spending projections through 2015. Health Aff (Millwood). 2006;25:W61–73.

9. Hiller BE, Kirkwood JM, Agarwala SS. Burden of illness associated with metastatic melanoma. Cancer. 2001;91:1814–21.
10. Hussussian CJ, Struewing JP, Goldstein AM, et al. Germ line p16 mutations in familial melanoma. Nat Genet. 1994;8:15–21.
11. Carey Jr WP, Thompson CJ, Synnestvedt M, et al. Dysplastic nevi as a melanoma risk factor in patients with familial melanoma. Cancer. 1994;74:3118–25.
12. Goldstein AM, Martinez M, Tucker MA, Demenais F. Gene-covariate interaction between dysplastic nevi and the CDKN2A gene in American melanoma-prone families. Cancer Epidemiol Biomarkers Prev. 2000;9:889–94.
13. Greene MH, Clark Jr WH, Tucker MA, Kraemer KH, Elder DE, Fraser MC. High risk of malignant melanoma is melanoma-prone families with dysplastic nevi. Ann Intern Med. 1985;102:458–65.
14. Tsao H, Pehamberger H, Sober AJ. Precursor lesions and markers of melanoma. In: Balch CM, Houghton AN, Sober AJ, Soong S-J, editors. Cutaneous melanoma. St. Louis, MO: Quality Medical Publishing, Inc; 1998. p. 65–79.
15. Clark Jr WH, Reimer RR, Greene M, Ainsworth AM, Mastrangelo MJ. Origin of familial malignant melanoma from heritable melanocytic lesions: the B-K mole syndrome. Arch Dermatol. 1978;114: 732–8.
16. Goldstein AM, Chan M, Harland M, et al. High-risk melanoma susceptibility genes and pancreatic cancer neural system tumors and uveal melanoma across GenoMEL. Cancer Res. 2006;66:9818–28.
17. Council ML, Gardner JM, Helms C, Liu Y, Cornelius LA, Bowcock AM. Contribution of genetic factors for melanoma susceptibility in sporadic US melanoma patients. Exp Dermatol. 2009;18:485–7.
18. Valverde P, Healy E, Jackson I, Rees JL, Thody AJ. Variants of the melanocyte-stimuating hormone receptor gene are associated with red hair and fair skin in humans. Nat Genet. 1995;11:328–30.
19. van der Velden PA, Sandkuijl LA, Bergman W. Melanocortin-1 receptor variant R151C modifies melanoma risk in Dutch families with melanoma. Am J Hum Genet. 2001;69:774–9.
20. Kefford RF. Counseling and DNA testing for individuals perceived to be genetically predisposed to melanoma: a consensus statement of the Melanoma Genetics Consortium. J Clin Oncol. 1999;17: 3245–51.
21. Fears T. Average midrange ultraviolet radiation flux and time outdoors predict melanoma risk. Cancer Res. 2002;62:3992–6.
22. Ghissassi F, et al. Special report: policy. A review of human carcinogens. Lancet. 2009;10:751–2.
23. Langley R, Sober A. A clinical review of the evidence for the role of ultraviolet radiation in the etiology of cutaneous melanoma. Cancer Invest. 1997;15:561–7.
24. Davies H, Bignell GR, Cox C, et al. Mutations of the BRAF gene in human cancer. Nature. 2002;417:949–54.
25. Maldonado JL, Fridlyand J, Patel H, et al. Determinants of BRAF mutations in a primary melanomas. J Natl Cancer Inst. 2003; 95:1878–80.
26. DiFronzo LA, Wanek LA, Elashoff R, Morton DL. Increased incidence of second primary melanoma in patients with a previous cutaneous melanoma. Ann Surg Oncol. 1999;6:705–11.
27. Bhatia S, Estrada-Batres L, Maryon T, Bogue M, Chu D. Second primary tumors in patients with cutaneous malignant melanoma. Cancer. 1999;86:2014–20.
28. Goggins W, Tsao H. A population-based analysis of risk factors for a second primary cutaneous melanoma among melanoma survivors. Cancer. 2003;97:639–43.
29. Puig S, Malvehy J, Badenas C, et al. Role of the CDKN2A locus in patients with multiple primary melanomas. J Clin Oncol. 2005;23:3043–51.
30. McMasters KM, Reintgen DS, Ross MI, et al. Sentinel lymph node biopsy for melanoma: controversy despite widespread agreement. J Clin Oncol. 2001;19:2851–5.
31. Gershenwald JE, Thompson W, Mansfield PF, et al. Multi-institutional melanoma lymphatic mapping experience: the prognostic value of sentinel lymph node status in 612 stage I or II melanoma patients. J Clin Oncol. 1999;17:976–83.
32. Morton DL, Thompson JF, Cochran AJ, et al. Sentinel-node biopsy or nodal observation in melanoma. N Engl J Med. 2006;355:1307.
33. Balch CM, et al. Final version of the American joint committee on cancer staging system for cutaneous melanoma. J Clin Oncol. 2001;19:3635–48.
34. Thomas JM, A'Hern RP, Grichnik JM, et al. Sentinel-node biopsy in melanoma. N Engl J Med. 2007;356:418–21.
35. Cancer AJCO. Melanoma of the skin. In: Ecbrsdge SB, Byrd DR, Compton CC, Fritz AG, Greene FL, Trotti A, editors. AJCC staging manual. 7th ed. New York, NY: Springer; 2010.
36. Balch CM, Gershenwald JE, Soong SJ, et al. Final version of 2009 AJCC melanoma staging and clarification. J Clin Oncol. 2010;27: 6199–206.
37. Spanknebel K, Coit DG, Bieligk SC, Gonen M, Rosai J, Klimstra DS. Characterization of micrometastatic disease in melanoma sentinel lymph nodes by enhanced pathology: recommendations for standardizing pathological analysis. Am J Surg Pathol. 2005;29: 412–4.
38. Carlson GW, Murray DR, Lyles RH, Staley CA, Hestley A, Cohen C. The amount of metastatic melanoma in a sentinel lymph node: does it have prognostic significance? Ann Surg Oncol. 2003;10: 575–81.
39. Ranieri JM, Wagner JD, Azuaje R. Prognostic importance of lymph node tumor burden in melanoma patients staged by sentinel node biopsy. Ann Surg Oncol. 2002;9:975–81.
40. Thomas JM. Prognostic false-posivity of the sentinel node in melanoma. Nat Clin Pract Oncol. 2008;5:18–23.
41. Francken AB, Accortt NA, Shaw HM, et al. Prognosis and determinants of outcome following locoregional or distant recurrence in patients with cutaneous melanoma. Ann Surg Oncol. 2008;15: 1476–84.
42. Pawlik TM, Ross MI, Thompson JF, et al. The risk of in-transit melanoma metastasis depends on tumor biology and not the surgical approach to regional lymph nodes. J Clin Oncol. 2005;23: 4588–90.
43. Thompson J, de Wilt J. Isolated limb perfusion in the management of patients with recurrent limb melanoma: an important but limited role. Ann Surg Oncol. 2001;8:564–5.
44. Garbe C, Paul A, Kohler-Späth H, et al. Prospective evaluation of a follow-up schedule in cutaneous melanoma patients: recommendations for an effective follow-up strategy. J Clin Oncol. 2003;21: 520–9.
45. Yancovitz M, Finelt N, Warycha MA, et al. Role of radiologic imaging at the time of initial diagnosis of stage T1b–T3b melanoma. Cancer. 2007;110:1107–14.
46. Fazel R, Krumholz HM, Wang Y, et al. Exposure to low-dose ionizing radiation from medical imaging procedures. N Eng J Med. 2009;361:849–57.
47. Ahmadzadehfar H, Singh B, Ezziddin S, et al. Preoperative FDG-PET/CT imaging in the detection of regional lymph node metastases in stages I and II of malignant melanoma. Nucl Med. 2008;49(Supp 1):145P.
48. Beyer T, Townsend DW, Brun T, et al. A combined PET/CT scanner for clinical oncology. J Nucl Med. 2000;41:1369–79.
49. Fawzy FI, Fawzy NW, Hyun CS, et al. Malignant melanoma: effects of an early structured psychiatric intervention, coping and affective state on recurrence and survival 6 years later. Arch Gen Psychiatry. 1993;50:681–9.
50. Gutman M, Shafir R, Rozin RR, et al. Are malignant melanoma patients at higher risk for a second cancer? Cancer. 1991;68: 660–5.

51. Kang S, Barnhill RL, Mihm Jr MC, Sober AJ. Muliple primary cutaneous melanoma. Cancer. 1992;70:1911–6.
52. Dicker TJ, Kavanagh GM, Herd RM, et al. A rationale approach to melanoma follow-up in patients with primary cutaneous melanoma. Br J Dermatol. 1999;140:249–54.
53. Francken AB, Shaw HM, Accortt NA, Soong SJ, Hoekstra HJ, Thompson JF. Detection of first relapse in cutaneous melanoma patients: implications for the formulation of evidence-based follow-up guidelines. Ann Surg Oncol. 2006;14:1924–33.
54. Ollila DW, Caudle A. Surgical management of distant metastases. Surg Oncol Clin N Am. 2006;15:385–98.
55. Ollila D, Morton D. Surgical resection as the treatment of choice for melanoma metastatic to the lung. Chest Surg Clin N Am. 1998;8:1.
56. Meier F, Will S, Ellwanger U, et al. Metastatic pathways and time courses in the orderly progression of cutaneous melanoma. Br J Dermatol. 2002;147:62–70.
57. Kalady MF, White RR, Johnson JL, Tyler DS, Seigler HF. Thin melanomas: predictive lethal characteristics from a 30-year clinical experience. Ann Surg. 2003;121:221–30.
58. Voit C, Mayer T, Kron M, et al. Efficacy of ultrasound B-scan compared with physical examination in follow-up of melanoma patients. Cancer. 2001;91:2409–16.
59. Thompson JF, Shaw H. Benefits of sentinel node biopsy for melanoma. ANZ J Surg. 2006;76:100–3.
60. Sirott MN, Bajorin DF, Wong GYC, et al. Prognostic factors in patients with metastatic malignant melanoma. A multivariate analysis. Cancer. 1993;72:3091–8.
61. Beyeler M, Waldispuhl S, Strobel K, et al. Detection of melanoma relapse: first comparative analysis on imaging techniques versus S100 protein. Dermatology. 2006;213:187–91.
62. Marks R. Melanoma prevention: is it possible to change a population's behavior in the sun? Pigment Cell Res. 2006;7:104–6.
63. Swerdlow AJ, Weinstock MA. Do tanning lamps cause melanoma? An epidemiologic assessment. J Am Acad Dermatol. 1998;38:89–98.
64. Lazovich D, Vogel RI, Berwick M, Weinstock MA, Anderson KE, Warshaw EM. Indoor tanning and risk of melanoma: a case-control study in a highly exposed population. Cancer Epidemiol Biomarkers Prev. 2010;19:1557.
65. Mayer JA, Hoerster KD, Pichon LC, Rubio DA, Woodruff SI, Forster JL. Enforcement of state indoor tanning laws in the United States. Prev Chronic Dis. 2008;5:1–10.
66. Feit N, Dusza S, Marghoob AA. Melanomas detected with the aid of total cutaneous photography. Br J Dermatol. 2004;150:706–14.
67. Patel JK, Konda S, Perez OA, Amini S, Elgart G, Berman B. Newer technologies/techniques and tools in the diagnosis of melanoma. Eur J Immunol. 2008;18:617–31.
68. Geller AC, Miller DR, Swetter SM, Demierre MF, Gilchrest BA. A call for the development and implementation of a targeted national melanoma screening program. Arch Dermatol. 2006;142:504–7.

Cutaneous Melanoma Surveillance Counterpoint: Australia

51

Michael A. Henderson

Keywords

Gene • Invasive melanoma • Australia • Primary melanoma • Freckle

Melanoma has been referred to as the Australian malignancy, and unfortunately this epithet is justified. The incidence in Australia (and New Zealand) is approximately three times higher than in the United States and four times higher than in the UK and Europe [1]. The reasons for this disparity in incidence for populations with a similar genetic background (predominantly Caucasian/Anglo Saxon) are multifactorial but include high ambient UV levels (Australia is located in comparatively low latitudes, close to the equator) and a favourable climate that predisposes to extended periods outdoors and, until recently, poor understanding of the importance of sun avoidance behaviours. Cutaneous malignancy (including squamous cell carcinoma and basal cell carcinoma as well as melanoma) is a major public health issue for Australia. Surveillance involves large numbers of patients who, in addition to the risks from their index primary lesion, remain at significantly increased risk for the subsequent development of both melanoma and non-melanoma skin cancer.

The estimated population of Australia on December 30, 2008 was approximately 21,500,000 persons according to the Australian Bureau of Statistics (http//www.abs.gov.au/). In 2003, melanoma (excluding in situ melanoma and non-melanoma skin cancer) was the fourth commonest cancer diagnosed in Australia after bowel, breast, and prostate cancer with nearly 10,000 cases. The lifetime risk to age 85 for all persons for developing melanoma in Australia is 1 in 19 (1 in 15 for males and 1 in 25 for females). There is considerable variation in the incidence of melanoma throughout the country reflecting the amount of UV exposure with Queensland (the most northerly state and closest to the equator) having an annualised standard rate of 65.3 cases per 100,000 people compared to Victoria (the most southerly mainland state) with a rate of 35.4 per 100,000. Over the 10 years from 1993 to 2003, the incidence increased by 14% (19% for males, 7% for females) [2]. In the state of Victoria (population approximately five million), which has led the country in sun avoidance programs, the incidence in persons under the age of 60 has started to fall but for older persons the incidence has increased, particularly for males. Probably because of greater public awareness of melanoma, melanoma in situ is now a common diagnosis, which has implications for rational planning of follow-up programs. In the state of Victoria, there were 2,347 cases of invasive melanoma and 1,466 cases of melanoma in situ diagnosed in 2005 [3]. Synchronous and metachronous melanoma also add to the burden of the disease. In the state of New South Wales, there were 3,402 new diagnoses of melanoma as well as 440 cases of new primary or simultaneous melanoma in 2004 [4].

Melanoma is now the tenth commonest cause of death due to cancer in Australia. In 2004, there were 1,200 deaths among 9,722 new cases. In contrast to the significant increase in incidence over the period from 1993 to 2003, the increase in mortality was much smaller at 4.4% [2]. Analysis of more recent data from the State of Victoria shows that in recent years mortality rates have stabilised and may actually be starting to fall for females [3]. Nationally, the 5-year survival probability for patients with localised disease plateaued in 2004 at 92% [2]. This figure compares favourably with results from the United States, UK, and Europe.

The median age at diagnosis of invasive melanoma is 60 years, and approximately three-quarters of melanomas

M.A. Henderson, M.B.B.S., B.M.ed.Sc., M.D., F.R.A.C.S. (✉)
Division of Cancer Surgery, Peter MacCallum Cancer Center, St Andrew's Place, Locked Bag 1 A'Beckett St, East Melbourne 3002, VIC 8006, Australia
e-mail: Michael.Henderson@petermac.org

F.E. Johnson et al. (eds.), *Patient Surveillance After Cancer Treatment*, Current Clinical Oncology,
DOI 10.1007/978-1-60327-969-7_51,

are good-prognosis lesions less than 1 mm in thickness [3]. The burden of melanoma in the community potentially requiring follow-up is best described by the prevalence of a condition. Data from the Australian Institute of Health and Welfare shows that for all persons diagnosed with melanoma between 1980 and 2003 there were 116,182 persons still alive in 2004 and, after breast cancer, melanoma is the second most prevalent cancer [2].

In summary, melanoma is a major health issue for Australia in terms of the number of patients presenting with melanoma. Most patients have a favourable prognosis because of early diagnosis. The net result is a large population living with a past history of melanoma who are at risk not just for recurrence of their melanoma but also the development of a new primary melanoma and a significant risk of development of non-melanoma skin cancer. The follow-up regimen used at the author's institution (Peter MacCallum Cancer Centre, Melbourne) as well as other major centres in Australia including the Sydney Melanoma Unit (John Thompson, personal communication) are consistent with those in the Clinical Practice Guidelines for the Management of Melanoma in Australia and New Zealand published in 2008 [5]. Although these best practice guidelines are predominantly evidence-based, the absence of any high-quality data on follow-up (e.g., valid randomised trials) means that the guidelines are consensus recommendations only based on the opinions of a group of experts supported by two recent systematic reviews [6,7]. The basis for the current timing of surveillance visits is based on studies going back for several decades which may not be appropriate for current practice. Francken et al. point out that the magnitude of the risk and pattern of recurrent disease are modified by the use of treatments such as elective lymph node dissection, which predominated in previous studies, and sentinel node biopsy, which predominate in more recent studies of the natural history of melanoma [8]. The surveillance schedules described in Tables 51.1–51.5 reflect the likely time course and risk of recurrence with the aim of identifying potentially treatable disease, specifically loco-regional recurrence, at an early stage. More intense follow-up is therefore justified in the first 2–3 years, declining by 5 years to an annual follow-up which is directed predominantly at detection of new cutaneous malignancy. The conundrum as demonstrated in a recent Australian report is that most recurrences are detected by the patient and there was no difference in outcome attributable to who found the local recurrence [9]. Clearly an area for future evaluation is the role of patient education in detecting recurrences. In contrast to the detection of recurrent disease, the identification of a new primary melanoma by patients is less frequent. A recent study from the Sydney Melanoma Unit showed that, while 59% of first primary melanomas were detected by the patient, only 46% of second melanomas were detected by the patient [10]. Most studies of new melanomas developing after excision of the first melanoma have short follow-up and suggest that the risk of a new melanoma declines quite rapidly in the first few years after the first diagnosis. A large and important study of 52,997 patients with melanoma followed over 20 years in Queensland indicated that the rate of development of subse-

Table 51.1 Surveillance after curative-intent treatment for in situ melanoma at Peter MacCallum Cancer Centre, Melbourne

	Year					
	1	2	3	4	5	>5
Office visit	1	1	1	1	1	1

Consider educating patient to conduct monthly skin self-examinations
The physical examination should include skin inspection and palpation of primary tumour site
Lifetime surveillance by the patient's primary care practitioner for new cutaneous malignancy should occur after 5 years.
Patient should be advised to conduct lifelong, regular, self-examination of the skin
The patient should be instructed to avoid sunburns and extended unprotected solar or artificial UV exposure
The number in each cell indicates the number of times a particular modality is recommended during a particular post-treatment year

Table 51.2 Surveillance after curative-intent treatment for stage IA melanoma at Peter MacCallum Cancer Centre, Melbourne

	Year					
	1	2	3	4	5	>5
Office visit	2	2	2	2	2	1

Consider educating patient to conduct monthly skin self-examinations
The physical examination should include regional lymph node examination, skin inspection and palpation of primary tumour site
Lifetime surveillance by the patient's primary care practitioner for new cutaneous malignancy should occur after 5 years.
The patient should be instructed to avoid sunburns and extended unprotected solar or artificial UV exposure
The patient should be advised to conduct lifelong, regular, self-examination of the skin and peripheral lymph nodes
The number in each cell indicates the number of times a particular modality is recommended during a particular post-treatment year

Table 51.3 Surveillance after curative-intent treatment for stage IB-II melanoma at Peter MacCallum Cancer Centre, Melbourne

	Year					
	1	2	3	4	5	>5
Office visit	3–4	3–4	3–4	3–4	3–4	1

Consider educating patient to conduct monthly skin and lymph node self-examinations
The physical examination should include regional lymph node examination, skin inspection and palpation of primary tumour site
Total duration of follow-up is 10 years
Lifetime surveillance by the patient's primary care practitioner for new cutaneous malignancy should occur after 5 years.
The patient should be instructed to avoid sunburns and extended unprotected solar or artificial UV exposure
The patient should be advised to conduct lifelong, regular, self-examination of the skin and peripheral lymph nodes
The number in each cell indicates the number of times a particular modality is recommended during a particular post-treatment year

Table 51.4 Surveillance after curative-intent treatment for stage III melanoma at Peter MacCallum Cancer Centre, Melbourne

	Years post-treatment					
	1	2	3	4	5	>5
Office visit	3–4	3–4	3–4	3–4	3–4	1

The physical examination should include regional lymph node examination, skin inspection and palpation of primary tumour site
Total duration of follow-up is 10 years
Lifetime surveillance by the patient's primary care practitioner for new cutaneous malignancy should occur after 5 years.
The patient should be instructed to avoid sunburns and extended unprotected solar or artificial UV exposure
The patient should be advised to conduct lifelong, regular, self-examination of the skin and peripheral lymph nodes
The number in each cell indicates the number of times a particular modality is recommended during a particular post-treatment year

Table 51.5 Surveillance after curative-intent treatment for high-risk patients[+] at Peter MacCallum Cancer Centre, Melbourne

	Years post-treatment					
	1	2	3	4	5	>5
Office visit	4	4	1–2	1–2	1–2	1–2

[+] High-risk patients are those with sporadic or familial dysplastic nevus syndrome or a strong family history (≥2 first-degree relatives or ≥3 second-degree relatives) or multiple suspicious naevi and a past history of multiple melanomas
The physical examination should include regional lymph node examination, skin inspection and palpation of primary tumour site
Lifetime surveillance for new cutaneous malignancy should occur after 5 years.
The patient should be instructed to avoid sunburns and extended unprotected solar or artificial UV exposure
The patient should be advised to conduct lifelong, regular, self-examination of the skin and peripheral lymph nodes
The number in each cell indicates the number of times a particular modality is recommended during a particular post-treatment year

quent melanoma remained stable over this extended time period and the risk was higher for males, elderly patients, and patients with thicker lesions. Nevertheless, there was no difference in the risk of a second melanoma after diagnosis of an in situ, lentigo maligna or invasive melanoma [11]. These data in an Australian context strongly argue for lifetime surveillance for second melanoma (and non-melanoma skin cancer) regardless of whether the initial lesion was an invasive or an in situ lesion. Disappointingly, a survey of surveillance practices after a previous version of the guidelines had been published in 2001 found that only 9% of patients had a formal, planned skin examination as part of routine follow-up [12]. Anecdotal evidence suggests that this has improved, partly due to education but also because of better co-ordination of patient care. Because skin cancer is so common in Australia, many primary care practitioners have expertise in skin examination and management of low-risk cutaneous malignancy. In the author's institution, follow-up is often shared with the patient's primary care practitioner. Patients with in situ lesions are routinely referred back to the patient's primary care practitioner after 12 months; after 24 months for patients with stage I melanoma;and after 5 years for stage IIA melanoma. Patients receive information on sun avoidance behaviour and the need for long-term surveillance in view of the increased risk of new skin malignancy prior to discharge to their primary care practitioner. The patient's primary care practitioner is also provided with specific advice on the patient's follow-up.

The Australian and New Zealand surveillance guidelines are consensus recommendations in the absence of high-level evidence. In reviewing the evidence, the Dutch Guidelines Group also found no evidence to support the role of intensive surveillance (but neither can it be claimed that the absence of surveillance would not be associated with poorer outcome). In contrast, the Dutch took a more hardline view and recommended that patients with thin lesions (less then 1 mm in thickness) need no further follow-up. Against the evidence but mindful of possible harm to patients in an uneasy compromise, they recommended that patients with thicker lesions follow a relatively intense surveillance program. A recent retrospective review of patient outcomes from the Sydney Melanoma Unit found that the AJCC Staging System (2002) accurately predicted the risk and timing of recurrence [13]. Based on this data, an alternative surveillance regimen was proposed. Low-risk patients (stage I) need only be followed annually while stage IIB and IIC patients are followed three times per year for 2 years, twice in the third year and then annually. There is no conclusive evidence on whether follow-up should be performed by the patient's primary care provider or specialist medical practitioners or a combination. Both the new Australian and New Zealand Guidelines and the US National Comprehensive Cancer Network Guidelines amongst other guidelines recommend very close (and resource intensive) surveillance. Certainly in Australia, routine follow-up, particularly after the period of maximum likelihood of recurrence, is likely to fall more often on the patient's primary care provider.

The Australian and New Zealand guidelines do not recommend the use of any imaging or blood tests as part of routine follow-up of asymptomatic patients. The issue of imaging studies has been recently reviewed by Nieweg et al. [6]. No advantage for regular targeted screening for lung, liver, CNS, or bone metastases has been demonstrated convincingly and, on that basis, imaging is not recommended in the current Australian and New Zealand guidelines nor performed outside of clinical trials in the author's institution. In the absence of any definitive data supporting the role of PET or PET/CT scanning during surveillance, this imaging modality is not currently used. Routine blood tests (e.g., full blood examination and liver function tests) have not been found to be of value for follow-up and are not used. Similarly, serum lactate dehydrogenase concentration, which has prognostic significance and is now incorporated in the new AJCC staging classification for stage IV disease, has not been demonstrated to be of value in surveillance of asymptomatic patients, and its use is reserved for patients with stage IV disease only. Molecular techniques to identify patients at risk of metastatic disease by detection of circulating tumour cells or free tumour DNA are currently under evaluation and may represent an alternative follow-up strategy in years to come.

The current Australian and New Zealand Guidelines recommend that sentinel node biopsy should at least be discussed with appropriate patients with T2 or T3 melanoma. For patients declining this procedure, the role of serial sonography of the regional lymph node basins has received attention. There is consensus that sonography of lymph node basins is more sensitive than physical examination, although no survival advantage has been demonstrated [14]. In the author's institution, patients declining sentinel node biopsy are followed as for patients with stage II disease (Table 51.3) without the use of sonography of regional lymph node basins.

Hutchinson's melanotic freckle is a form of in situ disease predominantly affecting the head and neck in elderly patients. It presents considerable challenges for surveillance as careful histological examination often demonstrates atypical melanocytes close to or involving surgical margins, indicating widespread changes in adjacent sun-exposed skin. The protocol at the author's institution is to resect the invasive melanoma with an appropriate margin and any suspicious pigmented lesion. The presence of minimal residual in situ disease is closely monitored in a multidisciplinary team setting involving specialist dermatologists and surgeons at least twice per year with liberal use of serial photography, dermatoscopy, and punch biopsy.

Patients considered to be at increased risk of developing a new primary melanoma on the basis of a strong family history (two or more first-degree relatives, three second-degree relatives), personal history of multiple melanomas, or suspicious naevi (particularly multiple lesions) are managed by dermatological and surgical oncology review twice per year with liberal use of total body photography, dermatoscopy, and excision biopsy.

References

1. Ferlay J, Bray F, Pisani P, Parkin DM. GLOBOCAN2002: cancer, mortality and prevalence worldwide. IARC cancerbase No 5. version 2.0 2004. Lyon: IARC Press. http://www-dep.iarc.fr/
2. Australian Institute of Health and Welfare, Cancer Australia & Australasian Association of Cancer Registries 2008. Cancer survival and prevalence in Australia: cancers diagnosed from 1982 to 2004. Cancer Series no. 42. Cat. no. CAN 38. Canberra: AIHW. http//www.aihw.gov.au
3. Canstat: cancer In Victoria 2005. The Cancer Council Victoria Epidemiology Centre 2008 No 45, February 2008. http//www.cancervic.org.au.
4. Tracey EA, Baker D, Chen W, Stavrou E, Bishop J. Cancer in New South Wales: incidence, mortality and prevalence 2005. 2007. Sydney: Cancer Institute NSW Incidence
5. Australian Cancer Network Melanoma Guidelines Revision Working Party. Clinical Practice Guidelines for the Management of Melanoma in Australia and New Zealand. Cancer Council Australia and Australian Cancer Network, Sydney and New Zealand Guidelines Group, Wellington (2008). http//www.cancer.org.au
6. Nieweg OE, Kroon BB. The conundrum of follow-up: should it be abandoned? Surg Oncol Clin N Am. 2006;15(2):319–30.
7. Francken AB, Bastiaannet E, Hoekstra HJ. Follow-up in patients with localised primary cutaneous melanoma. Lancet Oncol. 2005;6(8):608–21.
8. Francken AB, Accortt NA, Shaw HM, Wiener M, Soong SJ, Hoekstra HJ, et al. Prognosis and determinants of outcome following locoregional or distant recurrence in patients with cutaneous melanoma. Ann Surg Oncol. 2008;15(5):1476–84. Epub 2008 Jan 15.
9. Francken AB, Shaw HM, Accortt NA, Soong SJ, Hoekstra HJ, Thompson JF. Detection of first relapse in cutaneous melanoma patients: implications for the formulation of evidence-based follow-up guidelines. Ann Surg Oncol. 2007;14(6):1924–33.
10. Francken AB, Shaw HM, Thompson JF. Detection of second primary cutaneous melanomas. Eur J Surg Oncol. 2008;34(5):587–92.
11. McCaul KA, Fritschi L, Baade P, Coory M. The incidence of second primary invasive melanoma in Queensland, 1982–2003. Cancer Causes Control. 2008;19(5):451–8.
12. Kelly JW, Henderson MA, Thursfield VJ, Slavin J, Ainslie J, Giles GG. The management of primary cutaneous melanoma in Victoria in 1996 and 2000. Med J Aust. 2007;187(9):511–4.
13. Francken AB, Accortt NA, Shaw HM, Colman MH, Wiener M, Soong SJ, et al. Follow-up schedules after treatment for malignant melanoma. Br J Surg. 2008;95(11):1401–7.
14. Bafounta ML, Beauchet A, Chagnon S, Saiag P. Ultrasonography or palpation for detection of melanoma nodal invasion: a meta-analysis. Lancet Oncol. 2004;5(11):673–80.

52 Cutaneous Melanoma Surveillance Counterpoint: Japan

Yoichi Moroi

Keywords
Cutaneous melanoma • Dermatologist • Recurrence • 5-S-cysteinyldopa • Lactic dehydrogenase • Interferon-β • Melanoma inhibitory activityIntroduction

Although the number of patients with melanoma in Japan has increased, the incidence in Japan is still much lower than in Australia, the United States and Europe. The sex ratio of melanoma in Japan is male:female = 1:1.075. The slight preponderance of female patients has increased in recent years. The incidence of melanoma in Japan was estimated to be 1,500–2,500 new cases per year [1]. The overall 10-year survival rate for melanoma patients in Japan was estimated to be 61% from 1987 to 1991, 69% from 1992 to 1996, and 70% from 1997 to 2001 [1]. The 140-month survival rate was 71% for females and 60% for males in cases diagnosed from 1987 to 2001 [1]. The survival rate was significantly better for females ($p < 0.0001$). The survival rate in female melanoma patients is also reported to be higher than that of male patients in other Japanese series, whereas the sex ratio of white patients with melanoma varies among countries [2, 3]. Because of the low incidence in Japan, the public still lacks sufficient medical knowledge about this disease. Thus, most patients are at advanced stages when they visit hospitals, leading to a poor prognosis.

In Japan there is no report discussing follow-up of patients with this disease. The basic purpose of the follow-up of patients with cancer is early detection of recurrence, which permits a better chance of cure, although recurrence is not always curable. Because the incidence of second primary melanoma or familial melanoma is extremely low in Japan, follow-up for the detection of these has little significance. Patients are encouraged to take active responsibility for their own follow-up, and a program of patient education is provided to them. This education program includes self-examination, not only for primary cutaneous lesions, but also for regional nodal areas and areas between the primary tumor and regional nodes.

Dermatologists diagnose and treat patients with melanoma in Japan. This includes surgery (wide resection, reconstruction, and lymph node dissection) and chemotherapy. Therefore, dermatologists have the main responsibility for follow-up. Recently, the number of medical oncologists in Japan has gradually increased, and some of them may share responsibility for the treatment of patients with melanoma in the future.

The fundamental assumption in cancer follow-up is that early detection of recurrence improves long-term survival. The most important aim is to detect treatable local recurrence, since visceral metastases can rarely be treated successfully. The guideline for melanoma from The National Comprehensive Cancer Network also mentions that surveillance can permit the earlier detection of recurrent disease at a time when it might be more amenable to potentially curative surgical resection [4].

A rational formula of surveillance for patients treated definitively for their primary melanoma should be based on the natural history of the disease. An understanding of patterns of recurrence and time to recurrence should help to design panels of follow-up examinations and to determine the frequency with which those examinations and investigations should be performed. Physicians in Japan also classify patients with melanoma according to the TNM classification defined by International Union against Cancer [5]. A recent report from Japan showed that the overall survival rate is

Y. Moroi, M.D., Ph.D. (✉)
Department of Dermatology, Graduate School of Medical Science, Kyushu University, 3-1-1 Maidashi, Higashiku, Fukuoka, 812-8582, Japan
e-mail: ymoroi@dermatol.med.kyushu-u.ac.jp

F.E. Johnson et al. (eds.), *Patient Surveillance After Cancer Treatment*, Current Clinical Oncology,
DOI 10.1007/978-1-60327-969-7_52,

90% in stage I, 72% in stage II, 54% in stage III, and 7% in stage IV [1]. Recurrence occurred in 18% of patients, with melanoma in stages I and II. Of the stage I patients, 8% had recurrence, with 80% of these in regional lymph nodes and the remainder consisting of regional skin recurrence and in-transit metastasis. Of the stage II patients, 26% had recurrence, with 65% of these in regional nodes, and most of the remainder were visceral metastases. In patients with advanced disease at diagnosis, the initial sites of extranodal metastasis were the skin and subcutaneous tissue (53%), lung (26%), liver (9%), bone (9%), and brain (3%) [6].

The National Cancer Center Hospital in Japan reported the time course of recurrence [7]. Recurrences in stage I (UICC 1997) patients were found at a minimum of 19 months to a maximum of 9 years (median 6 years) after definitive treatment of the primary melanoma. This suggests that annual follow-up is sufficient. Whereas the National Comprehensive Cancer Network guidelines recommend annual surveillance for life [4], more than 5 years of surveillance for the patients with in situ or stage IA melanoma may not be needed because of the extremely low incidence of second primary melanomas in Japan. Recurrences in stage II patients were detected at a minimum of 2 months to a maximum of 12 years (median one and a half years) after treatment of the primary tumor; 58% of these were found within the first 2 years and 95% within the first 5 years. Therefore, the surveillance should include an office visit every 3 months for the first 2 years. Recurrences in stage III patients were detected at a minimum of 1 month to a maximum of 6 years (median 1 year) after treatment of the primary tumor; 62% of the recurrences were found within the first year, 79% within the first 2 years and 96% within the first 5 years. This indicates that an office visit every 3 months is warranted for the first 5 years.

In the National Comprehensive Cancer Network guidelines, skin examination and surveillance at least once a year for life is recommended for all patients with melanoma [4]. For patients with stage IA melanoma, a history and physical examination (with specific emphasis on the regional nodes and skin) are recommended every 3–12 months for 5 years and annually thereafter, as clinically indicated [4]. For patients with stages IB–IV melanomas, comprehensive history and physical examination (with emphasis on the regional lymph nodes and skin) should be performed every 3–6 months for 2 years, then every 3–12 months for 3 years, and annually thereafter, as clinically indicated [4].

The Japanese Skin Cancer Society published its "General rules for clinical and pathological studies on malignant neoplasms of the skin" in 2002 [8]. These rules recommend that physical examination should be performed every 1–3 month(s) after initial treatment for stage I–II patients and every month after initial treatment for stage III patients for 5 years after initial treatment. Now many physicians believe that physical examinations can be less frequent. The Japanese Skin Cancer Society released the first guideline for the management of skin cancer, including malignant melanoma, in 2007 [9]. Unfortunately, this guideline does not describe the frequency of follow-up for patients with melanoma. Two clinical questions for posttreatment surveillance after initial curative-intent treatment exist for melanoma in the Japanese guideline. One concerns the limited efficacy of the frequent imaging tests and the other emphasizes the importance of patient education.

As mentioned earlier, dermatologists are often responsible for the treatment of patients with melanoma. A systematic network for the treatment and follow-up of the patients is not well established in Japan, though radiation oncologists and some medical oncologists contribute to the follow-up of some patients. Although there is consensus among dermatologists and other contributors, closer cooperation of specialists is needed.

As indicated in the Japanese guidelines, an integral part of the follow-up of patients with melanoma is education. Education permits the patient's family and friends to understand the disease. In a report from Japan, 58% of regional nodal and cutaneous recurrences were detected by patients and the remaining 42% were detected by physicians [7]. The National Comprehensive Cancer Network guidelines also recommend educating patients about monthly self-examination of skin and lymph nodes [4].

The National Comprehensive Cancer Network guidelines recommend chest X-ray, serum lactic dehydrogenase level, and hematocrit every 6–12 months for patients with stages IB–IV [4]. In the Japanese guidelines, frequent imaging tests are not recommended since they do not improve the prognosis of patients with this cancer. It is well known that routine computed tomographic or nuclear medicine scans have an extremely low yield in the absence of clinical symptoms. Many physicians, however, obtain CT scans or nuclear medicine scans every 6–12 months for 5 years after initial treatment. Most patients also agree with the practice of performing frequent imaging tests in Japan. Laboratory tests play a limited role in the follow-up of patients with melanoma. In Japan the measurement of the serum 5-S-cysteinyldopa level is considered useful [10]. Measurement of the serum lactic dehydrogenase level may also be useful.

In Japan, monthly low-dose interferon-β (intradermally injected surrounding the primary site) is recommended as adjuvant therapy after definitive treatment of primary tumor, especially in stages IIC and III [11]. Although this treatment has not been shown to be effective in improving the prognosis, many physicians in Japan still offer it. This therapy also provides a good motive for the patients to come to the hospital.

There has been no report that Japanese patients with melanoma are at increased risk for other invasive noncutaneous malignancies. Screening systems are being organized in which citizens with high incidence of malignancies, such as

Table 52.1 Surveillance after curative-intent therapy for in situ and Stage IA melanoma at Kyushu University

	Posttreatment year					
Modality	1	2	3	4	5	>5
Office visit	2	2	1	1	1	0

The physical examination should include regional lymph node examination, skin inspection, and palpation of the primary tumor site
The patient should be advised to conduct lifelong, regular self-examination of the skin and peripheral lymph nodes
The numbers in the table indicate the number of times the modality is recommended during the indicated year posttreatment

lung, colorectal, gastric, breast, and uterine cancers, are screened in groups in the physician's office or the local community hospital. Because the incidence of second primary melanoma or familial melanoma is extremely low in Japan, surveillance to detect these lesions has little significance so taking whole-body photographs of the patients to track pigmented lesions is not routinely done.

The dermatologists also assess lymphedema or other consequences of therapy as well as recurrence in each physical examination after initial therapy. When lymphedema is found in patients after lymph node dissection, it is treated with compression bandages. Such patients are introduced to specialists who treat them with complex decongestive therapy. This is a method that combines manual lymphatic drainage, compression bandages, myolymphokinetic exercises, skin care, and precautions during daily activities.

Most dermatologists in Japan follow the "General rules for clinical and pathological studies on malignant neoplasms of the skin" and the "Clinical guidelines for melanoma" [8, 9]. Because medical insurance by the government supports clinical care, most patients are willing to visit the hospital frequently after an initial treatment.

For the majority of patients, detection of asymptomatic recurrence by a physician during routine follow-up does not improve survival, as compared to detection by the patient. A prospective, randomized study of close follow-up vs. a policy of trusting the patient to contact his physician when recurrence is detected is needed. Melanoma inhibitory activity appears promising as a serum marker for early detection of recurrence after definitive treatment of the primary tumor in melanoma patients, and a clinical trial is warranted [12].

There is no documentation of an optimal formula for the surveillance of patients with melanoma. Tables 52.1, 52.2, and 52.3 outline the follow-up schedules in use at Kyushu University. These are based on "General rules for clinical and pathological studies on malignant neoplasms of the skin" and the "Clinical guidelines for melanoma" [8, 9]. Of course, decisions about follow-up may be modified on an individual basis according to the patient's preference. Also, the follow-up schedule may be modified using existing data. For example, patients in stage IIIA with microscopic metastasis in a sentinel lymph node may require less frequent follow-up than a patient

Table 52.2 Surveillance after curative-intent therapy for stages IB–IIB melanoma at Kyushu University

	Posttreatment year					
	1	2	3	4	5	>5
Office visit	4–12[a]	4–12	4	1	1	1[b]
Chest X-ray, LDH, 5-S-CD	2–4	2–4	2–4	1	1	0–1

The physical examination should include regional lymph node examination, skin inspection, and palpation of the primary tumor site
[a]Monthly visits tend to coincide with monthly INF-ß injection at primary site for 2–3 years posttreatment
[b]The total duration of follow-up is 10 years
LDH = serum lactic dehydrogenase level, 5-S-CD = serum 5-S-cysteinyldopa level
The patient should be advised to conduct lifelong, regular self-examination of the skin and peripheral lymph nodes
The numbers in the table indicate the number of times the modality is recommended during the indicated year posttreatment

Table 52.3 Surveillance after curative-intent therapy for Stages IIC–III at Kyushu University

	Years posttreatment					
	1	2	3	4	5	>5
Office visit	4–12[a]	4–12	4	1	1	1
Chest X-ray, LDH, 5-S-CD	2–4	2–4	2–4	1	1	0–1

The physical examination should include regional lymph node examination, skin inspection, and palpation of the primary tumor site
[a]Monthly visits tend to coincide with monthly INF-ß injection at primary site for 2–3 years posttreatment
Lifelong follow-up is advised
LDH = serum lactic dehydrogenase level, 5-S-CD = serum 5-S-cysteinyldopa level
The patient should be advised to conduct lifelong, regular self-examination of the skin and peripheral lymph nodes
The numbers in the table indicate the number of times the modality is recommended during the indicated year posttreatment

with bulky metastases. The optimal duration of follow-up is unknown. Late recurrences more than 10 years after treatment of localized melanoma are well recognized in Japan.

References

1. Ishihara K, Saida T, Ohtsuka F, Yamasaki N. The Prognosis and Statistical Investigation Committee of the Japanese Skin Cancer Society. Statistical profiles of malignant melanoma and other skin cancers in Japan: 2007 update. Int J Clin Oncol. 2008;13:33–41.
2. Ishihara K, Saida T, Yamamoto A. The Prognosis and Statistical Investigation Committee of the Japanese Skin Cancer Society. Updated statistical data for malignant melanoma in Japan. Int J Clin Oncol. 2001;6:109–16.
3. Garbe C, Leiter U. Melanoma epidemiology and trends. Clin Dermatol. 2009;27:3–9.
4. Coit DG, Andtbacka R, Bichakjian CK, Dilawari RA, Dimaio D, Guild V, Halpern AC, Hodi FS, Kashani-Sabet M, Lange JR, Lind A, Martin L, Martini MC, Pruitt SK, Ross MI, Sener SF, Swetter SM, Tanabe KK, Thompson JA, Trisal V, Urist MM, Weber J, Wong MK, NCCN Melanoma Panel. Melanoma. J Natl Compr Canc Netw. 2009;7:250–75.

5. Balch CM, Buzaid AC, Soong SJ, Atkins MB, Cascinelli N, Coit DG, et al. Final version of the American Joint Committee on Cancer staging system for cutaneous melanoma. J Clin Oncol. 2001;19:3635–48.
6. Yamamoto A, Ishihara K. A statistical study of 242 cases of malignant melanoma. Acta Sch Med Univ Gifu. 1987;35:207–37.
7. Yamamoto A. Cutaneous melanoma—counter point. In: Johnson FE, Virgo KS, editors. Cancer Patient Follow-up. St. Louis: Mosby-Year Book; 1997. p. 275–8.
8. The Japanese Skin Cancer Society. Malignant melanoma. In: Japanese Skin Cancer Society. General rules for clinical and pathological studies on malignant neoplasms of the skin (in Japanese), Tokyo: Kanehara & Co., Ltd.; 2002. p. 16–37.
9. Saida T, Manabe M, Takenouchi T, Kiyohara T, Yamamoto A, Kiyohara Y, Takata M, Yamasaki N, Moroi Y, Kamiya H, Hatta N, Uhara H, Kona K, Shikama N, Tsuchida T, Koga H on behalf of The Japanese Skin Cancer Society. The guideline for the management of skin cancer in Japanese only. Jpn J Dermatol. 2007; 117:1855–925. http://www.dermatol.or.jp/medical/guideline/skincancer/index.htm.
10. Wakamatsu K, Kageshita T, Furue M, Hatta N, Kiyohara Y, Nakayama J, Ono T, Saida T, Takata M, Tsuchida T, Uhara H, Yamamoto A, Yamazaki N, Naito A, Ito S. Evaluation of 5-S-cysteinyldopa as a marker of melanoma progression: 10 years' experience. Melanoma Res. 2002;12:245–53.
11. Kageshita T, Yamamoto A, Yamazaki N, Ishihara K, Ono T. Low frequency of neutralizing antibodies against natural interferon-β during adjuvant therapy for Japanese patients with melanoma. J Dermatol Sci. 1999;19:208–12.
12. Matsushita Y, Hatta N, Wakamatsu K, Takehara K, Ito S, Takata M. Melanoma inhibitory activity (MIA) as a serum marker for early detection of post-surgical relapse in melanoma patients: comparison with 5-S-cysteinyldopa. Melanoma Res. 2002;12:319–23.

Breast Carcinoma

53

David Y. Johnson, Shilpi Wadhwa, and Frank E. Johnson

Keywords
Breast • Carcinoma • Age • Obesity • Menopause

The International Agency for Research on Cancer (IARC), a component of the World Health Organization (WHO), estimated that there were 1,151,298 new cases of breast cancer worldwide in 2002 (1). The IARC also estimated that there were 410,712 deaths due to this cause in 2002 (1).

The American Cancer Society estimated that there were 180,510 new cases and 40,910 deaths (males and females) due to this cause in the United States in 2007(2). The estimated five-year survival rate (all races) in the United States in 2007 was 89 % for female breast cancer (2). Survival rates were adjusted for normal life expectancies and were based on cases diagnosed from 1996 to 2002 and followed through 2003.

Female sex is a dominant etiologic factor, as are advancing age, nulliparous status, early menopause, and obesity. A family history of breast cancer confers increased risk, acting through factors such as mutated p53, BRCA 1 and 2, and others. Ionizing radiation, particularly during youth, increases risk. The presence of premalignant changes in the breast, such as atypical hyperplasia, confers markedly increased risk (3, 4).

Geographic Variation Worldwide

There is considerable geographic variation in the incidence of breast cancer. The annual incidence is 70 per 100,000 women in western countries such as the United States, Canada, and large parts of Europe. The incidence is also high in South American countries such as Argentina and Uruguay, and in Australia and New Zealand (5). Geographic variation in the United States is also pronounced (6).

Surveillance Strategies Proposed by Professional Organizations or National Government Agencies and Available on the Internet

- National Comprehensive Cancer Network (NCCN, www.nccn.org)—NCCN guidelines were accessed on 1/28/12 (Tables 53.1–53.3). There were minor quantitative and qualitative changes compared to the guidelines accessed on 4/10/07.
- American Society of Clinical Oncology (ASCO, www.asco.org)—ASCO guidelines were accessed on 1/28/12 (Table 53.4). There were no significant changes compared to the guidelines accessed on 10/31/07.
- The Society of Surgical Oncology (SSO, www.surgonc.org)—SSO guidelines were accessed on 1/28/12. No quantitative guidelines exist for breast cancer surveillance, including when first accessed on 10/31/07.
- European Society for Medical Oncology (ESMO, www.esmo.org)—ESMO guidelines were accessed on 1/28/12. No quantitative guidelines currently exist for breast cancer surveillance, compared to the quantitative guidelines accessed on 10/31/07.
- European Society of Surgical Oncology (ESSO, www.esso-surgeonline.org)—ESSO guidelines were accessed on 1/28/12. No quantitative guidelines exist for breast cancer surveillance, including when first accessed on 10/31/07.

D.Y. Johnson • S. Wadhwa
Department of Internal Medicine, Saint Louis University Medical Center, Saint Louis, MO, USA

F.E. Johnson (✉)
Saint Louis University Medical Center and Saint Louis Veterans Affairs Medical Center, Saint Louis, MO, USA
e-mail: frank.johnson1@va.gov

F.E. Johnson et al. (eds.), *Patient Surveillance After Cancer Treatment*, Current Clinical Oncology,
DOI 10.1007/978-1-60327-969-7_53, © Springer Science+Business Media New York 2013

Tables 53.1 Breast cancer: lobular carcinoma in situ (Obtained from NCCN (www.nccn.org) on 1/28/12 breast cancer)

	Years posttreatment[a]					
	1	2	3	4	5	>5
Office visit	1–2	1–2	1–2	1–2	1–2	1–2
Mammogram	1	1	1	1	1	1
Breast awareness[b]						
Consider risk reduction strategies[c]						

NCCN guidelines were accessed on 1/28/12. There were minor qualitative changes compared to the guidelines accessed on 4/10/07

[a]The numbers in the table indicate the number of times the modality is recommended during the indicated year posttreatment

[b]Women should be familiar with their breasts and promptly report changes to their healthcare provider. Periodic, consistent breast self-examination may facilitate breast self-awareness. Premenopausal women may find breast self-examination most informative when performed at the end of menses

[c]See NCCN Breast Cancer Risk Reduction Guidelines

Table 53.2 Breast cancer: ductal carcinoma in situ (Obtained from NCCN (www.nccn.org) on 1/28/12)

	Years posttreatment[a]					
	1	2	3	4	5	>5
Office visit	1-2	1-2	1-2	1-2	1-2	1
Mammogram[b]	1–2	1–2	1–2	1–2	1–2	1–2

If treated with tamoxifen, monitor per NCCN Breast Cancer Risk Reduction Guidelines

NCCN guidelines were accessed on 1/28/12. There were minor quantitative and qualitative changes compared to the guidelines accessed on 4/10/07

[a]The numbers in the table indicate the number of times the modality is recommended during the indicated year posttreatment

[b]Mammogram every 12 months (and 6–12 month postradiation therapy if breast conserved)

- Cancer Care Ontario (CCO, www.cancercare.on.ca)—CCO guidelines were accessed on 1/28/12. No quantitative guidelines exist for breast cancer surveillance, including when first accessed on 10/31/07.
- National Institute for Clinical Excellence (NICE, www.nice.org.uk)—NICE guidelines were accessed on 1/28/12 (Table 53.5). There are new quantitative guidelines compared to the qualitative guidelines accessed on 10/31/07.

Table 53.3 Breast cancer: invasive breast cancer (Obtained from NCCN (www.nccn.org) on 1/28/12)

	Years posttreatment[a]					
	1	2	3	4	5	>5
Office visit[b]	2–3	2–3	2–3	2–3	2–3	1
Mammogram	1	1	1	1	1	1
Women on aromatase inhibitor or who experience ovarian failure secondary to treatment should have monitoring of bone health with a bone mineral density determination at baseline and periodically thereafter[c]						

Assess and encourage adherence to adjuvant endocrine therapy

Evidence suggests that active lifestyle and achieving and maintaining an ideal body weight (20-25 BMI) may lead to optimal breast cancer outcomes

NCCN guidelines were accessed on 1/28/12. There were minor qualitative changes compared to the guidelines accessed on 4/10/07

[a]The numbers in the table indicate the number of times the modality is recommended during the indicated year posttreatment

[b]Women on tamoxifen: annual gynecologic assessment every 12 months if uterus present

[c]The use of estrogen, progesterone, or selective estrogen receptor modulators to treat osteoporosis or osteopenia in women with breast cancer is discouraged. The use of a bisphosphonate is generally the preferred intervention to improve bone mineral density. Optimal duration of bisphosphonate therapy has not been established. Factors to consider for duration of anti-osteoporosis therapy include bone mineral density, response to therapy, and risk factors for continued bone loss or fracture. Women treated with a bisphosphonate should undergo a dental examination with preventive dentistry prior to the initiation of therapy and should take supplemental calcium and vitamin D

- The Cochrane Collaboration (CC, www.cochrane.org)—CC guidelines were accessed on 1/28/12. No quantitative guidelines exist for breast cancer surveillance, including when first accessed on 11/24/07.
- The American Society of Breast Surgeons (ASBS, www.breastsurgeons.org)—ASBS guidelines were accessed on 1/28/12. No quantitative guidelines exist for breast cancer surveillance, including when first accessed on 12/13/07.
- The M.D. Anderson Surgical Oncology Handbook also has follow-up guidelines, proposed by authors from a single National Cancer Institute-designated Comprehensive Cancer Center, for many types of cancer (7). Some are detailed and quantitative, others are qualitative.

Table 53.4 Breast cancer (Obtained from ASCO (www.asco.org) on 1/28/12)

	Years posttreatment[a]					
	1	2	3	4	5	>5
Office visit[b,c]	2–4	2–4	2–4	1–2	1–2	1
Mammogram[d]	1–2	1–2	1–2	1–2	1–2	1–2

Women at high risk for familial breast cancer syndromes should be referred for genetic counseling in accordance with clinical guidelines recommended by the US Preventive Services Task Force[e]

All women should be counseled to perform monthly breast self-examination

Regular gynecologic follow-up is recommended for all women[f]

CBC, automated chemistry studies, chest x-ray, bone scan, ultrasound of the liver, CT scan, FDG-PET scan, breast MRI, CA 15-3 or CA 27.29, and carcinoembryonic antigen testing are not recommended for surveillance

ASCO guidelines were accessed on 1/28/12. There were no significant changes compared to the guidelines accessed on 4/10/07

[a] The numbers in the table indicate the number of times the modality is recommended during the indicated year posttreatment

[b] Physicians should counsel patients about the symptoms of recurrence including new lumps, bone pain, chest pain, dyspnea, abdominal pain, or persistent headaches

[c] The risk of breast cancer recurrence continues through 15 years after primary treatment and beyond. Continuity of care for breast cancer patients is recommended and should be performed by a physician experienced in the surveillance of cancer patients and in breast examination, including the examination of irradiated breasts. Follow-up by a primary care physician (PCP) seems to lead to the same health outcomes as specialist follow-up with good patient satisfaction

[d] Women treated with breast-conserving therapy should have their first post-treatment mammogram no earlier than 6 months after definitive radiation therapy. Mammography should be performed yearly if stability of mammographic findings is achieved after completion of locoregional therapy

[e] Criteria to recommend referral include the following: Ashkenazi Jewish heritage; history of ovarian cancer at any age in the patient or any first- or second-degree relatives; any first-degree relative with a history of breast cancer diagnosed before the age of 50 years; two or more first- or second-degree relatives diagnosed with breast cancer at any age; patient or relative with diagnosis of bilateral breast cancer; and history of breast cancer in a male relative

[f] Patients who receive tamoxifen therapy are at increased risk for developing endometrial cancer and should be advised to report any vaginal bleeding to their physicians. Longer follow-up intervals may be appropriate for women who have had a total hysterectomy and oophorectomy

Table 53.5 Early and locally advanced breast cancer (Obtained from NICE (www.nice.org.uk) on 1/28/12)

	Years posttreatment[a]					
	1	2	3	4	5	>5
Office visit[b]	1	1	1	1	1	0
Mammogram[c,d]	1	1	1	1	1	0

After completion of adjuvant treatment (including chemotherapy, and/or radiotherapy where indicated) for early breast cancer, discuss with patients where they would like follow-up to be undertaken. They may choose to receive follow-up care in primary, secondary, or shared care

Patients treated for breast cancer should have an agreed, written care plan, which should be recorded by a named healthcare professional (or professionals), a copy sent to the GP, and a personal copy given to the patient[e]

Do not offer ultrasound or MRI for routine posttreatment surveillance in patients who have been treated for early invasive breast cancer or DCIS

NICE guidelines were accessed on 1/28/12. These are new quantitative guidelines compared to the qualitative guidelines accessed on 10/31/07

[a] The numbers in the table indicate the number of times the modality is recommended during the indicated year posttreatment

[b] Mammography was the only quantitative recommendation given. We inferred that office visit would be recommended as frequently as this

[c] On reaching the NHS Breast Screening Programme or Breast Test Wales Screening Programme (NHSBSP/BTWSP) screening age or after 5 years of annual mammography follow-up, NICE recommends that the NHSBSP/BTWSP stratify screening frequency in line with patient risk category

[d] Do not offer mammography of the ipsilateral soft tissues after mastectomy

[e] This plan should include designated named healthcare professionals; dates for review of any adjuvant therapy; details of surveillance mammography; signs and symptoms to look for and seek advice on; contact details for immediate referral to specialist care; contact details for support services, for example support for patients with lymphedema

Summary

This is a common cancer with significant variability in incidence worldwide. We found guidelines based on consensus as well as high-quality evidence (8, 9).

References

1. Parkin DM, Whelan SL, Ferlay J, Teppo L, Thomas DB. Cancer incidence in five continents. IARC Scientific Publication 155, vol. VIII. Lyon: IARC; 2002. ISBN 92-832-2155-9.
2. Jemal A, Seigel R, Ward E, Murray T, Xu J, Thun MJ. Cancer statistics, 2007. CA Cancer J Clin. 2007;57:43–66.
3. Schottenfeld D, Fraumeni JG. Cancer epidemiology and prevention. 3rd ed. New York, NY: Oxford University Press; 2006. ISBN 13:978-0-19-514961-6.
4. DeVita VT, Hellman S, Rosenberg SA. Cancer. 7th ed. Philadelphia, PA: Lippincott Williams & Wilkins; 2005. ISBN 0-781-74450-4.
5. Mackay J, Jemal A, Lee NC, Parkin M. The Cancer Atlas. 2006 American Cancer Society 1599 Clifton Road NE, Atlanta, Georgia 30329, USA. Can also be accessed at www.cancer.org. ISBN 0-944235-62-X.
6. Devesa SS, Grauman DJ, Blot WJ, Pennello GA, Hoover RN, Fraumeni JF Jr. Atlas of cancer mortality in the United States. NIH Publication No. 99–4564. National Institutes of Health, National Cancer Institute; September 1999.
7. Feig BW, Berger DH, Fuhrman GM. The M.D. Anderson surgical oncology handbook. 4th ed. Philadelphia, PA: Lippincott Williams & Wilkins; 2006 (paperback). ISBN 0-7817-5643-X.
8. The GIVO. Investigations. Impact of follow-up testing on survival and health-related quality of life in breast cancer patients: a multicenter randomized controlled trial. JAMA. 1994;271: 1587–92.
9. Rosselli Del Turco M, Palli D, Cariddi A, Ciatto S, Pacini P, Distane V. Intensive diagnostic follow-up treatment of primary breast cancer: a randomized trial. JAMA. 1994;271:1593–7.

54 Breast Carcinoma Surveillance Counterpoint: USA

Kelli Pettit and Julie A. Margenthaler

Keywords
Breast cancer • Follow-up strategy • Staging

Historically, the incidence of breast cancer has been increasing. However, the incidence of breast cancer in the USA decreased by 2.2% per year from 1999 to 2005 [1]. The increasing population in the USA means the absolute number of women diagnosed with breast cancer continues to increase yearly, with an estimated 192,370 new cases in 2009 [1]. This, in combination with decreasing mortality rates, has now led to an increase in the number of breast cancer survivors who need long-term follow-up [2]. There has been significant debate over what tests should be obtained, how often they should be obtained, how long surveillance should be continued, and by whom this should be performed. The National Comprehensive Cancer Network guidelines recommend interval history and physical examination every 4–6 months for 5 years and then annually thereafter, with mammogram every 12 months (the first posttreatment mammogram to be obtained 6–12 months following the completion of chemotherapy). For women on tamoxifen or aromatase inhibitors, annual gynecologic examinations are recommended. Regular bone mineral density examinations are recommended for women on aromatase inhibitors. No other routine laboratory and/or imaging modalities are currently recommended for routine surveillance. Further testing is only recommended when abnormalities are detected by history, physical examination, or mammography, as routine testing has not been shown to improve overall or disease-free survival [3, 4]. Surveillance recommendations are not stratified based on stage of cancer at time of initial diagnosis or treatment. The American Society of Clinical Oncology guidelines are similar: history and physical examination every 3–6 months for the first 3 years, every 6–12 months for years 4 and 5, and then annually thereafter, with further testing only if symptoms arise. Annual mammography, gynecologic examination, and bone mineral density examination recommendations mirror the National Comprehensive Cancer Network guidelines [5].

Traditionally, physicians have considered breast cancer recurrence to occur most commonly within the first 5 years after initial treatment. Therefore, as suggested by the National Comprehensive Cancer Network and the American Society of Clinical Oncology guidelines, many of these women have had intensive follow-up with de-escalation after 5 years. However, recently published data suggest that women with hormone-receptor-positive breast cancer have a steady, more gradual rate of recurrence over a 10-year period, raising the question of whether we should be tailoring our follow-up strategies based on tumor biology, rather than stage at diagnosis [6, 7]. Currently, practice guidelines, including our own institutional practice, do not stratify surveillance intensity based on tumor biology but rather by the extent of disease at the time of diagnosis and treatment. Standard follow-up practice for patients who have undergone curative intent treatment for Stage 0–III breast cancer at the Siteman Cancer Center at Washington University School of Medicine and Barnes-Jewish Hospital is based on a multidisciplinary model. Patients are seen by their surgeon, radiation oncologist (if radiation was received), and medical oncologist (if systemic chemotherapy or endocrine therapy was received). To the extent possible, the surveillance for male patients is the same as for female patients.

K. Pettit, M.D. • J.A. Margenthaler, M.D. (✉)
Department of Surgery, Washington University School of Medicine, Siteman Cancer Center, 660 S. Euclid Avenue, Campus Box 8109, St. Louis, MO 63110, USA
e-mail: kelli.pettit@gmail.com; margenthalerj@wudosis.wustl.edu

F.E. Johnson et al. (eds.), *Patient Surveillance After Cancer Treatment*, Current Clinical Oncology, DOI 10.1007/978-1-60327-969-7_54, © Springer Science+Business Media New York 2013

All patients are followed by their respective surgeon or their surgeon's physician extender within the breast surgery center twice (typically at 6-month intervals) during the first year following completion of surgery and then annually thereafter. This is not altered by stage and is continued indefinitely. We do not release patients back to their primary care physicians after 5 years, as is the practice of many surgeons. Annual screening or diagnostic mammography is coordinated with this visit. Women who have had breast-conserving therapy undergo bilateral diagnostic mammograms, which are read immediately on site by our dedicated breast radiologists. Women who have had unilateral mastectomy undergo contralateral screening mammography. Women who have had bilateral mastectomy undergo clinical examination only. If any change or concern is found by the patient and/or surgeon during the clinical breast examination, the patient is able to immediately be evaluated with full diagnostic imaging. Follow-up screening with magnetic resonance imaging is reserved for those women who qualified for screening magnetic resonance imaging (BRCA mutation carriers, unknown BRCA status with a first-degree relative BRCA carrier, lifetime risk >20%, or prior chest irradiation) prior to their diagnosis of breast cancer but did not receive bilateral mastectomies. To date, studies do not support the use of routine breast magnetic resonance imaging in follow-up after breast-conserving therapy [8, 9]. Our surveillance magnetic resonance imaging utilization is based on these data.

All of our patients who undergo breast-conserving therapy are referred to radiation oncology. With the exception of a minority of women over 70 years old with small, hormone-receptor-positive tumors, all of our patients who receive breast-conserving surgery also undergo adjuvant radiation therapy. Patients who receive mastectomy are also considered for adjuvant radiation when the pathology report demonstrates tumor characteristics placing them at high risk for local recurrence (positive or close margins, extensive lymphovascular invasion, tumor size >5 cm, >3 positive axillary lymph nodes). Patients who receive conventional external beam radiation therapy are seen by the radiation oncologist 6 weeks following completion of the radiation, 6 months post-radiation, every 6–12 months for 5 years and annually thereafter. Their first post-radiation mammogram is obtained between 3 and 6 months after completion of radiation (coordinated through the surgeon's office as described above). Those patients who receive accelerated partial breast radiation are typically enrolled in a clinical study and are followed more closely with history and physical examinations performed every 3–6 months for 5 years and then annually thereafter. The radiation oncology follow-up after 5 years tends to be on a more self-selected basis. The patients who have had a more difficult course of treatment (locally advanced disease, significant postradiation clinical skin changes), as determined by the radiation oncologist, are followed annually in their office. Otherwise, our radiation oncologists release the patient at 5 years and follow-up is continued by the patient's surgeon and/or medical oncologist.

Nearly all of our patients have some form of treatment directed by a medical oncologist, either chemotherapy with or without endocrine therapy or endocrine therapy alone. The exception to this is for patients who have had only Stage 0 ductal carcinoma in situ. Patients with ductal carcinoma in situ are followed and treated with endocrine therapy (when appropriate) every 6 months for 5 years (or more) during the treatment phase by their surgeon or by a designated internal medicine specialist who has a practice focusing on high-risk breast cancer patients and patients with ductal carcinoma in situ. The determination of who is going to follow patients with ductal carcinoma is made by the surgeon; those surgeons comfortable with prescribing and following patients on endocrine therapy do so, and the others refer to the internal medicine specialist. Currently, about 50% of our patients with ductal carcinoma are followed by their surgeon and about 50% are followed by the internal medicine specialist. The majority of patients with ductal carcinoma in situ are treated with tamoxifen. Annual gynecologic examinations are coordinated through the patient's primary care physician.

All patients with invasive breast cancer are referred to a medical oncologist. Those who do not require chemotherapy and those who receive endocrine therapy only are followed every 6 months for the 5 years (or more) of treatment. This includes a history and physical examination. An overall health assessment is performed, focusing not only on breast health but bone health as well. Patients on aromatase inhibitors receive a baseline bone densitometry measurement, which is repeated every 2 years. The medical oncologist generally releases low-risk patients (i.e., those who did not receive chemotherapy or those who did receive chemotherapy but did not have bulky axillary disease) back to the primary care physician for annual history and physical examination after 5 years of follow-up. Patients at high risk for recurrence (i.e., those with inflammatory cancer or stage III disease) are seen every 3 months or 5 years and then every 6 months for a variable amount of time (typically years 5–10) and then annually thereafter. Aside from history and physical examination, the only other routine test used in follow-up by a select number of our medical oncologists (~30–50%) is the serum CA 15-3 level. While there are no studies demonstrating improved survival duration or quality of life attributable to routine CA 15-3 screening, some of our medical oncologists feel that increasing levels can indicate asymptomatic disease progression and a normal level may provide some reassurance for both the patient and the physician. Although early detection of recurrence does not alter survival outcomes [4], treatment of asymptomatic recurrences may decrease total symptoms long-term. If a patient develops signs or symptoms concerning for disease progression, such as bone or abdominal pain or neurologic symptoms, or if the serum CA 15-3 level is elevated or progressively increasing over baseline, further imaging is performed. At our institution, the choice of imaging is typically limited to computed tomography scan of the head, chest, abdomen/pelvis, and bone scan. Positron emission tomography is rarely utilized, except in the course of research or for patients with widely metastatic disease. With the exception of yearly gynecologic examinations for patients on tamoxifen or aromatase inhibitors and biennial bone densitometry for patients on aromatase inhibitors, no specific follow-up testing is performed to identify any long-term sequel of treatment.

Among the various physicians caring for the patient (surgeon, radiation oncologist, medical oncologist, primary care physician, gynecologist), we try to coordinate the visits such that the patient is being seen every 3–6 months for the first 5 years, depending on how many people are active in the care of the patient and how far they travel to have the visits. Once the patient has survived for 5 years following initial treatment without cancer recurrence, we coordinate at least annual visits. Some of our patients travel a long distance for their surgical care and often have a medical or radiation oncologist closer to home to continue follow-up care. If no specialist is close to home, a dedicated primary care physician may assume that role. Of course, if patients desire to have continued follow-up in all three clinics, they are not turned away.

In addition, as mentioned earlier, our institution utilizes physician extenders to offload the volume burden as more patients are requiring follow-up. This works well for us, as the surgeon is usually immediately available to see any patients who have new or active issues that the physician extender may need help solving, and the patients are happy to see someone yearly. This does not address the issue of cost of follow-up visits. We feel that all breast cancer patients should still have yearly follow-up by a primary care physician as most patients treated for early breast cancer die of an unrelated disease. Rather than utilizing physician extenders to decrease the volume burden on surgical oncologists, there is increasing literature to support referral of patients back to their primary care physician for annual history and physical examination and symptom-directed imaging [3, 4]. Multiple papers have shown that care provided by a specialist is not superior to that by a primary care physician when looking at morbidity, mortality, or patient satisfaction [10–13]. However, one complaint by patients is the lack of communication between the specialist and the primary care physician, and poor planning for transfer of care. The result is that primary care physicians sometimes feel unqualified to provide adequate care. In addition, those studies have been performed in countries with a national health care system [10–13]. To date, no studies have evaluated primary care physician follow-up care in the United States to determine if the same is true. We do not have any specific information regarding the relationship between the cost of surveillance and adequacy of care at our institution.

Table 54.1 Surveillance after curative-intent treatment for early stage/low-risk disease (tumor size <5 cm and <4 lymph nodes involved) at Siteman Cancer Center, USA

Posttreatment year	1	2	3	4	5	>5
History and physical examination[a]						
Surgeon	2	1	1	1	1	1[a]
Radiation Oncologist	4	2	2	2	2	1[a]
Medical Oncologist	2–6	2	2	2	2	1[a]
Mammogram[b]	2	1	1	1	1	1[a]
Magnetic resonance imaging of breast[c]	1	1	1	1	1	1
Serum CA 15-3 level[a]	2	2	2	2	2	1
Gynecologic examination[d]	1	1	1	1	1	1
Bone mineral density[e]	1		1		1	Biennial

The number in each cell is the number of times a particular modality is obtained during a particular posttreatment year

Computed tomography of chest/abdomen/pelvis and/or bone scan is obtained when indicated by a change in history and physical examination or rising serum CA 15-3 levels

[a] After 5 years, the patient is referred back to his/her primary care physician for annual examinations, but he/she may continue annual follow-up with the specialist, if desired

[b] First ipsilateral mammogram 6 months postsurgical therapy or 3 months following completion of radiation therapy

[c] For women who were previously at high risk and did not receive bilateral mastectomy, alternating every 6 months with mammography

[d] For women who are being treated with tamoxifen or an aromatase inhibitor

[e] For women who are being treated with an aromatase inhibitor. After 5 years, the patient undergoes biennial bone mineral density for the duration of treatment if such duration is >5 years

From our experience, patients appreciate our system of care. The close clinical follow-up with a surgeon or surgeon extender, in coordination with yearly mammography (when indicated), is convenient for the patient and allows instant results. We are able to reassure patients we consider to be free of recurrence, and we are able to quickly investigate new abnormalities. For patients who travel a long distance to our institution, coordination of visits between the specialties is taken into consideration to minimize the number of trips as much as possible. There are, of course, patients who have been lost to follow-up who return only when symptoms arise. The exact proportion of patients who are compliant with our recommended follow-up strategy is difficult to determine, though we estimate that the number is approximately 70% or greater of the total population treated.

Tables 54.1 and 54.2 summarize the follow-up care at our institution. In alignment with nationally published guidelines, most of our surveillance relies on history, physical examination, and regular mammography.

Table 54.2 Surveillance after curative-intent treatment for late stage/ high-risk disease (tumor size ≥5 cm or ≥4 lymph nodes involved, or inflammatory breast cancer) at Siteman Cancer Center

Posttreatment year	1	2	3	4	5	>5
History and physical examination[a]						
Surgeon	2	1	1	1	1	1[a]
Radiation oncologist	4	2	2	2	2	1[a]
Medical oncologist	2–6	2–4	2–4	2–4	2–4	1-2[a]
Mammogram[b]	2	1	1	1	1	1[a]
Magnetic resonance imaging of breast[c]	1	1	1	1	1	1[a]
Serum CA 15-3 level[a]	2	2	2	2	2	1[a]
Gynecologic examination[d]	1	1	1	1	1	1
Bone mineral density[e]	1		1		1	Biennial

The number in each cell is the number of times a particular modality is obtained during a particular posttreatment year

[a]After 5 years, the patient is referred back to his/her primary care physician for annual examinations, but he/she may continue annual follow-up with the specialist, if desired

[b]First ipsilateral mammogram 6 months postsurgical therapy or 3 months following completion of radiation therapy

[c]For women who were previously at high risk and did not receive bilateral mastectomy, alternating every 6 months with mammography

[d]For women who are being treated with tamoxifen or an aromatase inhibitor

[e]For women who are being treated with an aromatase inhibitor. After 5 years, the patient undergoes biennial bone mineral density for the duration of treatment if such duration is >5 years

Computed tomography of chest/abdomen/pelvis and/or bone scan is obtained when indicated by a change in history and physical examination or rising serum CA 15-3 levels

References

1. American Cancer Society. Cancer facts & figures 2009. Atlanta: American Cancer Society; 2009.
2. Ries LAG, Melbert D, Krapcho M, et al., editors. SEER cancer statistics review, 1975–2005. Bethesda, MD: National Cancer Institute, seer.cancer.gov/csr/1975_2005/, 2008.
3. National Comprehensive Cancer Network. NCCN clinical practice guidelines in oncology (NCCN Guidelines), Breast Cancer, vol. 1. Fort Washington, PA: NCCN; 2009.
4. Rojas MP, Telaro E, Russo A, Moschetti I, Coe L, Fossati R, et al. Follow-up strategies for women treated for early breast cancer. Cochrane Database Syst Rev 2000. 2000;(4). Art. No.: CD001768.
5. Khatcheressian JL, Wolff AC, Smith TJ, et al. American Society of Clinical Oncology 2006 update of the breast cancer follow-up and management guidelines in the adjuvant setting. J Clin Oncol. 2006;24:5091–7.
6. Pagani O, Price KN, Gelber RD, et al. International Breast Cancer Study Group (IBCSG). Patterns of recurrence of early breast cancer according to estrogen receptor status: a therapeutic target for a quarter of a century. Breast Cancer Res Treat. 2009;11(2):319–24; Epub ahead of print January 10, 2009.
7. Early Breast Cancer Trialists' Collaborative Group. Effects of chemotherapy and hormonal therapy for early breast cancer on recurrence and 15 year survival: An overview of the randomized trials. Lancet. 2005;365:1687–717.
8. Gorechlad JW, McCabe EB, Higgins JH, et al. Screening for Recurrences in Patients Treated with Breast-Conserving Surgery: Is there a Role for MRI? Ann Surg Oncol. 2008;15(6):1703–9.
9. Rebner M, Grills I, Vicini F. Should screening MRI be included in surveillance for patients treated with breast-conserving therapy? Nat Clin Pract Oncol. 2009;6(1):8–9.
10. Sheppard C, Higgins B, Yiangou C, et al. Breast cancer follow up: A randomized controlled trial comparing point of need access versus routine 6-monthly clinical review. Eur J Oncol Nurs. 2009;13(1):2–8.
11. Beaver K, Tysver-Robinson D, Campbell M, et al. Comparing hospital and telephone follow-up after treatment for breast cancer: randomized equivalence trial. BMJ. 2009;338:a3147.
12. Cameron DA. Extended follow-up of breast cancer patients in clinic wastes time for both patients and doctors: the case against. Breast Cancer Res. 2008;10 Suppl 4:S8.
13. Chapman D, Cox E, Britton PD, Wishart GC. Patient-led breast cancer follow up. Breast. 2009;18(2):100–2.

Breast Carcinoma Surveillance Counterpoint: Europe

55

Stefano Ciatto

Surveillance for early detection of distant metastases in their asymptomatic phase by various modalities was a routine procedure until the 1990s. Physical examination, chest X-ray and bone scan were performed at varying intervals, possibly combined with liver ultrasonography and serum markers. Uncontrolled studies of the clinical impact of detection of asymptomatic M1 disease, followed by two controlled randomized trials [1, 2], provided convincing evidence that such practices have no significant impact on prognosis, and presently there seems to be general agreement that such regimens have no efficacy. Most European authorities and scientific societies recommend no surveillance for this purpose (Table 55.1). Based on these recommendations and the existing evidence, the common practice of intensive follow-up for the early detection of metastases is disappearing, although slowly [3].

The issue has been authoritatively addressed by a Cochrane systematic review in 2000 [4], updated in 2005 [5], clearly stating that there is no evidence of improved prognosis with early detection of metastases in the medical literature. The statement that early detection of asymptomatic metastases has no impact on prognosis was mainly based on two Italian randomized studies [1, 2], although the GIVIO study [1] failed to obtain data that would permit an estimation of a possible impact on prognosis due to early diagnosis. The study of Rosselli Del Turco et al. (National Research Council Project) did document a substantial diagnostic anticipation in the intensive follow-up study arm compared to controls, but it also showed no association of early diagnosis of metastases with improved overall prognosis.

Even if we assume that such evidence is sufficient to show a lack of efficacy of intensive follow-up, some limitations should be briefly discussed. The findings of the Roselli del Turco study refer to an unselected cohort of T1-3 N ± operable breast cancer patients. The study design had inadequate power to demonstrate whether there was any subset of patients (selected by age, stage, disease free interval or metastatic site) who might benefit from early detection of distant metastases. The study conclusions are true for the state of art of diagnosis of distant metastases in the late 1980s, but the study used only chest X-ray and bone scintigraphy to detect asymptomatic M1 disease. Diagnostic tests have greatly improved since, and several new diagnostic tools are available today (e.g., total body CT, MRI, PET [6]) that are likely to have a greater accuracy compared with tests used in that study. These might allow for earlier detection and treatment and possibly greater efficacy. What is true for diagnostic tools is also true for treatment available today compared to the 1980s. New drugs and molecular agents might allow for a more effective management of metastases detected early through intensive follow-up.

Overall, diagnosis and treatment of metastatic breast cancer have substantially improved since the National Research Council Project study and, while we may agree that, based on the existing evidence, intensive follow-up for the early detection of asymptomatic M1 disease is still not justified, it is definitely time for new controlled studies to test the efficacy of a follow-up regimen based on these new diagnostic tools and new therapeutic regimens. Surprisingly, there is no evidence that such new studies are in progress.

No controlled studies have been carried out so far on the prognostic impact of early detection of local recurrences. There is evidence from retrospective studies, including a recent Cochrane systematic review [7, 8], that patients with less advanced (asymptomatic) local recurrences have a longer survival duration that those with more advanced (symptomatic) cases. This is true also when survival is measured from primary treatment, to adjust for detection lead time, which would bias comparisons of survival measured from the diagnosis of recurrence. Although such evidence may be affected by length-biased sampling, with slow-growing recurrences more likely to be detected in the asymptomatic phase, and at the same time being associated with longer

S. Ciatto (✉)
ISPO—Istituto per lo Studio e la Prevenzione Oncologica,
Viale A. Volta 171, 50131 Florence, Italy
e-mail: stefano.ciatto@gmail.com

F.E. Johnson et al. (eds.), *Patient Surveillance After Cancer Treatment*, Current Clinical Oncology,
DOI 10.1007/978-1-60327-969-7_55, © Springer Science+Business Media New York 2013

Table 55.1 Recent recommendations for breast cancer surveillance from Europe

Country	Year	Source	Recommended periodic screening for asymptomatic metastases[a]
Europe	2008	ESMO European Society of Medical Oncology [14]	None
Spain	2005	Consejería de Salud, Junta de Andalucia [15]	None
Europe	1998	International Society of Technology Assessment in Health Care [16]	None
Italy	2006	Italian National Task Force for Breast Cancer (FONCAM) [17]	None
UK	2008	National Institute for Health and Clinical Excellence (NICE) in England and Wales [18]	None
Scotland	2008	Scottish Intercollegiate Guidelines Network (SIGN) [19]	None
Europe	2003	European Society of Mastology (EUSOMA) [20]	None

[a]Symptoms suggestive of recurrence should be investigated according to the physician's preference.
Screening for in-breast recurrence and metachronous primary breast cancer should be based on the best available evidence [1, 2]

Table 55.2 Surveillance after curative-intent treatment for breast cancer at *Istituto per lo Studio e la Prevenzione Oncologica, Italy*

	Years posttreatment					
	1	2	3	4	5	>5
Office visit[a]	2	2	2	2	2	1
Mammogram[b]	1	1	1	1	1	1

The numbers in the table indicate the number of times the modality is recommended during the indicated year posttreatment
No changes in the surveillance procedure are recommended for patients who have received tamoxifen therapy. Patients should be advised to promptly report any abnormal vaginal bleeding to their physicians
Use of bone scan, chest X-ray, liver sonogram, CT scan, FDG-PET (fluorodeoxyglucose positron emission tomography) scan, breast MRI, serum CEA (carcinoembryonic antigen) level and other breast cancer tumour markers is not recommended
[a]Physicians should counsel patients about the symptoms of recurrence including new lumps, bone pain, dyspnea, abdominal pain or persistent headaches. Women should also be advised to perform monthly breast self-examinations, but these should not replace mammography as a breast cancer screening tool
[b]After the fifth year of surveillance, mammography should be performed every 2 years

survival duration, the common observation that at least some patterns of local recurrence (e.g., axillary nodes, isolated nodules at the chest wall mastectomy scar) are associated with long-term survival after simple excision justifies the adoption of periodic surveillance with physical examination as a part of follow-up. This is particularly true for ipsilateral breast recurrence after breast-conserving treatment. Controlled randomized studies have demonstrated the equivalence of breast-conserving surgery and radical mastectomy as measured by survival duration. This implies that recurrence in the breast alone has no significant prognostic impact if properly detected and treated.

Although contralateral metachronous breast carcinoma cannot be regarded as a recurrence of the index cancer, its early detection is often included among the goals of surveillance. The evidence of screening efficacy for primary breast cancer applies to contralateral metachronous lesions, and retrospective studies have shown a better survival (measured from the first breast cancer, to avoid lead-time bias) of subjects in whom asymptomatic contralateral metachronous cancer is detected compared to the symptomatic phase.

Adjuvant tamoxifen treatment has been associated with increased risk of endometrial carcinoma and active surveillance, including gynecological clinic visits, endometrial cytology, or transvaginal ultrasound scans have been suggested. Few studies have addressed the efficacy of such surveillance, and most have evaluated ultrasound imaging only [9–11]. These suggest that such a policy is not warranted, due to its low sensitivity and specificity. This is related to the fact that abnormal endometrial thickness is commonly induced by tamoxifen, which triggers many invasive assessment procedures, such as hysteroscopy. Considering that endometrial cancer is associated with low lethality and is very often curable when detected at the time symptoms appear, no gynecologic follow-up is recommended, though patients are advised to report any abnormal vaginal bleeding to their physicians.

Overall, the practice of surveillance by periodic physical examination and mammography for the early diagnosis of asymptomatic local recurrences and contralateral breast cancer seems a reasonable option and, although this is based only on evidence from uncontrolled series, it is commonly adopted worldwide. Our scheme for periodic surveillance is shown in Table 55.2. Ideally, mammographic screening frequency should be determined by the expected detection lead time. Evidence from retrospective studies comparing recurrences detected in the asymptomatic or symptomatic phase suggests that detection lead time is relatively short (about 3 months) for local recurrences [7, 12] and much longer (about three years) for contralateral metachronous cancers [13]. A progressive increase in surveillance interval over time may be justified with length bias sampling as slow-growing recurrences are more likely to be associated with longer detection lead time and to surface late. In the absence of controlled studies comparing different surveillance regimens, however, the choice of the interval between mammograms is largely arbitrary.

References

1. The GIVO Investigators. Impact of follow-up testing on survival and health-related quality of life in breast cancer patients: a multicenter randomized controlled trial. JAMA. 1994;271:1587–92.
2. Rosselli M, Palli D, Cariddi A, Ciatto S, Pacini P, Distane V. Intensive diagnostic follow-up treatment of primary breast cancer: a randomized trial; National Research Council Project on Breast Cancer Follow-up. JAMA. 1994;271:1593–7.
3. Ciatto S, Muraca MG, Rosselli Del Turco M. Survey of the practice of follow-up for the early detection of distant metastases in breast cancer patients in Europe. Breast. 1998;7:72–4.
4. Rojas MP, Telaro E, Russo A, Fossati R, Confalonieri C, Liberati A. Follow-up strategies for women treated for early breast cancer. Cochrane Database Syst Rev. 2000;(4):CD001768.
5. Rojas MP, Telaro E, Russo A, Moschetti I, Coe L, Fossati R, Palli D, del Roselli TM, Liberati A. Follow-up strategies for women treated for early breast cancer. Cochrane Database Syst Rev. 2005;(1):CD001768. http://www.cochrane.org/reviews/en/ab001768.html. Accessed February 12, 2009.
6. Dose J, Bleckmann C, Bachmann S, Bohuslavizki KH, Berger J, Jenicke L, et al. Comparison of fluorodeoxyglucose positron emission tomography and "conventional diagnostic procedures" for the detection of distant metastases in breast cancer patients. Nucl Med Commun. 2002;23:857–64.
7. Ciatto S, Rosselli Del Turco M, Pacini P, De Luca Cardillo C, Bastiani P, Bravetti P. Early detection of local recurrences in the follow-up of primary breast cancer. Tumori. 1984;70:179–83.
8. Lu WL, Jansen L, Post WJ, Bonnema J, Van de Velde JC, De Bock GH. Impact on survival of early detection of isolated breast recurrences after the primary treatment for breast cancer: a meta-analysis. Breast Cancer Res Treat. 2008;114(3):403–12 [Epub ahead of print].
9. Cecchini S, Ciatto S, Bonardi R, et al. Screening by ultrasonography for endometrial carcinoma in postmenopausal breast cancer patients under adjuvant Tamoxifen. Gynecol Oncol. 1996;60:409.
10. Love CD, Muir BB, Scrimgeour JB, Leonard RC, Dillon P, Dixon JM. Investigation of endometrial abnormalities in asymptomatic women treated with Tamoxifen and an evaluation of the role of endometrial screening. J Clin Oncol. 1999;17:2050–4.
11. Fung MF, Reid A, Faught W, et al. Prospective longitudinal study of ultrasound screening for endometrial abnormalities in women with breast cancer receiving Tamoxifen. Gynecol Oncol. 2003;91:154–9.
12. Ciatto S. Rosselli Del Turco M, Pacini P, et al. Early detection of breast cancer recurrences through periodic follow-up. Is it useless? Tumori. 1985;71:325–9.
13. Ciatto S, Miccinesi G, Zappa M. Prognostic impact of the early detection of metachronous contralateral breast cancer. Eur J Cancer. 2004;40:1496–501.
14. ESMO. European Society of Medical Oncology—clinical recommendations for diagnosis, treatment and follow-up. Pestalozzi B, Castiglione M on behalf of ESMO guidelines Working Group. Ann Oncol. 2008;19:7–10.
15. de Salud C, de Andalucia J. Càncer de Mama. Detecciòn Precoz de Càncer de Mama. 2nd ed. Sevilla: Junta; 2005.
16. Roy T, Mille D, Ferdjaoui N, Spath HM, Ray I, Carrere MO, et al. International Society of Technology Assessment in Health Care Meeting, Lyon, France. Health policy and the use of clinical guidelines: economic impact assessment in the breast cancer follow-up. Annu Meet Int Soc Technol Assess Health Care Int Soc Technol Assess Health Care Meet. 1998;14:52.
17. Italian National Task Force for Breast Cancer. (FONCAM) 2006 revised guidelines. www.foncam.it. Accessed July 2008.
18. National Institute for Health and Clinical Excellence (NICE) in England and Wales. www.nice.org.uk. Accessed July 2008.
19. Scottish Intercollegiate Guidelines Network (SIGN). www.sign.ac.uk. Accessed July 2008.
20. Perry NM. on behalf of EUSOMA working party. 2003 revised version of EUSOMA position paper. Eur J Cancer. 2001;37:159–72.

Breast Carcinoma Surveillance Counterpoint: Australia

56

Andrew J. Spillane and Meagan E. Brennan

Keywords
Breast cancer • Follow-up • Survivorship • Guidelines • Australia

Australia has a population of 21 million people spread across a land area roughly 15% smaller than the United States of America. Most people live in the eastern part of the continent, particularly along the costal rim. In Australia, breast cancer is the most common invasive cancer diagnosed in women and is also the leading cause of cancer death in females. The incidence is increasing. In 2004, there were 12,235 new cases of breast cancer, at an age-standardized rate in females of 112.8 per 100,000. The incidence of breast cancer in Australia is higher than in many developed countries in the world but it is slightly lower than the incidence in the United States, New Zealand, United Kingdom, and Canada. The death rates are also slightly lower than in these countries. The 5-year relative survival rate in New South Wales at the end of 2005 was 88% [1, 2].

There are over 113,000 Australian women who have had a diagnosis of breast cancer in the last 20 years. Over 80% of these women are still alive and the numbers are increasing each year [1]. Given the size of the country and the geographic challenges, Australian oncologists have a range of issues that need to be considered when making recommendations about frequency of surveillance. As there has been an increasing incidence, better survival statistics, and an oncology workforce that is not proportionally increasing in numbers, Australia faces significant challenges to providing high-quality care that meets patient expectations and best practice medical requirements. The issue of the large area of Australia and the relatively well-educated but sparse population distribution outside major cities increases these challenges and leads to problems of equity of resource distribution. Several Australian studies have shown that women who have treatment in rural areas have a lower rate of breast conservation than women treated in metropolitan areas, highlighting the discrepancies in quality of care between urban and rural areas [3–7]. Practical access to radiotherapy is a particular challenge for women in rural areas. Rural women may be faced with the choice of leaving their family to travel to metropolitan area for 5–6 weeks of radiotherapy treatment. As a result, some choose to undergo mastectomy for very early disease. The implementation of partial breast radiotherapy is in its infancy in Australia and is still considered investigational. Breast reconstruction and nuclear medicine facilities that enable lymphatic mapping for sentinel lymph node biopsy are also frequently unavailable in the rural-remote setting. This may be seen as adding to the complexity of treatment decisions or alternatively limiting options for these women. In addition, the support of a breast care nurse, a nurse specialized in meeting the specific needs of women undergoing breast cancer treatment and providing support and care coordination, may not be available to women outside metropolitan centers [8, 9]. Attempts to address these

A.J. Spillane, M.D., F.R.A.C.S. (✉)
The University of Sydney, Northern Clinical School, Sydney, Australia

Mater Hospital, The Poche Centre, 40 Rocklands Road, North Sydney, NSW 2060, Australia

Royal North Shore Hospital, Westbourne Street, St. Leonards, Sydney 2065, Australia

Sydney Cancer Centre, Royal Prince Alfred Hospital, Missenden Road, Camperdown, NSW 2050, Australia
e-mail: andrew.spillane@melanoma.org.au

M.E. Brennan, F.R.A.C.G.P., F.A.S.B.P.
The University of Sydney, Northern Clinical School, Sydney, Australia

Mater Hospital, The Poche Centre, 40 Rocklands Road, North Sydney, NSW 2060, Australia

F.E. Johnson et al. (eds.), *Patient Surveillance After Cancer Treatment*, Current Clinical Oncology,
DOI 10.1007/978-1-60327-969-7_56, © Springer Science+Business Media New York 2013

inequities are being made by funding agencies and consumer support groups [10, 11].

There is much political debate in Australia about equity of access and maintaining the quality of regional hospitals. There has been a tendency to focus skills in major regional centers, creating "base hospitals" that can have an adequate throughput to support specialist practices. This means people from smaller towns may only have to travel 200–300 km for care rather than 500–700 km or more to a major metropolitan center. Breast surgeons in some base hospital settings are developing high-standard oncoplastic practices that serve to improve opportunities for women in these localities. A problem, however, is that, even in the base hospital setting, the caseload may not be high enough to support specialized breast practice and oncologists may not be willing to leave larger metropolitan centers and live in rural areas. This has led to the development of outreach clinics where medical and radiation oncologists travel to more remote areas on a weekly (or less frequent) basis and chemotherapy is administered by remote supervision. The challenge for the medical profession is to balance the maintenance of high standards of practice that maximize outcomes, including survival duration (known to be caseload dependent [12, 13]) and providing adequate supportive care with the desire or need for women to be treated in a center close to their homes.

There are several major breast cancer consumer groups active in Australia. These groups provide support and education to women who are being treated for breast cancer or are living with a history of breast cancer [14–16]. They are also increasingly working with health professionals, politicians, and health policymakers, having input into research projects and the development of agendas of research priorities, and collaborating to develop clinical practice guidelines and promoting participation in clinical trials [17]. Consumer representation has made significant contributions to the national guidelines for the management of breast cancer and these groups are supportive of the recommendations in these documents [8, 9, 18–20] (Fig. 56.1).

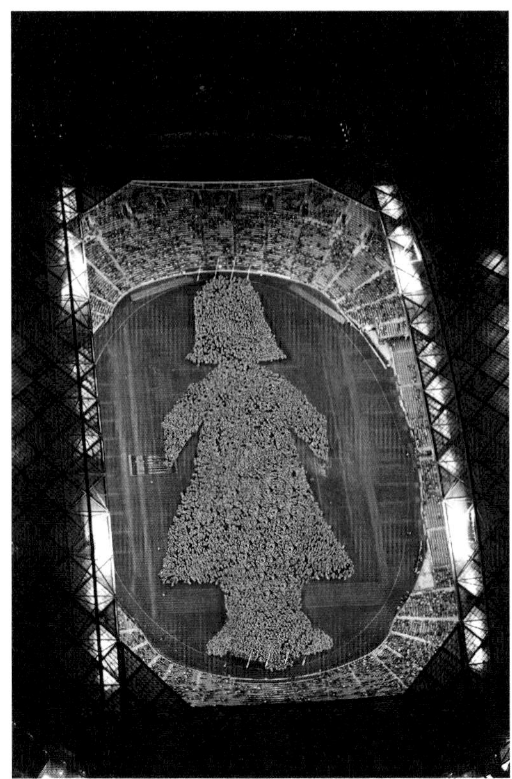

Fig. 56.1 Field of Women, 2005 [15]. Breast Cancer Network Australia, the national voice for Australians affected by breast cancer, brings to life the national annual breast cancer statistics in the *Field of Women LIVE*, Sydney, Australia. 13,000 women in pink (and 100 men in blue) stood together on a football field to represent the number of Australians diagnosed with breast cancer in 2007 (Publication of image approved by BCNA)

Survivorship is now considered a distinct phase of the cancer experience and may be defined as life from the moment of cancer diagnosis and thereafter. The concept of survivorship care acknowledges that a woman's life is forever changed physically and psychologically when she is diagnosed with breast cancer, whether she is cured or develops metastatic disease. Many women have lifelong needs related to their breast cancer or its treatment. Survivorship care is an extension of traditional follow-up care. It is a comprehensive form of long-term care that aims to maximize health and well-being, including maintenance of maximal quality of life for women living with metastatic disease. Survivorship care may be delivered by an individual medical practitioner, such as a surgeon or family physician, or may be provided by a team of health professionals that may include a breast care nurse, physiotherapist or lymphedema therapist, psychologist, dietitian and others, depending on patient need.

How to best care for the large number of breast cancer survivors is an area of increasing interest in Australia and around the world. In the past, surveillance has focused on the detection of cancer recurrence or second primary breast cancer. It is now acknowledged that there are many other issues to be addressed, including detection and care of treatment-related side effects such as menopausal symptoms, sexual dysfunction, psychological issues, and lymphedema. Many of the adverse effects from breast cancer treatment may be prevented or their impact minimized with appropriate assessment and early evidence-based intervention [21] (Box 56.1).

Endocrine treatment may now continue for 10 or more years. Therefore, ongoing consideration needs to be given to commencing, continuing, or changing therapy years after diagnosis and monitoring for ongoing toxicity, such as osteoporosis caused by aromatase inhibitors [22–25]. Numerous Australian and international clinical trials are currently addressing the issue of extended adjuvant hormonal therapy (outlined below) so consideration of eligibility for clinical trials is also an important issue during long-term care.

Box 56.1: Potential Late Effects of Breast Cancer and its Treatment, with Causes and Interventions

Detection and treatment of these effects must be incorporated into follow-up care (Adapted from Hewitt et al. [38])

Late effect	Possible cause(s)	Intervention
Cancer recurrence	Cancer biology	Annual mammography ± breast ultrasound Clinical examination
Second primary cancer	Genetic factors	Annual mammography ± breast ultrasound Clinical examination Patient education
Psychosocial distress	Cancer experience Body image issues Relationship/sexuality issues Menopausal symptoms (adjuvant chemo or endocrine therapy, including ovarian ablation/oophorectomy in premenopausal women)	Assessment for distress Some psychosocial interventions are effective in reducing distress
Arm lymphedema	Axillary dissection Axillary radiotherapy Sentinel lymph node biopsy (uncommon cause of lymphedema)	Early detection (bioimpedance measurements) Massage and exercise (manual lymphatic drainage), use of elastic compression garments, complex decongestive therapy
Premature menopause and related infertility	Adjuvant chemo or endocrine therapy including ovarian ablation/oophorectomy in premenopausal women	New reproductive technologies for infertility Diagnostic and preventive strategies for osteoporosis Assessment of sexual function
Osteoporosis	Postmenopausal women—effect of aromatase inhibitors for adjuvant endocrine therapy Premenopausal women—effect of premature menopause due to adjuvant chemo or endocrine therapy (including ovarian ablation/oophorectomy)	Calcium, vitamin D, exercise Monitoring of bone density Treatment of osteoporosis with bisphosphonates
Symptoms of estrogen deprivation (e.g., hot flushes, sweats, vaginal discharge or vaginal dryness)	Menopause caused by adjuvant chemo or endocrine therapy (including ovarian ablation/oophorectomy)	Possible non-hormone treatments include antidepressants, dietary changes, and exercise Local vaginal therapy (moisturizer, lubricant or topical estrogen therapy) Systemic estrogen-replacement therapy contraindicated unless severe disabling symptoms
Weight gain (associated with poorer prognosis)	Menopause Adjuvant chemo or endocrine therapy	Diet/exercise interventions
Cardiovascular disease	Normal ageing population health issue, including cancer survivors Some adjuvant treatments can cause cardiac problems (e.g., anthracycline chemotherapy, tamoxifen therapy)	Symptomatic women should have a symptom-directed cardiac workup; routine screening of cardiac function is not recommended Preventive strategies for heart disease
Fatigue	Common after cancer treatment, particularly chemotherapy	Exercise programs appear promising
Cognitive impairment	Common after cancer treatment, particularly chemotherapy	Evidence lacking
Risk to family members	Genetic factors	Genetic counseling and testing for BRCA gene mutations where family history indicates potential high risk

The majority of women with breast cancer have their case discussed and managed within a multidisciplinary team. This is true both in public hospitals and increasingly in the private health system as well. The majority of follow-up care in Australia is shared between the primary medical specialists who were involved in this multidisciplinary treatment. This usually involves the breast surgeon, radiation oncologist and/or medical oncologist. These specialist oncologists spend a large proportion of their clinical time (11–50% in one study [26]) providing follow-up care to women after breast cancer treatment. Despite the increasingly heavy burden on their practices, most specialists believe that such care is an important part of their role as a breast cancer specialist and most feel that the amount of time they spend on this is about right. Sustainability, however, has been identified as an issue [26]. Specialists are open to the idea of sharing follow-up care with primary care physicians, breast physicians (specially trained family physicians [27, 28] and breast care nurses [8, 9]).

Breast surgeons in Australia fall into two main categories: the larger group with breast and endocrine surgical expertise and the smaller group with breast surgical oncology expertise. There is a growing group of breast surgeons who are involved in oncoplastic breast surgical procedures to varying degrees. Currently, the primary group that represents the interests of breast surgeons is the Royal Australasian College of Surgeons Breast Surgery Section. The training of breast surgeons involves receiving appropriate subspecialty experience and training after completing general surgery training. This has not been as part of a prescribed training program but there are plans to develop this in the future. In the past the majority of practicing breast surgeons has gone overseas for 1–2 years to receive added experience and training. However, this is happening less often these days as fewer training posts are available. As many breast surgeons have an interest in breast surgery, but also do a wide range of general surgical procedures, there is also a wide range of caseloads and expertise. There is also a wide range of commitment to breast-related continuing medical education and there may be a tendency by some to deflect surveillance and management decisions to other oncology colleagues.

Breast physicians are unique to Australasia, sharing only few similarities with breast clinicians in the United Kingdom and having no counterparts in North America. A breast physician is a medical practitioner, usually from a family medicine (general practice) background, who undertakes additional specialized training in the diagnosis and management of breast disease [27, 28]. The skill mix varies from person to person but most breast physicians have skills that add value at all stages of the breast disease spectrum, including breast cancer diagnosis, ultrasound biopsy techniques, counseling, assisting at surgery, multidisciplinary involvement, and ongoing follow-up. This relatively small group of specialized clinicians has a unique and constantly expanding role in multidisciplinary breast teams in Australia and New Zealand and many breast surgeons work closely with breast physicians to enhance the quality of care they provide and to share follow-up care. A formal training program, examination process, fellowship, and set of competency standards have been developed for Australasian breast physicians [29].

Breast care nurses are specialist nurses who undertake further training and education in the area of support for breast cancer patients. They tend to specialize in coordination of care and providing a more tailored approach to support and treatment, enhancing medical specialist care during the diagnosis and treatment phases of the breast cancer journey. However, increasingly, the advanced qualifications of clinical nurse specialists and clinical nurse consultants are leading to the development of nurse-led clinics. These clinics have been successful in other specialist areas of medicine, such as midwifery and diabetes clinics, and may well extend to involve breast cancer surveillance and survivorship clinics in the future.

The use of a formal written Survivorship Care Plan (in the form of a standard follow-up program that could be modified for individual patient needs) has been recommended by some bodies [30]. There is limited evidence that a Survivorship Care Plan may increase confidence in shared care programs [26]. A Survivorship Care Plan suitable for the issues specific to the local environment is currently being developed for trial in Australia.

Guidelines for surveillance after treatment for early breast cancer have been developed by the National Breast and Ovarian Cancer Centre (NBOCC) and these are in widespread use. Updated guidelines were released in 2009 [18]. These guidelines include recommendations for holistic survivorship care. In addition, guidelines for the psychosocial care of women with cancer are available [31]. The guidelines are summarized in Tables 56.1.

They provide a framework for follow-up care and they may be adapted for individualized, tailored care through discussion with the patient and the multidisciplinary team. The framework is broadly followed by the majority of oncology multidisciplinary teams. The combination of specialists managing the patient varies, depending on the adjuvant therapy program. For instance, in a case with a low risk tumor with no chemotherapy, the surgeon and radiotherapist may alternate follow-up visits for the first 5 years so that someone reviews the person according to the recommended schedule but not the same person each visit. The general acceptance of this schedule by the oncology team members is high with many getting personal benefit and reassurance from the experience and finding such care rewarding in that it provides a balance to the poor outcomes and more advanced cases that many oncologists manage [26]. There also seems to be patient acceptance of this program with a reduction in frequency of contacts over the years following diagnosis.

Table 56.1 Australian national guidelines for surveillance care after breast cancer [18]

Purpose of follow-up care includes
The early detection of local, regional, or distant recurrence
Screening for a new primary breast cancer
Detection and management of treatment-related side effects
Detection and management of psychosocial distress, anxiety, or depression
Review and updating of family history
Observation of outcomes of therapy
Review of treatment, including new therapies that may be potentially relevant to the patient
Method of detection of recurrence or new breast cancer
Following breast conservation, women should have annual bilateral mammography with or without breast ultrasound
Follow-up with chest X-ray, bone scan, CT scan, PET scan, MRI, blood count, and biochemistry or tumor markers are not part of standard follow-up and are recommended only if clinically indicated
Follow-up care provider
Provider should be determined by the multidisciplinary team, including the general practitioner and the patient at the end of treatment
The profession of the health care provider who is responsible for follow-up care does not influence survival outcomes or psychosocial or quality of life outcomes and may include a medical oncologist, radiation oncologist, surgeon, breast care nurse and general practitioner
A patient held follow-up schedule should be provided to assist with coordination of the patient care plan as per NICE guidelines 2008
Other follow-up considerations
Psychosocial well-being and quality of life must be considered and appropriate referral offered when needed
Other disease, treatment, and patient factors may influence the requirements for follow-up and should be considered. These include
Long-term hormonal therapy
Age and hormonal status
Genetic factors
Accessibility of services
Clinical trial participation
Long-term effects of systemic therapy
Side effects of active treatment such as secondary lymphedema
Patient preference
Comorbidities
Management of interval presentation for investigation of symptoms
Bone health
Sexuality and body image
Fertility
Advice about lifestyle factors that may reduce risk of recurrence

Table 56.2 A surveillance program commonly utilized in Australia after treatment with curative-intent treatment for breast cancer

	Year posttreatment[b]					
Modality	1	2	3	4	5	>5
Office visit	2-4	2-4	1-2	12	1-2	1
Mammogram[a]	1	1	1	1	1	1

Women taking an aromatase inhibitor should have monitoring of bone health

Chest X-ray, bone scan, CT scan, PET, MRI, blood count, biochemistry, tumor markers, and pelvic examination are not routinely recommended

[a]First mammogram performed 12 months after diagnosis; bilateral mammography may be supplemented with breast ultrasound

[b]The numbers in the table indicate the number of times the modality is recommended during the indicated year posttreatment

Most patients seem to want the reassurance of these consultations with their treating team and it is unusual for patients not to attend. A surveillance program commonly utilized in Australia after treatment with curative-intent treatment is shown in Table 56.2. Particular things that may influence type and frequency of surveillance include.

1. Distance
   Women who live in remote area and need to travel to have breast imaging and to see their treatment team may have less frequent surveillance by a specialist and may instead have local surveillance with their family physician.
2. TNM Stage
   Women with noninvasive disease (DCIS only) or small low-grade cancers who are not experiencing any ongoing side effects of treatment may be managed with less frequent appointments with a medical specialist. They would still have yearly mammography, with or without ultrasound, in the majority of cases.
3. Type of Surgery for Primary Cancer
   An argument can be made for less intensive surveillance for women who had early breast cancer and were treated with mastectomy rather than breast preservation. Women who have had bilateral mastectomy, for example, are at very low risk of local recurrence. They remain at risk of systemic relapse and require appropriate monitoring for this as well as management of the consequences of therapy.

4. Type of Adjuvant Therapies
   Adjuvant therapy recommendations influence surveillance recommendations. Women undergoing chemotherapy with particular agents may require specific surveillance. For example, cardiac monitoring may be needed for women who experienced a decline in cardiac function during treatment with anthracyclines. Adjuvant endocrine therapy for estrogen-receptor (ER-positive) women has become more complicated in recent years (see below.) The previous standard 5 years of tamoxifen may now be replaced by a combination of sequential tamoxifen and upfront aromatase inhibitor treatment in various combinations. The therapy may extend beyond 5 years and may require monitoring and treatment for different side effects such as osteopenia/osteoporosis (Table 56.2).

The current standard of care for ER-positive breast cancer is 5 years of adjuvant endocrine therapy. This has been challenged by the MA 17 Study [32] that demonstrated a disease-free survival advantage for postmenopausal women continuing on an aromatase inhibitor (letrozole in this study) after completing 5 years of tamoxifen. It is well known that, after 5 years postsurgery, 30% of relapses occur in the subsequent 10 years [33]. For a woman who has had breast cancer and completed her treatment, there is still a substantial ongoing risk of her developing another breast cancer, or having the original breast cancer return. For these women, that chance can be up to 1 in 25 per year [34].

The Australian and New Zealand Breast Cancer Trials Group (ANZBCTG) is the largest breast cancer collaborative trials group in Australasia. [17] The ANZBCTG developed the study protocol for the ANZ 0501 (LATER) study to investigate the possible benefits of letrozole usage beyond 5 years in postmenopausal women who have completed a 5-year course of adjuvant endocrine therapy and have had a gap of more than 1 year without adjuvant endocrine therapy. The LATER study aims to determine whether recommencing adjuvant endocrine therapy in the form of letrozole can prevent or delay recurrence of breast cancer or prevent new breast cancers from developing [17]. The LATER study is a randomized double-blind trial and is an example of the high-quality collaborative clinical trials being developed in Australia and New Zealand.

The ANZBCTG is also participating in the IBCSG 35-07/BIG 1-07 SOLE Study. This study is interested in continuous versus intermittent letrozole in women after 4–6 years of adjuvant endocrine therapy. The theory is that the reintroduction of estrogen may help to sensitize cells to further exposure of an aromatase inhibitor drug [35]. Collaboration with other international trialists is occurring in Australia. This is encouraging many of the developing nations in the Asia-Pacific region to contribute participants to these large, multicenter international clinical trials.

Chemoprevention is in its infancy in Australia. It is an uncommon part of most management strategies. High-risk clinics exist in some centers and it is more often utilized in this setting.

As there may be a desire in rural-remote areas to form links with larger centers but the distances of travel are not practical, there is increasing investment in video-teleconferencing or web-based conferencing facilities. The practical issues of multiple specialists and paramedical staff meeting at the same time for a multidisciplinary meeting are significantly increased by these additional complexities but the effort can be rewarding for those involved and certainly adds to the confidence of patients managed in remote environments.

On June 30, 2006 the estimated Indigenous population of Australia was 517,200, or 2.5% of the total population. In the period 1996–2001, the life expectancy at birth for Indigenous Australians was estimated to be 59 years for males and 65 years for females, compared with 77 years for all males and 82 years for all females for the period 1998–2000, a difference of approximately 17 years for both males and females [36].

In 2006, more Indigenous people in Australia lived in major cities than in other areas (31%). The remaining Indigenous population was evenly distributed across Inner Regional (22%), Outer Regional (23%) and remote/very remote Australia (24%). Some of these Indigenous people are living in the most remote of environments, in some cases thousands of kilometers from medical assistance. Breast cancer is the most common cancer experienced by Aboriginal and Torres Strait Islander women but the incidence is lower than for the non-Indigenous population. There is evidence of later presentation and poorer outcomes. Aboriginal and Torres Strait Islander women had 9% higher rates of breast cancer mortality than the Australian female population as a whole, based on the age-standardized rates for the 2000–2004 period for Queensland, Western Australia, South Australia, and Northern Territory registered deaths [37].

In conclusion, survivorship care for women after treatment for early breast cancer must aim to maximize long-term quality of life, detect recurrent or new breast cancer, detect and manage treatment- related side effects and review options to commence, change, or continue ongoing treatments such as endocrine therapy. The majority of Australian people live in major well-resourced cities or large towns but the environment and rural-remote indigenous and nonindigenous populations add complexity to the challenge of providing equity of access and care.

References

1. Australian Institute of Health and Welfare, National Breast Cancer Centre. Breast cancer in Australia: an overview (cat. no. CAN 29.), Cancer series, vol. 34. Canberra: AIHW; 2006.
2. Tracey E, Baker D, Chen W, Stavrou E, Bishop J. Cancer in New South Wales: incidence, mortality and prevalence, 2005. Sydney: Cancer Institute NSW; 2007.
3. Hall SE, Holman CD, Hendrie DV, Spilsbury K. Unequal access to breast-conserving surgery in Western Australia 1982-2000. ANZ J Surg. 2004;74:413–9.

4. Kok DL, Chang JH, Erbas B, Fletcher A, Kavanagh AM, Henderson MA, et al. Urban-rural differences in the management of screen-detected invasive breast cancer and ductal carcinoma in situ in Victoria. ANZ J Surg. 2006;76:996–1001.
5. Spilsbury K, Semmens JB, Saunders CM, Hall SE, Holman CD. Subsequent surgery after initial breast conserving surgery: a population based study. ANZ J Surg. 2005;75:260–4.
6. Thompson B, Baade P, Coory M, Carrière P, Fritschi L. Patterns of surgical treatment for women diagnosed with early breast cancer in Queensland. Ann Surg Oncol. 2008;15:443–51.
7. Mitchell KJ, Fritschi L, Reid A, McEvoy SP, Ingram DM, Jamrozik K, et al. Rural-urban differences in the presentation, management and survival of breast cancer in Western Australia. Breast. 2006;15:769–76.
8. Centre NBC. Specialist breast nurse competency standards and associated educational requirements. Camperdown: National Breast Cancer Centre; 2005.
9. National Breast Cancer Centre (NBCC). Specialist Breast Nurses: an evidence-based model for Australian practice. Kings Cross: iSource National Breast Cancer Centre; 2000.
10. Cancer Institute NSW. Successful grants, 2008. http://www.cancer-institute.org.au/cancer_inst/grants/successful.html#ctnctn.
11. The McGrath Foundation. www.mcgrathfoundation.com.au. Accessed January 2009.
12. Sainsbury R, Haward B, Rider L, Johnston C, Round C. Influence of clinician workload and patterns of treatment on survival from breast cancer. Lancet. 1995;345(8960):1265–70.
13. Ingram DM, McEvoy SP, Byrne MJ, Fritschi L, Joseph DJ, Jamrozik K. Surgical caseload and outcomes for women with invasive breast cancer treated in Western Australia. Breast. 2005;14:11–7.
14. Breast Cancer Action Group. www.bcag.org.au. Accessed January 2009.
15. Breast Cancer Network Australia. www.bcna.org.au. Accessed January 2009.
16. Cancer voices Australia. www.cancervoicesaustralia.org.au. Accessed January 2009.
17. Australian New Zealand Breast Cancer Trials Group. www.anzbctg.org. Accessed January 2009.
18. National Breast Cancer Centre (NBCC). Recommendations for follow-up of women with early breast cancer. Camperdown: National Breast Cancer Centre; 2008.
19. National Breast Cancer Centre (NBCC). Clinical practice guidelines for the management of early breast cancer. 2nd ed. Camperdown: National Breast Cancer Centre; 2001.
20. National Breast Cancer Centre (NBCC). Clinical practice guidelines for the management of advanced breast cancer. Camperdown: National Breast Cancer Centre; 2001.
21. Demark-Wahnefried W, Pinto B, Gritz ER. Promoting health and physical function among cancer survivors: potential for prevention and questions that remain. J Clin Oncol. 2006;24:5125–31.
22. Ganz PA, Kwan L, Stanton AL, Krupnick JL, Rowland JH, Meyerowitz BE, et al. Quality of life at the end of primary treatment of breast cancer: first results from the moving beyond cancer randomized trial. JNCI J Natl Cancer Inst. 2004;96:376–837.
23. Broeckel JA, Jacobsen PB, Balducci L, Horton J, Lyman GH. Quality of life after adjuvant chemotherapy for breast cancer. Breast Cancer Res Treat. 2000;62:141–50.
24. Holzner B, Kemmler G, Kopp M, Moschen R, Schweigkofler H, Dünser M, et al. Quality of life in breast cancer patients-not enough attention for long-term survivors? Psychosomatics. 2001;42:117–23.
25. Winer EP, Lindley C, Hardee M, Sawyer WT, Brunatti C, Borstelmann NA, et al. Quality of life in patients surviving at least 12 months following high dose chemotherapy with autologous bone marrow support. Psychooncology. 1999;8:167–76.
26. Brennan ME, Butow P, Spillane AJ, Boyle FM. Follow-up care after treatment for early breast cancer- practices and attitudes of Australian health professionals. Asia Pac J Clin Oncol. 2008;4 Suppl 2:A108.
27. Brennan ME, Spillane AJ. The evolving role of the breast physician in the multidisciplinary breast team ANZJS. 2007;77:846–9.
28. Brennan ME, Spillane AJ. The breast physician-an example of specialisation in general practice. Med J Aust. 2007;187:111–4.
29. The Australasian Society of Breast Physicians. Standards for Training and Competency of Breast Physicians. Sydney: Australasian Society of Breast Physicians; 2007.
30. Hewitt M, Greenfield S, Stovall E. From cancer patient to cancer survivor: lost in transition: National Academics Press; 2006.
31. National Breast Cancer Centre (NBCC), National Cancer Control Initiative (NCCI). Clinical practice guidelines for the psychosocial care of adults with cancer. Camperdown: National Breast Cancer Centre; 2003.
32. Goss PE, Ingle JN, Pater JL, Martino S, Robert NJ, Muss HB, et al. Late extended adjuvant treatment with letrozole improves outcome in women with early-stage breast cancer who complete 5 years of tamoxifen. J Clin Oncol. 2008;26:1948–55.
33. Early Breast Cancer Trialists' Collaborative Group (EBCTCG). Effects of chemotherapy and hormonal therapy for early breast cancer on recurrence and 15-year survival: an overview of the randomised trials. Lancet. 2005;365(9472):1687–717.
34. Saphner T, Tormey DC, Gray R. Annual hazard rates of recurrence for breast cancer after primary therapy. J Clin Oncol. 1996;14:2738–46.
35. Jordan VC, Lewis JS, Osipo C, Cheng D. The apoptotic action of estrogen following exhaustive antihormonal therapy: a new clinical treatment strategy. Breast. 2005;14:624–30.
36. Australian Bureau of Statistics. Population distribution, Aboriginal and Torres Strait Islander Australians. Canberra: Commonwealth of Australia; 2006.
37. National Breast Cancer Centre (NBCC). Statistics. www.nbcc.org.au/bestpractice/statistics.
38. Hewitt M, Greenfield S, Stovall E. From cancer patient to cancer survivor: lost in transition: National Academies Press; 2006.

Breast Carcinoma Surveillance Counterpoint: Japan

57

Eriko Tokunaga and Yoshihiko Maehara

Keywords
Breast cancer • NCCN • Genetic counseling • Japan • Early detection

In Japan, the incidence of breast cancer and the number of breast cancer-related deaths are increasing. Many Japanese doctors who have a major interest in breast cancer acknowledge the importance of evidence-based management of breast cancer, including surveillance after primary therapy. The Japanese Breast Cancer Society (JBCS) has published guidelines about systemic therapy, surgery, radiation therapy, screening, diagnosis, and epidemiology of breast cancer since 2004. The guidelines are written in Japanese and they are updated periodically. The JBCS guidelines refer to international professional organizations such as The American Society of Clinical Oncology (ASCO). The principles of surveillance after primary therapy are described in one of the guidelines. In our hospital, we perform surveillance based on the JBCS guidelines. We also refer to the guidelines of ASCO and the National Comprehensive Cancer Network (NCCN). Thus, the practice of surveillance is similar to that in the United States.

Genetic counseling is increasingly important. Mutation rates of BRCA1 and BRCA2 have been studied in Japanese breast cancer families. Early studies conducted on a few patients reported that the mutation rate for BRCA1 was 10% and that of BRCA2 was 15% [1, 2]. Later, mutation analysis of BRCA1 and BRCA2 was conducted on 113 breast cancer patients with at least 1 breast cancer or 1 ovarian cancer patient in their first-degree relatives [3]. Fifteen deleterious mutations (13.3%) were identified in BRCA1, and 21 deleterious mutations (18.6%) were identified in BRCA2. In site-specific breast cancer families, the mutation frequency of BRCA1 or BRCA2 was high in families with three or more breast cancer patients (36%, 9/25), early onset (40< or = years old) breast cancer patients (38%, 19/50), and bilateral breast cancer patients (40%, 6/15). Haplotype analysis suggests that carriers of each of these mutations have common ancestors. These results demonstrate that family profiles are important determinants of the risk for carrying a BRCA1 or BRCA2 mutation and that the cumulative frequency of BRCA1 and BRCA2 mutations in Japanese breast cancer families (31.9%) is within the range observed in Caucasian breast cancer families. The US Preventive Services Task Force published a systemic evidence review on genetic risk assessment and BRCA mutation testing for breast and ovarian cancer susceptibility [4]. Risk assessment, genetic counseling, and mutation testing did not cause adverse psychological outcomes, and counseling improved distress and risk perception in the highly selected populations studied. However, because there are no mature systems for genetic counseling and testing in Japan, it is not currently recommended for women with a family history of breast cancer to have screening for mutations of BRCA1 and BRCA2.

Pregnancy after a diagnosis of breast cancer has not been shown to affect the prognosis. We generally support patients who wish to become pregnant after breast cancer treatment. We usually recommend delaying pregnancy for at least 2 years after completion of cytotoxic therapy. However, we also respect the wishes of the patient and her family.

Surveillance for toxicity and complications of treatment is routinely done. Endometrial cancer screening is included in the surveillance of all patients taking tamoxifen. We question all women taking tamoxifen at each visit about

E. Tokunaga, M.D., Ph.D. (✉) • Y. Maehara, M.D., Ph.D., F.A.C.S.
Department of Surgery and Science, Graduate School of Medical Sciences, Kyushu University, 3-1-1 Maidashi, Higashi-ku, Fukuoka 812-8582, Japan
e-mail: eriko@surg2.med.kyushu-u.ac.jp; maehara@surg2.med.kyushu-u.ac.jp

F.E. Johnson et al. (eds.), *Patient Surveillance After Cancer Treatment*, Current Clinical Oncology,
DOI 10.1007/978-1-60327-969-7_57,

Table 57.1 Surveillance after curative-intent treatment for ductal carcinoma in situ at Kyushu University, Japan

	Year posttreatment[$]					
Modality	1	2	3	4	5	>5
Office visit	2–4	2	2	2	2	1
Mammography	1	1	1	1	1	1
Breast ultrasound	1	1	1	1	1	1

If patient is treated with tamoxifen, gynecological assessment is performed annually or biannually
The numbers in the table indicate the number of times the modality is recommended during the indicated year posttreatment

Table 57.2 Surveillance after curative-intent treatment for invasive breast carcinoma at Kyushu University, Japan

	Year posttreatment					
Modality	1	2	3	4	5	>5
Office visit	2–4	2–4	2–4	2–4	2–4	1
Liver function tests[a]	2–4	2–4	2–4	2–4	2–4	1
Mammography	1[b]	1	1	1	1	1
Breast ultrasonography	1[b]	1	1	1	1	1
Serum CEA level	2–4	2–4	2–4	2–4	2–4	2–4
Serum CA15-3 level	2–4	2–4	2–4	2–4	2–4	2–4

- Women on tamoxifen should have gynecological assessment annually or biannually if the uterus is present.
- Women on an aromatase inhibitor or who experience ovarian failure secondary to treatment should have monitoring of bone health, according to current standard local practice.
- Chest X-ray, bone scintigram, abdominal CT, chest CT, and abdominal ultrasonography are performed only if clinically indicated.
- *CEA* carcinoembryonic antigen, *CT* computed tomography.
- The numbers in the table indicate the number of times the modality is recommended during the indicated year posttreatment.

[a]Consists of serum alkaline phosphatase and lactic dehydrogenase levels
[b]Mammogram and breast ultrasonography again at 6–12 months postradiation if the breast is conserved

symptoms related to gynecological disorders such as abnormal bleeding. We recommend a prompt visit to a gynecologist if abnormal bleeding or other gynecological symptoms occur. We recommend regular pelvic examination and screening for endometrial cancer by a gynecologist. In the NCCN guidelines, gynecologic assessment every 12 months is recommended for women with an intact uterus. However, many Japanese gynecologists recommend the screening for endometrial cancer every 6 months for patients taking tamoxifen.

The use of aromatase inhibitors or ovarian failure induced by treatment may cause bone loss. We monitor bone health with a bone mineral density determination at baseline and periodically thereafter for women on an aromatase inhibitor or who experience ovarian failure secondary to treatment.

The pattern of breast cancer recurrence, including the time frame, is similar in western countries and Japan. In our hospital, we perform postoperative surveillance based on the guidelines published by JBCS, as mentioned earlier. This includes a careful history and physical examination and inspection and palpation of the local region (ipsilateral chest wall, axillary region, supraclavicular region, and contralateral breast). Blood tests (liver function tests and serum CEA and CA15-3 levels) are obtained at each visit. Patients with invasive breast carcinoma are seen two to four times a year for 5 years. For patients with noninvasive ductal carcinoma, we recommend office visits two to four times for year 1 and then two times each year. We recommend that patients receiving adjuvant endocrine therapy visit us more frequently than those not receiving such therapy. We perform mammography and breast ultrasound annually to detect recurrence in the contralateral breast and the ipsilateral breast after the breast-conserving therapy, as well as nodal recurrence.

Berg and colleagues reported that there is a benefit of adding breast ultrasound to screening mammography for women with an elevated baseline risk of breast cancer [5]. Adding a single screening ultrasound to mammography yields an additional 1.1–7.2 cancer diagnoses per 1,000 high-risk women. However, it also substantially increases the number of unnecessary biopsies. There are few high-quality reports that have shown the utility of ultrasound, but we feel that breast ultrasound is very useful and effective to detect a new primary lesion in patients who have had breast cancer, especially for young women with dense breasts on mammography and for women after breast-conserving surgery for cancer.

We do not routinely perform chest X-ray, chest and abdominal computed tomography (CT), bone scintigraphy, liver ultrasonography, MRI, and FDG-PET, as these are not recommended in either the JBCS guidelines or international expert guidelines.

Previous studies have reported that the combination of serum CA15-3 and CEA levels is potentially more sensitive than radiographic imaging in detecting early disease recurrence. Elevation of these markers has been shown to predict breast cancer relapse with an average lead time of 5–6 months [6], but they are neither sensitive nor specific for breast cancer relapse. Since serum CA15-3 and CEA levels are not elevated in all patients with metastatic breast cancer, we consider that the clinical utility of serial serum tumor marker measurement is not fully defined. However, we feel that following CA15-3 and CEA levels is a useful and inexpensive method for detecting tumor recurrence, particularly hormone receptor-positive breast cancer. If there is a sustained elevation of these markers, patients are screened for metastatic disease using other modalities. Similarly, elevated serum alkaline phosphatase and lactic dehydrogenase levels sometimes predict liver and/or bone metastasis, so we now measure them at each visit.

To summarize, the goals of surveillance after primary treatment for breast cancer are early recognition and treatment of potentially curable recurrences and second primary breast cancers, evaluation for therapy-related complications, and detection of symptoms consistent with metastatic disease. In Japan, intensive surveillance was regularly performed until several years ago. Many patients believe that intensive follow-up and early detection of tumor recurrence leads to a longer survival, but evidence from well-controlled trials indicates that it has little impact on patient prognosis. In addition, excessive medical procedures have financial implications. In Japan, 70–90% of medical costs are reimbursed by the health insurance system supported by the government. Rising costs have become a major economic problem in Japan. We now appreciate the importance of the patient education about breast cancer, its treatment, and appropriate surveillance testing. We explain to our patients the importance of evidence-based surveillance after primary breast cancer therapy. We believe that this educational effort leads to improved quality of life.

References

1. Inoue R, Fukutomi T, Ushijima T, Matsumoto Y, Sugimura T, Nagao M. Germline mutation of BRCA1 in Japanese breast cancer families. Cancer Res. 1995;55:3521–4.
2. Inoue R, Ushijima T, Fukutomi T, Fukami A, Sugimura H, Inoue S, et al. BRCA2 germline mutations in Japanese breast cancer families. Int J Cancer. 1997;74:199–204.
3. Ikeda N, Miyoshi Y, Yoneda K, Shiba E, Sekihara Y, Kinoshita M, et al. Frequency of *BRCA1* and *BRCA2* germline mutations in Japanese breast cancer families. Int J Cancer. 2001;91:83–8.
4. Nelson HD, Huffman LH, Fu R, Harris EL, U.S. Preventive Service Task Force. Genetic risk assessment and BRCA mutation testing for breast and ovarian cancer susceptibility: systemic evidence review for the U.S. Preventive Services Task Force. Ann Inter Med. 2005;143:362–79.
5. Berg WA, Blume JD, Cormack JB, Mendelson EB, Lehrer D, Bohm-Velez M, et al. Combined screening with ultrasound and mammography vs. mammography alone in women at elevated risk of breast cancer. JAMA. 2008;299:2151–63.
6. Molina R, Zanon G, Filella X, Moreno F, Jo J, Daniels M, et al. Use of serial carcinoembryonic antigen and CA 15.3 assays in detecting relapses in breast cancer patients. Breast Cancer Res Treat. 1995;36:41–8.

Endometrial Carcinoma

58

David Y. Johnson, Shilpi Wadhwa, and Frank E. Johnson

Keywords
Corpus uteri • Estrogen • Surveillance • Tamoxifen • Obesity • Hypertension

The International Agency for Research on Cancer (IARC), a component of the World Health Organization (WHO), estimated that there were 198,783 new cases of cancer of corpus uteri (cornu of uterus, endometrium, fundus, myometrium, but excluding isthmus of uterus), worldwide in 2002 [1]. The IARC also estimated that there were 50,327 deaths due to this cause in 2002 [1].

The American Cancer Society estimated that there were 39,080 new cases and 7,400 deaths due to this cause in the United States in 2007 [2]. The estimated 5-year survival rate (all races) in the USA in 2007 was 84 % for corpus uteri [2]. Survival rates were adjusted for normal life expectancies and were based on cases diagnosed from 1996 to 2002 and followed through 2003.

Women with elevated estrogen levels have an increased likelihood of developing endometrial cancer. Use of tamoxifen is also associated with increased risk. Obesity, consumption of a high-fat diet, diabetes mellitus, hypertension, gallbladder disease, and prior pelvic radiation also confer increased risk [3, 4].

D.Y. Johnson • S. Wadhwa
Department of Internal Medicine, Saint Louis University Medical Center, Saint Louis, MO, USA

F.E. Johnson (✉)
Saint Louis University Medical Center and Saint Louis Veterans Affairs Medical Center, Saint Louis, MO, USA
e-mail: frank.johnson1@va.gov

Geographic Variation Worldwide

The incidence of endometrial cancer is highest in white women as compared to other races. However, in the United States women of various ethnicities experience the highest rates in the world [3]. Geographic variation in the United States is also pronounced [5].

Surveillance Strategies Proposed By Professional Organizations or National Government Agencies and Available on the Internet

National Comprehensive Cancer Network (NCCN, www.nccn.org)

NCCN guidelines were accessed on January 28, 2012 (Table 58.1). There were minor qualitative changes compared to the guidelines accessed on April 10, 2007.

American Society of Clinical Oncology (ASCO, www.asco.org)

ASCO guidelines were accessed on January 28, 2012. No quantitative guidelines exist for endometrial cancer surveillance, including when first accessed on October 31, 2007.

F.E. Johnson et al. (eds.), *Patient Surveillance After Cancer Treatment*, Current Clinical Oncology,
DOI 10.1007/978-1-60327-969-7_58,

Table 58.1 Uterine neoplasms: endometrial carcinoma

	Years posttreatment[a]					
	1	2	3	4	5	>5
Office visit	2–4	2–4	1–2	1–2	1–2	1–2
Vaginal cytology	2	2	1	1	1	1
Chest X-ray	1	1	1	1	1	1
Patient education regarding symptoms						
CA-125 optional						
CT/MRI as clinically indicated						
Consider genetic counseling/testing for young patients (<55 years old) with a significant family history and/or selected pathologic risk features[b,c]						

Source: Obtained from NCCN (www.nccn.org) on January 28, 2012

NCCN guidelines were accessed on January 28, 2012. There were minor qualitative changes compared to the guidelines accessed on April 10, 2007

[a] The numbers in the table indicate the number of times the modality is recommended during the indicated year posttreatment

[b] Screening with immunohistochemistry should be considered in all patients, but especially in patients younger than 55 years

[c] See Lynch syndrome/HNPCC in NCCN Colorectal Cancer Screening Guidelines

Table 58.2 Endometrial cancer

	Years posttreatment[a]					
	1	2	3	4	5	>5
Office visit	3–4	3–4	2	2	2	0[b]
The utility of Pap smears for detection of local recurrences has not been demonstrated						

Source: Obtained from ESMO (www.esmo.org) on January 28, 2012

ESMO guidelines were accessed on January 28, 2012. These are new quantitative guidelines compared to the guidelines accessed on October 31, 2007

[a] The numbers in the table indicate the number of times the modality is recommended during the indicated year posttreatment

[b] Further investigations after 5 years can be performed if clinically indicated

The Society of Surgical Oncology (SSO, www.surgonc.org)

SSO guidelines were accessed on January 28, 2012. No quantitative guidelines exist for endometrial cancer surveillance, including when first accessed on October 31, 2007.

European Society for Medical Oncology (ESMO, www.esmo.org)

ESMO guidelines were accessed on January 28, 2012 (Table 58.2). There are new quantitative guidelines compared to the guidelines accessed on October 31, 2007.

Table 58.3 Endometrial cancer: low risk of recurrence (stage IA or IB, grade 1 or 2)

	Years posttreatment[a]					
	1	2	3	4	5	>5
Office visit[b]	1–2	1–2	1–2	1	1	1
It is recommended that all patients receive counseling about the potential symptoms of recurrence of endometrial cancer[c]						
There is insufficient evidence to inform the routine use of Pap smear, chest X-ray, abdominal ultrasound, computed tomography (CT) scan, of CA-125 testing to detect asymptomatic recurrences						
Where treatment with radiotherapy is involved, it is recommended that patients be counseled on the potential adverse effects of radiotherapy[d]						

Source: Obtained from CCO (www.cancercare.on.ca) on January 28, 2012

CCO guidelines were accessed on January 28, 2012. There were no significant changes compared to the guidelines accessed on October 31, 2007

[a] The numbers in the table indicate the number of times the modality is recommended during the indicated year posttreatment

[b] Including a complete history and a pelvic-rectal examination

[c] Symptomatic signs of possible recurrence can include, but are not limited to, unexplained vaginal bleeding or discharge, detection of a mass, abdominal distension, persistent pain, especially in the abdomen or pelvic region, fatigue, diarrhea, nausea or vomiting, persistent cough, swelling, or weight loss

[d] Include complications with the rectum, urinary bladder, vagina, skin, subcutaneous tissue, bones, and other sites

European Society of Surgical Oncology (ESSO, www.esso-surgeonline.org)

ESSO guidelines were accessed on January 28, 2012. No quantitative guidelines exist for endometrial cancer surveillance, including when first accessed on October 31, 2007.

Cancer Care Ontario (CCO, www.cancercare.on.ca)

CCO guidelines were accessed on January 28, 2012 (Tables 58.3 and 58.4). There were no significant changes compared to the guidelines accessed on October 31, 2007.

National Institute for Clinical Excellence (NICE, www.nice.org.uk)

NICE guidelines were accessed on January 28, 2012. No quantitative guidelines exist for endometrial cancer surveillance, including when first accessed on October 31, 2007.

Table 58.4 Endometrial cancer: high risk of recurrence (stage IA or IB, grade 3, or stage IC or advanced stage)

	Years posttreatment[a]					
	1	2	3	4	5	>5
Office visit[b]	2–4	2–4	2–4	2	2	1

It is recommended that all patients receive counseling about the potential symptoms of recurrence of endometrial cancer[c]

There is insufficient evidence to inform the routine use of Pap smear, chest X-ray, abdominal ultrasound, computed tomography (CT) scan, of CA-125 testing to detect asymptomatic recurrences

Where treatment with radiotherapy is involved, it is recommended that patients be counseled on the potential adverse effects of radiotherapy[d]

Source: Obtained from CCO (www.cancercare.on.ca) on January 28, 2012

CCO guidelines were accessed on January 28, 2012. There were no significant changes compared to the guidelines accessed on October 31, 2007

[a]The numbers in the table indicate the number of times the modality is recommended during the indicated year posttreatment

[b]Including a complete history and a pelvic-rectal examination

[c]Symptomatic signs of possible recurrence can include, but are not limited to, unexplained vaginal bleeding or discharge, detection of a mass, abdominal distension, persistent pain, especially in the abdomen or pelvic region, fatigue, diarrhea, nausea or vomiting, persistent cough, swelling, or weight loss

[d]Include complications with the rectum, urinary bladder, vagina, skin, subcutaneous tissue, bones, and other sites

Table 58.5 Gynecologic malignancies: endometrial cancer, low risk (stage IA grade 1 or 2)

	Years posttreatment[a]					
	1	2	3	4	5	>5
Office visit	2	1	1[b]	1[b]	1[b]	1[b]

Papanicolaou test/cytologic evidence, cancer antigen 125, radiographic imaging (chest X-ray, positron emission tomography/computed tomography, magnetic resonance imaging) not recommended for routine use

Computed tomography and/or positron emission tomography scan ± cancer antigen 125 recommended if recurrence suspected

Source: Obtained from SGO[c] (www.sgo.org) on January 28, 2012

SGO guidelines were accessed on January 28, 2012. These are new quantitative guidelines compared to no guidelines found on December 13, 2007

[a]The numbers in the table indicate the number of times the modality is recommended during the indicated year posttreatment

[b]May be followed by a generalist or gynecologic oncologist

[c]These guidelines were obtained from the SGO website but are from the American Journal of Obstetrics and Gynecology (www.ajog.org)

The Cochrane Collaboration (CC, www.cochrane.org)

CC guidelines were accessed on January 28, 2012. No quantitative guidelines exist for endometrial cancer surveillance, including when first accessed on November 24, 2007.

Table 58.6 Gynecologic malignancies: endometrial cancer, intermediate risk (stage IB or II)

	Years posttreatment[a]					
	1	2	3	4	5	>5
Office visit	4	2	2[b]	2[b]	2[b]	1[c]

Papanicolaou test/cytologic evidence, cancer antigen 125, radiographic imaging (chest X-ray, positron emission tomography/computed tomography, magnetic resonance imaging) not recommended for routine use

Computed tomography and/or positron emission tomography scan ± cancer antigen 125 recommended if recurrence suspected

Source: Obtained from SGO[d] (www.sgo.org) on January 28, 2012

SGO guidelines were accessed on January 28, 2012. These are new quantitative guidelines compared to no guidelines found on December 13, 2007

[a]The numbers in the table indicate the number of times the modality is recommended during the indicated year posttreatment

[b]Consider alternating visits with a generalist and gynecologic oncologist

[c]May be followed by a generalist or gynecologic oncologist

[d]These guidelines were obtained from the SGO website but are from the American Journal of Obstetrics and Gynecology (www.ajog.org)

Table 58.7 Gynecologic malignancies: endometrial cancer, high risk (stage III/IV, serous or clear cell)

	Years posttreatment[a]					
	1	2	3	4	5	>5
Office visit	4	4	2	2	2	1[b]

Papanicolaou test/cytologic evidence, cancer antigen 125, radiographic imaging (chest X-ray, positron emission tomography/computed tomography, magnetic resonance imaging) not recommended for routine use

Computed tomography and/or positron emission tomography scan ± cancer antigen 125 recommended if recurrence suspected

Source: Obtained from SGO[c] (www.sgo.org) on January 28, 2012

SGO guidelines were accessed on January 28, 2012. These are new quantitative guidelines compared to no guidelines found on December 13, 2007

[a]The numbers in the table indicate the number of times the modality is recommended during the indicated year posttreatment

[b]May be followed by a generalist or gynecologic oncologist

[c]These guidelines were obtained from the SGO website but are from the American Journal of Obstetrics and Gynecology (www.ajog.org)

Society of Gynecologic Oncologists (SGO, www.sgo.org)

SGO guidelines were accessed on January 28, 2012 (Tables 58.5–58.7). There are new quantitative guidelines compared to no guidelines found on December 13, 2007.

The M.D. Anderson Surgical Oncology Handbook also has follow-up guidelines, proposed by authors from a single National Cancer Institute-designated Comprehensive Cancer Center, for many types of cancer [6]. Some are detailed and quantitative, others are qualitative.

Summary

This is a relatively common gynecologic cancer with the highest rate of incidence in white women and women of multiethnic origin residing in the United States. We found consensus-based guidelines but none based on high-quality evidence.

References

1. Parkin DM, Whelan SL, Ferlay J, Teppo L, Thomas DB. Cancer incidence in five continents, Vol. VIII, International Agency for Research on Cancer, 2002. (IARC Scientific Publication 155). Lyon, France: IARC Press; 2002. ISBN 92-832-2155-9.
2. Jemal A, Seigel R, Ward E, Murray T, Xu J, Thun MJ. Cancer Statistics, 2007. CA Cancer J Clin. 2007;57:43–66.
3. Schottenfeld D, Fraumeni JG. Cancer epidemiology and prevention. 3rd ed. New York, NY: Oxford University Press; 2006. ISBN 13:978-0-19-514961-6.
4. DeVita VT, Hellman S, Rosenberg SA. Cancer. 7th ed. Philadelphia, PA: Lippincott Williams & Wilkins; 2005. ISBN 0-781-74450-4.
5. Devesa SS, Grauman DJ, Blot WJ, Pennello GA, Hoover RN, Fraumeni JF Jr. Atlas of cancer mortality in the United States. National Institutes of Health, National Cancer Institute. NIH Publication No. 99-4564; 1999.
6. Feig BW, Berger DH, Fuhrman GM. The M.D. Anderson surgical oncology handbook. 4th ed. Philadelphia, PA: Lippincott Williams & Wilkins; 2006. paperback. ISBN 0-7817-5643-X.

Endometrial Cancer Surveillance Counterpoint: USA

59

Amit Bhate, Eric Donnelly, John Lurain, Julian Schink, and William Small Jr.

Keywords
Endometrium • Gynecologic cancer • Posttreatment • Surveillance • Women • Recurrence

Endometrial cancer is the most common gynecologic cancer in the United States, comprising 6% of diagnosed cancers and accounting for 3% of all cancer deaths in women annually. Over 40,000 new cases of endometrial cancer are diagnosed in the USA every year [1]. On presentation, the vast majority are confined to the uterus. Treatment generally entails a hysterectomy and bilateral salpingo-oophorectomy, as well as peritoneal cytology with or without pelvic and/or para-aortic lymphadenectomy. Patients deemed to be at risk for recurrence may receive postoperative adjuvant radiation therapy and/or chemotherapy. The 5-year survival rate is 95% for localized endometrial cancer and 83% for all stages combined. Overall, the recurrence rate is approximately 15%. The majority occur within the first 3 years [1].

There are no evidence-based guidelines regarding post-treatment surveillance for patients with endometrial cancer. Surveillance has largely been established by institutional preferences. The main motivation is the premise that early detection improves outcomes. However, there is no definitive evidence that frequent surveillance in this patient population with favorable outcomes appreciably improves survival. Since most patients have early-stage disease with relatively low recurrence rates, modifications in surveillance should be made based on individual patient characteristics. With the ever-rising cost of health care, it is imperative to use a cost-effective approach for surveillance based on risk of recurrence.

The issue of postsurgical surveillance in patients with endometrial cancer has been a topic of discussion in several publications [2–7]. Fung-Kee-Fung et al. performed a systematic review of 16 noncomparative retrospective studies that reported data on the strategies for patients who had received potentially curative treatment for endometrial cancer. The overall recurrence rate was 13%, with 61% of recurrences being distant metastases. The majority of recurrences were detected within 3 years across all studies, ranging from 68 to 100%. The most commonly performed tests were physical examination, vaginal vault cytology, and chest X-rays. All of the studies emphasized physical examination and vaginal vault cytology at every visit, except one in which vaginal vault cytology was done at every other visit [6].

Likewise, Agboola et al. reported a retrospective review of 432 patients with endometrial cancer who were treated with curative intent. The median follow-up duration was 54.5 months. Fifty patients had a recurrence (19 local and 31 distant). Asymptomatic recurrences were noted in 20 patients (10 local and 10 distant). There was no difference in overall survival duration between symptomatic and asymptomatic patients [7].

Currently, the National Comprehensive Cancer Network (NCCN) recommends that follow-up include a focused history and physical examination, vaginal cytology, chest

A. Bhate, M.D. • E. Donnelly, M.D.
Department of Radiation Oncology, The Robert H. Lurie Comprehensive Cancer Center of Northwestern University, 10 Health Services Drive, DeKalb, IL 60115, USA
e-mail: ambhate@hotmail.com; eric-donnelly@md.northwestern.edu

J. Lurain, M.D. • J. Schink, M.D.
Department of Obstetrics and Gynecology, Division of Gynecologic Oncology, The Robert H. Lurie Comprehensive Cancer Center, Northwestern University Feinberg School of Medicine, 250 East Superior Street, Suite 05-2168, Chicago, IL 60611, USA
e-mail: jlurain@nmff.org; jschink@nmff.org

W. Small Jr., M.D. (✉)
Department of Radiation Oncology, The Robert H. Lurie Comprehensive Cancer Center of Northwestern University, Radiation Oncology, Galter LC-178, 251 E. Huron Street, Chicago, IL 60611, USA
e-mail: wsmall@nmff.org

F.E. Johnson et al. (eds.), *Patient Surveillance After Cancer Treatment*, Current Clinical Oncology, DOI 10.1007/978-1-60327-969-7_59, © Springer Science+Business Media New York 2013

X-ray, and (optional) serum CA-125 level [8]. These recommendations and data from the recent studies by Fung-Kee-Fung et al. and Agboola et al. and other classic studies [2–5] are discussed in the following sections.

History and physical examination is the most effective method of follow-up. In the studies evaluated by Fung-Kee-Fung et al., physical examination found asymptomatic recurrences in 5–33% of patients. When the data were pooled, 53% of recurrences were found on physical examination alone. Similarly, Agboola et al. reported that, of 50 recurrences, 21 (42%) were detected by physical examination. These numbers compare well to other classic studies in which approximately 52% of asymptomatic patients with recurrence had the recurrence detected by physical examination [2–5]. Approximately two-thirds of patients with recurrence were symptomatic, indicating that patient education about the signs and symptoms associated with recurrent disease is an important part of a routine follow-up program. These studies strongly support the importance of a focused history and physical examination in routine follow-up visits.

Fung-Kee-Fung et al. reported that 4% or less of asymptomatic recurrences was detected by vaginal vault cytology. Agboola et al. noted that, of 4,830 Pap smears performed routinely on 410 patients, cancer was detected in only 6 Pap smears (0.1%). In the four classic surveillance series [2–5], only 13 (6.9%) of the 188 patients with recurrent disease had abnormal vaginal cytology. Based on these findings, the benefit of Pap smears in patients treated for endometrial cancer appears to be minimal, calling into question its routine use. Several other recent studies have also addressed its value for surveillance in endometrial cancer patients, finding it to be costly and ineffective, benefiting less than 1% of patients [9, 10]. In addition, patients treated with postoperative radiation and/or chemotherapy for endometrial cancer often have subsequent Pap smears that demonstrate inconclusive results secondary to treatment-related changes. These patients are then frequently subjected to further examinations, such as colposcopy with biopsies. This practice leads to higher health care costs and increased psychological stress for patients. In conclusion, the authors recommend the elimination or reduction of infrequency of vaginal cytology for the majority of patients.

In the four historical studies cited earlier, of 188 patients, 17 (9%) with recurrence had disease detected by chest X-ray [2–5]. In their reviews, Fung-Kee-Fung et al. [6] reported that 0 to 14% of asymptomatic recurrences were detected by chest X-ray and Agboola et al. [7] noted that recurrences were detected in only 7 of 2,057 (0.3%) routine chest X-rays. In addition to the low likelihood of detecting recurrences by routine chest X-rays, the survival rate for patients found to have recurrent, metastatic endometrial cancer is extremely poor [11]. A major goal of any surveillance strategy is to detect recurrence early, so that therapy may be initiated in a timely fashion with the intent of improving outcomes. Even with the use of current multiagent chemotherapeutic regimens, the median survival duration for this subset of patients is approximately 1 year.

Serum CA-125 levels obtained preoperatively have been shown to correlate with postsurgical pathologic findings, including histologic grade, stage, depth of myometrial invasion, and lymph node status [12]. The role for posttreatment CA-125 levels has yet to be determined. Rose et al. found that 55% of women with high-risk disease (stage II–IV, grade 3, or serous or clear cell histology) had serum CA-125 levels >35 U/mL (upper limit of normal) when recurrence was noted [13]. Reddoch et al. detected recurrence in 26% of asymptomatic patients by an elevated CA-125 level [3]. Likewise, Pastner et al. noted that among 13 women with stage I–II disease that recurred within the pelvis, abdomen, or lungs, 7 had elevated serum CA-125 levels. The six women with normal CA-125 levels had recurrences isolated to the vagina. Of note, four women were found to have elevated CA-125 levels without detectable recurrence [14].

To summarize, the recurrence rate in endometrial cancer is low: approximately 15% overall and less than 5% for low-risk disease [1]. Thus, the majority of women who are followed will not have recurrence of disease regardless of the surveillance strategy utilized. The primary goal of any surveillance strategy is to detect recurrence early so that appropriate salvage therapy can be initiated with the goal of improving morbidity and mortality. Intensive follow-up does not change survival in patients with early stage endometrial cancer. Therefore, simplified follow-up programs tailored for patient subsets with different recurrence risks are recommended [15]. The modality that seems to have the most value is history and physical examination. Current data demonstrate that routine Pap testing and chest X-rays have minimal value. Most recurrences occur within 3 years from the time of diagnosis [6], questioning the value of long-term follow-up. In addition, approximately two-thirds of recurrences are symptomatic and would be detected regardless of the follow-up strategy, highlighting the importance of patient education of signs and symptoms of recurrence for prompt recognition. Another significant component of a follow-up visit that often goes unaddressed is the psychological and emotional support that it can provide. This type of end point is difficult to measure objectively. Regardless, it is the physician's duty to provide this type of support and reassurance. In addition to cancer surveillance, oncologists can have a major impact on non-oncologic related health care issues, including further cancer screening, routine health maintenance, and lifestyle recommendations.

The NCCN currently recommends the following: physical examination every 3–6 months for the first 2 years, then 6 months or annually thereafter; vaginal cytology every 6 months for 2 years and annually thereafter; chest X-ray annually, although this recommendation is based on lower-

Table 59.1 Surveillance after curative-intent treatment for endometrial carcinoma at Northwestern University

	Year					
Modality	1	2	3	4	5	>5
Office visit[a]	4	4	2	2	2	1
Chest X-ray	1	1	1	0	0	0

[a]History and physical examination, with attention to vaginal cuff
In patients with papillary serous carcinoma and in patients with elevated serum CA-125 levels prior to treatment, serum CA-125 levels should be monitored according to clinical details
The number in each cell indicates the number of times a particular modality is recommended during a particular posttreatment year

level evidence with a nonuniform consensus; and an optional serum CA-125 level at each office visit [16]. Currently, at Northwestern our practice follows NCCN guidelines but is modified based on the data from the aforementioned follow-up studies (Table 59.1). We commonly perform a history and physical examination every 3 months for the first 2 years, every 6 months for 3–5 years, and then annually thereafter. Vaginal cytology and serum CA-125 levels are not routinely obtained. Vaginal cytology/biopsies are obtained if symptoms arise or an abnormality is detected on physical examination. The serum CA-125 level is followed in patients with papillary serous carcinoma and in patients with an elevated serum CA-125 level prior to treatment. Annual chest X-rays are obtained for 2–3 years.

Until further data are available from either large prospective studies or randomized controlled trials, there will continue to be disagreement about which strategies should be employed in which patient populations. With the current rise in health care costs, evaluation needs to be undertaken that is mindful of not only the risk of recurrence but also resource availability and cost.

References

1. American Cancer Society 2009 Cancer Facts and Figures available online at http://www.cancer.org/downloads/STT/500809web.pdf (Accessed 22 Aug 2009).
2. Berchuck A, Anspach C, Evans AC, Soper JT, Rodriguez GC, Dodge R, et al. Postsurgical surveillance of patients with FIGO stage I/II endometrial adenocarcinoma. Gynecol Oncol. 1995;59:20–4.
3. Reddoch JM, Burke TW, Morris M, Tornos C, Levenback C, Gershenson DM. Surveillance for recurrent endometrial carcinoma: development of a follow-up scheme. Gynecol Oncol. 1995;59:221–5.
4. Shumsky AG, Stuart GC, Brasher PM, Nation JG, Robertson DI, Sangkarat S. An evaluation of routine follow-up of patients treated for endometrial carcinoma. Gynecol Oncol. 1994; 55:229–33.
5. Podczaski E, Kaminski P, Gurski K, MacNeill C, Stryker JA, Singapuri K, et al. Detection and patterns of treatment failure in 300 consecutive cases of "early" endometrial cancer after primary surgery. Gynecol Oncol. 1992;47:323–7.
6. Fung-Kee-Fung M, Dodge J, Elit L, et al. Follow-up after primary therapy for endometrial cancer: a systematic review. Gynecol Oncol. 2006;101:520.
7. Agboola OO, Grunfeld E, Coyle D, Perry GA. Costs and benefits of routine follow-up after curative treatment for endometrial cancer. CMAJ. 1997;157:879–86.
8. Greer BE, Koh WJ, Abu-Rustum N, et al. Uterine neoplasms. Clinical practice guidelines in oncology. J Natl Compr Canc Netw. 2009;7:498–531.
9. Cooper AL, Dornfeld-Finke JM, Banks HW, et al. Is cytologic screening an effective surveillance method for detection of vaginal recurrence of uterine cancer? Obstet Gynecol. 2006;107:171.
10. Bristow RE, Purinton SC, Santillan A, et al. Cost-effectiveness of routine vaginal cytology for endometrial cancer surveillance. Gynecol Oncol. 2006;103:709.
11. Ray M, Fleming G, et al. Management of advanced-stage and recurrent endometrial cancer. Semin Oncol. 2009;36:145–54.
12. Gadducci A, Cosio S, Capri A, et al. Serum tumor markers in the management of ovarian, endometrial and cervical cancer. Biomed Pharmacother. 2004;58:24–38.
13. Rose PG, Sommers RM, Reale FR, Hunter RE, Fournier L, Nelson BE. Serial serum CA 125 measurements for evaluation of recurrence in patients with endometrial carcinoma. Obstet Gynecol. 1994;84:12–6.
14. Patsner B, Orr Jr JW, Mann Jr WJ. Use of serum CA 125 measurement in posttreatment surveillance of early-stage endometrial carcinoma. Am J Obstet Gynecol. 1990;162:427–9.
15. Gadducci A, Cosio S, Fanucchi A, et al. An intensive follow-up does not change survival of patients with clinical stage I endometrial cancer. Anticancer. 2000;20(3B):1977–84.
16. NCCN practice guidelines for endometrial carcinoma. 2012.

Endometrial Cancer Surveillance Counterpoint: USA

60

Summer B. Dewdney and Premal H. Thaker

Keywords
Endometrium • Gynecologic cancer • Posttreatment • Surveillance • Women • Recurrence

In the United States, endometrial cancer is the most common malignancy of the female genital tract. It is estimated that 43,470 women were diagnosed with endometrial cancer in 2010 and 7,950 died of their cancer [1]. Fortunately, the majority of endometrial cancers are diagnosed at an early stage due to abnormal uterine bleeding, and most of these women are cured. Approximately 70% are diagnosed with localized disease, with a corresponding 5-year survival rate of 95% [1]. Although there has been a decrease in the death rate of endometrial cancer by a small percentage since 1991, there has been an increase in incidence over the past few years [1], likely attributable to the increasing prevalence of obesity. Other risk factors for endometrial cancer include diabetes, hypertension, endogenous or exogenous excess estrogen, nulliparity, family history, and endometrial hyperplasia.

Most endometrial cancers are initially surgically staged. According to the National Comprehensive Cancer Network (NCCN) and the American College of Obstetricians and Gynecologists (ACOG), standard definitive treatment includes a hysterectomy, bilateral salpingo-oophorectomy, and pelvic/paraaortic lymphadenectomy [2, 3], although the impact on survival of pelvic/paraaortic lymphadenectomy for the staging of endometrial cancer has been called into question by recent findings of the ASTEC trial [4]. Management after surgery depends on a patient's risk factors for recurrence. Options may include vaginal vault brachytherapy or pelvic external-beam radiation and/or chemotherapy. Risk factors considered in any decision for adjuvant therapy include high-grade histology (serous, clear cell, or grade 2/3 endometrioid), myometrial invasion greater than 50%, tumor extension beyond the uterine fundus, and lymphovascular space invasion. Depending on these risk factors, patients are categorized as being at low, intermediate, or high risk for recurrence. The Gynecologic Oncology Group (GOG) did a phase III trial evaluating whether adjuvant external beam radiation lowers the risk of recurrence and death in women with stages IB, IC, and II according to International Federation of Gynecology and Obstetrics (FIGO) staging of 1988. The authors found that radiotherapy does decrease the risk of recurrence but does not improve survival duration. Post-hoc analysis suggested that adjuvant therapy should be limited to high-intermediate risk patients, based on age and a number of risk factors [5]. It is important to note that others have found similar outcomes; in early-stage endometrial cancer, adjuvant radiotherapy improves locoregional control but not overall survival duration [5, 6]. A recent report from the ASTEC/EN.5 Study Group [7] showed no benefit of external beam radiotherapy for the overall survival in patients with intermediate or high risk for recurrence. Hence, controversy exists about which subset, if any, may benefit from adjuvant therapy.

Overall, the risk of recurrence for endometrial cancer is approximately 10–15% [8–11]. The first 3 years after diagnosis is the most critical for recurrence as that is when approximately 68–100% of patients with endometrial cancer who will recur do so [8]. The risk of recurrence is less than 5% in low-risk patients. Most patients who recur have symptoms: pooled

S.B. Dewdney
Department of Obstetrics and Gynecology, Rush University Medical Center, 1725 W. Harrison Street, Suite 1010, Chicago, IL 60612, USA
e-mail: Summer_Dewdney@rush.edu

P.H. Thaker (✉)
Division of Gynecologic Oncology, Department of Obstetrics and Gynecology, Washington University School of Medicine, 4911 Barnes-Jewish Hospital Plaza, 4th Floor Maternity Building Campus, Box 8064, St. Louis, MO 63110, USA
e-mail: thakerp@wudosis.wustl.edu

F.E. Johnson et al. (eds.), *Patient Surveillance After Cancer Treatment*, Current Clinical Oncology,
DOI 10.1007/978-1-60327-969-7_60,

data from 11 retrospective studies [8] demonstrated that 70% (95% CI, 65–75%) of recurrences were symptomatic. Survival of patients with recurrence depends on the location of recurrence. Some 35–40% of recurrences occur locally, while 55–60% occur at distant sites [8]. The 3-year survival rates after vaginal, pelvic, and distant recurrences are 73%, 8%, and 14%, respectively [12]. These figures contrast the excellent prognosis of isolated vaginal recurrence with the poor prognosis associated with pelvic or distant recurrences.

The main purpose of surveillance after curative-intent treatment is to improve overall survival through early diagnosis of asymptomatic recurrence. Appropriate surveillance must take into account the natural history of the disease, the efficacy of surveillance tests, and the life-prolonging potential of available treatments for a recurrence if one is detected. In part, surveillance is used to detect asymptomatic recurrence, assuming that a patient with recurrence eventually will present with a symptom. One important aspect of surveillance is patient education regarding symptoms of recurrence. Finally, with the escalating cost of health care, cost-effectiveness is an important factor when considering routine diagnostic testing and frequency of clinic visits.

Surveillance of patients with endometrial cancer who have completed their treatment entails close follow-up for the first 2–3 years and then less intensively in following years. This time schedule is based on our understanding of the natural history of the disease. Our ability to detect a recurrence is fairly good, given that the majority of recurrences are detected by clinical examination or patient symptoms. The routine use of diagnostic tests, including vaginal cytology and imaging, has been called into question because of low yield and cost-effectiveness. Life-prolonging therapy available for recurrent endometrial cancer is limited, especially with distant metastasis. If recurrence does occur, only patients with local vaginal recurrences are likely to be salvaged. Such patients have a high response rate (89%) with radiation therapy [12]. This group of patients benefits the most from surveillance because a treatment with a high response rate exists. However, this population usually presents with vaginal bleeding or pelvic pressure symptoms, so screening for detection of an asymptomatic recurrence may have limited value.

There is no current protocol that is based on level 1 evidence for surveillance of patients who have been potentially cured of their endometrial cancer. Guidelines recommend that patients be monitored with physical examination, vaginal cytology, chest X-rays, and sometimes cancer antigen CA-125 serum levels. The current schedule of surveillance is based on physician preferences and traditions. The NCCN recommends the following surveillance schedule [2]: physical examination every 3–6 months for 2 years and then every 6–12 months annually; vaginal cytology every 6 months for 2 years and then annually; and a chest X-ray annually, as well as patient questioning regarding symptoms of recurrence. There are a number of retrospective studies and three systematic reviews regarding surveillance for patients with endometrial cancer, but a prospective randomized trial would be difficult to conduct, given the low rate of recurrence in this population; hence, the number of patients needed to adequately power such a trial would be large.

In 2006, Fung-Kee-Fung et al. [8] did an excellent systematic review identifying 16 retrospective studies and 2 systematic reviews. Of the retrospective studies, 12 evaluated surveillance programs, and 4 evaluated the role of serum CA-125 level in detecting disease recurrence. The pooled data of the 12 studies included 2,922 patients who were followed from 26 to >120 months, with a total of 398 recurrences and a recurrence rate of 13% (11–14, 95%CI). They found no evidence to support the concept that intensive follow-up with routine diagnostic testing improves survival over less intensive follow-up. These authors presented one illustrative example based on their data regarding the lack of benefit of surveillance. Based on their pooled analysis, the recurrence rate for low-risk patients was 3%. Within this group of 3%, approximately two-thirds would present with a symptomatic recurrence whereas the remaining one-third would be diagnosed with an asymptomatic recurrence. Hence, approximately 1% of all patients in surveillance would benefit from surveillance by detection of a recurrence. However, of this 1% identified with an asymptomatic recurrence, more than half would have distant disease. Identification of this group would not benefit from early detection, because early detection of a distant recurrence has shown no overall survival benefit. Of the remaining patients with a local recurrence, only about half of them would benefit from salvage therapy. In conclusion, the authors estimated that, in the low-risk population, only 2 of 1,000 patients would benefit by surveillance. Applying current NCCN guidelines for surveillance, identifying these two women would require 7,000–11,000 examinations, 7,000 Pap tests, and 5,000 chest radiographs. The number benefited increases to 7 out of 1,000 if surveillance were applied only in the high-risk group. Both of these numbers are very low and provide evidence against intense surveillance after initial curative-intent therapy for endometrial cancer.

Smith and colleagues recently performed a retrospective evaluation of 2,637 patients with endometrial cancer and identified 280 patients with recurrence and records sufficiently detailed for analysis [13]. Their surveillance schedule included clinical examination every 3 months for 2 years with vaginal vault cytology performed twice a year, and then clinical examination every 6 months until 5 years with vaginal vault cytology annually. They found that the majority of the recurrences were symptomatic (71.1%), and the overall survival probability at 5 years in the low/intermediate risk population, defined as stage I or II with endometrioid histological type, was 38.0% and 25.7% for asymptomatic and symptomatic patients, respectively ($p=0.05$). This statistical difference seen in the low/intermediate asymptomatic population was an important finding in this study. These authors concluded that patients who have low/intermediate risk may benefit from intensive follow-up, including physical examinations, routine vaginal vault cytology, and imaging, although the difference between the asymptomatic and symptomatic patient groups in this study may have been identified secondary to lead-time bias.

Table 60.1 shows a summary of selected studies that reported information on how an asymptomatic recurrence was diagnosed. As previously stated, protocols for surveillance have not been strictly established. Next we discuss the evidence for each of the aspects of care during surveillance.

Fung-Kee-Fung et al. [8] found a wide range of frequency of clinic visits in the analysis of the 12 retrospective studies (Table 60.1). The range of visits in the first 2 years after primary treatment was from three to twelve visits per year, with the majority averaging four visits per year for the first 2 years. For the subsequent years up to 5 years post primary treatment, clinic visits ranged from one to four per year. In their discussion they stated that there was no discernible difference in outcomes between the various surveillance schedules.

Tjalma et al. [18] performed a systematic analysis and identified 11 retrospective studies. They did a cost analysis and suggested tailoring clinic visits based on risk of recurrence. Patients with low risk for recurrence could be seen every 6 months for 3 years and then annually; whereas, high-risk patients should be seen every 3 months for 2 years and then every 6 months for the following 3 years. They found a significant cost reduction in stratifying patients into these two groups. See Tables 60.1 and 60.2 for our recommendations on the frequency of surveillance.

There have been a number of studies that include information regarding detection of recurrence by clinical examination. Approximately 55% of the asymptomatic recurrences were found on clinical examination in a large retrospective study [13]. In the literature review performed by Tjalma et al. [18], more than 80% of the recurrences were detected either with clinical examination alone or patient symptoms. Fung-Kee-Fung et al. [8] found a range of 5–33% detection of asymptomatic recurrences with physical examination alone.

The physical examination has been found to be useful in detecting both asymptomatic and symptomatic recurrences. The clinical examination and history should evaluate known symptoms of recurrence. These include vaginal bleeding, abdominal or pelvic pain, persistent cough, or weight loss. Any symptoms need to be evaluated promptly. In addition, patient education is of great importance, because the majority of recurrences are symptomatic.

Although many gynecologic oncologists use vaginal vault cytology for surveillance in this patient population, there is little evidence to support it. Detection of asymptomatic recurrence with cytology ranged from 0–4% [8] of the total recurrences. In addition, it has not been found to be cost-effective. Bristow et al. [14] found that vaginal cytology had a detection rate of 0.5%; 1,067 vaginal cytologies needed to be performed for detection of one asymptomatic vaginal recurrence. This corresponded to cumulative charges of over $44,000 calculated in 2005 health dollars. Bristow et al. [14] concluded that a Pap smear as a surveillance test for endometrial cancer recurrence is costly and inefficient, and benefits a very small percentage of patients. Therefore, the use of routine vaginal cytology as a surveillance tool for endometrial cancer recurrence does not seem to be beneficial or cost-effective.

The use of serum CA-125 levels for detection of endometrial cancer recurrence was studied by Rose et al. [19]. They found 33 recurrences among 266 patients. Of those 33 recurrences, 27 were in the high-risk category, which was defined as stage II or greater, grade 3 endometrioid or serous or clear cell histologies. The serum CA-125 level was elevated in 19 of the 33 (58%) patients with a recurrence. They noted false elevations in 13 patients, 12 of whom had received radiation therapy. The authors concluded that the use of serum CA-125 levels is most beneficial in a high-risk population. In addition, it seems to be a good marker for patients who have an elevated serum CA-125 level at diagnosis. The routine use of this test for surveillance of recurrence of endometrial cancer cannot be recommended.

Chest X-rays have been used as a routine tool to detect distant recurrences in endometrial cancer. The clinical utility of this test for surveillance is called into question because of the poor prognosis of patients who have lung metastasis. Isolated lung metastases can be resected and lung metastases may respond well to chemotherapy or hormonal therapy, but survival benefits from these interventions are questionable. Nevertheless, chest X-rays are recommended annually by the NCCN for surveillance. In the pooled series of retrospective studies analyzed by Fung-Kee-Fung et al. [8], chest X-rays were performed as part of a follow-up program in eight studies. Detection of asymptomatic recurrences ranged from 0 to 14% in these studies, and no improvement of survival was found. In a more recent large retrospective study [13], imaging showed an 11.8% detection rate in asymptomatic patients, although this study included all imaging modalities (chest X-ray, CT scan, and ultrasound) as one group. In the high-risk population of patients in this study, they found a 31.0% detection rate in asymptomatic recurrences with all imaging modalities. The authors of this study concluded that, because high-risk patients tend to have distant disease at time of recurrence, the high yield suggests that imaging may be useful in this subgroup. However, given the limited evidence

Table 60.1 Summary of selected studies about detection of recurrences in endometrial cancer patients

Author (ref. no.)	Year of publication	Number of patients	Number of recurrences (%)	Number of asymptomatic recurrences (%)	Method for detection of asymptomatic recurrences (% of asymptomatic recurrences)				
					Clinical exam	Vaginal cytology	Chest X-ray	Other imaging	CA-125
Smith et al. [13]	2007	2,922	280[a]/438 (15)	81 (3)	44 (54)	8 (10)	–	15 (17)	11 (14)
Bristow et al. [14]	2006	377	61 (16)	2[b]	–	2	–	–	–
Morice et al. [15]	2001	390	27 (7)	5 (1)	3 (60)	0 (0)	0 (0)	1 (20)	0 (0)
Agboola et al. [16]	1997	432	50 (12)	20 (5)	13/25[c]	2/25[c]	7/25[c]	3/25[c]	–
Berchuck et al. [9]	1995	354	44 (12)	17 (5)	30/44[d]	11/44[d]	9/44[d]	–	–
Reddoch et al. [11]	1995	398	39[e]/44 (11)	23 (6)	13 (57)	1 (4)	1 (4)	2 (9)	6 (26)
Shumsky et al. [17]	1994	317	53 (17)	13 (4)	6 (11)	0 (0)	7 (13)	–	–
Total		5,190	717 (14)	159 (3)[f]					

[a]Data analysis was only complete on 280 patients
[b]Only vaginal recurrences
[c]Twenty-five recurrences detected during routine exams, not grouped by asymptomatic vs. symptomatic
[d]Detection methods were not grouped by asymptomatic vs. symptomatic
[e]Five patients did not have records available for recurrence detection
[f]Calculation is without Bristow et al.

Table 60.2 Surveillance after curative-intent initial treatment for patients with endometrial carcinoma at low risk for recurrence at Washington University School of Medicine.

	Posttreatment year					
Modality	1	2	3	4	5	>5
Office visit[a]	2	2	1	1	1	1
Vaginal cytology	1	1	1	1	1	1

[a]Includes vaginal speculum examination and rectovaginal examination Evaluation of overall health status, including detection and management of late treatment effects is part of the office visit.
The number in each cell indicates the number of times a particular modality is recommended during a particular posttreatment year.

Table 60.3 Surveillance after curative-intent initial treatment for patients with endometrial carcinoma at high risk for recurrence at Washington University School of Medicine.

	Posttreatment year					
Modality	1	2	3	4	5	>5
Office visit[a]	4	4	2	2	2	2
Vaginal cytology	2	2	1	1	1	1

[a]Includes vaginal speculum examination and rectovaginal examination Evaluation of overall health status, including detection and management of late treatment effects is part of the office visit.
The number in each cell indicates the number of times a particular modality is recommended during a particular posttreatment year.

of survival benefit from early detection and the poor prognosis, if a distant metastasis is detected, we cannot recommend chest X-rays for the routine screening for early-stage endometrial cancer recurrences.

There have not been any studies looking specifically at quality of life outcomes or emotional impact associated with intense surveillance following completed treatment for endometrial cancer. However, a randomized clinical trial in breast cancer patients [20] failed to show an impact on survival with intense follow-up versus symptomatic follow-up. In this study they randomized 214 patients to point of need (or patient initiated appointments) versus control (semi-annual appointments) and found no difference in multiple quality of life assessments or number of recurrences. Despite little evidence to show an improved survival with an intense surveillance model, one cannot discount the possible positive psychosocial impact of clinic appointments on a patient's quality of life. If a prospective trial were performed, this aspect of care should be accounted for in the study.

There have been many advances in the understanding of molecular events in endometrial carcinogenesis. Associations with different molecular features have been found in type I and type II endometrial cancer, including MSI, PTEN, K-ras, β-catenin, HER-2/neu, and ploidy [21, 22]. PTEN, β-catenin, and MSI have been found to be associated with type I cancers, whereas aneuploidy, HER-2/neu and p53 have been found to be associated with type II cancers. Yurkovetsky et al. [23] explored a panel of 64 serum biomarkers for early detection of endometrial cancer and found prolactin to accurately discriminate between cancer and control groups. However, for patients who are under posttherapy surveillance, there are no candidate molecular markers. Identification of a reliable marker would be invaluable in detecting recurrent disease, although this marker would need to be evaluated against the current standard of detection.

PET/CT has been shown to be predictive of survival in posttherapy surveillance of cervical cancer patients [24]. Sironi et al. [25] have shown in a preliminary study that PET/CT may be an accurate method for evaluation of recurrence if there is indication of recurrence with other modalities. Ryu et al. performed a feasibility study of 127 patients with predominantly early-stage endometrioid endometrial cancer undergoing PET scans as posttreatment surveillance, and could detect 15% of recurrences not detected by other methods [26]. Currently, given the expense of PET/CT, it should not have a role in routine surveillance for endometrial cancer outside of clinical trials.

With the current evidence, it is not clear whether intense surveillance improves survival rates. Only two of the multiple retrospective studies show a survival benefit in asymptomatic patients, and this may represent bias rather than a true benefit of screening. Gordon et al. [27] showed a significant survival advantage in asymptomatic recurrences, although the study has been criticized for its statistical analysis and methodology [8, 15]. The other retrospective study that showed a benefit was that of Smith et al. [13], and their survival difference was limited to the low/intermediate-risk population. This suggests that a surveillance program might provide a survival benefit in this population, although this study is limited by its retrospective design. Conversely, all of the other retrospective studies failed to show a difference in survival between asymptomatic patients and symptomatic patients. Definitive assessment of surveillance requires a prospective trial to accurately evaluate the benefit of intense surveillance after treatment for patients with endometrial cancer.

As previously stated, there have been no prospective clinical investigations to evaluate the proper frequency and diagnostic testing for surveillance of patients treated for endometrial cancer. With the current data, the surveillance of patients at Washington University can be seen in Tables 60.2 and 60.3. Without prospective trial data, NCCN guidelines remain the best guidance on surveillance at present.

References

1. Jemal A, Siegel R, Ward E, Xu J, Ward E. Cancer Statistics, 2010. CA Cancer J Clin. 2010;60(5):277–300.
2. National Comprehensive Cancer Network (NCCN) Guidelines. Available online at http://www.nccn.org. (Accessed 10 Jan 2010).
3. ACOG practice bulletin No.65. (2005) Clinical management guidelines for obstetrician-gynecologists, management of endometrial cancer.
4. ASTEC study group. Efficacy of systematic pelvic lymphadenectomy in endometrial cancer (MRC ASTEC trial): a randomised study. Lancet. 2009;373:125–36.
5. Keys HM, Roberts JA, Brunetto VL, et al. A phase III trial of surgery with or without adjunctive external pelvic radiation therapy in intermediate risk endometrial adenocarcinoma: a Gynecologic Oncology Group Study. Gynecol Oncol. 2004;92:744–51.
6. Creutzberg CL, van Putten WL, Koper PC, et al. Surgery and post-operative radiotherapy versus surgery alone for patients with stage-1 endometrial carcinoma: multicentre randomized trial. PORTEC study group. Post Operative Radiation Therapy in Endometrial Carcinoma. Lancet. 2000;355:1404–11.
7. ASTEC/EN 5 Study Group, Blake P, Swart AM, et al. Adjuvant external beam radiotherapy in the treatment of endometrial cancer (MRC ASTEC and NCIC CTG EN.5 randomised trials): pooled trial results, systematic review, and meta-analysis. Lancet. 2009; 373:137–46.
8. Fung-Kee-Fung M, Dodge J, Elit L, Lukka H, Chambers A, Oliver T. Follow-up after primary therapy for endometrial cancer: a systematic review. Gynecol Oncol. 2006;101:520–9.
9. Berchuck A, Anspach C, Evans AC, et al. Postsurgical surveillance of patients with FIGO stage I/II endometrial adenocarcinoma. Gynecol Oncol. 1995;59:20–4.
10. Podczaski E, Kaminski P, Gurski K, et al. Detection and patterns of treatment failure in 300 consecutive cases of 'early' endometrial cancer after primary surgery. Gynecol Oncol. 1992;47:323–7.
11. Reddoch JM, Burke TW, Morris M, Tornos C, Levenback C, Gershenson DM. Surveillance for recurrent endometrial carcinoma: development of a follow-up scheme. Gynecol Oncol. 1995;59:221–5.
12. Creutzberg CL, van Putten WL, Koper PC, et al. Survival after relapse in patients with endometrial cancer: results from a randomized study. Gynecol Oncol. 2003;89:201–9.
13. Smith CJ, Heeren M, Nicklin JL, et al. Efficacy of routine follow-up in patients with recurrent uterine cancer. Gynecol Oncol. 2007;107:124–9.
14. Bristow RE, Purinton SC, Santillan A, Diaz-Montes TP, Gardner GJ, Giuntoli RL. Cost-effectiveness of routine vaginal cytology for endometrial cancer surveillance. Gynecol Oncol. 2006;103:709–13.
15. Kew FM, Roberts AP, Cruickshank DJ. The role of routing follow-up after gynecological malignancy. Int J Gynecol Cancer. 2005;15: 413–9.
16. Morice P, Levy-Piedbois C, Ajaj S, et al. Value and cost evaluation of routine follow-up for patients with clinical stage I/II endometrial cancer. Eur J Cancer. 2001;37:985–90.
17. Agboola OO, Grunfeld E, Coyle D, Perry GA. Costs and benefits of routine follow-up after curative treatment for endometrial cancer. Can Med Assoc J. 1997;157:879–86.
18. Tjalma WAA, Van Dam PA, Makar AP, Cruickshank DJ. The clinical value and the cost-effectiveness of follow-up in endometrial cancer patient. Int J Gynecol Cancer. 2004;14:931–7.
19. Rose PG, Sommers RM, Reale FR, Hunter RE, Fournier L, Nelson BE. Serial serum CA 125 measurements for evaluation of recurrence in patients with endometrial cancer. Obstet Gynecol. 1994; 84:12–6.
20. Sheppard C, Higgins B, Wise M, Yiangou C, Dubois D, Kilburn S. Breast cancer follow up: a randomized controlled trial comparing point of need access versus routine 6-monthly clinical review. Eur J Oncol Nurs. 2009;13:2–8.
21. Hecht JL, Mutter GL. Molecular and pathologic aspects of endometrial carcinogenesis. J Clin Oncol. 2006;24:4783–91.
22. Prat J, Gallardo A, Cuatrecasas M, Catasus L. Endometrial carcinoma: pathology and genetics. Pathology. 2007;39:72–87.
23. Yurkovetsky Z, Ta'asan S, Skates S, et al. Development of multi marker panel for early detection of endometrial cancer. High diagnostic power of prolactin. Gynecol Oncol. 2007;107:58–65.
24. Schwarz JK, Siegel BA, Dehdashti F, Grigsby PW. Association of posttherapy positron emission tomography with tumor response and survival in cervical carcinoma. JAMA. 2007;298:2289–95.
25. Sironi S, Picchio M, Landoni C, et al. Posttherapy surveillance of patients with uterine cancers: value of integrated FDG PET/CT in the detection of recurrence. Eur J Nucl Med Mol Imaging. 2007;34:472–9.
26. Ryu SY, Kim K, Kim Y, et al. Detection of recurrence by F-FDG PET in patients with endometrial cancer showing no evidence of disease. J Korean Med Sci. 2010;25:1029–33.
27. Gordon AF, Owen P, Chien PFW, Duncan ID. A critical evaluation of follow-up of women treated for endometrial adenocarcinoma. J Obstet Gynaecol. 1997;17:386–9.
28. Schumsky AG, Stuart GCE, Brasher PM, Nation JG, Robertson DI, Sangkarat S. An evaluation of routine follow-up of patients treated for endometrial carcinoma. Gynecol Oncol. 1994;55:229–33.

Carcinoma of the Endometrium Surveillance Counterpoint: Japan

61

Yousuke Ueoka, Hiroaki Kobayashi, and Norio Wake

Keywords
Health insurance system • Chemotherapy • Lymphadenectomy • Laparoscopy • Medroxyprogesterone acetate (MPA) • Positron emission tomography (PET) • Vaginal cytology

Endometrial carcinoma is the third most common female genital tract carcinoma in Japan and its incidence is increasing. According to the Center for Cancer Control and Information Services at the National Cancer Center, endometrial cancer accounted for 6,625 new cancer cases in Japan in 2002 [1]. The incidence of endometrial cancer recurrence is also increasing proportionately. In 2006, the number of endometrial cancer-related deaths was 1,481, over three times higher than that reported 20 years ago. Recently, the incidence of endometrial cancer among younger patients, under 39 years of age, has also increased in Japan (from 75 patients in 1975 to 355 patients in 2002 [1]). In younger patients, hormone therapy has been attempted at several institutions in order to preserve fertility. Endometrial cancer generally has a favorable prognosis because about 80% of cases are diagnosed in stage I. For endometrial cancer, routine surgicopathological staging, including lymph node examination, has been recommended by the Cancer Committee of the International Federation of Gynecology and Obstetrics (FIGO) since 1988. With early-stage endometrial cancer, only approximately 10–15% of patients will experience recurrence. The primary aim of the follow-up strategy for endometrial cancer patients is thus to facilitate the early detection of recurrent lesions. It is generally assumed that detecting recurrence before symptoms have developed will permit earlier treatment and hence improve prognosis and survival rate. The goals of follow-up are to improve overall survival duration and to improve quality of life. However, a standard program for the follow-up of endometrial cancer patients has not yet been established. Generally, the risk of endometrial cancer recurrence depends on surgicopathological factors, including histological type and grade, depth of myometrial invasion, presence of lymph node metastasis, and the presence of extrauterine disease. Differences in operative technique and adjuvant therapy between Japan and the West may influence the type of recurrence.

Japan has a unique health insurance system. In Japan, everyone has medical insurance, as dictated by health insurance law. The majority of people pay 30% of the medical costs, and the national health insurance pays 70%. The national health insurance covers 90% of the medical cost for elderly patients over 70 years of age, except for patients with sufficient income who must contribute 30%. Thus, every Japanese citizen can get uniform medical services at a low cost. As a result, comparatively expensive examinations, such as magnetic resonance imaging (MRI) and positron emission tomography (PET)/CT, are frequently ordered, and those expensive medical procedures are popular in Japan. In addition to national health insurance, most Japanese people also have private health insurance.

Y. Ueoka (✉)
Hamanomachi Hospital, Maizuru 3-5-27, Chuou-ku, Fukuoka 810-8539, Japan
e-mail: ueoka-y@hamanomachi.jp

H. Kobayashi • N. Wake
Department of Obstetrics and Gynecology, Graduate School of Medical Sciences, Kyushu University Hospital,
Maidashi 3-1-1, Higashi-ku, Fukuoka 812-8582, Japan
e-mail: koba@med.kyushu-u.ac.jp; wake@med.kyushu-u.ac.jp

F.E. Johnson et al. (eds.), *Patient Surveillance After Cancer Treatment*, Current Clinical Oncology,
DOI 10.1007/978-1-60327-969-7_61, © Springer Science+Business Media New York 2013

The pattern of recurrence is affected by adjuvant therapy. In the FIGO annual report, radiotherapy is indicated roughly twice as often as chemotherapy for the postoperative patients with stage I/II endometrial cancers. In patients who receive radiation therapy in the form of pelvic external-beam radiation therapy and/or vaginal vault brachytherapy, the locoregional recurrence rate is significantly lower. However, radiotherapy does not prevent distant metastases and it increases treatment-related morbidity. No studies have reported a significant difference in the progression-free survival (PFS) and overall survival (OS) between adjuvant radiotherapy and chemotherapy. In Western countries, obese patients, for whom lymphadenectomy is difficult to perform, are common. Thus, pelvic radiotherapy is usually selected as adjuvant therapy. The Japanese Gynecologic Oncology Group (JGOG) conducted a randomized study comparing pelvic radiotherapy to platinum-based combined chemotherapy for endometrial cancer (JGOG2033 study). This study showed that chemotherapy significantly improved PFS and OS vs. pelvic radiation in high- to intermediate-risk patients [2]. In patients with low- to intermediate-risk endometrial cancer (defined as stage IC), patients under 70 years old with G1/2 endometrioid adenocarcinoma adjuvant therapy did not improve PFS and OS. In advanced-stage patients, the superiority of chemotherapy was demonstrated in the GOG-122 study. Because of this study, platinum-based combined chemotherapy is usually recommended for adjuvant therapy in Japan.

Table 61.1 Surgical procedures for endometrial cancer in the Japanese Gynecologic Oncology Group (JGOG)

	Number of institutions (%)
Total number of responders	139
Hysterectomy procedure	
TAH only	49 (35.3)
Class II only	42 (30.2)
Alternates based on clinicopathologic conditions	48 (34.5)
Radical hysterectomy	
Routinely performed	1 (0.7)
Performed based on clinicopathologic conditions	40 (28.8)
Never performed	98 (70.5)
Pelvic lymph node dissection	
Routinely performed	136 (97.8)
Performed based on clinicopathologic conditions	1 (0.7)
Never performed	2 (1.5)
Para-aortic lymph node treatment	
Routinely performed dissection	12 (8.6)
Routinely performed biopsy	5 (3.6)
Performed dissection based on clinicopathologic conditions	90 (64.7)
Performed biopsy based on clinicopathologic conditions	23 (16.5)
Never performed	9 (6.6)

TAH: abdominal simple total hysterectomy, Class II: extended hysterectomy (Piver), para-aortic lymph node biopsy: removal of three or fewer lymph nodes, para-aortic lymph node dissection: removal of four or more lymph nodes.
Modified from [4]

Pelvic MRI can accurately assess the depth of myometrial infiltration as well as the extent of cervical invasion. With MRI the presence of myometrial infiltration can be assessed as an interruption of the junctional zone on T2-weighted images or dynamic studies. For deep myometrial invasion, the sensitivity and specificity are reported to be 89% and 100%, respectively [3]. The diagnostic accuracy of cervical extension using MRI is also excellent [3]. For identification of enlarged pelvic and para-aortic lymph nodes, computed tomography (CT) scan is thought to be superior. Recent data from A Study in the Treatment of Endometrial Cancer (ASTEC) showed that, in early-stage endometrial cancer, addition of lymphadenectomy to hysterectomy and salpingo-oophorectomy does not improve survival. Lymphadenectomy lengthens the operation time and may cause operative complications such as deep vein thrombosis, bowel obstruction, lymphocysts, leg edema, and heavy bleeding. The deep myometrial, cervical invasion, and histological tumor grade are well known to correlate with lymph node metastases. In stage I of the disease, the incidence of lymph node metastases is usually considered to increase from 3% in patients with superficial myometrial invasion to 40% or more in those with deep invasion. A preoperative estimation of myometrial invasion and/or cervical involvement is very important to decide surgical procedures. In order to accurately estimate the extent of metastases, intraoperative consultation comparing gross visual inspection and pathological examination of frozen sections has been tried in some institutions. If the risk of lymph node metastases is pre/intraoperatively judged to be unlikely, lymphadenectomy may be excluded, reducing the chances of postoperative complications and facilitating an earlier recovery. However, the diagnostic assessment of superficial myometrial invasion is not yet sufficiently accurate. The presence of leiomyomas, deep tumor progression, and the presence of small isolated tumor foci are factors that tend to interfere with accurate diagnosis of myometrial invasion [3]. Even when intraoperative frozen sections are examined, the deepest invasion locus cannot always be evaluated precisely. Pathological grading is difficult to confirm using a preoperatively obtained specimen or via intraoperative frozen examination. Thus, the decision to omit lymphadenectomy cannot be made with confidence.

Abdominal total hysterectomy and bilateral salpingo-oophorectomy are cornerstones of the operative procedures of advanced endometrial cancer. In Japan, surgical treatment procedures for endometrial cancer vary by institution. The Japan Gynecologic Oncology Group (JGOG) reported that abdominal total hysterectomy was utilized by 35.3% of institutions, Piver class II extended hysterectomy was utilized by 30.2%, and radical hysterectomy was utilized by 29.5% of institutions as shown in Table 61.1 [4]. Radical hysterectomy is selected only in those patients with macroscopic cervical involvement in most JGOG institutions. According to this JGOG survey, pelvic and/or para-aortic lymphadenectomy are performed more aggressively in Japan than in other countries. The reasons for this discrepancy may be due to the fact that pelvic lymphadenectomy is routinely performed in radical hysterectomy for cervical cancer in Japan. Therefore, Japanese surgeons are familiar with the technique of lymphadenectomy and the additional morbidity of pelvic lymphadenectomy is within an acceptable range. In addition, severely obese patients, who are at high risk of postoperative complications, are less common among Japanese women when compared to Caucasians. Retrospective analyses reveal that prognoses are improved by performing retroperitoneal lymphadenectomy for endometrial cancer. Disease-specific survival and overall survival is significantly improved with lymphadenectomy in high-risk patients, (grade 3 endometrioid adenocarcinoma of stage I, and stage II or more advanced) relative to low-risk patients.

Laparoscopic lymphadenectomy has been introduced in some institutions for the treatment of gynecologic malignancies, such as cervical, endometrial, or ovarian cancer. Although laparoscopic approaches require higher technical skill, laparoscopic lymphadenectomy is reported to be as safe as laparotomy after an initial learning phase [5]. Using laparoscopic approaches in early-stage endometrial cancer, several groups report shorter hospitalization times and better quality of life. Systematic review of randomized controlled trials, however, reveals no significant difference between laparoscopic and laparotomic approaches in overall, disease-free, and cancer-related survival duration [6]. Although laparoscopic operations generally take longer, significantly lower intraoperative blood loss and lower postoperative complications are reported and the number of lymph nodes removed is equivalent to those removed in an open operation. Because no significant difference in therapeutic effect between laparoscopic and laparotomic approaches is reported in the literature, the recommended follow-up time is almost identical. In the laparoscopic procedure, however, some problems have been reported. Positive abdominal cytology may be promoted by using a uterine manipulator, and some recurrences at vaginal cuff or trocar site have been reported. Under current conditions and, at the present time, laparoscopic surgery for endometrial cancer has not been established as a standard procedure for gynecologic oncologists. In Japan, the cost of each procedure is defined by the governmental health insurance. For example, a standard laparotomy for endometrial cancer, including pelvic and para-aortic lymphadenectomy, costs 390,000 yen ($4,333). Laparoscopically assisted vaginal hysterectomy without lymphadenectomy costs 385,000 yen ($4,278). On the other hand, abdominal hysterectomy costs 176,000 yen ($1,956). This difference in cost is largely due to the fact that laparoscopic surgery requires many more disposable items of equipment. However, laparoscopic surgery for gynecologic malignancies is not yet covered by the health insurance in Japan and is therefore not performed generally but occasionally in a small number of hospitals.

Standard treatment for endometrial carcinoma includes hysterectomy and, after hysterectomy, patients cannot get pregnant. Endometrial carcinoma in women younger than 40 years of age usually has a more favorable outcome than in older patients. In younger patients, the incidence of myometrial invasion and lymph node metastasis is low. For these younger patients, fertility-preserving experimental treatment using Medroxyprogesterone Acetate (MPA) ranged between 200 and 800 mg per day, to avoid hysterectomy has been tried [7–9]. Ushijima et al. report a multicenter JGOG phase II study of conservative treatment [7]. Twenty-eight patients with presumed stage IA endometrial carcinoma and 17 patients with atypical endometrial hyperplasia were treated with 600 mg/day of MPA for 26 weeks. The toxicities of MPA are well known, the most serious one being thromboembolism. Because patients who have an abnormality in blood coagulation tests or a history of thromboembolism are thought to be at high risk of thromboembolism, MPA therapy is contraindicated. Patients whose body mass index is over 35 are also excluded for the same reason. Before starting this conservative treatment, the cases with myometrial invasion or any extrauterine lesions should be eliminated via imaging studies (CT and MRI). However, the diagnostic accuracy of imaging studies for myometrial invasion, especially in the case of superficial invasion, is limited, as described previously. Therefore, we should recognize that patients with myometrial invasion cannot be completely excluded without a hysterectomy. In the Ushijima study, a pathologically complete response was found in 55% of endometrial carcinomas and 82% of atypical endometrial hyperplasia. Seven deliveries were also achieved with MPA therapy [7]. On the other hand, eight recurrences of endometrial carcinoma were found [7]. In a review of 133 fertility-preserving cases after MPA treatment by Luis Chiva, approximately 50% of well-differentiated tumors showed a complete response to hormone treatment and 53 women achieved pregnancy [8]. On the other hand, 25% of patients suffered a relapse after a temporary response. A recurrent stage 1A endometrial carcinoma with pelvic lymph node metastasis after MPA therapy has also been reported [9]. Thus, conservative treatment for endometrial carcinoma is not safe enough to be considered standard treatment and remains a therapeutic challenge. Hence, patients should be informed of the risks and, after completing gestation, a standard surgical treatment must be considered. Chiva et al. advocated criteria for conservative treatment of endometrial carcinoma which consists of seven requirements [8]. Considering the risk of recurrence, strict and close follow-up is recommended for patients receiving conservative therapy. In Kyushu University Hospital, bimonthly examination, including an endometrial cytology

Table 61.2 Different costs according to Japanese standards (January 2009)

	In Japanese yen	In US dollars[a]
Clinical examination[b]	700	7.78
Vaginal vault cytology	2,960	32.89
Chest X-ray	2,860	31.78
Abdominal/pelvic ultrasound	5,300	58.89
Abdominal/pelvic CAT[c, d]	32,810	364.56
MRI[c, d]	43,480	483.11
Drip infusion pyelography[c, d]	16,120	179.11
FDG-PET/CT[b]	75,750	841.67
CA125[e]	3,600	40.00

[a]Converted into US dollar with the exchange rate at 1 US $=90 yen
[b]There may be small variations between institutions
[c]There may be small variations due to the type and volume of the enhancer
[d]There may be small variations due to digital analyzing methods and the use of scopolamine
[e]Including additional charge of cancer management

and an endometrial thickness measurement by transvaginal ultrasound (US), is conducted. In cases of atypical uterine bleeding or thickened endometrium, we examine endometrial biopsy, sometimes repeatedly. It is well known that the hyperestrogenic state tends to promote endometrial cancer and that women with an irregular menstrual cycle have an increased risk of endometrial cancer. After MPA treatment, we introduce active treatment for conception, including ovulatory stimulation. For patients who do not wish to conceive immediately, we administer cyclic estrogen-progestin to maintain regular withdrawal bleeding.

In follow-up after conventional surgery for endometrial cancer, many reports indicate that Pap test of the vaginal vault is inefficient at detecting localized recurrence. Although 5% of endometrial cancer patients experience a local recurrence of disease confined to the vagina and mid pelvis, most of them present with a vaginal bleeding and/or have a clinically apparent vaginal lesion. For general follow-up, careful examination for symptomatic patients may be enough. Because asymptomatic vaginal recurrence diagnosed by vaginal cytology alone is extremely rare [10, 11], the use of vaginal cytology for detecting recurrence may be of little significance and its omission can reduce costs. However, recurrence of isolated vaginal lesions can be successfully treated with surgery, radiotherapy, or a combination of both and has been shown to have a 50% 5-year survival rate, which is excellent when compared to a 6% 5-year survival rate in nonvaginal recurrences. Moreover, the cost of cytology is not a heavy burden for patients in Japan (Table 61.2). We feel that early detection of recurrence should improve survival rates, and thus we continue to perform a Pap test in addition to a pelvic examination at each follow-up visit.

Early and accurate detection of recurrence in patients has an important influence on additional therapy, and appropriate treatment has a significant impact on overall survival. With the exception of radiography and ultrasonography, conventional morphological imaging modalities, such as computed tomography (CT) and MRI, have been widely used for diagnosis of recurrent lesions. Though the improvement in equipment has brought the potential to detect smaller lesions, the conventional imaging modalities are still poor at visualizing small disseminated lesions or small lymph node metastases, especially micrometastasis. In the late 1990s, PET with ^{18}F-fluorodeoxyglucose (FDG) was widely used in the clinical imaging of various cancers. However, precise localization of recurrent endometrial carcinoma may be difficult with PET. To overcome this disadvantage of PET, an integrated PET/CT system, in which a full-ring detector clinical PET scanner and multidetector row helical CT scanner are combined, has been developed. PET/CT has made it possible to get both metabolic and anatomical imaging data using a single device. Currently, PET/CT equipment is widely available in Japan. In the follow-up of endometrial cancer, PET/CT has demonstrated superior sensitivity, specificity, and accuracy for the diagnosis of recurrence [12]. However, a tiny lymph node metastasis which could not be detected by PET/CT has been also reported [13]. PET/CT can detect lymph nodes which have a certain volume of malignant cells sufficient to change glucose metabolism, but is still not the perfect scanning modality for recurrent lesions. Patients with small recurrent lesions are sometimes found during follow-up. We treat them using chemotherapy, radiotherapy, and occasionally surgery. Recurrent lesions of endometrial cancer are often insensitive to chemotherapy and some statistical analyses reveal no survival advantage for patients with subclinical recurrences detected by CT scan [10].

A systematic review of papers reporting the follow-up of a total of 2,922 endometrial cancer patients revealed that there was an overall recurrence rate of 13% [14]. Seventy-seven percent of recurrent cases were associated with symptoms and 61% of recurrences involved distant metastases. Tjalma et al. reported similar results and demonstrated that 33% of recurrences are local, 57% are distant metastases, and 10% are both [10]. In detection of asymptomatic recurrences, 21% are detected by physical examination, 10% are detected by chest X-ray, and 2% are detected by vaginal vault cytology [14]. Physical examination is more helpful than other types of examination for the detection of recurrence. Most recurrent patients present with symptoms. The most frequently observed symptoms are abdominal or pelvic pain, followed by weight loss, lethargy, and vaginal bleeding [10]. Counseling, with careful attention to questioning about these symptoms, is important. Only one study reported that asymptomatic recurrent cases showed a significant survival advantage as compared with symptomatic recurrent cases [15]. In this report, however, there were only four cases of asymptomatic recur-

Table 61.3 Surveillance after curative-intent treatment for patient with endometrial carcinoma at lower risk of recurrence at Kyushu University Hospital

	Years posttreatment[a]					
	1	2	3	4	5	>5
Office visit[b]	4	3	2	2	2	1
Pap test	4	3	2	2	2	1
Tumor marker	4	3	2	2	2	1
Chest X-ray	2	1–2	2	2	2	1
Abdominal CT	2	1–2	1	1	1	0

Lower risk patients (In Kyushu University Hospital) are defined as stage IA or IB and grade 1 or 2 of endometrial adenocarcinoma cases, which are not indicated to adjuvant therapy after operation
[a]The numbers in the table indicate the number of times the modality is recommended during the indicated year posttreatment
[b]Should include pelvic exam and Pap smear. CBC, LFT (liver function test), KFT (kidney function test), and urinalysis are performed as clinically indicated

Table 61.4 Surveillance after curative-intent treatment for patient with endometrial carcinoma at higher risk of recurrence at Kyushu University

	Years posttreatment[a]					
	1	2	3	4	5	>5
Office visit[b]	6	4	3	2	2	1
Pap test	6	4	3	2	2	1
Tumor marker	6	4	3	2	2	1
Chest X-ray	3	2	1–2	1	1	1
Abdominal CT	2	2	1–2	1	1	0

Higher risk patients (In Kyushu University Hospital) cases indicated for adjuvant chemotherapy postsurgery. Such cases are as follows: (1) stage 1C, or more advanced stage; (2) any stage of grade 3 of endometrial adenocarcinoma; (3) any stage of serous adenocarcinoma or clear cell adenocarcinoma
[a]The numbers in the table indicate the number of times the modality is recommended during the indicated year posttreatment
[b]Should include pelvic exam and Pap smear. CBC, LFT (liver function test), KFT (kidney function test), and urinalysis are performed as clinically indicated

rence and other studies report no differences in survival rate. In conclusion, there seems to be no reliable difference in survival rates between patients with symptomatic and with asymptomatic recurrences.

Patients at a lower risk of recurrence had significantly fewer recurrences than patients at a higher risk of recurrence. Therefore, we divide the endometrial cancer patients into two groups as well as in National Comprehensive Cancer Network (NCCN) strategies. In Kyushu University Hospital, patients operatively diagnosed as stage 1A or 1B and grade 1 or 2 endometrioid adenocarcinoma are classified for the lower risk group and their treatment is completed by operation alone. The higher risk group consists of patients for whom adjuvant therapy is indicated. This group is defined as follows: (1) stage 1C or more advanced stage, (2) any stage of grade 3 endometrioid adenocarcinoma, and (3) any stage of serous adenocarcinoma or clear cell adenocarcinoma. As mentioned previously, chemotherapy is usually selected as adjuvant therapy for the higher risk group patients. In Japan, gynecologic oncologists, instead of medical oncologists, generally introduce adjuvant chemotherapy because the number of medical oncologists is not sufficient. Combination chemotherapy, using cyclophosphamide/epirubicin/cisplatin or paclitaxel/pirarubicin/carboplatin, was formerly used as the standard adjuvant treatment but, since 2006, a regimen combining paclitaxel and carboplatin has also been used. Although the patients who receive adjuvant radiation therapy are gradually decreasing in Japan, radiation oncologists introduce radiation therapy, if needed.

During the first follow-up year, we perform a clinical examination every 3 months for the lower risk group, and every 2 months for the higher risk groups (Tables 61.3 and 61.4). Our follow-up schedules request more frequent office visits than NCCN guidelines. One of the reasons is the low cost of medical services due to the unique national health insurance system in Japan. As far as the duration of follow-up is concerned, about half the reports cited in the literature are completed after 5 years, but annual follow-ups beyond 5 years are performed in some institutions for several years [14]. In Kyushu University Hospital, we perform routine follow-up led by gynecologic specialists for 5 years. After 5 years, we recommend patients visit a private gynecologic clinic annually.

In Kyushu University Hospital, gynecologic oncologists fundamentally have the responsibility for the patient's treatment. During the hospitalization, various clinicians communicate in the conference on the gynecological inpatient ward. Patients are educated regarding symptoms of recurrence as well as treatment complications, including later complications during their hospital stay. After the operation, gynecologic doctors inform patients about their disease, including stage or pathological grading. Patients are advised to pay close attention to certain symptoms (pain, bleeding, nausea, cough). In routine follow-up, careful physical examination, including pelvic, rectal, and breast examinations, is performed by a gynecologic oncologist. Although the consultation to medical oncologists or radiation oncologists is not routinely scheduled, it can be ordered, if required.

The use of routine tests (vaginal cytology, chest X-ray, abdominal ultrasound sonography, CT scan, CA 125) appears to be of low utility [10]. We do not employ vaginal or abdominal ultrasound scans as part of routine testing. We use them only in suspicious cases of recurrent lesion or ascites. Although a chest X-ray may detect pulmonary metastases or pleural effusion, this has little impact on outcome due to the poor effectiveness of systemic treatment for recurrent endometrial cancer. Because of the low cost of X-ray, we perform a chest X-ray every second visit for 3 years (Table 61.2).

We usually employ CT scans for screening recurrent lesions every second visit for the first 3 years in which period approximately 80% of recurrences are thought to occur. After 4 years, CT scans are not utilized as part of routine examinations.

Although PET/CT has become widespread in Japan, it is still too expensive to use in routine follow-up (Table 61.2). We utilize PET/CT for cases highly suspected recurrence in which no lesion is detected using conventional imaging modalities.

An abnormal serum CA 125 level is an important sign for recurrence. However, recurrent cases detected only by CA 125 testing are rare and about half of recurrent cases do not show CA 125 elevation. In CA 125 testing, false positive cases are frequent and adjuvant therapy is not usually indicated without additional evidence. Therefore, in Kyushu University Hospital, we include CA 125 in routine follow-up testing only in cases with preoperative CA 125 elevation.

Retrospective studies provide little evidence to inform us whether intensive follow-up schedules with multiple routine interventions result in overall survival benefits for postoperative endometrial cancer patients. From the view point of medical economy, reduction of follow-up visits and routine tests would mean an enormous reduction in costs. However, the aim of routine follow-up is not only to detect recurrent disease, but also to diagnose posttreatment complications. In addition, routine hospital visits are helpful for a patient's psychological well-being, a benefit not easily quantitated.

The most appropriate follow-up protocol is important to define, but precise evaluation of follow-up protocols is achieved only by prospective randomized trials. In the future, new medical technology may improve the diagnosis of recurrence, and new chemotherapeutic drugs may result in a more favorable outcome for recurrent patients. The Japan Gynecologic Oncology Group (JGOG) has just finished recruiting for a comparative phase II trial comparing three regimens of combined chemotherapy (paclitaxel/carboplatin vs. docetaxel/cisplatin vs. docetaxel/carboplatin). These results are forthcoming but for now we must content ourselves with continued contemporary follow-up examinations and hope for an improvement in the patient's quality of life.

References

1. National Cancer Center, Japan (http://ganjoho.jp/professional/statistics.html) (2009). Last Accessed on 23 Jan 2009. Center for Cancer Control and Information Services.
2. Susumu N, Sagae S, Udagawa Y, Niwa K, Kuramoto H, Satoh S, et al. Randomized phase III trial of pelvic radiotherapy versus cisplatin-based combined chemotherapy in patients with intermediate- and high-risk endometrial cancer: A Japanese Gynecologic Oncology Group Study. Gynecol Oncol. 2008;108:226–33.
3. Vasconcelos C, Félix A, Cunha TM. Preoperative assessment of deep myometrial and cervical invasion in endometrial carcinoma: comparison of magnetic resonance imaging and histopathologic evaluation. J Obstet Gynaecol. 2007;27(1):65–70.
4. Watanabe Y, Aoki D, Kitagawa R, Takeuchi S, Sagae S, Sakuragi N, et al. Status of surgical treatment procedures for endometrial cancer in Japan: results of a Japanese Gynecologic Oncology Group Survey. Gynecol Oncol. 2007;105:325–8.
5. Kfhlera C, Klemma P, Schaub A, Possoverc M, Kraused N, Tozzie R, et al. Introduction of transperitoneal lymphadenectomy in a gynecologic oncology center: analysis of 650 laparoscopic pelvic and/or para-aortic transperitoneal lymphadenectomies. Gynecol Oncol. 2004;95:52–61.
6. Palomba S, Falbo A, Mocciaro R, Russo T, Zullo F. Laparoscopic treatment for endometrial cancer: a meta-analysis of randomized controlled trials (RCTs). Gynecol Oncol. 2009;112(2):415–21.
7. Ushijima K, Yahata H, Yoshikawa H, Konishi I, Yasugi T, Saito T, et al. Multicenter phase II study of fertility-sparing treatment with medroxyprogesterone acetate for endometrial carcinoma and atypical hyperplasia in young women. J Clin Oncol. 2007;25:2798–803.
8. Chiva L, Lapuente F, González-Cortijo L, Carballo N, García JF, Rojo A, et al. Sparing fertility in young patients with endometrial cancer. Gynecol Oncol. 2008;111:S101–4.
9. Takahashi N, Hirashima Y, Harashima S, Takekuma M, Kawaguchi R, Yamada Y, et al. A patient with stage 1a endometrial carcinoma in whom a solitary recurrent lesion was detected in the external iliac lymph node after MPA therapy. Arch Gynecol Obstet. 2008;278:365–7.
10. Tjalma WAA, Vandam PA, Makar AP, Cruickshank DJ. The clinical value and the cost-effectiveness of follow-up in endometrial cancer patients. Int J Gynecol Cancer. 2004;14:931–7.
11. Santillan A, Govan L, Zahurak ML, Diaz-Montes TP, Giuntoli II RL, Bristow RE. Feasibility and economic impact of a clinical pathway for pap test utilization in Gynecologic Oncology Practice. Gynecol Oncol. 2008;109:388–93.
12. Kitajima K, Murakami K, Yamasaki E, Domeki Y, Kaji Y, Morita S, et al. Performance of integrated FDG-PET/contrast-enhanced CT in the diagnosis of recurrent uterine cancer: comparison with PET and enhanced CT. Eur J Nucl Med Mol Imaging. 2009;36(3):362–72. Epub 2008 Oct 18.
13. Kitajima K, Murakami K, Yamasaki E, Hagiwara S, Fukasawa I, Inaba N, et al. Performance of FDG-PET/CT in the diagnosis of recurrent endometrial cancer. Ann Nucl Med. 2008;22:103–9.
14. Fung-Kee-Fung M, Dodge J, Elit L, Lukka H, Chambers A, Oliver T. Follow-up after primary therapy for endometrial cancer: a systematic review. Gynecol Oncol. 2006;101:520–9.
15. Gordon F, Owen P, Chien PFW, Duncan ID. A critical evaluation of follow-up of women treated for endometrial adenocarcinoma. J Obstet Gynaecol. 1997;17(4):386–9.

Endometrial Carcinoma Surveillance Counterpoint: Canada

62

Michael Fung-Kee-Fung and Thomas K. Oliver

Keywords

Cancer • Cancer antigen (CA) 125 • Cancer detection • Cancer guidelines • Carcinoma • Computed tomography (CT) • Disease detection • Endometrial • Endometrium • Follow-up genetic counseling • Genetic testing • Examination • Physical examination • Pelvic examination • Recto-vaginal • Intravenous pyelography • Papanicolaou (PAP) • Quality of life (QOL) • Recurrence • Asymptomatic • Distant recurrence • High-risk recurrence • Local recurrence • Low-risk recurrence • Symptomatic surveillance • Survival • Survival disease-free • Overall survival • Tumor markers • Ultrasound • Vaginal vault cytology • X-ray • Chest X-ray

In Canada, approximately 4,400 women are diagnosed with endometrial cancer each year and approximately 800 die from the disease [1]. The majority of patients present with early-stage disease and this is reflected in an overall 5-year survival rate of approximately 85% [1]. Five-year survival rates range from approximately 96% for patients with local disease, 66% for those with regional disease, and 25% for those with more advanced disease [2]. Factors predictive of recurrence and survival include lymph node status, histological type, histological grade, stage of disease, depth of myometrial invasion, lymphovascular space involvement, and cervical involvement [3].

The optimum posttreatment surveillance of asymptomatic women with endometrial cancer has not been consistently defined or practiced in the clinical setting, nor has it been the target of rigorous investigation. This is evidenced by variations in surveillance schedules and tests, and also by the lack of prospective studies reported in the published literature. Due to the lack of high-quality evidence to guide surveillance, traditional approaches appear to be firmly entrenched in current practice. This is defined by a set number of visits by the treating physician using a variety of investigative modalities, usually well past year 5 after primary treatment [4–6].

Despite the limited evidence, there are known elements about relapse that can help guide posttreatment surveillance. The optimum schedule would be one that takes account of the risk of recurrence and the possibility of deriving a survival advantage by early detection and treatment. Such a surveillance schedule should take into account the risk of recurrence, symptoms and signs of disease recurrence, the likelihood of salvage, the timing of recurrence, the efficacy of follow-up tests, patient preferences and psychosocial well-being, and the type of practitioner conducting the surveillance, with the corresponding implications of limited resources.

Thus, a look at the literature, coupled with the known natural history of the disease, can be used to guide surveillance for patients who have been treated for endometrial cancer and who, in the majority of patients with early-stage disease, are likely to remain disease-free.

As seen in Table 62.1, a total of 14 studies have reported follow-up and outcome data on 2,647 patients treated for endometrial cancer [7–20]. Where reported, the majority of patients presented with Stage 1 disease (64–86%) [9, 12–17] and the rate of recurrence ranged from 8 to 19% [7–20]. In two studies, a smaller proportion of patients (approximately

M. Fung-Kee-Fung, MBBS, FRCS, MBA (✉)
Division of Gynecologic Oncology, Surgical Oncology Program, Department of Obstetrics and Gynecology, Ottawa Hospital/University of Ottawa, Ottawa, ON, Canada
e-mail: mfung@ottawahospital.on.ca

T.K. Oliver, BA
Department of Oncology, McMaster University, 711 Concession Street, Hamilton, ON L8V 1C3, Canada
e-mail: olivert@mcmaster.ca

F.E. Johnson et al. (eds.), *Patient Surveillance After Cancer Treatment*, Current Clinical Oncology,
DOI 10.1007/978-1-60327-969-7_62,

Table 62.1 Timing of routine follow-up visits

Patients			Recurrence				Number of follow-up visits per year					
		Total #	% with Stage 1	Overall rate %	% of symptomatic patients	% with distant disease	1	2	3	4	5	Total
MacDonald and Kidd [7]	1990	101	NR	19	100	NR	4	2	2	2	2	12
Podczaski et al [8].	1992	300	NR	16	49	38	4	4	2	2	2	14
Shumsky et al [9].	1994	317	82	16	75	53	4	3	2	2	2	13
Reddoch et al [10].	1995	398	NR	11	41	62	4	4	3	2	2	15
Berchuck et al [11].	1995	354	NR	12	61	45	4	3	3	2	2	14
Owen and Duncan [12]	1996	97	86	18	65	53	3–4	2	1	1	1	8–9
Agboola et al [13].	1997	432	79	12	60	62	4	3	2	2	2	13
Ng et al [14].	1997	86	64	14	86	86	6–12	6–12	4	2	2	20–32
Gordon et al [15].	1997	111	82	15	76	71	4	2	1	1	1	9
Salvesen et al [16].	1997	249	83	16	89	68	4	2	1	1	1	9
Gadducci et al [17].	2000	133	81	18	46	75	3–4	3–4	2	2	2	12–14
Morice et al [18].	2001	351	71	8	81	74	4	3	2	1	1	11
Sartori et al [19].	2007	84[a]	37	NR	52	58	4	3	2	1	1	13
Ueda et al [20].	2010	271	<34	11	45	45	12	4–6	4–6	2	2	24–28

Note: Ref, reference
[a]Only patients with recurrence were reported

one-third) presented with stage 1 disease [19, 20]. It should be noted that staging information in these reports was based on the International Federation of Gynecologists and Obstetricians 1998 staging system and not the current revision. The overall risk of recurrence was approximately 13% across all studies [7–20]. However, for patients at low risk (i.e., stages IA or IB, grades 1 or 2), the recurrence rate was approximately 3% in four studies that reported data on that outcome [10, 11, 17, 18]. The proportion of patients with symptoms at the time of recurrence ranged from 41 to 100% [7–20], with an overall average of approximately 65% across the series [7–20]. The lifetime risk of distant disease at the time of detection of recurrence (± local involvement) ranged from 38 to 86% [8–20] with an average distant recurrence rate of approximately 60% [4]. The follow-up schedules in these studies ranged from a low of 8 to 9 visits over a 5-year span to a high of 20–32 visits over a 5-year period [7–20]. Of the studies that reported data, follow-up was completed after 5 years in four [7, 10, 11, 15] and three studies specifically reported that follow-up continued for an additional 1 [20], 5 [12], or 8 [16] years beyond year 5. Five studies also reported that follow-up was continued on an annual [8, 13, 17, 18] or semi-annual [9] basis from the sixth year on, but no termination of surveillance was reported. Surveillance beyond year 5 is not supported by the natural history of the disease since, if a relapse is to occur, approximately 80% of patients do so by year 3 after treatment, and virtually all patients who ever have recurrence have done so by year 5 after treatment [7–20].

Physical examination was the most common clinical investigation employed for asymptomatic patients according to the schedule outlined in Table 62.1 [7–20]. Vaginal vault cytology was also regularly performed across the studies [7, 9–18, 20] with the exception of one study where Pap tests were scheduled semiannually [8], and one study that did not report the interval of Pap testing [19]. The use of chest X-ray was reported in 10 of the 14 studies [8–11, 13, 16–18, 20]. One study did not report the interval of chest X-rays performed [19]. Three studies reported the use of routine abdominal/pelvic ultrasound [17, 18, 20] and two studies reported the routine use of annual or semi-annual abdominal/pelvic computed tomography (CT) scans [17, 20]. Data on the routine collection of serum tumor markers, including cancer antigen (CA) 125, were reported in only one of the retrospective reviews where a subset of patients was tested one to four times annually [20]. In that study the use of tumor markers led to the detection of recurrent disease in three asymptomatic patients. Other retrospective studies have not reported any consistent benefit with routine testing for CA 125 [21–24].

The percentage of asymptomatic patients whose disease recurrence was detected through scheduled surveillance procedures is not well-defined in the identified literature. However, of the patients with recurrence who were asymptomatic (0–59% in the identified studies), it was reported that physical examination detected between 5 and 35% of recurrences, vaginal vault cytology detected 0–25% of recurrences, chest X-ray detected between 0 and 14% of recurrences, ultrasound detected 4–13% of recurrences, and CT detected 5–38% of recurrences [7–20]. Outside of one study that reported 25% of recurrences detected through the use of vaginal vault cytology [20], across the remaining studies a 0–4% detection rate was reported [7–19].

There were no studies that compared survival differences by type of follow-up strategy: less intensive vs. more intensive,

Table 62.2 Guidance on follow-up strategies by cancer guideline developers

Author year (Ref)	Recommended follow-up tests for asymptomatic patients: Physical exam	Pelvic exam	Vaginal vault cytology	X-ray	Ultrasound	CT	Other	Patient risk of recurrence	Recommended number of follow-up visits per year: Year 1	Year 2	Year 3	Year 4	Year 5	Year >5
NCCN 2010 [25]	Yes	NS	Yes[a]	Yes[b]	NI	NI	Yes[c, d]	NS	2–4	2–4	1–2	1–2	1–2	1–2
CCO 2009 [26]	Yes	Yes[c]	NI	NI	NI	NI	NI	Low	1–2	1–2	1–2	1–2	1–2	0
								High	2–4	2–4	2–4	2	2	0
BCCA 2006 [27]	Yes	Yes	NI	NI	NI	NI	NI	Low	4	2	1	1	1	1
								High	4	3	2	2	2	1
SCA 2005 [28]	Yes	Yes[e]	Yes	Yes[b]	NI	NI	NI	NS	3	3	2	2	2	2[f]

Note: Ref, reference; NS, Not specified, NI, Not indicated, NCCN, National Comprehensive Cancer Network, CCO, Cancer Care Ontario, BCCA, British Columbia Cancer Agency; SCA Saskatchewan Cancer Agency

[a]Every 6 months for 2 years, then annually thereafter

[b]Annual chest X-ray—optional

[c]CA-125 optional

[d]Consider genetic counseling for patients with a significant family history

[e]Including a recto-vaginal examination

[f]Follow-up to year 7

and there is little evidence to suggest that the earlier detection of asymptomatic disease leads to improvements in overall survival. Three of the 14 studies reported survival advantages in patients who were asymptomatic vs. symptomatic at the time of disease recurrence [15, 19, 20]. Due to the nature of the study designs, it is difficult to ascertain whether patients were truly asymptomatic at disease detection or if suspicion of disease prompted further targeted investigation that subsequently detected disease recurrence.

In the identified series, approximately 75% of patients presented with stage 1 disease [9, 12–18] and the overall risk of recurrence was approximately 13% [7–20]. For patients with features predicting a lower risk of recurrence (i.e., stage IA or IB, grade 1 or 2), the risk was less than 5% in four studies [10, 11, 17, 18]. Of the approximately 13% of patients who relapsed, about 65% experienced symptoms indicating recurrence outside of the planned follow-up visits [7–20]. Approximately 40% of women experienced a local recurrence and about 60% experienced a distant recurrence [7–20]. Most relapses occurred by the third year after treatment, and virtually all relapses occurred by the fifth year [7–20].

With this information, a follow-up algorithm illustrating the utility of surveillance can be used to help inform decision rules around follow-up strategies. For example, according to the identified evidence, and accounting for special circumstances, on average if 1,000 patients who were clinically disease-free after initial treatment for endometrial cancer were to be followed prospectively, approximately 87% or 870 patients would remain disease-free throughout the follow-up period and beyond, essentially cured of their disease. Approximately 13% or 130 patients would experience disease recurrence; most within 3 years of primary treatment and virtually all by year 5. Of those 130 patients, approximately 65% would present with symptomatic disease. This leaves approximately 45 asymptomatic patients for whom the early detection of recurrence through follow-up may be beneficial. Of those 45 patients, approximately 50% would experience a distant recurrence, where the early detection of recurrence has shown no overall survival benefit. That leaves a small proportion of patients with local disease recurrence of which about 50% are salvageable. For patients at a lower risk of recurrence, assuming a 3% recurrence rate, the absolute number of patients who would benefit from follow-up decreases to approximately two out of every 1,000 patients followed.

The utility of surveillance in improving survival outcomes is small but, for patients who do experience relapse, surveillance plays an important role in psychosocial health and is a major component of survivorship care planning. In addition, the early detection of recurrent disease provides essential information to alter the management strategy of patients and can have a substantial impact in terms of outcomes related to progression-free survival, morbidity, and/or quality of life. The cost implications of such a follow-up strategy for the benefits predicted are beyond the scope of this review, but would need to be considered in health technology assessments informing clinical policy.

Clinical guidance on the follow-up of patients with endometrial cancer has been developed by the National Comprehensive Cancer Network [25], Cancer Care Ontario (CCO) [26], the British Columbia Cancer Agency (BCCA) [27], and the Saskatchewan Cancer Agency (SCA) [28]. As seen in Table 62.2, physical and pelvic examinations are recommended as the primary surveillance strategies to detect disease recurrence. While not specifically reported in some of the guidelines, it is assumed that a speculum exam with bimanual and pelvic/rectal examination, as well as a complete patient history should comprise an integral component of the office visit. While only NCCN and CCO recommended that patients be counseled about signs and symptoms of disease recurrence, it is also assumed in remaining guidelines that counseling is an integral component of routine follow-up.

In contrast with the CCO and BCCA guidelines, the NCCN and SCA recommended vaginal vault cytology and optional chest X-ray as part of routine follow-up [24, 27]. The BCCA also recommended mammograms and colonoscopy every 2 years if patients are known to be or are suspected of being part of a Lynch Syndrome family [26], while the NCCN guideline recommended that CA-125 be optional and patients with a significant family history should be considered for genetic counseling [24].

Recommendations on the type of practitioner to conduct the follow-up were not consistent among the guideline documents. In the CCO guideline, the authors stated that surveillance should be conducted by either a physician knowledgeable about disease recurrence or by a specialist. If patients are followed by a specialist, they go on to suggest that it is reasonable for patients to be followed by a qualified general practitioner after 3–5 years of being disease-free [25]. The NCCN guideline did not specify the type of practitioner to conduct follow-up [24], while the BCCA recommended a follow-up visit 1 month after treatment by a BCCA specialist and routine follow-up through the family physician [26]. The SCA recommended follow-up through a family physician or gynecologist [27].

There was variation among the recommendations concerning the number of follow-up visits to year 5 and beyond. The recommended number of follow-up visits ranged from a potential low of five visits to a potential high of 16 visits over a 5-year period [24–27]. Targeted follow-up beyond year 5 was not recommended in one guideline [25], was recommended to year seven in one guideline [27], and guidance on the discontinuation of follow-up was not reported in two guidelines [24, 26].

Table 62.3 Surveillance after curative-intent treatment for endometrial carcinoma at the Ottawa Cancer Center

Surveillance modality	Patient risk of recurrence[a]	Time after primary treatment Year 1	Year 2	Year 3	Year 4	Year 5	Year >5
Physical examination[b, c]	Low	1–2	1–2	1–2	1	1	[d]
	High[e]	2–4	2–4	2–4	2	2	[d]

Follow-up by a general physician or gynecologist is encouraged for low-risk patients
Follow-up for high-risk patients is generally performed by the treating gynecologic oncologist or radiation oncologist
Targeted use of CT and/or US is used as appropriate in high-risk (advanced disease) cases
Vaginal vault cytology, chest X-ray, transvaginal ultrasonogram, CT, serum tumor marker levels, and other tests are used only if symptoms or signs of recurrence are noted
The number in each cell indicates the number of times a particular modality is recommended during a particular posttreatment year
[a]Low risk of recurrence = stage IA or IB, grade 1 or 2. High risk of recurrence = stage IA or IB, grade 3, stage IC or advanced stage
[b]Includes counseling on the signs and symptoms of disease recurrence, a complete history and pelvic-rectal examination
[c]The patient should be followed by a health care professional who is knowledgeable about the natural history of the disease and who is comfortable performing speculum and pelvic examinations. If a patient is initially followed by a specialist, it seems reasonable that she be followed by a qualified general practitioner after 3–5 years of recurrence-free follow-up
[d]Return to physical and pelvic examination as needed after 5 years of recurrence-free status
[e]Risk based on 1988 Fédération Internationale de Gynécologie Obstétrique (FIGO) staging system.

Patient Surveillance at the Ottawa Cancer Centre

As seen in Table 62.3, at the Ottawa Hospital, the follow-up of patients after primary treatment for endometrial cancer is conducted according to an Ontario clinical practice guideline [25]. Care is provided through a centralized multidisciplinary clinic where coordinated treatment planning and a common data system ensure that patients move through the system and are treated as efficiently as possible. Upon completion of treatment with curative intent, patients are counseled on the signs and symptoms of recurrence by the treating physician, and also by an oncology nurse upon discharge. As part of the survivorship care plan, all patients are given an information booklet on endometrial cancer at discharge with a copy sent to their primary physician. This includes a patient information sheet, which details their specific risk for recurrence, common sites and symptoms of recurrence, and a suggested examination protocol.

For patients at low risk of disease recurrence (Stage 1A or 1B, Grade 1 or 2), follow-up once or twice a year is encouraged and for those at a higher risk of recurrence (Stage 1A or 1B, Grade 3, or Stage 1C or more advanced stage), more intensive follow-up (10–16 visits over a 5 year span) is recommended. For patients at low risk who have not received adjuvant radiation therapy, their follow-up is directed to their family physician and/or a general gynecologist according to the standardized protocol. In addition, there is an established mechanism for rapid re-entry into the clinic which can be initiated by the physician or the patient herself. For all other patients, follow-up occurs in the cancer center by either a gynaecologic or radiation oncologist, who also use the common protocol.

For patients who receive radiotherapy, even though the pattern of recurrence may vary from those that do not receive radiotherapy, there is no evidence to suggest that different follow-up requirements are needed. Patients who have had radiation therapy as their primary modality are followed by the treating radiation oncologist and assessment is made not only for recurrence risk, but also for toxicities from radiation therapy.

After 5 years of being disease-free, those patients who have been followed in the cancer clinic are referred to their family doctor, again according to the standardized protocol. For patients that live at a distance, a sustainable follow-up strategy has not been implemented to date and patients are often followed by their primary care provider.

At the Ottawa Hospital, it is generally agreed that the evidence indicates that there is little utility for the routine use of Pap smear, chest X-ray, abdominal ultrasound, CT scan, or CA 125 testing in detecting potential recurrent disease in patients who are asymptomatic. Thus, these practices are generally not indicated as part of routine follow-up.

To date our surveillance strategies have been well received by both physicians and patients after a number of education awareness interventions, in particular those that focused on patient education and the benefits and limitations of routine follow-up.

Given that follow-up is a part of standard practice and it appropriately reflects a conservative approach to patient care, all strategies should attempt to balance the practical and resource considerations involved with following a large number of women who remain disease-free with that of the optimal cancer control strategy for those who do relapse.

Future Prospects

The retrospective evidence highlights the need for well-conducted prospective studies to further inform the most appropriate surveillance strategies for patients after treatment for endometrial cancer; most of whom are at a low risk of recurrence and who will remain disease-free throughout the surveillance period and beyond. Studies that stratify patients by risk of disease recurrence (low, intermediate, or high), by type of health care practitioner, and by comparing standard follow-up with more or less intense follow-up would be of great interest. Outcomes of interest would include obtaining a more accurate reflection of symptomatic vs. asymptomatic recurrence rates, rates of distant vs. local recurrences, the efficacy of investigative examinations, improvements or reductions in patients' quality of life, patient follow-up preferences, and in overall survival outcomes. Randomized trials comparing follow-up management strategies, such as the TOTem study (www.epiclin.cpo.it), are underway and will undoubtedly inform new models of effective surveillance. Until such time that prospective data are reported, the use of retrospective data and expert consensus opinion will continue to guide the discussion about the optimal surveillance strategy for patients who are clinically disease-free after treatment for endometrial cancer.

References

1. National Cancer Institute of Canada. Canadian Cancer Statistics 2009. Toronto (Canada): Canadian Cancer Society; National Cancer Institute of Canada; Statistics Canada; Provincial/Territorial Cancer Registries; Health Canada; 2009.
2. American Cancer Society. Cancer facts and figures 2006. Atlanta: American Cancer Society; 2006.
3. Uharcek P. Prognostic factors in endometrial carcinoma. J Obstet Gynaecol Res. 2008;34:776–83.
4. Fung-Kee-Fung M, Dodge J, Elit L, et al. Follow-up after primary therapy for endometrial cancer: a systematic review. Gynecol Oncol. 2006;101:520–9.
5. Kew FM, Roberts AP, Cruickshank DJ. The role of routine follow-up after gynecological malignancy. Int J Gynecol Cancer. 2005;15:413–9.
6. Tjalma WA, van Dam PA, Makar AP, Cruickshank DJ. The clinical value and the cost-effectiveness of follow-up in endometrial cancer patients. Int J Gynecol Cancer. 2004;14:931–7.
7. MacDonald JH, Kidd GM. An audit of endometrial carcinoma: the value of routine follow up. J Obstet Gynaecol. 1990;10:548–50.
8. Podczaski E, Kaminski P, Gurski K, et al. Detection and patterns of treatment failure in 300 consecutive cases of "early" endometrial cancer after primary surgery. Gynecol Oncol. 1992;47: 323–7.
9. Shumsky AG, Stuart GC, Brasher PM, Nation JG, Robertson DI, Sangkarat S. An evaluation of routine follow-up of patients treated for endometrial carcinoma. Gynecol Oncol. 1994;55:229–33.
10. Reddoch JM, Burke TW, Morris M, Tornos C, Levenback C, Gershenson DM. Surveillance for recurrent endometrial carcinoma: development of a follow-up scheme. Gynecol Oncol. 1995;59:221–5.
11. Berchuck A, Anspach C, Evans AC, et al. Postsurgical surveillance of patients with FIGO stage I/II endometrial adenocarcinoma. Gynecol Oncol. 1995;59:20–4.
12. Owen P, Duncan ID. Is there any value in the long term follow up of women treated for endometrial cancer? Br J Obstet Gynaecol. 1996;103:710–3.
13. Agboola OO, Grunfeld E, Coyle D, Perry GA. Costs and benefits of routine follow-up after curative treatment for endometrial cancer. Can Med Assoc J. 1997;157:879–86.
14. Ng TY, Ngan HYS, Cheng DKL, Wong LC. Vaginal vault cytology in the routine follow-up of patients treated for endometrial carcinoma: is it useful? Aust NZ J Obstet Gynaecol. 1997;37:104–6.
15. Gordon AF, Owen P, Chien PFW, Duncan ID. A critical evaluation of follow-up of women treated for endometrial adenocarcinoma. J Obstet Gynaecol. 1997;17:386–9.
16. Salvesen HB, Akslen LA, Iversen T, Iversen OE. Recurrence of endometrial carcinoma and the value of routine follow up. Br J Obstet Gynaecol. 1997;104:1302–7.
17. Gadducci A, Cosio S, Fanucchi A, Cristofani R, Genazzani AR. An intensive follow-up does not change survival of patients with clinical stage I endometrial cancer. Anticancer Res. 2000;20:1977–84.
18. Morice P, Levy-Piedbois C, Ajaj S, et al. Value and cost evaluation of routine follow-up for patients with clinical stage I/II endometrial cancer. Eur J Cancer. 2001;37:985–90.
19. Sartori E, Pasinetti B, Carrara L, Gambino A, Odicino F, Pecorelli S. Pattern of failure and value of follow-up procedures in endometrial and cervical cancer patients. Gynecol Oncol. 2007;107(1 Suppl 1):S241–7. Epub 2007 Sep 10.
20. Ueda Y, Enomoto T, Egawa-Takata T, et al. Endometrial carcinoma: better prognosis for asymptomatic recurrences than for symptomatic cases found by routine follow-up. Int J Clin Oncol. 2010;15:406–12. Epub 2010 Apr 28.
21. Patsner B, Orr Jr JW, Mann Jr WJ. Use of serum CA 125 measurement in posttreatment surveillance of early-stage endometrial carcinoma. Am J Obstet Gynecol. 1990;162:427–9.
22. Rose PG, Sommers RM, Reale FR, Hunter RE, Fournier L, Nelson BE. Serial serum CA 125 measurements for evaluation of recurrence in patients with endometrial carcinoma. Obstet Gynecol. 1994;84:12–6.

23. Lo SS, Khoo US, Cheng DK, Ng TY, Wong LC, Ngan HY. Role of serial tumor markers in the surveillance for recurrence in endometrial cancer. Cancer Detect Prev. 1999;23:397–400.
24. Price FV, Chambers SK, Carcangiu ML, Kohorn EI, Schwartz PE, Chambers JT. CA 125 may not reflect disease status in patients with uterine serous carcinoma. Cancer. 1998;82:1720–5.
25. National Comprehensive Cancer Network. Uterine neoplasms. http://www.nccn.org (2010). Accessed 20 Feb 2010.
26. Fung-Kee-Fung M, Dodge J, Elit L, et al. Follow-up after primary therapy for endometrial cancer: a clinical practice guideline. http://www.cancercare.on.ca/common/pages/UserFile.aspx?fileId=14108 (2010). Accessed 2 May 2010
27. BC Cancer Agency. Cancer management guidelines: gynecology. November 2008. http://www.bccancer.bc.ca/HPI/CancerManagementGuidelines/Gynecology/Endometrium/FU.html (2009). Accessed 27 March 2009.
28. Saskatchewan Cancer Agency. Follow-up guidelines: endometrial cancer. August 30, 2005. http://www.saskcancer.ca/ (2008). Accessed 10 Dec 2008.

Cervical Carcinoma

63

David Y. Johnson, Shilpi Wadhwa, and Frank E. Johnson

Keywords
Cervix • Immunosuppression • Sexual activity • HPV • Cervical cells

The International Agency for Research on Cancer (IARC), a component of the World Health Organization (WHO), estimated that there were 493,243 new cases of cervix cancer worldwide in 2002 [1]. The IARC also estimated that there were 273,505 deaths due to this cause in 2002 [1].

The American Cancer Society estimated that there were 11,150 new cases and 3,670 deaths due to this cause in the USA in 2007[2]. The estimated 5-year survival rate (all races) in the USA in 2007 was 10 % for cervical cancer [2]. Survival rates were adjusted for normal life expectancies and were based on cases diagnosed from 1996 to 2002 and followed through 2003.

Many risk factors for cervix cancer are known. HPV infection, particularly types 16, 18, 31, 33, and 45, is a major causative agent. Sexual promiscuity, including sexual activity with promiscuous males, smoking, and immunosuppression (particularly HIV-related immunosuppression) are risk factors. The risk increases with advancing age and lack of access to medical care, particularly Papanicolaou screening. Among women who have Papanicolaou screening, the risk of developing cervix cancer varies with cytological appearance of cervical cells [3, 4].

D.Y. Johnson • S. Wadhwa
Department of Internal Medicine, Saint Louis University Medical Center, Saint Louis, MO, USA

F.E. Johnson (✉)
Saint Louis University Medical Center and Saint Louis Veterans Affairs Medical Center, Saint Louis, MO, USA
e-mail: frank.johnson1@va.gov

Geographic Variation Worldwide

In Africa, the incidence of cervical cancer is reported to be highest in Tanzania, Swaziland, and Lesotho. Bolivia and Haiti also have very high incidence; Syria is reported to have the lowest incidence [5].

Geographic variation in the USA is also pronounced [6].

Surveillance Strategies Proposed by Professional Organizations or National Government Agencies and Available on the Internet

National Comprehensive Cancer Network (www.nccn.org)

National Comprehensive Cancer Network (NCCN) guidelines were accessed on 1/28/12 (Table 63.1). There were major quantitative and qualitative changes compared to the guidelines accessed on 4/10/07.

American Society of Clinical Oncology (www.asco.org)

American Society of Clinical Oncology (ASCO) guidelines were accessed on 1/28/12. No quantitative guidelines exist for cervical cancer surveillance, including when first accessed on 10/31/07.

F.E. Johnson et al. (eds.), *Patient Surveillance After Cancer Treatment*, Current Clinical Oncology,
DOI 10.1007/978-1-60327-969-7_63,

Table 63.1 Cervical carcinoma

	Years posttreatment[a]					
	1	2	3	4	5	>5
Office visit	2–4	2–4	1–2	1–2	1–2	1
Cervical/vaginal cytology	2–4	2–4	1–2	1–2	1–2	1
Chest X-ray	1	1	1	1	1	0
CBC, BUN, creatinine[b]	2	2	2	2	2	2

- PET-CT scan as clinically indicated[c]
- Recommend use of vaginal dilator after RT
- Patient education regarding symptoms

Obtained from NCCN (www.nccn.org) on 1-28-12
NCCN guidelines were accessed on 1/28/12. There were major quantitative and qualitative changes compared to the guidelines accessed on 4/10/07
[a]The numbers in the table indicate the number of times the modality is recommended during the indicated year posttreatment
[b]Optional
[c]PET-CT scan may be useful in detecting isolated recurrences or persistent disease that is amenable to potentially curative salvage therapy

Table 63.2 Cervical carcinoma

	Years posttreatment[a]					
	1	2	3	4	5	>5
Office visit	4	4	3	3	3	1
Pap smear	4	4	3	3	3	1

- SCC dosage in squamous cell carcinoma may be useful in patients' follow-up if initially increased
- PET/CT might have a role in early local recurrence and metastasis detection

Obtained from ESMO (www.esmo.org) on 1-28-12
ESMO guidelines were accessed on 1/28/12. These are new quantitative guidelines compared to the guidelines accessed on 10/31/07
[a]The numbers in the table indicate the number of times the modality is recommended during the indicated year posttreatment

Table 63.3 Cervical carcinoma

	Years posttreatment[a]					
	1	2	3	4	5	>5
Office visit[b]	3–4	3–4	1–2	1–2	1–2	1
Cervical/vaginal cytology[c]	1	1	1	1	1	1

- Patients need to be informed about symptoms of recurrence, because the majority of women have signs or symptoms of recurrence that occur outside of scheduled follow-up visits
- The routine use of other investigations in asymptomatic patients is not advocated as their role has yet to be evaluated in a definitive manner[d, e]

Obtained from CCO (www.cancercare.on.ca) on 1-28-12
CCO guidelines were accessed on 1/28/12. These are new quantitative guidelines compared to no guidelines found on 10/31/07
[a]The numbers in the table indicate the number of times the modality is recommended during the indicated year posttreatment
[b]Symptoms elicited during the patient history should include general performance status, lower back pain especially if it radiates down one leg, vaginal bleeding, or unexplained weight loss. A physical examination should attempt to identify abnormal findings related to general health and/or those that suggest vaginal, pelvic sidewall, or distant recurrence. Since central pelvic recurrences are potentially curable, the physical examination should include a speculum examination and bimanual and pelvic/rectal examination
[c]There is little evidence to suggest that vaginal vault cytology adds significantly to the clinical exam in detecting early disease recurrence. If cytology is performed as part of routine follow-up after surgery for cervical cancer, its role would be to detect new precancerous conditions of the vagina and should be no more frequent than once a year. An abnormal cytology result that suggests the possibility of neoplasia warrants colposcopic evaluation and directed biopsy for histologic confirmation
[d]The role of abdominal or pelvic computed tomography, magnetic resonance imaging scans, positron emission tomography, or ultrasound as part of routine follow-up has not been fully evaluated in prospective studies
[e]Use of serum markers such as squamous cell carcinoma antigen or cancer antigen 125 have shown promise in predicting surgical findings, or in the post-radiotherapy course when disease is present; however, their role in following patients' posttreatment has yet to be determined

The Society of Surgical Oncology (www.surgonc.org)

The Society of Surgical Oncology (SSO) guidelines were accessed on 1/28/12. No quantitative guidelines exist for cervical cancer surveillance, including when first accessed on 10/31/07.

European Society for Medical Oncology (www.esmo.org)

European Society for Medical Oncology (ESMO) guidelines were accessed on 1/28/12 (Table 63.2). There are new quantitative guidelines compared to the guidelines accessed on 10/31/07.

European Society of Surgical Oncology (www.esso-surgeonline.org)

European Society of Surgical Oncology (ESSO) guidelines were accessed on 1/28/12. No quantitative guidelines exist for cervical cancer surveillance, including when first accessed on 10/31/07.

Cancer Care Ontario (www.cancercare.on.ca)

Cancer Care Ontario (CCO) guidelines were accessed on 1/28/12 (Table 63.3). There are new quantitative guidelines compared to no guidelines found on 10/31/07.

National Institute for Clinical Excellence (www.nice.org.uk)

National Institute for Clinical Excellence (NICE) guidelines were accessed on 1/28/12. No quantitative guidelines exist for cervical cancer surveillance, including when first accessed on 10/31/07.

Table 63.4 Cervical carcinoma, low risk (early stage, treated with surgery alone, no adjuvant therapy)

	Years posttreatment[a]					
	1	2	3	4	5	>5
Office visit	2	2	1[b]	1[II]	1[II]	1[II]
Papanicolaou test/cytologic evidence[c]	1	1	1	1	1	1

- Chest X-ray, positron emission tomography/computed tomography, magnetic resonance imaging not recommended for routine use
- Computed tomography and/or positron emission tomography scan recommended if recurrence suspected

Obtained from SGO (www.sgo.org) on 1-28-12
SGO guidelines were accessed on 1/28/12. These are new quantitative guidelines compared to no guidelines found on 12/13/07
[a]The numbers in the table indicate the number of times the modality is recommended during the indicated year posttreatment
[b]May be followed by a generalist or gynecologic oncologist
[c]Insufficient evidence of value for cancer recurrence but may have value in the detection of other lower genital tract neoplasia

Table 63.5 Cervical carcinoma, high risk (advanced stage, treated with primary chemotherapy/radiation therapy or surgery plus adjuvant therapy)

	Years posttreatment[a]					
	1	2	3	4	5	>5
Office visit	4	4	2	2	2	1[b]
Papanicolaou test/cytologic evidence[c]	1	1	1	1	1	1

- Chest X-ray, positron emission tomography/computed tomography, magnetic resonance imaging not recommended for routine use
- Computed tomography and/or positron emission tomography scan recommended if recurrence suspected

Obtained from SGO (www.sgo.org) on 1-28-12
SGO guidelines were accessed on 1/28/12. These are new quantitative guidelines compared to no guidelines found on 12/13/07
[a]The numbers in the table indicate the number of times the modality is recommended during the indicated year posttreatment
[b]May be followed by a generalist or gynecologic oncologist
[c]Insufficient evidence of value for cancer recurrence but may have value in the detection of other lower genital tract neoplasia

The Cochrane Collaboration (CC, www.cochrane.org)

CC guidelines were accessed on 1/28/12. No quantitative guidelines exist for cervical cancer surveillance, including when first accessed on 11/24/07.

Society of Gynecologic Oncologists (www.sgo.org)

Society of Gynecologic Oncologists (SGO) guidelines were accessed on 1/28/12 (Tables 63.4 and 63.5). There are new quantitative guidelines compared to no guidelines found on 12/13/07.

The M.D. Anderson Surgical Oncology Handbook also has follow-up guidelines, proposed by authors from a single National Cancer Institute-designated Comprehensive Cancer Center, for many types of cancer [7]. Some are detailed and quantitative, others are qualitative.

Summary

This is the second most common cancer among women worldwide, and the most common gynecologic cancer in many developing countries. We found consensus-based guidelines but none based on high-quality evidence.

References

1. Parkin DM, Whelan SL, Ferlay J, Teppo L, Thomas DB. Cancer incidence in five continents, Vol. VIII, International Agency for Research on Cancer. (IARC Scientific Publication 155). Lyon, France: IARC Press; 2002. ISBN 92-832-2155-9.
2. Jemal A, Seigel R, Ward E, Murray T, Xu J, Thun MJ. Cancer statistics, 2007. CA Cancer J Clin. 2007;57:43–66.
3. Schottenfeld D, Fraumeni JG. Cancer epidemiology and prevention. 3rd ed. New York, NY: Oxford University Press; 2006. ISBN 13:978-0-19-514961-6.
4. DeVita VT, Hellman S, Rosenberg SA. Cancer. 7th ed. Philadelphia, PA: Lippincott Williams & Wilkins; 2005. ISBN 0-781-74450-4.
5. Mackay J, Jemal A, Lee NC, Parkin M. The Cancer Atlas. 2006 American Cancer Society 1599 Clifton Road NE, Atlanta, Georgia 30329, USA. Can also be accessed at www.cancer.org (2006). ISBN 0-944235-62-X.
6. Devesa SS, Grauman DJ, Blot WJ, Pennello GA, Hoover RN, Fraumeni JF Jr. Atlas of Cancer Mortality in the United States. National Institutes of Health, National Cancer Institute. NIH Publication No. 99-4564; Sep 1999.
7. Feig BW, Berger DH, Fuhrman GM. The M.D. Anderson Surgical Oncology Handbook. 4th ed. Philadelphia, PA: Lippincott Williams & Wilkins; 2006. ISBN 0-7817-5643-X (paperback).

Cervical Carcinoma Surveillance Counterpoint: USA

64

Joshua P. Kesterson and Shashikant Lele

Keywords
Cervical cancer • Pap smear • Chest X-ray • Human papillomavirus (HPV) • Smoking

Introduction

The role of follow-up surveillance for patients treated for cervical cancer with curative intent has not been fully defined. The National Comprehensive Cancer Network (NCCN) practice guidelines for surveillance recommend office visits and Pap tests every 3 months the first year, every 4 months the second year, every 6 months the third year, then annually (Table 64.1) [1]. They also recommend performing a chest X-ray annually with other imaging studies ordered as clinically indicated. The American College of Obstetricians and Gynecologists (ACOG) notes that patients treated for cervical cancer should be monitored regularly with thrice-yearly follow-up examinations the first 2 years and twice yearly, subsequently to year 5, with Pap tests and chest X-rays annually [2]. These recommendations are based primarily on expert opinion and consensus. Although evidence-based criteria for screening strategies are lacking and strict screening strategies are not uniformly implemented, the approach reported by most authors broadly consists of examinations every 3 months the year following treatment, with increasing intervals between screening the subsequent years. Pap smears, chest X-rays, and ultrasounds are used with varying frequency.

In order to justify screening for a particular disease, Wilson and Junger originally proposed that several criteria be met (Table 64.2) [3]. In this chapter we will address these criteria as they pertain to the follow-up surveillance of patients with a history of cervical cancer including: the incidence of recurrent cervical cancer; its natural history including usual presentation, timing, and sites of recurrence; methods currently implemented for screening; expected outcomes for those with recurrent disease; and an analysis of current studies assessing the benefit of current screening strategies. We will also discuss the risk of secondary malignancies in patients previously treated for cervical cancer.

Recurrent disease after treatment for cervical cancer is a clinically significant problem, affecting a considerable number of patients with cervical cancer. The risk of recurrence is dependent on several factors, including stage and type and treatment. Of patients with International Federation of Gynecology and Obstetrics (FIGO) stage IB cervical cancer treated with radical hysterectomy and pelvic lymphadenectomy, 11% will recur [4]. The addition of radiation therapy to radical surgery for patients with stage IB disease results in a similar percentage of recurrences [5, 6]. In their 1997 study, Landoni et al. reported equivalent 5-year overall and disease-free survival duration in women with Stage IB and IIA cervical carcinoma treated with radical surgery or radiotherapy [7]. Eighty-six (25%) of 343 patients developed recurrent disease. The risk of recurrence increases with more advanced stages of cancer. In a study consisting primarily of women with stage IIB and IIIB cervical cancer treated with a combination of external beam radiotherapy (EBRT) and brachytherapy, 21% of patients developed local relapse, 6.3% developed distant metastases, and 1.6% developed both local relapse and distant metastasis [8]. Failure rates after radiotherapy (RT) alone have been shown to be around 30% for patients with bulky stage IB-IIA and IIB disease, increasing to 50% for patients with stage III disease [9]. In a large study of 1,292 patients with stage I-IVA squamous cell carcinoma

J.P. Kesterson, M.D. • S. Lele, M.D. (✉)
Division of Gynecologic Oncology, Roswell Park Cancer Institute, Elm & Carlton Streets, Buffalo, NY 14263, USA
e-mail: joshua.kesterson@roswellpark.org; shashi.lele@roswellpark.org

F.E. Johnson et al. (eds.), *Patient Surveillance After Cancer Treatment*, Current Clinical Oncology, DOI 10.1007/978-1-60327-969-7_64, © Springer Science+Business Media New York 2013

Table 64.1 Surveillance after curative-intent treatment for cervical carcinoma at Roswell Park Cancer Institute (NCCN member)

	Years posttreatment					
	1	2	3	4	5	>5
Pap test and office visit	4	3	2	1	1	1
Chest X-ray	1	1	1	1	1	0

CBC, BUN, and serum creatinine levels every 6 months is optional
The number in each cell indicates the number of times in a particular year a particular surveillance modality is recommended
[a]NCCN Clinical Practice Guidelines in Oncology-Cervical Cancer (V.I.2009)

Table 64.2 Summary of criteria for screening[a]

The condition sought should be an important health problem for the individual and community
There should be an accepted treatment or useful intervention for patients with the disease
Facilities for diagnosis and treatment should be available
The natural history of the disease should be adequately understood
There should be a latent or early symptomatic stage
There should be a suitable and acceptable screening test or examination
There should be an agreed upon policy on whom to treat as patients
Treatment started at an early stage should be of more benefit than treatment started later
The cost should be economically balanced in relation to possible expenditure on medical care as a whole
Case findings should be a continuing process and not a once and for all project

[a]Wilson and Jungner [3]

(SCC) of the cervix treated with RT between 1990 and 1999, Hong et al. reported that 375 (29%) had either local or distant failure, including 35 (2.7%) with both pelvic and distant relapse [10]. In 1999, Morris et al. demonstrated improved survival in patients with locally advanced cervical cancer confined to the pelvis (stages IIB through IVA or stage IB or IIA with a tumor diameter ≥5 cm or involvement of pelvic lymph nodes) with the addition of chemotherapy to external beam and intracavitary radiation [11]. In the combined therapy group, the rate of locoregional recurrence was 19% and the rate of distant relapse was 14%. In summary, recurrent cervical cancer affects a significant number of patients with a history of cervical cancer, across all stages and treatment modalities.

In patients who do recur, a majority do so within the first several years following treatment [5, 6, 12–17]. Estimates of the rate of symptomatic relapse range from 50 to 87% [4, 5, 12, 18–22]. Symptoms of recurrent cervical cancer include: vaginal bleeding and/or discharge, pain, sciatica, lymphedema, anorexia, dyspnea, and cough. The outcomes for patients with recurrent cervical cancer have historically been very poor. In a series of 500 patients treated for cervical cancer at the University of Kentucky, 160 (31%) patients experienced recurrence and only 6% of patients with recurrent disease survived 3 or more years [23]. All recurrences are not equal with regard to their expected outcome. Patients who develop a resectable central pelvic recurrence after prior radiation therapy may be candidates for pelvic exenteration with expected 5-year survival rates between 30 and 60% [24]. Patients who relapse locally after primary surgery may be treated with either radiation or pelvic exenteration. However, recurrent disease beyond the pelvis is, with few exceptions, incurable. The widespread implementation of programs aimed at screening for recurrent cervical cancer can only be justified if currently available screening modalities are capable of identifying potentially curable cases of recurrence before they become symptomatic and that early detection allows for an intervention which confers an improved outcome when compared to those patients who are treated after their symptomatic presentation.

Studies vary as to the survival benefit, if any, of screening for recurrent cervical cancer [25]. Herein, we analyze published studies designed to determine the effectiveness of currently utilized screening programs including patients studied, surveillance strategies used, sites of recurrences (with a focus on locally recurrent and therefore potentially curable disease), and outcomes of those with symptomatic and asymptomatic disease recurrences. We also discuss the limitations of existing studies, including lead time and length time biases.

In 1996, investigators from the United Kingdom reported the results of their retrospective study to determine the effectiveness of follow-up surveillance in detecting recurrent disease following radical hysterectomy and lymphadenectomy for stage IB cervical cancer [26]. Their reported standard surveillance consisted of a history and physical examination 6 weeks postoperatively, every 3 months the first year, every 6 months during the second year, then annually until 10 years after treatment. Six-hundred seventy-four patients were treated with radical hysterectomy and lymphadenectomy from 1974 through 1994. One hundred-twelve patients (17%) developed recurrent disease. The mean interval from treatment to recurrence was 25 months with 69 (62%) of recurrences developing within 2 years and 84 (75%) within 3 years. A majority of patients (82%) were symptomatic at time of diagnosis. At time of analysis, 88% of patients with recurrent disease had died of their disease. Only eight patients (7%) with recurrent disease were alive and free of disease. Seven of those eight patients had developed a central pelvic recurrence. Of those eight patients, only three patients had their recurrence detected as a result of the screening program. Because only 3 of 674 patients who underwent radical hysterectomy and lymphadenectomy for stage IB cervical cancer had a favorable outcome after recurrence which was detected as a result of the screening program, the authors concluded that "routine clinical follow-up surveillance is ineffective in detecting recurrent disease or in achieving a more favorable outcome." Furthermore, they concluded that the continuation of current surveillance programs could only be justified if their effectiveness improved.

Researchers from the Netherlands conducted a similar retrospective study of patients with stage IB and IIA cervical carcinoma to determine the impact of routine surveillance visits on those patients with recurrent disease, but came to different conclusions [6]. Two hundred seventy-one patients with stage IB and IIA cervical cancer who were treated with radical hysterectomy and pelvic lymphadenectomy from 1982 through 1991 were analyzed. Follow-up included examinations every 3 months the first year, every 6 months for the following 2 years, then annually until 10 years from treatment. Unlike the study by Ansink et al., routine testing included vaginal cuff cytology, in addition to chest X-rays and renal ultrasounds in patients who had previously received adjuvant radiotherapy as part of their treatment. Twenty-seven (10%) patients recurred. Recurrence sites were as follows: pelvic site alone (11 patients), extrapelvic site (13 patients), and both pelvic and extrapelvic site (3 patients). Seventy-seven percent of recurrences occurred within the 3 years after initial treatment. Twenty-two of the 27 patients who recurred died of their disease. A majority (65%) of patients with recurrent carcinoma had symptoms. Only 36% of recurrences were detected by routine surveillance in asymptomatic patients. The proportion of symptomatic patients was similar between patients with pelvic recurrences and extrapelvic recurrences. However, those with a central pelvic recurrence were more often asymptomatic than those who had an extrapelvic or pelvic side-wall recurrence. This is interesting, especially when considering that three of the four patients with an isolated central pelvic recurrence survived compared to all seven patients with an isolated side-wall recurrence, all of whom died of their disease. The death rate from recurrent carcinoma in symptomatic patients was worse than those patients with an asymptomatic recurrence (94% vs. 56%; $P=0.04$). Despite the low overall percentage of asymptomatic recurrences detected via routine surveillance, three of the four patients who survived after their recurrences were asymptomatic, suggesting that recurrences diagnosed in the absence of symptoms is associated with an improved outcome, thereby possibly justifying early, frequent follow-up. This study suggests that the surveillance strategy used may have been useful in identifying patients with a central pelvic recurrence in the asymptomatic stage.

In another study from the Netherlands, investigators attempted to determine what percentage of cervical cancer recurrences were detected during routine surveillance and which diagnostic tools were the most useful [19]. Of 277 women with stage IB-IVA cervical cancer, 47 (17%) recurred. Thirty-two percent of recurrences were detected during routine follow-up which consisted of clinic visits every 3 months the first year, every 4 months the second year, and every 6 months the third through fifth year. The use of vaginal cytology and chest X-rays was not standardized. Recurrent disease was most often detected via self-referral secondary to symptoms. There was no difference in survival when comparing patients who were self-referred vs. those who were asymptomatic and diagnosed at routine follow-up. Although their study did not show a survival advantage for asymptomatic patients as a result of surveillance, it is difficult to extrapolate these findings to the clinical setting as the study did not routinely implement Pap tests and chest X-rays as are commonly used in clinical practice. Also, the authors did not subdivide the location of recurrence and subsequent treatment by those who were symptomatic and those who were asymptomatic, thus making it impossible to identify a subset of patients who may have had a benefit from early detection of their recurrence while asymptomatic and thus justify their surveillance approach.

In 2004, investigators from France reported the results of their study to determine the value of routine follow-up for the detection of recurrences in patients treated for cervical cancer [20]. The records of 583 women with stage I and II cervical cancer treated with combination surgery and radiation over a 13-year period were reviewed. Follow-up consisted of a pelvic examination and Pap smear every 3 months the first year, every 4 months the second year, every 6 months the third year, and annually thereafter. Chest X-ray and abdomen-pelvic ultrasound were performed annually for the first 9 years of the study period. Excluding patients with less than 6 months of follow-up or a recurrence within 6 months of treatment, 45 women experienced recurrence. Recurrence sites were as follows: local (with pelvic and/or paraaortic nodal metastases), 25 patients; distant metastases, 13 patients; and local plus distant metastases, seven patients. Among patients with recurrent disease, seven (16%) were asymptomatic and 38 (84%) were symptomatic. Of the seven asymptomatic patients, four were detected at routine office visit, two with pelvic recurrence diagnosed during pelvic examination. Three had their recurrence diagnosed via imaging performed for an unrelated indication, and two had their recurrence diagnosed during routine follow-up (one as a result of an abnormal Pap smear; the other secondary to a routine chest X-ray). The median survival duration was similar in asymptomatic and symptomatic patients. All seven patients with asymptomatic disease died within 26 months of their recurrence. Based on the equivalent outcomes for symptomatic and asymptomatic patients and the low yield of their screening program, the authors recommended against routine Pap smears in patients treated with a combination of radical hysterectomy and RT and against performing routine radiology in asymptomatic patients.

The largest study designed to determine the role of post-treatment surveillance in patients with cervical cancer was performed at M.D. Anderson Cancer Center by Bodurka et al. [18]. They reviewed the records of 1,096 patients with stage IB cervical cancer treated over a 10-year period. Forty-six percent of patients were treated with primary surgical therapy and 54% were treated with primary radiation. Forty-eight patients were excluded from analysis because of persistent disease and 55 patients were excluded because their follow-up was at another institution. Routine surveillance consisted of four physical and pelvic examinations with Pap smears the first year, decreasing to three times annually the second and third years, then two examinations per year the fourth and fifth years. A chest X-ray was performed the first year. One hundred thirty-three (13%) of 993 patients evaluated developed recurrent disease. Nineteen (14%) patients with recurrent disease did so without any preceding symptoms. Sites of recurrence in the asymptomatic patients were as follows: central pelvis, seven patients; pelvic wall, one patient; lung, eight patients; nodes, three patients. The seven asymptomatic patients with central pelvic recurrences were diagnosed by clinical pelvic examination. The median survival was improved in patients with asymptomatic central recurrence compared to those with symptomatic pelvic recurrences (74 vs. 14 months). None of the asymptomatic recurrences were detected by Pap smear. Patients with asymptomatic pulmonary recurrences diagnosed by chest X-ray lived approximately 2 years longer than patients with symptomatic pulmonary recurrences (3 vs. 1 year). Overall, the patients with asymptomatic recurrences lived significantly longer after recurrence than those with symptomatic recurrences (42 vs. 11 months).

In 2007, two separate groups of Italian investigators published the results of their studies evaluation the surveillance strategies of cervical cancer patients following treatment [21, 22]. Zola et al. retrospectively reviewed the records of women with recurrent cervical cancer treated from 1980 to 2005 [22]. A majority of patients were stage IB1-IIB. The strategy varied somewhat between the eight institutions in the study, but a majority utilized office visits every 3–4 months the first 2 years following treatment and increasing to every 6 months thereafter until 5 years after treatment, then annually. The use of Pap smear, chest X-ray, CT, and ultrasound varied between institutions. Of the 327 patients who recurred, 164 (50.2%) were asymptomatic and 163 (49.8%) were symptomatic. The median overall survival duration of asymptomatic patients was significantly longer than symptomatic patients. The median survival since recurrence was longer in asymptomatic patients. These findings must be considered in the context of the shorter disease-free interval from original diagnosis to recurrence in the asymptomatic group compared to the symptomatic group. It is possible that the screening implemented only provided a longer awareness of the recurrence, thus giving the implementation of the screening test the false appearance of prolonged survival since recurrence.

Sartori et al. retrospectively evaluated the records of 63 stage IB-IIA patients diagnosed with recurrent cervical cancer from 1981 to 2004 [21]. Their reported surveillance program consisted of office visits every 3 months the first year, every 4 months the second year, every 6 months the third through fifth year, and annually thereafter. Pap smears and chest X-rays were performed annually. Forty-one (65%) of 63 patients had symptomatic recurrences and 35% were asymptomatic at diagnosis. A majority (87%) of recurrences were within the first 3 years. When comparing symptomatic vs. asymptomatic patients, asymptomatic patients were more likely to have local relapse. Patients with local relapse had an improved survival after recurrence compared to those with a distant relapse. Local recurrences were more likely to be diagnosed by physical examination. Despite a greater percentage of asymptomatic patients recurring locally, there was no statistically significant difference in survival duration between those with symptomatic and asymptomatic recurrences. Considering that a majority of asymptomatic recurrences were diagnosed by clinical examination and/or CT, the authors questioned the utility of standard screening tests for diagnosing recurrent cervical cancer. Interestingly, patients with positive lymph nodes for metastatic disease at primary diagnosis were more likely to have distant recurrences when compared to those with negative initial lymph node evaluation and the authors recommended that follow-up strategies should be appropriately tailored. However, they did not describe how many additional screening tests would be required within their study population to diagnose those distant metastases. Considering the lack of proven survival advantage for those diagnosed with asymptomatic distant relapses, it would be difficult to endorse such a screening program.

While studies by Bodurka et al., Samlal et al., and Zola et al. appear to show a survival advantage for those asymptomatic patients diagnosed as a result of posttreatment surveillance, these findings must be considered in the context of the biases in these retrospective studies, specifically lead time bias and length time bias [6, 18, 22]. Lead time is the interval between the earlier detection of the disease as a result of the screening test and the time of usual clinical presentation. The possibility exists that the reported survival advantage conferred by screening is merely a product of diagnosing the recurrence earlier and adding that lead time to the time interval from clinical presentation secondary to symptoms until death, thereby giving the false impression of a greater interval from diagnosis to death. Length time bias occurs when less aggressive disease processes are overrepresented in a screening cohort. It is possible that those patients with slower growing tumors had a greater likelihood of being diagnosed with recurrent disease during the screening protocol. This group, with more indolent tumors, may have, by the nature of there recurrences, a better overall prognosis irrespective of any screening interventions. These biases may account for the survival advantage the authors attribute to screening in those patients with asymptomatic central pelvic recurrences.

While the widespread and routine use of Pap smears has served to reduce the number of deaths from cervical cancer, it is of uncertain benefit in the detection of asymptomatic recurrent cervical cancer. In an attempt to determine the accuracy of cytology in detecting recurrent cervical cancer, Shield et al. performed a retrospective study in which they correlated the clinical features of patients treated for cervical cancer, including advanced stages, with the cytology results after therapy [27]. They found that 48.9% (23/47) of patients with local recurrence had a cytological diagnosis of recurrent cancer and that a cytological diagnosis of recurrent cervical cancer preceded clinical signs in 24.6% of cases. Extrapolating their findings to clinical practice is difficult because the surveillance schedule and other screening modalities are not detailed and it is unclear how many patients with positive cytology actually represented disease persistence and not recurrence. The study also lacks, for comparison, a denominator of those patients who did not have recurrence after treatment and what their cytology was.

Soisson et al. reported on their study to determine the sensitivity and specificity of patient symptoms, physical examination, and vaginal cytology in detecting recurrent disease in patients treated for stage IB and IIA cervical cancer [28]. There were 31 (15%) recurrences among 203 women. Vaginal cytology was noted to be the least sensitive (13%) in detecting recurrent disease. However, of the three patients who recurred and were alive without evidence of disease, two had their pelvic recurrences diagnosed by malignant cells on cytologic examination. Based on this, the authors concluded that, although not sensitive, vaginal cytology had the highest yield in regards to detecting recurrences in patients who subsequently had favorable outcomes. However, 2,639 Pap smears would have to be performed in their study group to detect two recurrences that had the possibility of being cured. In the retrospective review of Bodurka et al. of stage IB patients, including 133 with recurrent disease, Pap smear did not detect any of the asymptomatic recurrences [18]. Similarly, Ansink et al. noted that, in their 20-year study of the effectiveness of routine follow-up in stage IB patients, they discontinued the practice of routine Pap smears after the first 14 years because no patients had a positive Pap smear in the absence of other signs or symptoms [26]. Samlal et al. also reported the low yield of routine vaginal cytology. In their study of 271 patients with early stage cervical cancer, including 27 recurrences, only one of nine asymptomatic recurrences was detected secondary to vaginal cytology [6]. By their calculations, 3,800 Pap smears would have to be performed to detect this single recurrence. Of the seven asymptomatic patients in the study of Morice et al., only one had her recurrence diagnosed secondary to a routine Pap smear [20]. Furthermore, two patients with recurrences detected during pelvic examination had normal Pap smears.

All these findings point to the low yield of Pap smears in the detection of recurrent cervical cancer. The Pap smear, although highly effective in detecting dysplastic lesions of the cervix with routine use, does not appear to be as beneficial in the detection of asymptomatic cervical cancer recurrences. The inability of the Pap smear to detect asymptomatic disease may be secondary to a need for the recurrent tumor to invade through the vaginal mucosa before cells will be present for capture during cytologic evaluation, at which point the patient would most likely have symptoms and/or a pelvic examination would detect the tumor [29].

In patients who do develop distant metastases, the most commonly observed distant site is the lung [17]. Chest X-rays are routinely employed to screen for recurrent cervical cancer. The focus on the role of the chest X-ray in screening for recurrent cervical cancer should not be based solely on its ability to diagnose distant recurrences, but also on the outcomes of these patients after their distant recurrences have been diagnosed by chest X-ray. Bodurka et al. advocated the routine use of chest X-ray as they noted a significant increase in median survival from the time of recurrence for asymptomatic vs. symptomatic pulmonary recurrences [18]. Barter et al. reviewed the records of 2,116 women with cervical cancer, including 77 patients with pulmonary recurrences [30]. They did not detect a difference in survival between those with symptomatic pulmonary recurrences and those with asymptomatic recurrences diagnosed on chest X-ray. Therefore, they did not advocate chest X-rays in the surveillance of patients treated for cervical cancer. However, their conclusions must be considered in light of the fact that only 11 of the 77 patients had a unilateral, isolated parenchymal nodule and in only two of these patients was the pulmonary recurrence the only sign of recurrence. This is in contrast to the subset of eight patients with asymptomatic pulmonary recurrences detected by chest X-ray in the study of Bodurka et al., six of whom underwent either wedge resection or a lobectomy, suggesting isolated disease responsive to surgical intervention. Samlal et al. reported in their 1998 study that two patients with a pulmonary recurrence were treated with surgery and were without evidence of disease after 4 and 8 years [6]. Definitive conclusions regarding the role of chest X-ray are difficult to arrive at secondary to the retrospective nature of available studies, the heterogeneity of treatment, and the confounding possibility of coexistent recurrent disease in addition to the pulmonary recurrence. It does appear that patients with asymptomatic isolated, solitary pulmonary recurrences can possibly be cured. The role of routine chest X-rays in identifying this subset of patients remains to be determined in a prospective, randomized trial.

When designing and implementing a long-term surveillance strategy for secondary malignancies, one must consider the patient's risk factors for subsequent malignancies as well as the treatment modality used to treat the patient's cervical cancer. Long-term survivors of cervical cancer are known to be at risk for secondary malignancies [31–35]. Considering the role of human papillomavirus (HPV) and cigarette smoking in the development of cervical cancer, patients need to be followed for diseases resultant from the same factors [36, 37]. The increased risk of vaginal, vulvar, and anal cancer in patients with cervical cancer suggests that HPV is able to exert a dysplastic effect on structures adjacent to the cervix, a so-called "field effect." Additionally, radiation and chemotherapy are carcinogenic themselves [38]. In a recently published report of over 100,000 survivors of cervical cancer, Chaturvedi et al. demonstrated that these patients were at increased risk for both HPV-related cancers (pharynx, genital sites, rectum/anus) and smoking-related cancers (pharynx, trachea/bronchus/lung, pancreas, and bladder) [32]. When dividing the patients into those who had and had not received radiation as part of their treatment, those who had previously been irradiated were at increased risk for second malignancies at those sites which had been heavily radiated, including the colon, rectum/anus, bladder, and ovary. This increased risk persisted for over 40 years. This persistence and proportional increase for radiated tissues has been observed in other studies [31].

Roswell Park Cancer Institute is an NCI-designated National Comprehensive Cancer Center and as such we try to adhere to NCCN practice guidelines where indicated. This consists of routine visits scheduled at increasingly longer intervals proportional to the time from initial therapy (Table 64.2). This allows us to maintain a close working relationship with the patient, to manage any therapy-related complications and to detect persistent disease. We perform a full physical examination and a Pap smear at every visit with a chest X-ray performed annually. We do not routinely obtain additional laboratory tests or imaging studies unless clinically indicated. As cervical cancer patients receive either surgery, radiation, chemotherapy, or some combination thereof, the gynecologic oncologist tends to serve as the initial implementer and coordinator of that care. The radiation oncology team generally sees the patient 1 week following radiation therapy to determine any possible acute reactions with a subsequent follow-up visit 6–8 weeks following treatment. At that time a CT and cytology will be obtained to evaluate for disease persistence. If no evidence of persistent disease exists, the patient continues her follow-up with the gynecologic oncology service. Recognizing that patients with a history of cervical cancer are at risk of comorbidities, besides recurrent cervical cancer, including other HPV-related diseases and smoking-induced malignancies and diseases, we try to tailor each patient's follow-up care individually, including referral to specialists as clinical suspicion or testing warrants.

The surveillance strategy utilized at our institution appears to be well-received by patients. The routine appointments at the same location, with the same group of providers, allows for a continuity of care with a team that is familiar with the patient's clinical course, from diagnosis to treatment to subsequent follow-up. In addition to evaluating the patient's medical condition, including the development of a cervical cancer recurrence or separate malignancy, we are able to inquire into treatment-related side effects and concerns. Issues such as altered body image and dyspareunia affect quality of life and should be addressed, but the patient may not feel that these concerns warrant their making an appointment to discuss.

Cervical cancer is a major global health concern. An estimated 493,100 women are diagnosed with the disease annually [39]. Recurrent cervical cancer represents a significant risk for all women treated for cervical cancer. The risk of recurrence increases with increasing stage at initial diagnosis. A majority of patients with recurrent disease are symptomatic and a majority who do ultimately recur will do so within the first 3 years following therapy. The goal of routine surveillance after therapy for cervical cancer is twofold. The first goal is to identify, via available screening modalities, early local recurrences prior to the onset of symptoms when intervention is likely to lead to an improved outcome when compared to patients diagnosed later, when symptomatic. With available treatment modalities, only those patients with central pelvic recurrence or isolated pulmonary recurrence have a reasonable chance of being cured of their recurrence via a radical intervention. Surveillance efforts should focus on identifying this particular subset of patients. The benefit of routine surveillance in identifying this patient subpopulation has not been definitively determined. Studies attempting to evaluate the role of routine follow-up are all retrospective and subject to biases which may overrepresent any benefit of screening, including lead time and length time biases. Conclusions are also difficult to make based on these studies secondary to the nonstandard surveillance methods and treatments for recurrences. Additionally, the commonly implemented Pap smear and chest X-ray appear to be of questionable utility. The second goal of surveillance is to screen for and identify secondary malignancies in patients who have been treated for cervical cancer as these patients are at increased risk for cancers resultant from smoking, HPV, and treatment, particularly radiation therapy. Prospective, randomized studies in women who have been treated for cervical cancer are needed to confirm or disprove any benefit to widespread, routine surveillance. Further research should also focus on newer screening tests for recurrent disease, including biomarkers, and on improved treatment options for patients with distant and more extensive recurrences.

References

1. NCCN Clinical Practice Guidelines in Oncology-Cervical Cancer (V.I.2009).
2. ACOG practice bulletin. Diagnosis and treatment of cervical carcinomas. Number 35, May 2002. American College of Obstetricians and Gynecologists. Int J Gynaecol Obstet. 2002;78:79–91.
3. Wilson JM, Jungner YG. Principles and practice of mass screening for disease. Bol Oficina Sanit Panam. 1968;65:281–393.
4. Larson DM, Copeland LJ, Stringer CA, et al. Recurrent cervical carcinoma after radical hysterectomy. Gynecol Oncol. 1988;30: 381–7.
5. Gerdin E, Cnattingius S, Johnson P, Pettersson B. Prognostic factors and relapse patterns in early-stage cervical carcinoma after brachytherapy and radical hysterectomy. Gynecol Oncol. 1994;53:314–9.
6. Samlal RA, Van Der Velden J, Van Eerden T, et al. Recurrent cervical carcinoma after radical hysterectomy: an analysis of clinical aspects and prognosis. Int J Gynecol Cancer. 1998;8:78–84.
7. Landoni F, Maneo A, Colombo A, et al. Randomised study of radical surgery versus radiotherapy for stage Ib-IIa cervical cancer. Lancet. 1997;350:535–40.
8. Ferrigno R, Campos de Oliveira Faria SL, Weltman E, et al. Radiotherapy alone in the treatment of uterine cervix cancer with telecobalt and low-dose-rate brachytherapy: retrospective analysis of results and variables. Int J Radiat Oncol Biol Phys. 2003;55:695–706.
9. Hong JH, Tsai CS, Chang JT, et al. The prognostic significance of pre- and posttreatment SCC levels in patients with squamous cell carcinoma of the cervix treated by radiotherapy. Int J Radiat Oncol Biol Phys. 1998;41:823–30.
10. Hong JH, Tsai CS, Lai CH, et al. Recurrent squamous cell carcinoma of cervix after definitive radiotherapy. Int J Radiat Oncol Biol Phys. 2004;60:249–57.
11. Morris M, Eifel PJ, Lu J, et al. Pelvic radiation with concurrent chemotherapy compared with pelvic and paraaortic radiation for high-risk cervical cancer. N Engl J Med. 1999;340:1137–43.
12. Krebs HB, Helmkamp BF, Sevin BU, et al. Recurrent cancer of the cervix following radical hysterectomy and pelvic node dissection. Obstet Gynecol. 1982;59:422–7.
13. Larson DM, Copeland LJ, Malone Jr JM, et al. Diagnosis of recurrent cervical carcinoma after radical hysterectomy. Obstet Gynecol. 1988;71:6–9.
14. Burke TW, Hoskins WJ, Heller PB, et al. Clinical patterns of tumor recurrence after radical hysterectomy in stage IB cervical carcinoma. Obstet Gynecol. 1987;69:382–5.
15. Look KY, Rocereto TF. Relapse patterns in FIGO stage IB carcinoma of the cervix. Gynecol Oncol. 1990;38:114–20.
16. Tinga DJ, Bouma J, Boonstra H, Aalders JG. Symptomatology, localization and treatment of recurrent cervical carcinoma. Int J Gynecol Cancer. 1992;2:179–88.
17. Fagundes H, Perez CA, Grigsby PW, Lockett MA. Distant metastases after irradiation alone in carcinoma of the uterine cervix. Int J Radiat Oncol Biol Phys. 1992;24:197–204.
18. Bodurka-Bevers D, Morris M, Eifel PJ, et al. Posttherapy surveillance of women with cervical cancer: an outcomes analysis. Gynecol Oncol. 2000;78:187–93.
19. Duyn A, Van Eijkeren M, Kenter G, Zwinderman K, Ansink A. Recurrent cervical cancer: detection and prognosis. Acta Obstet Gynecol Scand. 2002;81:351–5.
20. Morice P, Deyrolle C, Rey A, et al. Value of routine follow-up procedures for patients with stage I/II cervical cancer treated with combined surgery-radiation therapy. Ann Oncol. 2004;15:218–23.
21. Sartori E, Pasinetti B, Carrara L, Gambino A, Odicino F, Pecorelli S. Pattern of failure and value of follow-up procedures in endometrial and cervical cancer patients. Gynecol Oncol. 2007;107: S241–7.
22. Zola P, Fuso L, Mazzola S, et al. Could follow-up different modalities play a role in asymptomatic cervical cancer relapses diagnosis? An Italian multicenter retrospective analysis. Gynecol Oncol. 2007;107:S150–4.
23. van Nagell Jr JR, Rayburn W, Donaldson ES, et al. Therapeutic implications of patterns of recurrence in cancer of the uterine cervix. Cancer. 1979;44:2354–61.
24. Friedlander M, Grogan M. Guidelines for the treatment of recurrent and metastatic cervical cancer. Oncologist. 2002;7:342–7.
25. Kew FM, Roberts AP, Cruickshank DJ. The role of routine follow-up after gynecological malignancy. Int J Gynecol Cancer. 2005;15: 413–9.
26. Ansink A, de Barros Lopes A, Naik R, Monaghan JM. Recurrent stage IB cervical carcinoma: evaluation of the effectiveness of routine follow up surveillance. Br J Obstet Gynaecol. 1996;103:1156–8.
27. Shield PW, Wright RG, Free K, Daunter B. The accuracy of cervicovaginal cytology in the detection of recurrent cervical carcinoma following radiotherapy. Gynecol Oncol. 1991;41:223–9.
28. Soisson AP, Geszler G, Soper JT, Berchuck A, Clarke-Pearson DL. A comparison of symptomatology, physical examination, and vaginal cytology in the detection of recurrent cervical carcinoma after radical hysterectomy. Obstet Gynecol. 1990;76:106–9.
29. Owen P, Duncan ID. Is there any value in the long term follow up of women treated for endometrial cancer? Br J Obstet Gynaecol. 1996;103:710–3.
30. Barter JF, Soong SJ, Hatch KD, Orr JW, Shingleton HM. Diagnosis and treatment of pulmonary metastases from cervical carcinoma. Gynecol Oncol. 1990;38:347–51.
31. Boice Jr JD, Day NE, Andersen A, et al. Second cancers following radiation treatment for cervical cancer. An international collaboration among cancer registries. J Natl Cancer Inst. 1985;74:955–75.
32. Chaturvedi AK, Engels EA, Gilbert ES, et al. Second cancers among 104,760 survivors of cervical cancer: evaluation of long-term risk. J Natl Cancer Inst. 2007;99:1634–43.
33. Hemminki K, Dong C, Vaittinen P. Second primary cancer after in situ and invasive cervical cancer. Epidemiology. 2000;11:457–61.
34. Kleinerman RA, Boice Jr JD, Storm HH, et al. Second primary cancer after treatment for cervical cancer. An international cancer registries study. Cancer. 1995;76:442–52.
35. Fisher G, Harlow SD, Schottenfeld D. Cumulative risk of second primary cancers in women with index primary cancers of uterine cervix and incidence of lower anogenital tract cancers, Michigan, 1985-1992. Gynecol Oncol. 1997;64:213–23.
36. Rabkin CS, Biggar RJ, Melbye M, Curtis RE. Second primary cancers following anal and cervical carcinoma: evidence of shared etiologic factors. Am J Epidemiol. 1992;136:54–8.
37. Walboomers JM, Jacobs MV, Manos MM, et al. Human papillomavirus is a necessary cause of invasive cervical cancer worldwide. J Pathol. 1999;189:12–9.
38. Allan JM, Travis LB. Mechanisms of therapy-related carcinogenesis. Nat Rev Cancer. 2005;5:943–55.
39. Kamangar F, Dores GM, Anderson WF. Patterns of cancer incidence, mortality, and prevalence across five continents: defining priorities to reduce cancer disparities in different geographic regions of the world. J Clin Oncol. 2006;24:2137–50.

Cervical Carcinoma Surveillance Counterpoint: Japan

65

Kenzo Sonoda, Hiroaki Kobayashi, and Norio Wake

Keywords
Cervical cancer • Recurrence • Surveillance • Radiology • Quality of life

Clinical Features

Uterine cervical cancer is one of the most common malignancies affecting women in developing countries, with approximately 500,000 new cases diagnosed annually [1]. Approximately 11,270 new cases and 4,070 deaths are anticipated in the United States for 2009 [2]. In Japan, the cervical cancer incidence has remained stable with 8,832 cases diagnosed in 1975 and 8,779 cases reported in 2002. The number of deaths has increased slightly from 1,583 cases in 1958 to 2,481 cases in 2006 [3]. However, the number of new cases per year in Japan of the other female malignancies has annually increased to 249,643 and the number of deaths per year has increased to 131,262. Therefore, the number of deaths caused by cervical cancer comprises only 1.8% of the deaths from all kinds of female malignancies. Early detection of cervical cancer and its precursors is quite effective. Until the early 1970s, approximately 75–80% of cervical cancer cases in the United States were invasive at the time of diagnosis [4]. The national screening system for detecting cervical cancer and its precursors has dramatically reduced the incidence and mortality rate of this malignancy in Japan. Since 2004, biennial cervical cancer screening has been available to all Japanese women over the age of 20. The number of women screened was 3,538,132 in 2007; additional diagnostic testing was needed for 40,392, resulting in the identification of 1,921 cancer cases [5]. However, only 18.8% of eligible women were screened. Therefore, a significant number of cancers likely will be prevented by increasing the screening rate.

Squamous cell carcinoma is the most common type of malignancy of the cervix, but the incidence of adenocarcinoma is increasing [6]. Older reports indicated that adenocarcinomas represented approximately 5% of all cervical cancer, whereas more recent reports showed an incidence of 21%. Other histological types of cervical cancer include small cell carcinoma, sarcoma, lymphoma, and melanoma. Small cell carcinoma is uncommon, but has an unequivocally poor prognosis. The prognostic significance of adenocarcinoma is more controversial. An increasing number of centers are reporting adenocarcinoma histologic type as a poor prognostic factor in multivariate analysis, but others report no difference from squamous lesions with respect to outcome.

Human papilloma virus (HPV) is detectable in more than 90% of cervical cancers, and the viral genome is expressed in the tumor [7]. HPV plays an important role in the development of precursor lesions with genetic alterations that progress to cervical carcinoma [8]. Several chromosomal deletions and microsatellite instability have been associated with carcinogenesis in the uterine cervix [9, 10]. The age-specific prevalence of HPV infection among women with normal cytology in Japan is 23.1% in those aged 20–29, and 7.9% in those aged 30–49 [11]. HPV infection does not usually persist and only 5–10% of the population remains positive 2 years after the initial infection. While cervical cancer was once a disease affecting women in or beyond their fourth decade, cervical dysplasia and cancer are being identified with increasing frequency in younger women. This shift is thought to be related to a decrease in the age when women first become infected with HPV. The infection may lie dormant for years

K. Sonoda, MD, PhD (✉) • H. Kobayashi, MD, PhD
• N. Wake, MD, PhD
Department of Obstetrics and Gynecology, Graduate School of Medical Sciences, Kyushu University, Maidashi 3-1-1, Higashi-ku, Fukuoka 812-8582, Japan
e-mail: kenzo@med.kyushu-u.ac.jp; koba@med.kyushu-u.ac.jp; wake@med.kyushu-u.ac.jp

F.E. Johnson et al. (eds.), *Patient Surveillance After Cancer Treatment*, Current Clinical Oncology,
DOI 10.1007/978-1-60327-969-7_65, © Springer Science+Business Media New York 2013

Table 65.1 Number of patients with cervical cancer treated in 2007 in Japan

Distribution by Initial TNM Stage	
Stage	Number (%)
0	4,847 (50.0)
I	2,565 (26.4)
A1	655
A2	75
B1	1,427
B2	408
II	1,173 (12.1)
A	330
B	843
III	674 (7.0)
A	57
B	617
IV	435 (4.5)
A	159
B	276
Total	9,694 (100.0)

only to recur. Even women treated with hysterectomy for cervical neoplasia may develop HPV-related vaginal or vulvar dysplasia. Thus, routine Pap smears are also recommended for these women as this will theoretically increase the rate of early detection and improve the survival of these patients.

The number of cervical cancer patients treated in 2007 was reported by the Japan Society of Obstetrics and Gynecology (Table 65.1) [12]. Surgery was generally used for patients with Stage I lesions and patients with more advanced disease were generally treated with radiation with or without chemotherapy. The 5-year survival rates of cervical cancer patients treated in 1994 were 83.4%, 62.9%, 38.4%, and 17.9% for Stages I, II, III, and IV, respectively [13]. Tumor stage, lymphovascular space invasion, lymph node metastasis, histologic type, and tumor volume are all prognostic factors in surgically treated cervical cancer [14–17].

We here show our surveillance program after treatment of cervical cancer and discuss the difference compared with other follow-up programs advocated by other authors and the National Comprehensive Cancer Network.

After invading the stroma, cervical cancer extension proceeds through the lymph vessels [18]. Therefore, while pelvic recurrence is most common, extrapelvic spread is also found. van Nagell et al. reported that, of 526 invasive cervical cancer patients treated with radical hysterectomy and pelvic lymphadenectomy and/or radiation therapy, 160 patients had recurrence [19]. There were 136 pelvic recurrences and 81 extrapelvic recurrences. Thirty-six patients developed ureteral obstruction secondary to tumor compression. The most common sites of extrapelvic spread were the lung and lymph nodes. Twenty-two patients developed pulmonary metastases and an additional 18 patients developed recurrence in the paraaortic or supraclavicular lymph nodes. Fifty-eight percent of patients recurred in the first year following treatment and 76% recurred within 2 years of treatment. Look and Rocereto reported that, of 96 patients with International Federation of Gynecology and Obstetrics (FIGO) Stage IB cervical carcinoma treated with radical surgery, radiation therapy, or combination therapy, 21 patients recurred [20]. Ten out of 30 patients developed recurrence after radiation and 11 of 55 developed recurrence after surgery alone. The first recurrence was central in three patients, locoregional in nine, and distant in nine. The median disease-free interval was 11 months for surgically treated and 10.5 months for irradiated patients. The risk of distant metastases was significantly lower after radical surgery (3 of 55 total cases (5.4%)) than after radiation (six of 30 total cases (20%)). The median time to pelvic recurrence (10 months) was significantly shorter than that for distant recurrence (20 months). Therefore, the site of relapse is influenced by the primary therapeutic modality, and pelvic recurrence tends to manifest itself before distant recurrence. Bodurka-Bevers et al. reported results of treatment in 1,096 patients with FIGO Stage IB cervical cancer treated by surgery or radiation. There were 133 patients who developed recurrent disease [21]. Of these, 114 were symptomatic and 19 were asymptomatic at the time recurrence was detected. Thirty-seven patients recurred in the central pelvis, 21 in the lung or pelvic wall, 22 in the lymph nodes, and 35 in other sites. The median disease-free interval was 17 months for symptomatic patients and 16 months for asymptomatic patients. The median survival time from both the date of initial diagnosis and the date of detection of recurrence was significantly longer in asymptomatic (83 and 42 months, respectively) than in symptomatic (31 and 11 months, respectively) patients. Multivariate analysis revealed that symptom status at the time of recurrence was a significant predictor of survival. This is currently the largest study on recurrent cervical carcinoma, which may be why a difference was detected. However, it is impossible to completely exclude length-time bias as a contributor to this finding.

An understanding of the natural history of cervical cancer recurrence allows for the optimal allocation of resources used to follow patients to detect recurrence. There is increasing evidence in support of surveillance for recurrence both within and outside of the pelvis. Additionally, we believe that surveillance should be particularly intensive within the first 2 years after treatment in order to detect cases while they are still asymptomatic.

The two main objectives for the routine follow-up of cancer patients after treatment are to diagnose complications related to treatment and to detect recurrence earlier in order to improve patient survival. The follow-up procedure includes a history and physical examination and is guided by the results of supplementary studies (cytology, radiology, or tumor markers).

Several reports have been published to evaluate the effectiveness of routine follow-up surveillance for cervical cancer patients. Ansink et al. described the standard surveillance performed for Stage IB patients after radical hysterectomy and lymph node dissection [22]. Standard surveillance consisted of a clinical history and physical examination 6 weeks postsurgery, and subsequently every 3 months for the 1 year, every 6 months for the 2 year, and yearly thereafter until 10 years posttreatment. However, standard surveillance detected recurrent disease in only 29 of 112 patients (26%) who recurred, leading the authors to conclude that routine follow-up surveillance was ineffective in detecting recurrence. Duyn et al. reported on the outcomes of follow-up in 277 cervical cancer patients with Stages IB-IVA tumors who were treated with curative intent and scheduled for routine follow-up visits [23]. Their follow-up schedule included an office visit every 3 months in the first year after treatment, every 4 months in the 2 year, every 6 months from years 3 to 6, and annually after that. History and physical examination were done at every visit. Vaginal smears and blood tests were used to a varying extent. Of the 277 patients, 47 developed recurrent disease, and recurrence was detected during a routine follow-up visit in only 32%. In the majority of patients, recurrent cervical cancer was detected by symptoms (87%), making this the most important diagnostic tool to detect recurrent disease. Morice et al. reported outcomes in 583 women with Stages I and II cervical carcinoma treated with combined surgery and radiation therapy and followed with clinical examinations, systematic Pap smear and radiography (chest X-ray and abdomino-pelvic ultrasonography) [24]. Forty-five patients had recurrences: 38 had symptoms and seven were asymptomatic at the time of diagnosis. Among the asymptomatic patients, only two recurrences were diagnosed by routine examinations. The authors concluded that following patients treated for cervical cancer with routine Pap smears and systematic radiography does not result in earlier detection of recurrences and does not increase survival. Another report also suggested that the use of routine follow-up methods may, in fact, delay the detection of recurrences because some women delay reporting symptoms until their next routine appointment [25].

However, Bodurka-Bevers et al. argued that survival of asymptomatic patients detected during a surveillance program was increased, thereby confirming the benefit of follow-up examinations [21]. All asymptomatic pelvic recurrences were diagnosed by pelvic examination and all asymptomatic pulmonary recurrences were detected by chest radiographs. Therefore, the use of studies such as Pap smears, chest X-rays, intravenous pyelograms, and computed tomography (CT) scans increases the recurrence detection rate beyond what can be achieved by history and physical exam alone. Additionally, it is also recommended that patients with a high risk of recurrence, such as those with positive lymph nodes or a large tumor diameter, should be offered a more intensive follow-up program. However, these recommendations are based on retrospective studies. Prospective studies are urgently needed to determine the risks and benefits of different forms of follow-up surveillance.

Recurrent cervical carcinoma is comprised of four categories: (1) recurrence at the primary site, involving the intrapelvic organs, (2) extension to the pelvic sidewall, (3) metastases to pelvic and extrapelvic lymph nodes, or (4) metastases to distant organs. Recurrence which is extrapelvic or involves the pelvic sidewall is more common in patients who undergo radiation therapy only. This is probably due to the more advanced disease stage in such patients and the limited field within which the radiation is effective [26]. Therefore, more careful examinations are needed for the patients treated by radiation therapy alone. Conventional radiographic studies include chest radiography, excretory urography, barium enema, and occasionally, lymphangiography. However, improvements in cross-sectional imaging modalities such as CT or magnetic resonance (MRI) imaging offer distinct advantages over conventional radiographic techniques. Presently the majority of practitioners in Japan utilize these modalities. CT is an effective diagnostic tool for the detection of recurrence that has some advantages over MRI, including a rapid acquisition time, lack of bowel motion artifact, and fewer contraindications than MRI imaging. However, with CT, it may be difficult to differentiate recurrence from postoperative and postirradiation fibrosis. MRI is more useful for making the diagnosis of tumor recurrence in such cases. A recurrent lesion shows increased signal intensity on T2-weighted images. MRI is better than CT for imaging vaginal recurrences and defining the involvement of the pelvic floor muscles. The disadvantages of MRI compared with CT are its high cost and long imaging time. CT and MRI have become pivotal for evaluating postoperative complications prior to radiologic intervention and for determining the presence of recurrent tumors and their response to radiation therapy. Knowledge of the normal therapeutic changes and the spectrum of recurrent tumors in patients with cervical carcinoma is important for accurate interpretation of follow-up CT and MRI [27]. Chung et al. reported that the sensitivity, specificity, and accuracy of the whole-body 2-[^{18}F]-fluoro-2-deoxy-D-glucose (FDG) positron emission tomography (PET) scan in the assessment of recurrence in patients with cervical cancer were 96.1%, 84.4%, and 91.7%, respectively [28]. Asymptomatic patients with recurrent disease were treated with curative intent and a complete response was achieved in 30.5% (11 out of 36 total cases). The 3-year overall survival rate was 85.6%. Therefore, the authors concluded that whole-body FDG-PET scan was a sensitive posttherapy surveillance modality for the detection of recurrent cervical cancer, even in asymptomatic patients.

FDG-PET may be used to guide treatment plans and, eventually, may have a favorable impact on prognosis and survival.

Because the majority of cervical cancers are histologically diagnosed as being squamous cell [6], a potentially useful instrument in the early detection of recurrent disease is the assessment of serological markers, such as the squamous cell carcinoma antigen (SCC) [29]. Pras et al. reported that patients who have normal SCC levels after treatment experience a better clinical outcome when compared with those who do not. Thus, the presence of an elevated posttreatment serum level of SCC indicates the need for additional salvage therapy because of its high positive predictive value for recurrence. In the series reviewed by Bolli et al., SCC levels were elevated in 81% of patients with recurrence and the time between its detection of an elevated SCC level and the clinical diagnosis of recurrence was 7 months [30]. The authors concluded that SCC level accurately reflects the response to treatment in patients who have elevated levels prior to treatment. However, even if recurrence is detected by early monitoring of SCC levels, increased survival duration may not result [30, 31]. Esajas et al. claimed that most recurrences were suspected based on history and/or physical signs, rather than by serum SCC elevation alone. The elevation of serum tumor marker levels does not give any information about the location or extent of the disease recurrence and is not useful in all cases. Thus, this marker is not cost-effective in the absence of curative treatment for disseminated disease [32]. It may, however, have use in distinguishing patients with fibrosis from those with recurrent disease.

Because early adjuvant chemotherapy or radiation may improve patient prognosis [21], the early detection of recurrent disease is clinically pivotal in cervical cancer. We therefore believe that routine surveillance is important during follow-up to detect recurrence. A meticulous examination of the upper abdomen is required in addition to routine pelvic scanning. Additionally, the FDG-PET scan is effective to evaluate recurrence when there is discordance between an elevation of serum tumor markers and no evidence of recurrent disease on conventional workup.

The comprehensive care of the cervical cancer patient requires not only curative efforts, but also attention to the psychological needs of the patient and her family. Research into the unmet needs of cervical cancer patients has revealed deficiencies in several areas, including emotional support, discussion about possible sexual side effects, and infertility induced by treatment. We here describe the clinical countermeasures needed to improve the patient's quality of life.

While Esajas et al. claimed that the utility of any routine follow-up surveillance for the early detection of recurrent disease in cervical cancer is questionable, owing to a lack of effective therapy [31], other beneficial effects from these visits have been shown. These include reassurance, psychological support, and the detection and management of complications including social and sexual sequelae of cancer therapy. Herzog and Wright reported that a patient's diagnosis and treatment often adversely affected not only her daily life and emotional state but her partner's as well [33]. The emotional impact on couples affected by cervical cancer is not always balanced. When the patient and her partner have unequal responses to diagnosis and treatment, illness-induced disruptions in their relationship and intimacy can arise. Patients often minimize the threat of their illness and refuse to dwell on negative thoughts. The medical staff should support this positive thought process. The partner is often more upset than the patient. The presence of supportive, positive, caregivers is essential for reducing long-term emotional suffering. Additionally, patients should be encouraged to report any feelings of emotional or psychological distress in an empathic, supportive, and non-threatening environment.

Bergmark et al. described anatomic and physiological changes in women who were treated for cervical cancer [34]. A patient may have persistent vaginal changes that compromise sexual activity including a short vagina and reduced vaginal lubrication and elasticity. Frumovitz et al. interviewed cervical cancer survivors and compared quality of life and sexual functioning between patients treated with surgery and those treated with radiotherapy [35]. When compared with surgery patients and controls, radiation patients had significantly poorer scores on standardized questionnaires measuring health-related quality of life (physical and mental health), psychosocial distress, and sexual functioning. However, there were no significant differences between radical hysterectomy patients and controls on any of the outcome measures as mentioned above. Traditionally, oncologists have focused their efforts on maximizing the overall survival of their patients. Although many oncologists acknowledge that quality of life after cancer therapy is an important aspect of patient care, it is often not the main consideration when recommending cancer treatment. However, when competing treatment options result in equivalent clinical outcomes, quality of life considerations become particularly important. Physicians caring for women with cervical cancer should discuss treatment-related organ changes that may affect sexual function. This topic should be addressed before and after treatment. Since the assessment of sexual satisfaction and function as well as emotional well-being should be incorporated into the history obtained during follow-up visits, the timing of follow-up is very important. Surgical morbidity and sexual side effects improve during the first year after radical hysterectomy. In contrast, the chronic fibrotic changes in pelvic tissue after radiotherapy create persistent, or even worsening, vaginal atrophy.

Although screening programs have significantly reduced the incidence and death rates of cervical cancer in the Western world, social pressures have led to a delay in childbearing. This has resulted in an increasing number of patients who present at an early stage who desire future fertility. Standard treatment is either radical hysterectomy or radiotherapy to the pelvis, both of which inevitably render future childbearing impossible. This has led to a questioning of the rationale for extensive surgery in all cases of early stage cervical cancer. Accurate staging can precisely localize the tumor, allowing early stage tumors to be treated with wide local excision (trachelectomy). This permits conservation of the uterine corpus and maintains future fertility. Shepherd and Milliken reviewed over 900 cases of radical trachelectomy that included 790 vaginal and 116 abdominal procedures [36]. There have been over 300 pregnancies with 195 live births in patients treated in this way. Because the recurrence rate is 4%, radical trachelectomy is likely a safe procedure in well-selected cases when carried out in medical centers with appropriate. Even trachelectomy, however, also has effects on quality of life and may be associated with significant psychological distress particularly if followed by infertility or miscarriage. Therefore, support systems for women undergoing fertility sparing surgery for cervical cancer must also be in place.

Routine follow-up after cervical cancer remains our standard practice in Kyushu University Hospital, despite the limited evidence to support its use. Kew and Cruickshank performed a questionnaire survey regarding current practices for the follow-up of patients after gynecological malignancy treatment [37]. The most common follow-up patterns were office visits every 3 months for the first year, every 4 months for the 2 year, every 6 months for the third and fourth years, then annually thereafter. Esajas et al. reported a high incidence of recurrences detected at routine follow-up visits scheduled every 2–3 months over the first 2 years [31]. They speculated that some patients delayed reporting symptoms until their visits, which were probably planned on short notice. The National Comprehensive Cancer Network guidelines propose follow-up office visits as every 3–6 months for 2 years, every 6–12 months for 3–5 years, and then annually based on patient's risk of disease recurrence [38]. Shepherd and Milliken described a follow-up pattern for radical trachelectomy that featured office visits every 3 months for the 1 year, every 4 months for the 2 year, every 6 months from the third to fifth years, then annually for 5 years thereafter [36].

Follow-up visits are routinely scheduled after treatment in Kyushu University Hospital at intervals of every 2 months for the 1 year, every 3 months for the 2 year, every 4 months for the 3 year, and biannually for the fourth and fifth years, then annually for at least 3 years. Office visits are judiciously supplemented with radiological studies as directed by symptoms, physical examination, and primary therapeutic modalities (Table 65.2). We follow all patients at the same intervals regardless of the histologic subtypes. The kinds of serum markers are different among histologic subtypes, because the serum CA125 level has prognostic significance for adenocarcinoma [39].

In our system, patients are more closely followed than recommended by National Comprehensive Cancer Network guidelines. Posttherapy surveillance programs are directed toward asymptomatic patients in whom the early detection

Table 65.2 Surveillance after curative-intent treatment for cervical cancer at Kyushu University, Japan

	Year					
	1	2	3	4	5	>5
Office visit	6	4	3	2	2	1
Serum marker levels[a]	6	4	3	2	2	1
Chest X-ray	3	3	3	2	2	1
Computed tomography	1	1	1	1	1	1[b]

[a]Analyzed when elevated before treatment: SCC and CEA for squamous cell carcinoma; CA125, CA19-9, and CEA for adenocarcinoma

[b]Performed as clinically indicated

The number in each cell indicates the number of times a particular modality is recommended in a particular posttreatment year

Office visit includes history, physical examination, pelvic examination, and Pap smear

of recurrence may impact survival. Our proposed intense surveillance program is one of the first of its kind. It is designed not only to detect recurrence, but also to support patients psychologically at a point where therapeutic intervention may significantly prolong life and improve quality of life. When our patients are intensively followed by history, physical examination, pelvic examination, Pap smear, serum tumor marker level, and imaging studies, we detect recurrence without delay and also address mental and social problems of our patients. This system is working well and does not impose a burden on either medical staff or patients. We also collaborate with radiation oncologists, medical oncologists, and psychiatrists in the treatment and follow-up of patients. The gynecologic oncologists are mainly responsive for the care of patients in the follow-up periods, as mentioned above, but every staff member can access test results by using our medical computer systems. We delegate responsibility for further follow-up to the primary care doctor when a patient is healthy 9 years after treatment. However, further efforts should be targeted toward the prospective evaluation of surveillance strategies to assess the potential clinical and economic benefits of our system.

Although there is little research documenting the value of follow-up after treatment for patients with cervical carcinoma, many patients are routinely followed with clinical examinations and imaging studies. They should be followed for a minimum of 5 years following the end of treatment because of late recurrences. The development of new techniques, including PET, may also be helpful for evaluating recurrence. In addition to monitoring for recurrence, follow-up visits should address the impact that cervical cancer has on quality of life. This includes psychological effects, the financial burden on patients, their families, and society, and the years of life lost due to premature death. Women diagnosed with cervical cancer experience significant emotional distress and anxiety. Postoperatively, treatment for cervical cancer can have long-lasting effects, in terms of reproduction, fertility, physical pain, and intimate relationships. Therefore, those addressing the clinical care for these patients should consider their psychological and educational needs throughout treatment and follow-up. Effective psychological support for cervical cancer patients should be available not only to patients but to their partners as well. The efficacy of routine follow-up after curative-intent treatment is not supported by high quality evidence. Prospective controlled trials are urgently needed to determine the risks and benefits of alternative follow-up strategies, as measured by survival duration, cost, quality of life, and psychosocial outcomes.

References

1. Cannistra SA, Niloff JM. Cancer of the uterine cervix. N Engl J Med. 1996;334:1030–8.
2. American Cancer Society. Cancer Facts & Figures-2009. (http://www.cancer.org), Accessed 8 May 2009.
3. National Cancer Center, Japan. 2009. (http://ganjoho.jp/professional/statistics/statistics.html). Center for Cancer Control and Information Services. Accessed 8 May 2009.
4. National Cancer Institute. Statistics of cervix uteri cancer. Rockville, MD: National Cancer Institute; 2003.
5. Japanese Ministry of Health, Labour and Welfare. Health and welfare services for the elderly. The implementation status of health services. (2009) http://www.mhlw.go.jp. Accessed 8 May 2009.
6. Hacker NF. Cervical cancer. In: Berek JS, Hacker NF, editors. Practical gynecologic oncology. 3rd ed. Philadelphia: Lippincott Williams & Wilkins; 2000. p. 345–405.
7. Zur Hausen H. Human papillomaviruses in the pathogenesis of anogenital cancer. Virology. 1991;184:9–13.
8. Wentzensen N, Ridder R, Klaes R, Vinokurova S, Schaefer T, von Knebel Doeberitz M. Characterization of viral-cellular fusion transcripts in a large series of HPV16 and 18 positive anogenital lesions. Oncogene. 2002;21:419–26.
9. Srivatsan ES, Chakrabarti R, Zainabadi K, Pack SD, Benyamini P, Mendonca MS, et al. Localization of deletion to a 300 Kb interval of chromosome 11q13 in cervical cancer. Oncogene. 2002;21:5631–42.
10. Nishimura M, Furumoto H, Kato T, Kamada M, Aono T. Microsatellite instability is a late event in the carcinogenesis of uterine cervical cancer. Gynecol Oncol. 2000;79:201–6.
11. Inoue M, Sakaguchi J, Sasagawa T, Tango M. The evaluation of human papilloma virus DNA testing in primary screening for cervical lesions in a large Japanese population. Int J Gynecol Cancer. 2006;16:1007–13.
12. Annual report on cervical cancer treatment in 2007. Acta Obst Gynaec Jpn. 2009;61:914–38.
13. Five-year result of cervical cancer patients who received treatments in 1994. Acta Obst Gynaec Jpn. 2009;61:1042–54.
14. Burghardt E, Pickel H, Haas J, Lahousen M. Prognostic factors and operative treatment of Stages IB to IIB cervical cancer. Am J Obstet Gynecol. 1987;156:988–96.
15. Noguchi H, Schiozawa I, Sakai Y, Yamazaki T, Fukuta T. Pelvic lymph node metastasis of uterine cervical cancer. Gynecol Oncol. 1987;27:150–8.
16. Kamura T, Tsukamoto N, Tsuruchi N, Saito T, Matsuyama T, Akazawa K, et al. Multivariate analysis of the histopathologic prognostic factors of cervical cancer in patients undergoing radical hysterectomy. Cancer. 1992;69:181–6.
17. Pickel H, Haas J, Lahousen M. Prognostic factors in cervical cancer. Eur J Obstet Gynecol Reprod Biol. 1997;71:209–13.
18. Stehman FB, Perez CA, Kurman RJ, Thigpen JT. Uterine cervix. In: Hoskins WJ, Perez CA, Young RC, editors. Principles and practice of gynecologic oncology. 3rd ed. Philadelphia: Lippincott Williams & Wilkins; 2000. p. 841–918.
19. van Nagell Jr JR, Rayburn W, Donaldson ES, Hanson M, Gay EC, Yoneda J, Marayuma Y, Powell DF. Therapeutic implications of patterns of recurrence in cancer of the uterine cervix. Cancer. 1979;44:2354–61.
20. Look KY, Rocereto TF. Relapse patterns in FIGO stage IB carcinoma of the cervix. Gynecol Oncol. 1990;38:114–20.
21. Bodurka-Bevers D, Morris M, Eifel PJ, Levenback C, Bevers MW, Lucas KR, et al. Posttherapy surveillance of women with cervical cancer: an outcomes analysis. Gynecol Oncol. 2000;78:187–93.
22. Ansink A, de Barros Lopes A, Naik R, Monaghan JM. Recurrent stage IB cervical carcinoma: evaluation of the effectiveness of routine follow-up surveillance. Br J Obstet Gynaecol. 1996;103:1156–8.
23. Duyn A, Van Eijkeren M, Kenter G, Zwinderman K, Ansink A. Recurrent cervical cancer: detection and prognosis. Acta Obstet Gynecol Scand. 2002;81:351–5.
24. Morice P, Deyrolle C, Rey A, Atallah D, Pautier P, Camatte S, et al. Value of routine follow-up procedures for patients with stage I/II cervical cancer treated with combined surgery-radiation therapy. Ann Oncol. 2004;15:218–23.
25. Olaitan A, Murdoch J, Anderson R, James J, Graham J, Barley V. A critical evaluation of current protocols for the follow-up of women treated for gynecological malignancies: a pilot study. Int J Gynecol Cancer. 2001;11:349–53.
26. Choi JI, Kim SH, Seong CK, Sim JS, Lee HJ, Do KH. Recurrent uterine cervical carcinoma: spectrum of imaging findings. Korean J Radiol. 2000;1:198–207.
27. Jeong YY, Kang HK, Chung TW, Seo JJ, Park JG. Uterine cervical carcinoma after therapy: CT and MR imaging findings. Radiographics. 2003;23:969–81.
28. Chung HH, Kim SK, Kim TH, Lee S, Kang KW, Kim JY, et al. Clinical impact of FDG-PET imaging in post-therapy surveillance of uterine cervical cancer: from diagnosis to prognosis. Gynecol Oncol. 2006;103:165–70.
29. Pras E, Willemse PH, Canrinus AA, de Bruijn HW, Sluiter WJ, ten Hoor KA, et al. Serum squamous cell carcinoma antigen and CYFTA 21-1 in cervical cancer treatment. Int J Radiat Oncol Biol Phys. 2002;52:23–32.
30. Bolli JA, Doering DL, Bosscher JR, Day Jr TG, Rao CV, Owens K, et al. Squamous cell carcinoma antigen: clinical utility in squamous cell carcinoma of the uterine cervix. Gynecol Oncol. 1994;55:169–73.
31. Esajas MD, Duk JM, de Bruijn HW, Aalders JG, Willemse PH, Sluiter W, et al. Clinical value of routine serum squamous cell carcinoma antigen in follow-up of patients with early-stage cervical cancer. J Clin Oncol. 2001;19:3960–6.
32. Chang Y, Ng TY, Ngan HYS, Wong LC. Monitoring of serum squamous cell carcinoma antigen levels in invasive cervical cancer: is it cost effective? Gynecol Oncol. 2002;84:7–11.
33. Herzog TJ, Wright JD. The impact of cervical cancer on quality of life-the components and means for management. Gynecol Oncol. 2007;107:572–7.
34. Bergmark K, Avall-Lundqvist E, Dickman PW, Henningsohn L, Steineck G. Vaginal changes and sexuality in women with a history of cervical cancer. N Engl J Med. 1999;340:1383–9.
35. Frumovitz M, Sun CC, Schover LR, Munsell MF, Jhingran A, Wharton JT, et al. Quality of life and sexual functioning in cervical cancer survivors. J Clin Oncol. 2005;23:7428–36.
36. Shepherd JH, Milliken DA. Conservative surgery for carcinoma of the cervix. Clin Oncol. 2008;20:395–400.
37. Kew FM, Cruickshank DJ. Routine follow-up after treatment for a gynecological cancer: a survey of practice. Int J Gynecol Cancer. 2006;16:380–4.
38. National Comprehensive Cancer Network 2013. Practice guidelines in oncology cervical cancer version 2. http://www.nccn.org. Accessed on 2 Nov 2012.
39. Duk JM, De Bruijn HWA, Groenier KH, Fleuren GJ, Aalders JG. Adenocarcinoma of the cervix. Cancer. 1990;65:1830–7.

Cervical Carcinoma Surveillance Counterpoint: Canada

66

Michael Fung-Kee-Fung and Thomas K. Oliver

Keywords

Cancer • Cancer antigen 125 • Cancer guidelines • Carcinoma • Cervix • Cervical • Computed tomography • Disease detection • Follow-up • Examination • Examination, physical • Examination, pelvic • Examination, rectovaginal examination • Intravenous pyelography • Magnetic resonance imaging • Papanicolaou test • Positron emission tomography • Quality of life • Recurrence • Recurrence, asymptomatic • Recurrence, distant • Recurrence, local • Recurrence, asymptomatic • Surveillance • Survival • Survival, disease-free • Survival, overall • Tumor markers • Ultrasound • Vaginal vault cytology • X-ray • X-ray, chest

Cervical cancer is the second most common cancer worldwide, resulting in approximately 275,000 deaths yearly [1]. In Canada, approximately 1,350 Canadian women are diagnosed annually, and approximately 400 women per year die from their disease [2]. According to the SEER database, approximately 50% of patients are diagnosed with local disease (stage IA or IB) that is confined to the cervix, while 35% are diagnosed with locoregional disease that has extended beyond the cervix but not to the pelvic wall or the lower third of the vagina (stage IIA or IIB). The remaining patients represent those with more advanced disease (stage III or IV) that has spread to the lower third of the vagina, the pelvic wall, or beyond (11%). For a small proportion of patients (5%), staging information was not available [3]. The 5-year survival rates were approximately 92% for patients with local disease, 58% with locoregional disease, and 17% with distant disease [3].

M. Fung-Kee-Fung, MBBS, FRCS, MBA (✉)
Division of Gynecologic Oncology, Surgical Oncology Program, Department of Obstetrics and Gynecology, Ottawa Hospital/University of Ottawa, Ottawa, ON, Canada
e-mail: mfung@ottawahospital.on.ca

T.K. Oliver, B.A.
Department of Oncology, McMaster University, 711 Concession Street, Hamilton, ON, Canada L8V 1C3
e-mail: olivert@mcmaster.ca

The follow-up of patients is intended to facilitate the early detection of disease recurrence. It is generally believed that early detection of recurrence provides greater treatment or disease management options, with the potential for lower morbidity, improved quality of life, and perhaps improved survival. This general consensus is based on the assumption that surveillance tests perform well at detecting early recurrence and that effective management options are available. Generally, however, the prognosis for the majority of patients with recurrent disease is poor.

While surveillance strategies often vary, patients are typically followed either by a gynecologic oncologist, a gynecologist, or a primary care physician, according to a schedule that generally spans 5 or more years. Patients are exposed to a variety of surveillance modalities intended to detect disease recurrence; surveillance options may include the recording of detailed patient histories, physical examinations, pelvic examinations, vaginal cytology, ultrasound, magnetic resonance imaging (MRI), computed tomography (CT), fluoro-2deoxy-glucose positron emission tomography (PET), PET/CT, intravenous pyelography, and/or the use of tumor markers. Surveillance strategies are often based on an individual patient's risk of recurrence, patient and physician preferences, as well as complications related to primary therapy, such as the aftereffects of radiotherapy.

To avoid potentially harmful variations in clinical practice, as well as to promote best practice, responsible resource utilization, and the standardization of care, it is essential to

F.E. Johnson et al. (eds.), *Patient Surveillance After Cancer Treatment*, Current Clinical Oncology, DOI 10.1007/978-1-60327-969-7_66, © Springer Science+Business Media New York 2013

determine whether patient follow-up is effective at detecting disease recurrence, whether the early detection of disease improves patient outcomes related to survival, morbidity, or quality of life, what, if any, are the most effective surveillance strategies that should be routinely offered to patients, whether some follow-up strategies have the potential to produce greater harms in terms of false positive results and greater patient anxiety than benefits for a large proportion of patients who will remain disease-free, whether current surveillance strategies are an effective use of limited resources, and what patients prefer and what best promotes their psychosocial health and well-being.

As seen in Table 66.1, 17 retrospective studies provide the evidence base informing the role of follow-up for patients with cervical cancer treated with curative intent [4–20]. For a more in-depth analysis of the evidence on the follow-up of patients with cervical cancer, please refer to a recent systematic review of the evidence produced by the Cancer Care Ontario Genecology Disease Site Group [21].

With the exception of five studies that did not report staging data [7, 8, 10, 15, 18] and three studies that included a larger number of patients with more advanced disease [4, 12, 20], 9 studies reported that 71–100% of patients presented with stage IA or stage IB disease [5, 6, 9, 11, 13, 14, 16, 17, 19]. Where reported, the proportion of patients with stage II disease ranged from 9 to 40% of the study populations in eight studies [4, 5, 9, 12, 13, 16, 19, 20]. Patients with stage III or IV disease comprised 6–31% in 5 studies that reported data on stage of disease [4, 9, 12, 16, 20].

Where reported in 15 series, the overall rate of recurrence ranged from 8 to 49% of patients [4–18]. In the six studies in which 90% or greater of the patient population was diagnosed with stage IA or IB disease, the recurrence rate ranged from 11 to 18% [5, 6, 11, 13, 14, 17]. In patients with more advanced stage disease, the exact rates of recurrence by stage were not well defined. However, for these patients, the patients are usually followed closely for signs and symptoms of disease as rates of recurrence are higher.

In patients who experienced disease recurrence, the majority (62–89%) recurred within 2 years of primary treatment [4–8, 10, 11, 17, 18] and 89–99% of patients had recurred by year 5 after treatment [4–6, 8, 17, 18]. Overall, across all studies, the median time to recurrence ranged from 7 to 36 months after potentially curative treatment for cervical cancer [4–20]. Of the six studies that reported data for the time to recurrence by symptom status, the median time to recurrence for patients who presented with symptoms ranged from 14 to 36 months and 11 to 24 months for patients who were asymptomatic [6, 9, 14, 18–20].

The median overall survival after disease recurrence ranged between 7 and 12 months in 5 studies that reported recurrence data for the entire patient population [8, 10, 11, 15, 16]. For patients who were symptomatic at the time of recurrence detection, the median overall survival duration after recurrence ranged from 8 to 38 months [5–7, 14, 17–20]. Aside from two studies where the detection of asymptomatic disease was beneficial in terms of the median overall survival duration [4, 12], in 10 studies the median survival duration for patients with recurrence ranged from 7 to 17 months after detection of recurrence [5–8, 10, 11, 15, 16, 18,19].

In the retrospective series identified, central recurrences, which are potentially curable with total pelvic exenteration, ranged from 14 to 57%. The proportion of patients with sidewall recurrences ranged from 10 to 33% [4–7, 9, 10, 13, 14, 16, 18, 20], and the rate of distant disease (± local involvement), or disease detected at multiple sites, ranged from 15 to 61% in 15 of the 17 studies informing the topic [4–10, 12–16, 18–20].

Sixteen of the 17 retrospective studies reported the timing of the follow-up visits [5–20] with a generally consistent pattern of follow-up every 3 to 4 months within the first 2 years, every 6 months for the next 3 years, and then annually thereafter, or until year 10 or discharge, at the discretion of the treating physician. All but 1 of the 17 studies reported that follow-up extended beyond year 5 [4–20]. However, the rationale for termination of specialized follow-up often was not reported.

While not all data were consistently reported, the proportion of patients who presented with symptoms outside of regularly scheduled follow-up ranged from 46 to 87% in the 15 studies reporting the relevant data [5–11, 13–20]. Overall it appears that, in the series identified, approximately two thirds of patients presented with symptoms of disease recurrence, while one third experienced no symptoms prior to detection of recurrence [5–11, 13–20].

The detection of asymptomatic disease recurrence was not well or consistently reported in the retrospective studies. Due to the nature of the study designs, it is difficult to ascertain whether patients were truly asymptomatic at disease detection or if suspicion of disease prompted further targeted investigation that subsequently led to detection of recurrence.

Where reported, in approximately 15% of patients who relapsed, disease recurrence in asymptomatic patients was detected through physical examination in 0–75% in 11 studies [6, 7, 9, 10, 13, 14, 16–20], vaginal vault cytology in 0 to 17% in 11 studies [4, 6, 7, 9, 13, 14, 16, 18–20], chest X-ray in 20–47% in five studies [6, 9, 13, 14, 18], MRI in 0–9% in 3 studies [14, 18, 20], computed tomography in 0–100% in 5 studies [14, 17–20]. In the 1 study with 100% disease detection with CT, asymptomatic disease was

Table 66.1 Timing of routine follow-up visits

		Patients	Recurrence				Number of follow-up visits per year					
		Total # of Pts.	% With stage I disease	Overall rate (%)	% of Symptomatic patients	# With distant disease (%)	1	2	3	4	5	Total
Muram [4]	1982	323	45	15	NR	30	NR	NR	NR	NR	NR	NR
Krebs [5]	1982	312	91	13	75	35	12	3–4	3–4	3–4	3–4	24–28
Larson [6]	1988	249	100	11	63	40	4	3	2	2	2	13
Look [7]	1990	96	NR	22	67	43	5	4	2	2	2	15
Soisson [8]	1990	203	NR	15	71	58	4	3	2	2	2	13
Tinga [9]	1992	367	71	26	77	55	4	3	2	2	2	13
Gerdin [10]	1994	167	NR	11	84	23	4	3	2	2	2	13
Ansink [11]	1996	674	100	17	74	NR	4	2	1	1	1	9
Rintala [12]	1997	89	29	49	NR	61	4	4	2	2	2	14
Samlal [13]	1998	271	90	10	67	48	4	2	2	1	1	10
Bodurka-Bevers [14]	2000	993	100	13	86	56	4	3	3	2	2	14
Esajas [15]	2001	225	NR	16	46	37	6	4	3	2	2	17
Duyn [16]	2002	277	72	17	87	51	4	3	2	2	2	13
Lim [17]	2004	291	94	18	85	NR	4	2	1	1	1	9
Morice [18]	2004	583	NR	8	84	15	4	3	2	1	1	11
Sartori [19]	2007	NR	83	NR	65	43	4	3	2	2	2	13
Zola [20]	2007	NR	44	NR	50	33	3–4	3–4	2	2	2	12–14

Note: # of pts., number of patients, NR, not reported
The numbers in each cell indicate the number of times a particular modality is recommended during a particular posttreatment year

detected in two out of two patients [17]. Ultrasound detected 0–2% of recurrences in three studies [13, 18, 20]. Intravenous pyelography did not detect any recurrence in the two studies that reported data [6, 9]. Tumor markers detected 26% of recurrences in one study [15], but 0% in four other studies that reported data on the use of tumor markers [9, 13, 16, 18]. Six retrospective reviews reported that asymptomatic disease recurrence was detected in 11–33% of patients through other surveillance methods that were not specifically reported.

None of the studies reported on the efficacy of PET or PET/CT in the detection of recurrent disease. There is emerging evidence that surveillance with PET/CT aids in the detection of asymptomatic recurrences in patients with cervical cancer [22, 23]. In one small series, PET/CT results were used to alter the treatment plan, initiate unplanned treatment, and obviate the need for other planned diagnostic procedures [22]. Although, at this time, there is no firm evidence that PET/CT improves survival outcomes, as treatments improve over time, this modality will likely play a greater role in surveillance, especially among patients with asymptomatic disease.

It must again be noted that, in the retrospective studies, neither the sequence of surveillance testing nor the suspicion of disease recurrence prompting further tests were well defined. Further discussion on the utility of surveillance tests for asymptomatic disease can be found in greater detail elsewhere [21, 24].

The data from the retrospective studies are by no means definitive, but they can provide valuable insight when considering follow-up strategies for women treated for their cervical cancer who are now at a certain risk of recurrence and who are in need of surveillance. The data tell us that approximately 50% of patients present with stage I disease [3], and the risk of recurrence is approximately 15% [5, 6, 11, 13, 14, 17]. The overall survival duration for these patients at 5 years is approximately 92% [3]. For those with higher stage disease, rates of recurrence ranged up to 49% in the series identified [4–18], and it is well known that persistent or recurrent disease is much more common in more advanced stage disease. The percent of patients with advanced disease surviving for 5 years can be as low as 17% of patients [3].

Of the approximate 15% of stage I patients who relapse, about two thirds experience symptoms of disease recurrence. Of the remaining one third who were asymptomatic at the time of detection, physical examination was the most employed noninvasive method of detecting disease recurrence. The exact contribution of routine physical examination and/or other investigative modalities in detecting disease recurrence in this group is unknown.

Regardless of symptom status, if patients are going to relapse, most will do so within two years of primary treatment, and the median overall survival duration for these patients typically does not exceed 24 months. Central recurrences are amenable to further potentially curative surgery, but distant recurrence, for which there is no known cure, is experienced by approximately 33% of women who relapse. That is not to say that the early detection of distant disease is not of value in informing other important outcomes. Indeed, the early detection of disease recurrence provides critical information in determining the most appropriate disease management options for patients which can have direct quality of life implications. Treatment plans may change, patients may be spared further surgery if distant disease is detected, and an appropriate palliative approach may then be taken.

Thus, if 1,000 patients with early stage disease who were clinically disease-free after primary treatment for cervical cancer were to be followed prospectively, we would expect that with a recurrence rate of approximately 15%, about 85% or 850 patients would remain disease-free not only throughout the duration of the follow-up period but would be cured of their disease. Of the remaining 150 women that would experience disease recurrence, approximately two thirds would experience symptomatic disease recurrence outside of regularly scheduled follow-up.

Of the remaining asymptomatic women whose disease would be successfully detected through surveillance, approximately one third would experience distant/multiple site recurrence for which there is no known cure. For those patients the value of surveillance leading to early disease detection lies in the determination of the best disease management options, typically care with palliative intent. Of the remaining women who experience local disease recurrence, salvage therapy is successful in approximately 50% of cases [25].

In terms of an absolute survival benefit, it appears that, regardless of surveillance strategy employed, follow-up may only be truly beneficial to a very limited percentage of patients. For other important endpoints, such as progression-free survival, morbidity, and/or quality of life, the early detection of disease recurrence becomes a critical piece of information that cannot be dismissed because of a lack of an overall survival benefit. The early detection of disease recurrence may very well inform an optimum care strategy, whether it be through the route of further potentially curative therapy, entry into a clinical trial, a change in the treatment plan, or the recognition that prolongation of life is now the goal of managing the disease.

While the data from the 17 retrospective studies help inform practices on the optimum surveillance strategies for patients who are clinically disease-free after treatment for cervical cancer, it is also helpful to look at the expert consensus opinion of guideline groups who have developed recommendations on the topic. A search of Canadian and international cancer guideline developers revealed that five clinical practice guidelines were developed on the topic of the follow-up of patients with cervical cancer. The National Comprehensive Cancer Network (NCCN), Cancer Care Ontario (CCO), the Scottish Intercollegiate Guidelines Network (SIGN), the British Columbia Cancer Agency (BCCA), and the Saskatchewan Cancer Agency (SCA) have provided guidance on the topic of follow-up for patients with cervical cancer [26–30]. The recommended surveillance tests and schedules are provided in Table 66.2. The CCO guideline also recommended that patients be fully informed about symptoms of recurrence because the majority of patients have signs or symptoms of recurrence that occur outside of scheduled follow-up visits [27]. The BCCA recommended that other investigations such as CT scan may be requested as required for specific indications [29]. This would be assumed for all other appropriate surveillance tests if suspicion of recurrence warranted further investigation.

As seen in Table 66.3, physical examination and pelvic examination were recommended as the primary surveillance tests to detect asymptomatic disease recurrence. Where not specifically reported, it is assumed that the physical examination would include a complete patient history, and the pelvic exam would comprise a speculum examination and bimanual pelvic/rectal examination. Unless indicated, further follow-up tests or procedures are not recommended as part of routine follow-up. Recommendations on the type of practitioner to conduct the follow-up are not well defined and it is not clear which type of practitioner would be best suited to perform follow-up on this patient population. The recommended number of follow-up visits over a 5-year period were lowest in the Ontario and Saskatchewan setting with 9–14 visits over 5 years and the termination of routine follow-up after 5 years [27, 30]. The guideline from British Columbia included 7 follow-up visits during year 1, for a total of 16 visits over a 5-year period, and no specified termination of routine follow-up for cervical cancer recurrence [29].

Care is provided through a centralized multidisciplinary clinic where coordinated treatment planning and a common data system ensure that patients move through the system and are treated efficiently. Upon completion of treatment with curative intent, patients are counseled on the signs and symptoms of recurrence by the treating physician and also by an oncology nurse at discharge.

Follow-up generally consists of a complete physical and pelvic examination, including speculum with bimanual pelvic/rectal examination, patient history, and continued counseling about the signs and symptoms of recurrence (which includes lower back pain, pain radiating down one leg, leg edema, unexplained vaginal bleeding, and/or unexplained weight loss). For patients who have received radiation therapy, specific follow-up assessments by a radiation oncologist are done to assess for side effects of treatment, including gastrointestinal, genitourinary, and vaginal toxicities. In addition, assessment of menopausal effects is made and appropriate referrals are made to a general gynecologist with special interest in these issues.

The routine use of Pap testing or chest X-ray is generally not indicated in asymptomatic patients. Targeted investigations

Table 66.2 Follow-up strategies recommended by Canadian cancer agencies

	Recommended follow-up tests for Asymptomatic patients									Recommended number of follow-up visits per year						
Author Year (Ref)	Physical exam	Pelvic exam	Vaginal vault cytology	Chest x-ray	CT	MRI	PET	Tumor markers	Type of practitioner to conduct follow-up	Year 1	Year 2	Year 3	Year 4	Year 5	Total (Year 1–5)	Year 6+
NCCN 2010 [26]	Yes[a]	NS	Yes	Yes[h]	NI	NI	NI	NI	Not Specified	2–4	2–4	2	2	2	10–14	2[g]
CCO 2009 [27]	Yes[a]	Yes [b]	NI[e]	NI	NI	NI	NI	NI	Experienced in Cancer Surveillance	3–4	3–4	1–2	1–2	1–2	9–14	0[d]
SIGN [28] 2008	Yes[a]	NS	Yes	NI	NI	NI	NI	NI	Not Specified	3	3	3[h]	3[h]	3[h]	6–15	3[h]
BCCA 2006 [29]	Yes	Yes	Yes[c]	NI	NI	NI	NI	NI	Not specified[f]	7	3	2	2	2	16	1
SCA 2005 [30]	Yes[a]	Yes[b]	Yes	NI	NI	NI	NI	NI	Family Physician or Gynecologist	3–4	3–4	2	2	2	12–14	0

Note: *Ref* reference; *NS* not stated; *NI* not indicated as part of routine follow-up; *NCCN* National Comprehensive Cancer Network; *CCO* Cancer Care Ontario; *SIGN* Scottish Intercollegiate Guidelines Network; *BCCA* British Columbia Cancer Agency; *SCA* Saskatchewan Cancer Agency; *CT* computed tomography; *MRI* magnetic resonance imaging; *PET* positron emission tomography

The numbers in each cell indicate the number of times a particular modality is recommended during a particular posttreatment year

[a]Includes patient history

[B]Includes a speculum exam with bimanual pelvic/rectal examination

[c]After 3 months from primary treatment

[d]Return to primary care physician annual assessment (history, general physical, and pelvic examination with Pap)

[e]If cytology is performed as part of routine follow-up, it should be at a frequency of no more than once per year

[f]Initial follow-up examination by the Agency medical staff, and arrangements for follow-up by the referring physician

[g]Up to year 7, then once annually thereafter

[h]Optional

[i]Every 3–6 months for 2 years, every 6 months for another 3–5 years, and then annually

Table 66.3 Surveillance after curative-intent treatment for cervical cancer (asymptomatic patients) at the Ottawa Cancer Centre

Follow-up modality	Time after primary treatment					
	Year 1	Year 2	Year 3	Year 4	Year 5	Year >5
Office visit[a–c]	3–4	3–4	1–2	1–2	1–2	0[d]
Vaginal vault cytology	0	0	0	0	0	0
Ultrasound	0	0	0	0	0	0
CT[e]	0	0	0	0	0	0
MRI[e]	0	0	0	0	0	0
PET[e]	0	0	0	0	0	0
Tumor markers	0	0	0	0	0	0
Other	0	0	0	0	0	0

CT computed tomography; *MRI* magnetic resonance imaging; *PET* positron emission tomography

[a]Includes counseling on the signs and symptoms of disease recurrence

[b]Includes a complete history and a speculum exam with bimanual pelvic/rectal examination

[c]Followed by health care professional knowledgeable about the natural history of the disease and comfortable performing speculum and pelvic exams

[d]Return to annual population-based general physical and pelvic examination after 5 years of recurrence-free follow-up

[e]Imaging modality targeted to symptoms or high-risk sites of recurrence in special circumstances.

The numbers in each cell indicate the number of times a particular modality is recommended during a particular posttreatment year

based on symptoms and/or higher risk of disease recurrence typically include MRI or PET/CT scans after an explicit discussion of the limitations of these tests. The use of PET/CT is evolving and, at present, is limited to those patients in whom consideration for an extenterative procedure is part of an attempt at cure. At the Ottawa Hospital, we are currently embarking on a clinical trial to further define the role of PET/CT as part of a follow-up protocol. This follow-up strategy is consistent with the identified retrospective reviews and cancer guidelines. However, with this strategy, less emphasis is placed on the role of vaginal vault cytology in detecting disease recurrence.

After 5 years, disease-free patients are referred to their family doctor. For patients who live at a distance, a sustainable follow-up strategy has not been implemented to date and patients are often followed by their primary care provider.

To date our follow-up strategies have been well received by both physicians and patients after a number of education awareness interventions, in particular those that focus on patient education and the benefits of routine follow-up.

Surveillance at the Ottawa Hospital reflects an evidence-informed and conservative approach to patient care and is one that attempts to balance patient and physician preferences with the natural history of the disease and also the practical and resource considerations associated with follow-up programs.

There is currently no definitive evidence to inform the most appropriate follow-up strategy for patients who are clinically disease-free after receiving primary treatment for cervical cancer. To date no randomized controlled trials or prospective studies have been available to inform the topic of follow-up in this patient population. With the existing evidence, it is not clear that traditional surveillance strategies represent the most effective approach in detecting early recurrence, or if early detection leads to improvements in outcomes related to survival. More surveillance may lead to earlier detection of disease recurrence in some cases, but it may also lead to more false positive results and greater anxiety for a large proportion of patients who will remain disease-free. In addition, the obvious benefits of detecting early disease recurrence are limited by the existing treatment options for cure that are only successful in about 50% patients with localized central disease recurrence. In the majority of patients with sidewall or distant disease, the early detection of recurrence impacts disease management with quality of life and the extension of progression-free survival becoming the goal of therapeutic interventions.

As treatment options improve, the detection of asymptomatic recurrent disease, especially with promising modalities such as PET/CT, will no doubt have a great influence on the survival outcomes of patients. Until that time, posttreatment follow-up strategies for patients should continue with the explicit understanding of the limitations of the current test modalities and a clear expectation of the goals of any surveillance strategy.

References

1. Parkin DM, Bray F, Ferlay J, Pisani P. Global cancer statistics, 2002. CA Cancer J Clin. 2005;55:74–108.
2. National Cancer Institute of Canada. Canadian Cancer Statistics 2008. Toronto: Canadian Cancer Society; National Cancer Institute of Canada; Statistics Canada; Provincial/Territorial Cancer Registries; Health Canada; 2008.
3. National Cancer Institute Surveillance Epidemiology and End Results (SEER). Accessed March 27, 2009, at http://seer.cancer.gov/statfacts/html/cervix.html.
4. Muram D, Curry RH, Drouin P. Cytologic follow-up of patients with invasive cervical carcinoma treated by radiotherapy. Am J Obstet Gynecol. 1982;142:350–4.
5. Krebs HB, Helmkamp BF, Sevin BU, Poliakoff SR, Nadji M, Averette HE. Recurrent cancer of the cervix following radical hysterectomy and pelvic node dissection. Obstet Gynecol. 1982;59:422–7.
6. Larson DM, Copeland LJ, Malone Jr JM, Stringer CA, Gershenson DM, Edwards CL. Diagnosis of recurrent cervical carcinoma after radical hysterectomy. Obstet Gynecol. 1988;71:6–9.
7. Look KY, Rocereto TF. Relapse patterns in FIGO stage IB carcinoma of the cervix. Gynecol Oncol. 1990;38:114–20.
8. Soisson AP, Gaszler G, Soper JT, Berchuck A, Clarke-Pearson DL. A comparison of symtomatology, physical examination, and vaginal cytology in the detection of recurrent cervical carcinoma after radical hysterectomy. Obstet Gynecol. 1990;76:106–9.
9. Tinga DJ, Bouma J, Boonstra H, Aalders JG. Symptomatology, localization and treatment of recurrent cervical carcinoma. Int J Gynecol Cancer. 1992;2:179–88.

10. Gerdin E, Cnattingius S, Johnson P, Pettersson B. Prognostic factors and relapse patterns in early-stage cervical carcinoma after brachytherapy and radical hysterectomy. Gynecol Oncol. 1994;53:314–9.
11. Ansink A, de Barros LA, Naik R, Monaghan JM. Recurrent stage IB cervical carcinoma: evaluation of the effectiveness of routine follow-up surveillance. Br J Obstet Gynaecol. 1996;103:1156–8.
12. Rintala MA, Rantanen VT, Salmi TA, Klemi PJ, Grenman SE. PAP smear after radiation therapy for cervical carcinoma. Anticancer Res. 1997;17:3747–50.
13. Samlal RAK, Van D, Van Eerden T, Schilthuis MS, Gonzalez DG, Lammes FB. Recurrent cervical carcinoma after radical hysterectomy: An analysis of clinical aspects and prognosis. Int J Gynecol Cancer. 1998;8:78–84.
14. Bodurka-Bevers D, Morris M, Eifel PJ, Levenback C, Bevers MW, Lucas KR, et al. Posttherapy surveillance of women with cervical cancer: an outcomes analysis. Gynecol Oncol. 2000;78:187–93.
15. Esajas MD, Duk JM, de Bruijn HWA, et al. Clinical value of routine serum squamous cell carcinoma antigen in follow-up of patients with early-stage cervical cancer. J Clin Oncol. 2001;19:3960–6.
16. Duyn A, Van EM, Kenter G, Zwinderman K, Ansink A. Recurrent cervical cancer: detection and prognosis. Acta Obstet Gynecol Scand. 2002;81:759–63.
17. Lim KC, Howells RE, Evans AS. The role of clinical follow-up in early stage cervical cancer in South Wales. BJOG: Int J Obstet Gynaecol. 2004;111(12):1444–8.
18. Morice P, Deyrolle C, Rey A, et al. Value of routine follow-up procedures for patients with stage I/II cervical cancer treated with combined surgery-radiation therapy. Ann Oncol. 2004;15:218–23.
19. Sartori E, Pasinetti B, Carrara L, Gambino A, Odicino F, Pecorelli S. Pattern of failure and value of follow-up procedures in endometrial and cervical cancer patients. Gynecol Oncol. 2007;107(1 Suppl 1):S241–7.
20. Zola P, Fuso L, Mazzola S, et al. Could follow-up different modalities play a role in asymptomatic cervical cancer relapses diagnosis? An Italian multicenter retrospective analysis. Gynecol Oncol. 2007;107:S150–4.
21. Elit L, Fyles AW, Devries MC, Oliver TK, Fung-Kee-Fung M, The Gynecology Cancer Disease Site Group. Follow-up for women after treatment for cervical cancer: A systematic review. Gynecol Oncol. 2009;114:528–35.
22. Chung HH, Jo H, Kang WJ, et al. Clinical impact of integrated PET/CT on the management of suspected cervical cancer recurrence. Gynecol Oncol. 2007;104:529–34. Epub 2006 Oct 16.
23. Amit A, Beck D, Lowenstein L, et al. The role of hybrid PET/CT in the evaluation of patients with cervical cancer. Gynecol Oncol. 2006;100:65–9.
24. Zanagnolo V, Minig LA, Gadducci A, et al. Surveillance procedures for patients for cervical carcinoma: a review of the literature. Int J Gynecol Cancer. 2009;19:306–13.
25. Jain P, Hunter RD, Livsey JE, Coyle C, Swindell R, Davidson SE. Salvaging locoregional recurrence with radiotherapy after surgery in early cervical cancer. Clin Oncol (R Coll Radiol). 2007;19:763–8.
26. National Comprehensive Network. Head and Neck Cancers V2. 2010. Accessed October 1, 2010 at: http://www.nccn.org/professionals/physician_gls/PDF/head-and-neck.pdf.
27. Cancer Care Ontario. Follow-up for women after treatment for cervical cancer. Accessed June 4, 2009 at: http://www.cancercare.on.ca/common/pages/UserFile.aspx?fileId=45866.
28. Scottish Intercollegiate Guidelines Network. Management of Cervical Cancer. A National Clinical Guideline. Accessed May 1, 2010 at: http://www.sign.ac.uk/pdf/sign99.pdf.
29. BC Cancer Agency. Cancer Management Guidelines: Gynecology. January 31, 2006. Accessed December 10, 2008 at: http://www.bccancer.bc.ca/HPI/CancerManagementGuidelines/Gynecology/Endometrium/FU.htm.
30. Saskatchewan Cancer Agency. Follow-Up Guidelines: Endometrial Cancer. August 30, 2005. Accessed December 10, 2008 at: http://www.saskcancer.ca/adx/aspx/adxGetMedia.aspx?DocID=93,3,1,Documents&MediaID=1686&Filename=Endometrial+Cancer+Follow+Up+-+June+2009.pdf.

Vaginal and Vulvar Carcinoma

67

David Y. Johnson, Shilpi Wadhwa, and Frank E. Johnson

Keywords
Vagina • Vulva • Cervical intraepithelial neoplasia • HPV • Factors

The data for the estimated new cases and deaths worldwide in 2002 for vaginal and vulvar carcinoma were not available through International Agency for Research on Cancer (IARC), a component of the World Health Organization (WHO) [1].

The American Cancer Society estimated that there were 5,630 new cases and 1,670 deaths due to vagina, vulva, and other female genital tract cancers in the USA in 2007 [2]. The data for the estimated 5-year survival rate (all races) in the USA in 2007 were not available for these types of cancer [2].

Carcinomas of the vagina and vulva are rare. Advancing age, black race, and low socioeconomic status are risk factors. Vaginal intraepithelial neoplasia is believed to result from the same factors that cause cervical intraepithelial neoplasia, particularly HPV infection. Maternal diethylstilbestrol ingestion is known to cause clear cell carcinoma. Ionizing radiation (such as for treatment of cervix cancer) is a risk factor [3, 4].

Geographic Variation Worldwide

Vaginal and vulvar cancers are rare throughout the world. The country with highest reported incidence of vulvar cancer is Argentina, followed by Brazil and Portugal. The incidence of vaginal cancer is below 1.0 per 100,000 women in most parts of the world [3]. Geographic variation in the USA is also pronounced [5].

Surveillance Strategies Proposed by Professional Organizations or National Government Agencies and Available on the Internet

National Comprehensive Cancer Network (www.nccn.org)

National Comprehensive Cancer Network (NCCN) guidelines were accessed on January 28, 2012. No quantitative guidelines exist for vaginal and vulvar cancer surveillance, including when first accessed on April 10, 2007.

American Society of Clinical Oncology (www.asco.org)

American Society of Clinical Oncology (ASCO) guidelines were accessed on January 28, 2012. No quantitative guidelines exist for vaginal and vulvar cancer surveillance, including when first accessed on October 31, 2007.

The Society of Surgical Oncology (www.surgonc.org)

Society of Surgical Oncology (SSO) guidelines were accessed on January 28, 2012. No quantitative guidelines

D.Y. Johnson • S. Wadhwa
Department of Internal Medicine, Saint Louis University Medical Center, Saint Louis, MO, USA

F.E. Johnson, M.D., F.A.C.S. (✉)
Saint Louis University Medical Center and Saint Louis Veterans Affairs Medical Center, Saint Louis, MO, USA
e-mail: frank.johnson1@va.gov

F.E. Johnson et al. (eds.), *Patient Surveillance After Cancer Treatment*, Current Clinical Oncology,
DOI 10.1007/978-1-60327-969-7_67,

exist for vaginal and vulvar cancer surveillance, including when first accessed on October 31, 2007.

European Society for Medical Oncology (www.esmo.org)

European Society for Medical Oncology (ESMO) guidelines were accessed on January 28, 2012. No quantitative guidelines exist for vaginal and vulvar cancer surveillance, including when first accessed on October 31, 2007.

European Society of Surgical Oncology (www.esso-surgeonline.org)

European Society of Surgical Oncology (ESSO) guidelines were accessed on January 28, 2012. No quantitative guidelines exist for vaginal and vulvar cancer surveillance, including when first accessed on October 31, 2007.

Cancer Care Ontario (www.cancercare.on.ca)

Cancer Care Ontario (CCO) guidelines were accessed on January 28, 2012. No quantitative guidelines exist for vaginal and vulvar cancer surveillance, including when first accessed on October 31, 2007.

National Institute for Clinical Excellence (www.nice.org.uk)

National Institute for Clinical Excellence (NICE) guidelines were accessed on January 28, 2012. No quantitative guidelines exist for vaginal and vulvar cancer surveillance, including when first accessed on October 31, 2007.

The Cochrane Collaboration (www.cochrane.org)

Cochrane Collaboration (CC) guidelines were accessed on January 28, 2012. No quantitative guidelines exist for vaginal and vulvar cancer surveillance, including when first accessed on November 24, 2007.

Society of Gynecologic Oncologists (www.sgo.org)

Society of Gynecologic Oncologists (SGO) guidelines were accessed on January 28, 2012 (Tables 67.1 and 67.2). There are new quantitative guidelines compared to no guidelines found on December 13, 2007.

The M.D. Anderson Surgical Oncology Handbook also has follow-up guidelines, proposed by authors from a single National Cancer Institute-designated Comprehensive Cancer Center, for many types of cancer [6]. Some are detailed and quantitative, others are qualitative.

Table 67.1 Obtained from SGO[a] (www.sgo.org) on January 28, 2012

	Years posttreatment[b]					
	1	2	3	4	5	>5
Office visit	2	2	1[c]	1[c]	1[c]	1[c]
Papanicolaou test/cytologic evidence[d]	1	1	1	1	1	1

- Chest X-ray, positron emission tomography/computed tomography, magnetic resonance imaging not recommended for routine use
- Computed tomography and/or positron emission tomography scan recommended if recurrence suspected

Gynecologic malignancies: vulvar and vaginal cancer, low risk (early stage, treated with surgery alone, no adjuvant therapy)
SGO guidelines were accessed on January 28, 2012. These are new quantitative guidelines compared to no guidelines found on December 13, 2007
[a]These guidelines were obtained from the SGO website but are from the American Journal of Obstetrics and Gynecology (www.ajog.org)
[b]The numbers in the table indicate the number of times the modality is recommended during the indicated year posttreatment
[c]May be followed by a generalist or gynecologic oncologist
[d]Insufficient evidence of value for detecting index cancer recurrence but may have value in the detection of other lower genital tract neoplasia

Table 67.2 Obtained from SGO[a] (www.sgo.org) on January 28, 2012

	Years posttreatment[b]					
	1	2	3	4	5	>5
Office visit	4	4	2	2	2	1[c]
Papanicolaou test/cytologic evidence[d]	1	1	1	1	1	1

- Chest X-ray, positron emission tomography/computed tomography, magnetic resonance imaging not recommended for routine use
- Computed tomography and/or positron emission tomography scan recommended if recurrence suspected

Gynecologic malignancies: vaginal cancer, high risk (advanced stage, treated with primary chemotherapy/radiation therapy or surgery plus adjuvant therapy)
SGO guidelines were accessed on January 28, 2012. These are new quantitative guidelines compared to no guidelines found on December 13, 2007
[a]These guidelines were obtained from the SGO website but are from the American Journal of Obstetrics and Gynecology (www.ajog.org)
[b]The numbers in the table indicate the number of times the modality is recommended during the indicated year posttreatment
[c]May be followed by a generalist or gynecologic oncologist
[d]Insufficient evidence of value for detecting cancer recurrence but may have value in the detection of other lower genital tract neoplasia

Summary

Vulvar and vaginal cancers are uncommon. We found no guidelines proposed for this type of cancer by professional organizations or national government agencies.

References

1. Parkin DM, Whelan SL, Ferlay J, Teppo L, Thomas DB. Cancer incidence in five continents, vol. VIII, International Agency for Research on Cancer. Lyon, France: IARC Press; 2002. IARC Scientific Publication 155. ISBN 92-832-2155-9.
2. Jemal A, Seigel R, Ward E, Murray T, Xu J, Thun MJ. Cancer statistics, 2007. CA Cancer J Clin. 2007;57:43–66.
3. Schottenfeld D, Fraumeni JG. Cancer epidemiology and prevention. 3rd ed. New York, NY: Oxford University Press; 2006. ISBN 13:978-0-19-514961-6.
4. DeVita VT, Hellman S, Rosenberg SA. Cancer. 7th ed. Philadelphia, PA: Lippincott Williams & Wilkins; 2005. ISBN 0-781-74450-4.
5. Devesa SS, Grauman DJ, Blot WJ, Pennello GA, Hoover RN, Fraumeni JF Jr. Atlas of Cancer Mortality in the United States. National Institutes of Health, National Cancer Institute. NIH Publication No. 99-4564, September 1999.
6. Feig BW, Berger DH, Fuhrman GM. The M.D. Anderson Surgical Oncology Handbook. 4th ed. Philadelphia, PA: Lippincott Williams & Wilkins; 2006. paperback. ISBN 0-7817-5643-X.

Vaginal and Vulvar Carcinoma Surveillance Counterpoint: Japan

68

Shinji Ogawa, Hiroaki Kobayashi, and Norio Wake

Keywords
Vulvar cancer • Vaginal cancer • FIGO annual report • Lymphedema

Cancer of the vulva accounts for 5% of all female genital malignancies [1]. The ages of vulvar cancer patients are higher than those of other gynecological cancer patients. The incidence increases with age and the peak incidence is observed in the sixth decade of life [2]. In addition, it appears that the incidence has been increasing over the past few years, which is believed to be due to increases in female life expectancy. Vaginal cancer is less common, accounting for only 1–3% of gynecologic malignancies [1]. Most patients are in their fifth decade or older [3].

In Japan, carcinomas of the vulva and vagina are both rare. There have been no large-scale multi-institutional studies of vulvar or vaginal cancer in Japan, except for a report by the Gynecologic Tumor Committee of the Japan Society of Obstetrics and Gynecology [4]. There were 339 vulvar cancer patients treated in 139 institutions who were recruited for study during 3 years, between 1986 and 1988. The peak age distribution was 70–79 years, and squamous cell carcinoma (SCC) was the most common pathologic type (69%), which is similar to results of studies from other countries. However, there have been no large Japanese studies on vaginal cancer. In our recent 10-year experience at Kyushu University Hospital (1998–2007), among 1,468 gynecologic malignancies, there were 28 cases (1.9%) of vulvar and 15 cases (1.0%) of vaginal cancer treated, which indicates that the incidence of vulvar/vaginal cancer in Japan is lower than in other countries.

S. Ogawa (✉) • H. Kobayashi • N. Wake
Department of Obstetrics and Gynecology, Graduate School of Medical Sciences, Kyushu University, 3-1-1 Maidashi, Higashiku, Fukuoka 812-8582, Japan
e-mail: shogawa@gynob.med.kyushu-u.ac.jp; koba@gynob.med.kyushu-u.ac.jp; wake@gynob.med.kyushu-u.ac.jp

The most important epidemiological considerations of surveillance are survival and recurrence rates. In the latest International Federation of Gynecology and Obstetrics (FIGO) annual report on carcinoma of the vulva [2], the overall 5-year survival rates were reported to be 78.5% for stage I, 58.8% for stage II, 43.2% for stage III, and 13.0% for stage IV. Oonk et al. reported that 65 of 238 patients (27%) developed recurrent disease during a median follow-up time of 58 months; there were 49 local, 2 skin, 6 inguinal, and 8 distant recurrences, consisting of pelvic lymph node, bone, lung, and skin metastases [5]. Over 80% of recurrences occurred within 2 years after initial treatment.

The overall 5-year survival rates for carcinoma of the vagina, as reported in the FIGO annual report, were 77.6% for stage I, 52.2% for stage II, 42.5% for stage III, 20.5% for stage IVa, and 12.9% for stage IVb [3]. Frank et al. demonstrated excellent outcomes for patients with SCC of the vagina treated with definitive radiotherapy; the 5-year disease-specific survival rates were 85% for stage I, 78% for stage II, and 58% for stage III–IVa [6]. The recurrence sites were also listed; there were 11 patients recurring only in the vagina, 9 patients only in the pelvis, 13 patients only at a distant site, 4 patients in both the vagina and pelvis, 9 patients in the pelvis and at a distant site, and 3 patients in the vagina and a distant site. Of relapsed patients, 73% had a locoregional component, which indicates that follow-up examinations should take into consideration the possibility of distant recurrence.

An additional important consideration is detection of treatment complications. The most common long-term complication in patients treated for vulvar cancer is lymphedema of the lower extremities, especially in patients who have had inguinal and deep pelvic node dissection. Lymphedema diminishes patient quality of life and sometimes causes bacterial lymphangitis. It seems to be more prevalent among

F.E. Johnson et al. (eds.), *Patient Surveillance After Cancer Treatment*, Current Clinical Oncology,
DOI 10.1007/978-1-60327-969-7_68,

vulvar cancer patients than other gynecological cancer patients. A population-based cross-sectional mail survey revealed that there was a considerably higher prevalence (36%) of diagnosed lymphedema in vulvar cancer patients than in all other gynecologic cancer patients [7]. Undiagnosed symptomatic lower limb swelling was also reported in 15% of patients with vulvar cancer. Groin lymphocyst is another complication resulting from surgery for vulvar cancer. Lymphocysts were found in 7–15% of patients receiving a modified radical vulvectomy with bilateral inguinofemoral lymphadenectomy using separate groin incisions [8–11]; however, they often improve spontaneously [11].

The complications from radiotherapy for vaginal cancer were described by Frank et al. [6] They reported that the 5- and 10-year cumulative rates of major complications were 10% and 17%, respectively; there were 19 major gastrointestinal complications, including 7 cases of proctitis requiring transfusion, 5 fistulas, and 4 small bowel obstructions; 6 genitourinary complications, including 3 cases of hemorrhagic cystitis, 2 vesicovaginal fistulas, and 1 urethral stricture. Similarly, Tran et al. reported that 10 among 78 vulvar cancer patients treated with radiotherapy developed grade 3–4 complications, including 3 recto-vaginal fistulas, 2 small bowel obstructions, 2 cases of perineal skin breakdown, 1 bowel perforation, 1 rectal ulcer, 1 case of proctitis, and 1 case with pelvic bone necrosis [12]. Early detection of these complications does not necessarily improve the results; however, it is important to detect and manage these complications during follow-up visits.

Guidelines for posttreatment surveillance after initial treatment do not exist for either vulvar or vaginal cancer patients. Oonk et al. described a surveillance schedule for vulvar cancer patients [5]. Intervals between each follow-up visit were 3 months for 2 years, 6 months until the fifth year, and 12 months thereafter. They also showed that 65% of recurrences were found at a scheduled office visit. Local recurrences found during a scheduled visit tended to be smaller, but there was no survival difference seen between patients whose recurrences were detected at routinely scheduled follow-up visits and those whose recurrences were diagnosed at another time. They concluded that further studies should explore issues such as timing of routine follow-up visits and different follow-up schedules for patients at low and high risk for recurrence.

Follow-up intervals for patients with vaginal cancer have been described in two reports. Pingley et al. follow patients at 3–4 month intervals for 1 year, at 6 month intervals for the second and third years, and at yearly intervals thereafter [13]. Frank et al. reported on their routine schedule at MD Anderson Cancer Center, which is follow-up at 3-month intervals for 2–3 years, at 6-month intervals for an additional 2 years, and then yearly [6]. To our knowledge, the length of follow-up intervals appropriate for vaginal cancer patients has not yet been discussed.

Table 68.1 Surveillance after curative-intent treatment for vulvar or vaginal cancer patients (stages I–II treated without radiotherapy) at Kyushu University Hospital, Japan

	Year				
	1	2	3	4	5
Office visit[a]	4	3	2	2	2
Pap test	4	3	2	2	2
Tumor marker levels	4	3	2	2	2
Chest X-ray	3	3	2	2	2
Abdominal CT	1	1	1	1	1

[a]Includes history, physical examination, and pelvic examination
The number in each cell is the number of times in a particular posttreatment year a particular surveillance modality is recommended

Table 68.2 Surveillance after curative-intent treatment for vulvar or vaginal cancer patients (stages I–IV, treated with radiotherapy) at Kyushu University Hospital, Japan

	Year				
	1	2	3	4	5
Office visit[a]	6	3	2	2	2
Pap test	6	3	2	2	2
Tumor marker levels	6	3	2	2	2
Chest X-ray	3	3	2	2	2
Abdominal CT	2	1	1	1	1

[a]Includes history, physical examination, and pelvic examination
CT-computed tomography
The number in each cell is the number of times in a particular posttreatment year a particular surveillance modality is recommended

We have developed our own surveillance protocol for vulvar/vaginal cancer patients in our institute (Tables 68.1 and 68.2). They are based on retrospective analysis of the clinical experiences of our gynecologic oncologists. Vulvar and vaginal cancer patients are managed the same way, based on the staging and the types of treatment. Pelvic examinations, neck and inguinal lymph node palpation, and Papanicolaou smears are performed at every consultation. If a serum tumor marker level is elevated before the first treatment, it is also measured at every consultation. During the initial diagnostic examination of all gynecologic malignancies, we routinely measure serum SCC antigen and carcinoembryonic antigen (CEA) levels for patients with squamous cell cancer, or CA125, CA19-9, and CEA for those with adenocarcinoma. A chest radiograph is performed every 4 months or at longer intervals. We also schedule computed tomography at least once a year for the first 5 years. After 5 years, consultation is on an annual basis but computed tomography is not performed unless recurrence is suspected.

During surveillance, treatment-related complications should be taken into consideration. The most important complication is lower limb lymphedema. Treatment includes physiotherapy, use of elastic stockings, and/or massage methods, and referral to a specialist may be considered if improvement is insufficient.

Referrals to specialists are required for various other problems such as dysuria, fistula, cystitis, proctitis, and ileus.

Scheduled follow-up examinations are performed by several members of the gynecologic oncology team in our institute, and other specialists such as radiation oncologists or dermatologists who were concerned with treatments do not participate in surveillance. Our gynecologic oncologists believe that these intervals are suitable. Most patients are satisfied with our surveillance schedule. Although some patients would prefer to be examined at a local hospital, this is not feasible in many cases because there are few gynecologic oncologists and they are usually only in large urban hospitals.

Taking into consideration that the results reported by Oonk et al. did not clearly show that routine surveillance provides a beneficial effect on prognosis of vulvar cancer patients [5], our scheduled intervals seem to be rather short. However, the other benefits of surveillance include detection and management of complications and patient reassurance. We believe that a prospective randomized trial should be carried out to compare high-intensity and low-intensity protocols. Because accrual would be slow in any particular country, a multinational trial might be required.

References

1. Stehman FB. Invasive cancer of the vulva. Chapter 8. In: DiSaia PJ, Creasman WT, editors. Clinical gynecologic oncology. 7th ed. China: Elsevier Health Sciences, Inc; 2007. p. 235–64.
2. Beller U, Quinn MA, Benedet JL, Creasman WT, Ngan HY, Maisonneuve P, Pecorelli S, Odicino F, Heintz AP. Carcinoma of the vulva. FIGO 6th annual report on the results of treatment in Gynecological Cancer. Int J Gynaecol Obstet. 2006;95 Suppl 1:S7–27.
3. Beller U, Benedet JL, Creasman WT, et al. Carcinoma of the vagina. FIGO 6th annual report on the results of treatment in Gynecological Cancer. Int J Gynaecol Obstet. 2006;95 Suppl 1:S29–42.
4. Sugimori H, Kudo R. Acta Obstet Gynecol Jpn. 1995;47:685–93 [Japanese].
5. Oonk MH, de Hullu JA, Hollema H, Mourits MJ, Pras E, Wymenga AN, van der Zee AG. The value of routine follow-up in patients treated for carcinoma of the vulva. Cancer. 2003;98:2624–9.
6. Frank SJ, Jhingran A, Levenback C, Eifel PJ. Definitive radiation therapy for squamous cell carcinoma of the vagina. Int J Radiat Oncol Biol Phys. 2005;62:138–47.
7. Beesley V, Janda M, Eakin E, Obermair A, Battistutta D. Lymphedema after gynecological cancer treatment: prevalence, correlates, and supportive care needs. Cancer. 2007;109:2607–14.
8. Lin JY, DuBeshter B, Angel C, Dvoretsky PM. Morbidity and recurrence with modifications of radical vulvectomy and groin dissection. Gynecol Oncol. 1992;47:80–6.
9. Hopkins MP, Reid GC, Morley GW. Radical vulvectomy. The decision for the incision. Cancer. 1993;72:799–803.
10. Leminen A, Forss M, Paavonen J. Wound complications in patients with carcinoma of the vulva. Comparison between radical and modified vulvectomies. Eur J Obstet Gynecol Reprod Biol. 2000;93:193–7.
11. Gould N, Kamelle S, Tillmanns T, Scribner D, Gold M, Walker J, Mannel R. Predictors of complications after inguinal lymphadenectomy. Gynecol Oncol. 2001;82:329–32.
12. Tran PT, Su Z, Lee P, Lavori P, Husain A, Teng N, Kapp DS. Prognostic factors for outcomes and complications for primary squamous cell carcinoma of the vagina treated with radiation. Gynecol Oncol. 2007;105:641–9.
13. Pingley S, Shrivastava SK, Sarin R, Agarwal JP, Laskar S, Deshpande DD, Dinshaw KA. Primary carcinoma of the vagina: Tata Memorial Hospital experience. Int J Radiat Oncol Biol Phys. 2000;46:101–8.

Ovarian Carcinoma

69

David Y. Johnson, Shilpi Wadhwa, and Frank E. Johnson

Keywords
Ovaries • Surveillance • Epithelial ovarian carcinoma • Mutations • Rarity

The International Agency for Research on Cancer (IARC), a component of the World Health Organization (WHO), estimated that there were 204,499 new cases of ovarian carcinoma worldwide in 2002 [1]. The IARC also estimated that there were 124,860 deaths due to this cause in 2002 [1].

The American Cancer Society estimated that there were 22,430 new cases and 15,280 deaths due to this cause in the USA in 2007 [2]. The estimated 5-year survival rates (all races) in the USA in 2007 was 45% for ovarian carcinoma [2]. Survival rates were adjusted for normal life expectancies and were based on cases diagnosed from 1996 to 2002 and followed through 2003. Recent changes in the classification of ovarian cancer, namely excluding borderline tumors, have affected 1996–2002 survival rates.

Epithelial ovarian carcinoma is rare in girls, uncommon in young women, and increases rapidly with advancing age until menopause, then plateaus. Radiation, asbestos exposure, and nulliparity are felt to be causative factors. The presence of a germ line BRCA-1 mutation and other genetic abnormalities markedly increases risk [3, 4].

D.Y. Johnson • S. Wadhwa
Department of Internal Medicine, Saint Louis University Medical Center, Saint Louis, MO, USA

F.E. Johnson, M.D., F.A.C.S. (✉)
Saint Louis University Medical Center and Saint Louis Veterans Affairs Medical Center, St. Louis, USA
e-mail: frank.johnson1@va.gov

Geographic Variation Worldwide

The incidence for ovarian cancer varies greatly with geographic location. The incidence is highest in Denmark, Sweden, England, and the USA, intermediate in France, Spain, and Italy, and lowest in Japan, China, and Egypt [3]. Geographic variation in the USA is also pronounced [5].

Surveillance Strategies for Ovarian Cancer Patients [Stages I–IV (Complete Responders)] Proposed by Professional Organizations or National Government Agencies and Available on the Internet

National Comprehensive Cancer Network (www.nccn.org)

National Comprehensive Cancer Network (NCCN) guidelines were accessed on January 28, 2012 (Tables 69.1, 69.2, and 69.3). There were minor quantitative and qualitative changes as well as new quantitative guidelines compared to the guidelines accessed on April 10, 2007.

American Society of Clinical Oncology (www.asco.org)

American Society of Clinical Oncology (ASCO) guidelines were accessed on January 28, 2012. No quantitative guidelines exist for ovarian cancer surveillance, including when first accessed on October 31, 2007.

F.E. Johnson et al. (eds.), *Patient Surveillance After Cancer Treatment*, Current Clinical Oncology,
DOI 10.1007/978-1-60327-969-7_69,

Table 69.1 Obtained from NCCN (www.nccn.org) on January 28, 2012

	Years posttreatment[a]					
	1	2	3	4	5	>5
Office visit[b]	3–6	3–6	2–4	2–4	2–4	1
CA-125 or other tumor markers[c]	3–6	3–6	2–4	2–4	2–4	1

- CBC and chemistry profile as indicated
- Chest/abdominal/pelvic CT, MRI, PET–CT, or PET as clinically indicated
- Chest X-ray as indicated
- Consider family history evaluation, if not previously done[d]

Ovarian cancer: epithelial/fallopian tube/primary peritoneal
NCCN guidelines were accessed on January 28, 2012. There were minor quantitative and qualitative changes compared to the guidelines accessed on April 10, 2007
[a]The numbers in the table indicate the number of times the modality is recommended during the indicated year posttreatment
[b]Includes pelvic examination
[c]If initially elevated. There are data regarding the utility of CA-125 for monitoring of ovarian cancer after completion of primary therapy, see The Society of Gynecologic Oncology (SGO) position statement and Discussion from NCCN Ovarian Cancer Guidelines
[d]See NCCN Genetic/Familial High-Risk Assessment Guidelines and NCCN Colorectal Cancer Screening Guidelines

Table 69.2 Obtained from NCCN (www.nccn.org) on January 28, 2012

	Years posttreatment[a]					
	1	2	3	4	5	>5
Office visit[b]	2–4	2–4	2–4	2–4	2–4	1
CA-125 or other tumor markers[c]	2–4	2–4	2–4	2–4	2–4	1

- Ultrasound as indicated for patients with fertility-sparing surgery
- CBC and chemistry profile as indicated
- After completion of childbearing in patients who underwent unilateral salpingo-oophorectomy, consider completion surgery

Ovarian cancer: borderline epithelial (low malignant potential)
NCCN guidelines were accessed on January 28, 2012. These are new quantitative guidelines compared to the guidelines accessed on April 10, 2007
[a]The numbers in the table indicate the number of times the modality is recommended during the indicated year posttreatment
[b]Includes pelvic examination
[c]If initially elevated. There are data regarding the utility of CA-125 for monitoring of ovarian cancer after completion of primary therapy, see The Society of Gynecologic Oncology (SGO) position statement and discussion from NCCN Ovarian Cancer Guidelines

The Society of Surgical Oncology (www.surgonc.org)

Society of Surgical Oncology (SSO) guidelines were accessed on January 28, 2012. No quantitative guidelines exist for ovarian cancer surveillance, including when first accessed on October 31, 2007.

Table 69.3 Obtained from NCCN (www.nccn.org) on January 28, 2012

	Years posttreatment[a]					
	1	2	3	4	5	>5
Office visit[b]	3–6	3–6	0	0	0	0
Markers[c]	3–6	3–6	0	0	0	0

Ovarian cancer: malignant germ cell tumors
NCCN guidelines were accessed on January 28, 2012. These are new quantitative guidelines compared to the guidelines accessed on April 10, 2007
[a]The numbers in the table indicate the number of times the modality is recommended during the indicated year posttreatment
[b]Markers were the only quantitative recommendation given. We inferred that office visit would be recommended as frequently as this
[c]If initially elevated

Table 69.4 Obtained from ESMO (www.esmo.org) on January 28, 2012

	Years posttreatment[a]					
	1	2	3	4	5	>5
Office visit[b]	4	4	3	2	2	1[c]

- There is no benefit from early detection of relapse by routine CA-125 measurement and, even if CA-125 rises, chemotherapy can be delayed until signs or symptoms of tumor recurrence[d]
- CT scans should be performed if there is a clinical or CA-125 evidence for progressive disease[e]
- ESMO guidelines were accessed on 1/28/12. There were minor quantitative and qualitative changes compared to the guidelines accessed on 10/31/07

Epithelial ovarian carcinoma
[a]The numbers in the table indicate the number of times the modality is recommended during the indicated year posttreatment
[b]Includes pelvic examination
[c]Follow-up should continue until disease progression is documented
[d]It is important to offer women informed choices in follow-up and keep in mind that a potentially resectable occult macroscopic recurrence can be signaled by a CA-125 rise
[e]From data in the literature, PET-CT scans seem to be superior to CT scans in detecting more sites of tumor, especially nodal, peritoneal, and subcapsular liver disease. If a patient is considered for surgery, PET scan allows a more accurate selection of cases potentially candidates for secondary surgery

European Society for Medical Oncology (www.esmo.org)

European Society for Medical Oncology (ESMO) guidelines were accessed on January 28, 2012 (Table 69.4). There were minor quantitative and qualitative changes compared to the guidelines accessed on October 31, 2007.

Cancer Care Ontario (www.cancercare.on.ca)

Cancer Care Ontario (CCO) guidelines were accessed on January 28, 2012. No quantitative guidelines exist for ovarian cancer surveillance, including when first accessed on October 31, 2007.

Table 69.5 Obtained from NICE (www.nice.org.uk) on January 28, 2012

	Years posttreatment[a]					
	1	2	3	4	5	>5
Office visit[b]	4	4	4	1	1	1[c]

Ovarian cancer
NICE guidelines were accessed on January 28, 2012. These are new quantitative guidelines compared to the guidelines accessed on October 31, 2007
[a]The numbers in the table indicate the number of times the modality is recommended during the indicated year posttreatment
[b]Includes pelvic examination
[c]After every 3 months for the first 3 years, once a year for the following 5 years

Table 69.6 Obtained from SGO[a] (www.sgo.org) on January 28, 2012

	Years posttreatment[a]					
	1	2	3	4	5	>5
Office visit	4	4	2–3	2	2	1[b]

- Papanicolaou test/cytologic evidence, radiographic imaging (chest X-ray, positron emission tomography/computed tomography, magnetic resonance imaging) not recommended for routine use
- Cancer antigen 125 optional
- Computed tomography and/or positron emission tomography scan, cancer antigen 125 recommended if recurrence suspected

Gynecologic malignancies: ovarian cancer
SGO guidelines were accessed on January 28, 2012. These are new quantitative guidelines compared to the guidelines accessed on December 13, 2007
[a]These guidelines were obtained from the SGO website but are from the American Journal of Obstetrics and Gynecology (www.ajog.org)
[b]The numbers in the table indicate the number of times the modality is recommended during the indicated year posttreatment
[c]May be followed by a generalist or gynecologic oncologist

National Institute for Clinical Excellence (www.nice.org.uk)

National Institute for Clinical Excellence (NICE) guidelines were accessed on January 28, 2012 (Table 69.5). There are new quantitative guidelines compared to the guidelines accessed on October 31, 2007.

The Cochrane Collaboration (www.cochrane.org)

Cochrane Collaboration (CC) guidelines were accessed on January 28, 2012. No quantitative guidelines exist for ovarian cancer surveillance, including when first accessed on November 24, 2007.

Society of Gynecologic Oncologists (www.sgo.org)

Society of Gynecologic Oncologists (SGO) guidelines were accessed on January 28, 2012 (Tables 69.6, 69.7, and 69.8).

Table 69.7 Obtained from SGO[a] (www.sgo.org) on January 28, 2012

	Years posttreatment[b]					
	1	2	3	4	5	>5
Office visit	3–6	3–6	1	1	1	1
Serum tumor markers	3–6	3–6	0	0	0	0

- Radiographic imaging (chest X-ray, positron emission tomography/computed tomography, magnetic resonance imaging) not recommended for routine use, except for use in first 2 years if tumor marker normal at initial presentation
- Computed tomography and tumor markers recommended if recurrence suspected

Gynecologic malignancies: nonepithelial ovarian cancer (germ cell)
SGO guidelines were accessed on January 28, 2012. These are new quantitative guidelines compared to the guidelines accessed on December 13, 2007
[a]These guidelines were obtained from the SGO website but are from the American Journal of Obstetrics and Gynecology (www.ajog.org)
[b]The numbers in the table indicate the number of times the modality is recommended during the indicated year posttreatment

Table 69.8 Obtained from SGO[a] (www.sgo.org) on January 28, 2012

	Years posttreatment[b]					
	1	2	3	4	5	>5
Office visit	3–6	3–6	2	2	2	2
Serum tumor markers	3–6	3–6	2	2	2	2

- Radiographic imaging (chest X-ray, positron emission tomography/computed tomography, magnetic resonance imaging) not recommended for routine use
- Computed tomography and tumor markers recommended if recurrence suspected

Gynecologic malignancies: nonepithelial ovarian cancer (sex cord)
SGO guidelines were accessed on January 28, 2012. These are new quantitative guidelines compared to the guidelines accessed on December 13, 2007
[a]These guidelines were obtained from the SGO website but are from the American Journal of Obstetrics and Gynecology (www.ajog.org)
[b]The numbers in the table indicate the number of times the modality is recommended during the indicated year posttreatment

These are new quantitative guidelines compared to the guidelines accessed on December 13, 2007.

The M.D. Anderson Surgical Oncology Handbook also has follow-up guidelines, proposed by authors from a single National Cancer Institute-designated Comprehensive Cancer Center, for many types of cancer [6]. Some are detailed and quantitative, others are qualitative.

Summary

This is the third most common gynecologic cancer worldwide, and the fifth most common cancer among women in the USA [3, 7]. We found consensus-based guidelines but none based on high-quality evidence.

References

1. Parkin DM, Whelan SL, Ferlay J, Teppo L, Thomas DB. Cancer incidence in five continents, vol. VIII, International Agency for Research on Cancer. Lyon, France: IARC Press; 2002. (IARC Scientific Publication 155. ISBN 92-832-2155-9.
2. Jemal A, Seigel R, Ward E, Murray T, Xu J, Thun MJ. Cancer statistics, 2007. CA Cancer J Clin. 2007;57:43–66.
3. Schottenfeld D, Fraumeni JG. Cancer epidemiology and prevention. 3rd ed. New York, NY: Oxford University Press; 2006. ISBN 13:978-0-19-514961-6.
4. DeVita VT, Hellman S, Rosenberg SA. Cancer. 7th ed. Philadelphia, PA: Lippincott Williams & Wilkins; 2005. ISBN 0-781-74450-4.
5. Devesa SS, Grauman DJ, Blot WJ, Pennello GA, Hoover RN, Fraumeni JF Jr. Atlas of Cancer Mortality in the United States. National Institutes of Health, National Cancer Institute. NIH Publication No. 99-4564, September 1999.
6. Feig BW, Berger DH, Fuhrman GM. The M.D. Anderson Surgical Oncology Handbook. 4th ed. Philadelphia, PA: Lippincott Williams & Wilkins; 2006. paperback. ISBN 0-7817-5643-X.
7. Mackay J, Jemal A, Lee NC, Parkin M. The cancer atlas. Atlanta, GA: American Cancer Society; 2006. www.cancer.org. ISBN 0-944235-62-X.

Ovarian Carcinoma Surveillance Counterpoint: USA

70

Maurie Markman

Keywords
Ovaries • Surveillance • Epithelial ovarian carcinoma • Mutations • Rarity

It would be difficult to find another aspect of the management of epithelial ovarian cancer that is less evidence-based than any suggested statement regarding the "optimal" or "appropriate" follow-up strategy for patients who have completed their primary treatment program [1]. In the large majority of situations, primary treatment consists of an attempt at maximal surgical cytoreduction and a platinum/taxane-based combination chemotherapy regimen [2, 3].

In most patients this surgery is performed prior to the initiation of antineoplastic drug delivery, but in an increasing proportion of individuals this cytoreductive procedure may be undertaken after the administration of several cycles of a platinum-based neoadjuvant regimen [4, 5]. Depending on the specific clinical circumstances (e.g., "small volume" versus "large volume" residual cancer following primary surgery) and physician and patient choice, the chemotherapy may be administered entirely intravenously, or the platinum and paclitaxel may be delivered by the intraperitoneal route [6, 7].

Current data reveal that overall in about 50 % (or more) of patients who initially present with advanced (stages III/IV) epithelial ovarian cancer there is no clinical evidence of residual disease at the completion of approximately six cycles of platinum-based combination chemotherapy. The definition of a "clinical complete response" includes the following features: (a) normal physical examination; (b) normal CT scan of the abdomen and pelvis; (c) serum CA-125 antigen level within normal limits; (d) no symptoms or other laboratory abnormalities suggestive of persistent cancer.

M. Markman, M.D. (✉)
Department of Gynecologic Medical Oncology, The University of Texas, M.D. Anderson Cancer Center, 1515 Holcombe Boulevard, Houston, TX 77030, USA
e-mail: mmarkman@mdanderson.org

For many years it was standard practice to perform a surgical procedure at the completion of the planned chemotherapy program to determine if residual cancer was present [8]. It is important to emphasize that this diagnostic strategy was initially employed in an era devoid of even modestly effective biomarkers (e.g., CA-125) or radiographic imaging (e.g., CT scan). Further, there was genuine concern about the prolonged administration of cytotoxic treatment in a patient in a clinical complete response (whose cancer may potentially have been cured). This reflected the disquieting recognition that high cumulative doses of alkylating agents could result in the development of secondary (therapy-induced) acute leukemia [9, 10].

Unfortunately, data from several centers have revealed that, even in the presence of a negative "second-look" surgical procedure, the risk of relapse is quite high (i.e., >50% for patients with grade 3 ovarian cancers), raising serious questions regarding the utility of this approach [11, 12]. Further, reported experience from large nonrandomized databases has failed to reveal any impact of these second-look assessments on ultimate outcome [13].

It is important to appreciate that the current routine practice of considering six cycles of platinum-based chemotherapy to be the standard of care in the management of advanced ovarian cancer is not supported by solid data. Rather, this approach appears to have been adopted more than a decade ago based on the known substantial toxicity of cisplatin and the major difficulty associated with delivering >6 treatment cycles that include this agent [14]. However, to the best of this author's knowledge, a phase 3 trial specifically designed to define the optimal number of cycles of a carboplatin-based combination regimen administered as frontline treatment for advanced ovarian cancer has never been conducted.

F.E. Johnson et al. (eds.), *Patient Surveillance After Cancer Treatment*, Current Clinical Oncology,
DOI 10.1007/978-1-60327-969-7_70, © Springer Science+Business Media New York 2013

Thus, while patients with documented persistent disease (e.g., abnormal serum CA-125 level or abdominal/pelvic CT scan) after the completion of six cycles of a platinum/taxane regimen frequently continue treatment, it is considered routine practice to discontinue all antineoplastic drug therapy in patients with advanced ovarian cancer who have attained a clinical complete response. This decision is made despite the recognized fact that more than 60–70% of patients in this setting will ultimately experience a recurrence of their disease [15, 16].

Results of a somewhat controversial randomized phase 3 trial which explored the clinical utility of 12 cycles of single-agent monthly maintenance paclitaxel (compared to 3 cycles of monthly maintenance paclitaxel) in women with advanced ovarian cancer who attained a clinically defined complete response to a frontline platinum/paclitaxel regimen has raised further questions regarding the optimal number of treatment cycles to be delivered in the primary setting [16]. This study revealed a highly statistically significant improvement in progression-free survival in favor of continuation of single-agent paclitaxel for an additional year. Unfortunately, early closure of the trial (due to these positive results) by its independent Data Safety and Monitoring Committee prevented a definitive statement regarding the impact of this novel approach on overall survival.

The Gynecologic Oncology Group is currently conducting another phase 3 trial that is directly examining the potential impact on survival of a maintenance paclitaxel strategy. Other studies are exploring alternative approaches to maintenance therapy in ovarian cancer, including the delivery of antiangiogenic agents following the completion of cytotoxic chemotherapy and the use of tumor antigen-based vaccines. As a result, it is quite possible that within the next several years there will be a major change in the accepted standard paradigm of six cycles of antineoplastic drug therapy in the primary management of advanced ovarian cancer.

In the absence of evidence-based data that defines the optimal number of treatment cycles for a patient with advanced epithelial ovarian cancer who is responding to a platinum-based combination chemotherapy regimen, or a diagnostic test that is able to reliably define the risk of relapse for an individual patient, what is the most appropriate strategy for surveillance when a decision is made to discontinue treatment? Before attempting to answer this question, one additional issue must be addressed: What is the evidence that documenting recurrence relatively early results in a superior outcome, compared to discovering that recurrence somewhat later in the natural history of a particular patient's cancer? Stated somewhat differently, does it matter if a recurrent ovarian cancer is discovered 3 or 6 months earlier, based on the finding of a rising serum CA-125 antigen level or a newly enlarged retroperitoneal lymph node observed on an abdominal/pelvic CT scan (or PET scan) in an asymptomatic patient? Will such a discovery result in an improved overall survival, or delay (or even prevent) cancer-related symptoms? Conversely, will this earlier diagnosis result in treatment-related morbidity at a point in time when the patient would otherwise be experiencing a good quality of life, without producing a more favorable outcome, compared to delaying therapy until definite cancer-associated symptoms are present?

Table 70.1 Surveillance after curative-intent treatment for ovarian cancer following the attainment of a clinically defined complete response at M.D. Anderson Cancer Center

Modality	Posttreatment year				
	1	2	3	4	≥5
Office visit	6	3–4	3–4	2	1
CT scan (abdomen/pelvis)	[a]	[a]	[a]	[a]	[a]

[a]If the serum CA-125 antigen level is not a reliable tumor marker for a particular patient, it would be reasonable to obtain an abdominal/pelvic CT scan every 6–12 months for 1–2 years and only if clinically indicated thereafter

The number in each cell indicates the number of times a particular modality is recommended during a particular posttreatment year

The results of a randomized trial conducted in Europe provide important objective data regarding the optimal follow-up of women with ovarian cancer who have completed primary therapy. In this trial, all participants had a blood sample obtained on a protocol-defined follow-up schedule for evaluation of the serum CA-125 antigen level. All samples were sent to a regional reference laboratory for analysis. In the control arm of the study, the physicians of patients who experience a study-defined rise in this serum tumor marker were informed of these results. A decision regarding future treatment could then be made by the physician and patient based on this laboratory result. In the experimental arm, physicians were not informed of such an elevation, and retreatment was therefore based on other criteria (e.g., development of subsequent symptoms). The study end points include overall survival and impact of early initiation of therapy on the study population's overall duration of life and quality of life. This ambitious and novel trial clearly showed that tumor marker-based monitoring for recurrence of epithelial ovarian cancer does not result in clinical benefit [17].

Despite the current paucity of data, it is reasonable to propose a specific and detailed strategy for follow-up surveillance of women with advanced ovarian cancer, if for no other reason than to deal with the very real (and often profound) anxiety associated both with the objective risk, and disconcerting implications, of disease recurrence. Table 70.1 outlines one approach commonly utilized by many oncologists with experience in the management of epithelial ovarian cancer. Future research in this arena should provide more solid evidence upon which recommendations for surveillance in this difficult clinical setting can be based.

References

1. Markman M. Follow-up of the asymptomatic patient with ovarian cancer. Gynecol Oncol. 1994;55(3 Pt 2):S134–7.
2. Bristow RE, Tomacruz RS, Armstrong DK, Trimble EL, Montz FJ. Survival effect of maximal cytoreductive surgery for advanced ovarian carcinoma during the platinum era: a meta-analysis. J Clin Oncol. 2002;20:1248–59.
3. Covens A, Carey M, Bryson P, Verma S, Fung Kee FM, Johnston M. Systematic review of first-line chemotherapy for newly diagnosed postoperative patients with stage II, III, or IV epithelial ovarian cancer. Gynecol Oncol. 2002;85:71–80.
4. Vergote I, De Wever I, Tjalma W, Van Granberen M, Decloedt J, van Dam P. Neoadjuvant chemotherapy or primary debulking surgery in advanced ovarian carcinoma: a retrospective analysis of 285 patients. Gynecol Oncol. 1998;71:431–6.
5. Hou JY, Kelly MG, Yu H, et al. Neoadjuvant chemotherapy lessens surgical morbidity in advanced ovarian cancer and leads to improved survival in stage IV disease. Gynecol Oncol. 2007;105:211–7.
6. Armstrong DK, Bundy B, Wenzel L, et al. Intraperitoneal cisplatin and paclitaxel in ovarian cancer. N Engl J Med. 2006;354:34–43.
7. Trimble EL, Alvarez RD. Intraperitoneal chemotherapy and the NCI clinical announcement. Gynecol Oncol. 2006;103(2 Suppl 1):S18–9.
8. Podratz KC, Kinney WK. Second-look operation in ovarian cancer. Cancer. 1993;71(4 Suppl):1551–8.
9. Greene MH, Boice Jr JD, Greer BE, Blessing JA, Dembo AJ. Acute nonlymphocytic leukemia after therapy with alkylating agents for ovarian cancer: a study of five randomized clinical trials. N Engl J Med. 1982;307:1416–21.
10. Travis LB, Curtis RE, Boice Jr JD, Platz CE, Hankey BF, Fraumeni Jr JF. Second malignant neoplasms among long-term survivors of ovarian cancer. Cancer Res. 1996;56:1564–70.
11. Copeland LJ, Gershenson DM. Ovarian cancer recurrences in patients with no macroscopic tumor at second-look laparotomy. Obstet Gynecol. 1986;68:873–4.
12. Rubin SC, Randall TC, Armstrong KA, Chi DS, Hoskins WJ. Ten-year follow-up of ovarian cancer patients after second-look laparotomy with negative findings. Obstet Gynecol. 1999;93:21–4.
13. Greer BE, Bundy BN, Ozols RF, et al. Implications of second-look laparotomy in the context of optimally resected stage III ovarian cancer: a non-randomized comparison using an explanatory analysis: a Gynecologic Oncology Group study. Gynecol Oncol. 2005;99:71–9.
14. Hakes TB, Chalas E, Hoskins WJ, et al. Randomized prospective trial of 5 versus 10 cycles of cyclophosphamide, doxorubicin, and cisplatin in advanced ovarian carcinoma. Gynecol Oncol. 1992;45:284–9.
15. Ozols RF, Bundy BN, Greer BE, et al. Phase III trial of carboplatin and paclitaxel compared with cisplatin and paclitaxel in patients with optimally resected stage III ovarian cancer: a Gynecologic Oncology Group study. J Clin Oncol. 2003;21:3194–200.
16. Markman M, Liu PY, Wilczynski S, et al. Phase III randomized trial of 12 versus 3 months of maintenance paclitaxel in patients with advanced ovarian cancer after complete response to platinum and paclitaxel-based chemotherapy: a Southwest Oncology Group and Gynecologic Oncology Group trial. J Clin Oncol. 2003;21:2460–5.
17. Rustin GJ, van der Burg ME, Griffin CL, Guthrie D, Lamont A, Jayson GC, et al. Early versus delayed treatment of relapsed ovarian cancer (MRC OV05/EORTC 55955): a randomized trial. Lancet. 2010;376:1155–63.

Ovarian Cancer Surveillance Counterpoint: Europe

71

Andy Nordin

Keywords
BGCS • MRI • PET • Ovaries • United Kingdom

Abbreviations

BGCS	British Gynaecological Cancer Society
CT	Computerized tomography
EORTC	European Organization for Research in Treatment of Cancer
FIGURE	Follow-up for Gynaecological cancer Units: Randomized Evaluation
IOG	Improving outcomes guidance
MDT	Multidisciplinary team
MRI	Magnetic resonance imaging
NCCN	National Comprehensive Cancer Network
NCRI	National Cancer Research Institute
NICE	National Institute for Clinical Excell ence
NSSG	Cancer Network Site-Specific Group
PET	Positron emission tomography

Cancer follow-up has been a hot topic in the United Kingdom for almost 10 years. In 1999 an evidence-based document "Improving Outcomes Guidance (IOG): Gynaecological Cancer" was published by the National Health Service, providing a template for service reconfiguration with the establishment of gynecological cancer "centers" managing a population of around one million or more, fed by mainly diagnostic cancer "units." Service reconfiguration progressed during the early years of the new millennium, with formalized agreed referral and management pathways within a designated *cancer network* [1]. While the Improving Outcomes Guidance specified little regarding follow-up, the teams within the cancer networks identified it as a potential area for service improvement and improved clinical efficiency. In 2006, the group of cancer network gynecological lead clinicians [Network Site-Specific Group (NSSG) Leads Group] published the results of a national survey aiming to determine the mode of detection of recurrence of gynecological cancers by their respective multidisciplinary teams. This paper questioned the value of routine scheduled follow-up appointments and raised the suggestion that the diagnosis of recurrence may actually be delayed in many instances by patients waiting for their clinic appointment before reporting symptoms [2].

Before specifically addressing ovarian cancer, several major developments in the United Kingdom relating to the care of women following the completion of treatment for all gynecological cancers should be considered. The notion of patient-initiated follow-up has been discussed for a number of years and has been the subject of several small feasibility studies [3]. The principle involves a formalized educational consultation at the completion of treatment, with the provision of appropriate information documentation, explaining the nature of possible symptoms of disease recurrence and treatment-related side effects. Patients are given the contact details of a key worker, usually the clinical nurse specialist, who is at the heart of every multidisciplinary team. Women do not receive any routine follow-up appointments, but contact the key worker should they develop any concerns. The key worker triages the patient into an appropriate clinic, refers her to the general practitioner (family doctor), or reassures her, as appropriate [4]. A large-scale randomized controlled trial involving gynecological cancer centers throughout the United Kingdom [Follow-up for Gynaecological Cancer

A. Nordin (✉)
Cancer Services Collaborative, National Clinical Lead For Gynaecology, East Kent Gynaecological Oncology Centre, Queen Elizabeth The Queen Mother Hospital, University College London, St. Peter's Road, Margate, Kent, CT9 4AN, UK
e-mail: mail@andynordin.com

F.E. Johnson et al. (eds.), *Patient Surveillance After Cancer Treatment*, Current Clinical Oncology,
DOI 10.1007/978-1-60327-969-7_71, © Springer Science+Business Media New York 2013

Units: Randomized Evaluation (FIGURE)] was proposed and fully supported by all of the principal UK professional bodies, including the British Gynaecological Cancer Society, The NSSG Leads Group and the Gynaecological Group of the National Cancer Research Institute. For scientific reasons (to minimize heterogeneity of subjects) the trial design was modified from the initial proposal, which included all gynecological malignancies, to focus solely on endometrial cancer. It is hoped that the trial will commence in the UK shortly, as soon as funding issues have been resolved.

The second important development throughout the UK oncology community is an acceptance of a wider notion of survivorship, considering a holistic picture of the patient at the completion of treatment. The Government's recent document, entitled *Cancer Reform Strategy*, directing the course of cancer services over the next 5 years, highlights this as a major initiative [5]. Disease follow-up, in whatever format, will become integrated into comprehensive programs, including psychosocial support services, telephone follow-up, patient survivorship groups, community-based rehabilitation and physiotherapy services, counseling services, etc.

With specific reference to ovarian cancer, the National Institute for Clinical Excellence (NICE) is currently conducting a review of the management of ovarian cancer, with contributions from the British Gynaecological Cancer Society and the Cancer Network Site-Specific Group Leads Clinical Guidelines Group. The Cochrane Collaboration has also recently commissioned a large number of reviews in the field of gynecological cancer, including ovarian cancer, so evidence-based guidance may emerge in the near future from these initiatives.

Considering that this chapter relates to the follow-up of women who have completed treatment for ovarian cancer are in clinical remission and have not previously been diagnosed with disease recurrence, perhaps the most important factor to influence future practice is the OV05 Medical Research Council trial [6]. This trial was jointly initiated by the European Organization for Research in Treatment of Cancer (EORTC) as EORTC protocol 55955. It was designed to assess the value of monitoring CA-125 serum levels after the completion of treatment. Samples from recruited women are taken at three monthly intervals but the results are withheld from the patient and the managing clinician. If the CA-125 level rises to twice the normal level, the patient is randomized for either disclosure of this event to the clinician (for early investigation and treatment of probable early recurrence) or nondisclosure, in which case management continues as clinically indicated. There were 1,442 women recruited (1,144 by the MRC in the UK and 298 by EORTC centers). Recruitment is closed in 2005 and the trial remains open until 650 randomizations have been achieved. It is anticipated that preliminary results will be presented at the American Society of Clinical Oncology meeting in 2009.

Table 71.1 Surveillance after curative-intent treatment for ovarian cancer at Queen Elizabeth The Queen Mother Hospital, UK

	Years posttreatment					
	1	2	3	4	5	>5
Office visit[a]	4	4	2	1	1	±1
Serum CA-125 level[b]	4	4	2	1	1	±1

[a]Additional visits when required at discretion of clinician and patient
[b]CA-125 optional, depending on preference of patient and clinician
Physical examination (including pelvic examination) at office visit
Ultrasound/CT scan only as clinically indicated
The numbers in each cell indicate the number of times per year each modality is recommended during a particular year posttreatment

In the UK, all gynecological oncology patients traditionally undergo routine follow-up appointments (Table 71.1). This schedule is similar to the quoted US National Comprehensive Cancer Network guidelines. Scheduled office follow-up visits continue for minimum 5 years, as shown. The traditional follow-up schedule in the UK varies slightly from the National Comprehensive Cancer Network model in several aspects. The frequency of routine office visits decrease to once per year during the fourth and fifth years and many clinicians discontinue follow-up after 5 years for patients without evidence of recurrent disease or significant long-term treatment-related morbidity, on the assumption that the risk of recurrence is low beyond this time. Despite a lack of evidence of benefit, traditional follow-up practice in the UK includes routine pelvic examination, on the assumption that this intervention may identify early asymptomatic peritoneal disease recurrence. When different clinicians are involved in care (for example, surgical gynecological oncologist and medical oncologist), traditionally both review the patient independently on similar schedules.

In the absence of clinical trial data to support the full introduction of patient-initiated follow-up in 2004, the NSSG Leads Group discussed and supported a proposal for a hybrid follow-up schedule (Table 71.2). The protocol includes all aspects of patient-initiated follow-up, with a formal end-of-treatment interview, detailed printed information, and ready access to the multidisciplinary team via the clinical nurse specialist. It also includes a reduced schedule of five appointments at 6, 12, 18, 24, and 36 months, coordinated between appropriate clinicians (rather than duplicated). Patients are discharged at 3 years if they have not relapsed and they are free from treatment-related morbidity but retain access to the multidisciplinary team through the clinical nurse specialist. The protocol includes all gynecological malignancies but can be modified by the clinical team on the basis of clinical need such as management of disease recurrence or treatment-related side effects. On average, women free from clinical problems have 50–80 % fewer outpatient appointments under this system than they would have had under the former system.

Table 71.2 Hybrid scheduled/patient-initiated follow-up surveillance after curative-intent treatment for ovarian cancer at Queen Elizabeth The Queen Mother Hospital, UK

	Years posttreatment					
	1	2	3	4	5	>5
Office visit	2	2	1	a	a	a
Serum CA-125 level	2[b]	2[b]	1[b]	0	0	0

[a]Additional visits when required at discretion of clinician and patient
Access to team via clinical nurse specialist generates additional office visits as necessary
[b]CA-125 testing optional, depending on preference of patient and clinician (until results of OV05 trial published)
Physical examination (including pelvic examination) at each office visit
Ultrasound/CT scan only as clinically indicated
The numbers in each cell indicate the number of times per year each modality is recommended during a particular year posttreatment

In preparation for this book, the author surveyed the NSSG Leads Group in June 2008 in order to assess the degree of adoption of patient-initiated follow-up approach and the new hybrid model. Of 14 responses, only one cancer network reported complete conversion to the patient-initiated follow-up scheme, not offering any routine scheduled clinical follow-up appointments following the completion of the primary treatment episode. A second network is introducing this model piecemeal. Only one of the 14 networks practices the formal hybrid model, as described above for ovarian cancer follow-up. The remainder continue to practice variations on the traditional model for patients completing treatment for ovarian cancer, all utilizing a regimen similar to the National Comprehensive Cancer Network model with consultations every 3 months during the first 2 years and most progressing to appointments every 6 months until 5 years. Of the 11 networks practicing traditional follow-up, nine cease scheduled tests at 5 years while two continue for 10 years. Ten networks coordinate appointments between various specialties involved in care, most by the use of a multidisciplinary clinic. Of the 14 responding networks, 7 have either modified their follow-up protocol recently or intend to do so shortly. Ten of the 14 networks routinely check CA-125 levels during follow-up for asympasymptomatic women, but none perform routine ultrasound, CT, MRI, or PET imaging for asymptomatic women. Consistent with the National Comprehensive Cancer Network guidelines, all imaging modalities and blood tests but CA-125 are utilized only when clinically indicated.

These findings are supported by a publication of a national audit of follow-up practice in the UK [7]. The majority of cancer centers in this report practice routine clinic visits every 3 months for the first 2 years following completion of treatment for ovarian cancer, followed by clinic visits every 6 months for a further 3 years. Sixty-seven percent of centers use routine CA-125 surveillance to assess for evidence of preclinical disease recurrence.

From limited feedback from colleagues in continental Europe, it appears that traditional long-term scheduled follow-up protocols comparable to the NCCN guidelines remain commonplace. Colleagues in Belgium, Austria, and Spain report life-long follow-up after treatment for ovarian cancer, with initial clinic visits every 3 months, decreasing ultimately to annual surveillance. Serum CA-125 tests and frequent CT imaging are used routinely. Colleagues from a center in Sweden and three centers in the Netherlands report a five- to 10-year duration schedule similar to the National Comprehensive Cancer Network model, including CA-125 tests but not routine imaging. A colleague from Denmark reports a similar practice, but includes routine ultrasound in addition to CA-125 during 5-year surveillance.

References

1. Nordin AJ. Organisation of gynaecological oncology services. Obstet Gynaecol Reprod Med. 2007;17:91–4.
2. Nordin AJ (on behalf of the National Group of Gynaecology NSSG Leads). Mode of detection of recurrent gynaecological malignancy: Does routine follow-up delay diagnosis and treatment?. Int J Gynecol Cancer. 2006;16:1746–1748
3. Olaitan A, Murdoch J, Anderson R, et al. A critical evaluation of current protocols for the follow-up of women treated for gynecological malignancies: a pilot study. Int J Gynecol Cancer. 2001;11:349–53.
4. Nordin AJ. Gynaecological oncology hot topics. Follow-up. NHS Cancer Services Collaborative-Improvement Partnership, 2005. www.cancerimprovement.nhs.uk/View.aspx?page=/tumour_groups/gynaecology_docs/hot_topics.html. Last accessed 5 Sept 2008.
5. Cancer Reform Strategy. Department of Health, 2007. www.dh.gov.uk/en/Publicationsandstatistics/Publications/Publications-PolicyAndGuidance/dh_081006. Last Accessed 5 Sept 2008.
6. Medical Research Council OV05 trial summary. www.ctu.mrc.ac.uk/studies/OV05.asp. Last Accessed 5 Sept 2008.
7. Kew FM, Cruikshank DJ. Routine follow-up after treatment for a gynaecological cancer: a survey of practice. Int J Gynecol Cancer. 2006;16:380–4.

72 Ovarian Cancer Surveillance Counterpoint: Japan

Hiroaki Kobayashi and Norio Wake

Keywords
Ovarian cancer • Japanese Gynecologic Oncology Group • Second-look operation • CA-125 • Computed tomography • Integrated PET/CT • Surveillance guideline

The incidence of ovarian cancer is gradually rising in Japan. There are approximately 8,000 cases annually. There were 4,006 deaths from this disease in 1996 and 4,467 in 2005 [1]. The main reason for the increasing incidence in Japan is believed to be changes in the lifestyle of Japanese women. As in Western countries, childbearing now occurs later in life and the number of pregnancies per woman is decreasing. Moreover, oral contraceptives are not as popular in Japan as in Western countries. Although ovarian cancers are classified into various histological subtypes, most are common epithelial carcinoma. Germ cell, stromal, and borderline tumors are fairly rare. Therefore, this counterpoint focuses on common epithelial cancer.

It has the worst prognosis among common gynecologic cancers in Japan, as in other countries. Nearly half of the cases are detected in advanced stages (III and IV) [1]. Delayed diagnosis is related to lack of symptoms and signs in early stages and lack of affordable, safe, sensitive screening tests. For advanced cases, a staging laparotomy and maximal tumor resection is performed. Postoperative adjuvant chemotherapy is generally given except for low-risk cases (stages IA and IB).

Before cisplatin was available, the prognosis of advanced cases was poor and 5-year survivors were very rare. After introduction of cisplatin, approximately 30% of patients with advanced disease survived >5 years after primary treatment. In the 1980s, combination chemotherapy with cyclophosphamide, adriamycin, and cisplatin, given monthly for >6 cycles, was commonly used as postoperative first-line chemotherapy [2]. To reduce nephrotoxicity and cardiotoxicity of this regimen, carboplatin and 4 ′ epi-adriamycin were used later. In the late 1990s, paclitaxel was introduced into the first-line adjuvant chemotherapy and the standard combination was then paclitaxel and carboplatin, both of which were administered every 3–4 weeks for six cycles by infusion over 3 hours [3]. Now docetaxel plus carboplatin is used, but long-term results are not yet available so this regimen is not yet the standard first-line choice. However, it is useful for patients with drug-induced peripheral neuropathy. Recently, the Japanese Gynecologic Oncology Group (JGOG) reported the results of JGOG 3016 trial, indicating superiority of a dose-dense (weekly) paclitaxel + carboplatin regimen rather than the conventional adjuvant regimen [4]. Other regimens are also used, depending on the individual patient circumstances [5]. Clear cell carcinoma of the ovary is frequent in Asia. It is less chemosensitive and portends a poor prognosis [6].

After primary treatment (surgery plus adjuvant chemotherapy), a second-look operation may be performed. In Kyushu University Hospital, this was offered only to patients with no evidence of disease after suboptimal surgery in order to determine whether additional chemotherapy was required and to evaluate the pathological response to chemotherapy [7]. However, the utility of second-look surgery proved to be poor and it is no longer standard treatment.

In our long-term study of stage III–IV cases treated with surgery, followed by cisplatin-based chemotherapy during 1980–1993 in Kyushu University Hospital, 30% of the patients had progressive disease unresponsive to primary treatment, 27% were disease-free after 5 years, and the remaining 43% experienced recurrence after once obtaining disease-free status.

H. Kobayashi (✉) • N. Wake
Department of Obstetrics and Gynecology, Graduate School of Medical Sciences, Kyushu University, Maidashi 3-1-1, Higashi-ku, Fukuoka 812-8582, Japan
e-mail: koba@med.kyushu-u.ac.jp; wake@med.kyushu-u.ac.jp

F.E. Johnson et al. (eds.), *Patient Surveillance After Cancer Treatment*, Current Clinical Oncology,
DOI 10.1007/978-1-60327-969-7_72,

Table 72.1 Surveillance of patients with ovarian cancer after curative-intent initial therapy at Kyushu University Hospital, Japan

	Year					
Modality	1	2	3	4	5	>5
Office visit, including pelvic examination	6	4	3	2	2	1
Serum CA-125 level	6	4	3	2	2	1
Transvaginal ultrasonography	6	4	3	2	2	a
Chest X-ray	6	4	3	2	2	a
Abdominal and pelvic CT	3	2	1–2	1	1	a

[a]As clinically indicated
The number in each cell indicates the number of times a particular modality is recommended during a particular posttreatment year

There is a high probability of recurrence in advanced cases within 2 years after the initial treatment (approximately 20% and 50% within 1 year and 2 years, respectively) [9]. Therefore, we believe surveillance testing should be performed at least every 3–4 months for 2 years after the initial treatment, as suggested by NCCN guidelines [10].

Surveillance of ovarian cancer patients who achieve NED (no evident disease) status after initial therapy is the focus of this counterpoint. Since there are few relevant trials to determine the optimal surveillance intensity, Japanese guidelines are consensus-based [1]. Table 72.1 shows our strategy. We recommend office visits every 2–3 months for 2 years after primary treatment. Prudent surveillance continues for 5 years. After 5 years, some patients are released to their primary doctor.

As recommended by NCCN [10], we routinely perform pelvic examinations. The serum CA-125 level is an effective tumor marker for detecting recurrent ovarian cancer [11]. A retrospective multicentric study reported that the test establishing the diagnosis of recurrence in asymptomatic patients was clinical examination in 14.8%, an imaging technique in 27.2%, serum CA-125 level in 23.3%, and both serum CA-125 and an imaging technique in 34.7% [12]. A recent large randomized trial indicated that determining CA-125 levels does not improve overall survival [13]. This trial is changing surveillance practice worldwide.

Since initial recurrence tends to appear in distant organs, as mentioned before, our examinations in each office visit include various imaging modalities (ultrasonography, chest X-ray and abdominal and pelvic computed tomography). Chest X-ray and transvaginal ultrasonography are not sensitive for detecting recurrence but they are noninvasive and relatively inexpensive. Both are usually performed at every visit. When ovarian cancer recurs intraperitoneally, ascites typically is present. Transvaginal ultrasonography can detect even minimal pelvic ascites and ultrasonography is sometimes useful in diagnosis. Transabdominal ultrasonography is also useful to detect recurrence in parenchymal organs such as the liver, kidney, and spleen, but is not sensitive for detecting intraperitoneal masses without ascites. Therefore, abdominal and pelvic CT is preferred in our department. In fact, a retrospective multicentric study reported that the surveillance procedure to detect recurrence in asymptomatic patients was CT in 26.6% and ultrasonography in only 0.6% [12].

We usually obtain CT scans every second visit for the first 5 years, in which most recurrences occur. After 5 years, CT scans are not utilized routinely (Table). When the CT scan shows a questionable lesion without any sign of recurrence by all other examinations, we usually repeat the CT at monthly intervals until the diagnosis is clear. We also use magnetic resonance imaging, positron emission tomography (PET) with ^{18}F-fluorodeoxyglucose (FDG) or integrated PET/CT scans. Although PET and PET/CT equipment are widely available in Japan, these scans are too expensive to use for routine surveillance. We use MRI, PET, and PET/CT only for cases in which the diagnosis is unclear. In some cases, intravenous pyelography, Ga scintigraphy, bone scintigraphy, and laparoscopy are useful to establish a diagnosis. In practice, gynecologic oncologists at Kyushu University Hospital modify surveillance intervals and modalities depending on a variety of prognostic factors, including stage, histology, degree of residual disease after surgery, and so on.

Reducing the frequency of office visits and routine tests would mean an enormous reduction in costs. However, the aim of surveillance is not only to detect recurrent disease but also to diagnose posttreatment complications. We believe that routine office visits are helpful for a patient's psychological well-being although the benefit is not easily quantitated.

Randomized prospective trials of high-intensity vs. low-intensity surveillance are needed to rationalize clinical care. They are expensive to perform and require many years to complete. Without high-quality evidence, however, creating rational guidelines for patient care will not be possible.

References

1. Ovarian Cancer Treatment Guidelines 2007 (in Japanese). Japan Society of Gynecologic Oncology. http://www.jsgo.gr.jp/09_guideline/guideline/ransou2007-02.pdf.
2. Kamura T, Tsukamoto N, Suenaga T, Kaku T, Matsukuma K, Matsuyama T. Evaluation of the efficacy of cisplatin-based chemotherapy for epithelial ovarian cancer: comparison with treatments employed before cisplatin era (in Japanese). Gan To Kagaku Ryoho. 1987;14:1260–3.
3. Kuzuya K, Ishikawa H, Nakanishi T, et al. Optimal doses of paclitaxel and carboplatin combination chemotherapy for ovarian cancer: a phase I modified continual reassessment method study. Int J Clin Oncol. 2001;6:271–8.
4. Katsumata N, Yasuda M, Takahashi F, et al. Dose-dense paclitaxel once a week in combination with carboplatin every 3 weeks for advanced ovarian cancer: a phase 3, open-label, randomised controlled trial. Lancet. 2009;374:1303–5.
5. Sugiyama T, Yakushiji M, Kamura T, et al. Irinotecan (CPT-11) and cisplatin as first-line chemotherapy for advanced ovarian cancer. Oncology. 2002;63:16–22.
6. GCIG/JGOG3017 Version 3.1: Randomized Phase III Trial of Paclitaxel plus Carboplatin (TC) Therapy versus Irinotecan plus Cisplatin (CPT-P) Therapy as a First Line Chemotherapy for Clear

Cell Carcinoma of the Ovary. http://www.jgog.gr.jp/kaiin/kaiin2/enforcement_outline/jgog3017/pdf/pro/en/GCIG_JGOG3017_Protocol_English_Ver3.1.pdf.
7. Kamura T, Tsukamoto N, Saito T, Kaku T, Matsuyama T, Nakano H. Efficacy of second-look laparotomy for patients with epithelial ovarian carcinoma. Int J Gynaecol Obstet. 1990;33:141–7.
8. Creasman WT. Second-look laparotomy in ovarian cancer. Gynecol Oncol. 1994;55:122–7.
9. Heintz AP, Odicino F, Maisonneuve P, et al. Carcinoma of the ovary. J Epidemiol Biostat. 2001;6:107–38.
10. Ovarian Cancer Guideline (Version 2.2009). National Comprehensive Cancer Network. http://www.nccn.org/professionals/physician_gls/PDF/ovarian.pdf.
11. Rosman M, Hayden CL, Thiel RP, et al. Prognostic indicators for poor risk of epithelial ovarian carcinoma. Cancer. 1994;74:1323–8.
12. Gadducci A, Fuso L, Cosio S, et al. Are surveillance procedures of clinical benefit for patients treated for ovarian cancer?: a retrospective Italian multicentric study. Int J Gynecol Cancer. 2009;19:367–74.
13. Rustin GJ, van der Burg ME, et al. Early versus delayed treatment of relapsed ovarian cancer (MRC OV05/EORTC 55955): a randomized trial. Lancet. 2010;376:1155–63.

Renal Carcinoma

73

Shilpi Wadhwa, David Y. Johnson, and Frank E. Johnson

Keywords
Renal carcinoma • Chemical exposure • Tobacco • Kidney • Risk factors

The International Agency for Research on Cancer (IARC), a component of the World Health Organization (WHO), estimated that there were 208,480 new cases of renal cancer worldwide in 2002 (1). The IARC also estimated that there were 101,895 deaths due to this cause in 2002 (1).

The American Cancer Society estimated that there were 51,190 new cases and 12,890 deaths due to kidney and renal pelvis cancer in the USA in 2007(2). The estimated five-year survival rate (all races) in the USA in 2007 was 66% for kidney cancer (2). Survival rates were adjusted for normal life expectancies and were based on cases diagnosed from 1996 to 2002 and followed through 2003.

The dominant known etiologic factor for kidney cancer is tobacco smoking. Analgesic abuse, obesity, exposure to various chemicals (such as trichloroethylene, cadmium, and asbestos) is associated with increased risk. The risk of renal carcinoma is increased 100-fold in patients with end-stage renal disease. Genes causing renal cancer have been well documented, including VHL (clear cell carcinoma), Met (papillary carcinoma), fumarate hydratase (papillary carcinoma), BHD (chromophobe carcinoma or oncocytoma) (3, 4).

Geographic Variation Worldwide

Malignant tumors of the kidney account for about 2% of new cancer cases in the USA and worldwide (1). The incidence of renal cell cancer is high in several Western and Eastern European countries, North America, Taiwan, Australia, and New Zealand. The incidence of cancer of the renal pelvis and ureter is exceptionally high in parts of Bulgaria, Yugoslavia, and Romania due to a predisposing condition, Balkan nephropathy, which is endemic in the region. The incidence is reported to be lowest in Asia and Africa (3). Geographic variation in the USA is also pronounced, with higher incidence and mortality rates in urban than rural areas (3, 5).

Surveillance Strategies Proposed by Professional Organizations or National Government Agencies and Available on the Internet

National Comprehensive Cancer Network (NCCN, www.nccn.org)—NCCN guidelines were accessed on 1/28/12 (Table 73.1). There were no significant changes compared to the guidelines accessed on 4/10/07.

American Society of Clinical Oncology (ASCO, www.asco.org)—ASCO guidelines were accessed on 1/28/12. No quantitative guidelines exist for renal cancer surveillance, including when first accessed on 10/31/07.

The Society of Surgical Oncology (SSO, www.surgonc.org)—SSO guidelines were accessed on 1/28/12. No quantitative guidelines exist for renal cancer surveillance, including when first accessed on 10/31/07.

European Society for Medical Oncology (ESMO, www.esmo.org)—ESMO guidelines were accessed on 1/28/12.

S. Wadhwa • D.Y. Johnson (✉)
Department of Internal Medicine, Saint Louis University Medical Center, Saint Louis, MO, USA
e-mail: frank.johnson1@va.gov

F.E. Johnson
Saint Louis University Medical Center and Saint Louis Veterans Affairs Medical Center, Saint Louis, MO, USA
e-mail: frank.johnson1@va.gov

F.E. Johnson et al. (eds.), *Patient Surveillance After Cancer Treatment*, Current Clinical Oncology,
DOI 10.1007/978-1-60327-969-7_73,

Table 73.1 Kidney cancer (Stage I–III) (Obtained from NCCN (www.nccn.org) on 1/28/12)

	Years posttreatment[a]					
	1	2	3	4	5	>5
Office visit	2	2	1	1	1	1[b]
Comprehensive metabolic panel[c]	2	2	1	1	1	1^2
Chest and abdominal imaging[d]	1	0	0	0	0	0

NCCN guidelines were accessed on 1/28/12. There were no significant changes compared to the guidelines accessed on 4/10/07.

[a]The numbers in the table indicate the number of times the modality is recommended during the indicated year posttreatment.

[b]After every 6 months for 2 years, annually for 5 years.

[c]Including LDH.

[d]At 2–6 months, then as indicated.

No quantitative guidelines exist for renal cancer surveillance, including when first accessed on 10/31/07.

European Society of Surgical Oncology (ESSO, www.esso-surgeonline.org)—ESSO guidelines were accessed on 1/28/12. No quantitative guidelines exist for renal cancer surveillance, including when first accessed on 10/31/07.

Cancer Care Ontario (CCO, www.cancercare.on.ca)—CCO guidelines were accessed on 1/28/12. No quantitative guidelines exist for renal cancer surveillance, including when first accessed on 10/31/07.

National Institute for Clinical Excellence (NICE, www.nice.org.uk)—NICE guidelines were accessed on 1/28/12. No quantitative guidelines exist for renal cancer surveillance, including when first accessed on 10/31/07.

The Cochrane Collaboration (CC, www.cochrane.org)—CC guidelines were accessed on 1/28/12. No quantitative guidelines exist for renal cancer surveillance, including when first accessed on 11/24/07.

American Urological Association (AUA, www.auanet.org)—AUA guidelines were accessed on 1/28/12. No quantitative guidelines exist for renal cancer surveillance, including when first accessed on 12/13/07.

The M.D. Anderson Surgical Oncology Handbook also has follow-up guidelines, proposed by authors from a single National Cancer Institute-designated Comprehensive Cancer Center, for many types of cancer (6). Some are detailed and quantitative, others are qualitative.

Summary

This is a common cancer with significant variability in incidence worldwide. We found consensus-based guidelines but none based on high-quality evidence.

References

1. Parkin DM, Whelan SL, Ferlay J, Teppo L, Thomas DB. Cancer incidence in five continents. IARC Scientific Publication 155, vol. VIII. Lyon: IARC; 2002. ISBN 92-832-2155-9.
2. Jemal A, Seigel R, Ward E, Murray T, Xu J, Thun MJ. Cancer Statistics, 2007. CA Cancer J Clin. 2007;57:43–66.
3. Schottenfeld D, Fraumeni JG. Cancer epidemiology and prevention. 3rd ed. New York, NY: Oxford University Press; 2006. ISBN 13:978-0-19-514961-6.
4. DeVita VT, Hellman S, Rosenberg SA. Cancer. 7th ed. Philadelphia, PA: Lippincott Williams & Wilkins; 2005. ISBN 0-781-74450-4.
5. Devesa SS, Grauman DJ, Blot WJ, Pennello GA, Hoover RN, Fraumeni JF Jr. Atlas of cancer mortality in the United States. NIH Publication No. 99–4564. National Institutes of Health, National Cancer Institute; September 1999.
6. Feig BW, Berger DH, Fuhrman GM. The M.D. Anderson surgical oncology handbook. 4th ed. Philadelphia, PA: Lippincott Williams & Wilkins; 2006 (paperback). ISBN 0-7817-5643-X.

Renal Carcinoma Surveillance Counterpoint: Europe

74

Alessandro Antonelli, Claudio Simeone, and Sergio Cosciani Cunico

Keywords
Nonmetastatic kidney cancer • Kidney • Nephrectomy • Surveillance • Papillary carcinoma

Despite the increase in early diagnoses that took place in recent years, thanks to the increase in popularity of imaging techniques (ultrasonography and CT), the kidney neoplasm is still the urologic cancer with the highest mortality rate [1] due to the significant number of cases with distant metastases for which no systemic treatment with curative potential exists. The disease has a variable and often highly unpredictable biological behavior and recurrence is possible also after radical treatment of organ-confined disease. The most common sites of relapse are lung, adrenal, liver, bone, brain, lumbar fossa, and contralateral kidney, but the literature documents that kidney carcinoma can metastasize to virtually any organ. The absence of effective systemic therapy can justify adoption of the most accurate follow-up plan available to diagnose a relapse as quickly as possible and surgically remove it. As a matter of fact, surgical metastasectomy, wherever technically feasible, can be curative and/or lead to an increase in survival duration [2].

Several clinical, biochemical, pathological, and molecular factors have been analyzed for their prognostic value but today pathological staging according to the TNM system remains the most important single prognostic factor. In order to increase its accuracy, several authors have proposed some integrated staging systems in which the TNM stage is combined with other prognostic factors [3].

In our institution, over the last two decades, we have surgically treated more than 1,500 patients with renal cell carcinoma. In cases where radical surgery was applied to a nonmetastatic neoplasm (pN0/Nx M0), patients are followed with a surveillance plan independent of the disease stage. Periodic controls are done with blood tests (complete blood count, kidney and liver function tests), abdominal imaging examinations (ultrasonography or CT) and chest examinations (plain X-rays or CT) once each 6 months in the first 2 years after surgery and then again every year for an indefinite time. Additional examinations (brain CT and bone scintigraphy) have been, used only in the presence of specific symptoms. In light of this experience, which has allowed us to monitor these patients continuously, we have recently reviewed the results obtained and retrospectively applied an integrated staging system to assess which cases might require more intense surveillance and which cases might well be served by less intense surveillance [4].

Among the many integrated staging systems available, we have chosen the one developed at UCLA (UCLA Integrated Staging System, UISS [5]), which is based on two pathological factors (the stage according to TNM 1997 [6] and the cytonuclear grading according to Fuhrman [7]) plus a clinical factor (the performance status as defined by the ECOG score [8]) (see Table 74.1). The widespread availability of this information makes this staging system applicable in all institutions, which is one of its greatest assets. The combination of the three factors permits assignment to three risk classes, i.e., low risk (LR), intermediate risk (IR), and high risk (HR) (see Table 74.2).

We have reviewed data on 814 patients with nonmetastatic kidney cancer (pN0/Nx M0), 158 of which had undergone nephron-sparing surgery, the remaining 656 had undergone nephrectomy. Average follow-up duration for all patients was 76 months (minimum 24 months). Relapses have occurred in 193 cases, corresponding to 24% of the total. According to UISS, 140 cases were LR, 420 IR, and 254 HR. Relapse rate in the follow-up for the three risk

A. Antonelli (✉) • C. Simeone • S.C. Cunico
Department of Urology, University of Brescia, Spedali Civili Hospital, Piazzale Spedali Civili 1, Brescia 25123, Italy
e-mail: alxanto@hotmail.com

F.E. Johnson et al. (eds.), *Patient Surveillance After Cancer Treatment*, Current Clinical Oncology,
DOI 10.1007/978-1-60327-969-7_74, © Springer Science+Business Media New York 2013

Table 74.1 Prognostic systems

TNM 1997	
pT1	Tumor <= 7 cm in the greatest dimension, limited to the kidney
pT2	Tumor >7 cm in the greatest dimension, limited to the kidney
pT3	Tumor extends into major veins or directly invades the adrenal gland or perinephric fat tissues but not beyond the Gerota's fascia
pT4	Tumor directly invades beyond Gerota's fascia
Fuhrman's grading	
G1	Tumor cells with small (~10 μm) round uniform nuclei without nucleoli
G2	Tumor cells with larger nuclei (~15 μm) with irregularities in outline nucleoli when examined under high power (400)
G3	Tumor cells with even larger nuclei (~20 μm) with obviously irregular outline prominent larger nucleoli even at low power (100)
G4	Tumor cells with bizarre, multilobed nuclei heavy clumps of chromatin
ECOG score	
0	Fully active, able to carry on all predisease performance without restriction
1	Restricted in physically strenuous activity but ambulatory and able to carry out work of a light or sedentary nature, e.g., light housework, office work
2	Ambulatory and capable of all self care but unable to carry out any work activities. Up and about more than 50% of waking hours
3	Capable of only limited self-care, confined to bed or chair more than 50% of waking hours
4	Completely disabled. Cannot carry on any self-care. Totally confined to bed or chair

Table 74.2 UISS definitions

UISS risk class	pT	G	ECOG
Low risk	1	1–2	0
Intermediate risk	1	1–2	>0
	1	3–4	Any
	2	Any	Any
	3	1	Any
	3	>1	0
High risk	3	>1	>0
	4	Any	Any

classes was 10, 22, and 54%, respectively, with an average latency after surgery of 54, 36, and 30 months, respectively. The most common type of relapse was distant metastasis (73%), followed by local relapse (12%) and by the appearance of a new kidney neoplasm in the contralateral kidney (11%) or in the remaining kidney after nephron-sparing surgery (4%). Table 74.3 shows the distribution of relapses, with onset times, in the different UISS risk classes. It is

Table 74.3 Site of relapse

	latency (months)	All patients (%)	LR (%)	IR (%)	HR (%)
Operated kidney	23.4	4.1	11.6	5.4	0
Contralateral kidney	71.8	10.9	30.1	10.1	4.0
Local recurrence	26.4	11.9	3.9	7.6	20.0
Distant metastasis	29.5	73.0	53.8	76.1	76.0
Abdomen	32.8	15.6	7.2	17.1	15.8
Chest	29.5	48.3	35.7	50.0	49.1
Bone	14.9	11.3	21.4	12.9	7.0
Others	41.4	9.9	21.4	8.6	8.8
Multiple sites	24.1	14.9	14.3	11.4	19.3

Recurrence sites and time, as a percentage of asymptomatic patients, and the distribution of different types of recurrence in UISS risk groups (LR low risk, IR intermediate risk, HR high risk; the sum of percentages of each site of distant metastasis is 100%)

easy to note that the risk of relapse via a new renal neoplasm decreases gradually over time among the three risk classes (LR, IR, and HR) while the chance of local relapse or distant metastasis increases from LR to IR to HR class. From a biological point of view relapses in the kidney deserve to be viewed and dealt with differently from distant metastases or local relapses. Indeed, the development of a neoplasm in the kidney undergoing nephron-sparing surgery may be explained by the presence of unrecognized multifocal disease or by the lack of adequate surgical margins while a neoplasm in the contralateral kidney can be considered a new primary cancer. Patients with a relapse in the contralateral kidney, in the ipsilateral kidney after nephron-sparing surgery, with distant metastasis, and local recurrence have a 12-month survival rate after diagnosis of 96, 86, 70, and 44%, respectively. Figures 74.1 and 74.2 show the time distribution of the three risk classes of relapses in the chest and in the abdomen, including abdominal metastases, local relapses, and kidney relapses. Disease relapse in LR patients in the first 5 years of follow-up occurs chiefly at abdominal level, while the risk of lung recurrence is less serious. On the other hand, IR patients in the first 5 years after surgery have a higher risk of relapse in the lung, especially in the first 24–36 months, while risk of relapse in the abdomen is lower; the same happens, albeit at a significantly lower rate, for the subsequent 5 years. HR patients, during the earliest years of follow-up, show a high risk of relapse in the abdomen and a lower risk of lung metastasis. This risk, though still significant, decreases in the subsequent 5 years. All risk classes, after 10 years of follow-up, feature only rare relapses, chiefly in the abdominal area and in the contralateral kidney. As regards the imaging methods to be used for monitoring the chest and abdomen, from a cost/benefit point of view, it is preferable

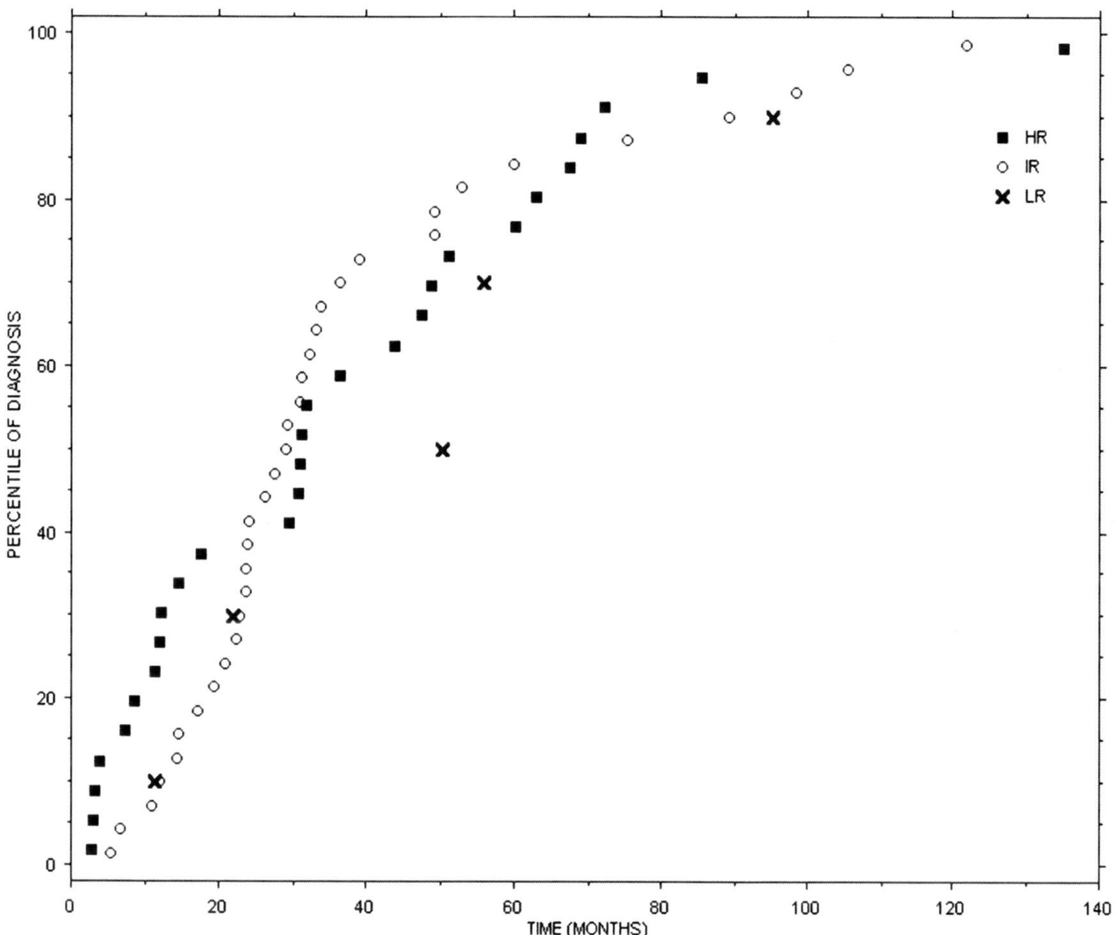

Fig. 74.1 Time distribution of thoracic relapses (LR low risk, IR intermediate risk, HR high risk; marks represent the events of recurrence as percentiles on overall recurrences in each specific site; zero point is the time of treatment of primary tumor)

to use cheaper and safer (for the patient) techniques like abdominal ultrasonography and chest radiography for lower-risk patients, using CT only for higher-risk patients. The risk of bone metastases is limited. It is higher in the time period closer to the surgery and it also pertains chiefly to HR cases. In light of these data, we think it is possible to offer different surveillance plans, depending on risk classes, as shown in Tables 74.4, 74.5, 74.6.

There is no significant difference in risk and relapse mode between patients subjected to nephrectomy and those subjected to nephron-sparing surgery. There is consequently no need to modify surveillance according to this factor.

One factor not included in the UISS but, in our opinion, worthy of consideration is the tumor histological subtype. Currently, according to the classification drafted in the Heidelberg and Rochester consensus conferences, there are four main histological subtype of kidney carcinoma: clear cell (80% of cases), papillary (in turn divided in type 1 and type 2), chromophobe, and collecting duct [9]. Although the independent prognostic role of the histotype has not been clearly demonstrated, it is quite evident that patients suffering with chromophobe and type 1 papillary renal cell carcinomas usually have a highly favorable prognosis, whereas patients with collecting duct carcinoma have an extremely unfavorable prognosis and the prognosis of patients with type 2 papillary carcinoma or conventional renal cell carcinoma is somewhere in between the extremes [10, 11]. Consequently, we propose to manage follow-up of patients with favorable histotype (chromophobe and type 1 papillary renal cell carcinoma) with the plan proposed for LR class patients and to apply the HR follow-up plan for patients with the unfavorable histotype (collecting duct carcinoma). The follow-up of patients with type 2 papillary carcinoma can be decided by stratification with the UISS.

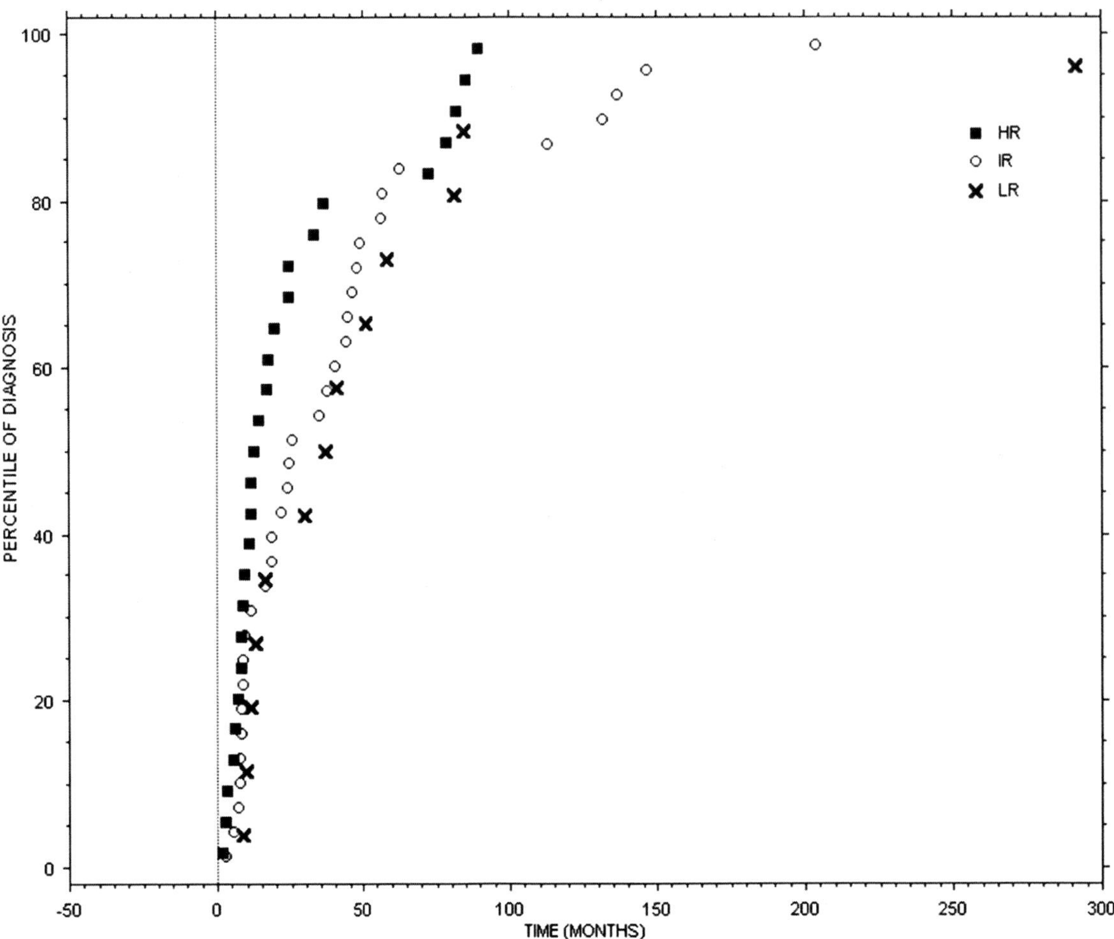

Fig. 74.2 Time distribution of abdominal relapses (LR low risk, IR intermediate risk, HR high risk; marks represent the events of recurrence as percentiles on overall recurrences in each specific site; zero point is the time of treatment of primary tumor)

Table 74.4 Surveillance after curative-intent treatment for renal cancer for LR patients at Spedali Civili Hospital

	years posttreatment						
	1	2	3	4	5	5–10	>10
Chest X-ray	0	1	0	1	0	0	0
Abdomen US	1	1	1	1	1	2	1
Abdomen CT	0	0	0	0	0	0	0
Chest CT	0	0	0	0	0	0	0
Bone scan	0	0	0	0	0	0	0

The number in each cell is the number of times a particular examination is recommended in a particular posttreatment year (LR, low risk)

Table 74.5 Surveillance after curative-intent treatment for renal cancer for IR patients at Spedali Civili Hospital

	years posttreatment						
	1	2	3	4	5	5–10	>10
Chest X-ray	1	1	2	1	1	5	0
Abdomen US	1	1	2	1	1	5	1
Abdomen CT	1	1	0	0	0	0	0
Chest CT	1	1	0	0	0	0	0
Bone scan	0	0	0	0	0	0	0

The number in each cell is the number of times a particular examination is recommended in a particular posttreatment year (IR intermediate risk)

Table 74.6 Surveillance after curative-intent treatment for renal cancer for HR patients at Spedali Civili Hospital

	years posttreatment						
	1	2	3	4	5	5–10	>10
Chest X-ray	0	1	1	2	2	5	0
Abdomen US	0	1	1	2	2	5	1
Abdomen CT	2	1	1	0	0	0	0
Chest CT	2	1	1	0	0	0	0
Bone scan	0	1	0	0	0	0	0

The number in each cell is the number of times a particular examination is recommended in a particular posttreatment year (HR high risk)

References

1. Jemal A, Tiwari RC, Murray T, et al. Cancer statistics 2004. CA Cancer J Clin. 2004;54:8–29.
2. Kuczyk MA, Anastasiadis AG, Zimmermann R, Merseburger AS, Corvin S, Stenzl A. Current aspects of the surgical management of organconfined, metastatic and recurrent renal cell cancer. BJU Int. 2005;96:721–7.
3. Furniss D, Harnden P, Ali N, et al. Prognostic factors for renal cell carcinoma. Cancer Treat Rev. 2008;34(5):407–26.
4. Antonelli A, Cozzoli A, Zani D, Zanotelli T, Nicolai M, Cosciani Cunico S, Simeone C. The follow-up management of nonmetastatic

renal cell carcinoma: definition of a surveillance protocol. BJU Int. 2007;99(2):296–300.

5. Zisman A, Pantuck AJ, Dorey F, et al. Improved prognostication of renal cell carcinoma using an integrated staging system. J Clin Oncol. 2001;19:1649–57.
6. Guinan P, Sobin LH, Algaba F, et al. TNM staging of renal cell carcinoma: workgroup no. 3. Union International Contre le Cancer (UICC) and the American Joint Committee on Cancer (AJCC). Cancer. 1997;80:992–3.
7. Fuhrman SA, Lasky LC, Limas C. Prognostic significance of morphologic parameters in renal cell carcinoma. Am J Surg Pathol. 1982;6:655–63.
8. Oken MM, Creech RH, Tormey DC, et al. Toxicity and response criteria of the Eastern Cooperative Oncology Group. Am J Clin Oncol. 1982;5:649–55.
9. Eble JN, World Health Organization. Pathology and genetics of tumours of the urinary system and male genital organs. Lyon, Oxford: IARC Press & Oxford University Press; 2004.
10. Cheville JC, Lohse CM, Zincke H, Weaver AL, Blute ML. Comparisons of outcome and prognostic features among histologic subtypes of renal cell carcinoma. Am J Surg Pathol. 2003;27: 612–24.
11. Patard JJ, Leray E, Rioux-Leclercq N, et al. Prognostic value of histologic subtypes in renal cell carcinoma: a multicenter experience. J Clin Oncol. 2005;23:2763–71.

Renal Carcinoma Surveillance Counterpoint: Japan

75

Masatoshi Eto, Wataru Takahashi, Yoshiaki Kawano, Jiro Honda, Juro Nakanishi, and Yoshihiro Wada

Keywords
Renal cell carcinoma • Surgery • Immunotherapy • Standard of care • VEGF

Huang et al. provide an excellent summary of contemporary renal cell carcinoma management, including the epidemiology, diagnosis, surgical treatment, systemic therapy, and strategies for follow-up [1]. We present our opinion, which slightly differs from that of Huang et al., based on recent reports and our experience at Kumamoto University, Japan.

Although Russo reported modification of the surgical treatment for small renal cell carcinoma detected incidentally, the trend toward partial nephrectomy for small renal cell carcinoma is well established, based on recent reports [1, 2]. In our institute, the first option of surgical treatment for T1a (<4 cm) renal cell carcinoma is now open or laparoscopic partial nephrectomy.

Metastatic renal cell carcinoma is currently one of the most treatment-resistant malignancies. Cytotoxic chemotherapy is reported to have little antitumor activity [3]. Although immunotherapy with interferon-alpha (IFN-α) or interleukin-2 (IL-2) is generally considered the standard of care, only a limited subset of patients obtain clinically meaningful benefit [4]. A growing understanding of the underlying biology has identified vascular endothelial growth factor (VEGF) as a logical therapeutic target. Therapy directed against VEGF has undergone clinical trials in metastatic renal cell carcinoma, with evidence of a substantial antitumor effect. Two multikinase inhibitors, sorafenib and sunitinib, were approved by the US Food and Drug Administration (FDA) for metastatic renal cell carcinoma [5, 6]. In addition, temsirolimus, an inhibitor of the mammalian target of rapamycin (mTOR), improves overall survival rates in such patients [7] and is also approved by the FDA.

The surveillance of patients after initial surgery should emphasize early detection of treatable recurrence and should be cost-effective. We have, therefore, modified our surveillance, as reported in AUA update series 2004 [8]. We have adopted two schedules, one for T1 disease and the other for T2–T4 disease. For T1 patients who have had radical or partial nephrectomy, we use the follow-up schedule shown in Table 75.1. Basically, we perform annual follow-up with simultaneous chest and abdominal CT for T1 patients. In Japan, high speed CT is now available in many institutes and, at annual follow-up, we recommend simultaneous chest and abdominal CT, instead of chest X-ray and abdominal CT, in order not to miss small lung nodules. Surveillance for patients with T2 and T3 disease who have undergone radical nephrectomy or those with T4 disease who have had complete resection of metastases (simultaneously with or subsequent to radical nephrectomy) is summarized in Table 75.2. This relies heavily on chest and abdominal CT for those patients.

M. Eto, M.D., Ph.D. (✉) • W. Takahashi • Y. Kawano • J. Honda • J. Nakanishi • Y. Wada
Department of Urology, Kumamoto University, 1-1-1, Honjo, Kumamoto-city, Kumamoto, 860-8556, Japan
e-mail: etom@kumamoto-u.ac.jp; tkhshwtr@kumamoto-u.ac.jp; yoshiaki.kawano@gmail.com; honjiro@fc.kuh.kumamoto-u.ac.jp; juronakanishi@fc.kuh.kumamoto-u.ac.jp; yoshiwad@kumamoto-u.ac.jp

F.E. Johnson et al. (eds.), *Patient Surveillance After Cancer Treatment*, Current Clinical Oncology,
DOI 10.1007/978-1-60327-969-7_75, © Springer Science+Business Media New York 2013

Table 75.1 Surveillance after radical or partial nephrectomy for stage T1 renal cell carcinoma

	Year					
Modality	1	2	3	4	5	>5
Office visit	1	1	1	1	1	1
Laboratory tests[a]	1	1	1	1	1	1
Urinalysis	1	1	1	1	1	1
CT of chest and abdomen	1	1	1	1	1	[b]

Table 75.1 is a modification of Appendix 1 of ref. [8]
The number in each cell indicates the number of times a particular modality is recommended in a particular posttreatment year
[a]Comprehensive metabolic panel, complete blood count, urinalysis
[b]Every other year

Table 75.2 Surveillance after radical nephrectomy for T2–4 renal cell carcinoma

	Year					
Modality	1	2	3	4	5	>5
Office visit	2–4	2	2	2	2	1
Laboratory tests[a]	2–4	2	2	2	2	1
Urinalysis	2–4	2	2	2	2	1
CT of chest and abdomen	2–4	2	2	2	2	1

Table 75.2 is a modification of Appendix 2 of ref. [8]
The number in each cell indicates the number of times a particular modality is recommended in a particular posttreatment year
[a]Blood tests: electrolyte panel, liver function tests, complete blood count

References

1. Huang WC, Elkin EB, Levey AS, Jang TL, Russo P. Partial nephrectomy versus radical nephrectomy in patients with small renal tumors-is there a difference in mortality and cardiovascular outcomes? J Urol. 2009;181:55–61.
2. Go AS, Chertow GM, Fan D, McCulloch CE, Hsu CY. Chronic kidney disease and the risks of death, cardiovascular events, and hospitalization. N Engl J Med. 2004;351:1296–305.
3. Motzer RJ, Russo P. Systemic therapy for renal cell carcinoma. J Urol. 2000;163:408–17.
4. Bukowski RM. Cytokine therapy for metastatic renal cell carcinoma. Semin Urol Oncol. 2001;19:148–54.
5. Escudier B, Eisen T, Stadler WM, et al. TARGET Study Group. Sorafenib in advanced clear-cell renal-cell carcinoma. N Engl J Med. 2007;356:125–34.
6. Motzer RJ, Hutson TE, Tomczak P, et al. Sunitinib versus interferon alfa in metastatic renal-cell carcinoma. N Engl J Med. 2007;356:115–24.
7. Hudes G, Carducci M, Tomczak P, et al. Global ARCC trial. N Engl J Med. 2007;356:2271–81.
8. Theodorescu D, Rabbani F, Donat SM. Follow-up genitourinary malignancies for the office urologist: a practical approach. Part 2: kidney cancer and germ cell cancer of the testis. AUA Update Series. 2004;23:309–315.

Renal Carcinoma Surveillance Counterpoint: Canada

76

Michael Leveridge, Robert Abouassaly, and Michael A.S. Jewett

Keywords
Kidney • RCC • Urothelial cancers • Protocols • Recurrence

Wadhwa and Johnson have provided an overview of the diagnosis and staging of renal cancers, and have detailed the risk factors for recurrence. These prognostic factors are used to determine optimal follow-up protocols. We present the rationale and surveillance protocol currently used at the Princess Margaret Hospital in Toronto, Canada, and recommended for Canadian urologists.

The Canadian Cancer Society and the National Cancer Institute of Canada indicate that about 4,800 new cases of kidney cancer occur annually in Canada, with about 1,650 deaths due to this cause [1]. The American Cancer Society estimates that over 58,000 new cases and over 13,000 deaths occur each year in the United States [2]. Reporting of kidney cancer includes urothelial cancers of the collecting system in addition to parenchymal renal cell carcinoma (RCC). We confine our discussion to RCC.

About 75% of new kidney cancers present as early or locally advanced tumors that can be treated by surgery with radical or partial nephrectomy. This is the standard of care for RCC. Despite complete excision with negative surgical margins, there remains a risk of recurrence, both locally and at distant sites, which carries a poor prognosis [3]. Early detection may reduce the burden of treatment and ultimate outcome but this is unproven with RCC. There are numerous studies of tumor and host characteristics that may influence recurrence. Of these, pathologic tumor stage has been the most reliable predictor of recurrence risk, including time to and location of recurrence. Other relevant variables include tumor grade, histologic subtype, necrosis, microvascular invasion, patient performance status, and molecular and genomic factors [4–7].

These correlative studies have been used to develop risk nomograms and surveillance protocols [7–12]. Signs, symptoms, and performance status can be gleaned from the history and physical examination; serological tests can assess renal function and provide information about bone health via alkaline phosphatase (ALP). Radiologic examination of the chest and abdominal imaging are recommended at regular intervals, according to risk, and other tests are indicated only for symptomatic patients.

The Canadian Urological Association (CUA) recently approved guidelines dealing with surveillance for patients following radical or partial nephrectomy for RCC [8]. The first and second Canadian Kidney Cancer Forums developed a consensus document for the treatment and follow-up of RCC patients that endorsed the CUA Guideline [13, 14]. The CUA protocol is stage-based and acknowledges the merit of protocols based on other patient and tumor characteristics (and also the lack of prospective validation). The protocol is presented in Table 76.1, 76.2, and 76.3 for pathologic stages T1, T2, and TxN+, respectively. It is recommended that patients with partial nephrectomy be followed similarly to pT1 patients after radical nephrectomy, though a CT of the abdomen to assess the operative site at 3 months could be considered. Beyond 6 years, CT of the abdomen is

M. Leveridge, M.D.
University of Toronto, Toronto, ON, Canada

Department of Urology, Queen's University, Kingston, ON, Canada

R. Abouassaly, M.D.
University of Toronto, Toronto, ON, Canada

Division of Urology, Department of Surgical Oncology, Princess Margaret Hospital and the University Health Network, University of Toronto, Toronto, ON, Canada

M.A.S. Jewett, M.D. (✉)
Division of Urology, University of Toronto, 610 University Avenue, 3-124, Toronto, ON, Canada M5G 2C4
e-mail: m.jewett@utoronto.ca

F.E. Johnson et al. (eds.), *Patient Surveillance After Cancer Treatment*, Current Clinical Oncology, DOI 10.1007/978-1-60327-969-7_76,

Table 76.1 Surveillance after curative-intent treatment for patients following radical or partial nephrectomy for renal cell carcinoma (pathologic stage pT1) at University of Toronto

	Year					
Modality	1	2	3	4	5	>5
Office visit	1	1	1	1	1	1
Blood tests	1	1	1	1	1	1
CXR or CT chest	1	1	1	1	1	1
CT or U/S abdomen	0	1	0	0	1	0

Blood tests = complete blood count, serum chemistry panel, liver function tests
U/S = ultrasound examination
The number in each cell indicates the number of times a particular modality is recommended during a particular posttreatment year

Table 76.2 Surveillance after curative-intent treatment for patients following radical or partial nephrectomy for renal cell carcinoma (pathologic stage pT2) at University of Toronto

	Year					
Modality	1	2	3	4	5	>5
Office visit	2	2	2	1	1	1
Blood tests	2	2	2	1	1	1
CXR or CT chest	2	2	2	1	1	1
CT or U/S abdomen	1	0	1	0	1	0

Blood tests = complete blood count, serum chemistry panel, liver function tests
CXR = can be alternated with chest CT
U/S = ultrasound examination
The number in each cell indicates the number of times a particular modality is recommended during a particular posttreatment year

Table 76.3 Surveillance after curative-intent treatment for patients following radical or partial nephrectomy for renal cell carcinoma (pathologic stage pT3/pTxNx) at University of Toronto

	Year					
Modality	1	2	3	4	5	6
Office visit	2[a]	2	2	1	1	1
Blood tests	2[a]	2	2	1	1	1
CXR or CT chest	2[a]	2	2	1	1	1
CT	2[a]	2	1[b]	0[c]	1	0[c]

Blood tests = complete blood count, serum chemistry panel, liver function tests
CXR = can be alternated with chest CT
CT abdomen = can be alternated with U/S in pT1-2N0
The number in each cell indicates the number of times a particular modality is recommended during a particular posttreatment year
[a]3 times/year for N+
[b]2 times/year for N+
[c]1 time/year for N+

recommended at 7 and 9 years postoperatively for pT2 disease, every 2 years for pT3 disease and yearly for patients with node-positive disease. History, physical examination, blood work, and chest X-ray are recommended yearly beyond 6 years in all patients [8].

It is noteworthy that these protocols are not used after cancer recurrence. We are aware of no specific protocol for following patients in the setting of salvage treatment for metastatic disease. This applies to the surveillance of known small-volume metastases, follow-up after metastasectomy (as long-term survival has been noted after resection of small-volume pulmonary or hepatic metastases) [15], or surveillance during systemic treatment with targeted or biological agents. It is also noteworthy that there are no proven effective adjuvant therapies to prevent or delay recurrence in patients with high-risk disease at this time. Trials are underway to assess newer biologic agents in the adjuvant setting. The results of these trials may alter the natural history of the disease after curative-intent initial treatment and, thus, the surveillance protocols.

Given the high mortality rate associated with the diagnosis of metastatic disease, clinical trials continue in the efforts to uncover more effective prevention and treatment options. Trials have protocols for patient surveillance, and these may not be based on the same variables as described above. If available, patients should be encouraged to enroll in clinical trials and the surveillance procedures that they recommend.

Acknowledgements The authors gratefully acknowledge the work of the Canadian Urology Association in creating guidelines for surveillance of patients treated surgically for clinically localized renal cell carcinoma, and in particular the lead author, Dr. Wassim Kassouf.

References

1. Canadian Cancer Society/National Cancer Institute of Canada. Canadian Cancer Statistics 2010. Toronto, Canada; 2010.
2. American Cancer Society. Cancer facts and figures 2010. Atlanta; 2010.
3. Motzer RJ, Mazumdar M, Bacik J, Berg W, Amsterdam A, Ferrara J. Survival and prognostic stratification of 670 patients with advanced renal cell carcinoma. J Clin Oncol. 1999;17:2530–40.
4. Sorbellini M, Kattan MW, Snyder ME, et al. A postoperative prognostic nomogram predicting recurrence for patients with conventional clear cell renal cell carcinoma. J Urol. 2005;173:48–51.
5. Kattan MW, Reuter V, Motzer RJ, Katz J, Russo P. A postoperative prognostic nomogram for renal cell carcinoma. J Urol. 2001;166: 63–7.
6. Frank I, Blute ML, Cheville JC, Lohse CM, Weaver AL, Zincke H. An outcome prediction model for patients with clear cell renal cell carcinoma treated with radical nephrectomy based on tumor stage, size, grade and necrosis: the SSIGN score. J Urol. 2002;168: 2395–400.
7. Zisman A, Pantuck AJ, Wieder J, et al. Risk group assessment and clinical outcome algorithm to predict the natural history of patients with surgically resected renal cell carcinoma. J Clin Oncol. 2002;20:4559–66.
8. Kassouf W, Siemens R, Morash C, et al. Follow-up guidelines after radical or partial nephrectomy for localized and locally advanced renal cell carcinoma. Can Urol Assoc J. 2009;3:73–6.
9. Levy DA, Slaton JW, Swanson DA, Dinney CP. Stage specific guidelines for surveillance after radical nephrectomy for local renal cell carcinoma. J Urol. 1998;159:1163–7.
10. Ljungberg B, Alamdari FI, Rasmuson T, Roos G. Follow-up guidelines for nonmetastatic renal cell carcinoma based on the

occurrence of metastases after radical nephrectomy. BJU Int. 1999;84:405–11.
11. Skolarikos A, Alivizatos G, Laguna P, de la Rosette J. A review on follow-up strategies for renal cell carcinoma after nephrectomy. Eur Urol. 2007;51:1490–500. discussion 1501.
12. Stephenson AJ, Chetner MP, Rourke K, et al. Guidelines for the surveillance of localized renal cell carcinoma based on the patterns of relapse after nephrectomy. J Urol. 2004;172:58–62.
13. Canadian Kidney Cancer Forum 2008. Management of kidney cancer: Canadian Kidney Cancer Forum Consensus Statement. Can Urol Assoc J. 2008;2:175–82.
14. Canadian Kidney Cancer Forum 2009. Management of kidney cancer: Canadian Kidney Cancer Forum Consensus Statement. Can Urol Assoc J. 2009;3:200–4.
15. Kavolius JP, Mastorakos DP, Pavlovich C, Russo P, Burt ME, Brady MS. Resection of metastatic renal cell carcinoma. J Clin Oncol. 1998;16:2261–6.

Urinary Bladder Carcinoma

77

David Y. Johnson, Shilpi Wadhwa, and Frank E. Johnson

Keywords
Bladder cancer • Bladder • Age • Tobacco • Risk factors

The International Agency for Research on Cancer (IARC), a component of the World Health Organization (WHO), estimated that there were 356,557 new cases of bladder carcinoma worldwide in 2002 [1]. The IARC also estimated that there were 145,009 deaths due to this cause in 2002 [1].

The American Cancer Society estimated that there were 67,160 cases and 13,750 deaths due to this cause in the USA in 2007 [2]. The estimated 5-year survival rate (all races) in the USA in 2007 was 82% for bladder cancer [2]. Survival rates were adjusted for normal life expectancies and were based on cases diagnosed from 1996 to 2002 and followed through 2003.

Bladder cancer is more common in whites than in blacks and more common in men than in women. The incidence rises markedly with advancing age. Tobacco smoking is an important cause, as is exposure to various chemicals such as aniline dyes and cyclophosphamide. Chronic irritation from indwelling bladder catheters, infection with Schistosoma haematobium, and pelvic radiation increases the risk of bladder cancer. Occupations involving aniline dyes and other carcinogens are also hazardous [3, 4].

D.Y. Johnson • S. Wadhwa
Department of Internal Medicine, Saint Louis University Medical Center, Saint Louis, MO, USA

F.E. Johnson, M.D., F.A.C.S. (✉)
Saint Louis University Medical Center and Saint Louis Veterans Affairs Medical Center, Saint Louis, MO, USA
e-mail: frank.johnson1@va.gov

Geographic Variation Worldwide

The highest incidence of bladder cancer among men is seen in southern Europe, followed by western and northern Europe, North America, and Oceania. There is a relatively low incidence in Eastern Europe, Central America, South America, and several areas in Asia. Among women, the highest incidence is seen in North America, Oceania, and Asia. Male-to-female incidence ratios generally range between three and five, but they are less than three in India, Thailand, and blacks in the USA; and ratio exceeds six in many areas of southern Europe [1, 3]. Geographic variation in the USA is also pronounced [5].

Surveillance Strategies Proposed by Professional Organizations or National Government Agencies and Available on the Internet

National Comprehensive Cancer Network (www.nccn.org)

National Comprehensive Cancer Network (NCCN) guidelines were accessed on January 28, 2012 (Tables 77.1, 77.2, 77.3, 77.4, 77.5, and 77.6). There were major quantitative and qualitative changes compared to the guidelines accessed on April 10, 2007.

F.E. Johnson et al. (eds.), *Patient Surveillance After Cancer Treatment*, Current Clinical Oncology,
DOI 10.1007/978-1-60327-969-7_77,

Table 77.1 Obtained from NCCN (www.nccn.org) on January 28, 2012

	Years posttreatment[a]					
	1	2	3	4	5	>5
Office visit[b,c]	4	4	4	4	4	4
Cystoscopy[c]	4	4	4	4	4	4

Bladder cancer, cTa, low grade
NCCN guidelines were accessed on January 28, 2012. There were major quantitative changes compared to the guidelines accessed on April 10, 2007
[a]The numbers in the table indicate the number of times the modality is recommended during the indicated year posttreatment
[b]Cystoscopy was the only quantitative recommendation given. We inferred that office visit would be recommended as frequently as this
[c]Increasing interval as appropriate

Table 77.2 Obtained from NCCN (www.nccn.org) on January 28, 2012

	Years posttreatment[a]					
	1	2	3	4	5	>5
Office visit[b,c]	2–4	2–4	2–4	2–4	2–4	2–4
Cystoscopy[c]	2–4	2–4	2–4	2–4	2–4	2–4
Urine cytology[c]	2–4	2–4	2–4	2–4	2–4	2–4

- Consider imaging of upper tract collecting system every 1–2 years for high-grade tumors
- Urinary urothelial tumor markers optional

Bladder cancer, cTa, high grade; cT1 low or high grade; any Tis
NCCN guidelines were accessed on January 28, 2012. There were major quantitative and qualitative changes compared to the guidelines accessed on April 10, 2007
[a]The numbers in the table indicate the number of times the modality is recommended during the indicated year posttreatment
[b]Cystoscopy and urine cytology were the only quantitative recommendations given. We inferred that office visit would be recommended as frequently as these
[c]Increasing interval as appropriate

American Society of Clinical Oncology (www.asco.org)

American Society of Clinical Oncology (ASCO) guidelines were accessed on January 28, 2012. No quantitative guidelines exist for bladder cancer surveillance, including when first accessed on October 31, 2007.

The Society of Surgical Oncology (www.surgonc.org)

Society of Surgical Oncology (SSO) guidelines were accessed on January 28, 2012. No quantitative guidelines exist for bladder cancer surveillance, including when first accessed on October 31, 2007.

European Society for Medical Oncology (www.esmo.org)

European Society for Medical Oncology (ESMO) guidelines were accessed on January 28, 2012 (Tables 77.7 and 77.8). There were minor qualitative changes compared to the guidelines accessed on October 31, 2007.

European Society of Surgical Oncology (www.esso-surgeonline.org)

European Society of Surgical Oncology (ESSO) guidelines were accessed on January 28, 2012. No quantitative guide-

Table 77.3 Obtained from NCCN (www.nccn.org) on January 28, 2012

	Years posttreatment[a]					
	1	2	3	4	5	>5
Office visit[b]	2–4	2–4	<4	<4	<4	<4
Liver function tests, creatinine, electrolytes[c]	1–2	1–2	1–2	1–2	1–2	1–2
Imaging of upper tracts, abdomen, and pelvis[d]	2–4	2–4	0	0	0	0
Cystoscopy + urine cytology ± selected mapping biopsy[e,f]	2–4	2–4	<4	<4	<4	<4

- If cystectomy, see follow-up after cystectomy (Tables 77.4 and 77.5)

Bladder cancer, muscle invasive and selected metastatic disease treated with curative intent
NCCN guidelines were accessed on January 28, 2012. There were major quantitative and qualitative changes compared to the guidelines accessed on April 10, 2007
[a]The numbers in the table indicate the number of times the modality is recommended during the indicated year posttreatment
[b]There were no explicit quantitative recommendations for office visit. Cystoscopy with urine cytology and selected mapping biopsy were the most frequent quantitative recommendations given. We inferred that office visit would be recommended as frequently as these
[c]Depending on risk of recurrence
[d]As clinically indicated after 2 years
[e]If bladder preservation
[f]Every 3–6 months for 2 years, then increasing intervals

Table 77.4 Obtained from NCCN (www.nccn.org) on January 28, 2012

	Years posttreatment[a]					
	1	2	3	4	5	>5
Office visit[b]	2–4	2–4	1–2	1–2	1–2	1–2
Urine cytology, creatinine, electrolytes[c]	2–4	2–4	0	0	0	0
Imaging of chest, abdomen, and pelvis[d]	1–4	1–4	0	0	0	0
Urethral wash cytology[e]	1–2	1–2	1–2	1–2	1–2	1–2
Vitamin B12[f]	1	1	1	1	1	1

Bladder cancer with radical cystectomy

NCCN guidelines were accessed on January 28, 2012. There were major quantitative and qualitative changes compared to the guidelines accessed on April 10, 2007

[a]The numbers in the table indicate the number of times the modality is recommended during the indicated year posttreatment

[b]There were no explicit quantitative recommendations for office visit. Urine cytology, creatinine, electrolytes, and urethral wash with cytology were the most frequent quantitative recommendations given. We inferred that office visit would be recommended as frequently as these

[c]As clinically indicated after 2 years

[d]Based on risk of recurrence and then as clinically indicated after 2 years

[e]Particularly if Tis was found within the bladder or prostatic urethra

[f]If a continent diversion was created

Table 77.5 Obtained from NCCN (www.nccn.org) on January 28, 2012

	Years posttreatment[a]					
	1	2	3	4	5	>5
Office visit[b,c]	2–4	2–4	<4	<4	<4	<4
Urine cytology, creatinine, electrolytes[d]	2–4	2–4	0	0	0	0
Imaging of chest, abdomen, and pelvis[e]	1–4	1–4	0	0	0	0
Urethral wash cytology[f]	1–2	1–2	1–2	1–2	1–2	1–2
Vitamin B12[g]	1	1	1	1	1	1
Cystoscopy + urine cytology ± selected mapping biopsy[h,h]	2–4	2–4	<4	<4	<4	<4

Bladder cancer with segmental (partial) cystectomy or bladder preservation

NCCN guidelines were accessed on January 28, 2012. There were major quantitative and qualitative changes compared to the guidelines accessed on April 10, 2007

[a]The numbers in the table indicate the number of times the modality is recommended during the indicated year posttreatment

[b]There were no explicit quantitative recommendations for office visit. Urine cytology, creatinine, electrolytes, and cystoscopy with selected mapping biopsy were the most frequent quantitative recommendations given. We inferred that office visit would be recommended as frequently as these

[c]Increasing intervals after 2 years

[d]As clinically indicated after 2 years

[e]Based on risk of recurrence and then as clinically indicated after 2 years

[f]Particularly if Tis was found within the bladder or prostatic urethra

[g]If a continent diversion was created

[h]If bladder preservation

Table 77.6 Obtained from NCCN (www.nccn.org) on January 28, 2012

	Years posttreatment[a]					
	1	2	3	4	5	>5
Office visit[b,c]	4	<4	<4	<4	<4	<4
Cystoscopy[c]	4	<4	<4	<4	<4	<4
Imaging of upper tract collecting system[d,e]	1–4	1–4	1–4	1–4	1–4	1–4

Bladder cancer: upper GU tract tumors

NCCN guidelines were accessed on January 28, 2012. These are new quantitative guidelines compared to the guidelines accessed on April 10, 2007

[a]The numbers in the table indicate the number of times the modality is recommended during the indicated year posttreatment

[b]There were no explicit quantitative recommendations for office visit. Cystoscopy was the most frequent quantitative recommendation given. We inferred that office visit would be recommended as frequently as this

[c]Every 3 months for 1 year, then at increasing intervals

[d]For pT0, pT1, if endoscopic resection

[e]May include one or more of the following: IVP, CT urography, retrograde pyelogram, ureteroscopy, or MRI urogram; ±CT scan or MRI ± chest X-ray

Table 77.7 Obtained from ESMO (www.esmo.org) on January 28, 2012

	Years posttreatment[a]					
	1	2	3	4	5	>5
Office visit[b]	4	4	2	2	2	2
Cystoscopy	4	4	2	2	2	2
Urinary cytology	4	4	2	2	2	2

Bladder cancer with bladder-preservation strategy

ESMO guidelines were accessed on January 28, 2012. There were minor qualitative changes compared to the guidelines accessed on October 31, 2007

[a]The numbers in the table indicate the number of times the modality is recommended during the indicated year posttreatment

[b]Cystoscopy and urinary cytology were the only quantitative recommendations given. We inferred that office visit would be recommended as frequently as these

Table 77.8 Obtained from ESMO (www.esmo.org) on January 28, 2012

	Years posttreatment[a]					
	1	2	3	4	5	>5
Office visit[b]	4	4	2	2	2	0
Cystoscopy	4	4	2	2	2	0
Urinary cytology	4	4	2	2	2	0

Bladder cancer with cystectomy

ESMO guidelines were accessed on January 28, 2012. There were minor qualitative changes compared to the guidelines accessed on October 31, 2007

[a]The numbers in the table indicate the number of times the modality is recommended during the indicated year posttreatment

[b]Cystoscopy and urinary cytology were the only quantitative recommendations given. We inferred that office visit would be recommended as frequently as these

lines exist for bladder cancer surveillance, including when first accessed on October 31, 2007.

Cancer Care Ontario (www.cancercare.on.ca)

Cancer Care Ontario (CCO) guidelines were accessed on January 28, 2012. No quantitative guidelines exist for bladder cancer surveillance, including when first accessed on October 31, 2007.

National Institute for Clinical Excellence (www.nice.org.uk)

National Institute for Clinical Excellence (NICE) guidelines were accessed on January 28, 2012. No quantitative guidelines exist for bladder cancer surveillance, including when first accessed on October 31, 2007.

The Cochrane Collaboration (www.cochrane.org)

Cochrane Collaboration (CC) guidelines were accessed on January 28, 2012. No quantitative guidelines exist for bladder cancer surveillance, including when first accessed on November 24, 2007.

American Urological Association (www.auanet.org)

American Urological Association (AUA) guidelines were accessed on January 28, 2012. No quantitative guidelines exist for bladder cancer surveillance, including when first accessed on December 13, 2007.

The M.D. Anderson Surgical Oncology Handbook also has follow-up guidelines, proposed by authors from a single National Cancer Institute-designated Comprehensive Cancer Center, for many types of cancer [6]. Some are detailed and quantitative, others are qualitative.

Summary

This is a common cancer with significant variability in incidence worldwide. We found consensus-based guidelines but none based on high-quality evidence.

References

1. Parkin DM, Whelan SL, Ferlay J, Teppo L, Thomas DB. Cancer incidence in five continents, vol. VIII, International Agency for Research on Cancer. Lyon, France: IARC Press; 2002. IARC Scientific Publication 155. ISBN 92-832-2155-9.
2. Jemal A, Seigel R, Ward E, Murray T, Xu J, Thun MJ. Cancer statistics, 2007. CA Cancer J Clin. 2007;57:43–66.
3. Schottenfeld D, Fraumeni JG. Cancer epidemiology and prevention. 3rd ed. New York, NY: Oxford University Press; 2006. ISBN 13:978-0-19-514961-6.
4. DeVita VT, Hellman S, Rosenberg SA. Cancer. 7th ed. Philadelphia, PA: Lippincott Williams & Wilkins; 2005. ISBN 0-781-74450-4.
5. Devesa SS, Grauman DJ, Blot WJ, Pennello GA, Hoover RN, Fraumeni JF Jr. Atlas of Cancer Mortality in the United States. National Institutes of Health, National Cancer Institute. NIH Publication No. 99–4564, September 1999.
6. Feig BW, Berger DH, Fuhrman GM. The M.D. Anderson Surgical Oncology Handbook. 4th ed. Philadelphia, PA: Lippincott Williams & Wilkins; 2006. paperback. ISBN 0-7817-5643-X.

Urinary Bladder Carcinoma Surveillance Counterpoint: Japan

78

Kentaro Kuroiwa

Herr presents an excellent overview of follow-up strategy for patients with bladder cancer, including non-muscle- and muscle-invasive cancer. We should take account of balance between tumor progression and cost-benefit for follow-up of bladder cancer. The surveillance schedules followed by urologists at Graduate School of Medical Sciences Kyushu University are shown in the tables.

We agree almost entirely with the recommendations by Herr regarding non-muscle-invasive bladder tumor. Based on our finding that the hazard of tumor recurrence in the first 3 years after transurethral resection (TUR) is twice as high as that during years 4–5, the number of cystoscopies and urine cytologies is decreased after 3 years at our institute [1]. We perform cystoscopy and urine cytology once a year after 5 years and cystoscopy is omitted for regular examination after 10 years. For upper urinary tract tumor progression, we recommend annual CT urography up to 10 years after TUR of a bladder tumor. We have abandoned intravenous pyelography for detecting upper urinary tract tumors. Since pathological interpretation based on TUR specimens is thought to be inaccurate, especially for patients with high-grade T1 bladder cancer, we routinely perform restaging TUR for such patients 2–6 weeks after the initial TUR, as described by Herr et al. [2]. A restaging TUR can identify patients with non-muscle-invasive bladder cancer who are at high risk of early tumor progression.

Our follow-up schedule for invasive bladder cancer is almost as same as that described by Herr (Table 78.1). While deciding whether to use an ileal conduit or orthotopic neobladder for reconstruction after cystectomy, we carefully evaluate the characteristics of the resected bladder cancer as well as patient comorbidities and motivation for receiving an orthotopic neobladder. For male patients, if tumor cells are found in the prostatic urethra by transurethral biopsy, we avoid the neobladder option. We perform orthotopic neobladder only for patients with negative intraoperative pathological assessment of the urethral stump. For female patients, the orthotopic neobladder option is abandoned if the bladder neck is involved by tumor. We have not experienced urethral recurrence in 30 patients after the current criteria for orthotopic neobladder construction were introduced. Since prophylactic urethrectomy is performed for all patients with ileal conduit or ureterocutaneostomy in our institute, routine surveillance urethral washings are not necessary. CT urography for upper urinary tract recurrence is also important for patients with cystectomy. The 3-year risk of upper tract recurrence is about 4–6% [3].

K. Kuroiwa (✉)
Department of Urology, Graduate School of Medical Sciences, Kyushu University, 3-1-1 Maidashi, Higashi-ku, Fukuoka 812-8582, Japan
e-mail: tenyu@uro.med.kyushu-u.ac.jp

F.E. Johnson et al. (eds.), *Patient Surveillance After Cancer Treatment*, Current Clinical Oncology,
DOI 10.1007/978-1-60327-969-7_78,

Table 78.1 Surveillance after curative-intent cystectomy for invasive bladder cancer at Kyushu University Hospital, Japan

	Year				
	1	2	3	4	5
Office visit[a]	4	4	4	2	2
Blood tests[b]	2	2	2	1	1
Voided urine or ileal conduit cytology	4	4	4	2	2
Chest X-ray	2	2	1	1	1
Abdominal-pelvic computed tomography	2	2	1	1	1
Renal ultrasonography	2	2	1	1	1

The numbers in each cell indicate the number of times a particular modality is recommended during a particular posttreatment year

[a]We assess urinary, stomal, sexual function, and the presence of hematuria, fever, weight loss, and back pain at each visit. We include physical examination of the abdomen, stoma, and groin lymph nodes

[b]Consists of complete blood count, serum electrolyte levels, blood urea nitrogen, and serum creatinine levels

References

1. Koga H, Kuroiwa K, Yamaguchi A, Osada Y, Tsuneyoshi M, Naito S. A randomized controlled trial of short-term versus long-term prophylactic intravesical instillation chemotherapy for recurrence after transurethral resection of Ta/T1 transitional cell carcinoma of the bladder. J Urol. 2004;171:153–7.
2. Herr HW, Donat SM, Dalbagni G. Can restaging transurethral resection of T1 bladder cancer select patients for immediate cystectomy? J Urol. 2007;177:75–9.
3. Tran W, Serio AM, Raj GV, Dalbagni G, Vickers AJ, Bochner BH, Herr H, Donat SM. Longitudinal risk of upper tract recurrence following radical cystectomy for urothelial cancer and the potential implications for long-term surveillance. J Urol. 2008;179:96–100.

Urinary Bladder Carcinoma Surveillance Counterpoint: Canada

79

Faysal A. Yafi and Wassim Kassouf

Keywords
Bladder • Transurethral biopsy • NCCN • EAU • Tumors

Bladder cancer is the sixth most common cancer in Canada, accounting for 6,700 new cases per year and is the ninth most common cause of cancer death in Canada, with 1,800 deaths per year. It accounts for 5.8% of new cancer cases and 3.3% of deaths in males and 2.1% of new cases and 1.5% of deaths in females in Canada. One in 28 males and 1 in 84 females will be diagnosed during their lifetime with bladder cancer [1].

Histologically, bladder cancer is urothelial in origin in 90%, squamous cell carcinoma (SCC) in 5%, and adenocarcinoma in 2%. The World Health Organization (WHO) classifies bladder cancer as low-grade (grades 1 and 2) or high-grade (grade 3); 70% are papillary, 20% sessile, and 10% nodular. At time of diagnosis, 75% of these tumors are nonmuscle invasive (NMIBC, superficial), 20% muscle invasive, and 5% have metastasized.

The diagnosis of bladder cancer is typically made from a transurethral biopsy and classified according to WHO grade [2]. Clinical staging should be accomplished by cystoscopic examination, transurethral resection (TURBT), and bimanual examination under anesthesia (EUA). A complete history, physical examination, blood work comprising a CBC and creatinine level, and voided urinary cytology are part of the routine workup. If the tumor is invasive, chest imaging (X-ray or CT) and CT of the abdomen and pelvis are performed. Bone scan is ordered for any clinical or laboratory suspicion of metastasis to bone.

Based on the WHO grade and TNM staging, an appropriate management plan is laid out. Stage I tumors are defined as invading into the submucosa and are usually treated conservatively with a complete TURBT followed by careful surveillance. Intravesical therapy with BCG can be offered to intermediate or high-risk patients with NMIBC [3]. Nonresponders should be offered radical cystectomy due to the high progression rates (up to 45%) to muscle-invasive and/or metastatic bladder cancer [4]. For muscle-invasive tumors, radical cystectomy remains the standard of care [4–7]. Cisplatin-based neoadjuvant chemotherapy has been shown to improve survival in patients with cT2-T4 disease [8, 9], while adjuvant therapy can be offered to high-risk patients prone to recurrence (≥pT3 or pN+) [10–12]. Bladder-preservation protocols consisting of TUR ± neoadjuvant chemotherapy, radiotherapy, partial cystectomy or chemoradiation are further options which can be considered in select patients [13].

Most surveillance guidelines reported in the literature are consensus-based rather than evidence-based. The National Comprehensive Cancer Network (NCCN) offers comprehensive surveillance and follow-up algorithms for all stages and grades of bladder cancer [5]. The European Association of Urology (EAU) set up risk tables looking at tumor characteristics (number of tumors and their diameter), prior recurrence rate, stage, grade, and presence of concomitant carcinoma in situ (cis) in order to estimate recurrence and progression risks and adapt follow-up schedules accordingly [4]. The European Society for Medical Oncology also offers useful follow-up recommendations for invasive bladder cancer after radical cystectomy or bladder-preservation therapy [3]. The Canadian Urological Association (CUA) and American Urology Association (AUA), on the other hand, do not offer clear guidelines but state that "a risk-adapted approach should be considered" [6, 7].

Designing a surveillance strategy for a patient with a noninvasive tumor requires an understanding of the usual clini-

F.A. Yafi • W. Kassouf, M.D., F.R.C.S.(C) (✉)
Division of Urology, McGill University Health Center
1650 Cedar Avenue, Rm L8-315, Montreal, Canada, H3G 1A4
e-mail: wassim.kassouf@muhc.mcgill.ca

F.E. Johnson et al. (eds.), *Patient Surveillance After Cancer Treatment*, Current Clinical Oncology,
DOI 10.1007/978-1-60327-969-7_79, © Springer Science+Business Media New York 2013

Table 79.1 Surveillance after curative-intent transurethral resection for carcinoma of the bladder [stage Ta low-grade] at McGill University Health Center

	Years posttreatment[a]					
	1	2	3	4	5	>5
Cystoscopy + cytology	2	2	1	1	1	1

The numbers in each cell indicate the number of times a particular modality is recommended during a particular posttreatment year

[a]First cystoscopy at 3 months after initial resection

Table 79.2 Surveillance after curative-intent initial treatment for patients with stages T1 or Ta high-grade bladder carcinoma at McGill University Health Center

	Years posttreatment					
	1	2	3	4	5	>5
Cystoscopy + cytology[a]	4	4	2	2	1	1
Imaging of upper tract[b]	1	1	1	1	1	1

The numbers in each cell indicate the number of times a particular modality is recommended during a particular posttreatment year

[a]First cystoscopy at 3 months

[b]Intravenous pyelogram, CT, or ultrasound

cal course of bladder cancer. NMIBCs include a wide spectrum of disease ranging from low-risk (low-grade Ta confined to the mucosa) to high-risk (high-grade Ta, T1 confined to the submucosa, or concomitant cis) superficial disease. Overall, 50–70% of patients with Ta tumors will experience recurrence or develop a new cancer in the first five posttreatment years, with 5–20% developing progression of disease. The more aggressive high-grade Ta tumors tend to recur most often within 2–3 years, with progression to more advanced disease at the rate of 20% at 5 years and 30–40% at 10 years. This is similar to the behavior of T1 tumors which recur at rates of up to 50%, 80%, and 90% at 1 year, 3 years, and 5 years, respectively. If treated with TURBT alone, 50% of the T1 tumors progress to muscle invasion at 5 years [14]. The risk of progression is significantly increased in the presence of concomitant cis. The risk of developing upper urinary tract (ureters, renal pelvis) tumors is 2.4% for low-grade Ta; however, the incidence increases in the higher risk tumors to 15%, 25%, and 33% at 5 years, 10 years, and 15 years, respectively. Prostatic urethral recurrence is reported in 10–15% and 20–40% of high-risk tumors at 5 years and 10 years, respectively [14].

For low-grade solitary Ta tumors, the NCCN recommends an initial follow-up cystoscopy at 3 months followed by gradually longer intervals between repeat cystoscopies [5]. These intervals can then be further increased if there is no recurrence after 1 year. The EAU advocates cystoscopy at 6 months for tumors at low risk of recurrence; if it is negative, it should be repeated at 9 months, then annually for 5 years [4]. At the McGill University Health Center (MUHC), we follow a more or less similar protocol for all Ta low-grade tumors with flexible cystoscopy and urinary cytology at 3 months from transurethral resection, then every 6 months for the first 2 years, then yearly (Table 79.1). Any recurrence resets the schedule. We do not follow the upper tracts unless clinically indicated (flank pain, gross hematuria, abnormal urinary cytology, or multiple recurrences).

For Ta high-grade or T1 tumors, the NCCN recommends follow-up after transurethral resection with cystoscopy and urine cytology every 3 months for the first 2 years, then every 6 months for the next 2 years, then annually. Additional imaging of the upper urinary tract with an intravenous pyelogram (IVP), CT, or ultrasound (US) is performed yearly [5]. The EAU guidelines are similar: for tumors considered at high risk for recurrence, the EAU recommends cystoscopy initially at 3 months, then every 3 months for 2 years, every 4 months in the third year, every 6 months for years 4 and 5, and yearly thereafter [4]. At the MUHC, a schedule similar to the NCCN guidelines is followed. We favor BCG induction and maintenance for this patient population with a similar surveillance strategy as that provided by the NCCN (Table 79.2). For patients with compromised renal function, or age >80, we often recommend an ultrasound for upper tract surveillance in order to avoid the use of nephrotoxic iodine contrast agents. For large T1 high-grade, multifocal T1 high-grade, or T1 high-grade tumors with concomitant cis, selected patients may undergo upfront radical cystectomy.

Following radical cystectomy for muscle-invasive tumors, the main goals of follow-up are the detection of local recurrence, upper urinary tract recurrences, and metastasis, as well as complications from urinary diversion. The literature reports 5–15% local recurrence rates, mostly within the first 2 years following cystectomy (highest within 6–18 months from definitive therapy) and ~50% distant recurrence rate (highest within the first 24 months). These rates are greatly influenced by nodal status and tumor stage. Urethral recurrence, on the other hand, occurs in 5–17% of patients and increases to 21–64% if there is prostatic stromal invasion in males [15]. In females, the rates are 3–15% and depend on bladder neck involvement [16]. Of interest, the urethral recurrence rate is higher in those who undergo a cutaneous (4–8%) compared to orthotopic diversion (2–4%). Finally, upper tract recurrence is quite rare following cystectomy, with 2–4% risk, mostly between 2 and 4 years (median time, 3.3 years) [14, 17].

As such, following surgical intervention (radical cystectomy), the ESMO recommends office visits every 3 months in the first 2 years, then every 6 months for 5 years. They do not, however, offer any details of their follow-up tests [3]. The NCCN recommends urine cytology, liver function tests, creatinine, electrolytes, and chest radiograph (CXR) every 3–6 months for 2 years, then as clinically indicated. The NCCN also recommends Vitamin B12 levels routinely every

Table 79.3 Surveillance after curative-intent treatment for ≤pT2N0 bladder carcinoma (radical cystectomy) at McGill University Health Center

	Years posttreatment[a]					
	1	2	3	4	5	>5
Office visit	4	1	1	1	1	1
Lab studies	4	1	1	1	1	0
Chest X-ray	1	1	1	1	1	0
Triphasic CT abdomen/pelvis	1	1	1	1	1	0
Urine cytology[a]	1	1	1	1	1	0

Serum vitamin B-12 level when clinically indicated
The numbers in each cell indicate the number of times a particular modality is recommended during a particular posttreatment year
[a] Urine washings/cytology once a year is optional

year when a cutaneous diversion is performed and urethral washings every 6–12 months, especially when there is concomitant cis. Furthermore, the NCCN recommends postoperative imaging of the abdomen and pelvis by CT every 3–6 months for 2 years, then every 12 months [5]. Other groups, such as the one at Memorial Sloan-Kettering Cancer Center, advocate a closer follow-up, especially in the first 2 years, even though they acknowledge the lack of effective salvage treatment. The recommended follow-up consists of office visits, complete blood count, electrolytes, multichannel blood tests, liver function tests, and voided urine or ileal conduit cytology five times in the first year, three times in the second year and twice yearly thereafter, urethral washings four to five times in the first year, then three to four times per year for the two subsequent years and twice yearly thereafter, CT abdomen and pelvis three times in the first year, then twice in the second year, then once yearly subsequently, and CXR and upper tract imaging twice yearly for the first year, then annually [18]. The EAU offers only general recommendations such as more frequent follow-up for higher stage tumors, lifelong monitoring for kidney function, and stopping oncological surveillance at 5 years, if there is no recurrence, and replacing it with renal function surveillance [4].

Our follow-up strategy following radical cystectomy is stage-specific (Tables 79.3, 79.4, and 79.5). It consists of office visits with liver function tests, creatinine, CBC, and electrolytes every 3 months for 1 year, then every 6–12 months for another 4 years, depending on stage. Chest X-rays are recommended on a yearly basis for patients with organ-confined node-negative tumors (≤pT2N0), then every 6 months for the first 2 years, then annually for another 4 years for nonorgan-confined node-negative tumors (pT3–4N0). Chest X-rays are recommended every 4 months for the first year, then every 6 months for another 4 years in patients with node-positive tumors (pTxN+). Triphasic CT to assess upper tracts, abdomen, and pelvis is also done at varying intervals depending on the pathology. For patients with ≤pT2N0 tumors, we usually perform CT annually for 5 years. For patients with pT3–4N0 tumors, CT is performed every 6

Table 79.4 Surveillance after curative-intent treatment for pT3–4N0 bladder carcinoma (radical cystectomy) at McGill University Health Center

	Years posttreatment[a]					
	1	2	3	4	5	>5
Office visit	4	2	1	1	1	1
Lab studies	4	2	1	1	1	0
Chest X-ray	2	2	1	1	1	1
Triphasic CT abdomen/pelvis	2	1	1	1	1	a
Urine cytology[b]	1	1	1	1	1	0

Serum Vitamin B-12 level when clinically indicated
The numbers in each cell indicate the number of times a particular modality is recommended during a particular posttreatment year
[a] Triphasic CT abdomen/pelvis or abdominal ultrasound every second year beyond the 5-year follow-up
[b] Urine washings/cytology once a year is optional

Table 79.5 Surveillance after curative-intent treatment for pTx N+bladder carcinoma (radical cystectomy) at McGill University Health Center

	Years posttreatment[a]					
	1	2	3	4	5	>5
Office visit	4	2	2	2	2	1
Lab studies	4	2	2	2	2	0
Chest X-ray	3	2	2	2	2	1
Triphasic CT abdomen/pelvis	2	2	1	1	1	a
Urine cytology[b]	1	1	1	1	1	0

Serum vitamin B-12 level when clinically indicated
The numbers in each cell indicate the number of times a particular modality is recommended during a particular posttreatment year
[a] Triphasic CT abdomen/pelvis or abdominal ultrasound every second year beyond the 5-year follow-up
[b] Urine washings/cytology once a year is optional

months for 1 year, then annually for 4 years, and every second year thereafter. Finally, for those with pTxN+tumors, CT is performed every 6 months for the first 2 years, then annually for another 3 years, then every second year thereafter. If the patient is unable to receive contrast due to compromised renal function, an upper tract assessment is done annually via a loopogram. We do not routinely check vitamin B12 levels or perform urethral washings unless clinically indicated; however, we recommend urine cytology once a year in patients with a neobladder.

For patients treated with bladder-preservation therapies, closer surveillance is recommended. The ESMO recommends cystoscopy and urine cytology every 3 months for the first 2 years and then every 6 months thereafter [3]. The NCCN guidelines are more or less similar; they advocate cystoscopy ± biopsy and urine cytology every 3 months during the first year, then at gradually increasing intervals. Due to the elevated risk of recurrence within the urothelial tract or distant site, closer surveillance than the postcystectomy group is followed with this group [5]. Our strategy (Table 79.6) is similar to the ESMO recommendations,

Table 79.6 Surveillance for patients after curative-intent organ preservation therapy for bladder carcinoma at McGill University Health Center

	Years posttreatment					
	1	2	3	4	5	>5
Cystoscopy + cytology, ± biopsy	3	3	2	2	2	1
Office visit	3	3	2	2	2	0
Lab studies	3	3	2	2	2	0
Chest X-ray	3	2	2	2	2	1
Triphasic CT abdomen/pelvis	3	2	2	1	1	[a]
Urine cytology[a]	2	2	2	2	2	1

The numbers in each cell indicate the number of times a particular modality is recommended during a particular posttreatment year
[a]Triphasic CT abdomen/pelvis or abdominal ultrasound every second year beyond the 5-year follow-up

consisting of cystoscopy with cytology ± biopsy every 3–4 months for the first 2 years, then every 6 months for the next 3 years, then annually. Imaging of the upper tract, abdomen, and pelvis with triphasic CT is done every 4 months for 1 year, then every 6 months for 2 years, then annually for 2 years, then every second year thereafter.

It is important to note that, although we believe that identifying recurrence early will yield better outcomes (based on level 3 evidence), there are no studies that compare outcomes of patients with asymptomatic recurrences versus symptomatic recurrences and, as such, all recommended surveillance strategies are considered grade C.

References

1. Marrett LD, De P, Dryer D, Steering Committee of Canadian Cancer Statistics 2008. Cancer in Canada in 2008. CMAJ. 2008;179: 1163–70.
2. Epstein JI, Amin MB, Reuter VR, Mostofi FK. The World Health Organization/International Society of Urological Pathology consensus classification of urothelial (transitional cell) neoplasms of the urinary bladder. Bladder Consensus Conference Committee. Am J Surg Pathol. 1998;22:1435–48.
3. Bellmunt J, Albiol S, Kataja V. Invasive bladder cancer: ESMO clinical recommendations for diagnosis, treatment and follow-up. Ann Oncol. 2008;19:47–8.
4. http://www.uroweb.org
5. http://www.nccn.org
6. Kassouf W, Kamat AM, Zlotta A, et al. Canadian guidelines for treatment of non-muscle invasive bladder cancer: a focus on intravesical therapy. Can Urol Assoc J. 2010;4:168–73.
7. http://www.auanet.org
8. Hall R. Updated results of neoadjuvant cisplatin (C), methotrexate (M) and vinblastine (V) chemotherapy for muscle-invasive bladder cancer. Proc Annu Meet Am Soc Clin Oncol. 2002;21:178.
9. Grossman H, Natale R, Tangen C, et al. Neoadjuvant chemotherapy plus cystectomy compared with cystectomy alone for locally advanced bladder cancer. N Eng J Med. 2003;349:859–66.
10. Freiha F, Reese J, Torti FM. A randomized trial of radical cystectomy versus radical cystectomy plus cisplatin, vinblastine and methotrexate chemotherapy for muscle invasive bladder cancer. J Urol. 1996;155:495–9.
11. Stöckle M, Meyenburg W, Wellek S, et al. Advanced bladder cancer (stages pT3b, pT4a, pN1 and pN2): improved survival after radical cystectomy and 3 adjuvant cycles of chemotherapy. J Urol. 1992;148:302–7.
12. Skinner D, Daniels J, Russell C, et al. The role of adjuvant chemotherapy following cystectomy for invasive bladder cancer: a prospective comparative trial. J Urol. 1991;145:459–64.
13. Yafi FA, Steinberg J, Kassouf W. Contemporary management of muscle-invasive bladder cancer. Int J Clin Oncol. 2008;13:504–9.
14. Malkowicz SB, van Poppel H, Mickisch G, et al. Muscle-invasive urothelial carcinoma of the bladder. Urology. 2007;69:3–16.
15. Freeman JA, Tarter TA, Esrig D, et al. Urethral recurrence in patients with orthotopic ileal neobladders. J Urol. 1996;156: 1615–9.
16. Stenzl A, Draxl H, Posch B, Colleselli K, Falk M, Bartsch G. The risk of urethral tumors in female bladder cancer: can the urethra be used for orthotopic reconstruction in the lower urinary tract? J Urol. 1995;153:950–5.
17. Sanderson KM, Cai J, Miranda G, Skinner DG, Stein JP. Upper tract urothelial recurrence following radical cystectomy for transitional cell carcinoma of the bladder: an analysis of 1,069 patients with 10-year follow-up. J Urol. 2007;177:2088–94.
18. Johnson FE, Virgo KS. Cancer patient follow-up. 1st ed. St. Louis: Mosby; 1997. ISBN ISBN-10: 0815149255.

Prostate Carcinoma

80

David Y. Johnson, Shilpi Wadhwa, and Frank E. Johnson

Keywords
Prostate • Incidence • Age • Risk factors • Surveillance

The International Agency for Research on Cancer (IARC), a component of the World Health Organization (WHO), estimated that there were 679,023 new cases of prostate carcinoma worldwide in 2002 [1]. The IARC also estimated that there were 221,002 deaths due to this cause in 2002 [1].

The American Cancer Society estimated that there were 218,890 new cases and 27,050 deaths due to this cause in the USA in 2007 [2]. The estimated 5-year survival rate (all races) in the USA in 2007 was 100 % for prostate cancer [2]. Survival rates were adjusted for normal life expectancies and were based on cases diagnosed from 1996 to 2002 and followed through 2003.

Prostate cancer is rare before age 40. The incidence increases rapidly with advancing age. There is a marked geographic variation in incidence. The incidence in black men in the USA is 30-fold higher than in some areas in Japan and China. A high-fat diet is associated with increased risk of prostate cancer [3, 4].

Geographic Variation Worldwide

The reported incidence of prostate cancer is highest in Western Europe, Australia, New Zealand, North America, many South American countries, and African countries such as South Africa, Namibia, Gabon, Nigeria, Guinea-Bissau, and Cote d'Ivoire. The lowest incidence is observed in the Far East and the Indian subcontinent [3, 5]. The incidence of prostate cancer varies dramatically across the USA. The incidence is highest in the District of Columbia, New Jersey, Maryland, and Michigan and lowest in Alabama, Nevada, Tennessee, and Indiana [3, 6].

D.Y. Johnson • S. Wadhwa
Department of Internal Medicine, Saint Louis University Medical Center, Saint Louis, MO, USA

F.E. Johnson (✉)
Saint Louis University Medical Center and Saint Louis Veterans Affairs Medical Center, Saint Louis, MO, USA
e-mail: frank.johnson1@va.gov

Surveillance Strategies Proposed by Professional Organizations or National Government Agencies and Available on the Internet

National Comprehensive Cancer Network http://www.nccn.org

National Comprehensive Cancer Network (NCCN) guidelines were accessed on 1/28/12 (Table 80.1 and 80.2). There were no significant changes to previous quantitative guidelines as well as new quantitative guidelines compared to the guidelines accessed on 4/10/07.

American Society of Clinical Oncology http://www.asco.org

American Society of Clinical Oncology (ASCO) guidelines were accessed on 1/28/12. No quantitative guidelines exist for prostate cancer surveillance, including when first accessed on 10/31/07.

F.E. Johnson et al. (eds.), *Patient Surveillance After Cancer Treatment*, Current Clinical Oncology,
DOI 10.1007/978-1-60327-969-7_80,

Table 80.1 Obtained from NCCN (http://www.nccn.org) on 1/28/12. Prostate cancer with initial definitive therapy

	Years posttreatment[a]					
	1	2	3	4	5	>5
Office visit[b]	1–2	1–2	1–2	1–2	1–2	1
PSA	1–2	1–2	1–2	1–2	1–2	1
DRE	1	1	1	1	1	1

NCCN guidelines were accessed on 1/28/12. There were no significant changes compared to the guidelines accessed on 4/10/07

[a]The numbers in the table indicate the number of times the modality is recommended during the indicated year posttreatment

[b]There were no explicit quantitative recommendations for office visit. PSA and DRE were the only quantitative recommendation given. We inferred that office visit would be recommended as frequently as these

Table 80.2 Obtained from NCCN (http://www.nccn.org) on 1/28/12. Prostate Cancer, N1 or M1

	Years posttreatment[a]					
	1	2	3	4	5	>5
Office visit	2–4	2–4	2–4	2–4	2–4	2–4
PSA	2–4	2–4	2–4	2–4	2–4	2–4
DRE	2–4	2–4	2–4	2–4	2–4	2–4

NCCN guidelines were accessed on 1/28/12. These are new quantitative guidelines compared to the guidelines accessed on 4/10/07

[a]The numbers in the table indicate the number of times the modality is recommended during the indicated year posttreatment

The Society of Surgical Oncology http://www.surgonc.org

The Society of Surgical Oncology (SSO) guidelines were accessed on 1/28/12. No quantitative guidelines exist for prostate cancer surveillance, including when first accessed on 10/31/07.

European Society for Medical Oncology http://www.esmo.org

European Society for Medical Oncology (ESMO) guidelines were accessed on 1/28/12. No quantitative guidelines exist for prostate cancer surveillance, including when first accessed on 10/31/07.

European Society of Surgical Oncology http://www.esso-surgeonline.org

European Society of Surgical Oncology (ESSO) guidelines were accessed on 1/28/12. No quantitative guidelines exist for prostate cancer surveillance, including when first accessed on 10/31/07.

Table 80.3 Obtained from NICE (http://www.nice.org.uk) on 1/28/12. Localized Prostate Cancer with Radical Treatment

	Years posttreatment[a]					
	1	2	3	4	5	>5
Office visit	≥2	≥2	≥1	≥1	≥1	≥1
PSA[b]	≥2	≥2	≥1	≥1	≥1	≥1

- Men with prostate cancer should be clearly advised about potential longer term adverse effects and when and how to report them
- Routine digital rectal examination (DRE) is not recommended in men with prostate cancer while the PSA remains at baseline levels
- After at least 2 years, men with a stable PSA and who have had no significant treatment complications, should be offered follow-up at an outside hospital (for example, in primary care) by telephone or secure electronic communications, unless they are taking part in a clinical trial that requires more formal clinic-based follow-up

NICE guidelines were accessed on 1/28/12. These are new quantitative guidelines compared to the qualitative guidelines accessed on 10/31/07

[a]The numbers in the table indicate the number of times the modality is recommended during the indicated year posttreatment

[b]At the earliest, 6 weeks following treatment

Cancer Care Ontario http://www.cancercare.on.ca

Cancer Care Ontario (CCO) guidelines were accessed on 1/28/12. No quantitative guidelines exist for prostate cancer surveillance, including when first accessed on 10/31/07.

National Institute for Clinical Excellence http://www.nice.org.uk

National Institute for Clinical Excellence (NICE) guidelines were accessed on 1/28/12 (Table 80.3). These are new quantitative guidelines compared to the qualitative guidelines accessed on 10/31/07.

The Cochrane Collaboration http://www.cochrane.org

Cochrane Collaboration (CC) guidelines were accessed on 1/28/12. No quantitative guidelines exist for prostate cancer surveillance, including when first accessed on 11/24/07.

American Urological Association http://www.auanet.org

American Urological Association (AUA) guidelines were accessed on 1/28/12. No quantitative guidelines exist for prostate cancer surveillance, including when first accessed on 12/13/07.

The M.D. Anderson Surgical Oncology Handbook also has follow-up guidelines, proposed by authors from a single National Cancer Institute-designated Comprehensive Cancer Center, for many types of cancer [7]. Some are detailed and quantitative, others are qualitative.

Summary

This is a common cancer with significant variability in incidence worldwide. We found consensus-based guidelines but none based on high-quality evidence.

References

1. Parkin DM, Whelan SL, Ferlay J, Teppo L, Thomas DB. Cancer incidence in five continents. Volume VIII. International Agency for Research on Cancer, 2002. (IARC Scientific Publication 155). Lyon, France: IARC Press, ISBN 92-832-2155-9.
2. Jemal A, Seigel R, Ward E, Murray T, Xu J, Thun MJ. Cancer statistics, 2007. CA Cancer J Clin. 2007;57:43–66.
3. Schottenfeld D, Fraumeni JG. Cancer epidemiology and prevention. 3rd ed. New York, NY: Oxford University Press; 2006. ISBN 13:978-0-19-514961-6.
4. DeVita VT, Hellman S, Rosenberg SA. Cancer. 7th ed. Philadelphia, PA: Lippincott Williams & Wilkins; 2005. ISBN 0-781-74450-4.
5. Mackay J, Jemal A, Lee NC, Parkin M. The cancer Atlas. USA: American Cancer Society; 2006. Can also be accessed from 28 Jan, 2012. http://www.cancer.org. ISBN 0-944235-62-X.
6. Devesa SS, Grauman DJ, Blot WJ, Pennello GA, Hoover RN, Fraumeni JF Jr. Atlas of Cancer Mortality in the United States. National Institutes of Health, National Cancer Institute. NIH Publication No. 99–4564; 1999.
7. Feig BW, Berger DH, Fuhrman GM. The M.D. Anderson surgical oncology handbook. 4th ed. Philadelphia, PA: Lippincott Williams & Wilkins; 2006. paperback. ISBN 0-7817-5643-X.

Prostate Carcinoma Surveillance Counterpoint: USA

81

Angela Smith and Raj Pruthi

Keywords
Prostate • Tumor • Surveillance • Prostatectomy • Radical prostatectomy

Surveillance strategies following curative therapy for prostate cancer have been debated in the literature. Many institutions have developed their own algorithms. In this counterpoint, we discuss our experience at the University of North Carolina-Chapel Hill. Predictors of prostate cancer recurrence along with surveillance strategies are outlined for various treatment modalities, including radical prostatectomy, radiation therapy, ablative therapies, and active surveillance.

Surveillance After Radical Prostatectomy

The majority of men with prostate cancer recurrence after radical prostatectomy are identified through physician-specific surveillance protocols using serial serum prostate-specific antigen (PSA) measurements. However, the definition of biochemical recurrence is not straightforward. PSA failure is considered to range anywhere from 0.01 to 0.4 ng/mL [1, 2]. Amling et al. [1] performed a retrospect- tive review to identify the postoperative PSA threshold which ultimately leads to subsequent PSA failure and concluded that a PSA of 0.4 ng/mL should be the minimum value to define recurrence. The majority of institutions, including the University of North Carolina, consider a PSA level of 0.2 a reasonable threshold of possible biochemical recurrence. However, it is not this value alone that provides the best definition of biochemical recurrence, but rather the rise in PSA level over time. At the University of North Carolina, we recheck an initial post-procedure PSA after radical prostatectomy 3 months following the procedure and continue to track the patient every 3 months for the first year post-procedurally. As PSA has a half-life of 2–3 days, 8–12 weeks provides ample time for PSA to clear from serum.

The National Comprehensive Cancer Network guidelines recommend PSA follow-up every 6–12 months for the first 5 years and annually thereafter [3]. However, given that 45% of men treated for prostate cancer with curative-intent experience recurrence within the first 2 years, 77% within the first 5 years, and 96% by 9 years [4], we feel that more stringent follow-up in the first 2 years is warranted for all patients. It is for this reason that we elect to follow all patients every 3 months for the first year, regardless of risk. During the second year, PSA values are obtained every 6 months for low-risk patients and every 3 months for those at high risk (the definition of each to be described later in this counterpoint) (Tables 81.1 and 81.2).

PSA doubling time has also been recognized as both a predictor of disease relapse as well as an indicator of relapse type (local recurrence versus metastatic disease) [5]. Retrospective studies have shown that patients with a PSA doubling time <6 months are more likely to exhibit metastatic failure whereas a PSA doubling time >6 months is more likely to indicate local recurrence. Okotie and colleagues found that patients with a PSA doubling time <6 months are more likely to have a positive bone scan or CT and therefore recommended incorporating PSA doubling time as a factor to determine the need for bone scan after PSA recurrence [6]. Indeed, our practice at the University of North Carolina takes into account PSA doubling time when determining the need for bone scan. More details are given below when describing imaging modalities in prostate cancer follow-up.

A. Smith, M.D. (✉) • R. Pruthi, M.D.
University of North Carolina Division of Urologic Surgery, 2113 Physicians Office Building, CB 7235, 170 Manning Drive, Chapel Hill, NC 27599-7235, USA
e-mail: angela_smith@med.unc.edu; raj_pruthi@med.unc.edu

F.E. Johnson et al. (eds.), *Patient Surveillance After Cancer Treatment*, Current Clinical Oncology, DOI 10.1007/978-1-60327-969-7_81, © Springer Science+Business Media New York 2013

Table 81.1 Surveillance after curative-intent radical prostatectomy or radiation therapy for patients with for low-risk prostate cancer at the University of North Carolina[a]

	Year				
Modality	1	2	3	4	>5
Office visit and serum PSA level	4	2	1	1	1

The numbers in each cell are the number of times a particular modality is recommended in a particular year

[a]Low risk: negative node and margin status, and Gleason score ≤ 6 or 3 + 4, and negative seminal vesicle invasion, stage pT2

Table 81.2 Surveillance after curative-intent radical prostatectomy or radiation therapy for patients with high-risk prostate cancer at the University of North Carolina[a]

	Year				
Modality	1	2	3	4	≥5
Office visit and serum PSA level	4	4	2	2	1

The numbers in each cell are the number of times a particular modality is recommended in a particular year

[a]High risk: positive node or positive margin status or Gleason score ≥ 7 (4 + 3) or positive seminal vesicle invasion, stage pT3 or higher

Historically, PSA determinations have been combined with a digital rectal examination when evaluating prostate cancer patients, both in diagnosis and follow-up. A digital rectal examination is currently recommended as an annual screening test by the American Urological Association for men older than 50 years without other known risk factors [7]. The 2009 National Comprehensive Cancer Network practice guidelines in oncology recommend an annual digital rectal examination to monitor for prostate cancer recurrence [3]. Despite this recommendation, there are several studies which suggest that a digital rectal examination does not provide any additional clinical information beyond what one would obtain with a PSA measurement. Chaplin et al. [8] performed a prospective analysis on 1,118 patients treated by radical prostatectomy. The median follow-up duration was 4 years with 50% of patients having follow-up of more than 5 years and 35% determined to have biochemical progression. These patients were followed with PSA levels and digital rectal examinations; PSA elevation prompted transrectal ultrasound-directed biopsy and bone scan to distinguish local from metastatic disease. No patient in this series had palpable disease on digital rectal examination before the PSA level became detectable, and therefore digital rectal examination did not assist in defining recurrence.

Warren et al. [9] provided a review of the current literature for digital rectal examination after localized therapy for prostate cancer with curative intent. Over 5,000 radical prostatectomy patients were followed in the reviewed studies, and there were no instances of disease recurrence with undetectable PSA. The authors concluded that digital rectal examination is superfluous in the modern era of PSA assays following radical prostatectomy. Based on this current evidence, we choose not to perform a digital rectal examination on our patients during routine surveillance.

Although serial serum PSA measurements have provided a minimally invasive method for detecting early prostate cancer recurrence, investigators are constantly searching for better methods of earlier detection. Several studies have evaluated the utility of various imaging strategies in surveillance following radical prostatectomy. The majority of these studies have focused on transrectal ultrasound, bone scan, and CT. Wasserman et al. [10] studied the appearance of postoperative vesicourethral anastomoses in patients with suspected local recurrence (elevated PSA level). In this study, 16 patients with rising PSA levels were compared to a group with undetectable PSA levels, and there was no significant difference in the appearance of these scans between the groups. In fact, different studies conclude that prostate cancer local recurrence can appear isoechoic, hyperechoic, or slightly hypoechoic in relation to fat, rendering these techniques ineffective in distinguishing local recurrence from normal findings.

Transrectal ultrasound examinations have been used to detect local recurrence and bone scans have been employed to detect bone metastasis over the past two decades. Investigations have been conducted to determine which patients would most benefit from these studies as the majority of those who have completed local therapy do not have metastatic cancer. Warren et al. [11] reported a study of data from the Early Prostate Cancer Trial in which patients were required to have routine bone scans regardless of PSA levels. The incidence of positive bone scans was low (<3%) at PSA levels <20 ng/mL. In the group treated with radiation therapy or radical prostatectomy, the incidence of positive bone scans continued to be low (<1%) at PSA levels <5 ng/mL. However, it should be noted that the sample sizes were lower at PSA levels >5, making it difficult to provide a clear recommendation regarding this issue.

An additional study was conducted by Gomez et al. [12] in which 1,197 patients undergoing radical retropubic prostatectomy were chosen. They then identified all subjects with biochemical recurrence (PSA > 0.4 ng/mL) who had also undergone a bone scan. One hundred fifty-three patients had recurrences and, of these, 35 had bone scans. Of those with a negative bone scan, mean PSA levels were 5.2 ng/mL (with the majority <7 ng/mL) whereas those with a positive bone scan had a mean PSA of 30.6 ng/mL (with all patients having a PSA >7 ng/mL, and the majority >20 ng/mL). In a similar study by Cher et al. [13], PSA was found to be the best predictor of a positive bone scan after radical prostatectomy. The probability of a positive bone scan was less than 5% until the PSA level increased to 40–45 ng/mL or the PSA doubling time was less than 6 months. Neither preoperative PSA nor time to recurrence was predictive of bone scan findings. Their recommendation was that a bone scan should be obtained in the setting of PSA recurrence >40 ng/mL.

CT scans are viewed similarly to bone scans. Kane et al. [14] described their experience with CT and bone scans in assessing biochemical failure after radical prostatectomy. One hundred and thirty two patients experienced biochemical recurrence and underwent bone scan and CT. The mean PSA levels of those with positive bone scans and CT were 61 and 27 ng/mL, respectively, whereas those with negative scans had associated mean PSA levels of 4.9 and 4.9 ng/mL, respectively. Based on the above studies, transrectal ultrasound is not indicated as it is ineffective in distinguishing benign tissue from recurrence. We feel that a bone scan and CT scan are only indicated in cases of PSA levels >20 ng/mL, doubling time of 6 months or less, or worrisome symptoms. Therefore, bone scan and CT are not routinely offered in our surveillance strategy at the University of North Carolina except in cases where patients exhibit elevated PSA levels, worrisome symptoms or increased doubling time.

After radical prostatectomy, it is important to recognize treatment failure and distinguish local recurrence from metastatic disease. In the past, there has been debate regarding tissue sampling from the vesicourethral anastomosis or prostatic fossa following radical prostatectomy. A study by Naya et al. [15] retrospectively reviewed 126 patients who underwent prostatic fossa biopsy after radical prostatectomy. This strategy detected local recurrence in 29% of men. The PSA velocity after radical prostatectomy in men with a positive biopsy was greater than that with a negative biopsy. A greater detection rate of local recurrence was associated with a greater serum PSA at biopsy with no positive biopsies found in men with a PSA level <0.5 ng/mL. These findings were confirmed by Doneux et al. [16]. Therefore, the current recommendation is to avoid transrectal ultrasound-guided prostatic fossa biopsy in men with PSA <0.5 ng/mL and a normal digital rectal examination. Anagnostou et al. [17] provided a review of transrectal ultrasound-guided anastomotic biopsy and confirmed that the presence of local recurrence proven by biopsy is unlikely if the PSA level is <0.5 ng/mL. While they feel that biopsy is a safe procedure, the fundamental problem relates to the fact that biopsy outcome alone does not reliably rule out local recurrence (if biopsy result is negative) or systemic disease (if biopsy result is positive or negative). Large prospective studies will be needed to establish the true sensitivity and specificity of transrectal ultrasound examinations and anastomotic biopsy. At present, they are not routinely recommended in initial surveillance schemes at the University of North Carolina.

The frequency with which patients should be monitored for biochemical recurrence is debatable and depends on stage, grade, and therapy modality, among many other factors. As mentioned above, PSA remains the most reliable predictor of prostate cancer recurrence following radical prostatectomy. Therefore, our surveillance protocol centers around this measurement. In addition, many studies have emphasized the importance of other disease-specific variables when creating post-prostatectomy surveillance strategies, including stage, grade, margin status, seminal vesicle invasion, and lymph node involvement.

Margin status is routinely considered in post-prostatectomy patients, and many studies have identified positive margin status as a predictor of prostate cancer progression. Pfitzenmaier et al. [18] recently reported a prospective study of 406 post-prostatectomy patients over 5 years. Tumor stage, grade, number, and location of positive surgical margins were analyzed with respect to prostate cancer-specific survival. For patients with positive surgical margins, the PSA recurrence rate was 64% compared to only 20% in patients with negative margins. These results did not differ based on the number of positive margins nor location. Surgical margin status was also found to be a statistically significant predictor of biochemical recurrence and the development of metastases. Consequently, we place these individuals into our high-risk category when choosing a follow-up protocol.

Other studies have been conducted to provide a postoperative nomogram to predict early disease recurrence after radical prostatectomy [19, 20]. Walz studied 2,911 patients and examined the most important predictors of prostate cancer recurrence (on multivariate analysis). Along with positive margin status, patients with Gleason score 7 were approximately three times more likely to have a recurrence versus those with a score of 6 or less (odds ratio = 3.37). Those with a Gleason score of 8 were much more likely to have a recurrence (odds ratio = 9.32). Seminal vesicle invasion conferred an odds ratio of 3.00 and lymph node invasion conferred an odds ratio of 2.12. Based on similar results from many other studies, we choose to place patients with Gleason score 8 or above (as well as 4+3 disease), seminal vesicle invasion, and lymph node invasion into the high-risk category of surveillance. Because two-thirds of biochemical recurrences occur within the first 2 years after radical prostatectomy, our most intensive surveillance occurs during this time frame [21].

Based on these data, we follow patients using a simple stratification scheme in which patients are categorized into low- and high-risk categories. These groupings are formed by assessing stage, grade, seminal vesicle invasion, margin status, and node status. Low-risk patients include those with low grade cancers (Gleason score ≤6 or 3+4) as well as pT2 stage, negative seminal vesicle invasion, and negative margins. High-risk patients are considered those with Gleason score 7 (4+3) or above, Stage pT3 or higher, positive seminal vesicle invasion, or positive margins.

Based on this classification scheme, Table 81.1 describes our basic surveillance strategy. Low-risk patients are followed with a serum PSA level every 3 months for the first year, every 6 months for the second year and annually for each year thereafter. High-risk patients are followed more closely with a serum PSA every 3 months for the first and second years, every 6 months for the third and fourth years and annually for the fifth year and beyond. PSA is considered detectable at a level of 0.2 ng/ml and at this point we would begin to consider the possibilities of salvage therapies.

Moreover, during each PSA check, the patient is seen for a clinic visit to assess for clinical symptoms and to discuss and treat potential functional issues, including postoperative incontinence or erectile dysfunction. As mentioned above, a digital rectal exam is not indicated in these follow-ups and is therefore not performed routinely. Bone scans and CT scans are only reserved for cases of highly elevated PSA levels (>20 ng/mL) or worrisome symptoms. Additionally, if biochemical recurrence is noted, a biopsy of the urethrovesical junction is no longer recommended as this adds no value to our treatment strategy.

Surveillance After Radiation Therapy Differs from Surveillance After Prostatectomy

The PSA level is used for determining the effectiveness of treatment but the interpretation of the PSA level after external beam radiation therapy is more complicated than after radical prostatectomy since the prostate remains in situ. In the initial treatment phase, an elevation of PSA is expected and explained by cell death, inflammation, and subsequent release of PSA into the circulation [22]. For defining biochemical failure, in 1996, the Board of the American Society for Therapeutic Radiology and Oncology (ASTRO) formed a committee to develop a standardized definition for biochemical failure after external beam radiation therapy [23]. Through this study, PSA failure was defined as three consecutive PSA rises after a nadir (defined as the lowest PSA achieved) with the date of failure defined as the point halfway between nadir date and first rise. Additionally, the committee recommended follow-up PSA values every 3–4 months during the first 2 years and every 6 months thereafter. There were several shortcomings to this consensus, and therefore the definition of PSA failure was recently revised in a conference jointly sponsored by ASTRO and the Radiation Therapy Oncology Group (RTOG). This is known as the Phoenix Definition and it defines PSA failure as a rise of 2 ng/mL or more above the nadir PSA [24]. Admittedly, the consensus definition has shortcomings including a potential for false positives due to "benign PSA bounces," a lack of correlation with clinical progression, and the fact that it was developed to address external beam radiation monotherapy. However, the definition continues to be used as it builds on a large body of published literature and is considered a conservative definition of biochemical failure. This prior work suggests that recurrence rates using external beam radiation therapy are comparable to those achieved by surgery when this definition is used.

The time to PSA nadir after radiation therapy has also been studied extensively. Not only has this been shown to be a dose-dependent predictor of disease-free survival [25], a lower nadir has also been identified as an independent predictor of freedom from distant metastasis [26]. For example, Kestin et al. [27] found that 92% of men whose PSA reached a nadir at 36 months or longer remained disease free whereas only 30% of those who reached a nadir in less than 12 months remained disease free. Similarly, Lee et al. [25] found that 25% of those who reached a PSA nadir in >12 months had distant metastasis at 5 years whereas 75% of those who reached nadir <12 months had distant metastasis at 5 years.

Median time to nadir in patients who continue to exhibit no evidence of disease is estimated to be ~22–34 months [28, 29]. Because the time to nadir is ~2–3 years, we follow patients slightly more intensively during the first 2–3 years. Although the National Comprehensive Cancer Network guidelines recommend follow-up every 6 months for all patients who undergo radiation therapy for the first 5 years [3], we prefer to stratify patients into low- and high-risk groups (similar to that of radical prostatectomy patients). We follow all patients more intensively during the 2 years post-therapy and then relax our schedule during the third year and beyond.

Based on the original ASTRO definition, we continue to follow the current recommendations of PSA follow-up every 3 months during the first 2 years and every 6 months thereafter with some minor variations as in Tables 81.1 and 81.2.

Although National Comprehensive Cancer Network guidelines support the annual use of a digital rectal examination during the first 5 years of follow-up after radiation therapy [3], we do not include this in our standard surveillance protocols. Two relatively recent studies support the notion that digital rectal examination after radiotherapy is unnecessary in the absence of an increasing PSA level. A study by Johnstone et al. [30] examined the efficacy of a digital rectal examination after radiotherapy for localized prostate cancer by prospectively following 235 patients after definitive radiotherapy with both PSA and digital rectal examination. The majority of abnormal digital rectal examinations were caused by bleeding and radiation proctitis, which would have been detected by a primary care physician. Only 0.5% of a total of 1,544 digital rectal examinations represented new nodules, but all were in the context of increasing PSA. Therefore, it was concluded that digital rectal examination in patients with localized prostate cancer after definitive treatment with radiation can be omitted from follow-up protocols as it does not add to the information that the PSA level provides. A similar study was performed by Doneux et al. [16] in which 899 patients undergoing radiotherapy and neoadjuvant hormone therapy were followed with PSA and digital rectal examination. No recurrences were detected with digital rectal examination alone.

These studies were examined in detail, along with several others, in a comprehensive review by Warren et al. which studied the evidence in favor of or against digital rectal examination for prostate cancer surveillance after radiotherapy. She found that there was no evidence favoring digital rectal examination after radiation therapy. Although there is no published literature about the usefulness of digital rectal examination after brachytherapy, it may be presumed it is not worthwhile, but no studies have confirmed this.

Despite these findings, the 2009 National Comprehensive Cancer Network practice guidelines recommend digital rectal examination at least once annually [3]. While we agree that digital rectal examination may be a tool for detecting colorectal carcinoma, we do not routinely include this in our surveillance strategy, and the case may be made that primary care physicians may assume this role for the purpose of colorectal cancer screening.

While the PSA level alone (even without digital rectal examination) is sufficient to detect prostate cancer recurrence, several studies have investigated the role of imaging in early detection. Warren et al. [11] reported a study from the Early Prostate Cancer trial in which patients were required to have routine bone scans regardless of PSA levels. The incidence of positive bone scans was low (<3%) at PSA levels <20 ng/mL. In the group treated with radiation therapy or radical prostatectomy, the incidence of positive bone scans continued to be low (<1%) at PSA levels <5 ng/mL. We consider that neither routine bone scan nor CT should be routinely recommended in surveillance strategies for radiation-treated prostate cancer unless there are worrisome symptoms or rapidly increasing PSA levels. The utility of surveillance prostate biopsy in radiation-treated patients has been examined. It appears to be ineffective for early detection. Based on a study by Cox et al. [31], the American Society for Therapeutic Radiology and Oncology produced a consensus panel recommendation that routine prostate biopsy should not be performed for evaluation of PSA recurrence after radiation unless salvage prostatectomy or other salvage procedure is being considered. Several studies in the literature support this recommendation. In a study by Crook et al. [32], 498 men were treated with conventional radiation therapy from 1987 to 1996 and followed prospectively with transrectal ultrasound-guided post-radiation prostate biopsies starting 12–18 months after treatment. If the initial posttreatment biopsy was positive, follow-up biopsies were repeated every 6–12 months, and if the initial post-radiation biopsy was negative, re-biopsies were performed at 36 months. Results revealed that post-radiation prostate biopsies are not a gold standard of treatment efficacy but rather an independent predictor of outcome.

Hammerer and colleagues [33] analyzed the role of prostate re-biopsies after radiation to evaluate treatment success. A Medline search was performed spanning 21 years and, based on this literature review, it was concluded that patients with a positive posttreatment biopsy had higher PSA levels and a higher rate of local recurrence compared to those with negative biopsies. However, a rising PSA level after radiation therapy proved to be a more rigorous endpoint for evaluation of treatment efficacy. Therefore, prostate biopsies after radiation therapy are considered to be unnecessary as a standard surveillance procedure as they do not add additional information to the data provided by PSA measurements. This was further corroborated by a study by Svetec et al. [34] which involved performing biopsies on radical prostatectomy specimens immediately after the procedure. This revealed a 46% false-negative rate, much too high to provide a reliable means to measure efficacy of external beam radiation therapy or brachytherapy. As biopsies appear to be unreliable, they are not included in our surveillance strategy for patients undergoing radiotherapy for localized prostate cancer. Biopsies are only performed in the radiation failure patient if salvage local therapies (e.g., prostatectomy or cryotherapy) are being considered after biochemical failure.

Based on the above evidence, we choose to follow patients treated with radiation like those treated with radical prostatectomy (Tables 81.1 and 81.2). All patients are classified into low- and high-risk categories, according to Gleason score. All patients are followed every 3 months with a PSA measurement and office visit in the first posttreatment year. In the following year, low-risk patients are followed every 6 months and annually from the third year and beyond. High-risk patients are followed every 3 months for the first 2 years, every 6 months for the third and fourth years, and annually from year 5 and beyond.

Surveillance After Ablative Therapies Has Been Evaluated but Long-Term Data Are Scanty

High-Intensity Focused Ultrasonography (also called HIFU) is an example. It is an alternative approach for treatment of organ-confined prostate cancer. This therapy involves target zone tissue destruction through the coagulation, cavitation, and heat of acoustic energy applied to the target area.

As a relatively new treatment modality, gaining clinical usage in the late 1990s, some clinicians are beginning to report long-term efficacy outcomes. Blana et al. [35] described their long-term experience with high-intensity focused ultrasonography. Patients were considered for high-intensity focused ultrasonography if they were not suitable for radical prostatectomy or refused this therapeutic modality. Only those with a minimal follow-up duration of 3 years were included in the analysis, leading to a sample size of 163. Surveillance examinations were based on the investigators' clinical practice, and involved transrectal ultrasound, digital rectal examination, and PSA measurements every 3

Table 81.3 Surveillance after high-intensity focused ultrasound, cryotherapy, or active surveillance at the University of North Carolina

	Year				
Modality	1	2	3	4	≥5
Office visit and serum PSA level	4	2	2	2	2
Digital rectal examination	2	2	2	2	2
Transrectal ultrasound-guided prostate biopsy	1	1	0	1	0

The numbers in each cell are the number of times a particular modality is recommended in a particular year

months during the first year and every 6 months thereafter. Sextant biopsies were performed at 3–6 month intervals following therapy, especially in the setting of an increasing PSA level. The authors reported a 5-year disease-free survival rate of 96%, with 86% of patients achieving a PSA nadir of <1 ng/mL and 93% with negative posttreatment biopsy findings.

Despite these positive results, several questions remain regarding the true efficacy of high-intensity focused ultrasonography in the treatment of prostate cancer. First, the definition of biochemical recurrence continues to be debated. Most studies employ the ASTRO definition of biochemical failure, which is not an approved indication for high-intensity focused ultrasonography treatment. Furthermore, no literature exists regarding the surveillance of patients who undergo high-intensity focused ultrasonography. Therefore, we cannot provide an evidence-based follow-up recommendation for this treatment modality. However, it seems prudent to be conservative, in our opinion. We therefore recommend a strategy similar to that of active surveillance (Table 81.3).

Cryotherapy is another ablative therapy. It involves the localized destruction of prostate tissue by extremely low temperature and subsequent thawing. It was first applied to prostate cancer in the 1960s by Soanes [36]. Early reports revealed a host of complications, including rectovesical fistulas, urethral sloughing, erectile dysfunction, urinary retention, and lower urinary tract symptoms.

However, many advances have been made since that time, and complications are much less frequent. Fistula rates are now reported at 0–0.5%, urinary incontinence up to 7.5%, urinary retention 13% and erectile dysfunction up to 95% [37]. A Cochrane review focused on prostate cryotherapy for prostate cancer as a primary intervention for localized disease was published in 2009 [38]. The main concern regarding the use of cryotherapy for localized prostate cancer is the lack of any randomized controlled trials. Instead, the literature is filled with small case series. These studies indicate that 66–89% of patients achieve a PSA nadir of <1 ng/mL following cryotherapy. Additionally, 87–99% have a negative biopsy posttreatment. The overall 5-year survival rate appears to be about 89–100% with a disease-specific survival rate of about 94–99% [38].

Many earlier studies describe the use of surveillance biopsies as part of the protocol after prostate cryosurgery [39]. These biopsies were performed 6–12 months after treatment or for cause (such as rising PSA levels). However, the incidence of negative biopsies is high, ranging from 87 to 98%. A negative posttreatment biopsy decreases the probability of treatment failure, but does not guarantee eradication of disease, leaving the predictive utility of posttreatment biopsies uncertain at the present time.

In general, patients are followed with clinical examinations and serial PSA measurements. PSA measurements are obtained in 3-month intervals during the first 2 years and 6-month intervals thereafter. Immediately after the cryotherapy procedure, PSA levels rise dramatically due to tissue necrosis. The PSA nadir generally occurs at 3–6 months and this should therefore be taken into account during the first year measurements [40, 41]. An established definition of biochemical failure is yet to be determined; PSA level cutoffs of anywhere from 0.3 to 1.0 ng/mL have been used. Although there is no definitive evidence of reliability, the ASTRO definition of failure (three consecutive increases in PSA level) has also been used although this definition was recently changed (as described above). If the patient is hormone-naïve, the lowest postoperative PSA level is considered the nadir whereas the nadir in hormone-treated patients is defined as the 6-month postoperative PSA level [41].

A definitive surveillance scheme is still being developed for this new treatment. As for patients undergoing high-intensity focused ultrasonography, our patients are followed with the protocol employed for active surveillance (Table 81.3).

Active surveillance is growing in popularity. Given that autopsy studies show a 60–70% rate of prostate cancer in unselected men and a mere 3% risk of death from prostate cancer, the large disparity of the two numbers may point some patients toward the option of so-called watchful waiting. A more accurate description of this method is "active surveillance" or "expectant management with curative intent." This involves close monitoring of favorable-risk prostate cancer patients with PSA kinetics and serial biopsy, with subsequent curative-intent treatment used for those with aggressive or progressive disease. Favorable-risk prostate cancer involves a Gleason score ≤6, a PSA level ≤10 ng/mL, and T1c-T2a disease [42]. As described in a recent update by Klotz [43], there are currently eight prospective Phase 2 active surveillance trials ongoing. The primary endpoint (prostate cancer survival) is expected to be reached by 2025. In the meantime, Klotz has described his current follow-up protocol for those patients undergoing active surveillance [44, 45]. This includes close monitoring with serial serum PSA level determinations and digital rectal examinations every 3 months for 2 years, then every 6 months if the PSA level remains stable. Periodic prostate re-biopsies are performed at 1 year, then every 3–5 years until age 80.

Intervention is offered for a PSA doubling time <3 years or for grade progression on biopsy (Gleason score ≥ 7(4 + 3)). Other urologists have similar protocols with differences mainly involving prostate re-biopsy rates. For instance, Carter et al. [46] recommends surveillance biopsies every 1–2 years. Urologists must individually define a sufficiently conservative surveillance regimen to follow indolent disease and treat progressive disease based on their patient's characteristics. At the University of North Carolina, our usual strategy is similar to that of University of California-San Francisco and involves PSA measurement every 3 months, digital rectal examination every 3 months, and prostate biopsy after 1 year, then every 1–2 years depending on PSA level and digital rectal examination findings (Table 81.3).

With the advent of serum PSA testing, which is both convenient (as a simple blood draw) and inexpensive, follow-up of prostate cancer patients has been tremendously simplified for both patient and provider alike. PSA is not only one of the most sensitive and specific ways of detecting recurrence, but also one of the most simple and convenient ways. Patients have embraced this test which having avoids complicated strategies of imaging and physical examinations. PSA testing has given providers a straightforward and cost-effective surveillance tool.

Although PSA is the most important surveillance modality, follow-up of post-therapy prostate cancer patients requires additional knowledge of the efficacy of imaging modalities, physical examination utility (digital rectal examination), and treatment options once biochemical recurrence has been confirmed. The simplified scheme that we propose classifies patients into low- and high-risk categories based on knowledge of margin and node status, Gleason score, and seminal vesicle involvement. Although this has been our experience at the University of North Carolina, there is clearly no single correct surveillance strategy. An understanding of the literature and personal experience is therefore necessary.

References

1. Amling CL, Bergstralh EJ, Blute ML, Slezak JM, Zincke H. Defining prostate specific antigen progression after radical prostatectomy: what is the most appropriate cut point? J Urol. 2001;165:1146–51.
2. Han M, Partin AW, Zahurak M. Biochemical (prostate specific antigen) recurrence probability following radical prostatectomy for clinically localized prostate cancer. J Urol. 2003;169:517–23.
3. National Comprehensive Cancer Network Clinical Practice Guidelines in Oncology: Prostate Cancer. http://www.nccn.org/professionals/physician_gls/PDF/prostate.pdf. Accessed 12 Feb 2009
4. Pound CR, Partin AW, Epstein JI. Prostate-specific antigen after anatomic radical retropubic prostatectomy—patterns of recurrence and cancer control. Urol Clin North Am. 1997;24:395–8.
5. D'Amico AV. How to compare results after surgery or radiation for localized prostate carcinoma—prostate specific antigen (PSA) outcome (no), posttreatment PSA doubling time (maybe), or survival (yes)? Cancer. 2002;95:2041–3.
6. Okotie OT, Aronson WJ, Wieder JA. Predictors of metastatic disease in men with biochemical failure following radical prostatectomy. J Urol. 2004;171:2260–4.
7. AUA. Prostate-specific antigen (PSA) best practice policy. Oncology. 2000;14:267–70.
8. Chaplin BJ, Wildhagen MF, Schroder FH. Digital rectal examination is no longer necessary in the routine follow-up of men with undetectable prostate specific antigen after radical prostatectomy: the implications for follow-up. Eur Urol. 2005;48:906–10.
9. Warren KS, McFarlane JP. Is routine digital rectal examination required for the follow-up of prostate cancer? J Urol. 2007;178: 115–9.
10. Wasserman NF, Kapoor DA, Hildebrandt WC, Zhang G, Born KM, Eppel SM, Reddy PK. Transrectal US in evaluation of patients after radical prostatectomy. Part I. Normal postoperative anatomy. Radiology. 1992;185:361–6.
11. Warren KS, Chodak GW, See WA. Are bone scans necessary in men with low prostate specific antigen levels following localized therapy? J Urol. 2006;176:70–3.
12. Gomez P, Manoharan M, Kim SS. Radionuclide bone scintigraphy in patients with biochemical récurrence after radical prostatectomy: when is it indicated? BJU Int. 2004;94:299–302.
13. Cher ML, Bianco FJ, Lam JS. Limited role of radionuclide bone scintigraphy in patients with prostate specific antigen elevations after radical prostatectomy. J Urol. 1998;160:1387–91.
14. Kane CJ, Amling CL, Johnstone PAS, Pak N, Lance RS, Thrasher JB, Foley JP, Riffenburgh RH, Moul JW. Limited value of bone scintigraphy and computed tomography in assessing biochemical failure after radical prostatectomy. Urology. 2003;61:607–11.
15. Naya Y, Okihara K, Evans RB, Babaian RJ. Efficacy of prostatic fossa biopsy in detecting local recurrence after radical prostatectomy. Urology. 2005;66:351–5.
16. Doneux A, Parker CC, Norman A, Eeles R, Howich A, Huddart R. The utility of digital rectal examination after radical radiotherapy for prostate cancer. Clin Oncol. 2005;17:172–3.
17. Anagnostou T, Doumas K, Remzi M, Djavan B. Post-radical prostatectomy TRUS-guided anastomotic biopsy. Where do we stand today? Prostate Cancer Prostatic Dis. 2004;7:302–10.
18. Pfitzenmaier J, Pahernik S, Tremmel T, Haferkamp A, Buse S, Hohenfellner M. Positive surgical margins after radical prostatectomy: do they have an impact on biochemical or clinical progression? BJU Int. 2008;102:1413–8.
19. Walz J, Chun FKH, Klein EA, Reuther A, Saad F, Graefen M, Huland H, Karakiewicz PI. Nomogram predicting the probability of early recurrence after radical prostatectomy for prostate cancer. J Urol. 2009;181:601–7.
20. Kattan MW, Wheeler TM, Scardino PT. Postoperative nomogram for disease recurrence after radical prostatectomy for prostate cancer. J Clin Oncol. 1999;17:1499–507.
21. Dillioglugil O, Leibman BD, Kattan MW, Seale-Hawkins C, Wheeler TM, Scardino PT. Hazard rates for progression after radical prostatectomy for clinically localized prostate cancer. Urology. 1997;50:93.
22. Zagars CK, Poolack A. The fall and rise of PSA. Kinetics of serum PSA levels after radiation therapy for prostate cancer. Cancer. 1993;72:832.
23. ASTRO. Consensus statement: guidelines for PSA following radiation therapy. Int J Radiat Oncol Biol Phys. 1997;37:1035–41.
24. Roach M, Hanks G, Thames H, Schellhammer P, Shipley WU, Sokol GH, Sandler H. Defining biochemical failure following radiotherapy with or without hormonal therapy in men with clinically localized prostate cancer: recommendations of the RTOG-ASTRO phoenix consensus conference. Int J Radiat Oncol Biol Phys. 2006;65:965–74.

25. Lee WR, Hanlon AL, Hanks GE. Prostate specific antigen nadir following external beam radiation therapy for clinically localized prostate cancer: the relationship between nadir level and disease-free survival. J Urol. 1996;156:450–3.
26. Hanlon AL, Diratzouian H, Hanks GE. Posttreatment prostate-specific antigen nadir highly predictive of distant failure and death from prostate cancer. Int J Radiat Oncol Biol Phys. 2002;53: 297–303.
27. Kestin LL, Vicini FA, Ziaja EL. Defining biochemical cure for prostate carcinoma patients treated with external beam radiation therapy. Cancer. 1999;86:1557–66.
28. Hanlon AL, Diratzouian H, Hanks GE. Posttreatment prostate-specific antigen nadir highly predictive of distant failure and death from prostate cancer. Int J Radiat Oncol Biol Phys. 2002;53:297–303.
29. Pollack A, Zagars GK, Antolak JA. Prostate biopsy status and PSA nadir level as early surrogates for treatment failure: analysis of a prostate cancer randomized radiation dose escalation trial. Int J Radiat Oncol Biol Phys. 2002;54:677–85.
30. Johnstone PAS, McFarland JT, Riffenburgh RH. Efficacy of digital rectal examination after radiotherapy for prostate cancer. J Urol. 2001;166:1684–7.
31. Cox JD, Gallagher MJ, Hammand EH. Consensus statements on radiation therapy of prostate cancer: guidelines for prostate re-biopsy after radiation and for radiation therapy with rising prostate-specific antigen levels after radical prostatectomy. J Clin Oncol. 1999;17:1155–63.
32. Crook J, Malone S, Perry G, Bahadur Y, Robertson S, Abdolell M. Postradiotherapy prostate biopsies: what do they really mean? Results for 498 patients. Int J Radiat Oncol Biol Phys. 2000;48:355–67.
33. Hammerer P, Graefen M, Palisaar J, Huland H. Prostatic biopsy after radiotherapy: when and how? Eur Urol Suppl. 2002;1:83–8.
34. Svetec D, McCabe K, Peretsman S. Prostate rebiopsy is a poor surrogate of treatment efficacy in localized prostate cancer. J Urol. 1998;159:1606–8.
35. Blana A, Rogenhofer S, Ganzer R, Lunz JC, Schostak M, Wieland WF, Walter B. Eight years' experience with high-intensity focused ultrasonography for treatment of localized prostate cancer. Urology. 2008;72:1329–33.
36. Soanes WA, Gonder MJ. Use of cryosurgery in prostatic cancer. J Urol. 1968;99:793.
37. Han KR, Belldegrun AS. Third-generation cryosurgery for primary and recurrent prostate cancer. BJU Int. 2004;93:14–8.
38. Shelley M, Wilt TJ, Coles B. Cryotherapy for localized prostate cancer. Cochrane Database Syst Rev. 2007;3:CD005010.
39. Bahn DK, Lee F, Badalament R. Targeted cryoablation of the prostate: 7-year outcomes in the primary treatment of prostate cancer. Urology. 2002;60:S3–11.
40. Wieder J, Schmidt JD, Casola G. Transrectal ultrasound-guided transperineal cryoablation in the treatment of prostate carcinoma-preliminary results. J Urol. 1995;154:435–41.
41. Hubosky SG, Tepera CM, Fabrizio MD. Single center experience with third generation cryosurgery for treatment of localized prostate cancer: a critical evaluation of short term outcomes and complications. J Endourol. 2006;20:A65.
42. D'Amico AV, Whittington R, Malkowicz SB, Schultz D, Blank K, Broderick GA, Tomaszewski JE, Renshaw AA, Kaplan I, Beard CJ, Wein A. Biochemical outcome after radical prostatectomy, external beam radiation therapy, or interstitial radiation therapy for clinically localized prostate cancer. JAMA. 1998;280:969–74.
43. Klotz L. Active surveillance for prostate cancer: trials and tribulations. World J Urol. 2008;26:437–42.
44. Klotz L. Active surveillance for prostate cancer: for whom? J Clin Oncol. 2005;23:8165–9.
45. Klotz L. Active surveillance for favorable-risk prostate cancer: who, how, and why? Nat Clin Pract Oncol. 2007;4:692–8.
46. Carter HB, et al. Expectant management of prostate cancer with curative intent: an update of the Johns Hopkins experience. J Urol. 2007;178:2359–64.

Prostate Cancer Surveillance Counterpoint: USA

82

Erik T. Goluboff and Matthew Wosnitzer

Keywords
PSA • PSA failure • PSA nadir • PSA doubling time • Nomogram • Radiation therapy • Cryosurgery • High-intensity focused ultrasound • Recurrent prostate cancer • Surveillance • ASTRO criteria • Phoenix criteria

Aside from the NCCN guidelines described in the primary chapter, no guidelines exist for the follow-up of patients after treatment for prostate cancer. What follows here is what is commonly done in our urology practice and likely in most urology practices in the United States. Patient follow-up is guided by risk stratification for risk of recurrence.

Prostate cancer is the most common nonskin epithelial malignancy among American men, with 186,320 new cases and 28,660 deaths, the second leading cause of cancer mortality in that group for 2008 [1]. The number of new cases of prostate cancer per year has stabilized recently following the surge in new cases after prostate specific antigen (PSA) screening was introduced in the 1980s [2]. The number of annual prostate cancer deaths has decreased by 25% over the last 10 years [3, 4]. This is also thought to be due to the advent and adoption of widespread PSA screening. More than 90% of new cases of prostate cancer diagnosed now are driven by abnormalities in PSA blood tests.

Although PSA screening for prostate cancer is associated with poor specificity (i.e., there are three to four negative biopsies for every cancer found), various ways of manipulating PSA have been found to increase the specificity. PSA density is used to try to normalize the PSA level for the volume of the prostate [5, 6]. Since benign prostatic epithelium also makes PSA, a large benign prostate could be associated with elevated PSA levels in the absence of prostate cancer. Generally, an abnormal PSA density is one that is greater than 0.15 ng/dl/cm^3. Free PSA testing has also helped increase specificity in PSA screening for prostate cancer. PSA circulates in the blood in a bound and in a free form; the lower the percent-free PSA (out of the total PSA) the higher the risk of prostate cancer [7, 8]. The cutoff for a normal percent-free PSA is around 25%, with increasing risk as the percent-free goes down. Those with single digit percent-free PSA levels have the greatest risk. Age-adjusted PSA levels attempt to correct for the known growth in prostate size with age; as men get older, higher levels of PSA are "allowed [9]." PSA velocity, or kinetics, has been shown to increase specificity; those men with rapidly rising PSA levels over time have a greater risk of prostate cancer than those with stable PSA levels [10]. Finally, although not FDA approved, Prostate Cancer Gene 3 (PCA3) testing for mRNA transcripts in urine has been shown to increase specificity in PSA screening for prostate cancer [11–13].

While PSA screening for prostate cancer is not very specific, use of PSA in follow-up of patients who have been treated for prostate cancer is exceedingly so. The presence of PSA in the serum after radical prostatectomy, or rises in PSA levels after radiation therapy, cryosurgery, high-intensity focused ultrasound, or active surveillance reliably indicate failure of primary therapy and possible need for additional treatment [14]. More than 50,000 men annually in the United States relapse after surgery or radiation therapy [15]. While definitions of failure differ among the different therapies, and among investigators, changes in PSA levels are invariably a major part of that definition. Other parameters that are used to define failure after prostate cancer treatment include changes in digital rectal examination findings, serial prostate biopsies for residual/recurrent prostate cancer, and imaging

E.T. Goluboff, M.D., F.A.C.S. (✉) • M. Wosnitzer, M.D.
Beth Israel Medical Center, 10 Union Square East #3A, New York NY 10003, USA
e-mail: erik.goluboff@gmail.com

F.E. Johnson et al. (eds.), *Patient Surveillance After Cancer Treatment*, Current Clinical Oncology,
DOI 10.1007/978-1-60327-969-7_82,

studies such as abdominal/pelvic CT scans, bone scans, PET scans, and ProstaScint® scans [16–20]. The ProstaScint® scan is a site-specific murine monoclonal antibody (radiolabeled with Indium 111) test directed against a transmembrane glycoprotein (Prostate Specific Membrane Antigen: PSMA) expressed by prostate epithelial cells.

In following men after prostate cancer treatment, which studies are used in which patients and with what frequency is dependent on the degree of risk in a given patient. Various risk calculators have been developed from the D'Amico criteria [21] that assigns low, moderate, or high risk to patients based on serum PSA level, Gleason score, and clinical stage to the San Francisco criteria (Cancer of the Prostate Risk Assessment score from the University of California, San Francisco: CAPRA) which assigns a point score based on these and other criteria, to nomograms by Kattan, et al., Partin, et al. and other groups that can predict the risk of recurrence both before and after various forms of therapy [22–29]. As most patients with prostate cancer do not die of disease, it is important to stratify patients in terms of risk in order to know how to follow them. Those with higher risk disease need to be followed more frequently and with more extensive testing while those with lower risk disease can be spared the expense and worry associated with unnecessary testing. The use of molecular technology will likely improve our ability to predict risk in a given patient; unfortunately, none is FDA approved at the moment [30]. One promising example is the use of systems pathology that incorporates histopathology, nuclear structures, and molecular biology techniques to create a score for patients with prostate cancer to gauge their risk [31, 32].

Radical Prostatectomy

Radical prostatectomy is the surgical removal of all prostate tissue along with the seminal vesicles and parts of the vasa. Total surgical removal of the prostate is the only treatment for localized prostate cancer that has been shown in randomized controlled trials to decrease metastatic progression and disease-related mortality [33, 34]. Usually, some form of pelvic lymph node dissection is done as well but this can be tailored to patient risk [35]. In low-grade, low-stage patients with low PSA levels (low-risk patients), lymphadenectomy can be omitted altogether. In high-grade, high-stage patients with high PSA levels, extended lymph node dissections have been associated with improved outcomes [36]. Radical prostatectomy can be performed in various ways: retropubic, perineal, or laparoscopic. There were approximately 40,000 radical prostatectomies performed in 2008 in the US. More than 50% of the radical prostatectomies performed are now done laparoscopically with robotic assistance. Regardless of the method used for prostate removal, prostate cancer recurrence rates are similar [37–39]. Again, risk stratification based on pretreatment PSA level, pathologic tumor stage, and Gleason score is important in deciding how to follow these patients [27].

Table 82.1 Surveillance after curative-intent treatment for patients after primary treatment with surgery of prostate cancer

Parameter	Year 1	Year 2	Year 3	Year 4	Year 5 and after
History and Physical Examination	3	3	2	2	1
Serum PSA level	3	3	2	2	1

This is a general follow-up guide. Specific follow-up should be based on the patient's risk of recurrence

Physical examination includes digital rectal examination

Imaging (CT, bone scan, PET scan, and ProstaScint® scan) is done in specific patient situations, not as a routine

Anastomotic biopsy is done in specific patient situations, not as a routine

The number in each cell indicates the number of times a particular modality is recommended during a particular posttreatment year

In addition to following these patients for prostate cancer recurrence, common side effects after radical prostatectomy need to be monitored. These include urinary incontinence, erectile dysfunction, and stricture of the vesicourethral anastomosis.

A follow-up schema for post-prostatectomy patients is shown in Table 82.1. Post-prostatectomy, the first PSA level, is generally taken between 6 and 8 weeks. Earlier testing has led to false positive results. Detectable PSA at this time generally represents persistent disease, either in the prostatic fossa or, more likely, distant disease [40]. Definitions of failure after radical prostatectomy differ but the basic concept is that any detectable PSA after prostate removal signifies recurrence or persistence of disease. One common definition of failure is a PSA of $>=0.2$, either as a stand-alone result or rising on subsequent occasions at least 8 weeks following radical prostatectomy [41, 42]. The PSA doubling time post-prostatectomy (when detectable) has been shown to be predictive of distant failure and risk of prostate cancer-related mortality [14]. Cutoffs for high-risk patients, in terms of PSA doubling time, have been quoted as less than 6 months or less than 10 months [14, 43].

Assuming that the PSA level remains undetectable, post-prostatectomy patients should have follow-up visits that include history taking, physical examination (including digital rectal examination) and PSA testing three times a year for the first 2 years, then twice a year for 2 years, and then annually thereafter. There is no consensus as to when follow-up should stop; recurrences have been reported as long as 10 years after surgery [14]. In high-risk patients, 4 visits per year for the first 3 years are not unreasonable. The history taking should concentrate on systemic symptoms such as weight loss and bone pain as well as voiding symptoms such as urinary incontinence and pad use. Erectile function should also be assessed. Standardized quality of life questionnaires that encompass bladder, erectile, and overall functioning such as the Sexual Health Inventory for Men (SHIM) score, American Urological Association symptom score, University of California-Los Angeles Prostate Cancer Inventory score, and SF-36 are used, when possible [44–47].

When a patient is declared a failure after radical prostatectomy, the important differentiation is between local and distant failure. Local failure is associated with a longer time for PSA to begin rising postsurgery, slowly rising PSA (long PSA doubling time), positive margins on the prostatectomy specimen, and lower Gleason scores (seven or less). It can also be associated with an abnormal rectal examination. Distant failure is associated with a short time before PSA is detectable postsurgery, quickly rising PSA (short PSA doubling time), advanced stage such as positive seminal vesicles and positive lymph nodes on the prostatectomy pathology, and higher Gleason scores (8–10) [21, 48]. Patients can have both local and distant failure. PSA failure has been shown to predate clinically and radiographically detectable recurrent disease by 5–10 years [14]. For patients with abnormal rectal examinations or failure in the presence of positive margins, transrectal ultrasound guided anastomotic biopsy can be performed. Imaging studies such as abdominal/pelvic CT scans, bone scans, and ProstaScint® scans can be helpful, if positive, in differentiating local from distant failure [16–20]. In general, local failure can be treated with radiation therapy while distant failure can be treated with hormonal therapy [49, 50]. Therapeutic radiation therapy for prostatectomy failures can have durable long-term undetectable PSA rates in the 25% range, improve prostate cancer-specific survival, and should be initiated before the PSA rises much above 0.5 ng/ml [51, 52]. Hormonal therapy is not curative but can help control disease for long periods of time.

Three recent studies have looked at adjuvant radiation therapy for high-risk patients (stage T3 disease and/or positive margins) who had radical prostatectomies but who had not yet failed [53]. One retrospective cohort study [53] and two randomized controlled studies [54, 55] indicate that early adjuvant radiation therapy, following a waiting period of 3–4 months postoperatively, leads to longer PSA recurrence-free survival in these patients compared with observation only.

Radiation Therapy

Radiation therapy has long been a mainstay of treatment for prostate cancer [56]. Whether given as external beam radiation therapy or radioactive seeds (brachytherapy), as intensity-modulated or image-guided, success rates are similar and are dependent on PSA level, Gleason grade, and stage. Risk groupings, as described above, have also been used in the radiation therapy population [21, 57]. Nearly one-third of men with newly diagnosed prostate cancer are treated with external beam radiation therapy and/or brachytherapy as primary therapy [58]. The goal of radiation therapy is to eradicate all functioning epithelium in the prostate. Many studies have shown that combining radiation therapy with pre-, intra-, and posttreatment hormone ablation leads to better cancer outcomes [54, 59–62].

Since the prostate is not removed and remains in situ, PSA levels do not become undetectable as after prostatectomy. PSA levels usually nadir approximately 12–18 months after therapy; the depth of the nadir is predictive of subsequent outcome. For example, patients who nadir at an undetectable level do better than those who nadir with PSA levels above 1 ng/ml [63]. The use of hormone ablation can muddy the issue some as this can cause PSA levels to become undetectable on its own, without radiation therapy.

Definitions of failure after radiation therapy are also based on PSA levels. PSA failures in radiation therapy patients also predate clinical and radiographic failures by many years. The American Society for Radiation Oncology (ASTRO) has used various definitions of failure, including three consecutive rises and nadir plus 2 ng/ml [64]. The most current is the Phoenix definition: nadir plus 2 ng/ml [65]. In either case, the serum testosterone level (in patients who also were treated with hormone ablation) needs to be considered. For example, if the PSA level rises in a patient who was treated with radiation and hormonal therapy, and the hormone therapy has ceased, is it because the testosterone level is normalizing in the presence of functioning prostatic epithelium without tumor recurrence or is there tumor recurrence? Most would agree that, before declaring a failure, the serum testosterone level should be stable over the time course of the PSA levels. The PSA doubling time also plays a role in predicting outcome in patients who fail radiation therapy; shorter PSA doubling times are associated with worse outcomes [48, 66, 67].

Side effects after radiation therapy include voiding dysfunction, rectal toxicity, erectile dysfunction, and development of secondary malignancies. Since the 1990s, conformal radiation, in which radiation beams conform to the treatment target, have reduced radiation dose and side effects of surrounding tissues, especially rectal toxicity [68–70]. With intensity-modulated radiation therapy, the doses to surrounding tissues are further decreased when compared with conformal radiation [71]. Rigorous follow-up after radiation therapy for prostate cancer should assess these domains as well.

Assuming that treatment failure has not occurred, post-radiation therapy patients should have follow-up visits that include history taking, physical examination (including

Table 82.2 Surveillance after curative-intent treatment for patients after primary treatment with radiation for prostate cancer

Parameter	Year 1	Year 2	Year 3	Year 4	Year 5 and after
History and Physical Examination	3	3	2	2	1
Serum PSA level	3	3	2	2	1
Urinalysis	3	3	2	2	2
FOBT	3	3	2	2	2

This is a general follow-up guide. Specific follow-up should be tailored based on the patient's risk of recurrence
Physical examination includes digital rectal examination
Imaging (CT, bone scan, PET scan, and ProstaScint® scan) is done in specific patient situations, not as a routine
Prostate biopsy is done in specific patient situations, not as a routine
FOBT = fecal occult blood test
The number in each cell indicates the number of times a particular modality is recommended during a particular posttreatment year

digital rectal examination), PSA level, urinalysis, and fecal occult blood testing three times per year for the first 2 years, then twice a year for 2 years, and then annually thereafter (Table 82.2). Urinalysis and fecal occult blood testing are included to check for the development of second malignancies such as bladder and colorectal cancers. There is no consensus as to when follow-up should stop; recurrences have been reported as long as 10 years after radiation. In high-risk patients, 4 visits per year for the first 3 years is not unreasonable. The history taking should concentrate on systemic symptoms such as weight loss and bone pain as well as voiding symptoms, such as urinary incontinence, pad use, hematuria, and obstructive and irritative voiding symptoms. Bowel toxicity and erectile function should also be assessed [68, 69]. Standardized quality of life questionnaires that encompass bladder, bowel, erectile, and overall functioning, such as the SHIM score, American Urological Association symptom score, University of California-Los Angeles Prostate Cancer Inventory score, and SF-36, are used when possible [44–47].

When a patient is declared a failure after radiation therapy, it is important to differentiate between local and distant failure. Apart from changes in digital rectal examination findings and PSA doubling time, it is difficult to differentiate these in this population. Occasionally, posttreatment prostate biopsies can be useful in determining local failure [72, 73]. Patients with higher Gleason scores and pretreatment PSA levels tend to recur in distant sites [21–27]. Imaging studies such as abdominal/pelvic CT scans, bone scans, and ProstaScint® scans can be helpful, if positive, in differentiating local from distant failure. In general, treatment options for local failure include salvage prostatectomy (associated with significantly more toxicity than primary radical prostatectomy) and cryosurgery while distant failure can be treated with hormone therapy [4–6].

Cryosurgery

Cryosurgery involves the application of cryoprobes to freeze the prostate. The probes are placed through the perineum and are guided with transrectal ultrasound. Since its first application to the prostate in 1964, cryosurgery had been described as investigational [74].

The American Urological Association removed the "investigational" label from cryotherapy in 1996. Primary cryosurgery of the prostate, with or without hormone ablation, has become another option for treatment of men with localized prostate cancer [75–77]. Approximately 5,000 primary cryosurgeries of the prostate were performed in 2008 in the US. Advances in cryotherapy equipment and technique have permitted more accurate treatment with less damage to the adjacent rectum, urethra, and urinary sphincter. The use of gas rather than liquid systems, multiple cryoprobes, double rather than single freeze-thaw cycles, transrectal ultrasound, and urethral warming have all contributed to improved outcomes. These outcomes have been comparable to those after radiation therapy and need to be stratified for risk similarly [78, 79]. Unlike radiation and hormone therapy, which induce mitotic arrest and apoptosis, coagulative necrosis is the hallmark of cryosurgery.

In selected patients with low-grade, low-stage prostate cancers that are localized to one prostate lobe after extended prostate biopsy, focal cryosurgery can be performed to that lobe, only to further spare urinary and erectile dysfunction. Cryosurgery is also useful in prostate cancer that is not amenable to surgical resection [79]. As with other local therapies for prostate cancer, treatment outcome is dependent on grade and stage of cancer. Extensive periurethral disease (near the warming catheter) is a contraindication. Primary cryotherapy should be considered as an alternative to external beam radiation therapy and for men with multiple medical comorbidities who cannot undergo radical prostatectomy. Patients with gross extracapsular extension, seminal vesicle invasion, or prostate volume greater than 50 g, may undergo neoadjuvant hormonal therapy to reduce tumor volume prior to cryotherapy [80]. The freezing zone of cryotherapy can extend beyond the prostate capsule to capture extraprostatic disease. Cryotherapy is also an option for salvage treatment of radiorecurrent prostate cancer [81].

Since the prostate is not removed and remains in situ, PSA levels do not initially become undetectable as after prostatectomy. PSA levels first typically rise following cryosurgery, secondary to coagulative necrosis, which causes release of PSA [82]. PSA levels should be followed every 3 months for the first year and then every 6 months during the second year.

PSA levels usually nadir approximately 3–6 months after cryosurgery; the depth of the nadir is predictive of subsequent outcome [83]. For example, patients who nadir at an undetectable level do better than those who nadir with PSA levels above 1 ng/ml. There is no universal cutoff for PSA failure following cryotherapy. PSA values ranging from 0.2 to 1 ng/ml have been used in multiple studies as well as the American Society for Radiation Oncology and Phoenix criteria [84, 85]. Overall, 76% of men with low-risk prostate cancer (Gleason ≥ 6, PSA ≤ 10 ng/ml, ≤cT2) remained free from biochemical progression at 1 year. Men with high-risk prostate cancer (PSA ≥ 10 ng/ml and/or a Gleason score ≥ 8) have 1-, 5-, and 10-year biochemical-failure-free disease rates of 81.7, 50, and 35%, according to American Society for Radiation Oncology failure criteria [79–86]. PSA doubling time also plays a role in predicting outcome in patients who fail cryosurgery; shorter PSA doubling times are associated with worse outcomes.

PSA failures in cryosurgically treated patients predate clinical and radiographic failures by many years. In the setting of biochemical failure, biopsies may be performed but one must wait at least 6 months posttreatment to permit resolution of acute inflammation. The positive biopsy rate postcryotherapy is 7.7–25%, with recurrence most common at apex and seminal vesicles [78]. When a patient is declared a failure after cryosurgery, it is important to differentiate between local and distant failure. Apart from changes in digital rectal examination findings and the PSA doubling time, it is difficult to differentiate these in this population. Patients with higher Gleason scores and pretreatment PSA levels tend to recur more distantly. Imaging studies such as abdominal/pelvic CT scans, bone scans, and ProstaScint® scans can be helpful, if positive, in differentiating local from distant failure. The use of hormone ablation can muddy the issue some as this can cause PSA levels to become undetectable on its own, without cryosurgery. Testosterone levels also have to be considered, as in radiation therapy patients. Although limited data exist, treatment options for patients with recurrence include repeat cryoablation, hormonal ablation, radiation therapy, or salvage prostatectomy [87–89]. Radiation therapy and salvage prostatectomy in postcryosurgical patients are not generally offered due to significant morbidity.

In addition to following these patients for prostate cancer recurrence, common side effects after cryosurgery need to be monitored with a routine follow-up schedule. These include urinary incontinence, urethral sloughing, erectile dysfunction, and rectourethral fistulas. Assuming that treatment failure has not occurred, postcryosurgery patients should have follow-up visits that include history taking, physical examination (including digital rectal examination), and PSA levels three times per year for the first 2 years, twice a year for 2 years, and then annually thereafter (Table 82.3). There is no consensus as to when follow-up should stop; recurrences have been reported as long as 10 years after cryosurgery. In high-risk patients, four visits per year for the first 3 years is not unreasonable.

Table 82.3 Surveillance after curative-intent treatment for patients after primary treatment with cryotherapy for prostate cancer

Parameter	Year 1	Year 2	Year 3	Year 4	Year 5 and after
History and Physical Examination	3	3	2	2	1
Serum PSA level	3	3	2	2	1

This is a general follow-up guide. Specific follow-up should be tailored based on the patient's risk of recurrence

Physical examination includes digital rectal examination

Imaging (CT, bone scan, PET scan, and ProstaScint® scan) is done in specific patient situations, not as a routine

Prostate biopsy is done in specific patient situations, not as a routine

The number in each cell indicates the number of times a particular modality is recommended during a particular posttreatment year

The history taking should concentrate on systemic symptoms, such as weight loss and bone pain, as well as voiding symptoms such as urinary incontinence, pad use, hematuria, fecaluria, and obstructive and irritative voiding symptoms. Bowel toxicity and erectile function should also be assessed. Standardized quality of life questionnaires that encompass bladder, bowel, erectile, and overall functioning such as the SHIM score, American Urological Association symptom score, University of California-Los Angeles Prostate Cancer Inventory score, and SF-36 are used, when possible [44–47].

High-Intensity Focused Ultrasound

High-intensity focused ultrasound has not been approved for use in the United States but has been used for years in Europe and elsewhere. Guided by transrectal ultrasound, focused ultrasound waves converge in the prostate and generate heat (up to 100 °C) to ablate focal lesions or the entire gland [90]. Long-term outcomes after high-intensity focused ultrasound have not been well studied [91]. The procedure is generally well tolerated, requiring general anesthesia for 1–4 h. Most patients require a urethral or suprapubic catheter for several days. Prostate volume should not exceed 40 cm^3, and bladder neck incision is sometimes performed prior to procedure to reduce the possibility of postoperative urinary retention.

High-intensity focused ultrasound has been utilized as primary treatment for prostate cancer (T1-T2N0M0) with results similar to those of other minimally invasive therapies in men who are not surgical candidates for radical prostatectomy due to significant comorbidity and/or life expectancy of less than 10 years, or for patients who refuse surgery and external beam radiation [92, 93]. High-intensity focused ultrasound has also been used following radiation failure as salvage therapy, with efficacy rates of 17–57%, but data in this setting are too limited at this time to draw firm conclusions [94, 95]. Since the prostate is not removed and remains in situ, PSA levels do not become undetectable as after prostatectomy. PSA failures in high-intensity focused ultrasound-treated patients also predate clinical and radiographic failures by many years, and PSA has been found to be the major predictor of disease-free survival [92, 96, 97]. PSA levels usually nadir approximately 6 months after high-intensity focused ultrasound and this data provides early evidence of possible success with high-intensity focused ultrasound [96]. A definition of biochemical failure is lacking currently, and will require large data sets with longer-term follow-up. For now, the American Society for Radiation Oncology criteria have been used with a post-high-intensity focused ultrasound biochemical disease-free survival rate of about 78%. The Phoenix failure criteria have revealed a biochemical disease-free survival rate of about 75% [92–97]. Initial reports describe a 70% progression-free survival rate, and mean follow-up as long as 4.8 years has shown that 86% of patients reach a PSA nadir of <1 ng/ml [91, 92].

In addition to following these patients for prostate cancer recurrence, common side effects after high-intensity focused ultrasound need to be monitored. These include obstruction secondary to necrosis or scarring of the prostate which has been found in some studies to be reduced by incision of the bladder neck or transurethral resection of the prostate [96, 97]. Urinary incontinence and erectile dysfunction (27–60%), urinary fistula, urinary retention, bladder neck stenosis, urethral stricture, and perineal pain have also been identified [98].

Assuming that treatment failure has not occurred, post-high-intensity focused ultrasound patients should have follow-up visits that include history taking, physical examination (including digital rectal examination), and PSA levels three times per year for the first 2 years, twice a year for 2 years, and then annually thereafter. There is no consensus as to when follow-up should stop. In high-risk patients, 4 visits per year for the first 3 years are not unreasonable. The history taking should concentrate on systemic symptoms such as weight loss and bone pain as well as voiding symptoms such as urinary incontinence, obstructive and irritative voiding symptoms. Erectile function should also be assessed. Standardized quality of life questionnaires that encompass bladder, bowel, erectile, and overall functioning, such as the SHIM score, American Urological Association symptom score, University of California-Los Angeles Prostate Cancer Inventory score, and SF-36 are used, when possible [44–47] (Table 82.4).

When a patient is declared a failure after high-intensity focused ultrasound, it is important to differentiate between local and distant failure. Apart from changes in digital rectal examination findings and PSA doubling time, it is difficult to differentiate these in this population. Occasionally, posttreatment prostate biopsies can be useful in determining local failure. Patients with higher Gleason scores and pretreatment PSA levels tend to recur more distantly. Imaging studies such as abdominal/pelvic CT scans, bone scans, and ProstaScint® scans can be helpful, if positive, in differentiating local from distant failure. In general, as with failure after other primary therapies, treatment options for failure include radiation therapy and hormonal ablation.

Table 82.4 Surveillance after curative-intent treatment for patients after primary treatment with high frequency ultrasound for prostate cancer

Parameter	Year 1	Year 2	Year 3	Year 4	Year 5 and after
History and Physical Examination	3	3	2	2	1
Serum PSA level	3	3	2	2	1

This is a general follow-up guide. Specific follow-up should be tailored based on the patient's risk of recurrence
Physical examination includes digital rectal examination
Imaging (CT, bone scan, PET scan, and ProstaScint® scan) is done in specific patient situations, not as a routine
Prostate biopsy is done in specific patient situations, not as a routine
The number in each cell indicates the number of times a particular modality is recommended during a particular posttreatment year

Summary

Primary prostate cancer can be treated with radical prostatectomy, radiation therapy, cryosurgery, or high-intensity focused ultrasound. Intensity and duration of follow-up depend upon risk stratification by initial PSA level, grade, and stage. PSA testing is essential and reliable in assessing failure. Standardized questionnaires to evaluate quality of life should be used whenever possible in these patients. Overall, the algorithms described for surveillance of prostate cancer patients following primary treatment is easily employed in daily practice and has been well received by colleagues and patients. The impact of these algorithms on quality of life and mortality has not been well studied.

Definitions

HIFU: High-intensity focused ultrasound; focused ultrasound waves converge in the prostate and generate heat (up to 100 °C) to ablate focal lesions or the entire gland

ProstaScint® scan: ProstaScint® (Indium-labeled Capromab Pendetide) is a site-specific murine monoclonal antibody (radiolabeled by Indium 111) test directed against a transmembrane glycoprotein, PSMA, expressed by prostate epithelial cells. The antibody is strongly reactive with both primary and metastatic prostate cancer. Several days after antibody injection, imaging is completed using a whole body scan with dual detector head gamma camera. This is followed by a dual isotope single photon emission computed tomography (SPECT) scan of the pelvis and abdomen. The isotopes used are Indium 111-ProstaScint® and Tc-99 m labeled red blood cells which uses labeled red blood cells as an anatomic marker to aid in the localization of lymph nodes and the prostate bed. Fusion imaging, combining ProstaScint® imaging with CT or MRI imaging, co-registers the images to provide a uniquely detailed fusion image of improved diagnostic quality. Early results indicate that this fusion technique may significantly enhance detection of nodal disease, eliminate some of the false positive results from bowel activity, and accurately map the prostate gland for tumor distribution.

PET scan: Positron emission tomography: nuclear medicine imaging technique which reveals functional processes including cellular level metabolic changes occurring in an organ or tissue by detecting pairs of gamma rays emitted indirectly by a positron-emitting radionuclide (tracer) which is injected in to the patient. Fluorine-18 fluorodeoxyglucose (FDG), a glucose analog, is a commonly used tracer in oncologic studies resulting in intense radiolabeling of tissues with high glucose uptake, such as the brain, the liver, and most cancers. Images of tracer concentration in 3-dimensional space within the body are then reconstructed by computer analysis.

AUA symptom score: Patient evaluation questionnaire developed by the American Urologic Association with seven specific questions which ask the patient to rate the occurrence of various voiding characteristics secondary to enlarged prostate including: incomplete emptying, frequency, intermittency, urgency, weak stream, straining, nocturia, and quality of life if voiding symptoms persisted indefinitely. Questions rated on 0 (not at all) to 5 (almost always) scale.

SHIM: Sexual Health Inventory for Men: Patient evaluation questionnaire with five questions to rate sexual health in the past 6 months: confidence in erection, rigidity adequate for sexual intercourse, maintaining erection after penetration, maintaining erection until completion of intercourse, satisfaction with intercourse. Questions rated on zero (very low, or did not attempt intercourse) to five (almost always and without difficulty).

PSA DOUBLING TIME: Prostate Specific Antigen doubling time: PSA DOUBLING TIME has been evaluated in patients with a rising PSA after local treatment with either RP or RT [99]. In these settings, PSA DOUBLING TIME has been significantly shorter in patients who developed metastases, than in those who did not develop metastatic disease.

CAPRA: Cancer of the Prostate Risk Assessment score from the University of California, San Francisco. A preoperative index designed to predict the risk of prostate cancer recurrence following RP. The CAPRA score was developed based on a national database of men treated at large community practices across the United States. The CAPRA score ranges from zero to ten and is determined based on Gleason score, clinical T stage, age, PSA, and percent positive cores of at least a sextant biopsy. Median follow-up in the dataset was 34, and 26% of patients experienced recurrence (defined as two consecutive PSA values >0.2 or any second treatment). The 5-year actuarial recurrence-free survival ranged from 86% for CAPRA 0–1 patients to 21% for CAPRA 7–10 patients. The authors concluded that UCSF-CAPRA can accurately predict outcome in men following prostatectomy for prostate cancer.

SF-36: The SF-36 is a multipurpose, short-form health survey with 36 questions [100]. It includes an 8-scale profile of functional health and well-being scores and psychometrically based physical and mental health summary measures and a preference-based health utility index. It is a generic measure, as opposed to one that targets a specific age, disease, or treatment group. Accordingly, the SF-36 has proven helpful in studies of general and specific populations, comparing the relative burden of diseases, and in differentiating the health benefits derived from a wide range of different treatments.

References

1. Jemal A, Siegel R, Ward E, et al. Cancer statistics, 2008. CA Cancer J Clin. 2008;58:71–96.
2. Kuriyama M, Wang MC, Lee CI, et al. Use of human prostate-specific antigen in monitoring prostate cancer. Cancer Res. 1981;41:3874–6.
3. Pound CR, Walsh PC, Epstein JI, et al. Radical prostatectomy as treatment for prostate-specific antigen-detected stage T1c prostate cancer. World J Urol. 1997;15:373–7.
4. Polascik TJ, Oesterling JE, Partin AW. Prostate specific antigen: a decade of discovery–what we have learned and where we are going. J Urol. 1999;162:293–306.
5. Seaman EK, Whang IS, Cooner W, et al. Predictive value of prostate-specific antigen density for the presence of micrometastatic carcinoma of the prostate. Urology. 1994;43:645–8.
6. Benson MC, Whang IS, Olsson CA, et al. The use of prostate specific antigen density to enhance the predictive value of intermediate levels of serum prostate specific antigen. J Urol. 1992;147:817–21.
7. Christensson A, Bjork T, Nilsson O, et al. Serum prostate specific antigen complexed to alpha 1-antichymotrypsin as an indicator of prostate cancer. J Urol. 1993;150:100–5.
8. Lilja H, Christensson A, Dahlen U, et al. Prostate-specific antigen in serum occurs predominantly in complex with alpha 1-antichymotrypsin. Clin Chem. 1991;37:1618–25.
9. Oesterling JE, Cooner WH, Jacobsen SJ, et al. Influence of patient age on the serum PSA concentration. An important clinical observation. Urol Clin North Am. 1993;20:671–80.
10. Carter HB, Pearson JD, Waclawiw Z, et al. Prostate-specific antigen variability in men without prostate cancer: effect of sampling interval on prostate-specific antigen velocity. Urology. 1995; 45:591–6.
11. Groskopf J, Aubin SM, Deras IL, et al. APTIMA PCA3 molecular urine test: development of a method to aid in the diagnosis of prostate cancer. Clin Chem. 2006;52:1089–95.

12. Marks LS, Fradet Y, Deras IL, et al. PCA3 molecular urine assay for prostate cancer in men undergoing repeat biopsy. Urology. 2007;69:532–5.
13. van Gils MP, Hessels D, van Hooij O, et al. The time-resolved fluorescence-based PCA3 test on urinary sediments after digital rectal examination; a Dutch multicenter validation of the diagnostic performance. Clin Cancer Res. 2007;13:939–43.
14. Pound CR, Partin AW, Eisenberger MA, et al. Natural history of progression after PSA elevation following radical prostatectomy. JAMA. 1999;281:1591–7.
15. Moul JW. Prostate specific antigen only progression of prostate cancer. J Urol. 2000;163:1632–4.
16. Cher ML, Bianco Jr FJ, Lam JS, et al. Limited role of radionuclide bone scintigraphy in patients with prostate specific antigen elevations after radical prostatectomy. J Urol. 1998;160:1387–91.
17. Israeli RS, Powell CT, Fair WR, et al. Molecular cloning of a complementary DNA encoding a prostate-specific membrane antigen. Cancer Res. 1993;53:227–30.
18. Moul JW, Kane CJ, Malkowicz SB. The role of imaging studies and molecular markers for selecting candidates for radical prostatectomy. Urol Clin North Am. 2001;28:459–72.
19. Schettino CJ, Kramer EL, Noz ME, et al. Impact of fusion of indium-111 capromab pendetide volume data sets with those from MRI or CT in patients with recurrent prostate cancer. AJR Am J Roentgenol. 2004;183:519–24.
20. Schoder H, Herrmann K, Gonen M, et al. 2-[18 F]fluoro-2-deoxyglucose positron emission tomography for the detection of disease in patients with prostate-specific antigen relapse after radical prostatectomy. Clin Cancer Res. 2005;11:4761–9.
21. D'Amico AV, Moul JW, Carroll PR, et al. Surrogate end point for prostate cancer-specific mortality after radical prostatectomy or radiation therapy. J Natl Cancer Inst. 2003;95:1376–83.
22. Cooperberg MR, Pasta DJ, Elkin EP, et al. The University of California, San Francisco cancer of the prostate risk assessment score: a straightforward and reliable preoperative predictor of disease recurrence after radical prostatectomy. J Urol. 2005;173:1938–42.
23. Nam RK, Toi A, Klotz LH, et al. Assessing individual risk for prostate cancer. J Clin Oncol. 2007;25:3582–8.
24. Kattan MW, Eastham JA, Stapleton AM, et al. A preoperative nomogram for disease recurrence following radical prostatectomy for prostate cancer. J Natl Cancer Inst. 1998;90:766–71.
25. Kattan MW, Wheeler TM, Scardino PT. Postoperative nomogram for disease recurrence after radical prostatectomy for prostate cancer. J Clin Oncol. 1999;17:1499–507.
26. D'Amico AV, Whittington R, Malkowicz SB, et al. A multivariate analysis of clinical and pathological factors that predict for prostate specific antigen failure after radical prostatectomy for prostate cancer. J Urol. 1995;154:131–8.
27. Partin AW, Mangold LA, Lamm DM, et al. Contemporary update of prostate cancer staging nomograms (Partin tables) for the new millennium. Urology. 2001;58:843–8.
28. Kattan MW, Potters L, Blasko JC, et al. Pretreatment nomogram for predicting freedom from recurrence after permanent prostate brachytherapy in prostate cancer. Urology. 2001;58:393–9.
29. Stephenson AJ, Scardino PT, Eastham JA, et al. Postoperative nomogram predicting the 10-year probability of prostate cancer recurrence after radical prostatectomy. J Clin Oncol. 2005;23:7005–12.
30. Gurel B, Iwata T, Koh CM, et al. Molecular alterations in prostate cancer as diagnostic, prognostic, and therapeutic targets. Adv Anat Pathol. 2008;15:319–31.
31. Cordon-Cardo C, Kotsianti A, Verbel DA, et al. Improved prediction of prostate cancer recurrence through systems pathology. J Clin Invest. 2007;117:1876–83.
32. Donovan MJ, Hamann S, Clayton M, et al. Systems pathology approach for the prediction of prostate cancer progression after radical prostatectomy. J Clin Oncol. 2008;26:3923–9.
33. Bill-Axelson A, Holmberg L, Ruutu M, et al. Radical prostatectomy versus watchful waiting in early prostate cancer. N Engl J Med. 2005;352:1977–84.
34. Holmberg L, Bill-Axelson A, Helgesen F, et al. A randomized trial comparing radical prostatectomy with watchful waiting in early prostate cancer. N Engl J Med. 2002;347:781–9.
35. Allaf ME, Palapattu GS, Trock BJ, et al. Anatomical extent of lymph node dissection: impact on men with clinically localized prostate cancer. J Urol. 2004;172:1840–4.
36. Cadeddu JA, Partin AW, Epstein JI, et al. Stage D1 (T1–3, N1–3, M0) prostate cancer: a case-controlled comparison of conservative treatment versus radical prostatectomy. Urology. 1997;50:251–5.
37. Tewari A, Srivasatava A, Menon M. A prospective comparison of radical retropubic and robot-assisted prostatectomy: experience in one institution. BJU Int. 2003;92:205–10.
38. Menon M, Tewari A, Baize B, et al. Prospective comparison of radical retropubic prostatectomy and robot-assisted anatomic prostatectomy: the Vattikuti Urology Institute experience. Urology. 2002;60:864–8.
39. Han M, Partin AW, Pound CR, et al. Long-term biochemical disease-free and cancer-specific survival following anatomic radical retropubic prostatectomy. The 15-year Johns Hopkins experience. Urol Clin North Am. 2001;28:555–65.
40. Scher HI, Heller G. Clinical states in prostate cancer: toward a dynamic model of disease progression. Urology. 2000;55:323–7.
41. Oesterling JE. Prostate specific antigen: a critical assessment of the most useful tumor marker for adenocarcinoma of the prostate. J Urol. 1991;145:907–23.
42. Han M, Partin AW, Zahurak M, et al. Biochemical (prostate specific antigen) recurrence probability following radical prostatectomy for clinically localized prostate cancer. J Urol. 2003;169:517–23.
43. Roberts SG, Blute ML, Bergstralh EJ, et al. PSA doubling time as a predictor of clinical progression after biochemical failure following radical prostatectomy for prostate cancer. Mayo Clin Proc. 2001;76:576–81.
44. Clark JA, Rieker P, Propert KJ, et al. Changes in quality of life following treatment for early prostate cancer. Urology. 1999;53:161–8.
45. Ramanathan R, Mulhall J, Rao S, et al. Predictive correlation between the International index of erectile function (IIEF) and the sexual health inventory for men (SHIM): implications for calculating a derived SHIM for clinical use. J Sex Med. 2007;4:1336–44.
46. Schwartz EJ, Lepor H. Radical retropubic prostatectomy reduces symptom scores and improves quality of life in men with moderate and severe lower urinary tract symptoms. J Urol. 1999;161:1185–8.
47. White WM, Sadetsky N, Waters WB, et al. Quality of life in men with locally advanced adenocarcinoma of the prostate: an exploratory analysis using data from the CaPSURE database. J Urol. 2008;180:2409–13.
48. Freedland SJ, Humphreys EB, Mangold LA, et al. Risk of prostate cancer-specific mortality following biochemical recurrence after radical prostatectomy. JAMA. 2005;294:433–9.
49. Byar DP, Corle DK. Hormone therapy for prostate cancer: results of the Veterans Administration Cooperative Urological Research Group studies. NCI Monogr. 1988;7:165–70.
50. Schally AV, Arimura A, Baba Y, et al. Isolation and properties of the FSH and LH-releasing hormone. Biochem Biophys Res Commun. 1971;43:393–9.
51. Cox JD, Gallagher MJ, Hammond EH, et al. Consensus statements on radiation therapy of prostate cancer: guidelines for pros-

tate re-biopsy after radiation and for radiation therapy with rising prostate-specific antigen levels after radical prostatectomy. American society for radiation oncology consensus panel. J Clin Oncol. 1999;17:1155.
52. Trock BJ, Han M, Freedland SJ, et al. Prostate cancer-specific survival following salvage radiotherapy vs. observation in men with biochemical recurrence after radical prostatectomy. JAMA. 2008;299:2760–9.
53. Leibovich BC, Engen DE, Patterson DE, et al. Benefit of adjuvant radiation therapy for localized prostate cancer with a positive surgical margin. J Urol. 2000;163:1178–82.
54. Bolla M, van Poppel H, Collette L, et al. Postoperative radiotherapy after radical prostatectomy: a randomised controlled trial (EORTC trial 22911). Lancet. 2005;366:572–8.
55. Thompson Jr IM, Tangen CM, Paradelo J, et al. Adjuvant radiotherapy for pathologically advanced prostate cancer: a randomized clinical trial. JAMA. 2006;296:2329–35.
56. Roach M, Lu J, Pilepich MV, et al. Four prognostic groups predict long-term survival from prostate cancer following radiotherapy alone on Radiation Therapy Oncology Group clinical trials. Int J Radiat Oncol Biol Phys. 2000;47:609–15.
57. Pisansky TM, Kahn MJ, Rasp GM, et al. A multiple prognostic index predictive of disease outcome after irradiation for clinically localized prostate carcinoma. Cancer. 1997;79:337–44.
58. Mettlin CJ, Murphy GP, Rosenthal DS, et al. The National cancer data base report on prostate carcinoma after the peak in incidence rates in the US. The American college of surgeons commission on cancer and the American cancer society. Cancer. 1998;83: 1679–84.
59. Crook J, Ludgate C, Malone S, et al. Report of a multicenter Canadian phase III randomized trial of 3 months vs. 8 months neoadjuvant androgen deprivation before standard-dose radiotherapy for clinically localized prostate cancer. Int J Radiat Oncol Biol Phys. 2004;60:15–23.
60. Hanks GE, Pajak TF, Porter A, et al. Phase III trial of long-term adjuvant androgen deprivation after neoadjuvant hormonal cytoreduction and radiotherapy in locally advanced carcinoma of the prostate: the Radiation Therapy Oncology Group Protocol 92–02. J Clin Oncol. 2003;21:3972–8.
61. Lawton CA, Winter K, Grignon D, et al. Androgen suppression plus radiation versus radiation alone for patients with stage D1/ pathologic node-positive adenocarcinoma of the prostate: updated results based on national prospective randomized trial Radiation Therapy Oncology Group 85–31. J Clin Oncol. 2005;23:800–7.
62. Pilepich MV, Winter K, Lawton CA, et al. Androgen suppression adjuvant to definitive radiotherapy in prostate carcinoma–long-term results of phase III RTOG 85–31. Int J Radiat Oncol Biol Phys. 2005;61:1285–90.
63. Hanlon AL, Diratzouian H, Hanks GE. Posttreatment prostate-specific antigen nadir highly predictive of distant failure and death from prostate cancer. Int J Radiat Oncol Biol Phys. 2002;53: 297–303.
64. Consensus statement: guidelines for PSA following radiation therapy. American Society for Radiation Oncology Consensus Panel. Int J Radiat Oncol Biol Phys. 1997;37:1035–1041.
65. Roach 3rd M, Hanks G, Thames Jr H, et al. Defining biochemical failure following radiotherapy with or without hormonal therapy in men with clinically localized prostate cancer: recommendations of the RTOG-ASTRO Phoenix Consensus Conference. Int J Radiat Oncol Biol Phys. 2006;65:965–74.
66. Lee WR, Hanks GE, Hanlon A. Increasing prostate-specific antigen profile following definitive radiation therapy for localized prostate cancer: clinical observations. J Clin Oncol. 1997;15:230–8.
67. D'Amico AV, Moul J, Carroll PR, et al. Prostate specific antigen doubling time as a surrogate end point for prostate cancer specific mortality following radical prostatectomy or radiation therapy. J Urol. 2004;172:S42–6.
68. Beard CJ, Propert KJ, Rieker PP, et al. Complications after treatment with external-beam irradiation in early-stage prostate cancer patients: a prospective multiinstitutional outcomes study. J Clin Oncol. 1997;15:223–9.
69. Fraass BA. The development of conformal radiation therapy. Med Phys. 1995;22:1911–21.
70. Koper PC, Stroom JC, van Putten WL, et al. Acute morbidity reduction using 3DCRT for prostate carcinoma: a randomized study. Int J Radiat Oncol Biol Phys. 1999;43:727–34.
71. Luxton G, Hancock SL, Boyer AL. Dosimetry and radiobiologic model comparison of IMRT and 3D conformal radiotherapy in treatment of carcinoma of the prostate. Int J Radiat Oncol Biol Phys. 2004;59:267–84.
72. Crook JM, Perry GA, Robertson S, et al. Routine prostate biopsies following radiotherapy for prostate cancer: results for 226 patients. Urology. 1995;45:624–32.
73. Bocking A, Auffermann W. Cytological grading of therapy-induced tumor regression in prostatic carcinoma: proposal of a new system. Diagn Cytopathol. 1987;3:108–11.
74. Gonder MJ, Soanes WA, Smith V. Experimental prostate cryosurgery. Invest Urol. 1964;1:610–9.
75. Han KR, Belldegrun AS. Third-generation cryosurgery for primary and recurrent prostate cancer. BJU Int. 2004;93:14–8.
76. Pisters LL, Perrotte P, Scott SM, et al. Patient selection for salvage cryotherapy for locally recurrent prostate cancer after radiation therapy. J Clin Oncol. 1999;17:2514–20.
77. Vaidya A, Soloway MS. Salvage radical prostatectomy for radiorecurrent prostate cancer: morbidity revisited. J Urol. 2000;164:1998–2001.
78. Shinohara K, Connolly JA, Presti Jr JC, et al. Cryosurgical treatment of localized prostate cancer (stages T1 to T4): preliminary results. J Urol. 1996;156:115–21.
79. Prepelica KL, Okeke Z, Murphy A, et al. Cryosurgical ablation of the prostate: high risk patient outcomes. Cancer. 2005;103:1625–30.
80. Pisters LL, von Eschenbach AC, Scott SM, et al. The efficacy and complications of salvage cryotherapy of the prostate. J Urol. 1997;157:921–5.
81. Touma NJ, Izawa JI, Chin JL. Current status of local salvage therapies following radiation failure for prostate cancer. J Urol. 2005;173:373–9.
82. Leibovici D, Zisman A, Lindner A, et al. PSA elevation during prostate cryosurgery and subsequent decline. Urol Oncol. 2005;23:8–11.
83. Shinohara K, Rhee B, Presti Jr JC, et al. Cryosurgical ablation of prostate cancer: patterns of cancer recurrence. J Urol. 1997;158:2206–9.
84. Donnelly BJ, Saliken JC, Ernst DS, et al. Role of transrectal ultrasound guided salvage cryosurgery for recurrent prostate carcinoma after radiotherapy. Prostate Cancer Prostatic Dis. 2005;8:235–42.
85. Koppie TM, Shinohara K, Grossfeld GD, et al. The efficacy of cryosurgical ablation of prostate cancer: the University of California, San Francisco experience. J Urol. 1999;162:427–32.
86. Han KR, Cohen JK, Miller RJ, et al. Treatment of organ confined prostate cancer with third generation cryosurgery: preliminary multicenter experience. J Urol. 2003;170:1126–30.
87. Bahn DK, Lee F, Badalament R, et al. Targeted cryoablation of the prostate: 7-year outcomes in the primary treatment of prostate cancer. Urology. 2002;60:3–11.
88. Grampsas SA, Miller GJ, Crawford ED. Salvage radical prostatectomy after failed transperineal cryotherapy: histologic findings from prostate whole-mount specimens correlated with intraoperative transrectal ultrasound images. Urology. 1995;45:936–41.

89. McDonough MJ, Feldmeier JJ, Parsai I, et al. Salvage external beam radiotherapy for clinical failure after cryosurgery for prostate cancer. Int J Radiat Oncol Biol Phys. 2001;51:624–7.
90. Madersbacher S, Pedevilla M, Vingers L, et al. Effect of high-intensity focused ultrasound on human prostate cancer in vivo. Cancer Res. 1995;55:3346–51.
91. Blana A, Walter B, Rogenhofer S, et al. High-intensity focused ultrasound for the treatment of localized prostate cancer: 5-year experience. Urology. 2004;63:297–300.
92. Blana A, Murat FJ, Walter B, et al. First analysis of the long-term results with transrectal HIFU in patients with localised prostate cancer. Eur Urol. 2008;53:1194–201.
93. Rebillard X, Soulie M, Chartier-Kastler E, et al. High-intensity focused ultrasound in prostate cancer; a systematic literature review of the French Association of Urology. BJU Int. 2008;101:1205–13.
94. Chalasani V, Martinez CH, Lim D, et al. Salvage HIFU for recurrent prostate cancer after radiotherapy. Prostate Cancer Prostatic Dis. 2009;12:124–9. Published online October 2008.
95. Gelet A, Chapelon JY, Poissonnier L, et al. Local recurrence of prostate cancer after external beam radiotherapy: early experience of salvage therapy using high-intensity focused ultrasonography. Urology. 2004;63:625–9.
96. Poissonnier L, Chapelon JY, Rouviere O, et al. Control of prostate cancer by transrectal HIFU in 227 patients. Eur Urol. 2007;51:381–7.
97. Uchida T, Illing RO, Cathcart PJ, et al. To what extent does the prostate-specific antigen nadir predict subsequent treatment failure after transrectal high-intensity focused ultrasound therapy for presumed localized adenocarcinoma of the prostate? BJU Int. 2006;98:537–9.
98. Pickles T, Goldenberg L, Steinhoff G. Technology review: high-intensity focused ultrasound for prostate cancer. Can J Urol. 2005;12:2593–7.
99. Fowler Jr JE, Pandey P, Braswell NT, et al. Prostate specific antigen progression rates after radical prostatectomy or radiation therapy for localized prostate cancer. Surgery. 1994;116: 302–5.
100. Turner-Bowker DM, Bartley PJ, Ware Jr JE. SF-36® health survey & "SF" bibliography: Third Edition (1998–2000). Lincoln, RI: QualityMetric Incorportated; 2002.

Prostate Carcinoma Surveillance Counterpoint: Europe

83

Stefano Ciatto

Keywords
Surveillance • PSA • Prostate • TRUS • Recurrence

Before the prostate-specific antigen (PSA) era, surveillance of asymptomatic patients after primary radical treatment for prostate cancer was essentially based on digital rectal examination. When measurement of the serum PSA level became available, its superiority for detection of recurrent disease was clearly evident and follow-up became much easier, particularly in comparison to follow-up for other types of cancer. PSA is highly sensitive. Rising PSA levels in patients with asymptomatic untreated prostate cancer antedate the development of symptoms by greater than 10 years, according to current evidence [1]. Thus, it is not a surprise that serum PSA concentration is the only test currently used to monitor patients after primary treatment [2–4]. Other diagnostic tests are performed on demand but, even in the presence of symptoms that may suggest recurrence, the probability of any other test revealing a recurrence remains very low if no rise in PSA level is evident.

Some question may arise as to the cutoff in PSA level that defines a significant rise. After radical surgery it usually drops to almost null values and small elevations are considered to be evidence of recurrence, even in the absence of symptoms and even if other diagnostic tests do not demonstrate the site ("chemical recurrence"). After prostatectomy, having a very low baseline PSA value confers a substantial advantage compared to the detection of primary prostate cancer because abnormal PSA levels in a man with an intact prostate may be due to benign conditions such as benign prostate hyperplasia or prostatitis. This allows for a much higher specificity of PSA elevation in patients who have had a prostatectomy. Suggested cutoffs for chemical recurrence are 0.2 or 0.4 ng/ml, with evidence of a rising trend [3, 4]. Systemic treatment is commonly administered on the strength of this evidence alone. If bone scintigraphy is negative, radical radiotherapy to the surgical bed may be attempted when digital rectal examination and/or transrectal ultrasonography (TRUS) show evidence of local recurrence and TRUS-directed biopsy confirms recurrence.

After radical radiotherapy or hormonal treatment, with the prostate being left in situ, the serum PSA level may not drop to almost null values. A PSA plateau (nadir) is reached after some months, which is used as a reference baseline for judging PSA levels at subsequent assay points. When the PSA level postradiation reaches the nadir level and then rises by at least 2 ng/ml, systemic treatment is commonly administered [3, 4]. If bone scintigraphy is negative, radical surgery with curative intent may be attempted when digital rectal examination and/or TRUS shows evidence of cancer recurrence. Due to radiotherapy-induced fibrosis, digital rectal examination and TRUS are rather nonspecific and TRUS-directed biopsy is usually required to confirm recurrence.

No controlled evidence of a favorable prognostic impact of early detection of recurrence is available thus far in the literature. This is not surprising, considering that evidence of a beneficial effect is lacking also for the early detection of primary prostate cancer. The magnitude of detection lead time, using PSA level as the detection tool, is estimated to be around 12 years [1]. The competing mortality from other causes in elderly males, and the recent availability of highly effective palliative hormone therapies, explain the large overdiagnosis effect of screening by PSA. More than 50 % of screen-detected cancers have been estimated to be overdiagnosed [5], which means that the cancer would not have

S. Ciatto (✉)
ISPO–Istituto per lo Studio e la Prevenzione Oncologica,
Viale A. Volta, 171-50131 Florence, Italy
e-mail: stefano.ciatto@gmail.com

F.E. Johnson et al. (eds.), *Patient Surveillance After Cancer Treatment*, Current Clinical Oncology,
DOI 10.1007/978-1-60327-969-7_83, © Springer Science+Business Media New York 2013

become symptomatic during the patient's lifetime in the absence of screening. The same phenomenon might also affect patients with recurrence, as PSA may have a similar detection lead time for either local or distant recurrence, and life expectancy is shorter, considering that age at recurrence is higher than at first diagnosis. This does not mean that prostate cancer patients should not be followed up with periodic PSA assays, but the probability that such a follow-up policy may not be beneficial should be kept in mind when designing the follow-up protocol. It may even be detrimental for the quality of life because of the patient's knowledge of disease recurrence, side effects of treatments given for recurrence, etc. Detecting recurrence as early as possible is clearly not always useful and reasonable caution in defining chemical recurrence (e.g., waiting for a rising PSA trend to be unequivocal) should be adopted.

Overall, the practice of surveillance by periodic PSA assay aimed at early diagnosis of asymptomatic local or distant recurrences seems a reasonable option, even in absence of high-quality evidence of its efficacy. It is commonly practiced worldwide. Our scheme for periodic surveillance is shown in Table 83.1. Ideally, screening frequency should be determined by the expected detection lead time. PSA is definitely much more sensitive in detecting recurrent prostate cancer than any other test, including digital rectal examination, TRUS, and bone scan. Evidence from screening experiences suggests that the lead time for detection of recurrence by PSA level alone is well over 1 year [4]. One year, therefore, seems a reasonable interval between PSA assays once the nadir has been reached after primary treatment. A progressive increase in the surveillance interval over time may be justified. Due to length bias in sampling, slow-growing recurrences are more likely to surface late and to be associated with a longer detection lead time, thus increasing the risk of overdiagnosis. In the absence of controlled studies comparing different surveillance regimens, however, the optimal choice of the interval between PSA tests is somewhat arbitrary.

Table 83.1 Surveillance after curative-intent treatment for prostate cancer at *Istituto per lo Studio e la Prevenzione Oncologica*

	Years posttreatment					
	1	2	3	4	5	>5
Office visit[a]	1	1	1	1	1	1
PSA level	1–2	1–2	1–2	1–2	1–2	1

The number in each cell indicates the number of times a particular modality is recommended in a particular year posttreatment

This scheme does not consider patients managed only with active surveillance and deferred treatment

[a]Including digital rectal examination

References

1. European Society for Medical Oncology (ESMO). PSA surveillance after radical surgery. http://www.esmo.org. Last accessed July 2008.
2. National Institute for Clinical Excellence (NICE). http://www.nice.org.uk. Last accessed July 2008.
3. European Association of Urology (EAU). http://www.uroweb.org. Last accessed July 2008.
4. Draisma G, Boer R, Otto SJ, van der Cruijsen IW, Damhuis RAM, Schroder FH, de Koning HJ. Lead times and overdetection due to prostate-specific antigen screening: estimates from the European randomized study of screening for prostate cancer. J Natl Cancer Inst. 2003;95:868–78.
5. Zappa M, Ciatto S, Bonardi R, Mazzotta A. Overdiagnosis of prostate carcinoma by screening: an estimate based on the results of the Florence Screening Pilot Study. Ann Oncol. 1998;9:1297–300.

Prostate Carcinoma Surveillance Counterpoint: Japan

84

Akira Yokomizo

Keywords
Prostate cancer • Japan • PSA • PSA doubling time (PSADT) • PSA velocity (PSAV) • Radical prostatectomy • Radiation therapy • Hormone therapy

In Japan, the follow-up schedule for prostate cancer patients treated for cure tends to be more intensive than that in Western countries because all the Japanese patients are primarily covered by the health insurance. A schema for the follow-up schedule of the patients after definitive therapy (i.e., radical prostatectomy or external beam radiation therapy or brachytherapy) is shown in Table 84.1. National Comprehensive Cancer Network (NCCN, http://www.nccn.orc) practice guidelines describe that, for patients initially treated with intent to cure, a serum PSA (prostate-specific antigen) level should be measured every 6–12 months for the first 5 years and then rechecked annually. In our institute, initial PSA value is measured at 1 month after definitive therapy. However, this measurement alone should not be used to determine salvage treatment. Surveillance following salvage treatment should employ PSA kinetics such as PSA doubling time (PSADT) and PSA velocity (PSAV) [1, 2]. A histopathological diagnosis and measures to define whether recurrence is localized or distant is warranted [3]. Also, the definition of biochemical recurrence for radical prostatectomy is different from that for radiation therapy. For example, a specific PSA kinetic value ("PSA bounce") is sometimes observed in surveillance after radiation therapy.

The summarized follow-up schedule performed in our institute is described in Table 84.1.

A. Yokomizo, M.D., Ph.D. (✉)
Department of Urology, Graduate School of Medical Sciences, Kyushu University, Maidashi 3-1-1, Higashi-ku, Fukuoka 812-8582, Japan
e-mail: yokoa@uro.med.kyushu-u.ac.jp

In Japan, posttreatment surveillance is usually performed by the urologist only. Only a limited number of the medical oncologists are available in Japan. There are too few to see all prostate cancer patients. For patients treated with external beam radiation therapy. The radiation oncologist sees the patient during the treatment period to check on early adverse events. After finishing the radiation therapy, the patient usually returns to the urologist for surveillance.

Follow-Up After Radical Prostatectomy

After radical prostatectomy, the PSA level is measured every 3 months for 3 years, then every 6 months through 5 years in our institute, as shown in Table 84.1. The PSA measurement enables us to calculate the precise PSADT and PSAV if the patient has an increase in PSA level. This surveillance schedule is also described in the JCOG 040 I study, which evaluated radiotherapy and endocrine therapy for PSA failure after radical prostatectomy [4]. There is no consensus about the PSA criteria that define clinically significant biochemical recurrence. Definitions in the literature include single or multiple PSA values between 0.2 and 0.6 ng/ml [I]. When the PSA value is >0.1 ng/ml, PSA measurement is performed every month. This interval is decided based on evidence that a PSADT <3 months is significantly associated with time to prostate cancer-specific mortality [5, 6] and that patients treated with salvage radiation therapy at PSA levels of 0.5 ng/ml or lower have improved disease-free survival duration [2]. Monthly PSA testing enables us to find patients with a rapidly rising PSA who have a poor prognosis.

F.E. Johnson et al. (eds.), *Patient Surveillance After Cancer Treatment*, Current Clinical Oncology, DOI 10.1007/978-1-60327-969-7_84, © Springer Science+Business Media New York 2013

Table 84.1 Surveillance after curative-intent treatment for prostate cancer at Kyushu University

	Year posttreatment					
	1	2	3	4	5	>5
Office visit	4	4	4	2	2	1
Serum PSA level	4	4	4	2	2	1

This schedule does not consider patients managed with active monitoring and potential future intervention

The number in each cell is the number of times a particular modality is recommended in a particular posttreatment year

Follow-Up After Definitive Radiation Therapy

After the initial definitive radiotherapy, the PSA level is measured as for patients treated with the radical prostatectomy (Table 84.1). We adopted the ASTRO Phoenix Consensus (the value of PSA nadir + 2 ng/ml) as evidence of biochemical recurrence after definitive radiation therapy [7]. However, "PSA bounce" should be distinguished from the biochemical recurrence during the PSA-based follow-up after radiotherapy. The PSA bounce is defined as a temporary increase in PSA levels after radiation therapy for prostate cancer, which does not reflect disease recurrence [8, 9]. The bounce rate (with a very liberal definition of bounce), was 58 % with EBRT and 84 % with brachytherapy [8].

Follow-Up After Beginning Hormone Therapy

NCCN practice guidelines recommend that follow-up evaluation of these patients should include a history and physical examination, digital rectal examination, and PSA determination every 3–6 months. In our institute, after starting hormone therapy, patients are seen in the clinic every month with PSA. This enables us to assess the treatment effect and to detect adverse events. Japanese Response Criteria are used for evaluation of hormonal therapy. They are essentially the same as those of the World Health Organization, except that the former includes an evaluation of serum PSA. When the PSA value reaches nadir without any adverse effects, monitoring every 3 months is employed.

Progression of disease is defined as an increasing PSA level on three successive occasions. For recurrent disease, bicaltamide or flutamide is used to achieve a maximum androgen blockade for the patients who receive luteinizing hormone-releasing hormone analogue monotherapy. Alternatively, luteinizing hormone-releasing hormone analogue monotherapy may be added to antiandrogen monotherapy. When progressive disease is evaluated after maximum androgen blockade, the antiandrogen withdrawal syndrome is routinely observed.

Antiandrogen withdrawal syndrome, first described by Kelly and Scher in 1993, is a manifestation of a PSA decrease with or without subjective or objective symptomatic improvement on discontinuation of an antiandrogen such as flutamide [10]. A decrease in PSA has also been observed after discontinuing bicaltamide [11]. The reported incidence of antiandrogen withdrawal syndrome after initial maximum androgen blockade is 15.5 % for bicaltamide and 12.8 % for flutamide [12]. If a patient relapses after having antiandrogen withdrawal syndrome, alteration of nonsteroidal antiandrogens (flutamide to bicaltamide or bicaltamide to flutamide) is often effective. Suzuki et al. [12] reported that 142 (61.2 %) of 232 patients showed a prostate-specific antigen decrease in response to an alternative antiandrogen. These responders had significantly better survival than nonresponders, suggesting that responsiveness to second line therapy predicts increased survival [12].

Optimal surveillance and treatment strategies for hormone-refractory patients have not yet been established, but TAX 327 and Southwest Oncology Group 99–16 studies showed significant survival benefit with docetaxel-based treatment [13–15].

References

1. Simmons I. MN, Stephenson AJ, Klein ·EA. Natural history of biochemical recurrence after radical prostatectomy: risk assessment for secondary therapy. Eur Urol. 2007;51:1175–84.
2. Stephenson AJ, Scardino PT, Kattan MW, et al. Predicting the outcome of salvage radiation therapy for recurrent prostate cancer after radical prostatectomy. J Clin Oncol. 2007;25:2035–41.
3. Naito S. Evaluation and management of prostate-specific antigen recurrence after radical prostatectomy for localized prostate cancer. Jpn J Clin Oncol. 2005;35:365–74.
4. Yokomizo A, Kawamoto H, Nihei K, et al. Randomized controlled trial to evaluate radiotherapy ± endocrine therapy versus endocrine therapy alone for PSA failure after radical prostatectomy: Japan Clinical Oncology Group Study JCOG 040 I. Jpn J Clin Oncol. 2005;35:34–6.
5. D'Amico AV, Moul JW, Carroll PR, Sun L, Lubeck D, Chen MH. Surrogate end point for prostate cancer-specific mortality after radical prostatectomy or radiation therapy. J Natl Cancer Inst. 2003;9S:1376–83.
6. Zhou P, Chen MH, Mcleod D, Carroll PR, Moul JW, D'Amico AV. Predictors of prostate cancer-specific mortality after radical prostatectomy or radiation therapy. J Clin Oncol. 2005;23:6992–8.
7. Roach 3rd M, Hanks G, Thames Jr H, et al. Defining biochemical failure following radiotherapy with or without hormonal therapy in men with clinically localized prostate cancer: recommendations of the RTOG-ASTRO Phoenix Consensus Conference. lnt J Radiat Oncol Biol Phys. 2006;65:965–74.
8. Pickles T. Prostate-specific antigen (PSA) bounce and other fluctuations: which biochemical relapse definition is least prone to PSA false calls? An analysis of 2030 men treated for prostate cancer with external beam or brachytherapy with or without adjuvant androgen deprivation therapy. lnt J Radiat Oncol Biol Phys. 2006;64:1355–9.
9. Satoh T, lshlyama H, Matsumoto K, et al. Prostate-specific antigen 'bounce' after permanent (125)1-implant brachytherapy in Japanese men: a multi-institutional pooled analysis. BJU Int. 2009;I03:I064–1068.

10. Kelly WK, Scher HI. Prostate specific antigen decline after antiandrogen withdrawal: the FLT withdrawal syndrome. J Urol. 1993;149:607–9.
11. Scher HI, Zhang ZF, Nanus D, Kelly WK. Hormone and antihormone withdrawal: implications for the management of androgen-independent prostate cancer. Urology. 1996;47:61–9.
12. Suzuki H, Okihara K, Miyake H, et al. Alternative nonsteroidal antiandrogen therapy for advanced prostate cancer that relapsed after initial maximum androgen blockade. J Urol. 2008;180:921–7.
13. Tannock IF, de Wit R, Berry WR, et al. Docetaxel plus prednisone or mitoxantrone plus prednisone for advanced prostate cancer. N Engl J Med. 2004;351:1502–12.
14. Petrylak DP, Tangen CM, Hussain MH, et al. Docecaxel and estramustine compared with mitoxantrone and prednisone for advanced refractory prostate cancer. N Engl J Med. 2004;351:1513–20.
15. Berthold DR, Pond GR, Soban F, de Wit R, Eisenberger M, Tannock IF. Docetaxel plus prednisone or mitoxantrone plus prednisone for advanced prostate cancer: updated survival in the TAX 327 study. J Clin Oncol. 2008;26:242–5.

Prostate Carcinoma Surveillance Counterpoint: Canada

85

Andrew Loblaw and Colin Tang

Keywords
Prostate cancer • Active surveillance • Watchful waiting • Follow-up

It is estimated that cancer will overtake cardiovascular disease as the number one cause of death in Canada [1], mainly due to a drop in cardiovascular mortality driven by the discovery and implementation of more effective primary and secondary preventative treatments. Fortunately, the mortality of prostate cancer is also falling, now representing the third highest cause of cancer deaths in men (surpassed by colorectal cancer) [2]. This is most likely due to greater efforts applied to early cancer detection, driven by the increasing use of the prostate-specific antigen (PSA); other contributions include better treatments and a better understanding of the benefits and timing of multimodal treatments.

It is currently estimated that one in seven men will have prostate cancer diagnosed in their lifetime [3], although as discussed below, this is poised to change dramatically. The risk of prostate cancer is low for men below the age of 40 but rises precipitously for men aged 40 and above. The European Randomized Study of Screening for Prostate Cancer (ERSPC) reported a 20% reduction in prostate cancer-specific survival for the screening cohort of 55–74 years but the efficacy was greatest for men ages 55–69 [4].

Other than age, there are several other risk factors for prostate cancer: ethnicity (African descent > Caucasian > Asian descent); serum PSA level (higher PSA worse); PSA free: total ratio (lower free: total ratio worse); PSA density (total PSA / prostate volume—higher densities worse); family history (two or more affected primary relatives—worse); prostate examination (nodule worse) [5]. Nomograms which include a number of predictors listed above are proving to be the most accurate way to estimate risk of prostate cancer and are easily accessible on the internet [6, 7].

In 2006, the annual incidence of prostate cancer in Canada was estimated to be 20,700 (mortality 4,200) [8]. Compared to 1993, this represents at 33% increase (incidence was 15,800). The challenge in the next decade is the potential for a dramatic rise in prostate cancer incidence. There are four main factors which will drive this increase in incidence. The first is inevitable in North America. Men born between 1945 and 1959 (the "baby boomers") represent about one-third of the North American male population. By 2020, we there will be a 40% increase in number of men between the ages of 50 and 80 years [9].

The second biggest driver has the largest potential impact on prostate cancer incidence. It is now recognized that there is no "normal serum PSA level," i.e., no PSA level for which there is a 0% risk of prostate cancer if a biopsy was done [10]. It was widely practiced that only men with a serum PSA level above 4.0 ng/mL or a prostatic nodule should be referred for transrectal ultrasound-guided biopsy of the prostate. A 50-year-old Caucasian male with no other risk factors has a 25–35% risk of prostate cancer (and a 6–11% risk of a potentially lethal form of the disease) on transrectal ultrasound biopsy using the two most popular nomograms [6, 7]. Dropping the PSA threshold for biopsy and/or using a nomogram to articulate an individual's risk could increase the incidence of prostate cancer by sevenfold. (R Nam, personal communication; 2008).

The other two factors are: improved sensitivity of the biopsy through better imaging or greater sampling; and

A. Loblaw (✉)
Department of Radiation Oncology, Odette Cancer Centre, Sunnybrook Health Sciences Centre, Rm T2-142, 2075 Bayview Avenue, Toronto, ON, Canada M4N 3M5
e-mail: andrew.loblaw@sunnybrook.ca

C. Tang
Department of Radiation Oncology, Calvary Mater Newcastle Hospital, Waratah, NSW, Australia

F.E. Johnson et al. (eds.), *Patient Surveillance After Cancer Treatment*, Current Clinical Oncology,
DOI 10.1007/978-1-60327-969-7_85,

increased uptake of PSA testing. Now that more provincial governments are starting to fund the PSA blood test, more men will likely be willing to get tested. Currently about one-third of Canadian men surveyed had a prior PSA blood test [11], and more men may be willing to get tested. Currently just over one-third of Canadian men surveyed had a PSA blood test done in the last year [11]. Autopsy data will give us an estimate of the upper limit of the lifetime risk of prostate cancer. Fifty percent of men age 50–80 years and 75% of men 80 years of age have prostate cancer identifiable in their prostates on autopsy [12].

The Canadian Cancer Society estimates that, in 2008, the incidence of prostate cancer will be 24,200 (a 22% rise from 2006) [13]. Extrapolating this rate to 2020, the incidence in Canada would rise 400% over 2006 levels to 88,000 men. Given complete penetrance of the above factors, the incidence could be substantially higher than that. This incidence in prostate cancer therefore has the potential to overwhelm the healthcare systems in North America.

More salient to this chapter is that, given the large number of men who will be living with prostate cancer, it is critical to identify the optimal management and surveillance of men diagnosed with this disease. This counterpoint will discuss the rationale and evidence (where it exists) informing our management strategies of men on conservative management (i.e., before radical treatment) and on posttreatment follow-up.

Conservative Management of Prostate Cancer

Several studies suggest that conservative management of prostate cancer provides 10-year survival rates and quality-adjusted life-years that are similar to those of radical prostatectomy or radiotherapy [14–16]. However, conservative management deprives some patients with potentially curable, life-threatening disease of the opportunity for cure [17].

The dilemma of clinically localized prostate cancer management stems from the heterogeneity of the natural history of prostate cancer. The challenge is to differentiate patients with biologically aggressive disease for which curative therapy is indicated from those with indolent malignancy for which conservative management is sufficient. Observation or radical therapy for all patients results in under treatment in some or overtreatment in others.

Watchful Waiting

Expectant or conservative management of prostate cancer falls into two general paradigms: watchful waiting and active surveillance. Watchful waiting is classically considered a palliative approach in which prostate cancer is observed clinically and androgen deprivation therapy instituted at the onset of symptomatic prostate cancer (either locally or distantly). The PSA is typically about 100 ng/mL when this occurs, although wide variations are seen clinically. One of our patients presented with only lassitude and yet a PSA of 26,647 ng/mL; other patients can have low PSAs and have widespread metastatic disease, although both of these situations are rare.

There are wide selection criteria and practice patterns for patients managed with watchful waiting. Typically patients tend to be older, live farther from regional cancer centers and have more comorbidities [18]. Tumors can be early, low-grade tumors in which the risk of prostate cancer death (even if untreated) is considered to be low; or patients can have advanced, aggressive tumors where curative-intent therapies are unlikely to add significantly to a patient's survival. Recent level 1 evidence has shed more light on this latter group and will be discussed briefly below.

The American Society of Clinical Oncology has addressed the topic of the initial hormonal management of androgen-dependent recurrent, progressive and metastatic prostate cancer [19]. In the 2006 update, a meta-analysis of the literature regarding the optimal timing of androgen deprivation therapy was presented (seven randomized controlled trials, $n=5{,}684$ patients). While there was a relative risk reduction of prostate cancer-specific mortality of 17% (RR 0.83, $p<0.003$), there was no difference in overall survival duration seen (RR 0.98, $p=0.18$) between immediate treatment and deferred treatment. Most often the trigger for deferred androgen deprivation therapy was the onset of symptomatic disease. One of the larger and better quality trials (EORTC 30891) reported an unplanned subgroup analysis suggesting that a survival benefit was seen for patients when the serum PSA level was above 50 ng/mL or if the PSA doubling time (PSAdt) is less than 12 months [20].

Our practice is to follow patients on watchful waiting every 6 months clinically with PSA determinations (see Table 85.1). We believe that six or more PSA determinations are needed to determine an accurate PSAdt so that interval PSAs may be performed to derive a more accurate PSAdt [21], particularly if the doubling time appears to be close to 1 year (where we consider androgen deprivation therapy if PSAdt < 12 months) [20]. Androgen deprivation therapy is recommended if the PSA level reaches 50 ng/mL or if the patient develops symptomatic prostate cancer [19, 20, 22]. Restaging investigations (bone scan, CT abdomen/pelvis, CXR) are done to investigate symptoms. Prostate biopsies are repeated if radical treatment (i.e., with curative intent) is being considered, although arguably if the patient's PSA level is above 20 ng/mL, this will be of prognostic significance only as the treatment approach would not likely change.

There are a number of randomized clinical trials that demonstrate improved overall survival, cause-specific survival, distant

Table 85.1 Surveillance during watchful waiting for prostate cancer at Sunnybrook Health Sciences Centre

	Year posttreatment					
Modality	1	2	3	4	5	>5
Office visit + digital rectal examination	2	2	2	2	2	2
Serum PSA level	2	2	2	2	2	2
Transrectal ultrasound biopsy	1[a]	1[a]	1[a]	1[a]	1[a]	1[a]
Bone scan	[b]	[b]	[b]	[b]	[b]	[b]
CT abdomen/pelvis	[b]	[b]	[b]	[b]	[b]	[b]
Chest X-ray	[b]	[b]	[b]	[b]	[b]	[b]

The number in each cell indicates the number of times a particular modality is recommended during a particular posttreatment year
PSA prostate-specific antigen
[a]If radical treatment is considered
[b]If symptoms, signs, or other evidence suggest metastatic cancer

Table 85.2 Surveillance during active surveillance for prostate for prostate cancer at Sunnybrook Health Sciences Centre

	Year posttreatment					
Modality	1	2	3	4	5	>5
Office visit + digital rectal examination	2	2	2	2	2	2
Serum PSA level	4	4	2–4	2–4	2–4[a]	2–4[a]
Transrectal ultrasound biopsy	1	0	1	0	0	0
Bone scan	[b]	[b]	[b]	[b]	[b]	[b]
CT abdomen/pelvis	[b]	[b]	[b]	[b]	[b]	[b]
Chest X-ray	[b]	[b]	[b]	[b]	[b]	[b]

The number in each cell indicates the number of times a particular modality is recommended during a particular posttreatment year
PSA prostate-specific antigen
[a]If PSA doubling time is >5 years (or patient has low risk of progression based on ASURE.ca model), then serum PSA level should be measured every 6 months
[b]If symptoms, signs, or other evidence suggests metastatic cancer

metastatic disease-free survival, and/or biochemical disease-free survival for long-term adjuvant androgen deprivation therapy (2.5 years or greater) when added to radiation vs. radiation therapy and short-course androgen deprivation therapy or radiation therapy alone for patients with high-risk disease (T3, Gleason 8–10 and/or PSA>20 ng/mL) [23–26]. There are a number of randomized clinical trials which have addressed the additive role of radiation therapy. The Scandinavian Prostate Cancer Group 7 study has been reported and shows an improvement in 10-year overall survival probability (70% vs. 61%), cause-specific survival (88% vs. 76%) and PSA control (74% vs. 25%) favoring the combination approach [27]. Recently the Canadian NCIC PR3 and French randomized studies have been presented showing similar benefits for the addition of radiation to hormone therapy for patients with high-risk localized disease. For patients with advanced disease (mainly in nonscreened populations), surgery has been shown to improve overall survival over watchful waiting (5% absolute at 10 years) [17], underscoring the importance of considering radical therapy for patients even with advanced disease, particularly those with an aggressive tumor biology.

Active Surveillance

Active surveillance was originally called watchful waiting with selected delayed intervention [28]. This strategy developed approximately 15 years ago and only recently have these cohorts gained enough size and maturity to cautiously embrace this approach. The key is patient selection—selecting patients with favorable-risk localized prostate cancer identified in screened populations and surveilling them carefully for a few years to determine their biologic potential.

A few groups have published their active surveillance experiences with mature follow-up [29–35]. Patients can be watched with: serial PSA and other blood work measurements; serial digital rectal examinations; serial biopsies; and serial transrectal ultrasound and other radiologic studies. Table 85.2 shows Sunnybrook Health Science Centre's surveillance schedule.

PSA kinetics are generally believed to be the most important determinants of outcome. Various definitions can be used including: PSA velocity (first-last value or all values), PSA doubling time (first-last values or all values), and PSA thresholds (e.g., 10 or 20 ng/mL).

Since November 1995, 453 patients have been managed with active surveillance at Sunnybrook Health Sciences Centre. The median follow-up duration of survivors is 7.2 years (range 1–13 years). The overall survival percentage is 83%, and the prostate cancer-specific survival percentage is 99% (5 of 453 patients have died of prostate cancer). Thirty-five percent of patients have taken definitive therapy, 25% due to worrisome biologic factors (short PSAdt—14%; grade progression—6%; nodule growth—3%; or increase in percentage core involvement—2%); the other 10% were for other reasons such as patient preference (6%) and obstructive urinary symptoms (3%) [36].

In order to establish which method minimized the chances of unnecessary treatment, our group identified a subset of 135 patients who have remained under active surveillance, with no evidence that their cancer has spread. We have been following them for between 1 and 9 years (more than 50% of them for more than 5 years); 10% of the men died of other causes. According to their PSA results, if a PSA velocity of 2 ng/mL/year was used to define the need for treatment, 50% of the patients would have received treatment unnecessarily (recall that all patients have been well, with no evidence that their cancers have spread). Both PSAdt (either all values or only the first and last) and the 10 ng/mL threshold would have led to a false call for treatment in nearly 40% of cases. Of all the above methods, the threshold of 20 ng/mL was least likely to indicate treatment unnecessarily; only 10% of patients would be overtreated. But this may be misleading:

since all of these patients had PSA levels less than 15 ng/mL when they started and have slow-growing PSA trends, this number might go up with further follow-up [37].

We have developed a more sophisticated analysis technique based on the general linear mixed modeling method [21, 37]. This is available on the Sunnybrook website (www.ASURE.ca). While our method did not call for treatment in any of the above patients, further tests are needed to see if it can be validated by other patient groups managed with active surveillance.

In our hands, transrectal ultrasound offers little information. After a review of its utility, we no longer offer transrectal ultrasound by itself (only performing it at the time of transrectal ultrasound biopsy) [38]. Other groups have found it more useful [35].

In our group, digital rectal examination is done every 6 months. There is significant inter- and intraobserver variability for the digital rectal examination, particularly in serial assessments (hyperplastic nodules can become more or less prominent over time and the prostate consistency can also change). In our series, 2% of patients in the cohort were offered treatment due to nodule progression (defined as a doubling in its size when it was first identified).

Now that active surveillance appears to be an appropriate management paradigm for selected patients with favorable-risk localized prostate cancer, studies are underway to better define follow-up schedules, tests, and predictors that will better define those at low vs. high risk for progression. An international randomized clinical trial stewarded by the NCIC Clinical Trials Group is currently underway. In this trial, called START, 2,130 patients from North America, Europe, and Australasia are randomized to standard (either surgery, external radiation or brachytherapy) treatment vs. active surveillance.

Post-Radiotherapy Surveillance

After radiotherapy (with or without adjuvant or neoadjuvant hormone therapy), the PSA level and the clinical examination are the main parameters that are followed to determine whether a patient with prostate cancer is in remission. In fact, the serum PSA level has much greater sensitivity than the clinical examination in detecting relapse and is a surrogate predictor for prostate cancer-specific survival [39]. For a typical patient after radiotherapy, the PSA level will drop to a nadir and then fluctuate around that level.

PSA is not specific, however. There are situations in which the PSA level may be temporarily elevated, such as prostatitis, urolithiasis, or manipulation of the prostate during digital rectal examination. After internal radiation treatment (brachytherapy), a transient rise in PSA level ("benign PSA bounce") is common. The rise is usually observed during the second year after the brachytherapy implant, lasts 6–12 months and then returns to a low level. It can be challenging to distinguish a benign PSA bounce from true prostate cancer recurrence. However, one study documented that, at 4 years post-implant, the only patients who had persistently rising PSA levels were those who subsequently developed clinical recurrence [40].

A consistently rising PSA level after radiation is worrisome for recurrent prostate cancer following radiotherapy. Biochemical failure is most commonly determined by the American Society of Therapeutic Radiology and Oncology (ASTRO) consensus definition of three consecutive PSA rises [41]. However, shortcomings of this definition have been shown in numerous studies, and variations on the ASTRO definitions have been suggested [42]. The most recent ASTRO consensus definition defines biochemical failure as the PSA nadir +2 ng/mL (the Phoenix definition) [43]. A patient who does not fulfill the biochemical failure definition is defined as being in "biochemical control."

There are two philosophically different approaches after a patient has failed biochemically after primary radiotherapy. While a rising PSA level is a sensitive marker of recurrent prostate cancer, it does not reliably distinguish isolated local failure from distant failure. The patient with a positive prostate rebiopsy and negative restaging investigations (bone scan, CT scan, chest X-ray) is presumed to have local failure. Local salvage therapies such as radical prostatectomy brachytherapy, cryotherapy, high-intensity focused ultrasound, or thermal ablation may be offered to men who are believed to have isolated local failure. In each of these, cancer salvage rates are better with lower presalvage PSA levels. Therefore, in men for whom where a local salvage therapy is being considered, restaging should occur shortly after biochemical failure (unless the patient has had brachytherapy within 4 years of failure, in which case one may wish to observe to ensure it is not a benign bounce).

However, these therapies may not be technically possible. The patient may be medically unwell or may not want to accept the side effects or logistics of potentially curative treatment. Prostatectomy post-radiotherapy is also technically difficult due to radiation fibrosis, and complications such as urinary incontinence and bladder neck stricture are common. Therefore, systemic androgen deprivation therapy, which addresses local and distant failures, is the most commonly used first-line treatment in this situation. As per the ASCO guidelines described above, there is no good evidence informing the decision of when to start androgen deprivation therapy post-radiotherapy [19]. Such patients should be approached about entering clinical trials addressing this issue, if available. In Canada, there was a prospective multicenter randomized clinical trial called ELAAT open for accrual being conducted by the Ontario Clinical Oncology Group (OCOG). In Australasia, there was a similar trial named TOAD run by

Table 85.3 Surveillance after radical radiation therapy for prostate cancer at Sunnybrook Health Sciences Centre

	Year posttreatment					
Modality	1	2	3	4	5	>5
Office visit + digital rectal examination[a]	2	2[a]	2[a]	2[a]	2[a]	2[a]
Serum PSA level	2	2	2	2	2	2
Transrectal ultrasound-biopsy	[b]	[b]	[b]	[b]	[b]	[b]
Bone scan	[b]	[b]	[b]	[b]	[b]	[b]
CT abdomen/pelvis	[b]	[b]	[b]	[b]	[b]	[b]
Chest X-ray	[b]	[b]	[b]	[b]	[b]	[b]

The number in each cell indicates the number of times a particular modality is recommended during a particular posttreatment year
PSA prostate-specific antigen
[a]Digital rectal examination can be omitted if serum PSA level is <1.7 ng/mL
[b]If patient has a biochemical failure and local salvage is considered

the Trans-Tasman Radiation Oncology Group (TROG). Both are closed to accrual; first results are anticipated in 2014.

Our standard surveillance practice post-primary radiotherapy is shown in Table 85.3. We generally see the patient about 3 months post-radiotherapy, every 6 months until 5 years, then once a year after that. It would be reasonable to follow more closely a patient who had a benign bounce or rising PSA level due to unknown reasons.

At each office visit, the most important test is the serum PSA level. One study from the Royal Marsden Hospital followed 899 patients with T1-4 prostate cancer for a median of 5 years. The incidence of positive digital rectal examination was 4.3% (39/899). In no case was the digital rectal examination positive in the absence of a rising PSA level. The lowest serum PSA concentration at the time of clinically detectable local recurrence was 1.7 ng/mL [44]. This authors suggest that, with a PSA below 1.7 ng/mL, the digital rectal examination could be omitted.

This also opens the possibility that nonphysicians or nonspecialists could surveil patients once the PSA level is less than 1.7 ng/mL as the digital rectal examination is noncontributory—patients could simply be referred back if the PSA goes above this level. However, following the PSA is only one part of the follow-up post-radiotherapy. Visits with the radiation oncologist and his/her team also allow identification and optimal management of late radiation side effects to minimize their bother and maximize each patient's quality of life. Furthermore, patients may find these visits helpful in allaying anxiety (e.g., dealing with benign bounce).

Post-Prostatectomy Surveillance

The surveillance of patients after prostatectomy is very similar to that following radiotherapy. The major change in the last 2–3 years is the importance of adjuvant or salvage radiotherapy. There are now three randomized clinical trials demonstrating improved biochemical disease-free survival duration, decreased local recurrence rate, reduced need for (and increased time to) androgen ablation therapy with adjuvant radiotherapy for patients with extracapsular disease, or seminal vesicle involvement (pT3), or positive margins [23, 45, 46]. Most importantly, the SWOG 8794 study has recently published its 12-year follow-up results, now showing statistically significant improvements in overall survival duration (median 15.2y vs. 13.3y) and distant metastasis-free survival duration (14.7y vs. 12.9y) [45].

Before this evidence was available, many believed that radiotherapy was ineffective in high-risk subsets of patients, i.e., those with seminal vesicle involvement, those with high Gleason sums or those with a detectable PSA level at the time of adjuvant radiotherapy (defined as less than 0.2 ng/mL at the time this trial was started). The Thompson et al. update reports that for distant metastatis-free survival duration, the hazard ratio for each of these factors is less than one (suggesting a benefit of adjuvant radiation therapy) and that "The test of the interaction of each prognostic factor with radiotherapy was nonsignificant (interaction p values $p=1.0$ for PSA group, $p=0.20$ for Gleason category, $p=0.61$ for seminal vesicle factor), providing no evidence to suggest that any particular subset should not receive radiotherapy [45]."

A major criticism of the three randomized clinical trials is the lack of protocol for the control arms. There was a wide variation in treatments within the control arms with either observation, androgen ablation, salvage radiation (often too late and with inadequate dose), or a combination of the above.

As only half of prostatectomy patients with pT3 or positive surgical margins ever develop biochemical relapse, and there is the concern about added toxicities and cost with post-prostatectomy radiotherapy, the unanswered question is whether early salvage radiotherapy is just as effective as true adjuvant (immediate) radiotherapy in this high-risk subgroup of prostatectomy patients.

What is early salvage radiotherapy? Stephenson et al. published a multi-institutional study of the efficacy of salvage radiotherapy. In a recursive partitioning analysis, they reported predictive groups for 4-year biochemical distant metastasis-free survival duration. In addition, they showed that the PSA level at the time of radiotherapy (relapse PSA) was a strong predictor of biochemical disease-free survival (Fig. 85.1), with the lowest PSA group (defined as less than 0.5 ng/mL) faring best. Thompson et al. have also published relapse PSA values post-prostatectomy and prior to radiotherapy as a prognosticator in the recent update. They reported a statistically significant improvement in overall survival duration in the group of patients with undetectable PSA levels (defined as less than 0.2 ng/mL) vs. those with detectable PSA levels ($p=0.03$—Fig. 85.2).

While the evidence is mounting that patients have improved biochemical control which can lead to an improvement in

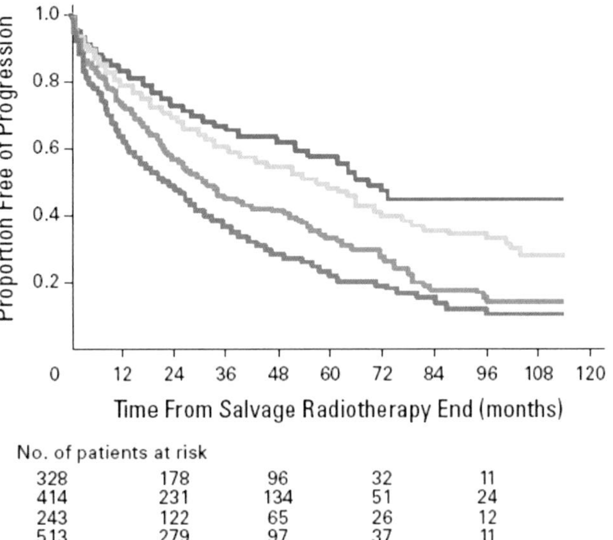

Fig. 85.1 Progression-free probability after salvage radiotherapy stratified by preradiotherapy prostate-specific antigen 0.50 or less (*blue*), 0.51–1.00 (*yellow*), 1.01–1.50 (*gray*), and more than 1.50 ng/mL (*red*). From Stephenson 2007

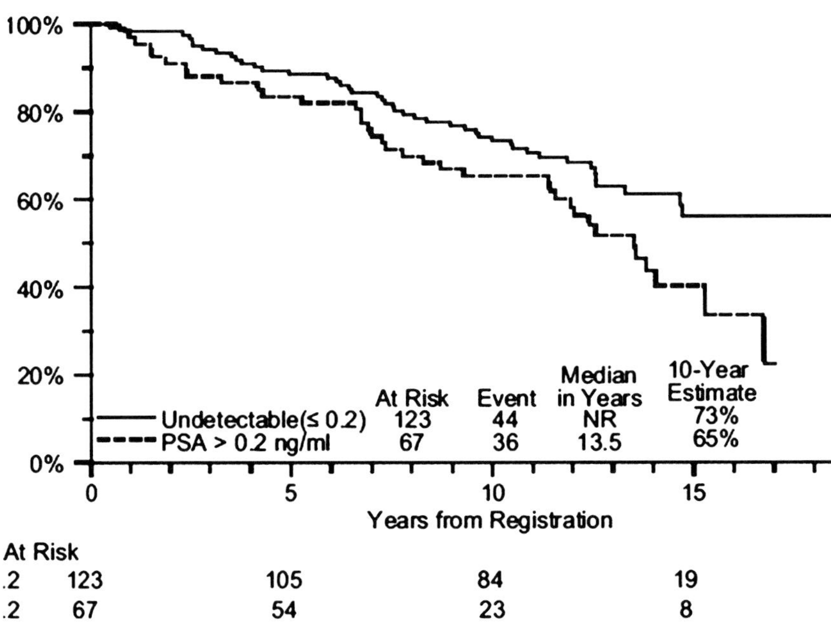

Fig. 85.2 Metastasis-free survival for radiotherapy arm stratified by PSA status after prostatectomy from SWOG 8794

overall survival when radiation therapy is started before PSA levels reach 0.2 ng/mL, both of these analyses were determined post-hoc. Therefore, is early salvage radiotherapy (e.g., when PSA level is ≤0.2 ng/mL) just as effective as true adjuvant (<16 weeks after surgery) radiotherapy in this high-risk subgroup of prostatectomy patients? Two randomized phase III studies are currently accruing patients with the aim of answering this question. RAVES (Radiotherapy Adjuvant Versus Early Salvage) run by TROG is a two-arm study looking at timing while the RADICALS (Radiotherapy and Androgen Deprivation In Combination After Local Surgery) coordinated by The Medical Research Council has two separate randomizations. The first randomization is performed immediately after radical prostatectomy in patients where there is clinical uncertainty about the timing of radiotherapy. The second randomization, performed shortly before the administration of radiotherapy, is between no androgen deprivation, short-term (4 months) and long-term (2 years) androgen deprivation.

What about patients with pT2 and negative margins but a rising PSA level on surveillance? The first question is to ask what the source of the PSA is, since the prostate has been removed. There are three potential sources. The first is a false negative margin. It is well recognized that the quality of pathologic evaluation is a strong predictor for margin status, whole mount sections requiring more time and therefore expense but detecting a positive margin if it exists [47].

The second is production of PSA by normal tissues of ectodermal origin, e.g., periurethral ducts. This is only possible now that the supersensitive PSA tests (some detecting PSA values as low as 0.01 ng/mL) have been widely implemented. We have a number of patients with PSA levels under 0.1 ng/mL who we continue to follow and who have had no clinical or PSA progression, even after years of follow-up.

The third is metastatic prostate cancer. This raises the issue of restaging investigations to rule out metastatic disease before proceeding with adjuvant (defined as within 16 weeks of surgery in the above trials) or salvage radiotherapy. A number of studies suggest that, since the chance of true positive scans is so low, these tests have no utility and simply delay the initiation of treatment, raise costs, and introduce worry if abnormalities (which are most likely to be false positives) are found. In our own practice audit, we performed 156 restaging investigations in 101 patients. Only one was a true positive test (0.6%)—this patient had a PSA level of 5 ng/mL and a PSAdt of approximately 1 month. 11.5% of the scans were false positive. Our practice at Sunnybrook Health Sciences Centre is to restage only patients who have symptoms suspicious for metastatic prostate cancer.

The final issue is when salvage radiotherapy should start. Stephenson et al. published a multi-institutional study of the efficacy of salvage radiotherapy [48]. In a recursive partitioning analysis, they reported predictive groups for 4-year biochemical disease-free survival. In addition, they showed that the PSA level at the time of radiotherapy (relapse PSA) was a strong predictor of disease-free survival (Fig. 85.1), with the lowest PSA group (defined as less than 0.5 ng/mL) faring best. Thompson et al. have also published relapse PSA as a prognosticator in the recent update. They reported a statistically significant improvement in overall survival in the group of patients with undetectable serum PSA levels (defined as less than 0.2 ng/mL) vs. detectable PSA levels ($p=0.03$—Fig. 85.2) [45].

While the evidence is mounting that patients have improved biochemical control which can lead to an improvement in overall survival when radiation therapy is started before the serum PSA level reaches 0.5 ng/mL, both of these analyses were determined post-hoc. There are intergroup randomized clinical trials open (MRC RADICALS) which will answer this question although the results are not expected for years as accrual is still ongoing.

Given that the recommendations for routine postoperative surveillance are still in evolution, the following would be reasonable. Two to four weeks postoperatively, the patient's pathology should be reviewed. PSA measurement is suggested at month 1 and every 3 months for the first year, every 6 months until 5 years, and annually thereafter. Table 85.4 summarizes this. PSA evaluation is not required if the patient has an absolute contraindication to radiotherapy (which is rare) or does not wish to have salvage radiotherapy, as patients should be referred for radiation before their PSA level reaches 0.2 ng/mL. As with post-radiotherapy follow-up, digital rectal examination is noncontributory when the PSA is "undetectable." This is confirmed by four retrospective post-prostatectomy series ($n=3,958$). There were no cases of local recurrence or metastatic disease in the setting of undetectable PSA [49–52]. Lattouf and Saad [50] found that a PSA level rise preceded positive digital rectal examination findings (when it was present) on average by 14 months. All authors do not recommend digital rectal examination in the presence of undetectable PSA. Due to the existence of ultrasensitive PSA testing, we recommend digital rectal examination in the post-prostatectomy patients only when PSA is >0.2 ng/mL [49, 53].

Table 85.4 Surveillance after curative-intent radical prostatectomy for prostate cancer at Sunnybrook Health Sciences Centre

	Year Posttreatment					
Modality	1	2	3	4	5	>5
Office visit + digital rectal examination[a]	2[a]	2[a]	2[a]	2[a]	2[a]	2[a]
Serum PSA level	4	2	2	2	2	1
Pathologic examination of surgical specimen	1					
Bone scan	[b]	[b]	[b]	[b]	[b]	[b]
CT abdomen/pelvis	[b]	[b]	[b]	[b]	[b]	[b]
Chest X-ray	[b]	[b]	[b]	[b]	[b]	[b]

The number in each cell indicates the number of times a particular modality is recommended during a particular posttreatment year

PSA prostate-specific antigen

[a]Digital rectal examination can be omitted if serum PSA level is undetectable (<0.2 ng/mL)

[b]If patient has a biochemical failure and local salvage is considered

For the asymptomatic patient who fails biochemically after adjuvant or salvage radiation, the assumption is that the patient has micrometastatic disease. The next line of therapy, outside of clinical trials, is androgen deprivation therapy and the surveillance would be the same for such patients as that for post-primary radiotherapy patients (Table 85.3).

Multi-institutional randomized clinical trials of differing follow-up schedules would be of academic interest only, i.e., not feasible to accrue to in a timely manner and funding would be difficult to obtain.

There is a great need for better staging investigations in the management of patients on active surveillance pre- or posttreatment. Measures utilizing radiolabeled PSA antibodies, positron emission tomography with prostate-specific isotopes, and ferromagnetic nanoparticles hold some promise but properly designed and conducted multicenter clinical trials would need to be completed. Magnetic resonance spectral imaging holds hope for identifying intraprostatic failures post-radiotherapy (either as an image-guidance system for directing biopsy needles or as a stand-alone test) but again would need further testing to be implemented widely.

Lastly, there is great hope that advances in molecular biology will enable clinicians to better prognosticate and/or stimulate the development of biologically targeted therapy agents. However, success to date has had limited impact outside of centers actively pursuing these research ideas.

References

1. CBC News. Cancer deaths set to exceed cardiovascular disease. StatsCan; 2007.
2. Canadian Cancer Statistics 2005. Toronto: Canadian Cancer Society/National Cancer Institute of Canada; 2005.
3. Canadian Cancer Society. Prostate Cancer Stats. Canadian Cancer Society; 2005.
4. Schroder FH, Hugosson J, Roobol MJ, et al. Screening and prostate-cancer mortality in a randomized European study. N Engl J Med. 2009;360:1320–8.
5. Nam RK, Toi A, Klotz LH, et al. Nomogram prediction for prostate cancer and aggressive prostate cancer at time of biopsy: utilizing all risk factors and tumor markers for prostate cancer. Can J Urol. 2006;13 Suppl 2:2–10.
6. Nam R. ProstateRIsk.ca; 2008.
7. National Cancer Institute. Early Detection Research Network: Cancer Risk Calculator—Forecasting the risk of disease.
8. Canadian Cancer Society/National Cancer Institute of Canada. Canadian Cancer Statistics 2006. Toronto; 2006.
9. Statistics Canada. Projected population by age group according to three projection scenarios for 2006, 2011, 2016, 2021, 2026 and 2031, at July 1, 2006.
10. Thompson IM, Ankerst DP. Prostate-specific antigen in the early detection of prostate cancer. CMAJ. 2007;176:1853–8.
11. Prostate Cancer Research Foundation of Canada. Report Card on prostate cancer knowledge and detection; 2007.
12. Sakr WA, Grignon DJ, Crissman JD, et al. High grade prostatic intraepithelial neoplasia (HGPIN) and prostatic adenocarcinoma between the ages of 20–69: an autopsy study of 249 cases. In Vivo. 1994;8:439–43.
13. Canadian Cancer Society/National Cancer Institute of Canada. Canadian Cancer Statistics 2008. Canada: Canadian Cancer Society/National Cancer Institute of Canada; 2008.
14. Fleming C, Wasson JH, Albertsen PC, et al. A decision analysis of alternative treatment strategies for clinically localized prostate cancer. JAMA. 1993;269:2650.
15. Johansson JE. Expectant management of early stage prostatic cancer: Swedish experience. J Urol. 1994;152:1753.
16. Wasson JH, Cushman CC, Bruskewitz RC, et al. A structured literature review of treatment for localized prostate cancer. Arch Fam Med. 1993;2:487.
17. Bill-Axelson A, Holmberg L, Ruutu M, et al. Radical prostatectomy versus watchful waiting in early prostate cancer. N Engl J Med. 2005;352:1977–84.
18. Taussky D, Liu A, Abrahamowicz M, et al. Factors influencing treatment decisions in patients with low risk prostate cancer referred to a brachytherapy clinic. Can J Urol. 2008;15:4415–20.
19. Loblaw DA, Virgo KS, Nam R, et al. Initial hormonal management of androgen-sensitive metastatic, recurrent, or progressive prostate cancer: 2006 update of an American Society of Clinical Oncology practice guideline. J Clin Oncol. 2007;25:1596–605.
20. Studer UE, Collette L, Whelan P, et al. Using PSA to guide timing of androgen deprivation in patients with T0-4N0-2 M0 prostate cancer not suitable for local curative treatment (EORTC 30891). Eur Urol. 2008;53:941–9.
21. Zhang L, Loblaw A, Klotz L. Modeling prostate specific antigen kinetics in patients on active surveillance. J Urol. 2006;176:1392–7; discussion 1397–8.
22. Loblaw DA, Mendelson DS, Talcott JA, et al. American Society of Clinical Oncology recommendations for the initial hormonal management of androgen-sensitive metastatic, recurrent, or progressive prostate cancer. J Clin Oncol. 2004;22:2927–41.
23. Bolla M, van Poppel H, Collette L, et al. Postoperative radiotherapy after radical prostatectomy: a randomised controlled trial (EORTC trial 22911). Lancet. 2005;366:572–8.
24. Hanks GE, Pajak TF, Porter A, et al. Phase III trial of long-term adjuvant androgen deprivation after neoadjuvant hormonal cytoreduction and radiotherapy in locally advanced carcinoma of the prostate: the Radiation Therapy Oncology Group Protocol 92–02. J Clin Oncol. 2003;21:3972–8.
25. Bolla M, De Reijke TM, Van Tienhoven GJ, et al. Six-month concomitant and adjuvant hormonal treatment with external beam irradiation is inferior to 3-years hormonal treatment for locally advanced prostate cancer: results of the EORTC randomized phase 3 trial 22961. Eur Urol Suppl. 2008;7:117 (abstract 186).
26. Pilepich MV, Winter K, Lawton CA, et al. Androgen suppression adjuvant to definitive radiotherapy in prostate carcinoma—long-term results of phase III RTOG 85–31. Int J Radiat Oncol Biol Phys. 2005;61:1285–90.
27. Widmark A, Klepp O, Solberg A, et al. Endocrine treatment, with or without radiotherapy, in locally advanced prostate cancer (SPCG-7/SFUO-3): an open randomised phase III trial. Lancet. 2009;373:301–8.
28. Choo R, DeBoer G, Klotz L, et al. PSA doubling time of prostate carcinoma managed with watchful observation alone. Int J Radiat Oncol Biol Phys. 2001;50:615–20.
29. Carter HB, Kettermann A, Warlick C, et al. Expectant management of prostate cancer with curative intent: an update of the Johns Hopkins experience. J Urol. 2007;178:2359–64; discussion 2364–5.
30. Khatami A, Aus G, Damber JE, et al. PSA doubling time predicts the outcome after active surveillance in screening-detected prostate cancer: results from the European randomized study of screening for prostate cancer, Sweden section. Int J Cancer. 2007;120:170–4.
31. Soloway MS, Soloway CT, Williams S, et al. Active surveillance; a reasonable management alternative for patients with prostate cancer: the Miami experience. BJU Int. 2008;101:165–9.
32. van As NJ, Norman AR, Thomas K, et al. Predicting the probability of deferred radical treatment for localised prostate cancer managed by active surveillance. Eur Urol. 2008;54:1297–305.
33. Roemeling S, Roobol MJ, de Vries SH, et al. Active surveillance for prostate cancers detected in three subsequent rounds of a screening trial: characteristics, PSA doubling times, and outcome. Eur Urol. 2007;51:1244–50; discussion 1251.
34. Loblaw DA, Choo R, Zhang L, et al. Updated Follow-up of Active Surveillance with Selected Delayed Intervention for Localized Prostate Cancer. Prostate Cancer Symposium Program/Proceedings. 2006:112 (abstract 37).
35. Dall'Era MA, Konety BR, Cowan JE, et al. Active surveillance for the management of prostate cancer in a contemporary cohort. Cancer. 2008;112:2664–70.
36. Klotz L, Zhang L, Lam A, et al. Clinical results of long term follow-up of a large active surveillance cohort. J Clin Oncol. 2010;28:126–31.
37. Loblaw A, Zhang L, Lam A, et al. Comparing prostate specific antigen triggers for intervention in men with stable prostate cancer on active surveillance. J Urol. 2010;84:1942–6.

38. Hruby G, Choo R, Klotz L, et al. The role of serial transrectal ultrasonography in a 'watchful waiting' protocol for men with localized prostate cancer. BJU Int. 2001;87:643–7.
39. Kim-Sing C, Pickles T. Intervention after PSA failure: examination of intervention time and subsequent outcomes from a prospective patient database. Int J Radiat Oncol Biol Phys. 2004;60:463–9.
40. Patel C, Elshaikh MA, Angermeier K, et al. PSA bounce predicts early success in patients with permanent iodine-125 prostate implant. Urology. 2004;63:110–3.
41. American Society for Therapeutic Radiology and Oncology Consensus Panel. Consensus statement: guidelines for PSA following radiation therapy. Int J Radiat Oncol Biol Phys. 1997;37:1035–41.
42. Thames H, Kuban D, Levy L, et al. Comparison of alternative biochemical failure definitions based on clinical outcome in 4839 prostate cancer patients treated by external beam radiotherapy between 1986 and 1995. Int J Radiat Oncol Biol Phys. 2003; 57:929–43.
43. Williams SG, Duchesne GM, Gogna NK, et al. An international multicenter study evaluating the impact of an alternative biochemical failure definition on the judgement of prostate cancer risk. Int J Radiat Oncol Biol Phys. 2006;65:351–7.
44. Doneux A, Parker CC, Norman A, et al. The utility of digital rectal examination after radical radiotherapy for prostate cancer. Clin Oncol (R Coll Radiol). 2005;17:172–3.
45. Thompson IM, Tangen CM, Paradelo J, et al. Adjuvant radiotherapy for pathological T3N0M0 prostate cancer significantly reduces risk of metastases and improves survival: long-term followup of a randomized clinical trial. J Urol. 2009;22:22.
46. Wiegel T, Bottke D, Willich N, et al. Phase III results of adjuvant radiotherapy (RT) versus "wait and see" (WS) in patients with pT3 prostate cancer following radical prostatectomy (RP)(ARO 96-02/AUO AP 09/95). J Clin Oncol. 2005 ASCO Annual Meeting Proceedings. 2005;23:abstract 4513.
47. Murphy GP, Busch C, Abrahamsson PA, et al. Histopathology of localized prostate cancer. Consensus Conference on Diagnosis and Prognostic Parameters in Localized Prostate Cancer. Stockholm, Sweden, May 12–13, 1993. Scand J Urol Nephrol Suppl. 1994;162:7–42; discussion 115–27.
48. Stephenson AJ, Scardino PT, Kattan MW, et al. Predicting the outcome of salvage radiation therapy for recurrent prostate cancer after radical prostatectomy. J Clin Oncol. 2007;25:2035–41.
49. Chaplin BJ, Wildhagen MF, Schroder FH, et al. Digital rectal examination is no longer necessary in the routine follow-up of men with undetectable prostate specific antigen after radical prostatectomy: the implications for follow-up. Eur Urol. 2005;48:906–10.
50. Lattouf JB, Saad F. Digital rectal exam following prostatectomy: is it still necessary with the use of PSA? Eur Urol. 2003;43:333–6.
51. Obek C, Neulander E, Sadek S, et al. Is there a role for digital rectal examination in the followup of patients after radical prostatectomy? J Urol. 1999;162:762–4.
52. Pound CR, Christens-Barry OW, Gurganus RT, et al. Digital rectal examination and imaging studies are unnecessary in men with undetectable prostate specific antigen following radical prostatectomy. J Urol. 1999;162:1337–40.
53. Warren KS, McFarlane JP. Is routine digital rectal examination required for the followup of prostate cancer? J Urol. 2007;178:115–9.

Testicle Carcinoma

86

David Y. Johnson, Shilpi Wadhwa, and Frank E. Johnson

Keywords
Sex cord-stromal tumors • Testes • Germ cell • Gonadotropin deficiency • Obesity

The International Agency for Research on Cancer (IARC), a component of the World Health Organization (WHO), estimated that there were 48,613 new cases of testicular cancer worldwide in 2002 [1]. The IARC also estimated that there were 8,878 deaths due to this cause in 2002 [1].

The American Cancer Society estimated that there were 7,920 new cases and 380 deaths due to this cause in the USA in 2007[2]. The estimated 5-year survival rate (all races) in the USA in 2007 was 96% for testicular cancer [2]. Survival rates were adjusted for normal life expectancies and were based on cases diagnosed from 1996 to 2002 and followed through 2003.

Most testicular cancers (95%) arise from germ cell elements. Sex cord-stromal tumors account for about 5%. In the U.S. the incidence and mortality rate are higher in whites than blacks. The highest incidence is in the upper socioeconomic strata. Cryptorchidism and syndromes of gonadotropin deficiency (obesity, Prader-Willi syndrome, among others) are strongly associated with testicular cancer. Exposure to various chemicals, particularly prenatal exposure to estrogens, has been implicated as a cause. Familial and hereditary factors have been described and others will probably be discovered in the future [3, 4].

D.Y. Johnson • S. Wadhwa
Department of Internal Medicine, Saint Louis University Medical Center, Saint Louis, MO, USA

F.E. Johnson (✉)
Saint Louis University Medical Center and Saint Louis Veterans Affairs Medical Center, Saint Louis, MO, USA
e-mail: frank.johnson1@va.gov

Geographic Variation Worldwide

There is considerable geographic variation in the incidence of testicular cancer. The highest incidence is seen in Scandinavia and western European populations and lowest in Africa and Asia [3, 5]. Within the USA, the incidence is low among blacks. The incidence among whites is more than five times that among blacks [6].

Surveillance Strategies Proposed by Professional Organizations or National Government Agencies and Available on the Internet

National Comprehensive Cancer Network (www.nccn.org)

National Comprehensive Cancer Network (NCCN) guidelines were accessed on 1/28/12 (Tables 86.1, 86.2, 86.3, 86.4, 86.5, 86.6, 86.7, and 86.8). There were major quantitative and qualitative changes compared to the guidelines accessed on 4/10/07.

American Society of Clinical Oncology (www.asco.org)

American Society of Clinical Oncology (ASCO) guidelines were accessed on 1/28/12. No quantitative guidelines exist for testicular cancer surveillance including when first accessed on 10/31/07.

F.E. Johnson et al. (eds.), *Patient Surveillance After Cancer Treatment*, Current Clinical Oncology,
DOI 10.1007/978-1-60327-969-7_86, © Springer Science+Business Media New York 2013

Table 86.1 Testicular cancer: pure seminoma (Stage IA, IB with surveillance for pT1, pT2 tumors)

	Years posttreatment[a]					
	1	2	3	4	5	>5
Office visit	3–4	3–4	1–2	1–2	1	1
AFP, beta-hCG, LDH	3–4	3–4	1–2	1–2	1	1
Abdominal/pelvic CT scan	2	2	1–2	1	1	0
• Chest X-ray as clinically indicated for years 1–5						

Obtained from NCCN (www.nccn.org) on 1-28-12
NCCN guidelines were accessed on 1/28/12. There were major quantitative and qualitative changes compared to the guidelines accessed on 4/10/07
[a]The numbers in the table indicate the number of times the modality is recommended during the indicated year posttreatment

Table 86.2 Testicular cancer: pure seminoma (Stage IA, IB with single agent carboplatin)

	Years posttreatment[a]					
	1	2	3	4	5	>5
Office visit	4	3	2	1	1	1
AFP, beta-hCG, LDH	4	3	2	1	1	1
Abdominal/pelvic CT scan	1	1	1	0	0	0
• Chest X-ray as clinically indicated						

Obtained from NCCN (www.nccn.org) on 1-28-12
NCCN guidelines were accessed on 1/28/12. There were major quantitative and qualitative changes compared to the guidelines accessed on 4/10/07
[a]The numbers in the table indicate the number of times the modality is recommended during the indicated year posttreatment

Table 86.3 Testicular cancer: pure seminoma (Stage IA, IB, IS with radiotherapy)

	Years posttreatment[a]					
	1	2	3	4	5	>5
Office visit	3	3	1	1	1	1[b]
AFP, beta-hCG, LDH	3	3	1	1	1	1[b]
Abdominal/pelvic CT scan[c]	1	1	1	0	0	0
• Chest X-ray as clinically indicated						

Obtained from NCCN (www.nccn.org) on 1-28-12
NCCN guidelines were accessed on 1/28/12. There were major quantitative and qualitative changes compared to the guidelines accessed on 4/10/07
[a]The numbers in the table indicate the number of times the modality is recommended during the indicated year posttreatment
[b]Annually for years 3–10
[c]For patients status post only para-aortic RT

The Society of Surgical Oncology (www.surgonc.org)

The Society of Surgical Oncology (SSO) guidelines were accessed on 1/28/12. No quantitative guidelines exist for testicular cancer surveillance including when first accessed on 10/31/07.

Table 86.4 Testicular cancer: pure seminoma (Stage IIA, IIB with radiotherapy[a])

	Years posttreatment[b]					
	1	2	3	4	5	>5
Office visit	4	2	2	2	2	1[c]
AFP, beta-hCG, LDH	4	2	2	2	2	1[c]
Chest x-ray	2	2	0	0	0	0
Abdominal/pelvic CT scan	1–2	1–2	1	0	0	0

Obtained from NCCN (www.nccn.org) on 1-28-12
NCCN guidelines were accessed on 1/28/12. There were major quantitative and qualitative changes compared to the guidelines accessed on 4/10/07
[a]To include para-aortic and ipsilateral iliac lymph nodes to a dose of 30–36 Gy
[b]The numbers in the table indicate the number of times the modality is recommended during the indicated year posttreatment
[c]Annually for years 6–10

Table 86.5 Testicular cancer: pure seminoma (Stage IIB, IIC, III after primary treatment with chemotherapy)

	Years posttreatment[a]					
	1	2	3	4	5	>5
Office visit	6	4	2	2	1	1
AFP, beta-hCG, LDH	6	4	2	2	1	1
Chest X-ray	6	4	2	2	1	1
Abdominal/pelvic CT scan[b, c, d]	2–4	0	0	0	0	0
• PET scan as clinically indicated						

Obtained from NCCN (www.nccn.org) on 1-28-12
NCCN guidelines were accessed on 1/28/12. There were major quantitative and qualitative changes compared to the guidelines accessed on 4/10/07
[a]The numbers in the table indicate the number of times the modality is recommended during the indicated year posttreatment
[b]Post RPLND
[c]Every 3–6 months, then as clinically indicated
[d]After all other primary management as clinically indicated

Table 86.6 Testicular cancer: nonseminoma (Stage IA, IB) with surveillance only

	Years posttreatment[a]					
	1	2	3	4	5	>5
Office visit	6–12	6	4	3	2	1
Markers	6–12	6	4	3	2	1
Chest X-ray	6–12	6	4	3	2	1
Abdominal/pelvic CT scan	3–4	2–3	1–2	1–2	1	0.5–1

Obtained from NCCN (www.nccn.org) on 1-28-12
NCCN guidelines were accessed on 1/28/12. There were major quantitative and qualitative changes compared to the guidelines accessed on 4/10/07
[a]The numbers in the table indicate the number of times the modality is recommended during the indicated year posttreatment

European Society for Medical Oncology (www.esmo.org)

European Society for Medical Oncology (ESMO) guidelines were accessed on 1/28/12 (Tables 86.9, 86.10, 86.11, 86.12,

Table 86.7 Testicular cancer: nonseminoma with RPLND only

	Years posttreatment[a]					
	1	2	3	4	5	>5
Office visit	4–6	4–6	2–4	2	1–2	1
Markers	4–6	4–6	2–4	2	1–2	1
Chest X-ray	4–6	4–6	2–4	2	1–2	1

• Baseline abdominal/pelvic CT scan, as indicated thereafter

Obtained from NCCN (www.nccn.org) on 1-28-12
NCCN guidelines were accessed on 1/28/12. There were major quantitative and qualitative changes compared to the guidelines accessed on 4/10/07
[a]The numbers in the table indicate the number of times the modality is recommended during the indicated year posttreatment

Table 86.8 Testicular cancer: nonseminoma with complete response to chemotherapy and RPLND

	Years posttreatment[a]					
	1	2	3	4	5	>5
Office visit	4–6	4–6	2–4	2	1–2	1
Markers	4–6	4–6	2–4	2	1–2	1
Chest X-ray	4–6	4–6	2–4	2	1–2	1
Abdominal/pelvic CT scan	2	1–2	1	1	1	0[b]

• Baseline abdominal/pelvic CT scan, as indicated thereafter

Obtained from NCCN (www.nccn.org) on 1-28-12
NCCN guidelines were accessed on 1/28/12. There were major quantitative and qualitative changes compared to the guidelines accessed on 4/10/07
[a]The numbers in the table indicate the number of times the modality is recommended during the indicated year posttreatment
[b]As clinically indicated

Table 86.9 Testicular seminoma, Stage I with surveillance only

	Years posttreatment[a]					
	1	2[b]	3	4	5[b]	>5[b]
Office visit	4	4	3	2	2	1
AFP, HCG, LDH	4	4	3	2	2	1
Chest X-ray	2	2	1	1	1	0
CT abdomen	2	2	1	1	1	0

Obtained from ESMO (www.esmo.org) on 1-28-12
ESMO guidelines were accessed on 1/28/12. There were major quantitative and qualitative changes compared to the guidelines accessed on 10/31/07
[a]The numbers in the table indicate the number of times the modality is recommended during the indicated year posttreatment
[b]Determination of late effects: urea and electrolytes, fasting cholesterol (HDL, LDL), triglycerides, fasting glucose, FSH, LH, testosterone

86.13, 86.14, 86.15, and 86.16). There were major quantitative and qualitative changes compared to the guidelines accessed on 10/31/07.

Table 86.10 Testicular seminoma, Stage I with carboplatin

	Years posttreatment[a]					
	1	2[b]	3	4	5[b]	>5[b]
Office visit	4	3	2	2	2	1[c]
AFP, HCG, LDH	4	3	2	2	2	1[c]
Chest X-ray	2	2	2	1	1	1[c]
CT abdomen	2	2	1	0	1	1[c]

Obtained from ESMO (www.esmo.org) on 1-28-12
ESMO guidelines were accessed on 1/28/12. There were major quantitative and qualitative changes compared to the guidelines accessed on 10/31/07
[a]The numbers in the table indicate the number of times the modality is recommended during the indicated year posttreatment
[b]Determination of late effects: urea and electrolytes, fasting cholesterol (HDL, LDL), triglycerides, fasting glucose, FSH, LH, testosterone
[c]Policies vary among countries and hospitals and there is no definitive evidence

Table 86.11 Testicular seminoma, Stage I with radiotherapy

	Years posttreatment[a]					
	1	2[b]	3	4	5[b]	>5[b]
Office visit	4	3	2	2	2	0
AFP, HCG, LDH	4	3	2	2	2	0
Chest X-ray	2	2	2	1	1	0
CT abdomen/pelvis	2	2	1	0	1	0

Obtained from ESMO (www.esmo.org) on 1-28-12
ESMO guidelines were accessed on 1/28/12. There were major quantitative and qualitative changes compared to the guidelines accessed on 10/31/07
[a]The numbers in the table indicate the number of times the modality is recommended during the indicated year posttreatment
[b]Determination of late effects: urea and electrolytes, fasting cholesterol (HDL, LDL), triglycerides, fasting glucose, FSH, LH testosterone

Table 86.12 Testicular seminoma, Stage IIA/B with radiotherapy, chemotherapy

	Years posttreatment[a]					
	1	2[b]	3	4	5[b]	>5[b]
Office visit	4	3	2	2	2	0
AFP, HCG, LDH	4	3	2	2	2	0
Chest X-ray	3	1	1	1	1	0
CT abdomen/pelvis	2	1	0	0	1	0

Obtained from ESMO (www.esmo.org) on 1-28-12
ESMO guidelines were accessed on 1/28/12. There were major quantitative and qualitative changes compared to the guidelines accessed on 10/31/07
[a]The numbers in the table indicate the number of times the modality is recommended during the indicated year posttreatment
[b]Determination of late effects: urea and electrolytes, fasting cholesterol (HDL, LDL), triglycerides, fasting glucose, FSH, LH, testosterone

European Society of Surgical Oncology (www.esso-surgeonline.org)

European Society of Surgical Oncology (ESSO) guidelines were accessed on 1/28/12. No quantitative guidelines exist

Table 86.13 Testicular seminoma, Stage IIC/III (good, intermediate) with chemotherapy

	Years posttreatment[a]					
	1	2[b]	3	4	5[b]	>5[b]
Office visit	6	3	2	2	2	0
AFP, HCG, LDH	6	3	2	2	2	0
Chest X-ray	3	3	1	1	1	0

- CT abdomen/pelvis 1–4× until CR with or without surgery, then according to chest X-ray plan

Obtained from ESMO (www.esmo.org) on 1-28-12
ESMO guidelines were accessed on 1/28/12. There were major quantitative and qualitative changes compared to the guidelines accessed on 10/31/07
[a]The numbers in the table indicate the number of times the modality is recommended during the indicated year posttreatment
[b]Determination of late effects: urea and electrolytes, fasting cholesterol (HDL, LDL), triglycerides, fasting glucose, FSH, LH testosterone

Table 86.14 Testicular nonseminoma, Stage I with surveillance only

	Years posttreatment[a]					
	1	2[b]	3	4	5[b]	>5[b]
Office visit	12	4	3	2	2	0[c]
AFP, HCG, LDH	12	4	3	2	2	0[c]
Chest X-ray	7	4	3	2	2	0[c]
CT abdomen	2	1	0	0	0	0[c]

- Follow-up beyond 5 years is probably relevant to detect late toxicities or secondary cancer for early intervention

Obtained from ESMO (www.esmo.org) on 1-28-12
ESMO guidelines were accessed on 1/28/12. There were major quantitative and qualitative changes compared to the guidelines accessed on 10/31/07
[a]The numbers in the table indicate the number of times the modality is recommended during the indicated year posttreatment
[b]Determination of late effects: urea and electrolytes, fasting cholesterol (HDL, LDL), triglycerides, fasting glucose, FSH, LH, testosterone
[c]Policies vary among countries and hospitals and there is no definitive evidence

Table 86.15 Testicular nonseminoma, Stage I with chemotherapy

	Years posttreatment[a]					
	1	2[b]	3	4	5[b]	>5[b]
Office visit	5	3	2	2	2	0[c]
AFP, HCG, LDH	5	3	2	2	2	0[c]
Chest x-ray	3	1	1	1	1	0[c]
CT abdomen	1	0	0	0	0	0[c]

- Follow-up beyond 5 years is probably relevant to detect late toxicities or secondary cancer for early intervention

Obtained from ESMO (www.esmo.org) on 1-28-12
ESMO guidelines were accessed on 1/28/12. There were major quantitative and qualitative changes compared to the guidelines accessed on 10/31/07
[a]The numbers in the table indicate the number of times the modality is recommended during the indicated year posttreatment
[b]Determination of late effects: urea and electrolytes, fasting cholesterol (HDL, LDL), triglycerides, fasting glucose, FSH, LH testosterone
[c]Policies vary among countries and hospitals and there is no definitive evidence

Table 86.16 Testicular nonseminoma, Stage IIA/B, IIC, III with chemotherapy

	Years posttreatment[a]					
	1	2[b]	3	4	5[b]	>5[b]
Office visit	6	3	2	2	2	0
AFP, HCG, LDH	6	3	2	2	2	0
Chest x-ray	3	3	1	1	1	0

- CT abdomen/pelvis 1–4× with or without surgery, then according to chest X-ray plan
- Follow-up beyond 5 years is probably relevant to detect late toxicities or secondary cancer for early intervention

Obtained from ESMO (www.esmo.org) on 1-28-12
ESMO guidelines were accessed on 1/28/12. There were major quantitative and qualitative changes compared to the guidelines accessed on 10/31/07
[a]The numbers in the table indicate the number of times the modality is recommended during the indicated year posttreatment
[b]Determination of late effects: urea and electrolytes, fasting cholesterol (HDL, LDL), triglycerides, fasting glucose, FSH, LH testosterone

for testicular cancer surveillance including when first accessed on 10/31/07.

Cancer Care Ontario (www.cancercare.on.ca)

Cancer Care Ontario (CCO) guidelines were accessed on 1/28/12 (Table 86.17). There are new quantitative guidelines compared to the inactive quantitative guidelines accessed on 10/31/07.

National Institute for Clinical Excellence (www.nice.org.uk)

National Institute for Clinical Excellence (NICE) guidelines were accessed on 1/28/12. No quantitative guidelines exist for testicular cancer surveillance including when first accessed on 10/31/07.

The Cochrane Collaboration (CC, www.cochrane.org)

CC guidelines were accessed on 1/28/12. No quantitative guidelines exist for testicular cancer surveillance including when first accessed on 11/24/07.

American Urological Association (www.auanet.org)

American Urological Association (AUA) guidelines were accessed on 1/28/12. No quantitative guidelines exist for

Table 86.17 Stage I seminoma

	Years posttreatment[a]					
	1	2	3	4	5	>5
Office visit[b]	3–4	3–4	3–4	<4	<4	<4
Chest X-ray[c]	1–2	1–2	1–2	<2	<2	<2
CT of abdomen, pelvis[d]	3–4	3–4	3–4	<4	<4	<4

- Follow-up should include appropriate investigations of sites at risk of relapse[e]
- When a primary surveillance approach is adopted, patients should be informed of their estimated risk of recurrence and the need for frequent surveillance

Obtained from CCO (www.cancercare.on.ca) on 1-28-12
CCO guidelines were accessed on 1/28/12. These are new quantitative guidelines compared to the qualitative guidelines accessed on 10/31/07
[a]The numbers in the table indicate the number of times the modality is recommended during the indicated year posttreatment
[b]Physical examination every 3–4 months in the first 3 years and then less often thereafter
[c]Chest X-ray every 6–12 months in the first 3 years and then less often thereafter
[d]CT of the abdomen and pelvis every 3–4 months in the first 3 years and then less often thereafter
[e]This approach can be based on the risk of relapse with the frequency as suggested in the evidence-based guidelines outlined by Martin et al. (Martin JM, Panzarella T, Zwahlen DR, Chung P, Warde P. Evidence-based guidelines for following stage I seminoma. Cancer. 2007;109(11): 2248–56.)

testicular cancer surveillance including when first accessed on 12/13/07.

The M.D. Anderson Surgical Oncology Handbook also has follow-up guidelines, proposed by authors from a single National Cancer Institute-designated Comprehensive Cancer Center, for many types of cancer [7]. Some are detailed and quantitative, others are qualitative.

Summary

This is a relatively uncommon cancer with significant variability in incidence worldwide. We found consensus-based guidelines but none based on high-quality evidence.

References

1. Parkin DM, Whelan SL, Ferlay J, Teppo L, Thomas DB. Cancer incidence in five continents, Vol. VIII, International Agency for Research on Cancer. (IARC Scientific Publication 155). Lyon, France: IARC Press; 2002. ISBN 92-832-2155-9.
2. Jemal A, Seigel R, Ward E, Murray T, Xu J, Thun MJ. Cancer statistics, 2007. CA Cancer J Clin. 2007;57:43–66.
3. Schottenfeld D, Fraumeni JG. Cancer epidemiology and prevention. 3rd ed. New York, NY: Oxford University Press; 2006. ISBN 13:978-0-19-514961-6.
4. DeVita VT, Hellman S, Rosenberg SA. Cancer. 7th ed. Philadelphia, PA: Lippincott Williams & Wilkins; 2005. ISBN 0-781-74450-4.
5. Mackay J, Jemal A, Lee NC, Parkin M. The Cancer Atlas. 2006 American Cancer Society 1599 Clifton Road NE, Atlanta, Georgia 30329, USA. Can also be accessed at www.cancer.org. ISBN 0-944235-62-X.
6. Devesa SS, Grauman DJ, Blot WJ, Pennello GA, Hoover RN, Fraumeni JF Jr. Atlas of Cancer Mortality in the United States. National Institutes of Health, National Cancer Institute. NIH Publication No. 99–4564; Sep 1999.
7. Feig BW, Berger DH, Fuhrman GM. The M.D. Anderson Surgical Oncology Handbook. 4th ed. Philadelphia, PA: Lippincott Williams & Wilkins; 2006. ISBN 0-7817-5643-X (paperback).

87 Testicle Carcinoma Surveillance Counterpoint: USA

Ian M. Thompson III and Sam S. Chang

Keywords
Testicular cancer • Seminoma • Nonseminomatous germ cell tumor (NSGCT) • Teratoma • Yolk sac tumor • Alpha fetoprotein AFP • Beta-HCG • Embryonal cell carcinoma • Retroperitoneal lymph node dissection (RPLND)

Testis cancer remains the most common solid tumor in males 20–35 years of age and accounts for approximately 1% of cancer cases in males. For unclear reasons, overall incidence has increased from 3.7/100,000 in 1975 to 5.4/100,000 in 2001 [1]. Fortunately, in the face of this trend, improved treatment success has resulted in a significant reduction in the mortality rate. In 2008, there were an estimated 8,000 new cases and 380 deaths from testis cancer in the United States [2]. The 5-year survival rate has increased from 83% in the 1970s to 96% by the end of the twentieth century due to the improvement in treatment [2].

We acknowledge the chapter introduction and the current institutional guidelines it cites. In addition to discussing our approach to surveillance, we have also expounded upon the background of this disease process to better contextualize current recommendations. The level of evidence in the literature regarding surveillance is somewhat lacking, though we feel our approach adequately addresses the surveillance needs for each stage/pathology of testis cancer while also being mindful of the patient's compliance with these regimens. Most patients are in fact agreeable and compliant with these treatment plans and surveillance strategies. As with all disease processes, patient education throughout the treatment process is essential.

Certain disease characteristics have aided in diagnosis and treatment. These include production of specific tumor markers, sensitivity to irradiation and chemotherapy, predictable pattern of spread from primary site, and the fact that most cases occur in younger, healthier men with few comorbidities who can tolerate treatments with potential side effects [3, 4]. Common to all types of germ cell tumor is the sequential and predictable lymphatic spread from the primary site to retroperitoneal lymph nodes. Understanding this lymphatic drainage has helped establish clinical staging paradigms and surveillance focused on the most common sites of spread of disease. Simplistically, the right testis drains to nodes in the interaortocaval region and has a tendency to spread to the contralateral left side, whereas left-sided tumors drain to the paraaortic and preaortic lymph nodes and are rarely associated with spread to contralateral (right) side [4–6].

Initial treatment of a suspected testis tumor includes radical inguinal orchiectomy. There is, historically, and for good reason, no role for transscrotal biopsy of a suspected testis tumor as this can disrupt normal lymphatic drainage of the testes and increase the rate of local recurrence [7]. Radical orchiectomy provides histopathological diagnosis, allows characterization of the tumor for TNM classification, is associated with minimal morbidity, and achieves excellent local control of the tumor [3, 5].

Histopathologic features of the orchiectomy specimen, such as presence of vascular or lymphatic invasion, presence or absence of certain histologic-tumor subtypes, and extent of tumor, yield prognostic information and assist in formulating appropriate management [8–11]. In addition, measurement of serum levels of tumor markers beta-HCG, alpha-fetoprotein, and lactate dehydrogenase provides essential staging and prognostic information and, if possible, should be done prior

I.M. Thompson III, M.D. • S.S. Chang, M.D. (✉)
Department of Urologic Surgery, Vanderbilt University Medical Center and Vanderbilt-Ingram Cancer Center, Nashville, TN 37232, USA
e-mail: ian.thompson@vanderbilt.edu; sam.chang@vanderbilt.edu

F.E. Johnson et al. (eds.), *Patient Surveillance After Cancer Treatment*, Current Clinical Oncology,
DOI 10.1007/978-1-60327-969-7_87, © Springer Science+Business Media New York 2013

to or at the time of orchiectomy. Continued elevation of tumor markers following radical orchiectomy often indicates either clinically evident or occult metastatic disease that should prompt further evaluation and systemic therapy [12]. Further evaluation should include physical examination and imaging of the abdomen, retroperitoneum, and chest. CT scan of the abdomen and pelvis, with sensitivity nearing 80%, is the primary imaging modality used to evaluate retroperitoneal lymph nodes [4, 5, 13, 14]. Posteroanterior and lateral chest radiographs are preferred for initial imaging of the chest as CT of the chest is highly sensitive, delineating lesions as small as 2 mm, of which 70% are benign [4]. In high-risk patients or if any abnormality is noted on chest X-ray, CT scan of the chest should be performed.

For all patients, it is essential to emphasize monthly self-examinations of the contralateral testis. In addition, the need, merits, and cost of sperm-banking are also discussed prior to any treatment choice.

Table 87.1 Surveillance after curative-intent treatment for patients with Stage I NSGCT at Vanderbilt-Ingram Cancer Center

	Year posttreatment					
Modality	1	2	3	4	5	>5
Office visit	12	6	4	3	2	1
Serum tumor marker levels	12	6	4	3	2	1
Chest X-ray	12	6	4	3	2	1
CT scan abdomen/pelvis	4	3	2	2	2	1

Tumor markers: alpha fetoprotein, beta-HCG, lactic dehydrogenase
The number in each cell is the number of times a particular surveillance modality is recommended in a particular posttreatment year

Table 87.2 Surveillance after curative-intent treatment for patients with Stage I NSGCT and pathologic Stage IIa after RPLND at Vanderbilt-Ingram Cancer Center

	Year posttreatment					
Modality	1	2	3	4	5	>5
Office visit	6	4	3	2	2	1
Serum tumor marker levels	6	4	3	2	2	1
Chest X-ray	6	4	3	2	2	1
CT scan abdomen/pelvis	1[a]	1	0	0	0	0

Tumor markers: alpha fetoprotein, beta-HCG, lactic dehydrogenase
The number in each cell is the number of times a particular surveillance modality is recommended in a particular posttreatment year
[a]Baseline, ~3 months after RPLND

Stage I Nonseminoma Germ Cell Tumors

In the United States, the current management options for clinical stage I nonseminoma germ cell tumors (NSGCT) following radical orchiectomy include retroperitoneal lymph node dissection (RPLND) and surveillance and, much less commonly, two cycles of bleomycin-etoposide-cisplatin chemotherapy [15]. There is some controversy regarding the optimal management of patients with stage I NSGCT as there are no prospective randomized control trials comparing these treatment options, and there have been reported >97% cure rates with RPLND or surveillance [15]. Adjuvant radiation therapy is not often used in treatment of stage I NSGCT in the United States [4].

The preferred treatment modality varies, based on disease and patient characteristics, and subsequent surveillance regimens differ. Patients with significant embryonal carcinoma component in the primary tumor, invasion of the epididymis or tunica albuginea, and/or presence of vascular or lymphatic invasion are at increased risk of relapse [9, 11]. These men should undergo RPLND, which provides not only further staging information regarding nodal status but also may be therapeutic with low volume disease. It also facilitates surveillance requirements by decreasing and even eliminating the need to frequently evaluate the abdomen by CT scans. Historically, the most important long-term complication of bilateral RPLND has been ejaculatory dysfunction and resulting infertility [5, 16]. The modified template RPLND approach and the nerve-sparing approach have significantly increased the likelihood of preserving ejaculatory function [17].

RPLND provides important staging information but patients followed in surveillance protocols after orchiectomy are understaged ~25% of the time. Conversely, ~70% of patients who undergo RPLND are found to have no nodal disease and therefore, theoretically, there is no therapeutic benefit [4]. However, as emphasized, RPLND provides important pathologic and staging information and decreases the complexity of surveillance by virtually eliminating the retroperitoneum as a site of relapse. Careful monitoring is required of patients in surveillance protocols, though Hao et al. demonstrated a compliance rate of 61% and 35% in the first and second years, respectively, in patients with clinical stage I NSGCT undergoing postorchiectomy surveillance [18]. These statistics are somewhat sobering, especially in the light of the fact that approximately 25–30% of patients will have disease recurrence, and that this most often occurs in the first 2 years [19]. It has been demonstrated that there is no significant economic advantage to either surveillance, primary chemotherapy, or RPLND [20].

Although not commonly accepted practice in the United States, several studies have demonstrated the success in treating patients with stage I NSGCT with two cycles of cisplatin-based combination chemotherapy; these studies have shown long-term survival rates of 95–100% [21–23]. True concern exists regarding the incidence and impact of late recurrences, as this regimen has not had long-term use. In addition, although a lower dose of chemotherapy is used, the possible overtreatment of the majority of patients is concerning. Further long-term evaluation will be necessary before this treatment paradigm can be accepted as safe and efficacious (see Tables 87.1 and 87.2).

Our surveillance recommendations match those put forth by the NCCN (Table 87.5 in the primary chapter). Compared to the ESMO recommendations, as demonstrated in Table 87.1, over the course of the 5-year surveillance period, we see these patients back slightly more frequently and continue to obtain CT scans throughout this period. The rationale is that tumor burden at recurrence can affect treatment success although recurrence is uncommon. We agree with the guidelines for stage I NSGCT surveillance espoused by Cancer Care Ontario (Table 87.2), although we recommend patient evaluation after year 5. This can be done by the patient's primary care physician.

Clinical and Pathologic Stage II NSGCT

Stage II NSGCT is defined as disease that has spread from the primary tumor to the retroperitoneum and is further divided into IIa (nodes <2 cm), IIb (nodes 2–5 cm), and IIc (nodes >5 cm). For Stage IIa and IIb tumors, RPLND has traditionally been the initial treatment approach as this yields further pathologic information and can direct subsequent therapy, if needed [24, 25]. Post-RPLND, chemotherapy may or may not be administered in patients with small volume pathologic Stage II disease. Williams and associates demonstrated a relapse rate of 49% in patients found to have any positive nodes who were observed after RPLND, though only ~6% of patients who received two postoperative cycles of chemotherapy relapsed [26]. Thus, the decision for these patients lies in weighing the morbidity of the chemotherapy vs. the inconvenience and expense of strict surveillance protocols.

Patients with clinical Stages IIa and IIb disease may benefit from primary chemotherapy, and, although philosophical differences exist among experts, in certain instances RPLND can be avoided [27]. Primary chemotherapy, as opposed to RPLND, is the treatment of choice for patients with clinical stage IIc disease (see Table 87.3).

As demonstrated, for those with Stage II NSGCT who have received RPLND with or without chemotherapy afterwards, we obtain CT of the abdomen/pelvis at year 1 after treatment and then elect to obtain subsequent CT imaging on an as-needed basis. This is a departure from the NCCN recommendations, but in line with those of ESMO. The likelihood of in-field retroperitoneal recurrences following a properly performed RPLND is low.

Clinical Stage III NSGCT

Patients with clinical stage III disease have significantly varied responses to primary chemotherapy. Therefore, patients are further classified as either low-risk (good prognosis), intermediate risk, or high-risk (poor prognosis) [28]. Characteristics of poor prognosis disease include nonseminomatous disease with a mediastinal primary, nonpulmonary visceral metastases, and/or significantly elevated serum tumor marker levels [28]. The therapeutic goal in low-risk patients is to achieve high cure rates while minimizing toxicity related to the treatment. Surveillance for these patients is outlined in Table 87.4.

Pure seminomas represent ~40% of germ cell tumors [29]. Seminomas are further classified as typical or classic seminoma (82–85%), anaplastic seminoma (5–15%), and spermatocytic seminoma (2–12%) [4]. Historically, the approach to treating low-stage seminoma has been adjuvant radiation therapy following inguinal orchiectomy.

Table 87.3 Surveillance after curative-intent RPLND/chemotherapy for patients with pathologic Stage III NSGCT at Vanderbilt-Ingram Cancer Center

	Year posttreatment					
Modality	1	2	3	4	5	>5
Office visit	4	3	2	2	2	1
Serum tumor marker levels	4	3	2	2	2	1
Chest X-ray	4	3	2	2	2	1
CT scan abdomen/pelvis	1	0	0	0	0	0

Tumor markers: alpha fetoprotein, beta-HCG, lactic dehydrogenase
The number in each cell is the number of times a particular surveillance modality is recommended in a particular posttreatment year

Table 87.4 Surveillance after curative-intent treatment for patients with Stage III NSGCT after chemotherapy with complete response at Vanderbilt-Ingram Cancer Center

	Year posttreatment					
Modality	1	2	3	4	5	>5
Office visit	4	3	2	2	2	1
Serum tumor marker levels	4	3	2	2	2	1
Chest X-ray	4	3	2	2	2	1
CT scan abdomen/pelvis	1	0	0	0	0	0

Tumor markers: alpha fetoprotein, beta-HCG, lactic dehydrogenase
The number in each cell is the number of times a particular surveillance modality is recommended in a particular posttreatment year

Stage I Seminoma

In Stage I seminoma, primary radiation therapy has historically been favored as the treatment of choice. Irradiation of the paraaortic and ipsilateral iliac lymph nodes, also known as "dog-leg" configuration, is typical and usually 25–35 Gy is administered [30]. Multiple studies have demonstrated 5-year survival rates of >94% for those treated with radiation therapy for stage I seminoma [31, 32]. The risk of developing second malignancies after radiation therapy is higher than that of age-matched controls [33]. Recently, a randomized trial comparing single-dose carbo-

Table 87.5 Surveillance after curative-intent treatment for patients with Stage I seminoma at Vanderbilt-Ingram Cancer Center

	Year posttreatment					
Modality	1	2	3	4	5	>5
Office visit	4	4	4	2	2	1
Serum tumor marker levels	4	4	4	2	2	1
Chest X-ray	4	4	4	2	2	1
CT scan abdomen/pelvis	4	4	4	2	2	1

Tumor markers: alpha fetoprotein, beta-HCG, lactic dehydrogenase
The number in each cell is the number of times a particular surveillance modality is recommended in a particular posttreatment year

Table 87.6 Surveillance after curative-intent treatment for patients with Stage I seminoma following surgery and radiation therapy at Vanderbilt-Ingram Cancer Center

	Year posttreatment					
Modality	1	2	3	4	5	>5
Office visit	4	3	2	1	1	1
Serum tumor marker levels	4	3	2	1	1	1
Chest X-ray	4	3	2	1	1	1
CT scan abdomen/pelvis	1	1	1	0	0	0

Tumor markers: alpha fetoprotein, beta-HCG, lactic dehydrogenase
The number in each cell is the number of times a particular surveillance modality is recommended in a particular posttreatment year

platin chemotherapy and radiation therapy after orchiectomy in patients with stage I seminoma demonstrated 5-year relapse rates of 5.3% for carboplatin and 4% for radiation. The authors of this study also demonstrated decreased acute toxicity with the single-dose carboplatin compared to radiotherapy [34, 35]. Over the past two decades there has been increased interest in surveillance. Approximately 17% of patients with stage I seminoma who do not receive adjuvant therapy relapse during mean follow-up period of 53 months, with median time to relapse of 15 months [4, 19, 36, 37]. Prognostic factors for relapse in patients with stage I seminoma managed with surveillance only include size of primary tumor and invasion of the rete testis [38]. Recent studies have shown a nearly 100% survival rate in stage I seminoma whether radiation or surveillance (and treatment at relapse) is chosen [39] (see Tables 87.5 and 87.6).

Our surveillance strategy for stage I seminoma after orchiectomy (Table 87.5) is in line with that recommended by NCCN, but we recommend more frequent imaging with CT than the surveillance schedule put forth by ESMO. Surveillance for stage I seminoma after radiation therapy requires less frequent imaging, as can be seen in Table 87.6. This is essentially consistent with the guidelines from both NCCN and ESMO. This is due to the treatment of the retroperitoneum that allows focus primarily on the chest and serum tumor marker levels.

Stage II Seminoma

In patients with minimal retroperitoneal disease, seminoma has been historically treated with radiation therapy to the ipsilateral external iliac, bilateral common iliac, paracaval, and paraaortic lymph nodes [4]. The radiated area should also include the contralateral inguinal region in cases when patient has history of orchiopexy or inguinal hernia repair, as these can potentially alter normal lymphatic drainage [4]. In patients with retroperitoneal node disease in close proximity to the kidney, radiation is often avoided due to renal toxicity, and chemotherapy is the treatment of choice [4].

Stage III Seminoma

In patients with advanced disease, cisplatin-based chemotherapy is regarded as first-line treatment and surgery or radiation is utilized for treatment failures [4]. After treatment with chemotherapy, many patients are not clear of radiographic masses on CT, often representing residual necrosis or fibrosis [4]. Among patients with advanced seminoma treated with chemotherapy, ~30% of those with residual mass >3 cm will have viable tumor within the residual retroperitoneal masses, and therefore we recommend resection when residual lesions >3 cm [40].

References

1. Sokoloff MH, Joyce GF, Wise M. Testis cancer. J Urol. 2007;177:2030–41.
2. Jemal A, Siegel R, Ward E, et al. Cancer statistics, 2008. CA Cancer J Clin. 2008;58:71–96.
3. Whitmore Jr WF. Surgical treatment of clinical stage I nonseminomatous germ gell tumors of the testis. Cancer Treat Rep. 1982; 66:5–10.
4. Richie JP. Neoplasms of the testis. In: Wein AJ, Kavoussi LR, Novick AC, Partin AW, Peters CA, editors. Campbell-Walsh urology. 9th ed. Philadelphia, PA: Saunders Elsevier; 2007. p. 893–935.
5. Sheinfeld J. Nonseminomatous germ cell tumors of the testis: current concepts and controversies. Urology. 1994;44:2–14.
6. Sogani PC. Evolution of the management of stage I nonseminomatous germ-cell tumors of the testis. Urol Clin North Am. 1991;18:561–73.
7. Capelouto CC, Clark PE, Ransil BJ, Loughlin KR. A review of scrotal violation in testicular cancer: is adjuvant local therapy necessary? J Urol. 1995;153(3 Pt 2):981–5.
8. Javadpour N, Young Jr JD. Prognostic factors in nonseminomatous testicular cancer. J Urol. 1986;135:497–9.
9. Freedman LS, Parkinson MC, Jones WG, et al. Histopathology in the prediction of relapse of patients with stage I testicular teratoma treated by orchidectomy alone. Lancet. 1987;2(8554):294–8.
10. Moriyama N, Daly JJ, Keating MA, Lin CW, Prout Jr GR. Vascular invasion as a prognosticator of metastatic disease in nonseminomatous germ cell tumors of the testis. Importance in "surveillance only" protocols. Cancer. 1985;56:2492–8.

11. Moul JW, McCarthy WF, Fernandez EB, Sesterhenn IA. Percentage of embryonal carcinoma and of vascular invasion predicts pathological stage in clinical stage I nonseminomatous testicular cancer. Cancer Res. 1994;54:362–4.
12. Lange PH, Raghaven D. Clinical applications of tumor markers in testicular cancer (Chapter 6). In: Donohue JP, editor. The management of testicular cancer. Baltimore, MD: Williams & Wilkins; 1983. p. 111–30.
13. Husband JE, Peckham MJ, Macdonald JS, Hendry WF. The role of computed tomography in the management of testicular teratoma. Clin Radiol. 1979;30:243–52.
14. Lien HH, Stenwig AE, Ous S, Fosså SD. Influence of different criteria for abnormal lymph node size on reliability of computed tomography in patients with non-seminomatous testicular tumor. Acta Radiol Diagn (Stockh). 1986;27:199–203.
15. Stephenson AJ, Sheinfeld J. Management of patients with low-stage nonseminomatous germ cell testicular cancer. Curr Treat Options Oncol. 2005;6:367–77.
16. Lange PH, Chang WY, Fraley EE. Fertility issues in the therapy of nonseminomatous testicular tumors. Urol Clin North Am. 1987;14:731–47.
17. Jewett MA, Torbey C. Nerve-sparing techniques in retroperitoneal lymphadenectomy in patients with low-stage testicular cancer. Semin Urol. 1988;6:233–7.
18. Hao D, Seidel J, Brant R, et al. Compliance of clinical stage I nonseminomatous germ cell tumor patients with surveillance. J Urol. 1998;160(3 Pt 1):768–71.
19. Sternberg CN. The management of stage I testis cancer. Urol Clin North Am. 1998;25:435–49.
20. Lashley DB, Lowe BA. A rational approach to managing stage I nonseminomatous germ cell cancer. Urol Clin North Am. 1998; 25:405–23.
21. Madej G, Pawinski A. Risk-related adjuvant chemotherapy for stage I non-seminoma of the testis. Clin Oncol (R Coll Radiol). 1991;3:270–2.
22. Cullen MH, Stenning SP, Parkinson MC, et al. Short-course adjuvant chemotherapy in high-risk stage I nonseminomatous germ cell tumors of the testis: a Medical Research Council report. J Clin Oncol. 1996;14:1106–13.
23. Oliver RT, Raja MA, Ong J, Gallagher CJ. Pilot study to evaluate impact of a policy of adjuvant chemotherapy for high risk stage 1 malignant teratoma on overall relapse rate of stage 1 cancer patients. J Urol. 1992;148:1453–55; discussion 1455–56.
24. Bredael JJ, Vugrin D, Whitmore Jr WF. Selected experience with surgery and combination chemotherapy in the treatment of nonseminomatous testis tumors. J Urol. 1983;129:985–8.
25. Walsh PC, Kaufman JJ, Coulson WF, Goodwin WE. Retroperitoneal lymphadenectomy for testicular tumors. JAMA. 1971;217: 309–12.
26. Williams SD, Stablein DM, Einhorn LH, et al. Immediate adjuvant chemotherapy versus observation with treatment at relapse in pathological stage II testicular cancer. N Engl J Med. 1987;317: 1433–8.
27. Horwich A, Norman A, Fisher C, Hendry WF, Nicholls J, Dearnaley DP . Primary chemotherapy for stage II nonseminomatous germ cell tumors of the testis. J Urol. 1994;151:72–7; discussion 77–8.
28. International Germ Cell Cancer Collaborative Group. International Germ Cell Consensus Classification: a prognostic factor-based staging system for metastatic germ cell cancers. J Clin Oncol. 1997;15:594–603.
29. Huddart R, Kataja V. Testicular seminoma: ESMO clinical recommendations for diagnosis, treatment and follow-up. Ann Oncol. 2008;19 Suppl 2:ii49–51.
30. Stephenson AJ. Current treatment options for clinical stage I seminoma. World J Urol. 2009;27:427–32.
31. Dosoretz DE, Shipley WU, Blitzer PH, et al. Megavoltage irradiation for pure testicular seminoma: results and patterns of failure. Cancer. 1981;48:2184–90.
32. Thomas GM, Rider WD, Dembo AJ, et al. Seminoma of the testis: results of treatment and patterns of failure after radiation therapy. Int J Radiat Oncol Biol Phys. 1982;8:165–74.
33. Travis LB, Curtis RE, Storm H, et al. Risk of second malignant neoplasms among long-term survivors of testicular cancer. J Natl Cancer Inst. 1997;89:1429–39.
34. Feldman DR, Bosl GJ. Treatment of stage I seminoma: is it time to change your practice? J Hematol Oncol. 2008;1:22.
35. Oliver RT, Oliver MD, Mead GM, et al. Radiotherapy versus single-dose carboplatin in adjuvant treatment of stage I seminoma: a randomised trial. Lancet. 2005;366:293–300.
36. Allhoff EP, Liedke S, de Riese W, Stief C, Schneider B, et al. Stage I seminoma of the testis. Adjuvant radiotherapy or surveillance? Br J Urol. 1991;68:190–4.
37. Horwich A, Alsanjari N, A'Hern R, Nicholls J, Dearnaley DP, Fisher C. Surveillance following orchidectomy for stage I testicular seminoma. Br J Cancer. 1992;65:775–8.
38. Warde P, Specht L, Horwich A, et al. Prognostic factors for relapse in stage I seminoma managed by surveillance: a pooled analysis. J Clin Oncol. 2002;20:4448–52.
39. Warde P, Jewett MA. Surveillance for stage I testicular seminoma. Is it a good option? Urol Clin North Am. 1998;25:425–33.
40. Herr HW, Sheinfeld J, Puc HS, et al. Surgery for a post-chemotherapy residual mass in seminoma. J Urol. 1997;157:860–2.

Testicle Carcinoma Surveillance Counterpoint: Australia

88

Michael Boyer and Kate Mahon

Keywords
Testicular germ cell tumours • Testes • Relapse • Male • NSGCT

Testicular germ cell tumours are the most common solid organ malignancies in young adult males between 20 and 40 years of age. The availability of potentially curative multimodality treatment, even in the context of metastatic disease, underscores the need for carefully considered surveillance protocols to detect early relapse.

Pure seminoma comprises approximately 50% of all germ cell tumours. Most (70%) present with clinical stage I disease [1]. For over 60 years, following orchiectomy, adjuvant extended field radiotherapy was considered standard treatment. The aim of radiotherapy was to eradicate occult para-aortic and inguinal nodal disease which causes the majority of relapses. This provided a >95% relapse-free rate and 99% overall survival probability. However, following the first published reports of surveillance in 1992, the issue of unnecessary treatment in the majority of patients was raised. This series of 103 patients with stage I seminoma post-orchiectomy undergoing surveillance revealed an 82% 5-year relapse-free survival probability with a 5-year overall survival probability in excess of 95% [2]. Since then, consensus regarding the need for adjuvant treatment or the form it will take has not been reached. The management options in this setting include surveillance alone, extended field radiotherapy, para-aortic radiotherapy and chemotherapy.

M. Boyer (✉)
Department of Medical Oncology, Sydney Cancer Centre, Royal Prince Alfred Hospital, Missenden Road, Camperdown, NSW 2050, Australia
e-mail: michael.boyer@lifehouserpa.org.au

K. Mahon
Garvan Institute, Sydney, NSW, Australia
e-mail: drkatemahon@gmail.com

While the risk of relapse following radical inguinal orchiectomy and high division of the spermatic cord is less than 20%, two main risk factors have been identified. Rete testis invasion and tumour size >4 cm are both independently associated with a higher rate of relapse. The risk of relapse is 12, 15 and >30% with 0, 1 and 2 risk factors, respectively [3]. These features may be helpful in guiding adjuvant treatment strategies though evidence from randomised trials for using this statification does not exist (Table 88.1).

Knowledge of the usual pattern of timing and first site of relapse helps in developing an appropriate surveillance protocol. Over 70% of relapses occur within 2 years post-diagnosis, but extended follow-up is required as up to 6.6% of relapses were seen after 6 years in a pooled analysis [3]. Anecdotal reports of first relapses occurring over 10 years from diagnosis have been published but a population-based study revealed this risk to be less than 0.5% [4]. At diagnosis of relapse, almost half of patients are asymptomatic and approximately 30% have elevated serum tumour markers [5]. Following surveillance alone, the vast majority of patients recur with abdominopelvic disease (15.5%) while only 0.5% relapse in the chest (pulmonary or mediastinal). Palpable lymph nodes are present in only 1.4% of patients with relapse [6]. In contrast, after adjuvant radiotherapy the overall risk of recurrence is around 5% with the majority of relapses occurring in the chest (1.8% failure risk) following extended field radiotherapy. After para-aortic radiotherapy, the risk of failure is similar but more relapses occur in the pelvis (1.9% failure risk) [6]. The use of adjuvant single agent carboplatin was shown to be non-inferior to radiotherapy in a large randomised trial in 2005 [7]. While relapse rates were similar (3-year relapse-free survival probability 95.9% vs. 94.8%, radiotherapy vs. carboplatin, respectively), the pattern of relapse was markedly different. The majority of relapses post-chemother-

F.E. Johnson et al. (eds.), *Patient Surveillance After Cancer Treatment*, Current Clinical Oncology,
DOI 10.1007/978-1-60327-969-7_88,

Table 88.1 Surveillance after curative-intent initial therapy (orchiectomy only) for patients with stage I seminoma at the Sydney Cancer Centre

	Years post-treatment					
Modality	1	2	3	4	5	>5
Office visit and serum tumour marker levels[a]	6	6	3	2	2	2
CXR	2	3	2	2	1	1
CT chest-abdomen-pelvis	4	3	1	0	1	1

The number in each cell is the number of times a particular modality is recommended in a particular post-treatment year
[a]AFP, beta HCG, LDH

Table 88.2 Surveillance after curative-intent initial therapy (orchiectomy + carboplatin) for patients with stage I seminoma at the Sydney Cancer Centre

	Years post-treatment					
Modality	1	2	3	4	5	>5
Office visit and serum tumour marker levels[a]	4	3	2	1	1	1
CXR	2	1	2	1	0	1
CT chest-abdomen-pelvis	1	1	1	0	1	0

The number in each cell is the number of times a particular modality is recommended in a particular post-treatment year
[a]AFP, beta HCG, LDH

Table 88.3 Surveillance after curative-intent initial therapy (orchiectomy + para-aortic radiotherapy) for patients with stage I seminoma at the Sydney Cancer Centre

	Years post-treatment					
Modality	1	2	3	4	5	>5
Office visit	2	2	2	1	1	1
Serum tumour marker levels[a]	2	2	2	0	0	0
CXR	1	1	1	1	1	1
CT pelvis	1	1	1	0	1	0

The number in each cell is the number of times a particular modality is recommended in a particular post-treatment year
[a]AFP, beta HCG, LDH

Table 88.4 Surveillance after curative-intent initial therapy (orchiectomy + extended-field radiotherapy) for patients with stage I seminoma at the Sydney Cancer Centre

	Years post-treatment					
Modality	1	2	3	4	5	>5
Office visit	2	2	2	1	1	1
Serum tumour marker levels[a]	2	2	2	0	0	0
CXR	1	1	1	1	1	1

[a]AFP, beta HCG, LDH
The number in each cell is the number of times a particular modality is recommended in a particular post-treatment year.

Table 88.5 Surveillance after curative-intent initial therapy (orchiectomy + platinum-based chemotherapy and/or radiotherapy) for patients with stage ≥ II seminoma at the Sydney Cancer Centre

	Years post-treatment					
Modality	1	2	3	4	5	>5
Office visit and serum tumour marker levels[a]	6	4	3	2	2	1
CXR	4	2	2	1	1	1
CT chest-abdomen-pelvis	2	2	1	1	1	0

[a]AFP, beta HCG, LDH
The number in each cell is the number of times a particular modality is recommended in a particular post-treatment year

apy occurred in para-aortic lymph nodes while most of the relapses after radiotherapy occurred in pelvic or supra-diaphragmatic nodal regions [7]. A recent update of long-term follow-up of these patients suggests that relapses after 5 years are rare and extended follow-up of patients who have received adjuvant treatment is not necessary [8]. Surveillance protocols must therefore be tailored to the adjuvant modality employed, as both frequency and site of relapse are heavily influenced by this factor (Tables 88.2, 88.3, 88.4).

Following a systematic review of prospective studies in stage I seminoma, it has been suggested that surveillance programs be developed according to the risk of relapse. Martin et al. advocate 4 monthly follow-up visits while the annual risk is over 5%, 6 monthly follow-up visits when the annual risk is 1–5%, annual follow-up if the annual risk is 0.3–1% and cessation of surveillance when the risk falls below 0.3% [6]. Clinical examination is included in every review while appropriate imaging is performed depending on the adjuvant treatment modality utilised (Tables 88.2, 88.3, 88.4).

Less than 20% of patients with seminoma present with more advanced disease (stage II, III) and, following treatment with chemotherapy and/or radiotherapy, there is little evidence to guide surveillance (Table 88.5). Due to small patient numbers there is wide variation in reported relapse rates with up to 25% risk of relapse following treatment. Relapses most commonly occur in the chest, particularly in those patients who have had para-aortic radiotherapy included in their primary treatment [9]. Relapses usually occur early and are rare more than 3 years following treatment [10].

Non-seminomatous germ cell tumours (NSGCT), including seminoma histology with elevated serum alpha fetoprotein levels, comprise around 50% of testicular tumours. Most have mixed elements that may include embryonal carcinoma, choriocarcinoma, yolk sac tumour, teratoma and seminoma. Around 50% of patients present with stage I disease.

With the introduction of cisplatin in the 1970s, NSGCT became curable, even in the presence of disseminated disease. Prior to this, adjuvant treatment following orchidectomy involved retroperitoneal lymph node dissection with the possible addition of radiotherapy for node-positive disease. This treatment was associated with significant

Table 88.6 Surveillance after curative-intent initial therapy (orchiectomy only) for patients with stage I non-seminoma germ cell tumour at the Sydney Cancer Centre.

	Years post-treatment					
Modality	1	2	3	4	5	>5
Office visit and serum tumour marker levels[a]	6	6	3	2	2	0
CXR	2	3	2	2	1	0
CT chest-abdomen-pelvis	4	3	1	0	1	0

The number in each cell is the number of times a particular modality is recommended in a particular post-treatment year

[a]AFP, beta HCG, LDH

Table 88.7 Surveillance after curative-intent initial therapy (orchiectomy + platinum-based chemotherapy) for patients with stage I non-seminoma germ cell tumour at the Sydney Cancer Centre

	Years post-treatment					
Modality	1	2	3	4	5	>5
Office visit and serum tumour marker levels[a]	4	2	2	1	1	0
CXR	2	1	1	1	0	0
CT chest-abdomen-pelvis	2	1	1	0	1	0

[a]AFP, beta HCG, LDH

The number in each cell is the number of times a particular modality is recommended in a particular post-treatment year

morbidity. Since then, post-orchiectomy surveillance with salvage chemotherapy at relapse has been investigated and shown to have equivalent long-term survival data (5-year overall survival 97–99%) [11–13]. Surveillance is now well-accepted, with adjuvant chemotherapy being generally reserved for patients with high-risk disease or where poor compliance is an issue.

Following orchiectomy, the overall risk of relapse for unselected patients with stage I NSGCT is around 30% [14]. The strongest independent predictor of relapse is evidence of vascular invasion in the orchiectomy specimen. The presence of embryonal carcinoma, high pathological stage and high proliferation rate are also associated with an increased risk of recurrence. Notably, pre-orchiectomy tumour marker levels have not proven useful in defining relapse risk [14]. In a prospective surveillance study involving 396 patients, 46% of those with 3 or more high-risk features developed recurrent disease [11]. In contrast, only 15–20% of patients at low risk (with 0 or 1 high-risk feature) develop recurrence. The development of risk stratification prompted the emergence of risk-adapted studies in which only high-risk patients (usually with 2 or more risk features present) received adjuvant platinum-based chemotherapy, reducing the risk of recurrence to 3% [14–18].

Eighty to 90% of recurrences occur within the first 12 months [11–13] and relapse is rare after 2 years. Very late relapses (beyond 5 years) are virtually never seen following stage I disease, hence surveillance may be ceased after this time. Most recurrences occur in the retroperitoneum (61%) but a substantial proportion present with lung metastases (25%). Fewer patients relapse with mediastinal and supraclavicular nodal disease (10%) and brain, bone or liver metastases (<1%). Over 40% of patients have normal serum tumour marker levels at relapse [11]. Notably there is marked discordance between tumour marker levels pre-orchiectomy and at relapse [19] emphasising the need to monitor serum tumour markers in all patients as part of a surveillance protocol (Table 88.7).

Surveillance protocols for stage I NSGCT vary widely and there is little consensus amongst centres [19]. The surveillance protocol attached reflects schedules used in the majority of surveillance studies performed to date (Table 88.6) [11–13, 19]. They reflect the need for intense surveillance during the initial 2 years when the risk of relapse is highest, ceasing at 5 years after which time recurrence is extremely rare. More recently, attempts have been made to reduce the intensity of the follow-up schedule, particularly in regard to imaging studies. Frequent radiological imaging has become a particular concern with the recognition that low-level radiation may cause other cancers. Data from prospective trials are not yet available [20]. A recent randomised study of 414 patients with stage I NSGCT was reported. Patients were randomised to a schedule involving either 2 (at 3 and 12 months) or 5 (at 3, 6, 9, 12 or 24 months) CT scans of the chest and abdomen. Other investigations including clinical examination, chest X-ray and tumour markers remained the same. With 40 months of follow-up, data on patients with intermediate-risk NSGCT, 2 patients in the 2-scan group compared to 1 patient in the 5-scan group were diagnosed with recurrence. No patients with poor prognosis disease have relapsed and no deaths are yet reported. The authors concluded that a 2-scan surveillance regimen should be considered in low-risk patients [19]. A retrospective review of 168 patients in which chest CT scans were omitted from the surveillance protocol has also suggested that this is safe. Of eight patients who relapsed with intrathoracic disease, all but one had another indicator of disease. This patient had disease evident on a chest X-ray. In this group, the only patient with poor-prognosis disease also had elevated serum tumour marker levels and it was postulated that routine chest CT scans would not have downstaged his disease at diagnosis of relapse [21]. While this evidence is compelling, the studies remain small and further minimisation of the surveillance schedule is not yet regarded as standard practice (Table 88.8).

Patients with advanced NSGCT (Stages II and III) have complete response rates of around 80% following platinum-based chemotherapy and surgery for residual masses. Relapse rates around 10% are seen and, as in stage I disease, the vast majority occur within 2 years of treatment (Tables 88.7,

Table 88.8 Surveillance after curative-intent initial therapy (orchiectomy + platinum-based chemotherapy ± retroperitoneal lymph node dissection) for patients with stage ≥ II non-seminoma germ cell tumour at the Sydney Cancer Centre

	Years Post-Treatment					
Modality	1	2	3	4	5	>5
Office visit and serum tumour marker levels[a]	6	4	3	2	2	1
CXR	4	2	2	1	1	1
CT chest-abdomen-pelvis	2	2	1	1	1	0

The number in each cell is the number of times a particular modality is recommended in a particular post-treatment year

[a]AFP, beta HCG, LDH

88.8) [22, 23]. Late recurrence is a small but significant risk in this group. A retrospective series of 1263 men with testicular tumours revealed late recurrences (beyond 2 years) in 6.7% of men with advanced NSGCT, with 3.1% relapsing beyond 5 years (with an estimated annual risk of 1% per year in years 5–10). Recurrences were seen up to 14 years post-treatment. Of very late recurrences, most (10 of 12) had teratomatous elements in either their original testicular specimen or in post-chemotherapy-resected masses [24]. This emphasises the need to continue surveillance in these patients for up to 10 years though, as the risk is small, intensive imaging is not generally required.

References

1. Bosl G, Bajorin D, Sheinfeld J, et al. Cancer of the testis. In: De Vita V, Hellman S, Rosenberg S, editors. Cancer: principles and practice of oncololgy. 7th ed. Philadelphia: Lippincott Williams & Wilkins; 2005. p. 1269–93.
2. Horwich A, Alsanjari N, A'Hern R, et al. Surveillance following orchidectomy for stage I testicular seminoma. Br J Cancer. 1992;65:775–8.
3. Warde P, Specht L, Horwich A, et al. Prognostic factors for relapse in stage I seminoma managed by surveillance: a pooled analysis. J Clin Oncol. 2002;20:4448–52.
4. Oldenburg J, Alfsen G, Waehre H, et al. Late recurrences of germ cell malignancies: a population based experience over three decades. Br J Cancer. 2006;94:820–7.
5. Dieckmann K, Albers P, Classen J, et al. Late relapse of testicular germ cell neoplasms: a descriptive analysis of 122 cases. J Urol. 2005;173:824–9.
6. Martin J, Panzarella T, Zwahlen D, et al. Evidence-based guidelines for following stage I seminoma. Cancer. 2007;109:2248–56.
7. Oliver R, Mason M, Mead G, et al. Radiotherapy versus single-dose carboplatin in adjuvant treatment of stage I seminoma: a randomized trial. Lancet. 2005;366:293–300.
8. Mead G, Fossa S, Oliver R et al. Relapse patterns in 2,466 stage I seminoma patients (pts) entered into Medical Research Council randomised trials. J Clin Oncol 2008; ASCO Annual Meeting Proceedings 26, 15S;5020.
9. Classen J, Schmidberger H, Meisner C, et al. Radiotherapy for stages IIA/B testicular seminoma: final report of a prospective multicenter clinical trial. J Clin Oncol. 2003;21:1101–6.
10. Chung P, Gospodarowicz M, Panzarella T, et al. Stage II testicular seminoma: patterns of recurrence and outcome of treatment. Eur Urol. 2004;45:754–9.
11. Read G, Stenning S, Cullen M, et al. Medical Research Council prospective study of surveillance for stage I testicular teratoma. J Clin Oncol. 1992;10:1762–8.
12. Gels M, Hoekstra H, Sleijfer D, et al. Detection of recurrence in patients with clinical stage I nonseminomatous testicular germ cell tumours and consequences for further follow-up: a single center 10-year experience. J Clin Oncol. 1995;13:1188–94.
13. Sogani P, Perrotti M, Herr H, et al. Clinical stage I testis cancer: long-term outcome of patients on surveillance. J Urol. 1998;159:855–8.
14. Vergouwe Y, Steyerberg E, Eijkemans M, et al. Predictors of occult metastasis in clinical stage I nonseminoma: a systematic review. J Clin Oncol. 2003;21:4092–9.
15. Oliver R, Raja M, Ong J, et al. Pilot study to evaluate impact of a policy of adjuvant chemotherapy for high risk stage I malignant teratoma on overall relapse rate of stage I cancer patients. J Urol. 1992;148:1453–6.
16. Klepp O, Dahl O, Flodgren P, et al. Risk-adapted treatment of clinical stage I non-seminoma testis cancer. Eur J Cancer. 1997;33:1038–44.
17. Ondrus D, Matoska J, Belan V, et al. Prognostic factors in clinical stage I nonseminomatous germ cell testicular tumours: Rationale for different risk-adapted treatment. Eur Urol. 1998;33:562–6.
18. Cullen M, Stenning S, Parkinson M, et al. Short course adjuvant chemotherapy in high-risk stage I nonseminomatous germ cell tumors of the testis: A medical research council report. J Clin Oncol. 1996;14:1106–13.
19. Rustin G, Mead G, Stenning S, et al. Randomized trial of two or five computed tomography scans in the surveillance of patients with stage I nonseminomatous germ cell tumors of the testis: Medical Research Council trial TE08, ISRCTN56475197 – The National Cancer Research Institute testis cancer clinical studies group. J Clin Oncol. 2007;25:1310–5.
20. Brenner D, Hall E. Computed tomography – an increasing source of radiation exposure. N Engl J Med. 2007;357:2277–84.
21. Harvey M, Geldart T, Duell R, et al. Routine computerized tomographic scans of the thorax in surveillance of stage I testicular noneminomatous germ-cell cancer – a necessary risk? Ann Oncol. 2002;13:237–42.
22. Gietema J, Meinardi M, Sleijfer D, et al. Routine chest X-rays have no additional value in the detection of relapse during routine follow-up of patients treated with chemotherapy for disseminated non-seminomatous testicular cancer. Ann Oncol. 2002;13:1616–20.
23. As N, Glilbert D, Money-Kyrle J, et al. Evidence-based pragmatic guidelines of the follow-up of testicular cancer: optimizing the detection of relapse. Br J Cancer. 2008;98:1894–902.
24. Shahidi M, Norman A, Dearnaley D, et al. Late recurrence in 1263 men with testicular germ cell tumors. Cancer. 2002;95:520–30.

Testicle Carcinoma Surveillance Counterpoint: Japan

89

Narihito Seki

Keywords
Testicular germ cell tumors • Testes • Relapse • Male • Japan

Introduction

The majority of testicular cancers (over 90%) are of germ cell origin. Germ cell tumors constitute 1–2% of all tumors in males and are the most common types of cancer in men 15–35 years of age. Advances in diagnostic radiology (computed tomography), coupled with the advent of serum tumor markers, have allowed for both more accurate staging and earlier diagnosis of recurrence of testicular cancer. Other developments in the management of testicular cancer include introduction of effective combination chemotherapy. Unlike many other cancers, recurrent and metastatic testicular cancer can be cured in the majority of cases. Therefore, defined protocols are needed in long-term surveillance of these patients. This counterpoint includes a follow-up schedule recommended in our department, focused on stages I and II (with retroperitoneal lymph node metastasis) testicular germ cell tumor (Table 89.1).

Seminoma (Clinical Stage I)

Following initial treatment, the relapse rate is significantly higher in patients without any adjuvant radiation therapy (15–20%) when compared to that observed in patients with adjuvant radiation (less than 5%). Therefore, our follow-up of clinical stage I seminoma distinguishes between the patients with and without postoperative adjuvant therapy after inguinal orchiectomy (Tables 89.2, 89.3. Although the majority of tumor relapses occur within 2 years (70%) postorchiectomy, 2–5% of the relapses are observed even at 5 years or later. Thus, these results suggest that long-term surveillance (over 10 years), in addition to close follow-up during the early postoperative period, is necessary. Because we have no specific tumor marker for the detection of tumor relapse, computed tomography scans of abdomen and pelvis, chest X-rays, and careful physical examination, are very important during surveillance. In patients without adjuvant radiation, the majority of relapses occur in the retroperitoneal space beneath the diaphragm, pelvic or inguinal lymph nodes, and lungs. Relapses occur mainly in supraclavicular or mediastinal lymph nodes and lungs in patients with prophylactic adjuvant retroperitoneal radiation after orchiectomy. Because good prognosis depends on early detection and treatment of relapse, lifelong meticulous follow-up is highly recommended.

Nonseminoma (Clinical Stage I)

Tumor relapse is observed in approximately 25–30% of the patients who receive orchiectomy for nonseminomatous germ cell tumor without any postoperative adjuvant therapy. Micrometastatic nodal involvement can be detected in about 30% of the patients with stage I nonseminoma who receive retroperitoneal lymph node dissection (RPLND). Although the majority of tumor relapses occur shortly after orchiectomy (approximately 50%, 80, and 90% within 6, 12, and 24 months, respectively), 4% of the relapses occur every year even at 3 years or later. They occur mainly in retroperitoneal lymph nodes and lungs. It has been suggested that vascular-lymphatic infiltration, advanced T-stage, and embryonal

N. Seki (✉)
Department of Urology, Graduate School of Medical Sciences, Kyushu University, 3-1-1 Maidashi, Higashi-ku, Fukuoka, 812-8582, Japan
e-mail: narihito@uro.med.kyushu-u.ac.jp

F.E. Johnson et al. (eds.), *Patient Surveillance After Cancer Treatment*, Current Clinical Oncology,
DOI 10.1007/978-1-60327-969-7_89, © Springer Science+Business Media New York 2013

Table 89.1 Stage classification of testicular cancer by the Japanese Urological Association

Stage			
I			No evidence of metastasis
II			Lymph node metastasis beneath diaphragm
	IIA		Retroperitoneal lymph node metastasis <5 cm in diameter
	IIB		Retroperitoneal lymph node metastasis ≥5 cm in diameter
III			Distant metastasis
	III0		Tumor marker positive (but metastasis site is unidentified)
	IIIA		Lymph node metastasis above diaphragm
	IIIB		Pulmonary metastasis
		B1	Number of metastases ≤4 and diameter of each metastasis <2 cm
		B2	Number of metastases ≥5 and diameter of any metastasis >2 cm
	IIIC		Metastasis other than lung

Table 89.2 Surveillance after curative-intent treatment for testicular cancer (stage I seminoma without adjuvant therapy) at Kyushu University Hospital

	Year				
Modality	1	2	3	4	≥ 5
Office visit	6	4	4	2	1
Chest X-ray	6	4	4	2	1
Tumor markers[a]	6	4	4	2	1
Abdominal/Pelvic CT	4	4	2	1	1

The number in each cell indicates the number of times a particular modality is recommended during a particular posttreatment year

[a]Serum beta-human chorionic gonadotropin, alpha-fetoprotein and lactic dehydrogenase levels

Table 89.3 Surveillance after curative-intent treatment for testicular cancer (stage I seminoma with adjuvant retroperitoneal irradiation) at Kyushu University Hospital

	Year				
	1	2	3	4	≥5
Office visit	6	4	4	2	1
Chest X-ray	6	4	4	2	1
Tumor markers[a]	6	4	4	2	1
Abdominal/Pelvic CT	2	2	1	1	1

The number in each cell indicates the number of times a particular modality is recommended during a particular posttreatment year

[a]Serum beta-human chorionic gonadotropin, alpha-fetoprotein and lactic dehydrogenase levels

cancer history are adverse prognostic factors. Therefore, adjuvant chemotherapy, including cisplatin and etoposide, is recommended for high-risk patients in order to prevent recurrence. The relapse rate is reduced to less than 5% by administration of two courses of cisplatin, etoposide, and bleomycin (BEP). Because 15–35% of tumor relapses are not accompanied by a significant elevation of any tumor marker, examination with computed tomography scans of abdomen and pelvis and chest X-rays are very important during surveillance (Tables 89.4 and 89.5).

Table 89.4 Surveillance after curative-intent treatment for nonseminoma (stage I without adjuvant therapy) at Kyushu University Hospital

	Year				
	1	2	3	4	≥ 5
Office visit	12	6	4	2	1
Chest X-ray	6	6	4	2	1
Tumor markers[a]	6	6	4	2	1
Abdominal CT/Pelvic CT	4	4	2	1	1

[a]Serum beta-human chorionic gonadotropin, alpha-fetoprotein and lactic dehydrogenase levels

The number in each cell indicates the number of times a particular modality is recommended during a particular posttreatment year

Table 89.5 Surveillance after curative-intent treatment for nonseminoma (stage I with adjuvant chemotherapy) at Kyushu University Hospital

	Year				
	1	2	3	4	≥ 5
Office visit	6	3	2	2	1
Chest X-ray	6	3	2	2	1
Tumor markers[a]	6	3	2	2	1
Abdominal/Pelvic CT	2	2	1	1	1

[a]Serum beta-human chorionic gonadotropin, alpha-fetoprotein and lactic dehydrogenase levels

The number in each cell indicates the number of times a particular modality is recommended during a particular posttreatment year

Seminoma (Clinical Stage II)

Approximately 15–20% of all seminoma patients have evidence of abdominal lymph node involvement on completion of a staging workup (stage II). Generally, three to four courses of cisplatin-based systemic chemotherapy (EP or BEP) or irradiation are recommended for patients with stage II seminoma. Follow-up examinations with computed tomography scans of abdomen and pelvis, in addition to chest X-rays and serum tumor marker levels, are very important for stage II seminoma. The interval between computed tomography during surveillance mainly depends on the response of each site of metastasis to treatment (Table 89.6).

Nonseminoma (Clinical Stage II)

Three to four courses of cisplatin-based systemic chemotherapy are recommended for the majority of patients with stage II nonseminomatous germ cell tumor. RPLND for stage II

Table 89.6 Surveillance after curative-intent treatment for nonseminoma (stage II after adjuvant chemotherapy) at Kyushu University Hospital

	Year				
	1	2	3	4	≥ 5
Office visit	12	6	3–4	3–4	1
Chest X-ray	12	6	3–4	3–4	1
Tumor markers[a]	12	6	3–4	3–4	1
Abdominal/Pelvic CT[b]	4	3	2	1	1
Chest CT	1	1	[c]	[c]	[c]
Brain CT	1	[d]	[d]	[d]	[d]

[a]Serum beta-human chorionic gonadotropin, alpha-fetoprotein and lactic dehydrogenase levels

[b]If recurrence is detected, repeat every 2–4 months until complete regression

[c]Recommended only if abnormality is suspected by chest X-ray. If recurrence is detected, repeat every 2–4 months until complete regression

[d]Recommended only if patient complains of headache or neurological symptoms

The number in each cell indicates the number of times a particular modality is recommended during a particular posttreatment year

nonseminomatous germ cell tumor should be restricted to patients with a retroperitoneal mass less than 2 cm in diameter and with normal levels of serum tumor markers. Surveillance consists of computed tomography scans of abdomen, pelvis and chest, chest X-rays, serum tumor markers, and careful physical examination. The interval between computed tomography scans during surveillance mainly depends on the response of each site of metastasis to treatment (Table 88.6).

Lymphoma

90

David Y. Johnson, Shilpi Wadhwa, and Frank E. Johnson

Keywords
Hodgkin's lymphoma • Incidence • Surveillance • Immune-deficiency • AIDS

The International Agency for Research on Cancer (IARC), a component of the World Health Organization (WHO), estimated that there were 362,900 new cases of lymphoma in 2002 (cases include Hodgkin's and non-Hodgkin lymphoma) [1]. The IARC also estimated that there were 194,632 deaths due to this cause in 2002 [1].

The American Cancer Society estimated that there were 71,380 new cases and 19,730 deaths due to this cause in the USA in 2007[2]. The estimated 5-year survival rate (all races) in the USA in 2007 was 86% for Hodgkin's lymphoma and 63% for non-Hodgkin lymphoma [2]. Survival rates were adjusted for normal life expectancies and were based on cases diagnosed from 1996 to 2002 and followed through 2003.

Hodgkin's lymphoma is uncommon. The incidence is bimodal with a peak in young adulthood and another in old age. There is considerable evidence for an infectious etiology; Epstein–Barr virus infection is a candidate agent. Occupational exposure has been implicated but the evidence is inconclusive. Several primary immunodeficiency disorders are risk factors for Hodgkin's lymphoma. Non-Hodgkin lymphomas comprise a heterogeneous group of diseases. Inherited immunodeficiency syndromes (severe combined immunodeficiency, Wiskott–Aldrich syndrome, ataxia–telangiectasia, and others) and acquired immune-deficiency states (solid organ transplantation, AIDS, rheumatoid arthritis, Sjögren's syndrome, celiac disease, and others) are important risk factors. Viral infections are strongly associated with lymphomas. Epstein–Barr virus infection is a cause of Burkitt's lymphoma and is implicated as a cause of other varieties. Human T-cell lymphotropic virus type I, human herpes virus-8, and simian virus 40 are also considered causative agents. Bacterial infection, particularly *Helicobacter pylori, Campylobacter jejuni, Chlamydia psittaci,* and *Borellia burgdorferi* are believed to be causative agents. Exposure to certain chemicals, particularly phenoxy herbicides, appears to be a risk factor. Treatment for cancer with various agents is clearly a cause of non-Hodgkin lymphoma. Dietary factors and use of illicit drugs and tobacco also are associated with non-Hodgkin lymphoma.

Geographic Variation Worldwide

The incidence of non-Hodgkin lymphoma is reported to be lowest in Asia and highest in Western Europe and North America. The geographic pattern of mortality within the USA from this cancer contrasts markedly with those of melanoma and other skin cancers, providing evidence against a strong association between ultraviolet radiation and lymphoma risk. In contrast, the incidence of Hodgkin's lymphoma is strongly associated with "westernized" style of economic development. The typical bimodal age incidence curve is seen in countries with strong western influence. Within the USA, Hodgkin's lymphoma mortality rates are higher in the eastern two-thirds of the country than in the west [3, 4].

D.Y. Johnson • S. Wadhwa
Department of Internal Medicine, Saint Louis University Medical Center, Saint Louis, MO, USA

F.E. Johnson (✉)
Saint Louis University Medical Center and Saint Louis Veterans Affairs Medical Center, Saint Louis, MO, USA
e-mail: frank.johnson1@va.gov

F.E. Johnson et al. (eds.), *Patient Surveillance After Cancer Treatment*, Current Clinical Oncology,
DOI 10.1007/978-1-60327-969-7_90, © Springer Science+Business Media New York 2013

Surveillance Strategies Proposed by Professional Organizations or National Government Agencies and Available on the Internet

Although treatment strategies for lymphoma may include hematopoietic cell transplant, quantitative surveillance recommendations that were accessed for lymphoma patients did not distinguish between those with or without transplant. The guidelines in this chapter should be considered applicable to all lymphoma patients, including those whose treatment includes transplant.

National Comprehensive Cancer Network (NCCN, www.nccn.org)—NCCN guidelines were accessed on 1/28/12 (Tables 90.1, 90.2, 90.3, 90.4, 90.5, 90.6). There were major quantitative and qualitative changes compared to the guidelines accessed on 4/10/07.

American Society of Clinical Oncology (ASCO, www.asco.org)—ASCO guidelines were accessed on 1/28/12. No quantitative guidelines exist for lymphoma surveillance including when first accessed on 10/31/07.

The Society of Surgical Oncology (SSO, www.surgonc.org)—SSO guidelines were accessed on 1/28/12. No quantitative guidelines exist for lymphoma surveillance including when first accessed on 10/31/07.

European Society for Medical Oncology (ESMO, www.esmo.org)—ESMO guidelines were accessed on 1/28/12 (Tables 90.7, 90.8, 90.9, 90.10, 90.11). There were major quantitative and qualitative changes and new quantitative guidelines compared to the guidelines accessed on 10/31/07.

Table 90.1 Hodgkin's lymphoma (Obtained from NCCN (www.nccn.org) on 1/28/12)

	Years posttreatment[a]					
	1	2	3	4	5	>5
Office visit	3–6	3–6	2–4	2–4	2–4	1
CBC, platelets, ESR[b]	3–6	3–6	2–4	2–4	2–4	1
TSH[c]	≥1	≥1	≥1	≥1	≥1	≥1
Chest X-ray or CT	1–2	1–2	0–2	0–2	0–2	1
Abdominal/pelvic CT	1–2	1–2	0–2	0	0	0

Annual influenza vaccine

Counseling: reproduction, health habits, psychosocial, cardiovascular, breast self-examination, skin cancer risk, end-of-treatment discussion

Surveillance PET should not be done routinely due to risk of false positives. Management decisions should not be based on PET scan alone; clinical or pathological correlation is needed

Additional quantitative guidelines for monitoring of late effects after 5 years. See NCCN Guidelines: Hodgkin's Lymphoma, p. HODG-11

NCCN guidelines were accessed on 1/28/12. There were major quantitative and qualitative changes compared to the guidelines accessed on 4/10/07

[a]The numbers in the table indicate the number of times the modality is recommended during the indicated year posttreatment

[b]If elevated at time of initial diagnosis

[c]If radiotherapy to neck

Table 90.2 Non-Hodgkin lymphomas: follicular lymphoma (Grade 1–2), Stage I, II, IIIX, III, IV; nodal marginal zone lymphoma; primary cutaneous marginal zone or follicle center cell lymphoma (Obtained from NCCN (www.nccn.org) on 1/28/12)

	Years posttreatment[a]					
	1	2	3	4	5	>5
Office visit	2–4	2–4	2–4	2–4	2–4	1[b]
CT scan[c]	0–2	0–2	0–1	0–1	0–1	0–1

Consider clinical trials appropriate for patients on observation

NCCN guidelines were accessed on 1/28/12. There were major quantitative and qualitative changes compared to the guidelines accessed on 4/10/07

[a]The numbers in the table indicate the number of times the modality is recommended during the indicated year posttreatment

[b]Annually or as clinically indicated

[c]Imaging should be performed whenever there are clinical indications

Table 90.3 Non-Hodgkin lymphomas: gastric MALT, nongastric MALT, extranodal marginal zone MALT, splenic marginal zone, mantle cell lymphoma

	Years posttreatment[a]					
	1	2	3	4	5	>5
Office visit	2–4	2–4	2–4	2–4	2–4	1[b]

For gastric MALT and extranodal marginal zone gastric lymphoma, optimal interval for follow-up endoscopy and imaging is not known. Follow-up endoscopy and imaging at NCCN institutions is driven by symptoms

For nongastric MALT, extranodal marginal zone nongastric, and splenic marginal zone lymphoma, follow-up includes diagnostic tests and imaging as clinically indicated

NCCN guidelines were accessed on 1/28/12. There were minor quantitative and qualitative changes compared to the guidelines accessed on 4/10/07

[a]The numbers in the table indicate the number of times the modality is recommended during the indicated year posttreatment

[b]Annually or as clinically indicated

Table 90.4 Non-Hodgkin lymphomas: diffuse large B-cell Lymphoma, Stage I, II, III, IV; primary cutaneous diffuse large B-cell lymphoma, leg type (Obtained from NCCN (www.nccn.org) on 1/28/12)

	Years posttreatment[a]					
	1	2	3	4	5	>5
Office visit	2–4	2–4	2–4	2–4	2–4	1[b]
CT scan[c]	0–2	0–2	0	0	0	0

NCCN guidelines were accessed on 1/28/12. There were major quantitative and qualitative changes compared to the guidelines accessed on 4/10/07

[a]The numbers in the table indicate the number of times the modality is recommended during the indicated year posttreatment

[b]Annually or as clinically indicated

[c]No more often than every 6 months for 2 years after completion of treatment, then only as clinically indicated

Table 90.5 Non-Hodgkin lymphomas: Burkitt lymphoma (Obtained from NCCN (www.nccn.org) on 1/28/12)

	Years posttreatment[a]					
	1	2	3	4	5	>5
Office visit	4–6	4	2	2	2	2

Relapse after 2 years is rare. Therefore, follow-up should be individualized according to patient characteristics
NCCN guidelines were accessed on 1/28/12. There were minor quantitative changes compared to the guidelines accessed on 4/10/07
[a]The numbers in the table indicate the number of times the modality is recommended during the indicated year posttreatment

Table 90.6 Non-Hodgkin lymphomas: peripheral T-cell lymphoma (Obtained from NCCN (www.nccn.org) on 1/28/12)

	Years posttreatment[a]					
	1	2	3	4	5	>5
Office visit	2–4	2–4	2–4	2–4	2–4	1[b]

NCCN guidelines were accessed on 1/28/12. There were minor quantitative changes compared to the guidelines accessed on 4/10/07
[a]The numbers in the table indicate the number of times the modality is recommended during the indicated year posttreatment
[b]Annually or as clinically indicated

Table 90.7 Hodgkin's lymphoma (Obtained from ESMO (www.esmo.org) on 1/28/12)

	Years posttreatment[a]					
	1	2	3	4	5	>5
Office visit	3	2	2	2	1	1
CBC, ESR, chemistry	3	2	2	2	1	1
TSH[b]	1	1	0	0	1	0

Testosterone and estrogen levels should be monitored, particularly in younger patients who received intensive chemotherapy
CT scans and previously pathological radiographic tests must be performed once to confirm the remission status. Thereafter, they are indicated if suspicious clinical symptoms occur
Patients should be asked about symptoms indicating the existence of long-term toxicity, particularly of heart and/or lung
Cancer screening (e.g., mammography in irradiated patients) should be conducted regularly due to the increased risk of hematological and solid secondary malignancies after HL treatment
ESMO guidelines were accessed on 1/28/12. There were major quantitative and qualitative changes compared to the guidelines accessed on 10/31/07
[a]The numbers in the table indicate the number of times the modality is recommended during the indicated year posttreatment
[b]If neck irradiated

European Society of Surgical Oncology (ESSO, www.esso-surgeonline.org)—ESSO guidelines were accessed on 1/28/12. No quantitative guidelines exist for lymphoma surveillance including when first accessed on 10/31/07.

Cancer Care Ontario (CCO, www.cancercare.on.ca)—CCO guidelines were accessed on 1/28/12. No quantitative guidelines exist for lymphoma surveillance including when first accessed on 10/31/07.

Table 90.8 Newly diagnosed and relapsed follicular lymphoma (Obtained from ESMO (www.esmo.org) on 1/28/12)

	Years posttreatment[a]					
	1	2	3	4	5	>5
Office visit	4	4	2–3	2–3	2–3	1[b]
CBC, chemistry[c]	2	2	0	0	0	0
TSH[d]	1	1	0	0	1	0
Radiologic or ultrasound examinations[e]	2	2	1	1	1	1

Minimal residual disease screening may be performed in clinical studies but should not guide therapeutic strategies
ESMO guidelines were accessed on 1/28/12. There were major quantitative and qualitative changes compared to the guidelines accessed on 10/31/07
[a]The numbers in the table indicate the number of times the modality is recommended during the indicated year posttreatment
[b]With special attention to transformation and secondary malignancies, including secondary leukemia
[c]Every 6 months for 2 years, then only as needed for evaluation of suspicious symptoms
[d]If neck irradiated
[e]Minimal adequate radiological or ultrasound examinations every 6 months for 2 years and annually thereafter. Regular CT scans are not mandatory outside of clinical trials

Table 90.9 Gastric marginal zone lymphoma of MALT type (Obtained from ESMO (www.esmo.org) on 1/28/12)

	Years posttreatment[a]					
	1	2	3	4	5	>5
Office visit	2	2	1	1	1	1
Endoscopy with multiple biopsies	2	2	1	1	1	1
CBC	1	1	1	1	1	1
Radiologic or ultrasound examinations	1	1	1	1	1	1

A preliminary breath test or stool antigen test should be performed at least 4 weeks after the cessation of antibiotic treatment to document H. pylori eradication
ESMO guidelines were accessed on 1/28/12. There were major quantitative and qualitative changes compared to the guidelines accessed on 10/31/07
[a]The numbers in the table indicate the number of times the modality is recommended during the indicated year posttreatment

National Institute for Clinical Excellence (NICE, www.nice.org.uk)—NICE guidelines were accessed on 1/28/12. No quantitative guidelines exist for lymphoma surveillance including when first accessed on 10/31/07.

The Cochrane Collaboration (CC, www.cochrane.org)—CC guidelines were accessed on 1/28/12. No quantitative guidelines exist for lymphoma surveillance including when first accessed on 11/24/07.

The M.D. Anderson Surgical Oncology Handbook also has follow-up guidelines, proposed by authors from a single National Cancer Institute-designated Comprehensive Cancer Center, for many types of cancer [5]. Some are detailed and quantitative, others are qualitative.

Table 90.10 Obtained from ESMO (www.esmo.org) on 1/28/12 diffuse large B-cell non-Hodgkin lymphoma

	Years posttreatment[a]					
	1	2	3	4	5	>5
Office visit[b]	4	2	2	1	1	1
CBC, LDH[c]	3	1	0	0	0	0
Radiologic examinations[d]	2	1	0	0	0	0

Routine surveillance with PET scan is not recommended
High-risk patients with curative options may potentially mandate more frequent controls
ESMO guidelines were accessed on 1/28/12. These are new quantitative guidelines compared to the guidelines accessed on 10/31/07
[a]The numbers in the table indicate the number of times the modality is recommended during the indicated year posttreatment
[b]With attention to development of secondary tumors or other long-term side-effects of chemotherapy
[c]At 3, 6, 12, and 24 months, then only as needed for evaluation of suspicious symptoms or clinical findings in those patients suitable for further therapy
[d]Minimal adequate radiological examinations at 6, 12, and 24 months after end of treatment. CT scan is usual practice but there is no definitive evidence that routine imaging in patients in complete remission provides any outcome advantage

Table 90.11 Obtained from ESMO (www.esmo.org) on 1/28/12 primary cutaneous lymphomas

	Years posttreatment[a]					
	1	2	3	4	5	>5
Office visit[b]	1–13	1–13	1–13	1–13	1–13	1–13

Additional testing (histology, blood examination, imaging, etc.) should only be performed if required
ESMO guidelines were accessed on 1/28/12. These are new quantitative guidelines compared to the guidelines accessed on 10/31/07
[a]The numbers in the table indicate the number of times the modality is recommended during the indicated year posttreatment
[b]The frequency of follow-up visits depends on the type of PCL and stage of disease. It may vary from every 6 or 12 months in patients with indolent types of PCL and stable disease or patients in complete remission to every 4–6 weeks in patients with active or progressive disease

Summary

This is a common cancer with significant variability in incidence worldwide. We found consensus-based guidelines but none based on high-quality evidence.

References

1. Parkin DM, Whelan SL, Ferlay J, Teppo L, Thomas DB. Cancer incidence in five continents. IARC Scientific Publication 155, vol. VIII. Lyon: IARC; 2002. ISBN 92-832-2155-9.
2. Jemal A, Seigel R, Ward E, Murray T, Xu J, Thun MJ. Cancer statistics, 2007. CA Cancer J Clin. 2007;57:43–66.
3. Schottenfeld D, Fraumeni JG. Cancer epidemiology and prevention. 3rd ed. New York, NY: Oxford University Press; 2006. ISBN 13:978-0-19-514961-6.
4. Devesa SS, Grauman DJ, Blot WJ, Pennello GA, Hoover RN, Fraumeni JF Jr. Atlas of cancer mortality in the United States. NIH Publication No. 99–4564. National Institutes of Health, National Cancer Institute; September 1999.
5. Feig BW, Berger DH, Fuhrman GM. The M.D. Anderson surgical oncology handbook. 4th ed. Philadelphia, PA: Lippincott Williams & Wilkins; 2006 (paperback). ISBN 0-7817-5643-X.

91 Lymphoma Surveillance Counterpoint: USA

Kenneth R. Carson and Nancy L. Bartlett

Keywords
Hodgkin lymphoma • non-Hodgkin lymphoma • Surveillance • CT scan • PET scan

The introduction provides a summary of the Hodgkin lymphoma and non-Hodgkin lymphoma surveillance screening guidelines promulgated by several clinical and governmental organizations throughout the world. Since the term non-Hodgkin lymphoma describes more than 40 histologically discrete diseases associated with wide variations in clinical aggressiveness, a single approach to surveillance based on stage is not appropriate [1]. Similarly, Hodgkin lymphoma can be divided into classical and lymphocyte-predominant subtypes, associated with somewhat more aggressive and indolent behaviors, respectively. To accommodate this clinical heterogeneity, surveillance guidelines are frequently vague, offering a wide range of suggested surveillance tests and testing intervals [2]. It is also important to point out that, for the most part, such guidelines are based upon expert opinion, and adherence to them has not been shown to improve clinical outcomes. Overall, current guidelines for surveillance serve best as a starting point for the discussion of cancer survivorship related to Hodgkin lymphoma and non-Hodgkin lymphoma, and do not represent an evidence-based approach. We hope future studies will allow rigorous evaluation of the clinical value and cost-effectiveness of various surveillance schedules and modalities. Until that time, in our practice we generally favor office visits consisting of clinical history, physical examination, patient education about possible symptoms of relapse, and periodic laboratory testing. We typically recommend radiologic imaging in asymptomatic patients annually for the first 2 years after treatment, or as dictated by symptoms, physical examination, and/or other findings. Such an approach minimizes radiology testing that may be costly, invasive, and anxiety-provoking for the patient.

When considering the surveillance for lymphoma patients (as in most other malignancies), four general questions must be asked:

1. Is evaluation necessary?
2. What is the appropriate evaluation interval?
3. How long should surveillance continue?
4. What diagnostic test(s) should be used?

The first question reflects a reasonable assessment of how results of a diagnostic test will be used before it is ordered. Patients who have no remaining treatment options, or are too sick for further intervention, receive minimal benefit from early detection of relapse. Determination of the appropriate interval (Question 2) should be based, in part, on the velocity of tumor growth. If a follow-up test is to be useful, it must detect growth before it is otherwise clinically apparent. Tumor masses in Burkitt lymphoma, for example, can double in size over a period of 24 h, while some indolent lymphomas will remain stable for many years in the absence of active therapy [3, 4]. Thus, patients with fast-growing tumors may require more frequent evaluation than those with indolent tumors. In indolent non-Hodgkin lymphoma, this task is complicated by the risk of transformation from indolent to aggressive histology [4]. Duration of testing (Question 3) is guided by the frequency of relapse over time. Since most diffuse large B-cell lymphoma relapses occur within 2 years of treatment, the utility of aggressive testing declines markedly after that [5]. Finally, the choice of diagnostic test

K.R. Carson
Section of Medical Oncology, Washington University School of Medicine, 4921 Parkview Place, St. Louis, MO, USA
e-mail: kcarson@dom.wustl.edu

N.L. Bartlett (✉)
Siteman Cancer Center, Washington University, 4921 Parkview Place, St. Louis, MO 63110, USA
e-mail: nbartlet@dom.wustl.edu

F.E. Johnson et al. (eds.), *Patient Surveillance After Cancer Treatment*, Current Clinical Oncology,
DOI 10.1007/978-1-60327-969-7_91, © Springer Science+Business Media New York 2013

modality should be based not only on the sensitivity and specificity of the particular test, but also on reasonable evidence that such surveillance improves clinical outcomes in a cost-effective fashion. We discuss each of these factors for selected types of lymphoma below.

In addition to evaluation for disease relapse, survivors of Hodgkin lymphoma in particular require consideration of long-term treatment-related toxicities and secondary cancers. While a recent article demonstrated that survivors of non-Hodgkin lymphoma have increased long-term risks for other, non-lymphoid malignancies, no additional screening is indicated for these patients [6]. Some of the long-term issues associated with Hodgkin lymphoma treatment are addressed in published guidelines mentioned before, and they should be rationally applied on a case-by-case basis based on clinician knowledge of treatment-related risks.

The most important evaluation for lymphoma patients is the history and physical examination. In Hodgkin lymphoma, history alone is responsible for detection of 55–81% of relapses [7, 8]. Physical examination, in conjunction with history, resulted in detection of 69–86% of relapses in these same studies. Symptoms such as fever, night sweats, and unintentional weight loss or signs such as lymphadenopathy or splenomegaly then prompt additional testing and/or restaging in patients with a previously documented complete remission. Similarly, studies evaluating routine surveillance in aggressive non-Hodgkin lymphoma have shown that 80% of relapses are discovered by history and physical examination [9].

In non-Hodgkin lymphoma, some experts advocate surveillance with complete blood count (CBC), serum metabolic panel and lactate dehydrogenase (LDH) testing at the time of clinical follow-up [10]. In Hodgkin lymphoma, the erythrocyte sedimentation rate (ESR) is often added to these [11]. Clinical evidence supporting use of these tests is relatively scant, however. The serum LDH level is the best-supported single test, based on its ability to detect preclinical relapse in non-Hodgkin lymphoma patients during the era before CT and positron emission tomography (PET) scans [12]. Components of the CBC and metabolic panel are included in the prognostic scores for Hodgkin and various non-Hodgkin lymphoma subtypes, so it is conceivable that these tests could be useful in the early detection of relapse, though this has not been proven [13–15]. ESR has been shown to have prognostic significance in early stage Hodgkin lymphoma, though its routine use as a surveillance tool is not supported by clinical studies [8, 16].

Some experts recommend routine surveillance of lymphoma patients by CT scan. Such an approach is associated with significant costs and considerable life-time radiation exposure [17]. Radiation exposure from CT scans may be associated with secondary malignancy later in life, and this risk should be considered in all surveillance strategies [18]. Furthermore, while most oncologists would assume that early detection of relapse is associated with improved survival in the setting of salvage therapy, the evidence supporting this conclusion is scant. One study demonstrated an improved overall survival duration among patients with preclinical relapse detected by CT scan compared to those with relapse detected by history and clinical examination, though this finding did not reach statistical significance (5-year survival 54% vs. 43%, $P=0.13$) [9]. It is quite conceivable that length-time bias (preferential detection of disease with less aggressive clinical behavior) was responsible for the modest survival difference. Cost-effectiveness analysis of annual CT scanning in asymptomatic patients demonstrated only a slight increase in quality adjusted survival, at a high cost, arguing against such a strategy [19]. Overall, the use of CT scanning to evaluate asymptomatic patients for lymphoma relapse remains controversial.

The introduction of 18-fluorodeoxyglucose PET scanning has improved the accuracy of pretreatment staging and response assessment of classical Hodgkin lymphoma and some types of non-Hodgkin lymphoma. Clinical trials are currently underway to evaluate the adaptation of treatment regimen based on early response observed by PET scan, though description of those trials is beyond the scope of this chapter [20]. Radiation exposure with combined PET/CT is approximately twice that seen with CT alone, again raising concerns about the safety of surveillance with PET or PET/CT [21]. Some authors suggest that this should be confined to clinical trials [22]. Zinzani et al. prospectively evaluated the use of PET scanning every 6 months for 2 years and annually thereafter for patients with Hodgkin lymphoma, diffuse large B-cell non-Hodgkin lymphoma, and follicular non-Hodgkin lymphoma who achieved complete remission by PET scan, following initial treatment [23]. While early and unsuspected relapses were detected in 10% of Hodgkin lymphoma patients, it is unclear if this impacted clinical outcomes significantly. In addition, patients with a positive PET and negative CT scan had a false positive rate of 42%. Thus, some patients underwent unnecessary and invasive biopsy procedures. Overall, the benefit of PET over clinical observation and/or CT scan remains unclear.

Hodgkin Lymphomas

Hodgkin lymphomas can generally be subclassified into classical and lymphocyte-predominant subtypes, classical representing 95% of new Hodgkin lymphoma diagnosis and lymphocyte-predominant the remaining 5% [24]. Classical Hodgkin lymphoma is a highly curable disease that is treated with combination chemotherapy such as ABVD (doxorubicin, bleomycin, vinblastine, dacarbazine), with or without external beam radiation [25]. In patients with relapsed or refractory disease, salvage chemotherapy and autologous hematopoietic stem cell transplant are the treatments of choice [26]. Most relapses occur within 5 years of the first treatment, though late relapses are not rare [27].

In asymptomatic patients in complete remission after initial treatment of classical Hodgkin lymphoma, our approach to assess for relapse is as follows: clinical visits with history and physical examination every 3 months for 2 years, every 6 months during years 3–5 after treatment, and annually thereafter. Approximately 1 month after completion of chemotherapy and 3 months after radiotherapy, a follow-up PET/CT scan is used to confirm complete remission. Thereafter, annual CT scan is performed for 2 years in asymptomatic patients, or as needed, based on symptoms. Laboratory testing with CBC, serum chemistry, and ESR are performed every 3 months for 2 years and every 6 months during years 3–5 in asymptomatic patients. Overall, this strategy reflects the availability of effective salvage therapy, the aggressive nature of the disease, the tendency for relapse to occur within 5 years, and conservative use of radiologic imaging and laboratory testing.

In addition to screening for relapsed Hodgkin lymphoma, surveillance is designed to detect long-term complications of treatment. Since radiation therapy remains a common treatment modality for either early-stage or bulky Hodgkin lymphoma, surveillance must consider damage to those organs exposed to significant radiation doses. Patients receiving neck radiation are screened annually for hypothyroidism with laboratory testing of thyroid stimulating hormone. Women who received radiation exposure to the breast between the ages of 10 and 30 receive annual breast cancer screening by mammography and MRI scan starting approximately 7 years after radiation exposure [28]. All other women should receive annual mammography starting at age 40. Some have suggested that annual low-dose CT scan screening for lung cancer may be useful in patients receiving significant lung irradiation, particularly smokers, though there is no consensus on the use of this technology. We do not routinely use it [29]. Patients receiving significant cardiac radiation exposure receive fractionated lipid screening every 5 years with initiation of lipid lowering therapy as needed to reduce the risk of premature coronary artery disease [30]. In addition, screening for asymptomatic cardiac ischemia with stress echocardiography should be considered every 5 years in these patients, starting 5–10 years after completion of therapy [31].

The long-term complications of chemotherapy, either alone or in combination with radiotherapy, do not lend themselves to a routine screening strategy. Anthracycline-induced cardiomyopathy is uncommon at the doses used in the treatment of Hodgkin lymphoma, and clinical signs and symptoms should guide decisions about further testing [32]. An increased risk of myeloid leukemia and myelodysplasia has been observed in patients treated with anthracyclines and/or alkylating agents, but additional screening beyond that listed above is not indicated. Previous bleomycin exposure can influence the oxygen concentration used during inhalational general anesthesia but does not warrant routine pulmonary function testing [33]. Lastly, alkylator-based combination chemotherapy may be associated with irreversible infertility but, again, there is no specific test that is indicated [34]. Overall, the long-term complications of chemotherapy are best followed with history, physical examination, and routine laboratory testing as part of follow-up screening for Hodgkin lymphoma, but inadequate follow-up remains a problem [35]. In an effort to address this, patients who leave our practice are given a letter detailing diagnosis and treatment, with suggestions for additional long-term follow-up testing required in the future.

In comparison to classical Hodgkin lymphoma, lymphocyte-predominant Hodgkin lymphoma is typically more indolent in nature and is characterized by slow progression of disease, with relapse occurring at a steady rate over many years [36]. The optimal initial therapy of lymphocyte-predominant Hodgkin lymphoma remains controversial, though chemotherapy and radiotherapy are both useful [37]. Since the malignant cells express CD20, rituximab is often used for relapse and clinical trials are underway to evaluate rituximab in the first-line setting. Treatment of relapse typically involves standard-intensity chemotherapy or immunotherapy with rituximab, as opposed to high-dose therapy and transplant as is used for classical Hodgkin lymphoma. As with indolent non-Hodgkin lymphoma, transformation from lymphocyte-predominant Hodgkin lymphoma into a more aggressive form of lymphoma (usually diffuse large B-cell non-Hodgkin lymphoma) is possible and must be considered in relapsed or rapidly progressive disease [38].

Surveillance of patients with lymphocyte-predominant Hodgkin lymphoma involves clinical visits every 3–4 months through 5 years and beyond, based on the slow but steady rate of disease progression. Screening tests include: office visit (with history and physical examination), CBC, metabolic panel, and periodic imaging. Given the constant rate of relapse, imaging may be required beyond 2 years from first treatment [36]. However, as emphasized earlier, repeated radiographic imaging increases the lifetime exposure to ionizing radiation and the associated long-term risks [18]. Given the rarity of death from lymphocyte-predominant Hodgkin lymphoma, we use radiographic imaging sparingly after the initial posttreatment assessment. Evaluation for long-term treatment complications is similar to that for classical Hodgkin lymphoma, as described above, and is largely determined by radiation exposure.

Table 91.1 Examples of lymphoma subtype

Highly aggressive non-Hodgkin lymphoma
Burkitt lymphoma
Precursor B-lymphoblastic lymphoma
Precursor T-lymphoblastic lymphoma
Aggressive non-Hodgkin lymphoma
Diffuse large B-cell lymphoma
Anaplastic large cell lymphoma
Peripheral T-cell lymphoma
Nasal NK-cell lymphoma
Indolent non-Hodgkin lymphoma
Follicular lymphoma
Mycosis fungoides
Chronic lymphocytic leukemia/small lymphocytic lymphoma
Lymphoplasmacytic lymphoma
Marginal zone B-cell lymphoma

Table 91.2 Surveillance after curative-intent treatment for diffuse large B-cell lymphoma at the Siteman Cancer Center

	Year					
	1	2	3	4	5	>5
Office visit	4	4	2	2	2	0
Blood tests[a]	4	4	2	2	2	0
Abdomen/pelvic CT[b]	1	1	0	0	0	0

After 5 years, patients who are clinically well are usually discharged to a primary care provider. We supply the designated physician a letter outlining the patient's diagnosis, treatment details, and other pertinent information

The number in each cell indicates the number of times a particular modality is recommended during a particular posttreatment year

[a]CBC (including platelet count), serum LDH level, and multichannel serum chemistry profile

[b]Despite the greater sensitivity of PET/CT, we do not advocate its use for surveillance of otherwise asymptomatic patients, as described in the text

Non-Hodgkin Lymphomas

Approximately 90–95% of non-Hodgkin lymphoma is of B-cell origin, and the remaining 5–10% are of T-cell or NK-cell origin [39]. To better conceptualize treatment and surveillance patterns for the various subtypes of non-Hodgkin lymphoma, some of the more common subtypes have been classified as indolent, aggressive, and highly aggressive forms (see Table 91.1). Such classification allows general statements to be made regarding surveillance. However, general principles may not apply in individual cases. For example, some patients with follicular lymphoma have a rapidly progressive disease course despite classification as an "indolent" non-Hodgkin lymphoma. Furthermore, some non-Hodgkin lymphoma subtypes, such as mantle cell lymphoma, exhibit characteristics of both indolent and aggressive forms of non-Hodgkin lymphoma.

Highly aggressive non-Hodgkin lymphoma requires rapid treatment with multi-agent chemotherapy, often at high doses associated with significant toxicity, frequently requiring hospitalization. Without treatment, newly diagnosed disease usually proves fatal in weeks or a few months. Treatment is administered with curative intent, and relapses are often observed within the first year after treatment is completed [40]. Salvage treatment typically consists of reinduction chemotherapy and autologous or allogeneic hematopoietic stem cell transplantation, depending upon donor availability and clinical status of the patient.

The utility of aggressive surveillance in frail or older patients can easily be questioned given the significant toxicity and low success rates associated with salvage therapy [41]. Therefore, goals of care should be carefully considered in these patients before diagnostic testing is ordered. In general, patients should be followed every 2 months for 1 year, every 3 months between years 1 and 2, and less frequently thereafter. With some treatment regimens, maintenance chemotherapy may dictate more frequent clinical visits. While relapses have been described after 2 years in patients with highly aggressive non-Hodgkin lymphoma, they are uncommon [42]. As a result, there is no clear indication for surveillance after 5 years. Testing that is performed at office visits includes history, physical examination, CBC, serum metabolic panel, and serum LDH level. The rapid growth of these tumors decreases the likelihood that imaging will detect asymptomatic disease, so imaging should largely be pursued based on history, physical examination, and blood tests.

Aggressive non-Hodgkin lymphoma also requires multi-agent chemotherapy, though usually this can be administered on an outpatient basis with manageable toxicity. Without treatment, newly diagnosed disease is usually fatal in a matter of months. Treatment is given with curative intent, and relapses are frequently seen within the first 2–3 years after treatment is completed. Salvage treatment usually consists of reinduction chemotherapy followed by autologous hematopoietic stem cell transplantation.

Surveillance involves history and physical examination every 3 months for the first 2 years, every 6 months during years 3–5, and as needed thereafter. Laboratory testing is performed every 3 months for the first 2 years and every 6 months during years 3–5. Radiologic imaging is performed annually in asymptomatic patients for 2 years and is based on symptoms, physical examination, or laboratory findings thereafter (Table 91.2). In our opinion, more aggressive imaging is associated with significantly higher costs, higher patient anxiety, and little associated benefit in terms of survival.

In some cases, indolent non-Hodgkin lymphoma can be observed and monitored without treatment, and some patients never require any treatment. Furthermore, attempts to utilize aggressive up-front therapy have not demonstrated improvement in overall survival duration [4]. In patients who require therapy, current recommendations are single-agent immunotherapy or combination chemoimmunotherapy.

Such treatments are generally not considered curative, though some patients may have prolonged relapse-free survival. After completion of induction therapy, most patients are then treated with maintenance immunotherapy [43]. Salvage treatment can involve use of the same agents as well as radioimmunotherapy, and may ultimately escalate to autologous or allogeneic hematopoietic stem cell transplantation. Transformation to a more aggressive histology which, in turn, requires more aggressive treatment, is a constant concern [4]. Evidence of marked progression between examination intervals should prompt rebiopsy to evaluate for disease transformation.

After initial diagnosis, patients who do not require therapy should be followed in the office every 3 months to evaluate the velocity of disease progression. Similarly, patients who receive treatment at diagnosis should be followed every 3 months to evaluate for relapse and/or progressive disease. Surveillance should include history, physical examination, and tests as in other types of non-Hodgkin lymphoma. The duration of surveillance should be considered indefinite, as this is not a curable disease (unless allogeneic hematopoietic stem cell transplantation is used). After 5 years, moving to a less intensive schedule can be considered in patients who clearly understand the possible symptoms of relapse and have no evidence of disease or a small volume of residual disease that does not threaten vital organ function. Imaging with CT scan can be performed every 6 months for the first year after diagnosis to evaluate disease velocity and annually thereafter, as relapse or disease progression is expected. PET scan can be used in the follow-up of indolent lymphoma when needed but, before the test is ordered, one should consider how the additional information obtained by PET (as opposed to CT scan without PET) will be used. For example, follicular lymphoma would be expected to be PET positive in any residual masses following initial therapy. In most circumstances, demonstrating continued PET avidity adds little to the treatment planning. On the other hand, a change in tumor size detectable by CT scan typically drives treatment plans. One other consideration with indolent non-Hodgkin lymphoma is that the risk of histologic transformation remains constant throughout the early follow-up period (8 years), arguing against discontinuation of surveillance or lengthening the testing interval to greater than 6 months though, in a patient with a long disease-free interval, this may be reasonable [44].

For most lymphoma subtypes, our follow-up approaches differ modestly from the published guidelines presented earlier in terms of surveillance strategies. Guidelines such as those proposed by NCCN remain vague, reflecting the clinically heterogeneous nature of lymphoma, and the need for flexibility. Most guidelines do not specify frequency of imaging or laboratory testing, reflecting the scant data supporting their use in the detection of preclinical disease. Our schedule of laboratory testing is probably more conservative than that of others. Our schedule of CT scanning during the initial follow-up period (the length of which is determined by disease subtype) is also more conservative than that of most physicians, since it is not clear that a more aggressive imaging schedule improves clinical outcomes. In our practice, PET scanning is reserved for evaluation of disease at the time of suspected relapse, given the associated increased cost and radiation exposure, without clear evidence of clinical benefit in the screening of asymptomatic patients.

References

1. Jaffe E, Harris N, Stein H, Isaacson P. Classification of lymphoid neoplasms: the microscope as a tool for disease discovery. Blood. 2008;112:4384–99.
2. NCCN Clinical Practice Guidelines in Oncology: Hodgkin Disease/Lymphoma. 2009. http://www.24hmb.com/UpLoad/Editor/2010/1/4/201001047125180l.pdf. Accessed 15 May 2009.
3. Evens AM, Gordon LI, Evens AM, Gordon LI. Burkitt's and Burkitt-like lymphoma. Curr Treat Options Oncol. 2002;3:291–305.
4. Gribben JG, Gribben JG. How I treat indolent lymphoma. Blood. 2007;109:4617–26.
5. Cabanillas F, Velasquez WS, Hagemeister FB, McLaughlin P, Redman JR. Clinical, biologic, and histologic features of late relapses in diffuse large cell lymphoma. Blood. 1992;79:1024–8.
6. Morton LM, Curtis RE, Linet MS, et al. Second malignancy risks after non-Hodgkin's lymphoma and chronic lymphocytic leukemia: differences by lymphoma subtype. J Clin Oncol. 2010;28:4935–44.
7. Radford JA, Eardley A, Woodman C, Crowther D. Follow-up policy after treatment for Hodgkin's disease: too many clinic visits and routine tests? A review of hospital records. BMJ. 1997;314:343–6.
8. Torrey MJ, Poen JC, Hoppe RT. Detection of relapse in early-stage Hodgkin's disease: role of routine follow-up studies. J Clin Oncol. 1997;15:1123–30.
9. Liedtke M, Hamlin PA, Moskowitz CH, Zelenetz AD. Surveillance imaging during remission identifies a group of patients with more favorable aggressive NHL at time of relapse: a retrospective analysis of a uniformly-treated patient population. [see comment]. Ann Oncol. 2006;17:909–13.
10. Armitage JO, Armitage JO. How I treat patients with diffuse large B-cell lymphoma. Blood. 2007;110:29–36.
11. Engert A, Dreyling M, Group EGW. Hodgkin's lymphoma: ESMO clinical recommendations for diagnosis, treatment and follow-up. Ann Oncol. 2008;19 Suppl 2:ii65–66.
12. Weeks JC, Yeap BY, Canellos GP, Shipp MA. Value of follow-up procedures in patients with large-cell lymphoma who achieve a complete remission. J Clin Oncol. 1991;9:1196–203.
13. Hasenclever D, Diehl V. A prognostic score for advanced Hodgkin's disease. International Prognostic Factors Project on Advanced Hodgkin's Disease. [see comment]. New Engl J Med. 1998;339: 1506–14.
14. Solal-Celigny P, Roy P, Colombat P, et al. Follicular Lymphoma International Prognostic Index. [see comment]. Blood. 2004;104: 1258–65.
15. Hoster E, Dreyling M, Klapper W, et al. A new prognostic index (MIPI) for patients with advanced-stage mantle cell lymphoma. [see comment]. Blood. 2008;111:558–65 [erratum appears in Blood. 2008 Jun 15;111(12):5761].
16. Friedman S, Henry-Amar M, Cosset JM, et al. Evolution of erythrocyte sedimentation rate as predictor of early relapse in posttherapy early-stage Hodgkin's disease. J Clin Oncol. 1988;6:596–602.

17. Ng AK, Constine L, Deming R, et al. ACR appropriateness criteria: follow-up of Hodgkin's disease. Reston, VA: American College of Radiology; 2005.
18. Brenner DJ, Hall EJ, Brenner DJ, Hall EJ. Computed tomography-an increasing source of radiation exposure.[see comment]. New Engl J Med. 2007;357:2277–84.
19. Guadagnolo BA, Punglia RS, Kuntz KM, et al. Cost-effectiveness analysis of computerized tomography in the routine follow-up of patients after primary treatment for Hodgkin's disease. J Clin Oncol. 2006;24:4116–22.
20. NCI. Rituximab and combination chemotherapy in treating patients with Stage II, Stage III or Stage IV diffuse large B-cell non-Hodgkin's lymphoma. Clinicaltrials.gov identifier: NCT00274924. http://clinicaltrials.gov/ct2/show/NCT00274924. Accessed 15 June 2009.
21. Juweid ME, Cheson BD, Juweid ME, Cheson BD. Positron-emission tomography and assessment of cancer therapy [see comment]. NEJM. 2006;354:496–507.
22. Cheson B, Cheson B. The case against heavy PETing. [comment]. J Clin Oncol. 2009;27:1742–3.
23. Zinzani PL, Stefoni V, Tani M, et al. Role of [18F]fluorodeoxyglucose positron emission tomography scan in the follow-up of lymphoma. [see comment]. J Clin Oncol. 2009;27:1781–7.
24. Morton LM, Wang SS, Devesa SS, Harge P, Weisenburger DD, Linet MS. Lymphoma incidence patterns by WHO subtype in the United States, 1992–2001. Blood. 2006;107:265–76.
25. Franklin JG, Paus MD, Pluetschow A, Specht L. Chemotherapy, radiotherapy and combined modality for Hodgkin's disease, with emphasis on second cancer risk. Cochrane Database Syst Rev. 2005;CD003187.
26. David KA, Mauro L, Evens AM, David KA, Mauro L, Evens AM. Relapsed and refractory Hodgkin lymphoma: transplantation strategies and novel therapeutic options. Curr Treat Options Oncol. 2007;8:352–74.
27. Herman TS, Hoppe RT, Donaldson SS, Cox RS, Rosenberg SA, Kaplan HS. Late relapse among patients treated for Hodgkin's disease. Ann Intern Med. 1985;102:292–7.
28. Saslow D, Boetes C, Burke W, et al. American Cancer Society guidelines for breast screening with MRI as an adjunct to mammography.[erratum appears in CA Cancer J Clin. 2007 May-Jun;57(3):185]. CA Cancer J Clin. 2007;57:75–89.
29. Das P, Ng AK, Earle CC, Mauch PM, Kuntz KM. Computed tomography screening for lung cancer in Hodgkin's lymphoma survivors: decision analysis and cost-effectiveness analysis. Ann Oncol. 2006;17:785–93.
30. Chen A, Punglia RS, Kuntz KM, Mauch PM, Ng AK. Cost-effectiveness of lipid screening in Hodgkin's disease survivors. Int J Radiat Oncol. 2006;66:S94–S95 (Abstract 168).
31. Heidenreich PA, Schnittger I, Strauss HW, et al. Screening for coronary artery disease after mediastinal irradiation for Hodgkin's disease. [see comment]. J Clin Oncol. 2007;25:43–9 [erratum appears in J Clin Oncol. 2007 Apr 20;25(12):1635].
32. Hequet O, Le QH, Moullet I, et al. Subclinical late cardiomyopathy after doxorubicin therapy for lymphoma in adults. J Clin Oncol. 2004;22:1864–71.
33. Hulbert JC, Grossman JE, Cummings KB. Risk factors of anesthesia and surgery in bleomycin-treated patients. J Urol. 1983;130: 163–4.
34. Jeruss JS, Woodruff TK, Jeruss JS, Woodruff TK. Preservation of fertility in patients with cancer. NEJM. 2009;360:902–11.
35. Oeffinger KC, Ford JS, Moskowitz CS, et al. Breast cancer surveillance practices among women previously treated with chest radiation for a childhood cancer.[see comment]. JAMA. 2009;301: 404–14.
36. Diehl V, Sextro M, Franklin J, et al. Clinical presentation, course, and prognostic factors in lymphocyte-predominant Hodgkin's disease and lymphocyte-rich classical Hodgkin's disease: report from the European Task Force on Lymphoma Project on Lymphocyte-Predominant Hodgkin's Disease.[see comment]. J Clin Oncol. 1999;17:776–83.
37. Nogova L, Reineke T, Brillant C, et al. Lymphocyte-predominant and classical Hodgkin's lymphoma: a comprehensive analysis from the German Hodgkin Study Group.[see comment]. J Clin Oncol. 2008;26:434–9.
38. Huang JZ, Weisenburger DD, Vose JM, et al. Diffuse large B-cell lymphoma arising in nodular lymphocyte predominant Hodgkin lymphoma: a report of 21 cases from the Nebraska Lymphoma Study Group. Leuk Lymphoma. 2004;45:1551–7.
39. Vose J, Armitage J, Weisenburger D, et al. International peripheral T-cell and natural killer/T-cell lymphoma study: pathology findings and clinical outcomes. J Clin Oncol. 2008;26:4124–30.
40. Ziegler JL, Bluming AZ, Fass L, Morrow Jr RH. Relapse patterns in Burkitt's lymphoma. Cancer Res. 1972;32:1267–72.
41. Sweetenham JW, Pearce R, Taghipour G, Blaise D, Gisselbrecht C, Goldstone AH. Adult Burkitt's and Burkitt-like non-Hodgkin's lymphoma–outcome for patients treated with high-dose therapy and autologous stem-cell transplantation in first remission or at relapse: results from the European Group for Blood and Marrow Transplantation. J Clin Oncol. 1996;14:2465–72.
42. Biggar RJ, Nkrumah FK, Henle W, Levine PH. Very late relapses in patients with Burkitt's lymphoma: clinical and serologic studies. J Natl Cancer Inst. 1981;66:439–44.
43. van Oers MH, Klasa R, Marcus RE, et al. Rituximab maintenance improves clinical outcome of relapsed/resistant follicular non-Hodgkin lymphoma in patients both with and without rituximab during induction: results of a prospective randomized phase 3 intergroup trial. Blood. 2006;108:3295–301.
44. Montoto S, Davies AJ, Matthews J, et al. Risk and clinical implications of transformation of follicular lymphoma to diffuse large B-cell lymphoma. J Clin Oncol. 2007;25:2426–33.

Lymphoma Surveillance Counterpoint: Japan

92

Kenjiro Kamezaki

Keywords
Malignant lymphoma • Adult T-cell leukemia/lymphoma • Non-Hodgkin's lymphoma • Hodgkin's lymphoma • Rituximab

The incidence of lymphoma in Japan is lower than that in the USA and Europe, but the incidence of T-cell lymphoma, particularly adult T-cell leukemia/lymphoma, is higher [1]. Kyushu University Hospital is in the Kyushu islands, a southwestern part of Japan where adult T-cell leukemia/lymphoma is endemic. Conventional chemotherapy regimens have been administered to adult T-cell leukemia/lymphoma patients, but the outcomes are very poor. Promising results of allogeneic stem cell transplantation for adult T-cell leukemia/lymphoma have recently been reported [2, 3].

The frequency and specific tests critical to the management of patients after treatment for lymphoma have never been firmly established. I generally agree with the follow-up strategies proposed by professional organizations and national government agencies, which are available on the Internet: The National Comprehensive Cancer Network (www.nccn.org), The European Society for Medical Oncology (www.esmo.org), and The National Guideline Clearinghouse (www.guideline.gov). Additional data are provided concerning the follow-up schedule at Kyushu University Hospital in Japan.

Rituximab has changed the treatment paradigm of CD20-positive lymphoma. It has shown improved response and survival rates in combination with conventional chemotherapy, and now rituximab-containing chemotherapy regimens are widely used for the initial standard treatment of patients with aggressive non-Hodgkin's lymphoma and low-grade non-Hodgkin's lymphoma at advanced stages [4–7].

Rituximab is a human/mouse chimeric monoclonal antibody that specifically targets the CD20 antigen expressed on normal and malignant B cells. A prolonged period of rituximab-induced normal B-cell depletion can compromise the immune system. This may cause an increase in serious viral infections. Reactivation of chronic hepatitis B virus, cytomegalovirus, and varicella-zoster virus infections have all been reported after rituximab treatment [8–10]. Reactivation of chronic hepatitis B virus is a well-recognized complication of chemotherapy in both HBs-Ag-positive inactive carriers and in individuals with chronic hepatitis B virus infection. Hepatitis B virus reactivation has been considered to be much less common in patients who have resolved hepatitis B virus (HBs-Ag negative, antibody to hepatitis B core antigen [anti-HBc] ±, and antibody to hepatitis B surface antigen [anti-HBs] positive). A recent paper reported that 23.8% of diffuse, large B-cell lymphoma patients who have resolved hepatitis B virus developed hepatitis B virus reactivation after rituximab treatment [10]. This report suggests that, for patients who are scheduled to receive rituximab, those patients who are HBs-Ag negative should further be screened for anti-HBc and anti-HBs. Patients who have resolved hepatitis B virus should be closely monitored for reactivation after rituximab therapy.

Late-onset neutropenia has been reported after chemotherapy combined with rituximab [11]. It usually occurs within 6 months after the last dose of rituximab and is usually self-limited. Life-threatening infections are rare. However, clinicians should be aware of it when following patients treated with rituximab-containing chemotherapy.

^{18}F-fluoro-deoxyglucose (FDG) positron emission tomography (PET) combined with computed tomography (CT) is a promising functional imaging test for patients with lymphoma

K. Kamezaki, M.D., Ph.D. (✉)
Medicine and Biosystemic Science, Graduate School of Medical Sciences, Kyushu University, 3-1-1 Maidashi, Higashi-ku Fukuoka 812-8582, Japan
e-mail: kamejiro@intmed1.med.kyushu-u.ac.jp

F.E. Johnson et al. (eds.), *Patient Surveillance After Cancer Treatment*, Current Clinical Oncology,
DOI 10.1007/978-1-60327-969-7_92,

Table 92.1 Surveillance after curative-intent treatment for lymphoma (Hodgkin's lymphoma or aggressive non-Hodgkin's lymphoma in complete remission) at Kyushu University Hospital, Japan

	Year					
	1	2	3	4	5	>5
Office visit	4–6	4	4	2–4	2–4	1–2
Complete blood count	4–6	4	4	2–4	2–4	1–2
Liver function tests	4–6	4	4	2–4	2–4	1–2
Chest X-ray	2	2	2	1–2	1–2	0–1
Site computed tomography	2	2	2	1–2	1–2	0–1
Positron emission tomography	1	0	0	0	0	0

The number in each cell indicates the number of times a particular modality is recommended in a particular posttreatment year

Table 92.2 Surveillance after curative-intent treatment for lymphoma (low-grade non-Hodgkin's lymphoma in complete remission) at Kyushu University Hospital, Japan

	Year					
	1	2	3	4	5	>5
Office visit	4–6	3	3	3	2	1–2
Complete blood count	4–6	3	3	3	2	1–2
Liver function tests	4–6	3	3	3	2	1–2
Chest X-ray	2	1	1	1	1	1
Site computed tomography	2	2	2	2	2	1–2
Positron emission tomography	1	0	0	0	0	0

The number in each cell indicates the number of times a particular modality is recommended in a particular posttreatment year

and has been shown to be useful for monitoring treatment response at completion of first-line treatment [12, 13]. FDG PET-CT scans are usually performed approximately 2 months after completion of therapy in our institution.

Tables 92.1 and 92.2 show the follow-up strategies recommended for non-Hodgkin's lymphoma patients treated with conventional treatment. During year 1 after completion of treatment patients are usually examined every 2–3 months because infectious complications, late-onset neutropenia, and hepatitis B virus reactivation occur frequently in year 1. Physical examination, complete blood count, and liver function tests are performed at each visit. CT is performed every 6–12 months during the first 5 years. Since patients with low-grade non-Hodgkin's lymphoma are at continuous risk for recurrence even after 10 years, they have CT every 6–12 months for 6–10 years. Since the risk of secondary malignancy such as solid tumors, myelodysplastic syndrome, and acute myelogenous leukemia seems to remain high even after 10 years, patients are examined every 6–12 months for over 5 years after completion of treatment, with specific diagnostic tests chosen on the basis of history and physical findings.

References

1. Tajima K. Malignant lymphomas in Japan: epidemiological analysis of adult T-cell leukemia/lymphoma (ATL). Cancer Metastasis Rev. 1988;7:223–41.
2. Okamura J, Utsunomiya A, Tanosaki R, et al. Allogeneic stem-cell transplantation with reduced conditioning intensity as a novel immunotherapy and antiviral therapy for adult T-cell leukemia/lymphoma. Blood. 2005;105:4143–5.
3. Kato K, Kanda Y, Eto T, et al. Allogeneic bone marrow transplantation from unrelated human T-cell leukemia virus-I-negative donors for adult T-cell leukemia/lymphoma: retrospective analysis of data from the Japan Marrow Donor Program. Biol Blood Marrow Transplant. 2007;13:90–9.
4. Coiffier B, Lepage E, Briere J, et al. CHOP chemotherapy plus rituximab compared with CHOP alone in elderly patients with diffuse large-B-cell lymphoma. N Engl J Med. 2002;346: 235–42.
5. Czuczman MS, Weaver R, Alkuzweny B, Berlfein J, Grillo-Lopez AJ. Prolonged clinical and molecular remission in patients with low-grade or follicular non-Hodgkin's lymphoma treated with rituximab plus CHOP chemotherapy: 9-year follow-up. J Clin Oncol. 2004;22:4711–6.
6. Habermann TM, Weller EA, Morrison VA, et al. Rituximab-CHOP versus CHOP alone or with maintenance rituximab in older patients with diffuse large B-cell lymphoma. J Clin Oncol. 2006;24: 3121–7.
7. Pfreundschuh M, Trumper L, Osterborg A, et al. CHOP-like chemotherapy plus rituximab versus CHOP-like chemotherapy alone in young patients with good-prognosis diffuse large-B-cell lymphoma: a randomised controlled trial by the MabThera International Trial (MInT) Group. Lancet Oncol. 2006;7: 379–91.
8. Suzan F, Ammor M, Ribrag V. Fatal reactivation of cytomegalovirus infection after use of rituximab for a post-transplantation lymphoproliferative disorder. N Engl J Med. 2001;345:1000.
9. Goldberg SL, Pecora AL, Alter RS, et al. Unusual viral infections (progressive multifocal leukoencephalopathy and cytomegalovirus disease) after high-dose chemotherapy with autologous blood stem cell rescue and peritransplantation rituximab. Blood. 2002;99: 1486–8.
10. Yeo W, Chan TC, Leung NW, et al. Hepatitis B virus reactivation in lymphoma patients with prior resolved Hepatitis B undergoing anticancer therapy with or without Rituximab. J Clin Oncol. 2009;27:605–11. Originally published as JCO Early Release 10.1200/JCO.2008.18.0182 on December 15, 2008.
11. Lemieux B, Tartas S, Traulle C, et al. Rituximab-related late-onset neutropenia after autologous stem cell transplantation for aggressive non-Hodgkin's lymphoma. Bone Marrow Transplant. 2004;33: 921–3.
12. Cheson BD, Pfistner B, Juweid ME, et al. Revised response criteria for malignant lymphoma. J Clin Oncol. 2007;25:579–86.
13. Juweid ME, Stroobants S, Hoekstra OS, et al. Use of positron emission tomography for response assessment of lymphoma: consensus of the Imaging Subcommittee of International Harmonization Project in Lymphoma. J Clin Oncol. 2007;25: 571–8.

Lymphoma (Following Autologous Stem Cell Transplant)

93

Shilpi Wadhwa, David Y. Johnson, and Frank E. Johnson

Keywords
Lymphoma • Hematopoietic cell transplant • Surveillance • Transplant • Evidence

Surveillance Strategies Proposed by Professional Organizations or National Government Agencies and Available on the Internet

Although treatment strategies for lymphoma may include hematopoietic cell transplant, quantitative surveillance recommendations that were accessed for lymphoma patients did not distinguish between those with or without transplant [1–5]. The guidelines in Chapter 26 should be considered applicable to all lymphoma patients, including those whose treatment includes transplant. The surveillance strategies related to immunosuppression are not discussed in this textbook.

National Comprehensive Cancer Network (NCCN, http://www.nccn.org)

NCCN guidelines were accessed on 1/28/12. No quantitative guidelines exist for lymphoma (following autologous stem cell transplant) surveillance including when first accessed on 4/10/07.

S. Wadhwa • D.Y. Johnson
Department of Internal Medicine, Saint Louis University Medical Center, Saint Louis, MO, USA

F.E. Johnson (✉)
Saint Louis University Medical Center and Saint Louis Veterans Affairs Medical Center, Saint Louis, MO, USA
e-mail: frank.johnson1@va.gov

American Society of Clinical Oncology (ASCO, http://www.asco.org)

ASCO guidelines were accessed on 1/28/12. No quantitative guidelines exist for lymphoma (following autologous stem cell transplant) surveillance including when first accessed on 10/31/07.

The Society of Surgical Oncology (SSO, http://www.surgonc.org)

SSO guidelines were accessed on 1/28/12. No quantitative guidelines exist for lymphoma (following autologous stem cell transplant) surveillance including when first accessed on 10/31/07.

European Society for Medical Oncology (ESMO, http://www.esmo.org)

ESMO guidelines were accessed on 1/28/12. No quantitative guidelines exist for lymphoma (following autologous stem cell transplant) surveillance including when first accessed on 10/31/07.

European Society of Surgical Oncology (ESSO, http://www.esso-surgeonline.org)

ESSO guidelines were accessed on 1/28/12. No quantitative guidelines exist for lymphoma (following autologous stem cell transplant) surveillance including when first accessed on 10/31/07.

F.E. Johnson et al. (eds.), *Patient Surveillance After Cancer Treatment*, Current Clinical Oncology,
DOI 10.1007/978-1-60327-969-7_93, © Springer Science+Business Media New York 2013

Cancer Care Ontario (CCO, http://www.cancercare.on.ca)

CCO guidelines were accessed on 1/28/12. No quantitative guidelines exist for lymphoma surveillance (following autologous stem cell transplant) including when first accessed on 10/31/07.

National Institute for Clinical Excellence (NICE, http://www.nice.org.uk)

NICE guidelines were accessed on 1/28/12. No quantitative guidelines exist for lymphoma surveillance (following autologous stem cell transplant) including when first accessed on 10/31/07.

The Cochrane Collaboration (CC, http://www.cochrane.org)

CC guidelines were accessed on 1/28/12. No quantitative guidelines exist for lymphoma surveillance (following autologous stem cell transplant) including when first accessed on 11/24/07.

The M.D. Anderson Surgical Oncology Handbook also has follow-up guidelines, proposed by authors from a single National Cancer Institute-designated Comprehensive Cancer Center, for many types of cancer [6]. Some are detailed and quantitative, others are qualitative.

Summary

This is a common cancer with significant variability in incidence worldwide. We found consensus-based guidelines but none based on high-quality evidence.

References

1. Parkin DM, Whelan SL, Ferlay J, Teppo L, Thomas DB. Cancer incidence in five continents, Vol. VIII, International Agency for research on cancer. (IARC Scientific Publication 155). Lyon, France: IARC Press; 2002: ISBN 92-832-2155-9.
2. Jemal A, Seigel R, Ward E, Murray T, Xu J, Thun MJ. Cancer statistics. CA Cancer J Clin. 2007;57:43–66.
3. Schottenfeld D, Fraumeni JG. Cancer epidemiology and prevention. 3rd ed. New York, NY: Oxford University Press; 2006: ISBN 13:978-0-19-514961-6.
4. DeVita VT, Hellman S, Rosenberg SA. Cancer. 7th ed. Philadelphia, PA: Lippincott Williams & Wilkins; 2005: ISBN 0-781-74450-4.
5. Devesa SS, Grauman DJ, Blot WJ, Pennello GA, Hoover RN, Fraumeni JF Jr. Atlas of cancer mortality in the United States. National Institutes of Health, National Cancer Institute. NIH Publication No. 99-4564; 1999.
6. Feig BW, Berger DH, Fuhrman GM. The M.D. Anderson surgical oncology handbook. 4th ed. Philadelphia, PA: Lippincott Williams & Wilkins; 2006: ISBN 0-7817-5643-X (paperback).

94 Lymphoma (Following Autologous Stem Cell Transplant) Surveillance Counterpoint: Japan

Toshihiro Miyamoto

Keywords
Lymphoma • Japan • Chemotherapy • High-dose chemotherapy • Rituximab

The Parma group study, a randomized multicenter trial of treatment for patients with chemotherapy-responsive, relapsed aggressive non-Hodgkin's lymphoma, has established the superiority of high-dose chemotherapy and autologous stem cell transplant over conventional salvage chemotherapy [1]. Subsequently, autologous stem cell transplant has become a standard approach for relapsed non-Hodgkin's lymphoma. Recent reports also have revealed that high-dose chemotherapy followed by autologous stem cell transplant is superior to standard chemotherapy as a primary treatment for newly diagnosed patients with aggressive non-Hodgkin's lymphoma [2, 3]. In our institution and the affiliated hospitals, the so-called Fukuoka Blood and Marrow Transplantation Group (upfront high-dose chemotherapy with autologous peripheral blood stem cell transplant after six cycles of the standard CHOP regimen) has been provided as consolidation for newly diagnosed patients as well as relapsed patients with aggressive non-Hodgkin's lymphoma since 1990 [4]. The specific disease entities that we consider are aggressive B-cell lymphomas, such as diffuse, large B-cell lymphoma and peripheral T-cell lymphomas, at the stage of high intermediate to high risk, according to the International Prognostic Index. The conditioning regimen consists of MCEC (ranimustine 200 mg/m^2 × 2, carboplatin 300 mg/m^2 × 4, etoposide 500 mg/m^2 × 3, cyclophosphamide 50 mg/kg × 2). In total, 3.6% of patients died of transplant-related causes. The estimated overall survival at 5 years following autologous stem cell transplant was 63% in aggressive B-cell lymphomas ($n = 252$) and 62% in peripheral T-cell lymphomas ($n = 39$) in the Fukuoka Blood and Marrow Transplantation Group experience. Five-year overall survival was significantly higher in patients transplanted at the first complete remission than in those with other disease status (79% vs. 50% in diffuse, large B-cell lymphoma and 83% vs. 49% in peripheral T-cell lymphomas, respectively).

Several reports have demonstrated a high incidence of second malignancies following high-dose therapy with autologous stem cell transplant. In the Fukuoka Blood and Marrow Transplantation Group experience, the cumulative incidence of developing a second cancer by 5 years after autologous peripheral blood stem cell transplant was 7.5%. In total, 1.7% of all patients developed acute myelogenous leukemia or myelodysplastic syndrome and 1.1% developed solid tumors at a median time of 56 (range 12–73) months following autologous peripheral blood stem cell transplant. Factors significantly associated with an increased risk of developing a second cancer were age >45 years ($p < 0.05$) and prior radiotherapy ($p < 0.01$). Therefore, patients who undergo autologous peripheral blood stem cell transplant are at a high risk for developing a second malignancy and should receive continuous follow-up.

Rituximab has changed the treatment paradigm of CD20-positive lymphoma and has improved response rate and overall survival duration in combination with chemotherapy [5–7]. Recent trials have focused on how to incorporate rituximab into high-dose chemotherapy regimens followed by autologous stem cell transplant as first-line treatment [8, 9], including the concept of in vivo purging of lymphoma cells from the circulation prior to the collection of blood for the autologous peripheral blood stem cell transplant [10, 11]. After September 2003, when rituximab was approved for the treatment of diffuse, large B-cell lymphoma in Japan, we

T. Miyamoto, M.D., Ph.D. (✉)
Medicine and Biosystemic Science, Kyushu University Graduate School of Medical Sciences, 3-1-1 Maidashi, Higashi-ku, Fukuoka 812-8582, Japan
e-mail: toshmiya@intmed1.med.kyushu-u.ac.jp

F.E. Johnson et al. (eds.), *Patient Surveillance After Cancer Treatment*, Current Clinical Oncology,
DOI 10.1007/978-1-60327-969-7_94, © Springer Science+Business Media New York 2013

Table 94.1 Surveillance after curative-intent treatment for lymphoma (following autologous stem cell transplant) at Kyushu University Hospital, Japan

	Years posttreatment				
	1	2	3	4	5
Office visit	6–8	4	4	2–4	2–4
Complete blood count	6–8	4	4	2–4	2–4
Liver function tests	6–8	4	4	2–4	2–4
Chest X-ray	3–4	2	2	1–2	1–2
Conventional CT	2	2	2	1–2	1–2
PET-CT	1	[a]	[a]	[a]	[a]

[a]only if clinically indicated. The numbers in each cell indicate the number of times per year each modality is recommended during a particular year posttreatment

conducted a trial consisting of rituximab plus CHOP as the front-line high-dose chemotherapy regimen with autologous peripheral blood stem cell transplant for patients with CD20-positive diffuse, large B-cell lymphoma and an age-adjusted International Prognostic Index score of 2 or 3 [4]. We have found no adverse effect of rituximab on the mobilization and engraftment of autologous peripheral blood stem cells so far [4]. However, late-onset neutropenia associated with rituximab has occurred more frequently following our rituximab-containing high-dose therapy regimen with autologous peripheral blood stem cell transplant compared to conventional treatment with rituximab plus CHOP (35% vs. 10%), as described elsewhere [12–14]. Late-onset neutropenia developed at a median of 5 months following autologous peripheral blood stem cell transplant in our series. Late-onset neutropenia episodes were self-limited and granulocyte-colony stimulating factor was administered in one patient without serious infectious complication. Therefore, clinicians should be aware of a high incidence of late-onset neutropenia when applying high-dose chemotherapy regimens along with rituximab.

Adult T-cell leukemia/lymphoma is endemic in southwestern Japan where our institution is located. Therapeutic trials using various combination chemotherapy regimens and autologous stem cell transplant to improve the poor prognosis of adult T-cell leukemia/lymphoma are unsatisfactory [15, 16]. Recently, a better therapeutic outcome has been obtained with allogeneic stem cell transplantation for adult T-cell leukemia/lymphoma [17, 18]. Prospective controlled studies by the Fukuoka Blood and Marrow Transplantation Group are underway to define the efficacy of, and clinical indications for, allogeneic stem cell transplantation in patients with adult T-cell leukemia/lymphoma.

Table 94.1 outlines the follow-up studies recommended for non-Hodgkin's lymphoma patients treated with high-dose therapy with autologous stem cell transplant. In our hospital, during year 1 after autologous peripheral blood stem cell transplant, patients are usually examined every 1–2 months because infectious complications, late-onset neutropenia, and disease relapse all occur more frequently during year 1 than thereafter. Since imaging with ^{18}F-fluorodeoxyglucose positron emission tomography combined with computed tomography (PET-CT) has been shown to be quite valuable for evaluating disease status and monitoring treatment response [19], PET-CT scans are usually performed at least at presentation, just before autologous peripheral blood stem cell transplant, and approximately 1 month after cessation of therapy. Physical examination, complete blood count, and liver function tests are performed at each visit. Conventional CT is performed every 6 months during the first 5 years.

References

1. Philip T, Guglielmi C, Hagenbeek A, et al. Autologous bone marrow transplantation as compared with salvage chemotherapy in relapses of chemotherapy-sensitive non-Hodgkin's lymphoma. N Engl J Med. 1995;333:1540–5.
2. Mangel J, Leitch HA, Connors JM, et al. Intensive chemotherapy and autologous stem-cell transplantation plus rituximab is superior to conventional chemotherapy for newly diagnosed advanced stage mantle-cell lymphoma: a matched pair analysis. Ann Oncol. 2004;15:283–90.
3. Milpied N, Deconinck E, Gaillard F, et al. Initial treatment of aggressive lymphoma with high-dose chemotherapy and autologous stem-cell support. N Engl J Med. 2004;350:1287–95.
4. Kamezaki K, Kikushige Y, Numata A, et al. Rituximab does not compromise the mobilization and engraftment of autologous peripheral blood stem cells in diffuse-large B-cell lymphoma. Bone Marrow Transplant. 2007;39:523–7.
5. Czuczman MS, Grillo-Lopez AJ, White CA, et al. Treatment of patients with low-grade B-cell lymphoma with the combination of chimeric anti-CD20 monoclonal antibody and CHOP chemotherapy. J Clin Oncol. 1999;17:268–76.
6. Vose JM, Link BK, Grossbard ML, et al. Phase II study of rituximab in combination with CHOP chemotherapy in patients with previously untreated, aggressive non-Hodgkin's lymphoma. J Clin Oncol. 2001;19:389–97.
7. Coiffier B, Lepage E, Briere J, et al. CHOP chemotherapy plus rituximab compared with CHOP alone in elderly patients with diffuse large-B-cell lymphoma. N Engl J Med. 2002;346:235–42.
8. Flinn IW, Lazarus HM. Monoclonal antibodies and autologous stem cell transplantation for lymphoma. Bone Marrow Transplant. 2001;27:565–9.
9. Nademanee A, Forman SJ. Role of hematopoietic stem cell transplantation for advanced-stage diffuse large cell B-cell lymphoma-B. Semin Hematol. 2006;43:240–50.
10. Buckstein R, Imrie K, Spaner D, et al. Stem cell function and engraftment is not affected by "*in vivo* purging" with rituximab for autologous stem cell treatment for patients with low-grade non-Hodgkin's lymphoma. Semin Oncol. 1999;26(5 Suppl 14):115–22.
11. Magni M, Di Nicola M, Devizzi L, et al. Successful *in vivo* purging of CD34-containing peripheral blood harvests in mantle cell and indolent lymphoma: evidence for a role of both chemotherapy and rituximab infusion. Blood. 2000;96:864–9.
12. Horwitz SM, Negrin RS, Blume KG, et al. Rituximab as adjuvant to high-dose therapy and autologous hematopoietic cell transplantation for aggressive non-Hodgkin lymphoma. Blood. 2004;103:777–83.

13. Lemieux B, Tartas S, Traulle C, et al. Rituximab-related late-onset neutropenia after autologous stem cell transplantation for aggressive non-Hodgkin's lymphoma. Bone Marrow Transplant. 2004;33:921–3.
14. Cairoli R, Grillo G, Tedeschi A, D'Avanzo G, Marenco P, Morra E. High incidence of neutropenia in patients treated with rituximab after autologous stem cell transplantation. Haematologica. 2004;89:361–3.
15. Shimoyama M, Ota K, Kikuchi M, et al. Chemotherapeutic results and prognostic factors of patients with advanced non-Hodgkin's lymphoma treated with VEPA or VEPA-M. J Clin Oncol. 1988; 6:128–41.
16. Tsukasaki K, Maeda T, Arimura K, et al. Poor outcome of autologous stem cell transplantation for adult T cell leukemia/lymphoma: a case report and review of the literature. Bone Marrow Transplant. 1999;23:87–9.
17. Okamura J, Utsunomiya A, Tanosaki R, et al. Allogeneic stem-cell transplantation with reduced conditioning intensity as a novel immunotherapy and antiviral therapy for adult T-cell leukemia/ lymphoma. Blood. 2005;105:4143–5.
18. Kato K, Kanda Y, Eto T, et al. Allogeneic bone marrow transplantation from unrelated human T-cell leukemia virus-I-negative donors for adult T-cell leukemia/lymphoma: retrospective analysis of data from the Japan Marrow Donor Program. Biol Blood Marrow Transplant. 2007;13:90–9.
19. Alousi AM, Saliba RM, Okoroji GJ, et al. Disease staging with positron emission tomography or gallium scanning and use of rituximab predict outcome for patients with diffuse large B-cell lymphoma treated with autologous stem cell transplantation. Br J Haematol. 2008;142:786–92.

Leukemia

95

David Y. Johnson, Shilpi Wadhwa, and Frank E. Johnson

Keywords
Leukemia • Lymphocytic leukemia • Age • Fanconi's syndrome • Bloom's syndrome • Trisomy 21

The International Agency for Research on Cancer (IARC), a component of the World Health Organization (WHO), estimated that there were 300,522 new cases leukemia worldwide in 2002 [1]. The IARC also estimated that there were 222,506 deaths due to this cause in 2002 [1].

The American Cancer Society estimated that there were 44,240 new cases and 21,790 deaths due to this cause in the USA in 2007 [2]. The estimated 5-year survival rate (all races) in the USA in 2007 was 49% for leukemia [2]. Survival rates were adjusted for normal life expectancies and were based on cases diagnosed from 1996 to 2002 and followed through 2003.

The molecular biology of leukemias has been extensively explored and many genetic events have been described. Acute leukemias are relatively rare. The incidence of acute lymphocytic leukemia peaks in childhood, with a secondary rise in old age, while the incidence of acute myelogenous leukemia increases steadily with age. Prior chemotherapy and/or radiation are causative factors, as is tobacco smoke. Occupational exposure to benzene is an established cause and perhaps other organic chemicals may be causative agents as well. Infection with human T-cell lymphoma virus type I and Epstein-Barr virus is a risk factor for leukemia. Specific genetic syndromes such as Fanconi's syndrome, Bloom's syndrome, and trisomy 21 are potent risk factors [3, 4].

D.Y. Johnson • S. Wadhwa
Department of Internal Medicine, Saint Louis University Medical Center, Saint Louis, MO, USA

F.E. Johnson (✉)
Saint Louis University Medical Center and Saint Louis Veterans Affairs Medical Center, Saint Louis, MO, USA
e-mail: frank.johnson1@va.gov

Geographic Variation Worldwide

Internationally, there is a distinct racial and geographic gradient for total leukemia incidence, with the highest incidence reported in white and Hispanic white populations of North America and in Oceania, Italy, and the United Kingdom. The incidence is low in African-Americans, Israeli Jews, and populations in Denmark, France, Sweden, and Spain, and lowest in Japanese in Osaka, Chinese in Shanghai, and Indians in Bombay [3]. Geographic variation in the USA is also pronounced [3, 5].

Surveillance Strategies Proposed by Professional Organizations or National Government Agencies and Available on the Internet

National Comprehensive Cancer Network (http://www.nccn.org)

National Comprehensive Cancer Network (NCCN) guidelines were accessed on 1/28/12 (Tables 95.1, and 95.2). There are new quantitative guidelines compared to the qualitative guidelines accessed on 4/10/07.

American Society of Clinical Oncology (http://www.asco.org)

American Society of Clinical Oncology (ASCO) guidelines were accessed on 1/28/12. No quantitative guidelines exist for leukemia surveillance, including when first accessed on 10/31/07.

F.E. Johnson et al. (eds.), *Patient Surveillance After Cancer Treatment*, Current Clinical Oncology,
DOI 10.1007/978-1-60327-969-7_95, © Springer Science+Business Media New York 2013

Table 95.1 Obtained from NCCN (http://www.nccn.org) on 1-28-12 Acute Myeloid Leukemia

	Years posttreatment[a]					
	1	2	3	4	5	>5
Office visit[b]	4–12	4–12	2–4	2–4	2–4	0
CBC, platelets	4–12	4–12	2–4	2–4	2–4	0

Bone marrow aspirate only if peripheral smear is abnormal or cytopenias develop
Alternative donor search (including cord blood) should be initiated at first relapse in appropriate patients concomitant with institution of other therapy if no sibling donor has been identified
NCCN guidelines were accessed on 1/28/12. These are new quantitative guidelines compared to the qualitative guidelines accessed on 4/10/07
[a]The numbers in the table indicate the number of times the modality is recommended during the indicated year posttreatment
[b]CBC and platelets were the only quantitative recommendations given. We inferred that office visits would be recommended as frequently as these

Table 95.2 Obtained from NCCN (http://www.nccn.org) on 1-28-12 Chronic Myelogenous Leukemia

	Years posttreatment[a]					
	1	2	3	4	5	>5
Office visit[b]	4	4	2	2	2	0
QPCR monitoring (peripheral blood)	4	4	2	2	2	0

NCCN guidelines were accessed on 1/28/12. These are new quantitative guidelines compared to the qualitative guidelines accessed on 4/10/07
[a]The numbers in the table indicate the number of times the modality is recommended during the indicated year posttreatment
[b]QPCR monitoring was the only quantitative recommendation given. We inferred that office visit would be recommended as frequently as this

The Society of Surgical Oncology (http://www.surgonc.org)

The Society of Surgical Oncology (SSO) guidelines were accessed on 1/28/12. No quantitative guidelines exist for leukemia surveillance, including when first accessed on 10/31/07.

European Society for Medical Oncology (http://www.esmo.org)

European Society for Medical Oncology (ESMO) guidelines were accessed on 1/28/12 (Tables 95.3, and 95.4). There are new quantitative guidelines and minor quantitative and qualitative changes to old guidelines accessed on 10/31/07.

European Society of Surgical Oncology (http://www.esso-surgeonline.org)

European Society of Surgical Oncology (ESSO) guidelines were accessed on 1/28/12. No quantitative guidelines exist for leukemia surveillance, including when first accessed on 10/31/07.

Table 95.3 Obtained from ESMO (http://www.esmo.org) on 1-28-12 Chronic Myeloid Leukemia

	Years posttreatment[a]					
	1	2	3	4	5	>5
Office visit[b]	8	2–4	2–4	2–4	2–4	2–4
Cytogenetics[c]	≥1–2	≥1–2	≥1–2	≥1–2	≥1–2	≥1–2
RT-Q-PCR[d]	2–4	2–4	2–4	2–4	2–4	2–4

Screening for BCR-ABL KD mutations is recommended only in the case of failure or suboptimal response
Measuring imatinib concentration in the peripheral blood is recommended only in the case of suboptimal response, failure, dose-limiting toxicity, or adverse events
ESMO guidelines were accessed on 1/28/12. These are new quantitative guidelines compared to the qualitative guidelines accessed on 10/31/07
[a]The numbers in the table indicate the number of times the modality is recommended during the indicated year posttreatment
[b]At the beginning, and during the first 3 months, clinical, biochemical, and hematological monitoring is recommended every 2 weeks to ensure the compliance of the patient. After this period, office visit recommendations based on quantitative cytogenetics and RT-Q-PCR recommendations
[c]Chromosome banding analysis of marrow cell metaphases is recommended at least every 6 months until a CCgR has been achieved and confirmed. Once a CCgR has been achieved and confirmed, cytogenetics can be performed every 12 months, but if the patient was high risk by Sokal, or was a suboptimal responder, more frequent monitoring is advisable
[d]BCR-ABL:ABL%, on blood cells is recommended every 3 months until MMoIR has been achieved and confirmed. Once an MMoIR has been achieved and confirmed, RT-Q-PCR can be performed every 6 months, but if the patient was high risk by Sokal, or was a suboptimal responder, more frequent monitoring is advisable

Table 95.4 Obtained from ESMO (http://www.esmo.org) on 1-28-12 Chronic Lymphocytic Leukemia

	Years posttreatment[a]					
	1	2	3	4	5	>5
Office visit[b]	1–4	1–4	1–4	1–4	1–4	1–4
CBC	1–4	1–4	1–4	1–4	1–4	1–4

Special attention should be paid to the appearance of autoimmune cytopenias as well as the development of a Richter's syndrome or prolymphocytic leukemia
Patients with CLL have a two to sevenfold increased risk of developing secondary malignancies, including secondary myelodysplastic syndromes or acute myelogenous leukemia as well as solid tumors
ESMO guidelines were accessed on 1/28/12. There were minor quantitative and qualitative changes compared to the guidelines accessed on 10/31/07
[a]The numbers in the table indicate the number of times the modality is recommended during the indicated year posttreatment
[b]Follow-up of asymptomatic patients should include a blood cell count, and the palpation of lymph nodes, liver, and spleen

Cancer Care Ontario (http://www.cancercare.on.ca)

Cancer Care Ontario (CCO) guidelines were accessed on 1/28/12. No quantitative guidelines exist for leukemia surveillance, including when first accessed on 10/31/07.

National Institute for Clinical Excellence (http://www.nice.org.uk)

National Institute for Clinical Excellence (NICE) guidelines were accessed on 1/28/12. No quantitative guidelines exist for leukemia surveillance, including when first accessed on 10/31/07.

The Cochrane Collaboration (CC, http://www.cochrane.org)

CC guidelines were accessed on 1/28/12. No quantitative guidelines exist for leukemia surveillance, including when first accessed on 11/24/07.

The M.D. Anderson Surgical Oncology Handbook also has follow-up guidelines, proposed by authors from a single National Cancer Institute-designated Comprehensive Cancer Center, for many types of cancer [6]. Some are detailed and quantitative, others are qualitative.

Summary

This is a common cancer with significant variability in incidence worldwide. We found consensus-based guidelines but none based on high-quality evidence.

References

1. Parkin DM, Whelan SL, Ferlay J, Teppo L, Thomas DB. Cancer incidence in five continents, Vol. VIII, International Agency for Research on Cancer. (IARC Scientific Publication 155). Lyon, France: IARC Press; 2002: ISBN 92-832-2155-9.
2. Jemal A, Seigel R, Ward E, Murray T, Xu J, Thun MJ. Cancer Statistics. CA Cancer J Clin. 2007;57:43–66.
3. Schottenfeld D, Fraumeni JG. Cancer epidemiology and prevention. 3rd ed. New York, NY: Oxford University Press; 2006: ISBN 13:978-0-19-514961-6.
4. DeVita VT, Hellman S, Rosenberg SA. Cancer. 7th ed. Philadelphia, PA: Lippincott Williams & Wilkins; 2005: ISBN 0-781-74450-4.
5. Devesa SS, Grauman DJ, Blot WJ, Pennello GA, Hoover RN, Fraumeni JF Jr. Atlas of cancer mortality in the United States. National Institutes of Health, National Cancer Institute. NIH Publication No. 99-4564; 1999.
6. Feig BW, Berger DH, Fuhrman GM. The M.D. Anderson surgical oncology handbook. 4th ed. Philadelphia, PA: Lippincott Williams & Wilkins; 2006: ISBN 0-7817-5643-X (paperback).

Leukemia Surveillance Counterpoint: USA

96

Olalekan Oluwole, Susan Greenhut, Bipin N. Savani, and Nishitha Reddy

Keywords
Malignancy • Leukemia • USA • Organ-specific toxicity • Cytopenias

Hematologic malignancies account for 6–8% of new cancers diagnosed in the USA annually. Over 40,000 new cases of leukemia and >20,000 deaths are attributed to leukemia of all types in the USA each year. Based on a recent National Cancer Institute report, the overall age-adjusted incidence of acute lymphoblastic leukemia in the USA is 1.5 in 100,000. The incidence in African–Americans is approximately one-half the incidence in Caucasians. The male-to-female ratio is 1.2:1.0. Among the approximately 4,000 new cases of acute lymphoblastic leukemia diagnosed each year in the USA, the incidence is highest in persons younger than 15 years old with a peak between ages 2 and 5. In the National Cancer Institute's 2000–2003 Surveillance Epidemiology and End Results Statistic Review (SEER), the median age at diagnosis was 13 years. The incidence of acute lymphoblastic leukemia decreases between the ages of 13–50; after age 50, it steadily rises. There are also geographic differences in the incidence, with higher rates in North America and Europe and lower rates in Africa and Asia [1].

The molecular biology of leukemia has been extensively explored and, as a result, many associated genetic events are known. Prior chemotherapy, radiation therapy, tobacco use, occupational exposure to benzene and other organic chemicals, infection with human T-cell lymphoma virus type I and Epstein–Barr virus, and specific genetic syndromes such as Fanconi's anemia, Bloom's syndrome, and Trisomy 21 are risk factors [1].

With improved survival duration after modern treatment, including hematopoietic stem cell transplantation (allo-HCT), there may be up to 500,000 long-term survivors worldwide who are at risk for treatment-related complications. These complications can result in significant morbidity and mortality. Most long-term survivors remain under the care of their hematologist–oncologist. Some are followed by a primary care physician who may not be familiar with specialized monitoring recommendations for this patient population. In this chapter, we describe practical approaches to detect and manage the late effects of allo-HCT, with the goal of reducing preventable morbidity and mortality in patients who are cured of their underlying disease.

There is no established surveillance schedule for patients who have been successfully treated for acute lymphoblastic leukemia. A major reason is that patients undergo a variety of chemotherapy regimens (i.e., both induction and consolidation therapies) in order to achieve remission. They then go through additional regimens as part of maintenance therapy. This heterogeneity in treatment leads to marked differences among patient subsets. Many patients, especially adults, also receive an allo-HCT [1, 2]. Survivors are at substantial risk for cardiovascular disease compared with the general population. Patients with acute lymphoblastic leukemia are treated with steroids either intermittently or continuously during the induction phase and are thus at risk for early development of elevated body mass index and high blood pressure, which places them at increased risk of adverse health conditions [3]. The incidence of complications increases with time from diagnosis and insures that the long-term impact of treatment on the health of survivors will be substantial.

O. Oluwole, M.D., M.P.H. • S. Greenhut, M.D.
• B.N. Savani, M.D. (✉) • N. Reddy, M.D., M.S.C.I.
Department of Medicine, Division of Hematology/Oncology, Hematology and Stem Cell Transplantation Section, Vanderbilt- Ingram Cancer Center, Vanderbilt University Medical Center, 1301 Medical Center Drive, 3927 TVC, Nashville, TN 37232-5505, USA
e-mail: Bipin.Savani@Vanderbilt.Edu

F.E. Johnson et al. (eds.), *Patient Surveillance After Cancer Treatment*, Current Clinical Oncology, DOI 10.1007/978-1-60327-969-7_96, © Springer Science+Business Media New York 2013

Surveillance after completion of maintenance therapy depends on several factors, including regimen-related toxicity, organ-specific toxicity, disease status, including measurement of minimal residual disease, and recommendations for allo-HCT recipients.

The specific agents, dose, and schedule determines which follow-up studies are needed to evaluate for regimen-related toxicity. Early identification of regimen-related toxicity allows for specific interventions that reduce long-term morbidity and mortality [4]. Regimen-related toxicity is traditionally divided into hematologic and organ-specific toxicity. Hematologic toxicity is common. There are no specific guidelines that specify how often acute lymphoblastic leukemia patients should be monitored for this [4]. In patients with other blood dyscrasias, such as chronic myelogenous leukemia and acute myelogenous leukemia, it is recommended that blood counts be checked every 3 months for the first 2 years [4–6]. We believe this is a reasonable recommendation to adopt in acute lymphoblastic leukemia patients in order to evaluate for marrow failure. Frequent monitoring of a patient's blood counts also allows for the detection of recurrent disease.

Chemotherapy-related marrow failure can be divided into three groups. Early cytopenias are due to cytotoxicity to progenitor and stem cells. This is usually self-limiting, although it can be prolonged. Intermediate cytopenias are usually due to a residual effect of chemotherapy, particularly if agents with a long half-life or that are known to be associated with cytopenias are used. For example, methotrexate can generate cytopenias that can be quite prolonged, especially if the patient received multiple courses and sustains stem cell damage as a result [7, 8]. The pattern of intermediate cytopenias is also perpetuated by the occurrence of graft-versus-host disease after allo-HCT [7, 8]. Both graft-versus-host disease and immunosuppressive therapy are clearly associated with prolonged cytopenias. In these instances, patients need to be monitored much more closely [7, 9].

Myelodysplasia is typically a late toxic effect. Many drugs, especially the alkylating agents and topoisomerase-2 inhibitors, lead to myelodysplastic syndrome [4]. This can occur from 6 months to >10 years after chemotherapy exposure. The pattern and time to onset of myelodysplasia ultimately depend on the treatment details. Since all patients receive combination chemotherapy, including alkylating agents, topoisomerase inhibitors, and antimetabolites, blood counts need to be periodically monitored for several years. We recommend measuring a CBC every 3 months for the first year following chemotherapy, every 3–6 months in year 2, and every 6 months thereafter for average-risk survivors.

Organ-specific toxicity is also common. There are several early and late effects of chemotherapy on various organs of the body. Many different chemotherapeutic agents are used to treat acute lymphoblastic leukemia, each with a unique late-toxicity spectrum. The frequency and type of examination done, therefore, depends on treatment details. In order to avoid expensive laboratory testing, routine monitoring of blood chemistry for organ-specific function is not recommended except for liver function testing in patients who have received a tyrosine kinase inhibitor [7].

Chemotherapy and radiation therapy can cause thyroid dysfunction [4, 10]. Tyrosine kinase inhibitors are well known to cause hypothyroidism [11]. The incidence of secondary thyroid carcinoma also increases markedly after radiation exposure; up to 30% of these patients develop hypothyroidism [10, 12]. We recommend measuring thyroid function at 1 year posttherapy, with subsequent testing based on abnormal thyroid hormone levels or patient symptoms. For those on tyrosine kinase inhibitor therapy, annual thyroid function testing while on the drug should be considered.

Patients who have been treated for acute lymphoblastic leukemia (especially those who have undergone allo-HCT) should be monitored for bone toxicity, particularly loss of bone mineral density. This is because myeloproliferative disease structurally weakens bone by infiltration of neoplastic cells. In addition, many transplant patients need to be on steroids for graft-versus-host disease; long-term steroid use can significantly reduce bone mineral density [13, 14]. Radiation treatment, either external beam or brachytherapy, can cause bone loss and result in pathologic fractures, especially when it involves the pelvic bones. Radiation can also affect epiphyseal plates, which lead to stunted growth in children, unstable epiphyses, and predisposition to scoliosis or kyphosis. Bone mineral density measurements are therefore recommended at 1 year post-allo-HCT. Subsequent monitoring depends on abnormal test results or new symptoms [14].

Practically all chemotherapeutic and radiation therapies affect gonadal function. Alkylating agents in particular are known to cause gonadal failure [4]. The result is loss of fertility and other symptoms which impair quality of life to varying degrees. Men often experience erectile dysfunction and fatigue. Hormone replacement therapy is available, and can easily be given to all those who need it. Even patients who are subclinically deficient benefit from hormone replacement therapy. It is therefore recommended that gonadal dysfunction be regularly evaluated with blood tests and evaluation of clinical symptoms [4, 15]. For prepubertal patients, we recommend assessment of gonadal function at 6 months following chemotherapy, and annually thereafter. For postpubertal men and women, we recommend starting at 1 year posttherapy.

Monitoring for toxic effects of particular drugs is now common. Patients who are Philadelphia chromosome positive receive imatinib and/or another tyrosine kinase inhibitor. They all have a variety of toxicities. Some may develop at initiation of drug therapy (during active treatment). Others may only be seen after active treatment. Since patients may remain on tyrosine kinase inhibitor therapy for years, it is necessary to monitor them for at least as long as the treatment is given. Patients on chronic tyrosine kinase inhibitor therapy need to be monitored for cytopenias, abnormal serum liver function tests, fluid retention (including pleural effusions), thyroid disease (both hypo- and hyperthyroidism), and cardiac toxicities (e.g., prolonged QT interval). It is recommended that such patients on tyrosine kinase inhibitors be monitored every 3 months with a physical examination and appropriate tests, as discussed earlier.

Adult survivors are at increased risk of a variety of cardiovascular problems such as congestive heart failure, valvular heart disease, myocardial infarction, and pericardial disease. These can be apparent as late as several decades after completion of therapy. This risk exists even at low exposures to anthracyclines and/or radiation therapy [16]. Therefore, as young patients approach middle age (in which cardiovascular disease is quite prevalent in the general population), very diligent monitoring is necessary. Optimal control of serum cholesterol and triglyceride levels and a focus on healthy lifestyle are recommended.

Minimal residual disease predicts relapses in patients with acute lymphoblastic leukemia [17, 29, 30, 31]. It is a molecular measurement that can detect one leukemic cell among 10^4–10^5 normal cells. A representative pattern of how the technology is currently used is outlined in the ECOG 2993 protocol. The test can be done on both peripheral blood (10 mL) and bone marrow (2 mL). Measurement should be done every 3 months during maintenance therapy. In patients with stem cell transplantation (SCT), it should be done every 3 months for the first year and every 6 months for second year. Beyond 2 years, there are no specific guidelines, but we recommend monitoring every 6 months.

Surveillance for allo-HCT recipients can be quite complex. Surveillance and management of late, non-disease-related effects have been recently reviewed [13, 18]. Transplant survivorship guidelines recommend checking thyroid function tests annually, or when symptoms are present. A large proportion of acute lymphoblastic leukemia patients are recipients of allo-HCT and thus at risk for marrow failure [19, 20]. Most graft failure occurs early (i.e., within months of transplant), and the risk decreases over time. Typically, patients with early recovery of blood counts after transplant become pancytopenic (with or without symptoms) [19–22]. This is ascribable to graft rejection. If identified early, graft rejection may be reversed by reducing the patient's immunosuppressive therapy and appropriately treating infections. Chimerism measurement in allo-HCT patients is an expected event after allo-HCT. Surveillance for chimerism is usually done at day 100 and every 30–90 days thereafter among such patients. Chronic graft-versus-host disease is common in patients with allo-HCT [23]. We recommend evaluation of allo-HCT patients for chronic graft-versus-host disease at day 30 posttransplant and at every subsequent clinic visit. Pulmonary, eye, otologic, hepatic, skin, and musculoskeletal issues problems are common. We recommend that allo-HCT patients have pulmonary function testing at 1 year and annually thereafter. Eye examinations are used to screen for cataracts and sicca symptoms among transplant and radiation recipients. Schirmer's testing is done for patients with graft-versus-host disease [24, 25]. Audiometry is recommended after total body irradiation because of the increased risk of sensorineural hearing loss [18, 26]. Many chemotherapy agents, including platinum agents and thiotepa, are also known to cause hearing loss. We therefore recommend audiometry for all acute lymphoblastic leukemia patients beginning at 1 year posttherapy. Liver function testing, a DEXA scan, and a detailed musculoskeletal examination should be done at 1 year for all acute lymphoblastic leukemia patients. Further annual testing is indicated only in the setting of abnormal test results or new symptoms. Skin evaluation is included in the graft-versus-host disease assessment among allo-HCT recipients. Detecting limitations in lifestyle is sometimes subtle. Performance status and psychosocial evaluation should be assessed for every patient at every clinic visit.

The effects of treatment of acute lymphoblastic leukemia should be assumed to be permanent. We recommend that a CBC should be done with every annual clinic visit. Immunodeficiency is essentially inevitable in survivors of acute lymphoblastic leukemia treatment. Immunizations can prevent infections. Therefore, varicella-zoster virus, pneumococcus, and Hemophilus influenzae vaccinations are potentially important, although the patient's antibody response is often suboptimal. This results in enhanced risk of recurrent bacterial infections and repeat hospitalizations in long-term survivors. About 20–50% of patients remain on immunosuppressive therapy >3 years after allo-HCT, with loss of protective vaccination titers if recipients are not repeatedly immunized. Metabolic and endocrine complications require long-term surveillance. Thyroid function, fasting serum lipid levels, gonadal function (including serum testosterone and estradiol levels), and serum parathyroid hormone levels should be routinely monitored. Pulmonary complications can be lethal. Annual pulmonary function tests and smoking cessation efforts are recommended. To assess risk of a dangerous bone density decrease, avascular necrosis, and subsequent major functional problems, bone mineral density testing should be done at 1 year. Subsequent screening intervals are variable, but repeat testing should be done every 2 years even in asymptomatic patients. To detect renal complications, serum creatinine level and BUN estimation should be checked at 6 months, 1 year, and annually thereafter. Annual history and physical examination should include screening for IQ, cognitive, psychosocial, and QOL

Table 96.1 Surveillance after initial curative-intent therapy for acute lymphoblastic leukemia at Vanderbilt-Ingram Cancer Center

	Year					
Modality	1	2	3	4	5	>5
Office visit (medical oncologist)	4	1	1	1	1	1
Office visit (gynecologist or urologist)	1[a]	1[a]	1[a]	1[a]	1[a]	1[a]
Office visit (ophthalmologist)	1[b]	1[b]	1[b]	1[b]	1[b]	1[b]
Office visit (audiologist)	1	1	[c]	[c]	[c]	[c]
CBC	4	2–4	2	2	2	2
Serum creatinine level + BUN	4	1	1	1	1	1
Serum T4 level and TSH level	1	[c]	[c]	[c]	[c]	[c]
Liver function tests	1	[c]	[c]	[c]	[c]	[c]
Serum sex hormone levels[d]	2	1	1	1	1	1
Serum parathormone level	1	[c]	[c]	[c]	[c]	[c]
Pulmonary function tests	1[b]	[c]	[c]	[c]	[c]	[c]
Chest X-ray	1[b]	[c]	[c]	[c]	[c]	[c]
Mammogram for women after age 40	1	1	1	1	1	1

[a]Pelvic examination with Pap test for females; testicular examination for males.

[b]For allotransplant patients; as clinically indicated for all others

[c]As clinically indicated only

[d]Testosterone for men; luteinizing hormone, follicle-stimulating hormone, and estradiol for women

BUN blood urea nitrogen level, *T4* Thyroxine, *TSH* Thyroid-stimulating hormone level, Pneumocystis carinii prophylaxis is recommended for allotransplant patients for 6 months posttransplant and whenever on therapy for graft-versus-host disease. Monitoring for cytomegalovirus every 6 months is recommended for allotransplant patients, those who have received alemtuzumab, and those with graft-versus-host disease. Colonoscopy for asymptomatic patients is recommended for all patients at age 50. The number in each cell indicates the number of times a particular modality is recommended during a particular posttreatment year

problems. For allo-HCT patients, cognitive screening should be done at 6 months and annually thereafter. Second malignancies are more common in the setting of allo-HCT than in age-matched controls. Patients with allo-HCT are at higher risk of second malignancies of the mouth, skin, breast, and gynecologic tract. Those who have received radiation therapy that included the breasts (e.g., total body irradiation) need annual mammograms beginning 8 years after radiation exposure or age 25, whichever comes first [27, 28]. Annual physical examinations should include a survey of specific organs to evaluate for signs of a second malignancy (Table 96.1).

To summarize, acute lymphoblastic leukemia is a common cancer with significant variability in incidence worldwide. There are consensus-based guidelines but none based on high-quality evidence. Given that there are no randomized trials testing diagnostic and treatment approaches for surveillance of the acute lymphoblastic leukemia population, and only limited published guidelines, our group has relied on extrapolation from general medicine resources for guidance, supplemented by our personal experiences. The rapidly growing population of acute lymphoblastic leukemia survivors creates an obligation to educate patients and physicians about potential problems that may occur in patients who have undergone therapy. High rates of second malignancies, as well as nonmalignant diseases involving virtually all organs, suggest that this population requires more frequent screening and earlier intervention than the general population. Since many survivors are cared for by their internists or primary oncologist, rather than the transplant specialist, we have tried to summarize our thoughts regarding appropriate screening and treatment of these common complications. Well-designed clinical trials are needed to design rational evidence-based surveillance guidelines. Clinicians, patient support groups, the public health community, and relevant professional societies such as the American Society of Clinical Oncology should advocate for the design and implementation of such trials. They are likely to be expensive and certain to take many years to complete. Subsequent trials will need to be devised and carried out periodically as new and better treatments enter clinical practice, better diagnostic tests emerge, and more effective salvage strategies become available.

Declaration of Commercial Interest: None

References

1. Itakura H, Coutre SE. Acute Lymphoblastic leukemia in adults. In: Greer JP, Foerster J, Rodgers GM, et al., editors. Wintrobe's clinical hematology. Philadelphia, PA: Wolters Kluwer/Lippincott Williams & Wilkins; 2009.
2. Kebriaei P, de Lima M. Acute leukemias. In: DeVita VT, Hellman S, Rosenberg SA, editors. Management of acute leukemias. Philadelphia, PA: Lippincott Williams & Wilkins (LWW); 2008.
3. Esbenshade AJ, Simmons JH, Koyama T, et al. Body Mass Index and Blood Pressure changes over the course of treatment of pediatric acute lymphoblastic Leukemia. Pediatr Blood Cancer. 2011; 56(3):372–8.
4. Brigden M, McKenzie M. Treating cancer patients. Practical monitoring and management of therapy-related complications. Can Fam Physician. 2000;46:2258–68.
5. Baccarani M, Dreyling M. Chronic myeloid leukaemia: ESMO Clinical Practice Guidelines for diagnosis, treatment and follow-up. Ann Oncol. 2010;21 Suppl 5:v165–7.
6. Fey MF, Dreyling M. Acute myeloblastic leukaemias and myelodysplastic syndromes in adult patients: ESMO Clinical Practice Guidelines for diagnosis, treatment and follow-up. Ann Oncol. 2010;21 Suppl 5:v158–61.
7. Ribera JM, Oriol A, Gonzalez M, et al. Concurrent intensive chemotherapy and imatinib before and after stem cell transplantation in newly diagnosed Philadelphia chromosome-positive acute lymphoblastic leukemia. Final results of the CSTIBES02 trial. Haematologica. 2010;95:87–95.
8. Tian H, Cronstein BN. Understanding the mechanisms of action of methotrexate: implications for the treatment of rheumatoid arthritis. Bull NYU Hosp Jt Dis. 2007;65:168–73.
9. Osterwalder B, Gratwohl A, Reusser P, Tichelli A, Speck B. Hematological support in patients undergoing allogenetic bone marrow transplantation. Recent Results Cancer Res. 1988;108: 44–52.

10. Sanders JE, Hoffmeister PA, Woolfrey AE, et al. Thyroid function following hematopoietic cell transplantation in children: 30 years' experience. Blood. 2009;113:306–8.
11. Torino F, Corsello SM, Longo R, Barnabei A, Gasparini G. Hypothyroidism related to tyrosine kinase inhibitors: an emerging toxic effect of targeted therapy. Nat Rev Clin Oncol. 2009;6: 219–28.
12. Savani BN, Koklanaris EK, Le Q, et al. Prolonged chronic graft-versus-host disease is a risk factor for thyroid failure in long-term survivors after matched sibling donor stem cell transplantation for hematologic malignancies. Biol Blood Marrow Transplant. 2009;15:377–81.
13. Savani BN, Donohue T, Kozanas E, et al. Increased risk of bone loss without fracture risk in long-term survivors after allogeneic stem cell transplantation. Biol Blood Marrow Transplant. 2007; 13:517–20.
14. Savani BN, Griffith ML, Jagasia S, Lee SJ. How I treat late effects in adults after allogeneic stem cell transplantation. Blood. 2011; 117(11):3002–9.
15. Hogervorst E, Bandelow S, Moffat SD. Increasing testosterone levels and effects on cognitive functions in elderly men and women: a review. Curr Drug Targets CNS Neurol Disord. 2005;4:531–40.
16. Mulrooney D, Yeazel MW, Kawashima T, et al. Cardiac outcomes un a cohort if adult survivors of childhood cancer: retrospective analysis of the Childhood Cancer Survivor Study cohort. BMJ. 2009;339:b4606.
17. Thorn I, Botling J, Hermansson M, et al. Monitoring minimal residual disease with flow cytometry, antigen-receptor gene rearrangements and fusion transcript quantification in Philadelphia-positive childhood acute lymphoblastic leukemia. Leuk Res. 2009;33: 1047–54.
18. Rizzo JD, Wingard JR, Tichelli A, et al. Recommended screening and preventive practices for long-term survivors after hematopoietic cell transplantation: joint recommendations of the European Group for Blood and Marrow Transplantation, the Center for International Blood and Marrow Transplant Research, and the American Society of Blood and Marrow Transplantation. Biol Blood Marrow Transplant. 2006;12:138–51.
19. Sebban C, Lepage E, Vernant JP, et al. Allogeneic bone marrow transplantation in adult acute lymphoblastic leukemia in first complete remission: a comparative study. French Group of Therapy of Adult Acute Lymphoblastic Leukemia. J Clin Oncol. 1994;12:2580–7.
20. Ram R, Gafter-Gvili A, Vidal L, et al. Management of adult patients with acute lymphoblastic leukemia in first complete remission: systematic review and meta-analysis. Cancer. 2010;116:3447–57.
21. Woolfrey A, Anasetti C. Allogeneic hematopoietic stem-cell engraftment and graft failure. Pediatr Transplant. 1999;3 Suppl 1:35–40.
22. Pulsipher MA, Bader P, Klingebiel T, Cooper LJ. Allogeneic transplantation for pediatric acute lymphoblastic leukemia: the emerging role of peritransplantation minimal residual disease/chimerism monitoring and novel chemotherapeutic, molecular, and immune approaches aimed at preventing relapse. Biol Blood Marrow Transplant. 2009;15:62–71.
23. Couriel D, Carpenter PA, Cutler C, et al. Ancillary therapy and supportive care of chronic graft-versus-host disease: national institutes of health consensus development project on criteria for clinical trials in chronic Graft-versus-host disease: V. Ancillary Therapy and Supportive Care Working Group Report. Biol Blood Marrow Transplant. 2006;12:375–96.
24. Bray LC, Carey PJ, Proctor SJ, Evans RG, Hamilton PJ. Ocular complications of bone marrow transplantation. Br J Ophthalmol. 1991;75:611–4.
25. Goldstone AH, Rowe JM. Transplantation in adult ALL. Hematology Am Soc Hematol Educ Program. 2009;:593–601.
26. Bertolini P, Lassalle M, Mercier G, et al. Platinum compound-related ototoxicity in children: long-term follow-up reveals continuous worsening of hearing loss. J Pediatr Hematol Oncol. 2004; 26:649–55.
27. Friedman DL, Rovo A, Leisenring W, et al. Increased risk of breast cancer among survivors of allogeneic hematopoietic cell transplantation: a report from the FHCRC and the EBMT-Late Effect Working Party. Blood. 2008;111:939–44.
28. Oeffinger KC, Ford JS, Moskowitz CS, et al. Breast cancer surveillance practices among women previously treated with chest radiation for a childhood cancer. JAMA. 2009;301:404–14.
29. Szczepanski T. Why and how to quantify minimal residual disease in acute lymphoblastic leukemia? Leukemia. 2007;21:622–6.
30. Cazzaniga G, Biondi A. Molecular monitoring of childhood acute lymphoblastic leukemia using antigen receptor gene rearrangements and quantitative polymerase chain reaction technology. Haematologica. 2005;90:382–90.
31. Elorza I, Palacio C, Dapena JL, et al. Relationship between minimal residual disease measured by multiparametric flow cytometry prior to allogeneic hematopoietic stem cell transplantation and outcome in children with acute lymphoblastic leukemia. Haematologica. 2010;95:936–41.

Leukemia Surveillance Counterpoint: Japan

97

Koji Nagafuji

Keywords
Leukemias • Hematology • Japan • Age • Cytogenetic response

Introduction

The age-standardized rates of leukemia in Japan seem to be lower than that in the USA. Rates in males (per/100,000) were 6.25 for acute myelogenous leukemia, 2.14 for acute lymphocytic leukemia, and 1.44 for chronic myelogenous leukemia in Japan. Those in females were 4.08, 1.4, and 1.14, respectively [1]. Chronic lymphocytic leukemia is rare in Japan [2] as compared to Western countries. Because of high human T-cell leukemia virus type-1 seropositivity, adult T-cell leukemia/lymphoma is more common in Japan than in Western countries [3]. Kyushu University Hospital is in the Kyushu islands, a southwestern part of Japan, which is an endemic region of adult T-cell leukemia/lymphoma. Adult T-cell leukemia/lymphoma is not discussed here in detail.

Here we describe the surveillance practices for patients after curative-intent therapy for leukemia at Kyushu University Hospital (Table 97.1).

For patients with acute leukemia who receive induction chemotherapy and autologous stem cell transplantation, the period of greatest risk of relapse is the first 12 months after completion of treatment [4, 5]. Thus, during the first year, patients are examined every 2–4 weeks. During the second and third years, patients are examined every 2–3 months. History, physical examination, complete blood count, liver function tests, and renal function tests are done at each follow-up visit. If these examinations reveal abnormal findings, a bone marrow examination is done as needed. The risk of relapse is much smaller after the fourth posttreatment year, but surveillance for adverse consequences of chemotherapy and/or autologous stem cell transplantation should be lifelong. Thus, such patients are followed once or twice a year for the remainder of their lives after year 4. We pay particular attention to the possibility of secondary malignancies, including myelodysplastic syndrome/acute myelogenous leukemia, and solid cancers [6].

Patients who receive induction chemotherapy and allogeneic stem cell transplantation are usually discharged at about 2 months post transplantation. At this time, they are at risk of developing acute graft-versus-host disease (GVHD) and opportunistic infections, including cytomegalovirus. Thus, in the first 3 months, patients are examined every 1–2 weeks. After 4 months, patients are examined every 2–3 weeks during the remainder of the first year. During years 2–4, patients are examined monthly. After the fourth year, patients are carefully evaluated one to two times per year for long-term consequences of therapy, including chronic GVHD and secondary malignancies such as oral, esophageal, colorectal, and breast cancers [4]. This schedule continues for the remainder of their lives.

Bronchiolitis obliterans (BO) is a pulmonary manifestation of GVHD with a very poor prognosis, if advanced. The onset of BO is often insidious. To detect BO early, we perform lung function tests, every 3 months for years 1–3 post-transplant [7].

Patients with chronic myelogenous leukemia are characterized by the presence of a BCR-ABL fusion gene, which is the result of a reciprocal translocation between chromosomes 9 and 22, cytogenetically visible as a shortened chromosome 22 (Philadelphia [Ph] chromosome). With the development

K. Nagafuji, MD. Ph.D. (✉)
Division of Hematology, Department of Medicine, Kurume University School of Medicine, 67 Asahi-machi, Kurume 830-0011, Japan
e-mail: knagafuji@med.kurume-u.ac.jp

F.E. Johnson et al. (eds.), *Patient Surveillance After Cancer Treatment*, Current Clinical Oncology,
DOI 10.1007/978-1-60327-969-7_97,

Table 97.1 Surveillance after curative-intent treatment for acute leukemia in first complete remission after treatment with chemotherapy and autologous stem cell transplantation incomplete remission at Kyushu University Hospital, Japan

	Year					
	1	2	3	4	5	>5
Office visit	12–16	4–6	4–6	2–4	1–2	1–2
Complete blood count	12–16	4–6	4–6	2–4	1–2	1–2
Serum liver function tests	12	4–6	4–6	2–4	1–2	1–2
Serum renal function tests	12	4–6	4–6	1–2	1–2	1–2

Bone marrow examinations are done as needed

The numbers in each cell indicate the number of times a particular modality is recommended during a particular posttreatment year

of tyrosine kinase inhibitors such as imatinib, the treatment outcome of chronic myelogenous leukemia has been dramatically improved [8]. Currently, patients with chronic-phase chronic myelogenous leukemia are treated as outpatients. During the first 3 months, the patient is examined every 2 weeks. This includes monitoring for adverse effects of imatinib carefully. If the patient's condition remains stable, he or she is followed four to six times per year lifelong. Physical examination, complete blood count, liver function tests, and renal function tests are performed at each follow-up visit. If these examinations reveal abnormal findings, a bone marrow examination is done, as necessary. Patients who achieve complete cytogenetic response (disappearance of the Philadelphia chromosome by conventional karyotype analysis) should be monitored for BCR/ABL chimeric mRNA by real-time quantitative polymerase chain reaction every 3–4 months for the remainder of their lives.

Conventional evaluation of leukemias is based on morphology and cytogenetics of bone marrow. This kind of analysis detects one leukemic cell among hundreds of nonleukemic cells. The progress of molecular hematology, using polymerase chain reaction method, has made sensitivity much higher (100 times or more) than that of morphology [9]. We can determine the degree of residual leukemic cells present in patients considered to be in morphological remission very early so treatment can begin promptly.

The developments of highly effective antileukemia drugs have made monitoring for minimal residual disease very useful for patient management, resulting in improved salvage rates. Progress in treatment resulting from improved surveillance methods has also been noted in acute promyelocytic leukemia (APL), a distinct subtype of acute myeloid leukemia. Morpho-logically, it is identified as the M3 subtype of acute myeloid leukemia by the French–American–British classification. Cytogenetically it is characterized by a balanced reciprocal translocation between chromosomes 15 and 17, which results in fusion between promyelocytic leukemia (PML) gene and retinoic acid receptor alpha (RARα). The effect of chemotherapy combined with all-trans retinoic acid for the treatment of APL is now monitored by real-time quantitative polymerase chain of PML/RARα [10]. For acute myelogenous leukemia other than APL, fusion transcripts and mRNA of Wilms' tumor 1 (WT-1) can be used as a target to monitor minimal residual disease. For acute lymphocytic leukemia, genes encoding immunoglobulin (Ig) and T-cell receptor (TCR) fusion transcripts can be used for evaluation of disease status. Minimal residual-disease-guided chemotherapy intensification (or intensification with hematopoietic stem cell transplantation) permits optimal and individualized treatment for each patient with leukemia.

References

1. Parkin D. Cancer incidence in five continents, vol. VIII. Lyon: IARC press; 2002.
2. Tamura K, Sawada H, Izumi Y, et al. Chronic lymphocytic leukemia (CLL) is rare, but the proportion of T-CLL is high in Japan. Eur J Haematol. 2001;67:152–7.
3. Shimoyama M. Diagnostic criteria and classification of clinical subtypes of adult T-cell leukaemia-lymphoma. A report from the Lymphoma Study Group (1984-87). Br J Haematol. 1991;79:428–37.
4. Ohno R, Asou N, Japan Adult Leukemia Study Group. The recent JALSG study for newly diagnosed patients with acute promyelocytic leukemia (APL). Ann Hematol. 2004;83 Suppl 1:S77–8.
5. Gondo H, Harada M, Miyamoto T, et al. Autologous peripheral blood stem cell transplantation for acute myelogenous leukemia. Bone Marrow Transplant. 1997;20:821–6.
6. Majhail. NS. Old and new cancers after hematopoietic-cell transplantation. Hematology Am Soc Hematol Educ Program. 2008: 142–149.
7. Tichelli A, Rovó A, Gratwohl A. Late pulmonary, cardiovascular, and renal complications after hematopoietic stem cell transplantation and recommended screening practices. Hematology Am Soc Hematol Educ Program. 2008;2008:125–33.
8. Goldman JM. How I, treat chronic myeloid leukemia in the imatinib era. Blood. 2007;110:2828–37.
9. Campana D. Status of minimal residual disease testing in childhood haematological malignancies. Br J Haematol. 2008;143:481–9.
10. Wang ZY, Chen Z. Acute promyelocytic leukemia: from highly fatal to highly curable. Blood. 2008;111:2505–15.

Multiple Myeloma

98

Shilpi Wadhwa, David Y. Johnson, and Frank E. Johnson

Keywords
Plasma cell • Radiation • Genetic factors • Exposure • Risk factors

Introduction

The International Agency for Research on Cancer (IARC), a component of the World Health Organization (WHO), estimated that there were 85,704 new cases of multiple myeloma worldwide in 2002 [1]. The IARC also estimated that there were 62,535 deaths due to this cause in 2002 [1].

The American Cancer Society estimated that there were 19,900 new cases and 10,790 deaths due to this cause in the USA in 2007 [2]. The estimated 5-year survival rate (all races) in the USA in 2007 was 33% for multiple myeloma [2]. Survival rates were adjusted for normal life expectancies and were based on cases diagnosed from 1996 to 2002 and followed through 2003.

Multiple myeloma is one of a group of related plasma cell syndromes. The most potent etiological agent is exposure to ionizing radiation. Occupational exposure to petroleum products such as benzene, organic herbicides, and pesticides, and metals such as nickel are considered possible risk factors. Genetic factors have been described. Premalignant conditions such as monoclonal gammopathy of unknown significance (MGUS) are well described and relatively common [3, 4].

S. Wadhwa • D.Y. Johnson
Department of Internal Medicine, Saint Louis University Medical Center, Saint Louis, MO, USA

F.E. Johnson (✉)
Saint Louis University Medical Center and Saint Louis Veterans Affairs Medical Center, Saint Louis, MO, USA
e-mail: frank.johnson1@va.gov

Geographic Variation Worldwide

Blacks have the highest incidence; European and North American Caucasians have intermediate incidence and Asians have low incidence [3]. Geographic variation in the USA is also pronounced with higher incidence reported in urban rather than rural areas [3, 5].

Surveillance Strategies Proposed by Professional Organizations or National Government Agencies and Available on the Internet

National Comprehensive Cancer Network (NCCN, www.nccn.org)—NCCN guidelines were accessed on 1/28/12 (Table 98.1). There were no significant changes compared to the guidelines accessed on 4/10/07.

American Society of Clinical Oncology (ASCO, www.asco.org)—ASCO guidelines were accessed on 1/28/12. No quantitative guidelines exist for multiple myeloma surveillance, including when first accessed on 10/31/07.

The Society of Surgical Oncology (SSO, www.surgonc.org)—SSO guidelines were accessed on 1/28/12. No quantitative guidelines exist for multiple myeloma surveillance, including when first accessed on 10/31/07.

European Society for Medical Oncology (ESMO, www.esmo.org)—ESMO guidelines were accessed on 1/28/12 (Table 98.2). There were minor quantitative changes compared to the guidelines accessed on 10/31/07.

F.E. Johnson et al. (eds.), *Patient Surveillance After Cancer Treatment*, Current Clinical Oncology,
DOI 10.1007/978-1-60327-969-7_98,

Table 98.1 Obtained from NCCN (www.nccn.org) on 1/28-12 Multiple Myeloma

	Years posttreatment[a]					
	1	2	3	4	5	>5
Office visit[b]	≥4	≥4	≥4	≥4	≥4	≥4
Quantitative immunoglobulins + quantitation of M protein	≥4	≥4	≥4	≥4	≥4	≥4
Bone survey[c]	1	1	1	1	1	1

Recommend obtaining CBC, differential, platelets, BUN, creatinine, calcium at each office visit
Bone marrow aspirate and biopsy as clinically indicated
Serum-free light-chain assay as clinically indicated
MRI as clinically indicated
PET/CT scan as clinically indicated
NCCN guidelines were accessed on 1/28/12. There were no significant changes compared to the guidelines accessed on 4/10/07
[a]The numbers in the table indicate the number of times the modality is recommended during the indicated year posttreatment
[b]There were no quantitative recommendations for office visits; quantitative immunoglobulins and quantitation of M protein were the most frequent quantitative recommendations given. We inferred that office visit would be recommended as frequently as these
[c]Annually or for symptoms

Table 98.2 Obtained from ESMO (www.esmo.org) on 1/28/12 Multiple Myeloma

	Years posttreatment[a]					
	1	2	3	4	5	>5
Office visit[b]	3–4	3–4	3–4	3–4	3–4	3–4
Full blood count, serum and urine electrophoresis, and/or serum-free light-chain determination, creatinine, calcium	3–4	3–4	3–4	3–4	3–4	3–4

In the case of bone pain, skeletal X-ray or MRI should be performed to detect new bone lesions
ESMO guidelines were accessed on 1/28/12. There were minor quantitative changes compared to the guidelines accessed on 10/31/07
[a]The numbers in the table indicate the number of times the modality is recommended during the indicated year posttreatment
[b]Full blood count, serum and urine electrophoresis, and/or serum-free light-chain determination, creatinine, and calcium were the only quantitative recommendations given. We inferred that office visit would be recommended as frequently as these

European Society of Surgical Oncology (ESSO, www.esso-surgeonline.org)—ESSO guidelines were accessed on 1/28/12. No quantitative guidelines exist for multiple myeloma surveillance, including when first accessed on 10/31/07.

Cancer Care Ontario (CCO, www.cancercare.on.ca)—CCO guidelines were accessed on 1/28/12. No quantitative guidelines exist for multiple myeloma surveillance, including when first accessed on 10/31/07.

National Institute for Clinical Excellence (NICE, www.nice.org.uk)—NICE guidelines were accessed on 1/28/12. No quantitative guidelines exist for multiple myeloma surveillance, including when first accessed on 10/31/07.

The Cochrane Collaboration (CC, www.cochrane.org)—ASCO guidelines were accessed on 1/28/12. No quantitative guidelines exist for multiple myeloma surveillance, including when first accessed on 11/24/07.

The M.D. Anderson Surgical Oncology Handbook also has follow-up guidelines, proposed by authors from a single National Cancer Institute-designated Comprehensive Cancer Center, for many types of cancer (6). Some are detailed and quantitative, others are qualitative.

Summary

This is a common cancer with significant variability in incidence worldwide. We found consensus-based guidelines but none based on high-quality evidence.

References

1. Parkin DM, Whelan SL, Ferlay J, Teppo L, Thomas DB. Cancer incidence in five continents. IARC Scientific Publication 155, vol. VIII. Lyon: IARC; 2002. ISBN 92-832-2155-9.
2. Jemal A, Seigel R, Ward E, Murray T, Xu J, Thun MJ. Cancer statistics, 2007. CA Cancer J Clin. 2007;57:43–66.
3. Schottenfeld D, Fraumeni JG. Cancer epidemiology and prevention. 3rd ed. New York, NY: Oxford University Press; 2006. ISBN 13:978-0-19-514961-6.
4. DeVita VT, Hellman S, Rosenberg SA. Cancer. 7th ed. Philadelphia, PA: Lippincott Williams & Wilkins; 2005. ISBN 0-781-74450-4.
5. Devesa SS, Grauman DJ, Blot WJ, Pennello GA, Hoover RN, Fraumeni JF Jr. Atlas of cancer mortality in the United States. NIH Publication No. 99–4564. National Institutes of Health, National Cancer Institute; September 1999.
6. Feig BW, Berger DH, Fuhrman GM. The M.D. Anderson surgical oncology handbook. 4th ed. Philadelphia, PA: Lippincott Williams & Wilkins; 2006 (paperback). ISBN 0-7817-5643-X.

Multiple Myeloma Surveillance Counterpoint: USA

99

Niyati Modi, G. David Roodman, and Suzanne Lentzsch

Keywords
MM • CRAB • USA • Relapse • Incurability

Multiple myeloma (MM) is characterized by neoplastic proliferation of a single clone of plasma cells producing monoclonal immunoglobulin, causing bone marrow infiltration which results in the replacement of normal marrow elements. The plasma cell clone invades the adjacent bone, leading to skeletal destruction with osteolytic lesions, osteopenia, and pathological fractures. Multiple myeloma accounts for approximately 10% of hematologic malignancies in the United States and 1% of all cancers [1]. In Olmsted County, Minnesota, the incidence rate was 4.6/100,000 between 1945 and 2001. Although most of the studies have reported the incidence of MM to be increased, the apparent increase is actually because of improved diagnosis secondary to better diagnostic tools and availability of medical facilities [2].

The incidence of MM increases with age. The median age of diagnosis is 66 years. MM is more common in males than females (1.4:1) [2]. Race and geographic location do not seem to affect the incidence of MM, but it varies by ethnicity, with African Americans and blacks from Africa being affected twice to thrice more than whites. However, race does not affect survival in MM [2–4].

To date, there is no curative therapy available for MM. Nonetheless, in the past decade, there has been increased overall survival due to availability of novel therapeutic agents such as thalidomide, lenalidomide and bortezomib. The goal of therapy in MM is to improve quality of life and to prolong survival. At initial diagnosis, it is important to decide whether the patient has monoclonal gammopathy of undetermined significance (MGUS) (Table 99.1), smoldering MM (Table 99.2), or symptomatic MM requiring active treatment. Only patients with newly diagnosed MM who meet CRAB criteria (Table 99.3) are started on an anti-MM regimen. Autologous stem cell transplant in MM is still standard of care for newly diagnosed transplant-eligible patients. Due to the excellent response rates to novel drugs with an outcome similar to that of autologous transplantation, the role of transplant needs to be reconsidered. The median overall survival duration of patients with myeloma is 5–6 years, with subsets of patients surviving over 10 years. Survival varies depending on individual patient's risk factors and eligibility for transplantation.

Determination of patient's response to treatment is made using IMWG uniform response criteria (Table 99.4) in outpatient settings. Response assessment should be performed as outlined in Table 99.5.

Surveillance of patients is determined by stage and activity of MM. Recommendations for symptomatic MM are different than those for MGUS, smoldering MM, and indolent MM (Table 99.6).

N. Modi, M.D.
Department of Medicine, West Penn Allegheny Health System, 4800 Friendship Avenue, Pittsburgh, PA 15224, USA
e-mail: modi_niyati@yahoo.com

G.D. Roodman, M.D., Ph.D. (✉)
University of Pittsburgh School of Medicine, Pittsburgh, PA 15240, USA

UPMC Health System, VA Pittsburgh Healthcare System, Research and Development (151-U), Room 2E-114, University Drive C, Pittsburgh, PA 15240, USA
e-mail: roodmangd@upmc.edu

S. Lentzsch, M.D., Ph.D.
Multiple Myeloma Program, Division of Hematology/Oncology, University of Pittsburgh, UPMC Cancer Pavilion, Pittsburgh, PA 15232, USA
e-mail: lentzschs@upmc.edu

F.E. Johnson et al. (eds.), *Patient Surveillance After Cancer Treatment*, Current Clinical Oncology, DOI 10.1007/978-1-60327-969-7_99,

Table 99.1 MGUS: monoclonal gammopathy of undermined significance diagnostic criteria: all three required [5]

Serum monoclonal protein and/or urine monoclonal protein level low*
Monoclonal bone marrow plasma cells < 10%
Normal serum calcium, hemoglobin level, and serum creatinine No bone lesions on full skeletal X-ray survey and/or other imaging if performed No clinical or laboratory features of amyloidosis or light chain deposition disease
Low is defined as
Serum IgG <3.5 g/dL Serum IgA <2.0 g/dL Urine monoclonal kappa or lambda <1.0 g/24 h

Table 99.2 Smoldering or indolent myeloma diagnostic criteria: all three required [5]

Monoclonal protein present in the serum and/or urine
Monoclonal plasma cells present in the bone marrow and/or a tissue biopsy
Not meeting criteria for MGUS, multiple myeloma, or solitary plasmacytoma of bone

Note: these criteria identify stage IA myeloma by Durie/Salmon stage

Table 99.3 Multiple myeloma diagnostic criteria: all three required [5]

Monoclonal plasma cells in the bone marrow >10% and/or presence of a biopsy-proven plasmacytoma
Monoclonal protein present in the serum and/or urine[a]
Myeloma-related organ dysfunction (one or more)[b]
[C] Calcium elevation in the blood. Serum calcium concentration >10.5 mg/L (or upper limit of normal)
[R] Renal insufficiency. Serum creatinine concentration >2 mg/dL [A] Anemia. Hemoglobin concentration <10 g/dL or 2 g<normal [B] Lytic bone lesions or osteoporosis[c]

Note: these criteria identify stage IB and stages II and III A/B myeloma by Durie/Salmon stage. Stage IA becomes smoldering or indolent myeloma (Table 99.2)

[a]If no monoclonal protein is detected (non-secretory disease), then >30% monoclonal bone marrow plasma cells and/or a biopsy-proven plasmacytoma is required

[b]A variety of other types of end-organ dysfunction can occasionally occur and lead to a need for therapy. Such dysfunction is sufficient to support classification of myeloma if proven to be myeloma-related

[c]If a solitary (biopsy-proven) plasmacytoma alone or osteoporosis alone (without fractures) is the sole defining criterion, then >30% plasma cells are required in the bone marrow

General recommendations for follow-up of MM patients:

1. The measurement of monoclonal (M) protein in the serum and/or urine remains the test of choice for the follow-up of the patients after autologous transplant. In the first year posttreatment, SPEP and/or UPEP is checked every month to monitor the response. Skeletal survey is only indicated if there is evidence of disease progression (weight loss, end organ damage, hypercalcemia, or pathological fracture) or to document disease status before treatment.
2. Serum free light chain measurement is used for patients who did not have a measurable M protein in the serum or urine with abnormal base line ratio (<0.26). We recommend a monthly FLC analysis post treatment for the first year.
3. BMB is required to confirm disease progression and before start of new therapies in order to document disease status and to have a baseline for response assessment.
4. A small subset of patients of MM lack measurable M protein and abnormal light chain ratio. In these patients, CBC and BMP should be followed every month with BMB and skeletal survey every year.

Elevated levels of serum creatinine (>2 mg/dL) and serum calcium (>11 mg/dL) also indicate poor prognosis. BM exam at diagnosis includes bone marrow aspirate, biopsy, FISH, and cytogenetic analyses. Karyotyping and FISH analyses are indispensable for evaluation of the prognosis of the patient.

We recommend flow cytometry only initially to rule out other malignancies associated with secretion of monoclonal protein, for example CLL or NHL, and to confirm the diagnosis of MM. Flow cytometry is not helpful for follow-up on disease status. Recently flow cytometry has been described to be very valuable to the estimation of prognosis [9].

Relapse within 12 months of initial therapy is associated with poor prognosis. There are still differing opinions regarding the treatment of relapsed MM, whether those patients can receive the same chemotherapeutic agents, a trial of new agent, or second transplant. The best approach is still unknown and decision of salvage therapy should be individualized per patient depending on the time of relapse after first treatment, response to the previous therapy, and patient's tolerance to the therapy. We consider a second transplant if the relapse occurs more than 12 months after the first transplant. If available, enrollment to a clinical trial should be encouraged.

Future Prospects

There are no standardized protocols for MM patients regarding first line of treatment, second line of treatment, and follow-up. It is currently unclear whether novel drugs such as lenalidomide or bortezomib should be used sequentially or in combination in order to achieve higher initial response rate. Due to the fact that patients survive a median 5–6 years [10], large multicenter randomized trials are required in order to define the optimal treatment resulting not only in high response rates or longer progression-free survival but also in significantly prolonged overall survival. In addition those trials also need to define the role of autologous transplant in light of achieving high response rates with novel drugs alone. Hopefully new insight into the pathogenesis of MM will help to create tailored treatments based on cytogenetic aberrations, especially for patients with poor prognosis.

Table 99.4 International myeloma working group (IMWG). Uniform response criteria for myeloma [6–8]

Response	IMWG criteria
sCR	CR as defined below plus normal FreeLite chain (FLC) ratio and absence of clonal cells in bone marrow[a] by immunohistochemistry or immunofluorescence[b]
CR	Negative immunofixation on the serum and urine and disappearance of any soft tissue plasmacytomas and ≤5% plasma cells in bone marrow[b]
VGPR	Serum and urine M-protein detectable by immunofixation but not on electrophoresis or ≥90% reduction in serum M-protein plus urine M-protein level <100 mg/24 h
PR	≥50% reduction of serum M-protein and reduction in 24 h urinary M-protein by ≥90% or to <200 mg/24 h
	If the serum and urine M-protein are not measurable,[c] a ≥50% decrease in the difference between involved and uninvolved FLC levels is required in place of the M-protein criteria If serum and urine M-protein are not measurable, and serum free light assay is also not measurable, ≥50% reduction in plasma cells is required in place of M-protein, provided baseline bone marrow plasma cell percentage was ≥30% In addition to the above listed criteria, if present at baseline, a ≥50% reduction in the size of soft tissue plasmacytomas is also required
MR	NA
No change/stable disease	Not meeting criteria for CR, VGPR, PR, or progressive disease
Plateau	NA
Progressive disease[c]	Increase of ≥25% from lowest response value in any one or more of the following
	Serum M-component and/or (the absolute increase must be ≥0.5 g/dL)[d] Urine M-component and/or (the absolute increase must be ≥200 mg/24 h) Only in patients without measurable serum and urine M-protein levels; the difference between involved and uninvolved FLC levels. The absolute increase must be >10 mg/dL Bone marrow plasma cell percentage; the absolute percentage must be ≥10%[e] Definite development of new bone lesions or soft tissue plasmacytomas or definite increase in the size of existing bone lesions or soft tissue plasmacytomas Development of hypercalcemia (corrected serum calcium >11.5 mg/dL or 2.65 mmol/L) that can be attributed solely to the plasma cell proliferative disorder
Relapse	Clinical relapse requires one or more of
	Direct indicators of increasing disease and/or end-organ dysfunction (CRAB features).[d] It is not used in calculation of time to progression or progression-free survival but is listed here as something that can be reported optionally or for use in clinical practice
	Development of new soft tissue plasmacytomas or bone lesions Definite increase in the size of existing plasmacytomas or bone lesions. A definite increase is defined as a 50% (and at least 1 cm) increase as measured serially by the sum of the products of the cross-diameters of the measurable lesion Hypercalcemia (>11.5 mg/dL) (2.65 mmol/L) Decrease in hemoglobin of ≥2 g/dL (1.25 mmol/L) Rise in serum creatinine by 2 mg/dL or more (177 mmol/L or more)
Relapse from CR[c] (to be used only if the end point studied is DFS)[f]	Any one or more of the following
	Reappearance of serum or urine M-protein by immunofixation or electrophoresis Development of ≥5% plasma cells in the bone marrow[e] Appearance of any other sign of progression (i.e., new plasmacytoma, lytic bone lesion, or hypercalcemia)

Note: A clarification to IMWG criteria for coding CR and VGPR in patients in whom the only measurable disease is by serum FLC levels: CR in such patients is defined as a normal FLC ratio of 0.26–1.65 in addition to CR criteria listed above. VGPR in such patients is defined as a >90% decrease in the difference between involved and uninvolved free light chain (FLC) levels

[a]Confirmation with repeat bone marrow biopsy not needed

[b]Presence/absence of clonal cells is based upon the kappa/lambda ratio. An abnormal kappa/lambda ratio by immunohistochemistry and/or immunofluorescence requires a minimum of 100 plasma cells for analysis. An abnormal ratio reflecting presence of an abnormal clone is kappa/lambda of >4:1 or <1:2

[c]All relapse categories require two consecutive assessments made at any time before classification as relapse or disease progression and/or the institution of any new therapy. In the IMWG criteria, CR patients must also meet the criteria for progressive disease shown here to be classified as progressive disease for the purposes of calculating time to progression and progression-free survival. The definitions of relapse, clinical relapse, and relapse from CR are not to be used in calculation of time to progression or progression-free survival

[d]For progressive disease, serum M-component increases of ≥1 g/dL are sufficient to define relapse if starting M-component is ≥5 g/dL

[e]Relapse from CR has the 5% cut-off vs. 10% for other categories of relapse

[f]For purposes of calculating time to progression and progression-free survival, CR patients should also be evaluated using criteria listed above for progressive disease

Table 99.5 Recommendations for surveillance of patients with MGUS and MM who are not on treatment

Disease	CBC, BMP, UPEP, SPEP	BMB	Skeletal survey
MGUS	1–2 times/year	Only if signs of disease progression[a]	Only if signs of disease progression[a]
Smoldering indolent MM	4–6 times/year	Only if signs of disease progression[a]	Only if signs of disease progression[a]
Postautologous transplant	Monthly	100 days after transplant	Only if signs of disease progression[a]
Symptomatic MM	Monthly	Before start of treatment and for response evaluation	Before start of treatment and for response evaluation

MGUS monoclonal gammopathy of undetermined significance; *CBC* complete blood count; *BMP* basal metabolic panel; *UPEP* urine protein electrophoresis; *SPEP* serum protein electrophoresis; *BMB* bone marrow biopsy

[a]M protein spike, weight loss, elevated serum calcium, elevated creatinine, pathological fracture

Table 99.6 International staging system and prognosis for multiple myeloma

Stage	Criteria	Median survival (months)
I	Serum β_2-microglobulin <3.5 mg/L	62
II	Serum albumin ≥3.5 g/dL	44
III	Not stage I or III[a]	29

[a]β_2-microglobulin is used as a prognostic marker independent from renal function. There are two categories for stage II: serum β_2-microglobulin <3.5 mg/L but serum albumin <3.5 g/dL; or serum β_2-microglobulin 3.5 to <5.5 mg/L irrespective of the serum albumin level

Table 99.7 Surveillance after curative-intent treatment for symptomatic multiple mylenoma posttreatment at the University of Pittsburgh Medical Center, Pittsburgh USA

	Posttreatment (year)				
	1	2	3	4	>5
Beta-microglobulin, SPEP, UPEP, CBC, BMP	12	6	3	3	3
FLC ratio	12	6	3	3	3
BMB	Day 100 posttransplant	1	[a]	[a]	[a]
Skeletal survey	1[a]	1[a]	[a]	[a]	[a]
PET/CT	[a]	[a]	[a]	[a]	[a]

The number in each cell indicates the number of times a particular modality is recommended during a particular posttreatment year

UPEP urine protein electrophoresis; *SPEP* serum protein electrophoresis; *CBC* complete blood count; *BMP* basal metabolic panel; *FLC* free light chain; *BMB* bone marrow biopsy

[a]If clinically indicated

Prognosis

Multiple myeloma is an incurable disease. Relapse is always expected. β_2-microglobulin and serum albumin are two markers which help to assess the prognosis. We follow ISS staging system for prognosis related to these two markers (Table 99.7).

References

1. Jemal A, Siegel R, Ward E, Hao Y, Xu J, Thun MJ (2009) Cancer statistics, 2009. CA Cancer J Clin 59:225–49
2. Kyle RA, Rajkumar SV (2007) Epidemiology of the plasma-cell disorders. Best Pract Res Clin Haematol 20:637–64
3. Kyle RA, Gertz MA, Witzig TE et al (2003) Review of 1027 patients with newly diagnosed multiple myeloma. Mayo Clin Proc 78:21–33
4. Baris D, Brown LM, Silverman DT et al (2000) Socioeconomic status and multiple myeloma among US blacks and whites. Am J Public Health 90:1277–81
5. Durie BGM. "CRAB" crawls into importance. International myeloma foundation. http://myeloma.org/ArticlePage.action?articleId=1045.
6. Durie BGM, Harousseau J-L, Miguel JS, et al. International uniform response criteria for multiple myeloma. International Myeloma Foundation. 2006. http://myeloma.org/ArticlePage.action?tabId=0&menuId=0&articleId=2994&aTab=–2991&tBack=&tDisplayBack=true.
7. Durie BG, Harousseau JL, Miguel JS et al (2006) International uniform response criteria for multiple myeloma. Leukemia 20:1467–73
8. Kyle RA, Rajkumar SV (2009) Criteria for diagnosis, staging, risk stratification and response assessment of multiple myeloma. Leukemia 23:3–9
9. Mateo G, Montalban MA, Vidriales MB et al (2008) Prognostic value of immunophenotyping in multiple myeloma: a study by the PETHEMA/GEM cooperative study groups on patients uniformly treated with high-dose therapy. J Clin Oncol 26:2737–44
10. Munshi NC, Longo DL, Anderson KC (2008) Plasma cell disorders. In: Fauci AS, Braunwald E, Kasper DL et al (eds) Harrison's principles of internal medicine, 17th edn. McGraw-Hill, New York

Multiple Myeloma Surveillance Counterpoint: Australia

100

Liane Khoo and Douglas Joshua

Keywords
Bence-Jones protein • Beta2 microglobulin • Bortezomib • Durie and Salmon staging system • Fluorescent in situ hybridization • Free light chain • Gene expression profiling • International Myeloma Working Group • International staging system • Kappa light chain • Lambda light chain • Lenalidomide • Light chain myeloma • Lytic bone lesions • Melphalan • Monoclonal gammopathy of undetermined significance • Monoclonal immunoglobulins (paraprotein) • Multiple myeloma • Myeloma cytogenetic abnormalities • Nonsecretory myeloma • Plasma cell labeling index • Plasma cells • Protein electrophoresis • Protein immunofixation • Smouldering myeloma • Autologous stem cell transplantation • Allogeneic stem cell transplantation • Thalidomide • Plasmacytoma

Multiple myeloma is a malignancy of plasma cells originating from the bone marrow. It is a clonal disorder with excess monoclonal immunoglobulins. It most commonly presents with bone lesions, renal failure, anemia, and hypercalcemia. Myeloma accounts for approximately 10% of all hematological malignancies. The annual incidence of myeloma in Australia is approximately 5 per 100,000. The median age of diagnosis is in the mid 60s [1]. There is variation in incidence among racial groups, with myeloma being twice as common in African Americans as in Caucasians [2] and less common in Asians [3]. The etiology of myeloma currently remains unknown. The major risk factor is the presence of monoclonal immunoglobulins (paraproteins) in the blood and the incidence of paraproteins increases with age. Plasma cell disorders related to myeloma include MGUS (monoclonal gammopathy of undetermined significance) and smouldering myeloma.

MGUS is defined by the presence of a monoclonal protein (<3 g/dL) without any end-organ damage or features of myeloma. The cause is currently unknown but this disorder can evolve into symptomatic myeloma. The risk of progression to myeloma is approximately 1% per year, with risk factors being a high monoclonal protein level, a high percentage of plasma cells in the bone marrow, IgA monoclonal protein, and an abnormal free light chain ratio [4]. The prevalence of MGUS increases with age (3.2% in persons over 50 years and 5.3% in persons over 70 years) [5].

Patients with smouldering myeloma have a serum monoclonal protein level of >3 g/dL and/or ≥10% bone marrow plasma cells with no end-organ damage from myeloma. It is an asymptomatic plasma cell dyscrasia with a higher risk of progression to symptomatic myeloma than MGUS [6].

Over the last 50 years there have been many advances in our understanding of the biology and treatment of myeloma. From the early 1960s, until early 2000s, melphalan plus steroids (prednisone/dexamethasone) formed the basis of treatment. Melphalan was also used in the conditioning regimens for autologous stem cell transplantation and in the treatment of patients deemed unsuitable for transplantation. Recently there has been progress in the treatment of myeloma with the development of new targeted therapies. These include thalidomide, lenalidomide, and bortezomib. These newer agents have significantly changed the treatment strategies.

Improved understanding of the biology of myeloma and the ability to risk stratify newly diagnosed patients has enabled individualized treatment approaches for both transplant-eligible and transplant-ineligible patients. This section

L. Khoo • D. Joshua (✉)
Institute of Haematology, Royal Prince Alfred Hospital, Camperdown, Sydney, NSW 2050, Australia
e-mail: Douglas.Joshua@sswahs.nsw.gov.au

F.E. Johnson et al. (eds.), *Patient Surveillance After Cancer Treatment*, Current Clinical Oncology, DOI 10.1007/978-1-60327-969-7_100, © Springer Science+Business Media New York 2013

Table 100.1 Diagnostic criteria for multiple myeloma and related disorders [7]

	Monoclonal gammopathy of undetermined significance (MGUS)	Smouldering "asymptomatic" myeloma	Symptomatic myeloma
Serum M protein level	<30 g/L	≥30 g/L	Presence of M protein
Bone marrow clonal plasma cell density	<10%	≥10%	Bone marrow plasma cells or plasmacytoma
Myeloma-related organ or tissue impairment, including lytic bone lesions	None	None	Present

Table 100.2 Definitions of myeloma-related organ or tissue impairment [7]

Increased calcium level: >0.25 mmol/L above the upper limit of normal or >2.75 mmol/L
Renal impairment: serum creatinine level above the upper limit of normal or estimated glomerular filtration rate below the lower limit of normal
Anemia: hemoglobin 2 g/dL below the lower limit of normal or hemoglobin <10 g/dL
Bone lesions: lytic lesions or osteoporosis with compression fractures
Others: symptomatic hyperviscosity, amyloidosis, recurrent bacterial infections (>2 episodes in 12 months)

Table 100.3 Investigations for a newly diagnosed myeloma patient [62]

Monoclonal protein: identification and measurement
Serum protein electrophoresis
Serum immunofixation
Quantitative immunoglobulin level
Serum free light chain level
24 h urine: total protein and Bence-Jones protein; with urine immunofixation
Bone marrow aspirate and trephine biopsy
Evaluating end organ damage
Full blood count
Serum creatinine level
Serum calcium level
Skeletal survey
Defining prognostic markers
Serum albumin level
Serum β(beta)2 microglobulin level
Serum LDH level
Bone marrow cytogenetics and FISH
Bone marrow plasma cell labeling index

will first look at the diagnosis of myeloma and risk stratification of newly diagnosed patients, including different staging systems and prognostic factors. The next section reviews new and evolving treatment options available for myeloma patients, together with the preferred surveillance strategies currently in use.

The diagnosis of myeloma is now standardized. The workup includes demonstration of a clonal plasma cell disorder and determination of end-organ damage. Conventional cytogenetics and FISH (fluorescent in situ hybridization) may also provide useful prognostic and staging information. The International Myeloma Working Group [7] has defined criteria for the classification of myeloma and related disorders (Table 100.1). Myeloma-related organ or tissue impairment can be related to hypercalcemia, renal impairment, anemia, and lytic bone disease (Table 100.2). The investigations for the workup of a newly diagnosed patient are summarized in Table 100.3. This involves characterizing the monoclonal protein, testing for end-organ damage, and defining prognostic markers. Detecting and quantitating the presence of a monoclonal protein with serum protein electrophoresis and immunofixation is a key initial laboratory investigation. The bone marrow biopsy determines the proportion of bone marrow infiltration with plasma cells and helps distinguish between MGUS, smouldering myeloma, and symptomatic myeloma.

The most common subtype of myeloma is IgG, observed in approximately 50% of patients; this is followed by IgA subtype (20%). IgD and IgE myeloma are very rare. Light chain myeloma (Bence-Jones myeloma—20%) is characterized by the excess of free light chains in the urine. Nonsecretory or oligosecretory myeloma occurs in approximately 1–2% of myeloma patients [1]. The serum free light chain assay (Freelite, The Binding Site, Birmingham, UK) is a marker for free light chains in the serum that are unbound to immunoglobulins [8]. The excess of κ (kappa) or λ (lambda) light chains can be used to demonstrate clonality. This is currently expressed as a ratio of kappa to lambda. The serum free light chain assay is useful in diagnosing and monitoring patients with nonsecretory myeloma and light chain myeloma [9, 10]; however, there have been some interlaboratory variations in the assay and this must be considered when evaluating and assessing serum free light chain ratios. The serum free light chain assay may provide prognostic information in newly diagnosed myeloma patients and an abnormal serum free light chain ratio could potentially be a risk factor for progression from MGUS to myeloma [11]. At present, the serum free light chain assay has not replaced the 24 h Bence-Jones protein measurement in light chain myeloma [12]. A recent set of guidelines by the International Myeloma Working Group for serum free light chain analysis in plasma cell disorders has been published [13].

Table 100.4 International staging system [15]

Stage	Criteria
I	serum β(beta)2 microglobulin level <3.5 mg/L and serum albumin level ≥3.5 g/dL
II	Neither stage I nor III
	Two categories: serum β(beta)2 microglobulin level <3.5 mg/L and serum albumin level <3.5 g/dL or serum β(beta)2 microglobulin level 3.5 to <5.5 mg/L, irrespective of the serum albumin level
III	Serum β(beta)2 microglobulin level ≥5.5 mg/L

Assessing prognostic variables allows for better risk stratification of the disease kinetics, individualization of therapeutic strategies and prediction of long-term outcomes. Prognostic markers can be divided firstly into those that reflect tumor burden: β (beta)2 microglobulin concentration, the number of lytic bone lesions, hemoglobin concentration, and percentage of bone marrow infiltration with plasma cells. Secondly, prognosis is related to tumor biology: plasma cell labeling index, conventional cytogenetics and FISH, and serum lactate dehydrogenase (LDH) level. Finally, patient-related factors also affect the progress of myeloma. These include serum albumin level, patient age, and performance status. There is ongoing research into using gene expression profiling as a prognostication tool.

Until recently, the Durie and Salmon staging system [14], utilizing clinical and laboratory parameters, was most commonly used in assessing myeloma patients. It was developed in 1975 and predicted outcomes after standard chemotherapy. Hemoglobin level, serum creatinine concentration, number of lytic lesions, and level of monoclonal paraprotein were used to classify patients into low, intermediate, or high cell mass.

With the development of new chemotherapeutic options and better understanding of disease biology, this staging system has been superseded by the International Staging System (Table 100.4) [15]. The International Staging System uses a combination of serum β (beta) 2-microglobulin level and serum albumin level to produce a three-stage classification (Stage I to III). The median survival durations in Stages I, II, III were 62 months, 44 months, and 29 months respectively. Future staging systems are likely to incorporate FISH, cytogenetics, and gene expression profiling to help stratify myeloma patients.

Chromosomal changes are common in myeloma. However, until fairly recently, it has been difficult to easily and routinely assess the chromosomal abnormalities of malignant plasma cells. Myeloma cells have low proliferative activity, making it difficult to assess metaphase cytogenetic changes. With the advent of fluorescence in situ hybridization, specific genetic changes can be detected in interphase cells, overcoming the problem of conventional cytogenetic methods which require dividing cells. The most common chromosomal translocation involves the site of the immunoglobulin heavy chain (IgH) located on chromosome 14q32. This results in upregulation of cyclin D [16, 17]. Using fluorescence in situ hybridization to analyzse over 1,000 newly diagnosed myeloma patients [18], the frequency of chromosomal changes was found to be ~90%. The most common abnormalities detected were: del (13)—48%; hyperdiploidy—39%; t(11;14) (IgH, Cyclin D1)—21%, t(4;14) (IgH, FGFR3)—14%; MYC translocations—13%, and inactivation of p53 (del 17p)—11%.

Several studies have looked at the prognostic information derived from cytogenetic studies. A study [19] of 350 myeloma patients treated with conventional chemotherapy stratified patients into three prognostic groups according to their cytogenetic characteristics. There was a high-risk group with poor prognosis (median survival 25 months): t (4;14); t(14;16), and del 17p. An intermediate prognosis group (median survival 42 months): del 13. And a good prognosis group (median survival 50 months): all other cytogenetic abnormalities. Other trials have also confirmed the poor prognosis conferred by the t(4;14) translocation despite intensive treatment [20, 21]. Interestingly, treatment with novel agents, especially bortezomib and lenalidomide, appear to be able to counter some of the consequences of the adverse cytogenetic markers [22].

The introduction of new agents—thalidomide, lenalidomide, and bortezomib—has resulted in major advances in the treatment of myeloma. These agents target both the malignant myeloma cell and the bone marrow microenvironment. They may not be available in all countries due to lack of government support for their use either as first-line agents or in patients with relapsed disease.

With the advent of new agents to treat myeloma, the International Myeloma Working Group has developed a set of widely accepted guidelines to assess response to treatment [23] (Table 100.5). These uniform response criteria are especially useful in allowing comparisons of the magnitude of response between clinical trials evaluating newer treatment options. Traditionally, melphalan and steroids have formed the basis of treating elderly patients and patients not suitable for stem cell transplantation. The introduction of novel agents has improved outcomes in this group of patients. Treatment goals for this group of patients include prolonging survival, maintaining quality of life, and minimizing treatment toxicities.

Treatment Options

After initial encouraging results from a phase II [24] study evaluating the addition of thalidomide to melphalan and prednisone, several phase III studies (GIMEMA [25], IFM 99-06 [26], IFM 01-01 [27] and Nordic Study [28]) were performed. Results from these trials showed that the addition

Table 100.5 International myeloma working group response criteria [23]

Response category	Response criteria
CR (complete response)	Negative immunofixation on the serum and urine and Disappearance of any soft tissue plasmacytomas and ≤5% plasma cells in bone marrow
VGPR (very good partial response)	Serum and urine M-protein detectable by immunofixation but not on electrophoresis or 90% or greater reduction in serum M-protein plus urine M-protein level <100 mg per 24 h
PR (partial response)	≥50% reduction of serum M-protein and reduction in 24 h M-protein by ≥90% or to <200 mg per 24 h
	If the serum and urine M-protein are unmeasurable, a ≥50% decrease in the difference between involved and uninvolved free light chain levels is required in place of the M protein criteria
	If serum and urine are unmeasurable, and serum free light assays is also unmeasurable, ≥50% reduction in plasma cells is required in place of M-protein, provided baseline bone marrow plasma cell percentage was ≥30%
	In addition to the above listed criteria, if present at baseline, a ≥50% reduction in the size of soft tissue plasmacytoma is also required
Progressive disease	Progressive disease : requires any one or more of the following
	Increase of ≥25% from baseline in serum M-component and/or (the absolute increase must be ≥0.5 g/dL)
	Urine M-component and/or (the absolute increase must be ≥200 mg/24 h)
	Only in patients without measurable serum and urine M-protein levels: the difference between involved and uninvolved free light chain levels. The absolute increase must be >10 mg/dL
	Bone marrow plasma cell percentage: the absolute % must be ≥10%
	Definite development of new bone lesions or soft tissue plasmacytomas or definite increase in the size of existing bone lesions or soft tissue plasmacytomas
	Development of hypercalcemia (corrected serum calcium >11.5 mg/dL or 2.65 mmol/L) that can be attributed solely to the plasma cell proliferative disorder

of thalidomide to melphalan and prednisone was superior to melphalan and prednisone alone. Both the GIMEMA study and IFM 99-06 trial showed that the melphalan-prednisone-thalidomide-treated group had higher complete response rates (15.5% vs. 2%; and 13% vs. 2%, respectively) and progression-free survival rates (54% vs. 27% at 2 years; and 27.5 vs. 17.8 months, respectively). There was nonsignificant improvement in overall survival duration in the melphalan-prednisone-thalidomide arm of the GIMEMA trial and the Nordic Study. However, both the IFM 99-06 and IFM 01-01 trials had significant improvements in overall survival duration with this regimen. Of interest, in the IFM 99-06 trial, melphalan-prednisone-thalidomide was also shown to be superior to autologous stem cell transplant in the elderly (over 75 years old). The addition of thalidomide resulted in significantly more side effects. Increased incidence of thrombosis, peripheral neuropathy, somnolence, and constipation were noted. In the GIMEMA trial, the addition of enoxaparin for anticoagulation prophylaxis did reduce the incidence of deep venous thrombosis. Venous thromboembolism prophylaxis has been recommended to prevent thalidomide and lenalidomide associated thrombosis in myeloma [29].

The addition of bortezomib to melphalan and prednisone has also shown promising results. The Spanish PETHEMA group undertook a phase I/II study [22] with bortezomib to melphalan and prednisone and had an overall response rate of 89% (32% complete response rate), with a median time to progression of 27.2 months. A large phase III trial (VISTA) with more than 600 patients has been published [30]. The bortezomib + melphalan + prednisone combination was found to be superior to melphalan-prednisone for all outcome measures—complete response rate, overall survival duration, progression-free survival duration, and time to progression [31]. The complete response rates were 30% vs. 4% in the bortezomib + melphalan + prednisone group vs. melphalan-prednisone group, respectively. There was also a statistically significant survival benefit in the bortezomib + melphalan + prednisone arm. The 3-year survival rates were 72% (bortezomib + melphalan + prednisone) and 59% (melphalan-prednisone) [32]. This combination has also proven to be well tolerated in patients with renal impairment, including those requiring dialysis [33].

Lenalidomide is a thalidomide analogue with immunomodulatory effects. A phase I/II study by the Italian GIMEMA group [34] added lenalidomide to melphalan and prednisone. The overall response rate was 81%, with a complete response rate of 17% and an 87% event-free survival rate at 16 months. Toxicities were common, with grade 3/4 neutropenia in about half the patients and thrombocytopenia in one quarter of patients. A study by the Eastern Cooperative Oncology Group (ECOG) compared high-dose dexamethasone to low-dose dexamethasone with lenalidomide. The complete response/very good partial response rates were 52% and 42%, respectively, but the 1-year overall percent survival rate better in the lower dose dexamethasone arm (96% vs. 87%) with significantly less toxicity (thromboembolism, infections, neutropenia) [35].

The current data shows that, in elderly patients (>65 years old) and patients not suitable for autologous stem cell transplant, any one of the new agents (thalidomide, lenalidomide, or bortezomib) with melphalan and prednisone is superior to melphalan and prednisone alone. Areas that need further study include evaluation of which novel agent or combination of novel agents offer the best safety/toxicity profile; the optimal length of induction treatment and whether there is a role for maintenance treatment [36].

In patients who are under 65 years old and not limited by severe comorbidities, the treatment of choice is chemotherapy followed by autologous stem cell transplantation. Induction chemotherapy is aimed at reducing both tumor burden and contamination of stem cell harvest by malignant cells. The aim of stem cell transplantation is to maintain better response rates and achieve a prolonged complete response. Longer-term studies suggest that a better response (complete or near-complete response) translates to a more durable response and longer overall survival duration.

Induction chemotherapy for patients with standard-risk myeloma who are candidates for stem cell transplant has evolved recently. Use of novel agents with conventional chemotherapy results in improved response rates prior to stem cell transplantation, compared to use of conventional chemotherapy alone. Thalidomide was the first such agent used in induction regimens. Thalidomide-containing regimens (thalidomide + dexamethasone) showed improved response rates with better progression-free survival duration [37, 38] when compared to vincristine, doxorubicin, and dexamethasone. Similarly, the Cavo et al. study showed that the overall response rate was higher in the thalidomide + dexamethasone group vs. the vincristine + doxorubicin + dexamethasone group (76% vs. 52%). However, there was an increase in thrombotic episodes in the thalidomide + dexamethasone group (15% vs. 2%). When thalidomide + dexamethasone was compared to dexamethasone alone in a Phase III trial [39], there were similar findings with improved outcomes in the thalidomide-containing group, with an overall response rate of 63% (thalidomide + dexamethasone) vs. 41% (dexamethasone alone). There was an increased rate of toxicities in the thalidomide-treated group, mainly thrombosis (17% vs. 3%) and peripheral neuropathy (7% vs. 4%).

Studies evaluating bortezomib (Velcade) have shown superior outcomes with bortezomib-containing regimens. A phase II study by the PETHEMA group [40] alternating bortezomib with dexamethasone showed an initial response rate (greater than partial response) of 65%, with an overall response rate of 88% (33% complete response) after autologous stem cell transplantation. Of interest, bortezomib appears to overcome adverse cytogenetic markers. Chromosome 13 deletion, t(4;14), and t(14;16) did not have a negative impact on response. The French IFM group in the IFM 2005/01 trial compared bortezomib + dexamethasone with vincristine + doxorubicin + dexamethasone as induction treatment prior to autologous stem cell transplantation [41]. The combination of bortezomib + dexamethasone also resulted in significantly improved response rates (complete response/very good partial response) compared to vincristine + doxorubicin + dexamethasone both before and after transplantation. The complete response and + near-complete response rates were 21% (bortezomib + dexamethasone) compared to 8% (vincristine + doxorubicin + dexamethasone) prior to transplantation; and 35% (bortezomib + dexamethasone) vs. 24% (vincristine + doxorubicin + dexamethasone) post-stem cell transplantation. However, there was a higher incidence of peripheral neuropathy in the bortezomib + dexamethasone group. Bortezomib can be used in patients with renal impairment without dose modification and has been shown to be both safe and efficacious [42].

Encouraging results are also seen using lenalidomide (Revlimid) in newly diagnosed myeloma patients. The Eastern Cooperative Oncology Group has already published the efficacy and safety profiles in newly diagnosed myeloma patients treated with lenalidomide and low-dose dexamethasone [35]. Studies by the Southwest Oncology Group [43] compared dexamethasone alone to lenalidomide + dexamethasone in newly diagnosed patients. There was significant improvement in progression-free survival duration (77% vs. 55%) but not in overall survival duration (93% vs. 91%) in the lenalidomide-containing arm. Due to its myelosuppressive effect, several studies have also looked at the effect of lenalidomide on stem cell harvest. It appears that lenalidomide-containing induction therapy may potentially impair stem cell mobilization [44]. However, this appears to be overcome when cyclophosphamide and granulocyte colony-stimulating factor are used for stem cell mobilization [45]. More studies are needed in evaluating the role of lenalidomide in induction chemotherapy prior to autologous stem cell transplantation.

There is a subgroup of newly diagnosed myeloma patients with high-risk features. These include stage III myeloma by International Staging System criteria; plasmablastic features (plasma cell leukemia, high plasma cell labeling index and adverse cytogenetics), as discussed earlier. Some of the newer agents appear to be able to overcome some of the effects of adverse cytogenetic markers [46]. Due to the poor prognosis of this group, they may benefit from risk-adapted treatment strategies to help improve outcomes [36, 47]. There are now trials using novel agents in this group for induction therapy prior to autologous stem cell transplantation. The role of allogeneic transplantation or tandem autologous stem cell transplantation in this group is still controversial, with no clear benefit documented at present [48].

Autologous stem cell transplant is considered the standard of care in younger patients. Studies in the mid 1990s showed that autologous stem cell transplantation is superior to conventional chemotherapy [49]. Induction chemotherapy (4–6 cycles) usually precedes autologous stem cell transplant.

As discussed before, there have been improvements in the induction regimen. Melphalan-containing induction regimens are avoided to prevent damage to hematopoietic stem cells and the risk of a low yield of hematopoietic stem cells. Granulocyte-colony stimulating factor, with or without cyclophosphamide, is the most common regimens used for mobilization. Conventionally, a minimum of 2×10^6 CD34 stem cells/kg body weight are required for a single autologous stem cell transplantation.

Single and tandem transplantation are both feasible options. Both the French IFM [50] and the Italian groups [51] showed that only patients with suboptimal response (less than very good partial response) to the first transplant benefited from a second transplant. In the Italian study, although there was higher complete response rate or near-complete response rate and event-free survival probability in the tandem transplant group, this did not translate to increase in overall survival duration.

At present, allogeneic stem cell transplantation, even with reduced-intensity conditioning regimens, has a fairly limited role in myeloma. This is mainly due to patient age (median age at diagnosis 60 years old), comorbid conditions of the group of myeloma patients, and the age of suitable sibling donors. There is also ongoing debate as to the benefit, given the high morbidity and mortality rates associated with allogeneic transplantation. Currently, there is no clear evidence for superior outcomes with allogeneic transplantation, although some studies show a trend toward improved event-free survival duration [52, 53].

The advent of novel agents has reintroduced the concept of maintenance treatment in myeloma in an attempt to prolong the duration of the response after transplantation. Initial results show promising results with thalidomide from several groups, including French [54] and Australian groups [55]. However, one needs to consider the long-term toxicities (such as peripheral neuropathy and thromboembolic disease) and potential drug resistance upon relapse. Obviously, some patients may be exposed to these effects without therapeutic benefit while on maintenance treatment. The French IFM group compared no maintenance, pamidronate or pamidronate + thalidomide. The thalidomide-containing arm of the group had improved event-free survival rate and overall survival duration (at 4-year follow-up). Interestingly, a Tunisian [56] group has shown that maintenance thalidomide, after single autologous transplantation, has superior outcomes compared to tandem transplantation (overall survival probability 85% vs. 65% at a median follow-up duration of 33 months). The use of bortezomib and lenalidomide as maintenance treatment is currently being investigated.

Relapse is very common. A recent review by San-Miguel et al. [36], on individualizing treatments for patients with myeloma in the era of novel agents, classified patients with relapsed myeloma into three groups. Patients with early relapse (<1 year) are considered to be in a high-risk group which may benefit from combination therapy to overcome drug resistance. The second group, with intermediate time to relapse (1–3 years), is one in which sequential therapy with novel agents is suggested. The third group with late relapse (>3 years) may benefit from a second stem cell transplant after repeat induction chemotherapy.

Table 100.6 Surveillance after curative intent treatment for myeloma patients after stem cell transplant at the Royal Prince Alfred Hospital

	Year					
Modality	1	2	3	4	5	>5
Blood tests[a]	4	1	1	1	1	1
Skeletal survey[b]	1	1	1	1	1	1
Bone marrow[c]	1[c]	1	1	1	1	1

Evaluation of neuropathy and other conditions as indicated by clinical findings
The number in each cell indicates the number of times a particular modality is recommended during a particular post-treatment year
[a]CBC; quantitative serum paraprotein, calcium, albumin, and beta-2 microglobulin levels
[b]Plain X-rays
[c]At 3 months post-transplant

Surveillance of a myeloma patient depends on his/her age and fitness for future treatments. As the majority of patients are not cured, we have developed a reasonable surveillance strategy for those who have obtained at least a very good partial response or better and received an autologous bone marrow transplant (Table 100.6). This works well in our practice as patients do need to be seen regularly and some of the investigations are not available via their local practitioners. This process is liked and well supported by our nursing and medical personnel. Nevertheless, we also encourage our patients to return to their local practitioners for ongoing care. The cost considerations of surveillance in Australia are met by the National Health Insurance Program and do not play a big role in determining where patients receive their ongoing surveillance. The key items we monitor are the serum paraprotein level, free light chain level, and urinary Bence-Jones protein level. Surrogate measures, such as the total IgG or IgA levels, may have to be used if the paraprotein spike overlies the normal beta globulin peak and cannot be adequately quantified. Quantification should be performed at two monthly intervals during induction therapy and immediately before high-dose therapy in the transplant-eligible group. In addition, monthly full blood counts, serum creatinine and calcium levels (together), and serum albumin and beta 2 microglobulin levels are needed to monitor disease progress and end-organ damage. In patients who have asymptomatic bony lesions, skeletal surveys should be repeated at 12- to 18-month intervals. MRI scanning is essential to document a true solitary plasmacytoma. It is useful to evaluate possible cord compression due to destructive vertebral column lesions, and plays a role in routine staging of patients with advanced disease.

A bone marrow biopsy is performed at diagnosis, after stem cell transplantation and if there is difficulty in monitoring response (such as the rare nonsecreting myeloma).

If novel agents are used [36], identifying possible additional toxicities such as neuropathy or thrombophilia should determine which agent is preferred. For example, neuropathy is a relative contraindication to bortezomib and a high risk of thrombosis is a contraindication to lenalidomide.

In the future, gene expression profiling [57] is likely to play an increasing role in our understanding of the molecular mechanisms. Large-scale RNA-based assays have given insights into the deregulation of cyclin D and its role in the pathogenesis of myeloma [58]. Such studies are also being used to develop a molecular-biology-based classification [59, 60]. At present, these studies are being performed in the research setting and are not yet available for routine clinical practice.

With the advent of novel agents, there are now trials of bortezomib plus lenalidomide. Such regimens are likely to be used in the first line setting as they have shown to yield durable response rates [61]. This will likely lead to improved overall survival.

References

1. Kyle R, Gertz M, Witzig T, et al. Review of 1027 patients with newly diagnosed multiple myeloma. Mayo Clin Proc. 2003;78:21–33.
2. Landgren O, Gridley G, Turesson I, et al. Risk of monoclonal gammopathy of undetermined significance (MGUS) and subsequent multiple myeloma among African American and white veterans in the United States. Blood. 2006;107:904–6.
3. Huang S, Yao M, Tang J, Lee W, et al. Epidemiology of multiple myeloma in Taiwan: increasing incidence for the past 25 years and higher prevalence of extramedullary myeloma in patients younger than 55 years. Cancer. 2007;110:896–905.
4. Kyle R, Therneau T, Rajkumar S, Offord J, et al. A long-term study of prognosis in monoclonal gammopathy of undetermined significance. N Engl J Med. 2002;346:564–9.
5. Kyle R, Therneau T, Rajkumar S, Larsen D, Plevak M, et al. Prevalence of monoclonal gammopathy of undetermined significance. N Engl J Med. 2006;354:1362–9.
6. Kyle R, Restein E, Therneau T, Dispenzieri A, et al. Clinical course and prognosis of smouldering (asymptomatic) myeloma. N Engl J Med. 2007;356:2582–90.
7. International Myeloma Working Group. Criteria for the classification of monoclonal gammopathies, multiple myeloma and related disorders: a report of the International Myeloma Working Group. Br J Haematol. 2003;121:749–57.
8. Bradwell AR, Carr-Smith HD, Mead GP, Harvey TC, Drayson MT. Serum testing for assessment of patients with Bence-Jones Myeloma. Lancet. 2003;361:489–91.
9. Mead G, Carr-Smith H, Drayson M, Morgan G, Child JA, Bradwell AR. Serum free light chains for monitoring multiple myeloma. Br J Haematol. 2004;126:348–54.
10. Drayson M, Tang LX, Drew R, Mead GP, Carr-Smith H, Bradwell AR. Serum free light-chain measurements for identifying and monitoring patients with nonsecretory multiple myeloma. Blood. 2001;97:2900–2.
11. Rajkumar S, Kyle R, Therneau T, et al. Serum free light chin ratio is an independent risk factor for progression in monoclonal gammopathy of undetermined significance. Blood. 2005;106:812–7.
12. Dispenzieri A, Zhang L, Katzmann J, et al. Appraisal of immunoglobulin free light chain as a marker of response. Blood. 2008;111:4908–19.
13. Dispenzieri A, Kyle R, San-Miguel J, et al. International Myeloma Working Group guidelines for serum free light chain analysis in multiple myeloma and related disorders. Leukemia. 2009;23:215–24.
14. Durie B, Salmon S. A clinical staging system for multiple myeloma. Cancer. 1975;36:842–54.
15. Greipp P, Miguel JS, Durie B, et al. International staging system for multiple myeloma. J Clin Oncol. 2005;23:3412–20.
16. Chesi M, Bergsagel PL, Brents LA, Smith CM, Gerhard DS, Kuehl WM. Dysregulation of cyclin D1 by translocation into an IgH gamma switch region in two multiple myeloma cell lines. Blood. 1996;88:674–81.
17. Fonseca R, Bargolie B, Bataille R, et al. Genetics and cytogenetics of multiple myeloma: a workshop report. Cancer Res. 2004;64:1546–58.
18. Avet-Loiseau H, Attal M, Moreau P, Charnbonnel C, et al. Genetic abnormalities and survival in multiple myeloma: the experience of the Intergroup Francophone du Myelome. Blood. 2007;109:3489–95.
19. Fonseca R, Blood E, Montserrat R, et al. Clinical and biological implications of recurrent genomic aberrations in myeloma. Blood. 2003;101:4569–75.
20. Chang H, Sloan S, Li D, et al. The t(4;14) is associated with poor prognosis in myeloma patients undergoing autologous stem cell transplant. Br J Hematol. 2004;125:64–8.
21. Gertz M, Lacy M, Dispenzieri A, et al. Clinical implications of t(11;14); t(4;114) and -17p13 in myeloma patients treated with high dose therapy. Blood. 2005;106:2837–40.
22. Mateos M, Hernandex J, Hernandex M, et al. Bortezomib plus melphalan and prednisone in elderly untreated patients with multiple myeloma; results of a multicentre phase I/II study. Blood. 2006;108:2165–72.
23. Durie B, Haroussau J, Miguel J, et al. International uniform response criteria for multiple myeloma. Leukemia. 2006;20:1467–73.
24. Palumbo A, Bertola A, Musto P, Caravita T. Oral melphalan, prednisone, and thalidomide for newly diagnosed patients with myeloma. Cancer. 2005;104:1428–33.
25. Palumbo A, Bringen S, Caravita T, et al. Oral melphalan and prednisone chemotherapy plus thalidomide compared with melphalan and prednisone alone in elderly patients with multiple myeloma: randomized controlled trial. Lancet. 2006;367:825–31.
26. Facon T, Mary J, Hulin C, et al. Melphalan and prednisone plus thalidomide versus melphalan and prednisone or reduced intensity autologous stem cell transplantation in elderly patients with multiple myeloma (IFM 99–06): a randomised trial. Lancet. 2007;370:1209–18.
27. Hulin C, Facon T, Rodon P, et al. Melphalan-prednisone-thalidomide demonstrated a significant survival advantage in elderly patients 75 years with multiple myeloma compared to melphalan-prednisone in a randomised double-blind placebo-controlled trial IFM 01/01 [abstract]. Blood. 2007;110:75a.
28. Waage A, Gimsing P, Juliusson G, et al. Melphalan-prednisone-thalidomide to newly diagnosed patients with multiple myeloma: a placebo controlled randomised Phase 3 trial. Blood. 2007;110:78a.
29. Palumbo A, Rajkumar S, Dimopoulos M, et al. Prevention of thalidomide and lenalidomide-associated thrombosis in myeloma. Leukemia. 2008;22:414–23.
30. San-Miguel J, Schlag R, Khuageva N, et al. Bortezomib plus melphalan and prednisone for initial treatment of multiple myeloma. N Engl J Med. 2008;359:906–17.
31. Harousseau J, Palumbo A, Richardson P, et al. Superior outcomes associated with complete response: analysis of the Phase III VISTA study of bortezomib plus melphalan–prednisone versus melphalan–prednisone. Blood. 2008;112:2778a.
32. Miguel JS, Schlag R, Khuageva N, et al. Updated follow-up and results of subsequent therapy in the phase III VISTA Trial: bortezomib

plus melphalan–prednisone versus melphalan–prednisone in newly diagnosed multiple myeloma. Blood. 2008;112:650a.
33. Dimopoulos M, Richardson P, Schlag R, et al. Bortezomib–melphalan–prednisone (VMP) in newly diagnosed multiple myeloma patients with impaired renal function: cohort analysis of the Phase III VISTA Study. Blood. 2008;112(11) Abstract 1727.
34. Palumbo A, Falco P, Corrandini P, et al. Melphalan, prednisone and lenalidomide treatment for newly diagnosed myeloma: a report from the GIMEMA-Italian Multiple Myeloma Network. J Clin Oncol. 2007;25:4459–65.
35. Rajkumar S, Jacobus S, Callander N, et al. A randomized trial of lenalidomide plus high dose dexamethasone (RD) versus lenalidomide plus low dose dexamethasone (Rd) in newly diagnosed multiple myeloma - a trial coordinated by the Eastern Cooperative Oncology Group. Blood. 2007;110:74a.
36. San-Miguel J, Harousseau J, Joshua D, et al. Individualizing treatment of patients with myeloma in the era of novel agents. J Clin Oncol. 2008;26:2761–6.
37. Marco M, Divine M, Uzunhan Y, et al. Dexamethasone+thalidomide (Dex/Thal) compared to VAD as pre-transplantation treatment in newly diagnosed multiple myeloma (MM): a randomized trial. Blood. 2006;108:57a.
38. Cavo M, Zamagni E, Tosi P, Tacchetti P, Cellini C, et al. Superiority of thalidomide and dexamethasone over vincristine-doxorubicin-dexamethasone (VAD) as primary therapy in preparation for autologous transplantation for multiple myeloma. Blood. 2005;106:35–9.
39. Rajkumar S, Blood E, Vesole D, Fonseca R, Greipp P. Phase III clinical trial of thalidomide plus dexamethasone compared with dexamethasone alone in newly diagnosed multiple myeloma: a clinical trial coordinated by the Eastern Cooperative Oncology Group. J Clin Oncol. 2006;24:431–6.
40. Rosinol L, Oriol A, Mateos M, et al. Phase II PETHEMA trial of alternating bortezomib and dexamethasone as induction regimen before autologous stem-cell transplantation in younger patients with multiple myeloma: efficacy and clinical implications of tumor response kinetics. J Clin Oncol. 2007;25:4452–8.
41. Harousseau J, Mathiot C, Attal M, et al. VELCADE/dexamethasone (Vel/D) versus VAD as induction treatment prior to autologous stem cell transplantation (ASCT) in newly diagnosed multiple myeloma (MM): updated results of the IFM 2005/01. Blood. 2007;110:139a.
42. Chanan-Khan A, Kaufman J, Mehta J, et al. Activity and safety of bortezomib in multiple myeloma patients with advanced renal failure: a multicentre retrospective study. Blood. 2007;109:2604–6.
43. Zonder J, Crowley J, Hussein M, et al. S2032: Dex +/- lenalidomide for previously untreated myeloma - updated results and impact of cytogenetics. J Clin Oncol. 2008;26:8521a.
44. Mazumder A, Kaufman J, Niesvizky R, Lonial S, Vesole D, Jagannath S. Effect of lenalidomide therapy on mobilization of peripheral blood stem cells in previously untreated multiple myeloma patients. Leukemia. 2008;22:1280–1.
45. Stern M, Furst J, Jayabalan D, et al. Stem cell mobilization with cyclophosphamide overcomes the suppressive effect of lenalidomide therapy on stem cell collection in multiple myeloma. Biol Blood Marrow Transplant. 2008;14:795–8.
46. Jagannath S, Richardson P, Sonneveld P, et al. Bortezomib appears to overcome the poor prognosis conferred by chromosome 13 deletion in phase 2 and 3 trials. Leukemia. 2007;21:151–7.
47. Stewart A, Bergsage P, Greipp P, et al. A practical guide to defining high risk myeloma for clinical trials, patients counselling and choice of treatment. Leukemia. 2007;21:529–34.
48. Garban F, Attal M, Michaellet M, et al. Prospective comparison of autologous stem cell transplantation followed by dose-reduced allograft (IFM99-03 trial) with tandem autologous stem cell transplantation (IFM99-04 trial) in high risk de novo multiple myeloma. Blood. 2006;107:3474–80.
49. Attal M, Harousseau J, Stoppa A, et al. A prospective, randomized trial of autologous bone marrow transplantation and chemotherapy in multiple myeloma. N Engl J Med. 1996;335:91–7.
50. Attal M, Harrousseau J, Facon T, et al. Single versus double autologous stem cell transplantation for multiple myeloma. N Engl J Med. 2003;349:2495–502.
51. Cavo M, Tosi P, Zamagni E, et al. Prospective, randomized study of single compared with double autologous stem-cell transplantation for multiple myeloma: Bologna 96 clinical study. J Clin Oncol. 2007;25:2434–41.
52. Garban F, Attal M, Michallet M, et al. Prospective comparison of autologous stem cell transplantation followed by dose-reduced allograft (IFM99-03 trial) with tandem autologous stem cell transplantation (IFM99-04 trial) in high-risk de novo multiple myeloma. Blood. 2006;107:3473–80.
53. Bruno B, Rotta M, Patriarca F, et al. A comparison of allografting with autografting for newly diagnosed myeloma. N Engl J Med. 2007;356:1110–20.
54. Attal M, Harousseau J, Leyvraz S, et al. Maintenance therapy with thalidomide improves survival in patients with multiple myeloma. Blood. 2006;108:3289–94.
55. Spencer A, Prince M, Rovers A, et al. First analysis of the Australian leukaemia and lymphoma group (ALLG) trial of thalidomide and alternate day prednisone followed by autologous stem cell transplantation (ASCT) for patients with multiple myeloma. Blood. 2006;108:58a.
56. Abdelkefi A, Ladeb S, Torjman L, et al. Single autologous stem cell transplantation followed by maintenance therapy with thalidomide is superior to double autologous transplantation in multiple myeloma: results of a multicentre randomized clinical trial. Blood. 2008;111:1805–10.
57. Davies F, Dring A, Li C, et al. Insights into the multistep transformation of MGUS to myeloma using micorarray expression analysis. Blood. 2003;102:4504–11.
58. Bergsagel D, Kuehl M, Zhan F, et al. Cyclin D dysregulation: an early and unifying pathogenic event in multiple myeloma. Blood. 2005;106:296–303.
59. Zhan F, Huang Y, Colla S, et al. The molecular classification of multiple myeloma. Blood. 2006;108:2020–8.
60. Shaughnessy J, Zhan F, Burington B, et al. A validated gene expression model of high-risk multiple myeloma is defined by deregulated expression of genes mapping to chromosome 1. Blood. 2007;109:2276–84.
61. Richardson P, Jagannath S, Jakubowiak A, et al. Lenalidomide, bortezomib, and dexamethasone in patients with relapsed or relapsed/refractory multiple myeloma (MM): encouraging response rates and tolerability with correlation of outcome and adverse cytogenetics in a Phase II study. Blood. 2008;112:1742a.
62. Smith A, Wislogg F, Samson D. Guidelines on the diagnosis and management of multiple myeloma 2005. On Behalf of the UK Myeloma Forum, Nordic Myeloma Study Group and British Committee for Standards in Haematology. Br J Haematol. 2005;132:410–51.

Multiple Myeloma Surveillance Counterpoint: Japan

101

Katsuto Takenaka

Keywords
Japan • Cytotoxic • Trials • Surveillance • Bone destruction • MRI

Multiple myeloma is the most common plasma cell disorder, with an estimated 3,785 deaths in Japan in 2005. The mortality rate due to multiple myeloma is increasing every year and reached 5.93 per 100,000 in 2005 [1].

Multiple myeloma is sensitive to various cytotoxic drugs. However, the responses are usually transient and multiple myeloma is not considered curable with current conventional treatment modalities. The prognosis of patients has been improved after the introduction of autologous stem cell transplantation and novel drugs, including thalidomide, lenalidomide, and bortezomib, into the initial treatment regimens and regimens for treatment of relapsed disease. Melphalan plus prednisone (MP) has been used since the 1960s and still remains the most widely accepted regimen for elderly patients or those ineligible for high-dose chemotherapy [2]. MP can induce objective responses in about 50% of patients, and the overall median survival with this regimen is about 3 years [3]. In the 1980s, high-dose chemotherapy followed by autologous stem cell transplantation was introduced, and randomized trials have demonstrated a survival advantage for this strategy compared with conventional chemotherapy [4–6]. Currently, transplantation is recommended for newly diagnosed multiple myeloma patients under 65 years of age. About 40–50% of patients can obtain complete responses after transplantation. However, relapses are usually seen, and the estimated overall median survival duration is 4 to 5 years after treatment. Recently, several novel drugs, including thalidomide, lenalidomide, and bortezomib, have been introduced, and their efficacy has been shown by clinical trials. Thalidomide and lenalidomide are now approved for multiple myeloma patients in Japan. However, bortezomib and lenalidomide are approved for only relapsed/refractory multiple myeloma patients. Based on these findings, at Kyushu University Hospital, the first step in evaluating a patient with newly diagnosed multiple myeloma is to determine whether he/she is a candidate for high-dose chemotherapy and autologous stem cell transplantation. For transplant candidates, the VAD (vincristine, doxorubicin, and dexamethasone) regimen (or bortezomib and dexamethasone) is used as induction therapy. Following induction, the patient is reevaluated for treatment response. Good transplant candidates undergo a peripheral blood stem cell harvest after completing a high-dose cyclophosphamide regimen. The preparative regimen for transplantation is high-dose melphalan (100 mg/m^2/day × 2 days). In our institute, patients who do not have at least a very good partial response after the first transplantation receive a second autologous stem cell transplantation after a 3-month interval [7]. The preparative regimen for tandem transplantation is also high-dose melphalan (100 mg/m^2/day × 2 days). After transplantation, we do not currently use maintenance therapy, but we will use lenalidomide in the near future. For nontransplant candidates, MP is usually used as induction chemotherapy, and is continued until a plateau is obtained or disease progression occurs.

Guidelines for posttreatment surveillance after treatment based on the high-quality evidence are not available for patients with multiple myeloma. However, since many of multiple myeloma patients relapse within several years after treatment, patients should remain under the care of a hematologist (Table 101.1).

In our institute, patients with a complete response are usually examined every 3–4 months for life after completion of treatment. Visits are frequent because of the continuous risk

K. Takenaka, M.D., Ph.D. (✉)
Medicine and Biosystemic Science, Kyushu University Graduate School of Medical Sciences, 3-1-1, Maidashi, Higashi-ku, Fukuoka 812-8582, Japan
e-mail: takenaka@intmed1.med.kyushu-u.ac.jp

F.E. Johnson et al. (eds.), *Patient Surveillance After Cancer Treatment*, Current Clinical Oncology, DOI 10.1007/978-1-60327-969-7_101, © Springer Science+Business Media New York 2013

Table 101.1 Surveillance after curative-intent treatment for multiple myeloma: initial therapy at Kyushu University Hospital, Japan

	Years posttreatment					
	1	2	3	4	5	>5
Office visit	4–6	4–6	4–6	3–4	3–4	3–4
Blood and urine tests[a]	4–6	4–6	4–6	3–4	3–4	3–4
Bone survey[b]	1	1	1	1	1	1

The numbers in each cell indicate the number of times a particular modality is recommended during a particular posttreatment year

[a]Complete blood count, quantitative serum immunoglobulin level, quantitative serum M protein level, serum protein electrophoresis, BUN. Also serum creatinine level, calcium level, LDH level, CRP level, beta-2 microglobulin level, and urinalysis

[b]In case of bone pain, skeletal X-ray and CT/MRI should be carried out to detect bone lesions

of recurrence. Many multiple myeloma patients after completion of treatment still have the disease in plateau phase or in partial response. Surveillance for those patients occurs every 2 months for the first 3 years and then every 3–4 months for life. The aim is to detect disease progression rather than relapse. Physical examination, complete blood count, kidney function tests, and urinalysis are done at each visit. Serum calcium, albumin, lactate dehydrogenase, C-reactive protein levels, and serum protein electrophoresis (SPEP) tests are also performed at each visit. Serum analysis including quantitative immunoglobulin levels of different types of antibodies (IgG, IgA, and IgM) and beta-2 microglobulin are examined every 4 months. Serum albumin, beta-2 microglobulin, lactate dehydrogenase, and C-reactive protein levels are prognostic factors [8, 9]. The level of beta-2 microglobulin is considered a standard measure of the tumor burden [9]. C-reactive protein level is a surrogate marker for interleukin-6, a stimulator of myeloma cell proliferation [10]. Assessing the amount of M protein by SPEP is useful to track the progression of the disease.

Almost all multiple myeloma patients develop osteolytic bone destruction that can cause pathologic bone fractures. However, it is not known whether routine follow-up radiographic imaging leads to earlier detection of relapsing disease or whether any advantage in patient outcome is gained by this. Therefore, in our institute, bone survey, including plain radiography and/or computed tomography (CT) and/or magnetic resonance imaging (MRI), is performed annually or as clinically indicated. CT is appropriate for the diagnosis of lytic bone changes and for assessment of fracture risk in multiple myeloma patients [11]. MRI is also well established as a useful tool for the diagnosis of bone lesions, especially for examination of the spine [12, 13]. Recently, many studies have shown the utility and excellent diagnostic accuracy of whole-body F18 FDG positron emission tomography (PET) or PET/CT in MM patients [14–16]. The choice of imaging modality for assessing disease status depends on the findings from the initial workup and clinical presentation.

References

1. Statistics and information department, Minister's secretariat, Ministry of Health, Labour and Welfare: Vital Statistics of Japan 2006. Health and Welfare Statistics Association.
2. Alexanian R, Haut A, Khan AU, et al. Treatment for multiple myeloma. Combination chemotherapy with different melphalan dose regimens. JAMA. 1969;208:1680–5.
3. Myeloma Trialists' Collaborative Group. Combination chemotherapy versus melphalan plus prednisone as treatment for multiple myeloma: an overview of 6,633 patients from 27 randomized trials. J Clin Oncol. 1998;16:3832–42.
4. McElwain TJ, Powles RL. High-dose intravenous melphalan for plasma-cell leukaemia and myeloma. Lancet. 1983;2:822–4.
5. Attal M, Harousseau JL, Stoppa AM, et al. A prospective, randomized trial of autologous bone marrow transplantation and chemotherapy in multiple myeloma. Intergroupe Francais du Myelome. N Engl J Med. 1996;335:91–7.
6. Child JA, Morgan GJ, Davies FE, et al. High-dose chemotherapy with hematopoietic stem-cell rescue for multiple myeloma. N Engl J Med. 2003;348:1875–83.
7. Attal M, Harousseau JL, Facon T, et al. Single versus double autologous stem-cell transplantation for multiple myeloma. N Engl J Med. 2003;349:2495–502.
8. Bataille R, Durie GM, Grenier J, Sany J. Prognostic factors and staging in multiple myeloma. A reappraisal. J Clin Oncol. 1986;4:80–7.
9. Greipp PR, San Miguel JF, Fonseca R, et al. Development of an International Prognostic Index (IPI) for myeloma: report of the International Myeloma Working Group. Hematol J. 2003;4 Suppl 1:S42–4.
10. Bataille R, Boccadoro M, Klein B, et al. C-reactive protein and beta-2 microglobulin produce a simple and powerful myeloma staging system. Blood. 1992;80:733–7.
11. Horger M, Claussen CD, Bross-Bach U, et al. Whole-body low-dose multidetector row-CT in the diagnosis of multiple myeloma: an alternative to conventional radiography. Eur J Radiol. 2005;54:289–97.
12. Walker R, Barlogie B, Haessler J, et al. Magnetic Resonance Imaging in Multiple Myeloma: Diagnostic and Clinical Implications. J Clin Oncol. 2007;25:1121–8.
13. Nosas-Garcia S, Moehler T, Wasser K, et al. Dynamic contrast-enhanced MRI for assessing the disease activity of multiple myeloma: a comparative study with histology and clinical markers. J Magn Reson Imaging. 2005;22:154–62.
14. Mulligan ME, Badros AZ. PET/CT and MR imaging in myeloma. Skeletal Radiol. 2007;36:5–16.
15. Breyer R, Mulligan M, Smith S, Line B, Badros A. Comparison of FDG PET/CT to other imaging modalities in myeloma. Skeletal Radiol. 2006;35:632–40.
16. Bredella M, Steinbach L, Caputo G, Segall G, Hawkins R. Value of FDG PET in the assessment of patients with multiple myeloma. Am J Roentgenol. 2005;184:1199–204.

Multiple Myeloma Surveillance Counterpoint: Canada

102

Matthew C. Cheung and Kevin R. Imrie

Keywords
Multiple myeloma • Practice guidelines • Free light chain assay • "Freelite" • Minimal residual disease • Serum protein electrophoresis • 24-h urine • Skeletal survey • Vaccinations • Magnetic resonance imaging • Positron emission tomography scan • Computed tomography scan

Abbreviations

BCCA	British Columbia Cancer Agency
NCCN	National Comprehensive Cancer Network
CCO	Cancer Care Ontario
IMF	International Myeloma Foundation
BCSH	British Committee for Standards in Haematology
ESMO	The European Society for Medical Oncology
FLC	Free light chain analysis

Multiple myeloma is a mature B-cell neoplasm originating in the bone marrow characterized by a serum monoclonal protein, plasma cell proliferation in the bone marrow, and skeletal destruction [1]. In 2008, the Canadian Cancer Society projected that 2,100 Canadians would be diagnosed with this cancer and that 1,350 would die from the disease [2]. Prior to the mid-1990s, myeloma was managed palliatively with steroids and oral alkylating agents. With such an approach, patients rarely attained prolonged remissions and were generally on active treatment for much of the time from diagnosis to death, which was typically only 2–4 years [3]. Given this, well follow-up visits were relevant to only a small proportion of patients, generally for short windows of time.

The management of myeloma has changed very significantly in the past 10–15 years. The standard of care for younger patients with myeloma is now autologous stem cell transplantation, which, despite not being curative therapy, is associated with durable remissions that can last for years [4]. In addition, the incorporation of novel agents such as thalidomide [5], bortezomib [6, 7], and lenalidomide [8–10] to current myeloma treatment regimens has resulted in improved survival duration with longer windows of time in remission [11].

Though current treatment approaches result in a greater proportion of patients experiencing durable remissions during which they could be eligible for periodic well follow-up visits, other changes in management may further influence the follow-up strategy. Maintenance therapy is making a resurgence after being largely abandoned in the early 1990s, when interferon alpha was shown not to be effective in this setting [12]. Maintenance therapy has implications for both the frequency and nature of follow-up visits. Recently, reports that maintenance therapy with thalidomide is associated with improved survival duration have led to a greater proportion of patients remaining on this agent after completing primary therapy [5]. Given the toxicities of this agent, which include peripheral neuropathy and venous thromboembolism, monitoring for toxicity is required. It is also standard practice for the majority of patients with myeloma who have bone disease to receive supportive treatment with bisphosphonates. These agents are typically administered intravenously monthly for at least 2 years [13]. While generally well tolerated, bisphosphonates

M.C. Cheung, M.D. (✉)
Sunnybrook Health Sciences, Odette Cancer Centre, 2075 Bayview Avenue, T2-031, Toronto, ON, Canada M4N 3M5

Department of Medicine, Division of Hematology/Medical Oncology, University of Toronto, Toronto, ON, Canada
e-mail: matthew.cheung@sunnybrook.ca

K.R. Imrie, M.D.
Department of Medicine, Sunnybrook Health Sciences Center, University of Toronto, 2075 Bayview Avenue, Room D474, Toronto, ON, Canada M4N 3M5

Department of Medicine, Division of Hematology/Medical Oncology, University of Toronto, Toronto, ON, Canada

F.E. Johnson et al. (eds.), *Patient Surveillance After Cancer Treatment*, Current Clinical Oncology, DOI 10.1007/978-1-60327-969-7_102,

are associated with rare but significant adverse events such as osteonecrosis of the jaw and renal failure, making monitoring for such toxicities necessary.

We conducted a systematic review of the literature as well as guidelines published on the Internet to evaluate and summarize current surveillance strategies in myeloma. MEDLINE (OVID) was searched from 1966 to September, week 4, 2008, with a broadly inclusive strategy for studies on follow-up in multiple myeloma. A systematic survey of guidelines published on the web was conducted by one author (MC) utilizing a listing of guideline databases and guideline developers maintained by the Program in Evidence-based Care of Cancer Care Ontario (www.cancercare.on.ca). Relevant articles and web publications were selected and reviewed by two reviewers and the reference lists from these sources were searched for additional trials. Articles with study designs of any type (including systematic reviews, meta-analyses, and evidence-based guidelines) were selected for inclusion in this systematic review if they were published as full articles or guidelines published on the web and if the following criteria were met: (1) addressed patients with multiple myeloma; and (2) reported on follow-up of patients after treatment, including chemotherapy, radiotherapy, or high-dose therapy, and stem cell transplantation. Studies were excluded if they were letters, comments, or editorial publication types or if they only reported on diagnostic test performance characteristics. Citations in the initial search of the literature were reviewed by two independent reviewers for inclusion. All discrepancies were resolved by consensus between the two reviewers and, if necessary, scored by a third reviewer.

Data were summarized descriptively and in tabular format. Data appropriate for pooling or meta-analysis were not expected. Recommendations on the use and duration of bisphosphonate therapy during the surveillance period were considered beyond the scope of this document; however, guideline recommendations that suggested appropriate surveillance and monitoring of individuals who continue on chronic bisphosphonate therapy were evaluated.

The primary literature search yielded a total of 954 citations for evaluation. Of 27 citations selected for further review, 14 publications were subsequently excluded for the following reasons: eight reported only on laboratory test performance characteristics, two reported on patients who had not received treatment, two reported only on response assessment upon completion of treatment, one did not report on testing during the surveillance period, and one was an earlier version of a guideline which was included. A total of 13 publications met inclusion criteria.

Of these 13 studies, two were practice guidelines (European Society for Medical Oncology, British Committee for Standards in Haematology) [14, 15]. Seven reported on minimal residual disease monitoring [16–22], three reported on free light chain assays [23–25], and one reported on vaccination [26]. The websites of 13 practice guideline development groups were searched for guidelines on multiple myeloma follow-up. Aside from the two guidelines found in the primary search, unique guidelines of relevance were available from the British Columbia Cancer Agency [27], National Comprehensive Cancer Network [28], Mayo Clinic [29], Cancer Care Ontario [30], and the International Myeloma Foundation [31]. A second guideline from the British Committee for Standards in Haematology website was found, reporting on the general management of myeloma [32]. A search of the National Guideline Clearing House, Canadian Medical Association Infobase, and Cochrane Database revealed a total of 69 guidelines for evaluation; however, no additional guidelines relevant to myeloma follow-up were found.

None of the practice guidelines or original publications provided recommendations or evidence to guide the frequency of clinical visits in individuals who have completed induction therapy. It is likely that physicians individualize the frequency of clinical visits for each patient, depending on achievement and depth of remission, need for adjunctive treatments, including bisphosphonate therapy, pain control requirements, and patient preferences. It should be noted that most guidelines suggest routine surveillance of laboratory and M-protein values in follow-up (described below); it is presumed that many physicians may align the clinical evaluations with the laboratory testing. None of the guidelines delineated the frequency of clinical visits for individuals receiving maintenance therapy. We appreciate that the role of maintenance therapy (including the use of prednisone/dexamethasone, interferon, thalidomide, and newer agents) is evolving, and that the frequency of clinical reevaluations will vary, depending on whether the patient is continuing on such therapy.

Practice guidelines from the National Comprehensive Cancer Network, the British Columbia Cancer Agency, the International Myeloma Foundation, and the European Society for Medical Oncology provide guidance on the frequency of laboratory reevaluations in follow-up [14, 27, 28, 31]. Recommendations from these groups were generally based on expert consensus. Laboratory testing is recommended as frequently as every 3 months (the National Comprehensive Cancer Network and the British Columbia Cancer Agency) to every 3–6 months (the International Myeloma Foundation and The European Society for Medical Oncology) and should generally include CBC with platelets, white cell differential, renal function (serum creatinine), calcium profile, and immunoquantitation with M-protein quantification by serum and/or urine protein electrophoresis (see Tables 102.1 and 102.2). The International Myeloma Foundation provides some guidance on M-protein quantification; serum protein and/or urine protein electrophoresis is preferred. However, nephelometric measurements are acceptable and may even be preferred in individuals with low level serum M-proteins or multimeric M-components

Table 102.1 Practice guidelines on patient surveillance in multiple myeloma

Guideline	General laboratory	Immuno-quant and M-protein quant	BM biopsy	Bone (skeletal) survey	Other imaging	Other recommendations
NCCN 2008 [28]	CBC with plts, differential, BUN, Cr, Ca (frequency NS)	q 3 mos[a]	As clinically indicated	Annually or as clinically indicated	Consider MRI and PET/CT (frequency NS)	–
BCSH 2007 [15] (Imaging Guideline) and BCSH 2006 [32]	–	–	–	*BCSH 2007*	*BCSH 2007*	*BCSH 2006*
				Insufficient evidence to recommend in untreated asymptomatic pts—recommended if evidence of disease progression (unless within 3 months of previous skeletal survey) (C)	Insufficient evidence to recommend PET/MIBI scanning (reasonable in select patients with extramedullary or nonsecretory disease)(C)	Vaccinations against influenza, streptococcus pneumonia, H influenza is recommended but efficacy not guaranteed (B)
					Insufficient evidence to recommend MR (C) or CT (C)	
					CT is reasonable to monitor soft tissue masses, unexplained symptoms, concern of on-going fracture, or lack of response (B)	
					BCSH 2006	In patients with recurrent infections, prophylactic immunoglobulins may be helpful in plateau phase (A)
					CT or MRI should be employed for evaluation of symptomatic areas when plain radiographs are negative (B)	
BCCA 2008 [27]	CBC with plts; Cr, Ca 24-h urine protein q 3 mos	q 3 mos	Frequency NS	Annually	–	–
Mayo Clinic 2006 [29]	–	–	–	–	–	After bisphosphonate therapy has been initiated, patients should see a dentist at least annually
						For patients who require a major oral surgical procedure, bisphosphonate therapy should be withheld for at least 1 month before and not resumed until full recovery
CCO 2007 [30]	Cr and 24-h urine protein in patients on bisphosphonate (frequency NS)	–	–	–	–	Patients on bisphosphonate should be followed by dentistry (frequency NS)
IMF 2003 [31]	Cr before bisphosphonate dose; 24-h urine protein q 3–6 mos	–	–	Regular reevaluation and follow-up testing (frequency NS)	–	Carefully selected exercises and avoidance of risky activities (risk of falling) are recommended
ESMO 2008 [14]	CBC, Cr, Ca, B2M q 3–6 mos	q 3–6 mos[b]	–	Skeletal X-ray (or MR) should be used in case of bone pain	Skeletal X-ray (or MR) should be used in case of bone pain	–

B2M beta-2-microglobulin; *NS* not specified; *mos* months

[a]Serum free light chain analysis can be considered (frequency not specified)

[b]Includes serum and urine electrophoresis or/and free light chain determination in serum or urine

Table 102.2 Quality of guidelines

Guideline	Guideline quality
NCCN 2008	(3)(5)
BCSH 2007 (Imaging Guideline)	BCSH 2006: BCSH 2007 vs. 2006? (1)(3)(5)(6)
BCSH 2006	(1)(2)(3)(4) (5)(6)
BCCA (2008 Update)	
Mayo Clinic 2006	(5)(6)
CCO 2007	(1)(2)(3)
IMF 2003	(1)(2)(4)(6)
ESMO 2008	(5)(6)

Guideline quality index:
(1) Systematic review of key literature clearly outlined
(2) Systematic review of previous guidelines
(3) External feedback from stakeholders/physicians
(4) External feedback from patients
(5) Grading of recommendations clearly outlined
Peer-reviewed publication

(particularly IgA subtypes). M-protein monitoring may include a 24-h urine protein electrophoresis if a serum M-component is not identified. Two guidelines (the British Columbia Cancer Agency and the International Myeloma Foundation) suggest the additional collection of a 24-h urine for total protein evaluation every 3–6 months. The International Myeloma Foundation and Cancer Care Ontario recommendations on 24-h urine collection for total protein quantitation are specific to the setting of chronic administration of bisphosphonate therapy to monitor for renal toxicity [30, 31].

In the absence of a detectable serum M-protein, the Freelite™ (Freelite, Binding Site, San Diego, CA) test can be applied to measure the levels of free kappa, free lambda, and the ratio of free kappa/lambda light chains. Free light chain analysis can provide a quantifiable marker in approximately 70 % of patients with nonsecretory disease or minimal residual disease [31]. The 2006 International Uniform Response Criteria for multiple myeloma has adopted the use of free light chain analysis in assessment of response in patients with non- or oligosecretory disease [33]. In the follow-up setting, guidelines from National Comprehensive Cancer Network and The European Society for Medical Oncology suggest that serum free light chain analysis be considered as part of the laboratory surveillance. The frequency of such monitoring is not delineated by these guidelines. Several small studies have suggested a role for free light chain analysis in early detection of progression but this remains to be validated [23–25].

Seven publications were identified to address minimal residual disease monitoring. These included three review articles [19–21], two comparisons of the sensitivity of flow cytometry with molecular monitoring with polymerase chain reaction [16, 18] and descriptive studies of molecular monitoring [22] and flow cytometry [17]. The identified publications report that both flow cytometry and molecular testing with polymerase chain reaction are sensitive measures of response and that minimal residual disease can predict shorter progression-free survival; however, none of the clinical studies provide evidence that earlier detection of relapse influences clinical outcomes.

No guidelines recommend a change in frequency of laboratory tests for individuals receiving maintenance therapy. Two guidelines (the National Comprehensive Cancer Network and the British Columbia Cancer Agency) indicate that bone marrow biopsies may play a role in surveillance with frequency dictated by clinical indication. The use of bone marrow biopsies as a means of following disease control in nonsecretory myeloma may be evolving (and potentially decreasing) in the era of sensitive free light chain analysis testing.

The frequency of skeletal (X-ray) surveys during myeloma follow-up was addressed by five of the practice guidelines and no original publications. Recommendations were generally based on expert consensus and differed among the various guideline groups. The British Columbia Cancer Agency suggested routine skeletal imaging on an annual basis. The International Myeloma Foundation also advocated for regular skeletal reevaluation but did not specify the frequency of testing. Skeletal surveys were recommended annually or as clinically indicated (for bone pain) by the National Comprehensive Cancer Network. The European Society for Medical Oncology guidelines favored the targeted use of skeletal imaging to investigate bone pain. Similarly, the British Committee for Standards in Haematology Imaging Guidelines (2007) [15] found insufficient evidence to recommend routine reimaging in asymptomatic patients; this group instead recommended that a repeat survey be completed only at the time of disease progression (unless within 3 months of previous skeletal survey). Thus, a spectrum of opinions is available to physicians ranging from routine reevaluation to directed imaging with symptoms or disease progression. We appreciate that the frequency of reevaluation may also be dependent on prior history and nature of bone disease, use of other imaging modalities (described below), and patient preference.

Magnetic resonance imaging, computed tomography scanning, and positron emission tomography are evolving technologies in the follow-up of patients with myeloma. No original studies were found documenting the utility of these imaging options in surveillance. However, expert consensus opinions were offered in four practice guidelines. As with skeletal survey X-rays, The European Society for Medical Oncology guidelines favored the targeted use of magnetic resonance imaging to investigate bone pain. The British Committee for Standards in Haematology myeloma guidelines (2006) suggest that computed tomography or magnetic resonance imaging be used to evaluate pain when plain X-rays are negative [32]. The British Committee for Standards in Haematology Imaging Guidelines (2007) do not recommend routine imaging but recognize that positron emission tomography imaging may be reasonable in select patients with extramedullary or nonsecretory disease and that computed tomography is reasonable to monitor soft tissue masses, unexplained symptoms, or concern of ongoing fracture or lack of response [15]. The National Comprehensive Cancer Network lists all three modalities as options to consider during the follow-up period but does not specify the frequency or indication for their use.

The Mayo Clinic guidelines specifically addressed the role of bisphosphonate therapy in myeloma, which was beyond the scope of this chapter to review [29]. However, the guidelines also discuss appropriate surveillance methods in those continuing on bisphosphonates. Specifically, patients should be seen by a dentist at least annually and if a major oral surgical procedure is recommended, bisphosphonate therapy should be withheld for at least 1 month before and not resumed until after full recovery. The Cancer Care Ontario guidelines are in agreement with the Mayo Clinic recommendations [4].

The British Committee for Standards in Haematology Guidelines (2006) highlight the ongoing increased risk of infection in this population [32]. This group recommended that vaccinations against influenza, streptococcus pneumonia, and *Haemophilus influenza* be completed. A single study of influenza vaccination in patients with chronic lymphoproliferative disorders and multiple myeloma is supportive of this approach [26]. In this study, 34 patients with lymphoproliferative disorders (including 6 patients with myeloma) were compared to 34 immunologically normal individuals who all received the same vaccine against influenza. One patient with chronic lymphocytic leukemia developed influenza; no patients with myeloma developed this infection. No significant toxicities were reported in either group.

Finally, the International Myeloma Foundation recommends that individuals with myeloma consider carefully selected exercises and avoidance of risky activities (risk of falling) [31].

Patient surveillance in multiple myeloma is an evolving concept that is unique in intent and design when compared to follow-up care in other malignancies. The idea of surveillance is a relatively new one, since it has only been in recent decades that longer remissions and improved survival have warranted recommendations during the plateau phase of care. The goals of follow-up are also different from those applied to curable malignancies in which the focus is often on preventing secondary complications of therapy and cancer survivorship. Despite major treatment advances, myeloma is still considered incurable with standard therapies and the prognosis for relapsed disease is poor. However, there are several reasons why close monitoring of patients in remission is warranted in myeloma. Progression in myeloma is frequently associated with devastating and potentially avoidable complications such as bone pain, fracture, renal failure, and hypercalcemia. The ability to detect disease recurrence with laboratory changes that precede clinical disease represents the underlying rationale for monitoring. While earlier detection of progression offers the potential to consider treatment at a time of low disease burden, it remains common practice, supported by randomized controlled trials, to defer initiation of treatment in myeloma until patients become symptomatic. Preventative measures, such as vaccinations, can further minimize the risk of complications associated with myeloma. Finally, surveillance for treatment of side effects will play an increasing role in the future as individuals continue on an increasing array of maintenance options.

There is a paucity of primary research on optimal patient surveillance in myeloma. In our review of the literature, only recent reports on the role of free light chain analysis monitoring and minimal residual disease surveillance are available. This evidence predominantly consists of small series of patients at various stages of disease followed retrospectively. Although both technologies appear to correlate with disease control and recurrence, the ability of these tests to change outcome in myeloma is as yet unproven. Given the preliminary nature of the evidence, a definitive recommendation on their use is difficult at this time. However, with regard to the free light chain analysis testing in particular, it may be reasonable to incorporate such testing into the monitoring of patients whose disease is primarily detectable by free light chain analysis.

Due to the lack of primary evidence on surveillance, it is not surprising the majority of guidelines on this topic base their recommendations on expert opinion. Despite differences in quality and methodology of the seven guidelines found in our review, there was general consensus on the most topics. Most guidelines suggest a 3–6 month frequency for laboratory and M-protein quantification. Most guidelines also support the use of skeletal surveys in monitoring, either annually or at the time of progression. The use of additional imaging modalities, including computed tomography, magnetic resonance imaging, and positron emission tomography/methoxyisobutyl isonitrile stress, are also considered reasonable, particularly for symptomatic areas or to follow extramedullary soft tissue disease. The guidelines were less explicit in other areas of follow-up. The frequency of clinical visits were generally not discussed, but could presumably be paired with the laboratory follow-ups (every 3–6 months). Guidelines were also silent on the timing of visits and laboratory reassessments in those on maintenance therapy. It is likely that physicians individualize the frequency of clinical visits for each patient depending on achievement and depth of remission, need for adjunctive treatments, including bisphosphonates and maintenance therapies, pain control requirements, and patient preferences.

Currently, the only Canadian-specific guidelines are those of the British Columbia Cancer Agency and Cancer Care Ontario [27, 30]. At our institution our practice reflects the

Table 102.3 Surveillance after curative-intent treatment for Multiple Myeloma at University of Toronto, Toronto, ON, Canada

	Years posttreatment					
	1	2	3	4	5	>5
Clinic visit[a]	4	4	4	4	4	4
Laboratory tests[a,b]	4	4	4	4	4	4
Immunoquantitation and M-protein quantitation[c]	4	4	4	4	4	4
Bone marrow biopsy	#	#	#	#	#	#
X-ray bone survey	0–1	0–1	0–1	0–1	0–1	0–1
Other Ω	1	1	1	1	1	1

Other imaging tests, as clinically indicated only. This includes computed tomography, magnetic resonance imaging, positron emission tomography/methoxyisobutyl isonitrile stress for symptomatic or extramedullary sites of disease

□ influenza vaccination bone marrow biopsy, as clinically indicated only, and dental examination for individuals on bisphosphonates

The numbers in each cell indicate the number of times per year each modality is recommended during a particular year posttreatment

[a]The frequency of clinical visits and general laboratory testing should be individualized for individuals on maintenance therapy, depending on regimen, side effects, and patient preference

[b]Complete blood count with differential, serum electrolyte levels, blood urea nitrogen, serum creatinine, and calcium levels. A 24-h urine protein determination is indicated if bisphosphonate therapy is continued.

[c]24-h urine or serum free light chain analysis is indicated if disease is predominantly monitored by these methods

recommendations outlined in these two documents (Table 102.3). We practice within a multidisciplinary team at an academic health sciences center affiliated with the University of Toronto. Our practice is guided by evidence-based treatment policies we develop locally and update every 2–3 years. These policies are available in printed form as well as via the web (www.hematology.utoronto.ca) and are distributed to team members, trainees, and to colleagues at affiliated institutions. Our policies are complimented by electronic order sets that are particularly useful in standardizing the ordering of testing with follow-up visits. This combination of standardized written policies and order sets facilitates communication between members and our patients appreciate the consistent messaging it provides.

For individuals who have completed induction therapy for myeloma, we recommend clinical and laboratory surveillance visits every 3 months. These follow-up visits are typically at the cancer center with the hematologist. While some patients coming from remote parts of the province may see their family physician for some of their myeloma follow-up, the complexity of the testing combined with the fact that most patients are receiving intravenous pamidronate at the time of their follow-up visit makes follow-up with the primary care provider impractical in many cases. Visits include history and physical examination, CBC, electrolytes, blood urea nitrogen (BUN)/creatinine, calcium profile, immunoquantitation, and M-protein quantitation (preferably by serum protein electrophoresis). Serum free light chain analysis (and/or 24-h urine collection for M-protein quantitation by urine protein electrophoresis) should also be included for those individuals who have disease predominantly detectable by these methods. Twenty-four urine collection for total protein should also be completed every 3 months for individuals on bisphosphonate therapy. Individuals continuing on bisphosphonates also warrant annual dental evaluation. We recommend annual skeletal survey screening and targeted imaging of symptomatic areas or extramedullary disease sites as clinically indicated. All patients should receive pneumococcal and annual influenza vaccinations. Finally, a proactive and multidisciplinary approach to pain management is warranted in all individuals with myeloma.

We recommend the same follow-up routine to individuals who are continuing on maintenance therapy. However, follow-up scheduling should be tailored towards the needs of these patients and may be more frequent to monitor for side effects of continued therapy (clinical visits ranging from 4 to 12 weeks). Additional interventions (e.g., thromboprophylaxis for individuals on maintenance thalidomide or lenalidomide) may be necessary, depending on the prescribed therapy, and should be individualized. Laboratory frequency (including M-protein quantitation) should follow the same schedule as for individuals who are not receiving maintenance. However, specific blood work to monitor for myelosuppression or other effects of maintenance therapy may be required more frequently.

In summary, despite the paucity of clinical trial evidence to guide the follow-up of patients with myeloma, practice guidelines from diverse jurisdictions are highly concordant. Follow-up practice will need to be periodically revisited with the increasing use of maintenance therapy, the availability of increasingly sophisticated laboratory testing for minimal residual disease, and the emergence of new active therapeutic agents that could offer the potential for use early in the course of disease progression. Well-designed clinical trials specifically addressing these questions are warranted.

Acknowledgements We are grateful to Drs. Christine Chen and Vishal Kukreti for their careful review of this manuscript and suggested revisions.

References

1. Jaffe ES. World Health Organization classification of tumours: pathology and genetics of tumors of haematopoietic and lymphoid tissues. Lyon: IARC; 2001.
2. Society CC, Canada NCIo. Canadian Cancer Statistics 2008. Toronto. www.cancer.ca.
3. Kyle RA, Rajkumar SV. Multiple myeloma. N Engl J Med. 2004;351:1860–73.
4. Imrie K, Esmail R, Meyer RM. The role of high-dose chemotherapy and stem-cell transplantation in patients with multiple myeloma: a practice guideline of the Cancer Care Ontario Practice Guidelines Initiative. Ann Intern Med. 2002;136:619–29.

5. Hicks LK, Haynes AE, Reece DE, et al. A meta-analysis and systematic review of thalidomide for patients with previously untreated multiple myeloma. Cancer Treat Rev. 2008;34:442–52.
6. San Miguel JF, Schlag R, Khuageva NK, et al. Bortezomib plus melphalan and prednisone for initial treatment of multiple myeloma. N Engl J Med. 2008;359:906–17.
7. Richardson PG, Sonneveld P, Schuster MW, et al. Bortezomib or high-dose dexamethasone for relapsed multiple myeloma. N Engl J Med. 2005;352:2487–98.
8. Fonseca R, Rajkumar SV. Consolidation therapy with bortezomib/lenalidomide/ dexamethasone versus bortezomib/dexamethasone after a dexamethasone-based induction regimen in patients with multiple myeloma: a randomized phase III trial. Clin Lymphoma Myeloma. 2008;8:315–7.
9. Weber DM, Chen C, Niesvizky R, et al. Lenalidomide plus dexamethasone for relapsed multiple myeloma in North America. N Engl J Med. 2007;357:2133–42.
10. Dimopoulos M, Spencer A, Attal M, et al. Lenalidomide plus dexamethasone for relapsed or refractory multiple myeloma. N Engl J Med. 2007;357:2123–32.
11. Kumar SK, Rajkumar SV, Dispenzieri A, et al. Improved survival in multiple myeloma and the impact of novel therapies. Blood. 2008;111:2516–20.
12. Myeloma Trialists' Collaborative Group. Interferon as therapy for multiple myeloma: an individual patient data overview of 24 randomized trials and 4012 patients. Br J Haematol. 2001;113:1020–34.
13. Berenson JR, Hillner BE, Kyle RA, et al. American Society of Clinical Oncology clinical practice guidelines: the role of bisphosphonates in multiple myeloma. J Clin Oncol. 2002;20:3719–36.
14. Harousseau JL, Dreyling M. Multiple myeloma: ESMO clinical recommendations for diagnosis, treatment and follow-up. Ann Oncol. 2008;19 Suppl 2:ii55–57.
15. D'Sa S, Abildgaard N, Tighe J, Shaw P, Hall-Craggs M. Guidelines for the use of imaging in the management of myeloma. Br J Haematol. 2007;137:49–63.
16. Lioznov M, Badbaran A, Fehse B, Bacher U, Zander AR, Kroger NM. Monitoring of minimal residual disease in multiple myeloma after allo-SCT: flow cytometry vs PCR-based techniques. Bone Marrow Transplant. 2008;41:913–6.
17. Liu H, Yuan C, Heinerich J, et al. Flow cytometric minimal residual disease monitoring in patients with multiple myeloma undergoing autologous stem cell transplantation: a retrospective study. Leuk Lymphoma. 2008;49:306–14.
18. Sarasquete ME, Garcia-Sanz R, Gonzalez D, et al. Minimal residual disease monitoring in multiple myeloma: a comparison between allelic-specific oligonucleotide real-time quantitative polymerase chain reaction and flow cytometry. Haematologica. 2005;90:1365–72.
19. Rasmussen T, Knudsen LM, Huynh TK, Johnsen HE. Molecular and clinical follow-up after treatment of multiple myeloma. Acta Haematol. 2004;112:105–10.
20. Fenk R, Haas R, Kronenwett R. Molecular monitoring of minimal residual disease in patients with multiple myeloma. Hematology. 2004;9:17–33.
21. Davies FE, Rawstron AC, Owen RG, Morgan GJ. Minimal residual disease monitoring in multiple myeloma. Best Pract Res Clin Haematol. 2002;15:197–222.
22. Cavo M, Terragna C, Martinelli G, et al. Molecular monitoring of minimal residual disease in patients in long-term complete remission after allogeneic stem cell transplantation for multiple myeloma. Blood. 2000;96:355–7.
23. Mosbauer U, Ayuk F, Schieder H, Lioznov M, Zander AR, Kroger N. Monitoring serum free light chains in patients with multiple myeloma who achieved negative immunofixation after allogeneic stem cell transplantation. Haematologica. 2007;92:275–6.
24. Mead GP, Carr-Smith HD, Drayson MT, Morgan GJ, Child JA, Bradwell AR. Serum free light chains for monitoring multiple myeloma. Br J Haematol. 2004;126:348–54.
25. Drayson M, Tang LX, Drew R, Mead GP, Carr-Smith H, Bradwell AR. Serum free light-chain measurements for identifying and monitoring patients with nonsecretory multiple myeloma. Blood. 2001;97:2900–2.
26. Rapezzi D, Sticchi L, Racchi O, Mangerini R, Ferraris AM, Gaetani GF. Influenza vaccine in chronic lymphoproliferative disorders and multiple myeloma. Eur J Haematol. 2003;70:225–30.
27. Agency BC. Multiple Myeloma. Cancer Management Guidelines 2008; http://www.bccancer.bc.ca/HPI/CancerManagementGuidelines/Lymphoma/plasma-cell-disorders/1.MultipleMyeloma.htm. Accessed November 24, 2008, 2008.
28. Anderson KC, Alsina M, Bensinger W, et al. Multiple myeloma. Practice guidelines in oncology [2008; v.2.2009]. http://www.nccn.org/professionals/physician_gls/PDF/myeloma.pdf. Accessed 24 November 2008.
29. Lacy MQ, Dispenzieri A, Gertz MA, et al. Mayo clinic consensus statement for the use of bisphosphonates in multiple myeloma. Mayo Clin Proc. 2006;81:1047–53.
30. Imrie K, Stevens A, Makarski J, et al. The role of bisphosphonates in the management of skeletal complications for patients with multiple myeloma: a clinical practice guideline. 2004. http://www.cancercare.on.ca/pdf/pebc6-4s.pdf. Accessed 24 November 2008, 2008.
31. Durie BG, Kyle RA, Belch A, et al. Myeloma management guidelines: a consensus report from the Scientific Advisors of the International Myeloma Foundation. Hematol J. 2003;4:379–98.
32. Smith A, Wisloff F, Samson D. Guidelines on the diagnosis and management of multiple myeloma 2005. Br J Haematol. 2008;132:410–51.
33. Durie BG, Harousseau JL, Miguel JS, et al. International uniform response criteria for multiple myeloma. Leukemia. 2006;20:1467–73.

Glioma of the Central Nervous System 103

David Y. Johnson, Shilpi Wadhwa, and Frank E. Johnson

Keywords
Gliomas • Survival rate • Epidemiology • Genetic disorders • Risk factors

The International Agency for Research on Cancer (IARC), a component of the World Health Organization (WHO), estimated that there were 189,485 new cases of CNS glioma (specified as cancer of the brain and other nervous system) worldwide in 2002 [1]. The IARC also estimated that there were 141,650 deaths due to this cause in 2002 [1].

The American Cancer Society estimated that there were 20,500 new cases and 12,740 deaths (males and females) due to this cause in the USA in 2007[2]. The estimated 5-year survival rate (all races) in the USA in 2007 was 34 % for brain cancer [2]. Survival rates were adjusted for normal life expectancies and were based on cases diagnosed from 1996 to 2002 and followed through 2003.

Gliomas are subdivided in various classification systems. The epidemiology is similarly complex. There are several known risk factors. Genetic disorders such as neurofibromatosis type I and Li-Fraumeni syndrome (p53 mutation) are well-established risk factors, but other sorts of risk factors are not [3, 4].

Geographic Variation Worldwide

There is considerable geographic variation in the incidence of this cancer. The incidence is reported to be high in Australia, Europe, Canada, and whites in USA, with a higher incidence in women than in men. Asian populations have relatively low rates, particularly in China, India, Japan, and the Chinese in Singapore [3]. Geographic variation in the USA is also pronounced with higher rates reported in white as compared to non-white populations [3, 5].

Surveillance Strategies Proposed by Professional Organizations or National Government Agencies and Available on the Internet

National Comprehensive Cancer Network (NCCN, www.nccn.org)—NCCN guidelines were accessed on 1/28/12 (Tables 103.1, 103.2, 103.3, 103.4, 103.5, and 103.6). There were major quantitative and qualitative changes compared to the guidelines accessed on 4/10/07.

American Society of Clinical Oncology (ASCO, www.asco.org)—ASCO guidelines were accessed on 1/28/12. No quantitative guidelines exist for glioma surveillance, including when first accessed on 10/31/07.

The Society of Surgical Oncology (SSO, www.surgonc.org)—SSO guidelines were accessed on 1/28/12. No quantitative guidelines exist for glioma surveillance, including when first accessed on 10/31/07.

European Society for Medical Oncology (ESMO, www.esmo.org)—ESMO guidelines were accessed on 1/28/12 (Table 103.6). There are new quantitative guidelines compared to no guidelines accessed on 10/31/07.

European Society of Surgical Oncology (ESSO, www.esso-surgeonline.org)—ESSO guidelines were accessed on 1/28/12. No quantitative guidelines exist for glioma surveillance, including when first accessed on 10/31/07.

D.Y. Johnson • S. Wadhwa
Department of Internal Medicine, Saint Louis University Medical Center, Saint Louis, MO, USA

F.E. Johnson (✉)
Saint Louis University Medical Center and Saint Louis Veterans Affairs Medical Center, Saint Louis, MO, USA
e-mail: frank.johnson1@va.gov

F.E. Johnson et al. (eds.), *Patient Surveillance After Cancer Treatment*, Current Clinical Oncology,
DOI 10.1007/978-1-60327-969-7_103, © Springer Science+Business Media New York 2013

Table 103.1 Central nervous system cancers: adult low-grade infiltrative supratentorial astrocytoma/oligodendroglioma[a] (obtained from NCCN (www.nccn.org) on 1-28-12)

	Years post-treatment[b]					
	1	2	3	4	5	>5
Office visit[c]	2–4	2–4	2–4	2–4	2–4	≥1
MRI	2–4	2-4	2–4	2–4	2–4	≥1

NCCN guidelines were accessed on 1/28/12. There were major quantitative changes compared to the guidelines accessed on 4/10/07
[a]Excluding pilocytic astrocytoma
[b]The numbers in the table indicate the number of times the modality is recommended during the indicated year post-treatment
[c]MRI was the only quantitative recommendation given. We inferred that office visit would be recommended as frequently as this

Table 103.2 Central nervous system cancers: anaplastic gliomas/glioblastoma[a] (obtained from NCCN (www.nccn.org) on 1-28-12)

	Years post-treatment[b]					
	1	2	3	4	5	>5
Office visit[c]	3–6	3–6	3–6	<6	<6	<6
MRI[d]	3–6	3-6	3–6	<6	<6	<6

NCCN guidelines were accessed on 1/28/12. There were major quantitative and qualitative changes compared to the guidelines accessed on 4/10/07
[a]This pathway includes the classification of mixed anaplastic oligoastrocytoma (AOA), anaplastic astrocytoma (AA), anaplastic oligodendroglioma (AO), and other rare anaplastic gliomas
[b]The numbers in the table indicate the number of times the modality is recommended during the indicated year post-treatment
[c]MRI was the only quantitative recommendation given. We inferred that office visit would be recommended as frequently as this
[d]MRI 2–6 weeks after radiotherapy, then every 2–4 months for 2–3 years, then less frequently

Table 103.3 Central nervous system cancers: adult intracranial ependymoma[a] (obtained from NCCN (www.nccn.org) on 1-28-12)

	Years post-treatment[b]					
	1	2	3	4	5	>5
Office visit[c]	3–4	2–3	1–2	1–2	1–2	1–2
Brain and spine MRI[d]	3–4	2–3	1–2	1–2	1–2	1–2

NCCN guidelines were accessed on 1/28/12. There were major quantitative and qualitative changes compared to the guidelines accessed on 4/10/07
[a]Excluding subependymoma and myxopapillary
[b]The numbers in the table indicate the number of times the modality is recommended during the indicated year post-treatment
[c]MRI was the only quantitative recommendation given. We inferred that office visit would be recommended as frequently as this
[d]If initially positive

Cancer Care Ontario (CCO, www.cancercare.on.ca)—CCO guidelines were accessed on 1/28/12. No quantitative guidelines exist for glioma surveillance, including when first accessed on 10/31/07.

National Institute for Clinical Excellence (NICE, www.nice.org.uk)—NICE guidelines were accessed on 1/28/12. No quantitative guidelines exist for glioma surveillance, including when first accessed on 10/31/07.

Table 103.4 Central nervous system cancers: adult medulloblastoma and supratentorial primitive neuroectodermal tumor[a] (obtained from NCCN (www.nccn.org) on 1-28-12)

	Years post-treatment[b]					
	1	2	3	4	5	>5
Office visit[c]	4	4	2	2	2	1
Brain MRI	4	4	2	2	2	1
Spine MRI	2	2	1	1	1	0

NCCN guidelines were accessed on 1/28/12. There were major quantitative and qualitative changes compared to the guidelines accessed on 4/10/07
[a]Excluding esthesioneuroblastoma
[b]The numbers in the table indicate the number of times the modality is recommended during the indicated year post-treatment
[c]MRI was the only quantitative recommendation given. We inferred that office visit would be recommended as frequently as this

Table 103.5 Central nervous system cancers: meningiomas (obtained from NCCN (www.nccn.org) on 1-28-12)

	Years post-treatment[a]					
	1	2	3	4	5	>5
Office visit[b c]	3	1–2	1–2	1–2	1–2	1–2
MRI[d]	3	1–2	1–2	1–2	1–2	1–2

NCCN guidelines were accessed on 1/28/12. There were major quantitative and qualitative changes compared to the guidelines accessed on 4/10/07
[a]The numbers in the table indicate the number of times the modality is recommended during the indicated year post-treatment
[b]MRI was the only quantitative recommendation given. We inferred that office visit would be recommended as frequently as this
[c]Less frequent surveillance after 5–10 years
[d]MRI at 3, 6, and 12 months, then every 6–12 months for 5 years, then every 1–3 years. More frequent imaging may be required for WHO Grade 3 meningiomas, and for meningiomas of any grade that are treated for recurrence or with chemotherapy

Table 103.6 High-grade malignant glioma (obtained from ESMO (www.esmo.org) on 1-28-12)

	Years post-treatment[a]					
	1	2	3	4	5	>5
Office visit[b]	3–4	3–4	3–4	3–4	3–4	3–4
MRI	3–4	3–4	3–4	3–4	3–4	3–4

Surveillance consists of a clinical evaluation with particular attention to neurological function, seizures, and corticosteroid use
Patients should be tapered off steroid use as early as possible
Venous thrombotic events occur frequently in patients with residual or recurrent tumors
Laboratory tests are not indicated unless the patient is receiving chemotherapy (blood counts), corticosteroids (glucose), or antiepileptic drugs (blood count, liver function tests)
ESMO guidelines were accessed on 1/28/12. These are new quantitative guidelines compared to no guidelines accessed on 10/31/07
[a]The numbers in the table indicate the number of times the modality is recommended during the indicated year post-treatment
[b]MRI was the only quantitative recommendation given. We inferred that office visit would be recommended as frequently as this

The Cochrane Collaboration (CC, www.cochrane.org)—CC guidelines were accessed on 1/28/12. No quantitative guidelines exist for glioma surveillance, including when first accessed on 11/24/07.

The M.D. Anderson Surgical Oncology Handbook also has follow-up guidelines, proposed by authors from a single National Cancer Institute-designated Comprehensive Cancer Center, for many types of cancer [6]. Some are detailed and quantitative, and others are qualitative.

Summary

This is a common cancer with significant variability in incidence worldwide. We found consensus-based guidelines but none based on high-quality evidence.

References

1. Parkin DM, Whelan SL, Ferlay J, Teppo L, Thomas DB. Cancer incidence in five continents. IARC Scientific Publication 155, vol. VIII. Lyon: IARC; 2002. ISBN 92-832-2155-9.
2. Jemal A, Seigel R, Ward E, Murray T, Xu J, Thun MJ. Cancer Statistics, 2007. CA Cancer J Clin. 2007;57:43–66.
3. Schottenfeld D, Fraumeni JG. Cancer epidemiology and prevention. 3rd ed. New York, NY: Oxford University Press; 2006. ISBN 13:978-0-19-514961-6.
4. DeVita VT, Hellman S, Rosenberg SA. Cancer. 7th ed. Philadelphia, PA: Lippincott Williams & Wilkins; 2005. ISBN 0-781-74450-4.
5. Devesa SS, Grauman DJ, Blot WJ, Pennello GA, Hoover RN, Fraumeni JF Jr. Atlas of cancer mortality in the United States. National Institutes of Health, National Cancer Institute. NIH Publication No. 99–4564; September 1999.
6. Feig BW, Berger DH, Fuhrman GM. The M.D. Anderson surgical oncology handbook. 4th ed. Philadelphia, PA: Lippincott Williams & Wilkins; 2006 (paperback). ISBN 0-7817-5643-X.

Glioma of the Central Nervous System Surveillance Counterpoint: Europe

104

Wolfgang Grisold, Stefan Oberndorfer, and Eefje Sizoo

Keywords
Astrocytomas • WHO • Glioblastoma • Tumor • Tumor treatment

Astrocytomas are conventionally graded according to WHO criteria. Patients with low-grade astrocytomas have a long survival and many features of chronic disease and will not be considered here. In comparison with other tumors, glioblastoma is rare [1]. Glioblastoma patients typically have a short survival duration.

Following initial tumor treatment with surgery, radiotherapy, and chemotherapy, patients decline due to tumor progression. Neurologic symptoms, particularly cognitive changes, mark the transition from active tumor treatment to symptomatic care. Our centers do not have any scheduled surveillance for glioblastoma patients as virtually all are incurable with current therapy (Table 104.1).

However, new glioblastoma treatment protocols are available. In most European countries, chemotherapy is given to patients in addition to surgery and radiation therapy. Costs are usually covered by national health insurance plans, which means that broad access to modern treatment options can be assumed in most European countries. Eventually virtually all glioblastoma patients deteriorate and palliative care is needed. Cognitive changes, neurologic deficits, and seizures dominate in gliomablastoma patients, whereas pain, fatigue, nausea, and asthenia are the main features in most other cancer patients [2–4]. Institutional care is provided in some countries, including hospice and palliative care. In other countries, glioblastoma patients in the final phases of their illness are taken care of by family, in-home caregivers, and family physicians.

When effective therapy permits long-term disease-free survival, surveillance strategies will undoubtedly be implemented. Most experts believe that the treatment of glioblastoma patients should involve an interdisciplinary tumor board which consists of all relevant specialists. However, the multidisciplinary field of neuro-oncology is not established in many European countries. Within the European Union of Medical Specialists (Union Européenne Des Médecins Spécialistes (UEMS) (www.uems.net), attempts are being made to establish neuro-oncology as a field of special competence in Europe. Another multidisciplinary European society, the European Association for Neuro-Oncology (www.EANO.eu), is also devoted to this field.

The UEMS has published a document (UEMS document D UEMS 2008/40), directed at the need for palliative care in neurology (www.uems.net), which can also be the basis for the development of papers and guidelines on palliative care in glioma patients.

In conclusion, the care of glioblastoma patients in Europe is heterogeneous, as are the various national health systems. Palliative care and end-of-life decision-making are important in glioblastoma care. Somatic, psychosocial, and spiritual needs are important for glioblastoma patients.

Organizations of Interest

1. *Societies* : In addition to the European Union of Medical Specialists (UEMS, www.uems.net), the European Federation of Neurological Societies (EFNS, www.efns.org), the

W. Grisold, MD, Prof. (✉) • S. Oberndorfer, MD, Doz.
Department of Neurology, Kaiser-Franz-Josef-Spital Hospital, Ludwig Boltzmann Institute for Neuro-Oncology, 1100 Vienna, Kundratstr. 1, Austria
e-mail: wolfgang.grisold@wienkav.at

E. Sizoo, MD.
Department of Neurology, Vrije Universiteit Medical Center, De Boelelaan 1117, Amsterdam, The Netherlands

F.E. Johnson et al. (eds.), *Patient Surveillance After Cancer Treatment*, Current Clinical Oncology, DOI 10.1007/978-1-60327-969-7_104, © Springer Science+Business Media New York 2013

Table 104.1

Surveillance for glioblastoma patients after curative-intent initial therapy.
In our centers we recognize that glioblastoma is virtually always fatal and do not carry out surveillance testing.
Tests are recommended in anticipation of patient decline and to manage specific treatable symptoms such as seizures

European Neurological Society (ENS, www.ensinfo.com), and the European Association of Neuro-Oncology (EANO, www.eano.eu), several other European activities, platforms, or journals are devoted to palliative care, for example, the European Association for Palliative Care (http://www.eapcnet.org/organisations/asseurope.html).

2. The Association of Neuro-Oncology Nurses (ANON) is a European organization of nurse specialists in neuro-oncology (www.ANON.org.uk). It organizes special sessions for nurses at EANO conferences. Nurse specialists from several European countries attend these sessions.
3. *Prominent European working groups*: Traditionally, much research into palliative care, quality of life (QOL), and cognitive function is provided by the Amsterdam group of Professor Heimans (including Drs. Klein, Taphoorn, and Sizoo). The Italian group of Professor Pace is very active in respect to palliative care in glioblastoma patients. Another Italian platform provides information and help (Brain Life (www.ilfondogio.it)). In Cologne, Germany, the German group of Professor Voltz (including Drs. Borasio and Ostgathe) publishes papers regarding palliative care for neurological patients. Many of these focus on neuro-oncological patients.
4. *Patient organizations*: This paper is not comprehensive, as several national organizations with different languages may exist. The worldwide International Brain Tumour Alliance (IBTA) (www.theibta.org/) is worthwhile mentioning, as is a UK activity (www.braintumouraction.org.uk) and a German patient-oriented group (http://www.hirntumorhilfe.de/en/home/projekte/brainstorm0/archiv/brainstorm-12.html). The European patient organization European Federation of Neurological Associations (EFNA) (http://www.efna.net/) has a link to the International Brain Tumour Alliance (www.teibta.org) on their website. In the Netherlands, there are two large foundations founded by patients (www.hersentumor.nl and www.STOPhersentumoren.nl). Both collect resources for brain tumor research and both have an extensive website providing information about brain tumors for patients, relatives, and health care professionals. The European Platform for Patients' Organisations, Science and Industry (EPPOSI) (www.epposi.org) is a European patient platform focusing on rare and/or chronic diseases.
5. *National guidelines*: a good example of thorough guidelines, and also extensively touching supportive care and palliative care are the National Institute for Clinical Excellence (NICE) (www.nice.org.uk/Guidance/CG/Published) guidelines.
6. *Death wish and euthanasia*: Several European countries have loosened restrictions about euthanasia: the Dutch association of voluntary euthanasia [5,6], a Belgian group [7], and the Swiss organization Dignitas (NGO). In France, the Association pour le Droit de Mourir dans la Dignité (ADMD) and the Spanish Fundacian Pro Derecho A. Morir Dignamente (DMD) (both associations for the right to die with dignity) have not been successful yet.
7. *Journals*: Although "Neuro-Oncology" is the official journal of the American Society for Neuro-Oncology, it is also strongly affiliated with the European Association for Neuro-Oncology (http://neuro-oncology.oxfordjournals.org/). The European Journal of Palliative care (http://www.ejpc.eu.com/ejpchome.asp?FR=1) is a European journal dealing with palliative care.
8. *EPPOSI*: European Platform for Patients' Organizations, Science and Industry (www.epposi.org) is a nonprofit partnership based multi-stakeholder think tank in Brussels. Several of their activities are directed towards rare and chronic diseases.

References

1. EPPOSI. Partnering for Healthcare Policy. http://www.epposi.org/. Accessed September 9.
2. Klein M, Taphoorn MJ, Heimans JJ, et al. Neurobehavioral status and health-related quality of life in newly diagnosed high-grade glioma patients. J Clin Oncol. 2001;19:4037–47.
3. Hilverda K, Bosma I, Heimans JJ, et al. Cognitive functioning in glioblastoma patients during radiotherapy and temozolomide treatment: initial findings. J Neurooncol. 2010;97:89–94.
4. Taphoorn MJ, Klein M. Cognitive deficits in adult patients with brain tumors. Lancet Neurol. 2004;3:159–68.

Glioma of the Central Nervous System Surveillance Counterpoint: Australia

105

Margot Lehman and Michael Barton

Keywords

Astrocytoma • Glioblastoma multiforme • Glioma • Magnetic resonance imaging • Positron emission tomography • Pseudo-progression

The median age at diagnosis of primary brain cancers in Australia was 55–59 years for males and 60–64 for females in 1999. Low-grade gliomas have a peak incidence in the fourth decade [1]. For high-grade gliomas the peak incidence occurs in the eighth decade. There were 1,369 people, or 6.8 per 100,000, diagnosed with primary brain cancer in 2004, the latest year for which national figures are available [2, 3]. In comparison, approximately 161 new cases of breast cancer and 64 new cases of colon cancer were diagnosed per 100,000 population that year. The Australian Institute of Health and Welfare ranks primary brain cancer as the 14th most common cancer. In the Australian States and Territories, the age-standardized incidence of brain cancer ranged from 6.3 per 100,000 in Western Australia and the Northern Territory to 7.5 per 100,000 in Victoria in 2001 (the most recent year for which State data are available) [4].

Malignant brain tumors make up only 2 % of all cancers but result in the fourth highest loss of potential years of life [5]. On average a patient with a malignant brain tumor loses 12 years of potential life, the highest average loss of life from any type of cancer [3]. Because of this, brain tumors cause the highest economic burden on Australian cancer patients' households with an average cost per patient estimated to be more than five times higher than for breast or prostate cancer patients [6]. Brain tumors "are among the most devastating to patients and their carers because they affect the organ that defines the self [7]."

While there are no high level data that examine the benefits of care coordination, it has become routine for most tumor sites. Brain tumor patients have a complex and difficult clinical course that involves multiple specialist clinical groups and repeated investigations. Care coordination is likely to significantly reduce the burden on patients and their caretakers.

Patterns of care studies [8, 9] have examined initial management but not patterns of follow-up practice.

There is no consensus about follow-up practice between or within professional groups. Current practice is ad hoc and has not been informed by guidelines or regulated by funding agencies. This is reflected in the lack of evidence-based recommendations in the guidelines listed in Chap. 103. There is considerable uncertainty among practitioners about the exact sequencing and timing of follow-up visits and investigations but there is general agreement that follow-up should be tailored to the patient's changing requirements. Patients often push for frequent imaging studies but clinicians realize that management is unlikely to change and that frequent imaging is not a good use of resources.

The main aim of follow-up for patients with either low- or high-grade astrocytoma is to evaluate tumor control, monitor and manage symptoms from tumor and treatment, and provide psychological support for the patient and the family. The optimal frequency of follow-up visits is unknown and should be determined by the patient's clinical condition. However, a routine schedule of one office visit every 1–3 months for patients with high-grade astrocytoma and one office visit every 3–6 months for patients with low-grade

M. Lehman
Princess Alexandra Hospital, 199 Ipswich Road, Woolloongabbo, QLD 4102, Australia
e-mail: Margot_lehman@health.qld.gov.au

M. Barton, OAM, MBBS, MD, FRANZCR (✉)
Liverpool Cancer Therapy Centre, Locked Bag 7103, Liverpool, BC NSW 1871, Australia
e-mail: Michael.Barton@sswahs.nsw.gov.au

F.E. Johnson et al. (eds.), *Patient Surveillance After Cancer Treatment*, Current Clinical Oncology,
DOI 10.1007/978-1-60327-969-7_105,

astrocytoma would appear reasonable. The exact schedule should vary according to the patient's condition.

There are many issues that need consideration during the follow-up of glioma patients, including dexamethasone and anticonvulsant dosage, rehabilitation, driving, imaging frequency, palliative and pastoral care. Dexamethasone is used to reduce intracerebral edema [10]. The dexamethasone dose should be gradually reduced and stopped when possible. Dexamethasone should not be stopped suddenly because severe and sometimes catastrophic cerebral edema can result. It may mimic tumor progression clinically and radiologically but can be rapidly reversed by reintroduction of dexamethasone. Dose reduction should be titrated to patient symptoms. It may take up to 1 week for a reduction in dexamethasone dose to result in cerebral edema so the titration must be undertaken slowly. Patients should be monitored for symptoms of the common side effects of dexamethasone, such as high blood sugar, osteoporosis, proximal myopathy, and gastric erosions. Anticonvulsants should only be discontinued after consultation with a neurologist. Patients should have a prolonged period without a seizure, stable disease, and a normal electroencephalogram. Anticonvulsants should be slowly withdrawn over a period of months.

Patients with brain tumors are only legally allowed to drive in Australia if they have no evidence of active tumor and are seizure free [11]. This is unusual in patients with grade IV gliomas. Cognitive changes that are not readily apparent in a clinical consultation may severely impede safe driving. It is recommended that all patients be assessed by a rehabilitation physician and occupational therapist before being certified as safe to drive.

The follow-up investigation of choice is MRI, which is reimbursed by Medicare, Australia's universal health insurance scheme for outpatients, or provided free by public hospitals. Positron emission tomography is also subsidized by Medicare. Standard MRI techniques with intravenous contrast are the most sensitive form of imaging intracranial lesions and show mass lesions such as low-grade gliomas that are poorly visualized with CT. Newer MRI techniques, such as spectroscopy, can measure the proportions of chemical compounds in small areas. These compounds, such as N-acetyl-aspartate, may be unique to glial tumors. Others may indicate the presence of necrosis.

CT may be useful for those with a contraindication to MRI. The role of positron emission tomography is controversial. It may delineate areas of increased or decreased uptake. Decreased tracer uptake may indicate areas of radionecrosis after radiotherapy but necrosis may also occur in high-grade gliomas and underlying malignancy may persist. The sensitivity and specificity of positron emission tomography for radiation necrosis are 75 and 81 %, respectively [12].

There is consensus that follow-up should involve multidisciplinary teams representative of all professional groups involved in care delivery. It is suggested that follow-up be undertaken in a setting where the patient has access to members of the multidisciplinary team involved in their care. The team should include the treating specialists, neurologists, social workers, nurses, radiologists, physiotherapy, occupational therapy rehabilitation, and palliative care specialists. A point of contact should be explicit. The general practitioner is also usually involved in patient care but, because gliomas are uncommon, the general practitioner's experience of gliomas is usually limited. They are usually reluctant to be involved in tumor-specific follow-up.

Nearly all gliomas recur at some stage. The median survival duration for high-grade gliomas is about 1 year [13] after surgery, chemotherapy, and radiotherapy, and only 25 % of patients survive 2 years. It is unusual to use a single modality unless the patient has a poor performance status or the tumor is deep and risky to biopsy. After treatment the MRI may be difficult to interpret because of the phenomenon of "pseudo-progression [14]." Edema and enhancement may occur after surgery, radiotherapy, and/or chemotherapy suggestive of tumor progression but may resolve with no further treatment. Similar appearances may be seen when dexamethasone dose is reduced. Low-grade gliomas, such as low-grade astrocytomas and oligodendrogliomas, may remain quiescent for many years. Follow-up schedules may be protracted with long intervals between clinic visits. However, nearly all tumors eventually recur and all patients should remain on active follow-up.

Salvage after recurrence is never possible but useful improvements in quality of life, and perhaps survival, can be obtained from further surgery or chemotherapy. Debulking may reduce mass effect but it is uncertain if debulking affects survival. Reirradiation has a high risk of causing necrosis because large areas of the brain will have been irradiated to tolerance dose. Second-line chemotherapy may reduce mass effect and slow tumor growth. The use of temozolomide [15], or carmustine wafers [16], has been shown to improve survival of patients with recurrence. New primary lesions are very rare. It is difficult to distinguish a new primary glioma from an intracerebral metastasis. Further surgery may be possible for diagnostic purposes.

Clinical trials in glioma are currently aimed at improving survival by augmenting treatment at diagnosis and identifying molecular markers, such as 1p19q loss of heterozygosity, that indicate better response to treatment. There are no trials planned at present which deal with posttreatment for surveillance strategies follow-up, treatment at diagnosis or after relapse (Tables 105.1 and 105.2).

Tables 105.1 Surveillance after curative-intent treatment for high-grade gliomas at Princess Alexandra Hospital, Australia

	Years posttreatment					
	1	2	3	4	5	>5
Office visit	8–12	4–8	4	2	1	[a]
MRI	3–4	2–4	2	1	1	[b]

The numbers in each cell indicate the number of times a particular modality is recommended in a particular year posttreatment

[a]Follow-up by general practitioner

[b]MRI only for new symptoms

Tables 105.2 Surveillance after curative-intent treatment for low-grade gliomas at Princess Alexandra Hospital, Australia

	Years posttreatment					
	1	2	3	4	5	>5
Office visit	2–3	2–3	2	2	1	1
MRI	2	2	1	1	1	1

[a]Follow-up by general practitioner

[b]MRI only for new symptoms

The numbers in each cell indicate the number of times a particular modality is recommended in a particular year posttreatment

Additional Guidelines

Australian Cancer Network Adult Brain Tumour Guidelines Working Party.

Clinical Practice Guidelines for the Management of Adult Gliomas: Astrocytomas and Oligodendrogliomas.

The Cancer Council Australia, Australian Cancer Network, and Clinical Oncological Society of Australia Inc., Sydney 2008. http://www.cancer.org.au/Healthprofessionals/clinicalguidelines/braintumours.htm.

References

1. Surveillance, Epidemiology and End Results SEER Program. SEER*Stat Database: Incidence—SEER 9 Regs Public-Use, Nov 2003 Sub (1973–2001), 1 April 2004. National Cancer Institute, DCCPS, Surveillance Research Program, Cancer Statistics Branch.
2. AIHW (Australian Institute of Health and Welfare) & AACR (Australasian Association of Cancer Registries). Cancer in Australia: an overview, 2006, No. 37, Cancer series. Canberra: AIHW; 2007.
3. Australian Institute of Health and Welfare. ACIM (Australian Cancer Incidence and Mortality) Books. Canberra: Australian Institute of Health and Welfare; 2007.
4. Australian Institute of Health and Welfare and Australasian Association of Cancer Registries. Cancer survival in Australia, 2001. Part 1: National summary statistics, 13. Cancer Series No. 18. Canberra: Australian Institute of Health and Welfare; 2001.
5. Australian Institute of Health and Welfare and Australasian Association of Cancer Registries. Cancer in Australia 2001, Cancer Series, vol. No. 28, CAN 23. Canberra: AIHW; 2004.
6. Access Economics. Cost of cancer in NSW, 15 June 2006. Sydney: Cancer Council NSW.
7. Kleihues P, Louis DN, Scheithauer BW, Rorke LB, Reifenberger G, Burger PC, et al. The WHO classification of tumors of the nervous system. J Neuropathol Exp Neurol. 2002;61:215.
8. Rosenthal MA, Drummond KJ, Dally M, Murphy M, Cher L, Ashley D, et al. Management of glioma in Victoria (1998–2000): retrospective cohort study. Med J Aust. 2006;184:270–3.
9. Chang SM, Parney IF, Huang W, Anderson FA, Asher AL, Bernstein M, et al. Patterns of care for adults with newly diagnosed malignant glioma. JAMA. 2005;293(5):557–64. Am Med Assoc. Ref Type: Generic.
10. Frappaz D, Chinot O, Bataillard A, Ben HM, Capelle L, Chanalet S, et al. Standards, options and recommendations 2002 for the management of adult patients with intracranial gliomas (summary report). Bull Cancer. 2003;90:873–86.
11. Australian Transport Council. Assessing fitness to drive for commercial and private vehicle drivers, and clinical management guidelines, vol. 3. Sydney: Austroads; 2003.
12. Chiro GD, Brooks A, Kornblith PL, Smith H. Issues in the in vivo measurement of glucose metabolism of human central nervous system tumors. Ann Neurol. 1984;15:S138–46.
13. Stupp R, Mason WP, van den Bent MJ, Weller M, Fisher B, Taphoorn MJ, et al. Radiotherapy plus concomitant and adjuvant temozolomide for glioblastoma. New Engl J Med. 2005;352:987–96.
14. Mason WP, Del Maestro R, Eisenstat D, Forsyth P, Fulton D, LaperriFre N, et al. Canadian recommendations for the treatment of glioblastoma multiforme. Curr Oncol. 2007;14:110.
15. Yung WK, Albright RE, Olson J, Fredericks R, Fink K, Prados MD, et al. A phase II study of temozolomide vs. procarbazine in patients with glioblastoma multiforme at first relapse. Br J Cancer. 2000;83:588–93.
16. Brem H, Piantadosi S, Burger PC, Walker M, Selker R, Vick NA, et al. Placebo-controlled trial of safety and efficacy of intraoperative controlled delivery by biodegradable polymers of chemotherapy for recurrent gliomas. Lancet. 1995;345:1008–12.

Glioma of the Central Nervous System Surveillance Counterpoint: Japan

106

Masahiro Mizoguchi, Koji Yoshimoto, and Tomio Sasaki

Keywords
Surgery • Cerebrospinal fluid • Gliomas • MRI • Tumor

Malignant gliomas are the most common and lethal primary brain tumors. This counterpoint focuses on treatment strategies and postoperative surveillance for patients with malignant glioma in Kyushu University Hospital. The clinical course of patients with malignant glioma varies depending on the biological aggressiveness of the tumor. The treatment strategy and postoperative surveillance should thus be based on biological characteristics. In our department, the initial therapeutic approach is surgical removal of the tumor for debulking and histological diagnosis (Table 106.1).

Recent advances in genetic analysis have revealed the genetic pathway of malignant glioma, facilitating further classification of this type of tumor based on genetic alterations. Most primary glioblastomas at our center have shown total loss of ch10, while 1p/19q co-deletion characterizes the oligodendroglial lineage. In particular, the subgroup of patients with 1p/19q co-deletion seems to show longer survival and better response to chemotherapy compared with patients lacking this deletion [1, 2]. We use a treatment protocol based on molecular genetic profiling. Patients with glioblastoma are treated with radiotherapy plus concomitant adjuvant temozolomide (TMZ), as previously reported [3]. The same regimen is applied to patients with anaplastic astrocytoma, anaplastic oligodendroglioma, or anaplastic oligo-astrocytoma (WHO grade 3) only when the tumor shows deletion of ch10. For patients with grade 3 glioma showing 1p/19q co-deletion, we start with chemotherapy alone using procarbazine, nimustine (ACNU), and vincristine (PAV regimen; a modification of the PCV regimen) [4]. At first progression, these patients are offered radiotherapy plus concomitant TMZ.

For patients with grade 3 glioma without 1p/19q co-deletion, we offer radiotherapy with ACNU and interferon β (IAR regimen), in accordance with the NCCN guidelines. Grade 3 gliomas without 1p/19q co-deletion are more likely than glioblastoma to respond to chemotherapy, so ACNU-based chemotherapy has been preferred in Japan. For patients with failure of prior chemotherapy, we offer chemotherapy with conventional TMZ on 5 consecutive days every 28 days. For these patients, repeat surgery should be considered before TMZ treatment.

Contrast-enhanced MRI is the gold standard for surveillance. We perform MRI every 2 months for a few years after surgery. More frequent MRI is recommended for patients with malignant glioma showing ch10 deletion, as this is the most aggressive genotype. MR spectroscopy, MR perfusion imaging, and positron emission tomography (PET) may be useful for distinguishing between tumor progression and necrosis when an enhanced lesion is detected. Currently, histological diagnosis using a surgical approach is highly recommended when the diagnosis remains unclear after attempting noninvasive evaluation. The frequency of distant recurrence and cerebrospinal fluid (CSF) spread is increased if local control is obtained.

The clinical course of patients with malignant glioma is varied. Frequent evaluation using MRI, sometimes combined with other noninvasive modalities, is necessary to detect recurrence. Genetic analysis may be useful to predict the clinical course in such patients. The postoperative surveillance strategy should be individualized based on histological classification, initial treatment, and genetic background.

M. Mizoguchi (✉) • K. Yoshimoto • T. Sasaki
Department of Neurosurgery, Graduate School of Medical Sciences, Kyushu University, 3-1-1 Maidashi, Higashi-ku, Fukuoka 812-8582, Japan
e-mail: mmizoguc@ns.med.kyushu-u.ac.jp; kyoshimo@ns.med.kyushu-u.ac.jp; tsasaki@ns.med.kyushu-u.ac.jp

F.E. Johnson et al. (eds.), *Patient Surveillance After Cancer Treatment*, Current Clinical Oncology,
DOI 10.1007/978-1-60327-969-7_106,

Table 106.1 Surveillance of patients after curative-intent treatment for glioma of central nervous system at Kyushu University Hospital

	Year					
Modality	1	2	3	4	5	>5
Office visit	6	6	6	6	6	6
MRI	6	6	6	6	6	6

The surveillance intensity may vary according to clinical evaluation, initial treatment, and genetic features
The number in each cell indicates the number of times a particular modality is recommended during a particular posttreatment year

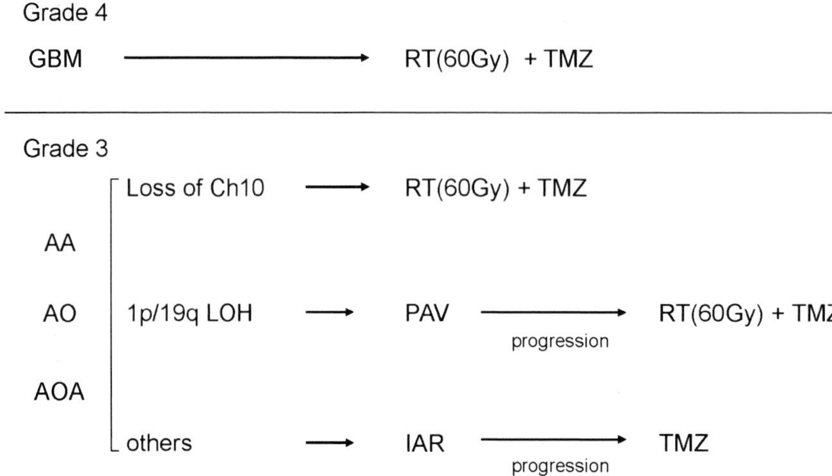

Grade 4
GBM
RT(60Gy) + TMZ
Grade 3
Loss of Ch10
RT(60Gy) + TMZ
AA
AO
1p/19q LOH
PAV
progression
RT(60Gy) + TMZ
AOA
others
IAR
progression
TMZ
GBM: glioblastoma, AA: anaplastic astrocytoma, AO: anaplastic oligodendroglioma,
AOA: anaplastic oligoastrocytoma, RT: radiotherapy, TMZ: temozolomide,
PAV: procarbazine + nimustine (ACNU) + vincristine
IAR: interferon-beta + nimustine (ACNU) + radiotherapy (60Gy)

Fig. 106.1 Treatment strategy based on genetic analysis

	Maintenance chemotherapy	Office visit	Labo check	Follow-up MRI
Grade4: GBM	TMZ every 28d x12-24	every 2-4wk	every 2-4wk	every 1-2mo
Grade3: AA, AO, AOA				
Loss of Ch10	TMZ every 28d x12	every 2-4wk	every 2-4wk	every 1-2mo for 2-3 y
1p/19q LOH	PCV(PAV) every 6-8wk x6	Day1, 8, 29	Day1, 8, 29	every 2-3mo for 2-3 y
others	ACNU every 6-8wk x6-12	every 2-4wk	every 2-4wk	every 2-3 mo for 2-3 y

Fig. 106.2 Postoperative surveillance based on genetic analysis

References

1. Mizoguchi M, Kuga D, Guan Y, et al. Loss of heterozygosity analysis in malignant gliomas. Brain Tumor Pathol. 2011;28:291–6.
2. Mizoguchi M, Yoshimoto K, Ma X, et al. Molecular characteristics of glioblastoma with 1p/19q co-deletion. Brain Tumor Pathol. 2012; 29:148–53.
3. Stupp R, Mason WP, van den Bent MJ, et al.; European Organisation for Research and Treatment of Cancer Brain Tumor and Radiotherapy Groups; National Cancer Institute of Canada Clinical Trials Group. Radiotherapy plus concomitant and adjuvant temozolomide for glioblastoma. N Engl J Med 2005; 352:987–96.
4. Lassman AB, Iwamoto FM, Cloughesy TF, et al.; International retrospective study of over 1000 adults with anaplastic oligodendroglial tumors. Neuro Oncol. 2011;13:649–59.

Index

A
Acquired immunodeficiency syndrome (AIDS), 235
Acute promyelocytic leukemia (APL), 486
Adenocarcinoma, 211–212
Aerodigestive tract carcinoma
geographic variation, 39
head and neck cancer, 40, 41
nasopharyngeal cancer, 41
surveillance strategies, 39–41
viral infections, 39
Agboola, O.O., 301, 302
Agency for Health Care Policy and Research (AHCPR), 2
Alkaline phosphatase (ALP), 383
Alpha-fetoprotein (AFP), 165
American Academy of Dermatology (AAD) Association, 253
American Cancer Society, 487
American College of Chest Physicians (ACCP), 73
American College of Obstetricians and Gynecologists (ACOG), 305, 327
American Head and Neck Society (AHNS), 40, 59
American Joint Committee on Cancer (AJCC), 236
American Society of Clinical Oncology (ASCO), 3, 13, 31, 39, 293, 469
anal carcinoma, 205
bladder cancer, 388
cervical cancer, 323
colon and rectum carcinoma, 179, 180
cutaneous melanoma, 251
endometrial carcinoma, 297
esophagus, 94
glioma, 511
leukemia, 475
liver and biliary tract carcinoma, 154
lung cancer, 72
lymphoma, 458, 469
multiple myeloma, 487
osteogenic sarcoma and dedifferentiated chondrosarcoma, 243
ovarian cancer, 357
pancreatic adenocarcinoma, 122
prostate cancer, 399
renal cancer, 373
soft tissue sarcoma, 227
stomach, 107
testicular cancer, 437
thyroid cancer, 58
vaginal and vulvar carcinoma, 349
American Society of Colon and Rectal Surgeons (ASCRS)
anal carcinoma, 206
colon and rectum carcinoma, 181, 182
American Society of Therapeutic Radiology and Oncology (ASTRO), 430
American Thyroid Association (ATA), 60, 65
American Urological Association (AUA), 395
bladder cancer, 390
prostate cancer, 400
renal cancer, 374
testicular cancer, 440, 441
Amling, C.L., 403
Anagnostou, T., 405
Anal carcinoma
Australia
active antiviral therapy, 217
CD4 count, 217
cost-effectiveness analysis, 218
cytology, 216
homosexual men, 215
PET scans, 216
physical examination, 216
risk factors, 215
salvage surgery, 217
SCCAg levels, 216
Canada
biopsy, 223
curative-intent treatment, 224
FDG-PET scan, 225
high-resolution anoscopy, 223
radiation therapy and chemotherapy, 224
squamous cell cancer, 223
survival duration, 224
geographic variation, 205
Japan
anal canal adenocarcinoma, 219
curative-intent treatment, 220
endorectal ultrasonography, 220
salvage surgery, 220
squamous cell carcinoma, 219
risk factors, 205
surveillance strategies
ASCO, 205
ASCRS, 206
CC, 205–206
CCO, 205
ESMO, 205, 206
ESSO, 205
NCCN, 205, 206
NICE, 205

F.E. Johnson et al. (eds.), *Patient Surveillance After Cancer Treatment*, Current Clinical Oncology, DOI 10.1007/978-1-60327-969-7, © Springer Science+Business Media New York 2013

Anal carcinoma (*cont.*)
SSAT, 206
SSO, 205
United States
adenocarcinoma, 211–212
HPV, 207
nodal status, 208
recurrence, 211
risk factors, 207
special populations, 211
squamous cell carcinoma, 208–209
surveillance, 209–211
treatment failure patterns, 208
Ansink, A., 337
Anticonvulsants, 518
Association of Community Cancer Centres (ACCC), 84
Association of Neuro-Oncology Nurses (ANON), 516
Association pour le Droit de Mourir dans la Dignité (ADMD), 516
Atypical adenomatous hyperplasia (AAH), 81
Australian and New Zealand Breast Cancer Trials Group (ANZBCTG), 290

B

Bakkevold, K.E., 133
Barcelona Clinic Liver Cancer staging system, 170
Bergmark, K., 338
Berg, W.A., 294
Bieri, S., 209
Bile duct cancer
adjuvant chemotherapy plus radiation, 174
cholangiocarcinoma, 174
postresection surveillance, 175
radiologic surveillance, 175
serum CA19-9 and carcinoembryonic antigen levels, 175
Bladder cancer
Canada
chest X-rays, 397
diagnosis, 395
ESMO recommendations, 397–398
low-grade solitary Ta tumors, 396
NCCN recommends, 396–397
radical cystectomy, 397
Ta high-grade, 396
urethral recurrence rate, 396
geographic variation, 387
Japan
curative-intent cystectomy, 393, 394
female patients, 393
male patients, 393
TUR, 393
surveillance strategies
ASCO, 388
AUA, 390
CC, 390
CCO, 390
ESMO, 388, 390
ESSO, 388, 390
NCCN, 387–390
NICE, 390
SSO, 388
Blana, A., 407
Blood urea nitrogen (BUN), 508
Bodurka, 329–331
Bodurka-Bevers, D., 337
Bohner, H., 111
Bolli, J.A., 338
Bone marrow. *See* Multiple myeloma (MM)
Borie, F., 17
Bortezomib, 501
Boysen, M., 45
Breast carcinoma
Australia
adjuvant therapies, 290
ANZBCTG, 290
base hospitals, 286
breast care nurses, 288
breast physicians, 288
categories, 288
causes and interventions, 286, 287
curative-intent treatment, 289
death rates, 285
diagnosis, 285
distance, 289
endocrine treatment, 286
Indigenous people, 290
medical oncologist, 288
multidisciplinary breast teams, 288
national guidelines, 286, 288, 289
primary cancer, 289
survivorship care, 286
TNM stage, 289
Europe
adjuvant tamoxifen treatment, 282
Cochrane systematic review, 281
contralateral metachronous lesions, 282
curative-intent treatment, 282
diagnostic tools, 281
intensive follow-up, 281
geographic variation, 273
Japan
aromatase inhibitors/ovarian failure, 294
BRCA1 and BRCA2, 293
ductal carcinoma, 294
gynecological symptoms, 294
invasive breast carcinoma, 294
JBCS guidelines, 293
mammography, 294
serum CA15-3 and CEA levels, 294
tamoxifen, 293–294
ultrasound, 294
risk factors, 273
surveillance strategies
ASBS, 274
ASCO, 273, 275
CC, 274
CCO, 274
ESMO, 273
ESSO, 273
NCCN, 273, 274
NICE, 274, 275
SSO, 273
United States
breast-conserving therapy, 278
curative-intent treatment, 279, 280
ductal carcinoma in situ, 278
follow-up strategy, 279
hormone-receptor-positive breast cancer, 277
mammogram, 277
radiation oncology, 278
Bristow, R.E., 307
British Columbia Cancer Agency (BCCA), 344, 504

British Committee for Standards in Haematology, 504
British Thyroid Association, 65
Bronchiolitis obliterans (BO), 485
Bronchioloalveolar cell carcinoma (BAC), 81
Buchler, T., 4
Buttrini, G., 145

C
Canadian Urological Association (CUA), 383, 395
Cancer
  AHCPR, 2
  bile duct cancer (*see* Bile duct cancer)
  bladder cancer (*see* Bladder cancer)
  cervical cancer (*see* Cervical cancer)
  cost-effective strategy, 5
  curative-intent primary therapy, 3
  cytotoxic chemotherapy, 1
  FDG-PET scans, 4
  guidelines, 2
  Institute of Medicine, 2
  ovarian cancer (*see* Ovarian cancer)
  patient treatment plan, 5
  postoperative surveillance, 1
  prostate cancer (*see* Prostate cancer)
  radiation therapy, 1
  rational screening program, 4
  soft-tissue sarcoma, 3
  testicular cancer (*see* Testicular cancer)
  thyroid cancer (*see* Thyroid cancer)
Cancer Care Ontario (CCO), 3, 40, 344, 470
  anal carcinoma, 205
  bladder cancer, 390
  cervical cancer, 324
  colon and rectum carcinoma, 181, 182
  cutaneous melanoma, 252
  endometrial carcinoma, 298
  esophagus, 94
  glioma, 512
  leukemia, 476
  liver and biliary tract carcinoma, 154
  lung cancer, 72
  lymphoma, 459, 470
  multiple myeloma, 488
  osteogenic sarcoma and dedifferentiated chondrosarcoma, 245
  ovarian cancer, 358
  pancreatic adenocarcinoma, 122
  prostate cancer, 400
  renal cancer, 374
  soft tissue sarcoma, 229
  stomach, 108
  testicular cancer, 440, 441
  thyroid cancer, 59
  vaginal and vulvar carcinoma, 350
Cancer of the Prostate Risk Assessment (CAPRA), 417
Cancer reform strategy, 366
Cancer surveillance strategies
  concerns
    patient, 10–11
    physician, 11
  duration of, 12
  goals, 10
  primary malignancy, 9
  prostate cancer, 10
  PSA, 9
  TNM staging system, 11
  USPSTF, 10
Cancer survivorship
  abdominal radiation, 33
  ASCO, 36
  bone radiation, 33
  chest radiation, 33
  consensus guidelines, 31
  cranial radiation, 33
  delayed wound healing, 33
  head and neck radiation, 33
  Hodgkin's disease, 32
  Institute of Medicine Treatment and Survivorship Care Plan, 32
  limb radiation, 33
  pelvic radiation, 33
  resources
    books, 33, 35
    journals, 35
    websites, 35
  second malignancies, 33
  skin radiation, 33
  surgical long-term effects, 32
  surveillance, 35
  systemic therapy, 34
  xerostomia, dental caries and periodontal disease, 33
Carbohydrate antigen 19–9 (CA19-9), 135
Carcinoembryonic antigen (CEA), 110, 166, 186, 189, 200, 354
Carter, H.B., 409
Cavo, M., 497
Cerebrospinal fluid (CSF), 521
Cervical cancer
  follow-up, Canada
    asymptomatic disease recurrence, 342, 343
    median survival, 342
    optimum surveillance strategies, 344
    PET/CT, 343, 346
    physical examination and pelvic examination, 344, 346
    recommended surveillance tests and schedules, 344, 345
    surveillance strategies, 341–342
    timing of, 342, 343
  geographic variation, 323
  Japan
    adenocarcinoma, 335
    asymptomatic pelvic recurrences, 337
    curative-intent treatment, 339
    follow-up procedure, 336–337
    HPV, 335–336
    incidence and mortality rate, 335
    pelvic and extrapelvic recurrences, 336
    posttherapy surveillance programs, 339
    quality of life and sexual functioning, 338–339
    recurrence, categories of, 337
    routine follow-up visits, 339
    SCC, 338
    surveillance program, 336
    survival rates, 336
  risk factors, 323
  surveillance strategies
    ASCO, 323
    CC, 325
    CCO, 324
    ESMO, 324
    ESSO, 324
    NCCN, 323, 324
    NICE, 324

Cervical cancer (*cont.*)
SGO, 325
SSO, 324
USA
chest X-rays, 329, 331
curative-intent treatment, 327, 328
cytological diagnosis, 330
HPV, 332
median survival, 330
pap smears, 329–331
pelvic exenteration, 328
radical hysterectomy and lymphadenectomy, 328–329
screening criteria, 327, 328
stage IB and IIA, 329
surveillance strategy, 332
survival advantage, 330
symptoms, 328
vaginal cytology, 331
Chan, A.O.O., 110
Chaplin, B.J., 404
Cher, M.L., 404
Chest radiograph (CXR), 236
Child-Turcotte-Pugh classification, 170
Chiva, L., 313
Chui, P., 98
Chung, H.H., 337
Cochrane Collaboration (CC), 40, 470
anal carcinoma, 205–206
bladder cancer, 390
cervical cancer, 325
colon and rectum carcinoma, 181
cutaneous melanoma, 252
endometrial carcinoma, 299
esophagus, 94
glioma, 512
leukemia, 477
liver and biliary tract carcinoma, 155
lung cancer, 73
lymphoma, 459, 470
multiple myeloma, 488
osteogenic sarcoma and dedifferentiated chondrosarcoma, 245
ovarian cancer, 359
pancreatic adenocarcinoma, 122
prostate cancer, 400
renal cancer, 374
soft tissue sarcoma, 229
stomach, 108
testicular cancer, 440
thyroid cancer, 59
vaginal and vulvar carcinoma, 350
Colon and rectum carcinoma
Australia
adjuvant therapy, 191
CEA level, 189
CSSANZ, 191
CT scan, 192
fecal occult blood test, 192
GILDA and FACS trial, 193
meta-analysis, 189
metachronous and luminal recurrence, 192
Norwegian surveillance protocol, 190
posttreatment surveillance, 193
QOL, 190
Canada
asymptomatic recurrent disease, 199
blood tests, 200
CT, MRI and PET scans, 200
endoscopy, 200
intense *vs.* less intense randomized trials, 201
liver metastases, 201
Ontario guidelines, 202
polypectomies, 199
routine surveillance, 202
surveillance bowel imaging, 201
TNM staging, 200
geographic variation, 179
Japan
CA19-9, 196
CEA level, 196
chest X-ray, 196
cost-effectiveness, 198
FDG-PET, 197
JSCCR, 195
liver metastasis, 197
pelvic CT, 197
recurrence sites, 195
standard surveillance schedules, 198
surveillance strategy, 195
risk factors, 179
surveillance strategies
ASCO, 179, 180
ASCRS, 181, 182
CC, 181
CCO, 181, 182
ESMO, 180, 181
ESSO, 180
NCCN, 179, 180
NICE, 181–182
SSAT, 182, 183
SSO, 180
United States
CEA level, 186
intensive surveillance, 185
PET/CT, 186
Colorectal surgical society of Australia and New Zealand (CSSANZ), 190
Complete blood count (CBC), 462
Computed tomography (CT), 47, 294, 467, 502
Cost-effectiveness analysis (CEA), 20
Cox, J.D., 407
Crook, J., 407
Cruickshank, D.J., 339
CT arterial portography (CTAP), 165
CT hepatic angiography (CTHA), 165
Cummings, B.J., 201, 224
Cutaneous melanoma
Australia
curative-intent treatment, 266, 267
follow-up, 266
imaging/blood tests, 267
intense surveillance program, 267
non-melanoma skin cancer, 266
sentinel node biopsy, 268
sonography, 268
synchronous and metachronous melanoma, 265
geographic variation, 251
Japan
curative-intent therapy, 271
lymphedema, 271
screening systems, 270
5-S-cysteinyldopa level, 270

survival rate, 269
TNM classification, 269
risk factors, 251
surveillance strategies
AAD, 253
ASCO, 251
CC, 252
CCO, 252
ESMO, 252
ESSO, 252
NCCN, 251, 252
NICE, 252
SSO, 252
United States
atypical nevi, 255
CDKN2A gene, 255
curative-intent treatment, 256
dermatologic surveillance, 258
digital photography/mole mapping, 260
disease-specific mortality rate, 259
distant metastases, 259
draining nodal basin, 260
FDG-PET, 258
follow-up strategies, 259
in-transit metastasis, 257
LDH level, 260
MSLT-1 interim analysis, 257
MSLT-2 trial, 261
nodal micrometastastic tumor, 257
sentinel lymph node biopsy, 256
ultraviolet radiation, 256
Cutili, 209

D

Das, P., 17, 208, 209
de Bekker-Grob, E.W., 17
Decision analytic models
cancer surveillance
internal and external validation, 25
recurrent disease, 24
sensitivity analysis, 25
simulation, 25–26
transition probabilities, 24–25
Cox proportional hazard regression models, 16
decision tree
clinical problem, 17–18
preferred clinical strategy, 18
presentation, 20
quantification of, 18
sensitivity analysis, 18, 20
implementation, 27
Kaplan–Meier curves, 16
lead time bias, 16
length time bias, 16
Markov models
constant transition probabilities, 21
fundamental matrix solution, 22
influence diagram, 21
Markov cohort analysis, 22
Monte Carlo simulation, 22, 23
mortality rate, 22
no memory, 21
one-cycle transition probabilities, 21
time horizon, 21
Medline database, 17
ovarian cancer, 23, 28
randomized controlled trial, 16
recurrences, 15
self-selection bias, 16–17
surveillance programs, 15
Deng, J.Y., 110
Des-gamma-carboxy prothrombin (DCP), 165
DeVisscher, A.V., 45
Dexamethasone, 518
Differentiated thyroid cancer, 60
Doneux, A., 405, 406

E

Earle, C., 201
Eastern Cooperative Oncology Group (ECOG), 496
Edelman, M.J., 83
Endometrial cancer, USA
asymptomatic recurrences, 302, 307, 308
chest X-rays, 302, 307, 309
curative-intent treatment, 303
gynecologic oncologists, 307
high risk, recurrence, 309
low risk, recurrence, 307, 309
pap smears, 302
patient's risk factors, 305
PET/CT, 309
physical examination, 307
recurrence rate, 301
recurrence, risk of, 305–306
serum CA-125 levels, 302, 303, 306, 307
Endometrial carcinoma
follow-up strategies, Canada
BCCA recommended, 320
clinical guidance, 319
NCCN guideline, 320
pap tests, 318
patient surveillance, 320–321
physical examination, 318
timing of, 317, 318
geographic variation, 297
Japan
cytology, cost of, 314
death rates, 311
gynecologic oncologist, 315
health insurance law, 311
higher risk group, 315
laparoscopic lymphadenectomy, 313
lower risk group, 315
lymph node metastases, 312
MPA therapy, 313
PET/CT system, 314, 316
PFS and OS *vs.* pelvic radiation, 312
radical hysterectomy, 312–313
radiotherapy, 312
serum CA 125 level, 316
surgical treatment procedures, 312
vaginal cytology, 314
surveillance strategies
ASCO, 297
CC, 299
CCO, 298, 299
ESMO, 298
ESSO, 298
NCCN, 297, 298
NICE, 298

Endometrial carcinoma (*cont.*)
SGO, 299
SSO, 298
Endoscopic mucosal resection (EMR), 115
Epidermal growth factor receptor (EGFR), 135
Erythrocyte sedimentation rate (ESR), 462
Esajas, M.D., 338, 339
Esaki, M., 104
Esophagogastroduodenoscopy (EGD), 110
Esophagogastroscopy, 117
Esophagus
Australia
anastomosis, 98
definitive chemoradiation therapy, 97
dysphagia, 98
endoscopy, 98
esophagectomy, 97
locoregional recurrences, 99
radiation pneumonitis, 99
surveillance, 100
geographic variation, 93
Japan
curative resections, 101
endoscopic mucosal resection, 104
follow-up schedule, 103, 104
intramural metastasis, 103
multimodal therapy, 104
PET-CT, 104
radical lymphadenectomy, 101
recurrence characteristics, 102
squamous cell carcinoma, 103
upper aerodigestive tract, 103
risk factors, 93
surveillance strategies, 93–94
European Association of Neuro-Oncology (EANO), 516
European Association of Urology (EAU), 395
European Consensus guidelines, 65
European Federation of Neurological Associations (EFNA), 516
European Neurological Society (ENS), 516
European Organization for Research and Treatment of Cancer (EORTC), 133, 149, 238, 366
European Platform for Patients' Organisations, Science and Industry (EPPOSI), 516
European Randomized Study of Screening for Prostate Cancer (ERSPC), 427
European Society for Medical Oncology (ESMO), 3, 39, 469, 506, 511
anal carcinoma, 205, 206
bladder cancer, 388, 390
cervical cancer, 324
colon and rectum carcinoma, 180, 181
cutaneous melanoma, 252
endometrial carcinoma, 298
esophagus, 94
high-grade malignant glioma, 511, 512
leukemia, 476
liver and biliary tract carcinoma, 154
lung cancer, 72, 73
lymphoma, 458, 469
multiple myeloma, 487, 488
osteogenic sarcoma and dedifferentiated chondrosarcoma, 244, 245
ovarian cancer, 358
pancreatic adenocarcinoma, 122
prostate cancer, 400
renal cancer, 373, 374
soft tissue sarcoma, 227, 229
stomach, 108
testicular cancer, 438–439
thyroid cancer, 59
vaginal and vulvar carcinoma, 350
European Society of Surgical Oncology (ESSO), 3, 40, 469
anal carcinoma, 205
bladder cancer, 388, 390
cervical cancer, 324
colon and rectum carcinoma, 180
cutaneous melanoma, 252
endometrial carcinoma, 298
esophagus, 94
glioma, 511
leukemia, 476
liver and biliary tract carcinoma, 154
lung cancer, 72
lymphoma, 459, 469
multiple myeloma, 488
osteogenic sarcoma and dedifferentiated chondrosarcoma, 244
pancreatic adenocarcinoma, 122
prostate cancer, 400
renal cancer, 374
soft tissue sarcoma, 229
stomach, 108
testicular cancer, 439, 440
thyroid cancer, 59
vaginal and vulvar carcinoma, 350
European Study Group of Pancreatic Cancer (ESPAC), 149
Examination under anesthesia (EUA), 395

F

Federation of Gynecology and Obstetrics (FIGO), 305
^{18}F-fluorodeoxyglucose (FDG), 314, 370, 467
^{18}F-fluorodeoxyglucose positron emission tomography (FDG-PET), 4, 258
Figueredo, A., 201
Food and Drug Administration (FDA), 381
Fox Chase Cancer Center, 186
Francken, A.B., 266
Frank, S.J., 353, 354
Frumovitz, M., 338
Fung-Kee-Fung, M., 301, 302, 306, 307

G

Gastrointestinal stromal tumors (GIST), 235
Gastrointestinal Tumor Study Group (GITSG), 149
Glioma
Australia
anticonvulsants, 518
clinical trials, 518
dexamethasone, 518
high-grade astrocytoma, 517, 519
low-grade astrocytoma, 517–519
MRI techniques, 518
Europe
interest, organizations of, 515–516
low-grade astrocytomas, 515
neurologic symptoms, 515
geographic variation, 511
Japan
MRI, 521
postoperative surveillance, 521, 522
1p/19q co-deletion, 521

TMZ, 521
treatment strategies, 521, 522
risk factors, 511
surveillance strategies
ASCO, 511
CC, 512
CCO, 512
ESMO, 511
ESSO, 511
NCCN, 511, 512
NICE, 512
SSO, 511
Gomez, P., 404
Gordon, A.F., 309
Graft-*versus*-host disease (GVHD), 481, 485
Guadagnolo, B.A., 17
Gynecologic Oncology Group (GOG), 305

H

Hammerer, P., 407
Hassan, C., 17
Hayman, J.A., 17
Helicobacter pylori 113
Hengge, U.R., 17
Herr, H.W., 393
Herzog, T.J., 338
High-intensity focused ultrasound (HIFU), 415–417
Hishinuma, S., 145
Hong, J.H., 328
Hopkins, M.L., 17
Howell, J., 192
Huang, W.C., 381
Human immunodeficiency virus (HIV), 207, 235
Human papilloma virus (HPV), 43, 207, 332, 335–336

I

Igaki, H., 103
Incremental cost-effectiveness ratio (ICER), 20
Interferon-alpha (IFN-α), 381
International Agency for Research on Cancer (IARC), 39, 57, 71, 323, 347, 357, 373, 387, 399, 457, 475, 487, 511
International Brain Tumour Alliance (IBTA), 516
International Myeloma Working Group (IMWG), 491, 495, 496
International staging system, 495
Intravenous pyelogram (IVP), 396

J

Jacobs, H.J., 17
Japanese Breast Cancer Society (JBCS), 293
Japanese Gynecologic Oncology Group (JGOG), 312, 316, 369
Japanese Skin Cancer Society, 270
Japanese Society for Cancer of the Colon and Rectum (JSCCR), 195
Johnstone, P.A.S., 406
Joypaul, B., 110
Junger, Y.G., 327

K

Kane, C.J., 405
Kaposi sarcoma, 235
Kattan, M.W., 412
Kent, M.S., 17
Kestin, L.L., 406
Kew, F.M., 339
Khanfir, K., 209
Kievit, J., 17
Kjeldsen, B.J., 201
Klatskin tumours, 162
Klotz, L., 408
Kobayashi, H., 196
Kodera, Y., 111
Korst, R.J., 85
Krug, B., 17
Kyushu University Hospital, 48, 69, 70, 81, 116, 117, 293–295, 313, 315, 316, 339, 353, 354, 369, 370, 394, 454, 467, 468, 472, 485, 486, 501, 521–522

L

Lachaine, J., 17
Lactate dehydrogenase (LDH), 260, 462, 495
Laparoscopic surgery, 115
Laryngeal cancer, 40
Lattouf, J.B., 433
Lee, J.H., 17
Lee, W.R., 406
Lenalidomide, 501
Leukemia
Japan
BO, 485
conventional evaluation, 486
curative-intent therapy, 485, 486
minimal residual disease, 486
PML/RARα, 486
molecular biology, 475
surveillance strategies
ASCO, 475
CC, 477
CCO, 476
ESMO, 476
ESSO, 476
NCCN, 475, 476
NICE, 477
SSO, 476
USA
acute lymphoblastic leukemia, 479
allo-HCT, 479, 480
annual pulmonary function tests, 481–482
audiometry, 481
cardiovascular problems, 481
chemotherapeutic and radiation therapies, 480
chimerism measurement, 481
clinical trials, 482
cytopenias, 480
eye examinations, 481
molecular biology, 479
myelodysplasia, 480
regimen-related toxicity, 480
tyrosine kinase inhibitors, 480, 481
Li-Fraumeni syndrome, 39
Liver and biliary tract carcinoma
Australia
AFP levels, 161
cholangiocarcinoma, 162
curative therapy, 162
gallbladder cancer, 163
HCC, 159
Klatskin tumours, 162
lead-time bias, 161

Liver and biliary tract carcinoma (*cont.*)
partial hepatectomy, 160
surgical removal, 159
TACE, 159
transplantation, 160
Canada
bile duct cancer, 174–176
cholangiocarcinoma, 176
gallbladder carcinoma, 176
HCC, 169–174
salvage therapy, 169
Europe
HCC, 157
OLT, 158
surgical resection/ablation, 157–158
geographic variation, 153
hepatocellular carcinoma, 154
Japan
CEA, 166
CTAP/CTHA, 165, 166
CT scan, 166
DCP level, 165
gallbladder cancer and extrahepatic/intrahepatic cholangiocarcinoma, 166
HCC, 165
hepatitis virus, 166
PET-CT, 167
portal venous invasion, 165
spiral-computed tomography, 165
risk factors, 153
surveillance strategies
ASCO, 154
CC, 155
CCO, 154
ESMO, 154
ESSO, 154
NCCN, 153
NICE, 155
SSAT, 155
SSO, 154
Lotan, Y., 17, 20
Lung carcinoma
Australia
clinic visits and CXR, 77
curative-intent primary therapy, 76
NSCLC, 75
PET scans, 76
pneumonitis, 75
postthoracotomy pain, 75
surveillance strategy, 77
Canada
combined modality therapy, 88
follow-up, 88
NSCLC, 83
posttreatment surveillance, 83
radical radiation therapy, 86–88
recurrent disease, 88
SCLC, 83
second primary cancers, 88
smoking cessation and surveillance, 88–90
surgical resection, 83–86
geographic variation, 71
Japan
AAH/BAC, 81
never-smoking patients, 80
NSCLC, 79
periodical surveillance, 79
pulmonary metastasis, 80
polycyclic aromatic hydrocarbons, 71
surveillance strategies
ACCP, 73
ASCO, 72
CC, 73
CCO, 72
ESMO, 72, 73
ESSO, 72
NCCN, 71–72
NICE, 72
SSO, 72
Lymphoma
ASCO, 469
CC, 470
CCO, 470
ESMO, 469
ESSO, 469
Japan
adult T-cell leukemia/lymphoma, 467, 472
B-cell lymphomas, 471
chronic hepatitis B virus, 467
curative-intent treatment, 472
Fukuoka Blood and Marrow Transplantation group, 470
high-dose chemotherapy, 471–472
late-onset neutropenia, 467
non-Hodgkin's lymphoma, 468, 471
peripheral T-cell lymphomas, 471
PET-CT scans, 472
rituximab, 467, 471–472
NCCN, 469
NICE, 470
SSO, 469
surveillance strategies, 469
ASCO, 458
CC, 459
CCO, 459
ESSO, 459
NCCN, 458
NICE, 459
SSO, 458
USA
anthracyclineinduced cardiomyopathy, 463
asymptomatic patients, 463
clinical trials, 462
CT scan, 462
diagnostic test, 461–462
Hodgkin lymphoma, 461, 462
lymphocyte-predominant hodgkin lymphoma, 463–465
non-Hodgkin lymphoma, 461, 462
PET scan, 462
testing period, 461
Lymphoproliferative disorders, 507

M

Magnetic resonance imaging (MRI), 47, 502
Makela, J., 192, 201
Marchant, F.E., 52
Marchet, A., 110
Maroun, J., 201
Marrelli, D., 110
Mataki, Y., 166
McLeod, R., 201
Medroxyprogesterone Acetate (MPA), 313

Medullary thyroid cancer, 60
Melanocortin 1 Receptor (MC1R) gene, 255
Melanoma Sentinel Lymph Node Trial-1 (MSLT-1), 257
Melphalan plus prednisone (MP), 501
Michel, P., 17
Milliken, D.A., 339
Minimal residual disease, 486
Moertel, C.G., 132
Monoclonal gammopathy of undetermined significance (MGUS), 489
Morice, P., 337
Morris, M., 328
Multiple myeloma (MM) (PM: Wrongly spelt as Multiple mylenoma in 6 occurrences in the text. Please correct it to Multiple myeloma.)
  American Cancer Society, 487
  bisphosphonate therapy, 504, 507
  chromosomal changes, 495
  clinical and laboratory surveillance, 508
  criteria, 504
  curative-intent treatment, 508
  cytogenetic changes, 495
  diagnosis, 489, 494, 499
  free light chain analysis, 506, 507
  geographic variation, 487
  IMWG uniform response criteria, 489, 491
  international staging system, 495
  international staging system and prognosis, 489, 492
  Japan
    autologous stem cell transplantation, 501
    curative-intent treatment, 501, 502
    high-dose chemotherapy, 501
    MP, 501
    osteolytic bone, 502
    PET/CT, 502
  laboratory testing, 504
  lymphoproliferative disorders, 507
  magnetic resonance imaging, 506–507
  maintenance therapy, 503
  Mayo clinic guidelines, 507
  melphalan, 493
  melphalan and steroids, 495
  MGUS, 489, 490, 493
  minimal residual disease, 506
  monoclonal protein level, 493
  M-proteins, 504, 506
  multimeric M-components, 504, 506
  myeloma-related organ/tissue impairment, 494
  nonsecretory/oligosecretory myeloma, 494
  patient surveillance, 507
  plasma cell clone, 489
  practice guidelines, 504, 505
  recommendations of, 489–490, 492
  risk factor, 493
  serum free light chain assay, 494
  skeletal surveys, 506
  smoldering/indolent myeloma diagnostic criteria, 489, 490
  surveillance strategies
    ASCO, 487
    CC, 488
    CCO, 488
    ESMO, 487
    ESSO, 488
    NCCN, 487
    NICE, 488
    SSO, 487
  treatment options
    autologous stem cell transplantation, 496–498
    bone marrow biopsy, 499
    bortezomib + melphalan + prednisone, 496
    lenalidomide, 496, 497
    melphalan-prednisone-thalidomide, 496
    single and tandem transplantation, 498
    vincristine + doxorubicin + dexamethasone group, 497
Munro, A.J., 17
Musculoskeletal Tumor Society Rating Scale (MSTS), 236

N
Nam, R.K., 17
Nasopharyngeal cancer, 39
National Breast and Ovarian Cancer Centre (NBOCC), 288
National Comprehensive Cancer Network (NCCN), 3, 39, 293, 301, 305, 315, 327, 344, 395, 469
  anal carcinoma, 205, 206
  bladder cancer, 387–390
  central nervous system cancers, 511–512
  cervical cancer, 323, 324
  colon and rectum carcinoma, 179, 180
  cutaneous melanoma, 251, 252
  endometrial carcinoma, 297
  esophagus, 93–94
  high-grade malignant glioma, 511, 512
  leukemia, 475
  liver and biliary tract carcinoma, 153, 154
  lung cancer, 71–72
  lymphoma, 458, 469
  multiple myeloma, 487
  osteogenic sarcoma and dedifferentiated chondrosarcoma, 243, 244
  ovarian cancer, 357, 358
  pancreatic adenocarcinoma, 121–122
  prostate cancer, 399, 400
  renal cancer, 373, 374
  soft tissue sarcoma, 227–229
  stomach, 107
  testicular cancer, 437–439
  thyroid cancer, 57–58
  vaginal and vulvar carcinoma, 349
National Comprehensive Cancer Network guidelines, 185
National Guideline Clearinghouse (NGC), 3
National Health and Medical Research Council, 190
National Institute for Clinical Excellence (NICE), 3, 40, 366, 470, 516
  anal carcinoma, 205
  bladder cancer, 390
  cervical cancer, 324
  colon and rectum carcinoma, 181–182
  cutaneous melanoma, 252
  endometrial carcinoma, 298
  esophagus, 94
  glioma, 512
  leukemia, 477
  liver and biliary tract carcinoma, 155
  lung cancer, 72
  lymphoma, 459, 470
  multiple myeloma, 488
  osteogenic sarcoma and dedifferentiated chondrosarcoma, 245
  ovarian cancer, 359
  pancreatic adenocarcinoma, 122
  prostate cancer, 400
  renal cancer, 374
  soft tissue sarcoma, 229

National Institute for Clinical Excellence (NICE) (*cont.*)
stomach, 108
testicular cancer, 440
thyroid cancer, 59
vaginal and vulvar carcinoma, 350
National Kyushu Cancer Center, 219
National Lung Screening Trial (NLST), 45
Naya, Y., 405
Newlin, H.E., 209
Niedergethmann, M., 145
Nieuwenhuis, E.J., 54
Nieweg, O.E., 267
Nigro, N.D., 207, 220
Nobuta, A., 113
Noji, T., 166
Nonseminoma germ cell tumors (NSGCT), 444, 450
Non-small cell lung cancer (NSCLC), 75, 79

O
Oettle, H., 134, 146
Ohlsson, B., 201
Ontario Clinical Oncology Group (OCOG), 430
Oonk, M.H., 354, 355
Orthotopic Liver Transplantation (OLT), 158
Osteogenic sarcoma and dedifferentiated chondrosarcoma
Canada
CT/MRI imaging, 250
curative-intent initial therapy, 250
metastatic disease, 249
screening, 249
geographic variation, 243
Japan
curative-intent initial treatment, 248
PET scan, 248
pre-and postoperative chemotherapy, 247
recurrent/metastatic lesion, 247
tumor necrosis, 247
risk factors, 243
surveillance strategies
ASCO, 243
CC, 245
CCO, 245
ESMO, 244, 245
ESSO, 244
NCCN, 243, 244
NICE, 245
SSO, 243
Osugi, H., 103
Ottawa Cancer Centre, 320–321
Ovarian cancer
Europe
cancer networks, 365
CA-125 serum levels, 366
hybrid follow-up schedule, 366, 367
Medical Research Council trial, 366
oncology community, 366
serum CA-125 tests, 367
traditional follow-up schedule, 366
women care, 365
geographic variation, 357
Japan
cisplatin, 369
curativeintent initial therapy, 370
docetaxel plus carboplatin, 369
PET/CT scans, 370
serum CA-125 level, 370
surveillance strategies
ASCO, 357
CC, 359
CCO, 358
ESMO, 358
NCCN, 357, 358
NICE, 359
SGO, 359
SSO, 358
USA
clinical complete response, 361
maintenance therapy, 362
platinum-based chemotherapy, 361
randomized trial, results of, 362

P
Pancreatic adenocarcinoma
Canada
adjuvant chemotherapy, 151
CA 19–9 level, 151
pancreaticoduodenectomy, 149
patient surveillance, 150
Europe
adjuvant chemotherapy, 136
CA19-9 levels, 136
chemotherapy, 133
computed tomography, 137
CONKO-01 study, 134
early follow-up period, 138
EGFR, 135
EORTC, 133
ESPAC-1, 133
extended lymphadenectomy, 130
external-beam radiation therapy, 132
gastrojejunostomy, 131
gemcitabine, 137
hepatectomy, 137
hepatojejunostomy, 131
malabsorption, 131
p53, 135
partial pancreatoduodenectomy, 131
pylorus-preserving procedures, 130
radical surgery, 130
resected pancreatic cancer, 134
risk factors, 129
SEER analysis, 129
smad4 expression, 135
surveillance, 138
tobacco smoking, 129
UKPACA-1 study, 132
geographic variation, 121
Japan
adjuvant therapy, 146
follow-up strategy, 146
PPPD, 145
surgical resection, 145
risk factors, 121
surveillance strategies, 121–122
United States
adjuvant therapy, 125
5-fluorouracil, 125
follow-up, 127
gemcitabine, 126

serum CA 19–9 level, 126
surgical intervention, 125
surveillance strategies, 127
Papillary thyroid microcarcinoma, 60
Papillon, J., 209
Park, K.C., 17
Park, S.M., 17
Partin, A.W., 412
Pastner, 302
Peiffert, D., 208, 209
Percutaneous ethanol injection (PEI), 165
Pfitzenmaier, J., 405
Pietra, N., 201
Pingley, S., 354
Plasma cell disorder. *See* Multiple myeloma (MM)
Positron emission tomography (PET), 47, 462, 467, 502, 521
Post-prostatectomy surveillance
clinical trials, 433–434
false negative margin, 432–433
metastatic prostate cancer, 433
positive margin, 433
PSA, 433
salvage radiotherapy, 431–432
Progression-free survival (PFS), 312
Promyelocytic leukemia (PML), 486
Prostate cancer
AUA symptom score, 417
Canada
active surveillance, 429–430
conservative management, 428
post-prostatectomy surveillance, 431–434
post-radiotherapy surveillance, 430–431
PSA level, 427–428
risk factors, 427
watchful waiting, 428–429
CAPRA, 417
cryosurgery, 414–415
Europe
periodic surveillance, 422
PSA level, 421
radical radiotherapy/hormonal treatment, 421
geographic variation, 399
HIFU, 415–417
Japan
definitive radiation therapy, 424
hormone therapy, 424
posttreatment surveillance, 423
radical prostatectomy, 423
PET scan, 417
PSA doubling time, 417
PSA level, 411
radiation therapy, 413–414
radical prostatectomy
local and distant failure, 413
post-prostatectomy patients, 412
SF-36, 417
SHIM, 417
surveillance strategies
ASCO, 399
AUA, 400
CC, 400
CCO, 400
ESMO, 400
ESSO, 400
NCCN, 399, 400
NICE, 400
SSO, 400
USA
ablative therapies, 407–409
radiation therapy, 406–407
radical prostatectomy, 403–406
Prostate Cancer Gene 3 (PCA3), 411
Prostate specific antigen (PSA), 9, 403–405, 411, 427
Pylorus-preserving PD (PPPD), 145

Q
Qin, X.L., 166
Quality-adjusted life years (QALYs), 18
Quality of life (QOL), 516

R
Radiation therapy
lung carcinoma, 86–88
prostate cancer, 406–407, 413–414
Radiation Therapy Oncology Group (RTOG), 207, 406
Radical prostatectomy
CT scans, 405
digital rectal examination, 404
low-and high-risk patients, 404–406
prostate specific antigen, 403–405
transrectal ultrasound examinations, 404
Reddoch, J.M., 302
Renal cancer
Canada
clinical trials, 384
CUA Guideline, 383
radical/partial nephrectomy, 383, 384
radiologic examination, 393
serological tests, 383
Europe
abdominal relapses, 376, 378
HR patients, 377, 378
IR patients, 377, 378
LR patients, 377, 378
nephron-sparing surgery, 376
prognostic systems, 375, 376
relapse, site of, 376
risk classes, 377
staging system, 375
thoracic relapses, 376, 377
UISS definitions, 375, 376
geographic variation, 373
Japan
cytotoxic chemotherapy, 381
T1 patients, 381, 382
T2–T4 disease, 381, 382
surveillance strategies
ASCO, 373
AUA, 374
CC, 374
CCO, 374
ESMO, 373, 374
ESSO, 374
NCCN, 373, 374
NICE, 374
SSO, 373
Renal cell carcinoma (RCC), 383
Retinoic acid receptor alpha (RARα), 486
Retroperitoneal lymph node dissection (RPLND), 444

Ritoe, S.C., 17, 52, 53
Rodriguez-Moranta, F., 191
Roehrborn, C.G., 20
Roohipour, R., 208
Rose, P.G., 307
Rosselli Del Turco, M., 281
Rumble, R., 201
Ryu, S.Y., 309

S
Saad, F., 433
Sakar, B., 110
Samlal, R.A.K., 330, 331
San-Miguel, J., 498
Sartori, E., 330
Saskatchewan Cancer Agency (SCA), 344
Sato, Y., 103
Schirmer's testing, 481
Schoemaker, D., 192, 201
Schwartz, E.J., 211
Scottish Intercollegiate Guidelines Network (SIGN), 344
Secco, G.B., 201
Serum protein electrophoresis (SPEP), 502
Sexual Health Inventory for Men (SHIM), 417
Shepherd, J.H., 339
Shield, P.W., 331
Shimada, H., 103
Shimizu, N., 110
Single photon emission computed tomography (SPECT) scan, 416–417
Siva, S., 4
Small-cell lung carcinoma (SCLC), 77
Smith, C.J., 306, 309
Smoking cessation, 88–90
Soanes, W.A., 408
Society for the Surgery of the Alimentary Tract (SSAT)
  anal carcinoma, 206
  colon and rectum carcinoma, 182, 183
  esophagus, 94
  liver and biliary tract carcinoma, 155
  pancreatic adenocarcinoma, 122
  stomach, 108
Society of Gynecologic Oncologists (SGO)
  cervical cancer, 325
  endometrial carcinoma, 299
  ovarian cancer, 359
  vaginal and vulvar carcinoma, 350
Society of Surgical Oncology (SSO), 3, 39, 469
  anal carcinoma, 205
  bladder cancer, 388
  cervical cancer, 324
  colon and rectum carcinoma, 180
  cutaneous melanoma, 252
  endometrial carcinoma, 298
  esophagus, 94
  glioma, 511
  leukemia, 476
  liver and biliary tract carcinoma, 154
  lung cancer, 72
  lymphoma, 458, 469
  multiple myeloma, 487
  osteogenic sarcoma and dedifferentiated chondrosarcoma, 243
  ovarian cancer, 358
  pancreatic adenocarcinoma, 122
  prostate cancer, 400
  renal cancer, 373
  soft tissue sarcoma, 227
  stomach, 108
  testicular cancer, 438
  thyroid cancer, 58
  vaginal and vulvar carcinoma, 349–350
Soft tissue sarcoma
  Canada
    adjuvant chemotherapy, 238
    AJCC staging system, 236
    clinical evaluation, 236
    core biopsy, 237
    GIST, 237
    Kaposi sarcomas, 235
    MRI, 236
    PET/CT, 236
    preoperative chemoradiation protocol, 237
    provincial cancer agencies, 235
    retroperitoneal tumors, 237
    surveillance, 238–240
  geographic variation, 227
  Japan
    chemotherapy, 233
    CT scan, 233
    curative-intent primary therapy, 234
    myxoid/round cell liposarcoma, 234
    PET scan, 233–234
  risk factors, 227
  surveillance strategies
    ASCO, 227
    CC, 229
    CCO, 229
    ESMO, 227, 229
    ESSO, 229
    NCCN, 227–229
    NICE, 229
    SSO, 227
  United States
    adjuvant chemotherapy, 231
    curative-intent therapy, 232
    MRI scan, 232
    surgical resection, 231
Soisson, A.P., 331
Spermon, J.R., 17
Splinter, T.A., 133
Squamous cell carcinoma (SCC), 327–328, 335, 338, 353
Stem cell transplantation (SCT), 481
Stephenson, A.J., 431–433
Stiggelbout, A.M., 17
Stomach cancer
  environmental factors, 107
  gastric cancer, 108
  geographic variation, 107
  Japan
    advanced gastric cancer, 116–118
    clinical treatment options, 114
    early gastric cancer, 115–116
    H. pylori 113
    treatment guidelines, 113
  surveillance strategies
    ASCO, 107
    CC, 108
    CCO, 108
    ESMO, 108
    ESSO, 108
    NCCN, 107

NICE, 108
SSAT, 108
SSO, 108
United States
CEA level, 110
curative-intent treatment, 110
E-cadherin, 110
EGD, 111
FDG-PET, 111
gastric cancer, 109
lymphatic spread, 110
Memorial Sloan-Kettering group, 109
TNM stage, 111
Sugiyama, T., 88
Sunnybrook Health Sciences Centre, 429
Suzuki, H., 424
Svetec, D., 407

T

Takada, A., 133, 134
Tan, I.T., 111
T-cell receptor (TCR), 486
Temozolomide (TMZ), 521
Testicular cancer
Australia
annual risk, 450
CT scans, 451
curative-intent initial therapy, 449, 450
NSGCT, 451, 452
orchiectomy, 450–451
palpable lymph nodes, 449
para-aortic lymph nodes, 450
geographic variation, 437
Japan
nonseminoma (clinical stage I), 453–454
nonseminoma (clinical stage II), 454–455
seminoma (clinical stage I), 453
seminoma (clinical stage II), 454
surveillance strategies
ASCO, 437
AUA, 440, 441
CC, 440
CCO, 440, 441
ESMO, 438–440
ESSO, 439, 440
NCCN, 437–439
NICE, 440
SSO, 438
USA
clinical and pathologic stage II NSGCT, 445
clinical stage III NSGCT, 445
germ cell tumor, 443
posteroanterior and lateral chest radiographs, 444
radical orchiectomy, 443–444
stage III seminoma, 446
stage II seminoma, 446
stage I nonseminoma germ cell tumors, 444–445
stage I seminoma, 445–446
Thalidomide, 501
Thyroglobulin (TG), 69
Thyroid cancer
American Cancer Society, 57
Australia
antithyroglobulin antibodies, 66
curative-intent treatment, 66
differentiated thyroid cancer, 64
follow-up surveillance, 65
long-term surveillance, 64
medullary thyroid cancer, 63
papillary thyroid carcinoma, 65
radioiodine scintigraphy, 63
serum calcitonin level, 67
serum thyroglobulin levels, 65
thyroxine suppression, 66
total thyroidectomy, 64
family history/follicular carcinoma, papillary of, 57
geographic variation, 57
Japan
AGES and AMES classification systems, 69
FDG-PET CT scan, 70
follicular carcinoma, 69
nodulectomy, 69
TG, 70
TSH-suppressive effect, 69
well-differentiated thyroid cancer, 70
surveillance strategies
AHNS, 59
ASCO, 58
ATA, 60
CC, 59
CCO, 59
ESMO, 59
ESSO, 59
NCCN, 57–58
NICE, 59
SSO, 58
Tjalma, W.A.A., 307
Tjandra, J.J., 189, 191, 192, 196
Toboul, 209
Toronto Extremity Salvage Score (TESS), 236
Transforming growth factor β (TGF-β), 118, 135
Transhepatic chemo-embolization (TACE), 159
Transrectal ultrasonography (TRUS), 421
Trans-Tasman Radiation Oncology Group (TROG), 431
Transurethral resection (TUR), 393
Trautmann, T.G., 208
Trede, M., 125
Tucker, M.A., 88

U

Ultrasonography (US), 47
Union Européenne Des Médecins Spécialistes (UEMS), 515
Upper aerodigestive tract carcinoma
Canada
curative-intent treatment, 53
distant metastases, 52
multimodality treatment plans, 51
oropharyngeal cancer, 51
routine chest radiographs, 53
salvage treatment, 52
second primary tumors, 52
squamous cell carcinoma, 52
surveillance guidelines, 53
Europe
curative-intent initial therapy, 44
ENT surgeon, 45
esophageal cancer, 44
head and neck cancer, 43–45
single-modality therapy, 43
squamous cell carcinoma, 43

Upper aerodigestive tract carcinoma (*cont.*)
surveillance strategies, 45
tobacco/alcohol consumption, 44
Japan
age-standardized mortality rate, 47
chemoradiation, 47, 48
curative-intent treatment, 48
FDG-PET scan, 48
primary cancer, 47
surgery and radiotherapy, 47
Urinary bladder carcinoma. *See* Bladder cancer
Ushijima, K., 313
US National Cancer Institute Surveillance Epidemiology and End Results, 129
US Preventive Task Force (USPSTF), 10

V
Vaginal and vulvar carcinoma
geographic variation, 349
Japan
curative-intent treatment, 354
follow-up intervals, 354
gynecologic malignancies, 354–355
lymphedema, 353–354
survival rates, 353
surveillance strategies
ASCO, 349
CC, 350
CCO, 350
ESMO, 350
ESSO, 350
NCCN, 349
NICE, 350
SGO, 350
SSO, 349–350
Vanderbilt-Ingram Cancer Center, 445, 446
van Loon, J., 17
Vascular endothelial growth factor (VEGF), 118, 135, 381

W
Warren, K.S., 404, 407
Wasserman, N.F., 404
Wattchow, D.A., 190
Whiting, J., 109
Wilms' tumor 1 (WT-1), 486
Wilson, J.M., 327
World Health Organization (WHO), 39, 57, 71
Worthington, T., 190
Wright, J.D., 338
Wu, B., 109

Y
Yamamoto, M., 115
Yang, I., 193
Yermilov, I., 145
Yoshioka, T., 111
Yurkovetsky, Z., 309

Z
Zinzani, P.L., 462
Zola, P., 330
Zuraw, L., 201
Zwall, C., 201

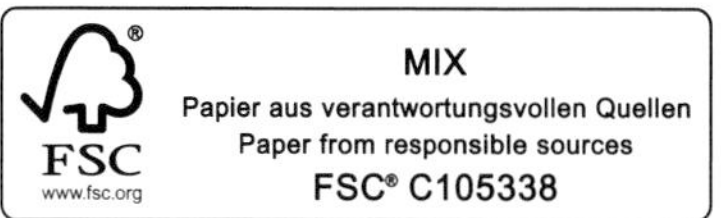

Printed by Books on Demand, Germany